Evidence-based practice
across the health professions
2nd edition

Evidence-based practice across the health professions
2nd edition

Tammy Hoffmann

Sally Bennett

Chris Del Mar

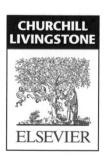

CHURCHILL LIVINGSTONE

ELSEVIER

Sydney   Edinburgh   London   New York   Philadelphia   St Louis   Toronto

Churchill Livingstone
is an imprint of Elsevier

Elsevier Australia. ACN 001 002 357
(a division of Reed International Books Australia Pty Ltd)
Tower 1, 475 Victoria Avenue, Chatswood, NSW 2067

ELSEVIER

eISBN: 9780729582278

Every attempt has been made to trace and acknowledge copyright, but in some cases this may not have been
possible. The publisher apologises for any accidental infringement and would welcome any information to redress
the situation.

This publication has been carefully reviewed and checked to ensure that the content is as accurate and current as
possible at time of publication. We would recommend, however, that the reader verify any procedures, treatments,
drug dosages or legal content described in this book. Neither the author, the contributors, nor the publisher
assume any liability for injury and/or damage to persons or property arising from any error in or omission from
this publication.

National Library of Australia Cataloguing-in-Publication Data

---

Author: Hoffmann, Tammy.

Title: Evidence-based practice across the health professions / Tammy Hoffmann, Sally Bennett, Chris Del Mar.

Edition: 2nd ed.

ISBN: 9780729541350 (pbk.)

Subjects: Clinical medicine–Decision making. Evidence-based medicine.

Other Authors/Contributors: Bennett, Sally. Del Mar, Chris.

Dewey Number: 616

Publisher: Melinda McEvoy
Developmental Editor: Amanda Simons
Project Coordinators: Liz Malcolm and Nayagi Athmanathan
Edited by Teresa McIntyre
Permissions editing by Sarah Johnson
Proofread by Tim Learner
Cover design by Georgette Hall
Internal design by Lisa Petroff
Index by Robert Swanson
Typeset by Toppan Best-set Premedia Limited
Printed in China by China Translation & Printing Services Limited

CONTENTS

Foreword

Paradigms change over time. The development of a new paradigm does not do away with the old one, but adapts and changes it. In the last three years we have seen increasing interest in fitting the evidence to the individual patient. Of course evidence-based practice, in addition to its focus on the evidence, also emphasises the need to relate the evidence to the unique condition and values of the individual patient. This emphasises two important aspects: the clinical condition of each patient and their values.

Wittgenstein said that every idea is a picture, and it may be, if we had used the picture below, that evidence-based medicine would not have been described and criticised as 'cookbook medicine' in its early years.

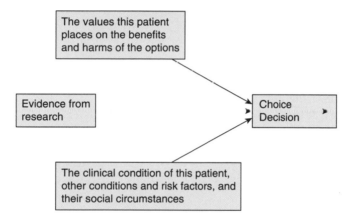

Throughout the new edition of this book the need to take all three of these factors, as well as a fourth, the practice context, into account when making decisions is emphasised and very clearly explained. One of the ways in which this has been achieved is by expanding the number of discipline-specific worked examples. The importance of this lies in making the practice of evidence—essential to getting the right information to the decision-making point—clearly relevant and achievable to *all* health professionals, whatever their unique role is in providing healthcare.

The editors have done a terrific job of clearing away the mystique of the subject matter to make the concepts and processes clear and accessible. Throughout it, this book keeps the focus on what it is that clinicians and patients really need to know to make decisions. This book should contribute to making sure we are all able to get the best available evidence to every patient choice and every clinical decision.

Professor Sir Muir Gray, CBE MD
Director, Better Value Healthcare
Formerly Chief Knowledge Officer of the National Health Service (NHS), UK

Contributors

Marilyn Baird BA, DCR, PhD

Associate Professor and Foundation Head, Department of Medical Imaging and Radiation Sciences, Monash University, Melbourne, Victoria, Australia

Marilyn created the curriculum for the degree of Bachelor of Radiography and Medical Imaging, which commenced in 1998, and subsequently supervised the introduction of an articulated masters degree in medical ultrasound and graduate-entry masters programs in radiation therapy and nuclear medicine. Marilyn is also the Associate Dean Teaching and Learning. Her research interests are primarily directed towards improving clinical teaching and learning. In June 2008 she was re-appointed by the Minister of Health (Victoria) as President of the Medical Radiation Practitioners Board of Victoria.

John W Bennett BMedSc, MBBS, BA(Hons), PhD, FRACGP, FACHI

Discipline of General Practice, School of Medicine, and The University of Queensland Health Service, The University of Queensland, Brisbane, Australia

John is a practice principal at the University Health Service, The University of Queensland, and regularly uses evidence-based medicine in his clinical practice. He has taught evidence-based medicine in Brisbane and Oxford (at the Centre for Evidence-Based Medicine) and has co-authored a number of articles relevant to evidence-based practice. He is on several Royal Australian College of General Practitioners' Quality Care committees and strives to use evidence in the production of resources for general practitioners.

Sally Bennett BOccThy(Hons), PhD

Senior Lecturer and Senior Research Fellow, Division of Occupational Therapy, School of Health and Rehabilitation Sciences, The University of Queensland, Brisbane, Australia

Sally is an occupational therapist with both clinical and research experience. She has designed a number of evidence-based practice curricula and taught evidence-based practice to occupational therapy, physiotherapy and speech pathology students for 11 years. She has undertaken research in evidence-based practice, including her PhD, and has authored multiple Cochrane reviews. She helped establish and currently manages the OTseeker database—an internationally-recognised occupational therapy evidence database. She is active in both national and international professional committees as an advisor on evidence-based practice and is also a member of the Critically Appraised Papers Advisory Board for the *Australian Occupational Therapy Journal*.

Malcolm Boyle ADipBus, ADipHSc(Amb Off), MICA Cert, BInfoTech, MClinEpi, PhD

Senior Lecturer, Department of Community Emergency Health and Paramedic Practice, Monash University, Victoria, Australia

Malcolm's primary teaching areas are trauma systems, pre-hospital clinical management, pre-hospital trauma management and evidence-based paramedic practice. His primary research interests include pre-hospital trauma triage, pre-hospital trauma management, the linking of ambulance datasets to other health-related datasets and subsequent analysis, workplace violence and its effects, and attributes and attitudes of undergraduate paramedic and allied health students. Malcolm has been a paramedic working in rural areas for over 24 years, with the last 20 years as a Mobile Intensive Care Ambulance Paramedic in Victoria.

Heather Buchan MBChB, Msc, FAFPHM

Director of Implementation Support, Australian Commission on Safety and Quality in Health Care

Heather is a public health doctor who has worked in medical management and policy positions in New Zealand, the UK and Australia. She was the Chief Executive Officer of the National Institute of Clinical Studies, established by the Australian government to help close gaps between evidence and clinical practice, from its beginnings in 2001 until it became part of the National Health and Medical Research Council in 2007. She was Vice-Chair of the Guidelines International Network from 2007 to 2009 and is currently co-chair of its Implementation Working Group.

Jeff Coombes BEd(Hons), BAppSc, MEd, PhD

Professor in Exercise Science, The University of Queensland, Brisbane, Australia

Jeff is also current Past-President of Exercise and Sports Science Australia, an accredited exercise physiologist and lectures to students on exercise prescription and programming and interprofessional education. He directs a research program that aims to improve the evidence base about the effects of exercise training on conditions such as cardiovascular disease, diabetes and kidney disease.

Chris Del Mar BSc, MA, MB BChir, MD, FRACGP, FAFPHM

Professor of Public Health and academic general practitioner, Centre for Research in Evidence-Based Practice, Faculty of Health Sciences and Medicine, Bond University, Gold Coast, Queensland, Australia

Chris was educated in science and medicine and worked as a general practitioner until commencing in an academic position at the University of Queensland in 1988, where he was Professor of General Practice from 1995 to 2004. He was Dean of Health Sciences and Medicine and also Pro-Vice-Chancellor of Research at Bond University from 2004 to 2009. He is an internationally-known evidence-based practice researcher, has led evidence-based practice workshops for over 20 years and has also conducted health services and clinical research. Chris has published four books and more than 300 research articles and book chapters. He has been Editor of the research section of the *Australian Family Physician*; Chair of the Royal Australian College of General Practitioners National Research Committee; President of the Australian Association for Academic General Practice, Visiting Professor of General Practice at Oxford University and Chair of the editorial committee of the Australian Government's health web portal, HealthInsite. He is a Coordinating Editor of the Cochrane Collaboration, and has been a member of the Editorial Board of the *BMJ* and a deputy editor of the *Medical Journal of Australia*.

Jenny Doust BA, BEcons, BMBS, Grad Dip Clin Epi, PhD, FRACGP

Professor of Clinical Epidemiology, Faculty of Health Sciences and Medicine, Bond University, Gold Coast, Queensland, Australia

Jenny has worked and trained as a general practitioner, clinical epidemiologist and economist. Since graduating in medicine, she has worked in positions that combine her interests in these three areas. Her main research areas of interest are diagnosis, screening and evidence-based practice in clinical practice. She is a member of the Cochrane Systematic Reviews of Diagnostic Accuracy Methods Working Group.

Susan Doyle MS, OTR/L, CFE

Occupational Therapist, Cascade Park Care Center, Vancouver, USA

Sue has worked as an occupational therapist for over three decades in a variety of practice settings in Australia and the USA. She has worked in clinical, management and program development roles. Sue was also Assistant Professor in the Occupational Therapy Department at Ithaca College, NY where she was involved with incorporating evidence-based practice into the curriculum and also taught the Research Methods and Thesis courses. Sue is an author for the Cochrane Stroke Group and has been invited to present on the Cochrane Colloquium, systematic reviews and evidence-based practice for the American Occupational Therapy Association Educational Program Director's meetings and various college clinical educator programs. Sue's post-professional master's degree research was in clinical reasoning and her PhD research includes exploring how therapists define and incorporate evidence into their reasoning process when working with people who have had a stroke.

Mark R Elkins BPhty, BA, MHSc, PhD

Senior Research Physiotherapist, Royal Prince Alfred Hospital, Sydney, New South Wales, Australia

As part of his research position Mark conducts original research and performs systematic reviews, primarily in the areas of physiotherapy and respiratory disease. He is a co-director of the Centre for Evidence-Based Physiotherapy, which maintains the Physiotherapy Evidence Database (PEDro). He is also a Clinical Senior Lecturer at the Central Clinical School of Medicine at the University of Sydney and has published and presented workshops in the area of evidence-based physiotherapy.

Edzard Ernst MD, PhD, F Med Sci, FRCP, FRCP(Ed)

Professor Ernst is an academic doctor and researcher who specialises in the study of complementary and alternative medicine. He was appointed as Professor of Complementary Medicine at the University of Exeter, the first such academic position in the world. His work has been awarded with 13 scientific prizes/awards and he served on the Medicines Commission of the British Medicines and Healthcare Products Regulatory Agency from 1994 to 2005. He has published more than 1000 papers in the peer-reviewed literature and more than 40 books.

Paul Glasziou MBBS, PhD, FRACGP, MRCGP

Professor of Evidence-Based Medicine and Director of the Centre for Research in Evidence-Based Practice, Bond University and NHMRC Australia Fellow, Gold Coast, Queensland, Australia

Paul was the director of Oxford University's Centre for Evidence-Based Medicine from 2003 to 2010 and is an international leader in evidence-based medicine. He is the author of seven books related to evidence-based practice and more than 190 peer-reviewed journal articles, and has led more than 100 evidence-based practice workshops in dozens of countries. Now at Bond University in Australia, his research focuses on improving the clinical impact of publications by reducing the more than $85 billion annual loss from unpublished and unusable research (see, for example, Chalmers I, Glasziou P. Avoidable waste in the production and reporting of research evidence. *Lancet* 2009; 374(9863):86–9). As a general practitioner, this work has particularly focused on the applicability and usability of published trials and reviews.

Karin Hannes MSc Med, PhD

Doctor-Assistant at the Centre for Methodology of Educational Research at KU Leuven (University of Leuven), Belgium

Karin has a background in social–cultural andragogics and medical social sciences, and now specialises in qualitative research methodology. She is the founder of the Belgian Campbell Group, co-convener of the Cochrane Qualitative Research Group, co-author of the Cochrane Handbook for systematic reviews of interventions and co-chair of the Campbell Process and Implementation Methods Group. Her most recent book addresses methods of qualitative evidence synthesis.

Joy Higgs AM, BSc, Grad Dip Phty, MHPEd, PhD

Strategic Research Professor in Professional Practice in The Research Institute for Professional Practice, Learning and Education and Director of The Education for Practice Institute, Charles Sturt University, New South Wales, Australia

Joy has worked in health sciences research and higher education for over 30 years. She has published widely, including 20 books, in her fields of expertise in professional practice, practice knowledge, clinical reasoning, qualitative research and professional education. In 2008 she published the third edition of *Clinical Reasoning in the Health Professions* with Mark Jones and colleagues. Joy is an experienced research supervisor and many of her students have researched clinical reasoning and professional practice. Joy has received a Member of the Order of Australia award for services to health sciences education, in recognition of her contributions to course development, scholarship, research and academic leadership.

Tammy Hoffmann BOccThy(Hons), PhD

Associate Professor of Clinical Epidemiology, Centre for Research in Evidence-Based Practice, Faculty of Health Sciences and Medicine, Bond University, Gold Coast, Queensland, Australia; and NHMRC/PHCRED Career Development Research Fellow, School of Health and Rehabilitation Sciences, The University of Queensland, Brisbane, Australia

Tammy is a clinical epidemiologist and occupational therapist with clinical, academic and research experience. Tammy's main research interests are in facilitators of evidence-based practice from the clinicians' perspective and communicating health information and evidence to patients, and she has researched and published widely in these areas. She has led many evidence-based practice workshops and coordinated and taught numerous undergraduate and postgraduate evidence-based practice courses to interdisciplinary groups of health professionals. Tammy is also a member of the team that developed and maintains the internationally-recognised occupational therapy evidence database, OTseeker (www.otseeker.com); an editorial board member of the Cochrane Stroke Group, *Topics in Stroke Rehabilitation,* and the Critically Appraised Papers department of the *Australian Occupational Therapy Journal*; and a member of the National Stroke Foundation Clinical Council.

Craig Lockwood RN, BN, GradDip, MNSc, PhD

Associate Director, Translation Science, The Joanna Briggs Institute, Faculty of Health Sciences, The University of Adelaide

Craig is the School Coordinator for higher degrees by research, and for the Institute's online resources for evidence-based policy and practice. His interests are in translation of evidence into policy and practice, supervision of higher-degree students and methods for the synthesis of qualitative research findings.

Annie McCluskey DipCOT, MA, PhD

Senior Lecturer (Occupational Therapy), Faculty of Health Sciences, The University of Sydney, New South Wales, Australia

Annie is an occupational therapist, health services researcher and co-developer of the freely available OTseeker evidence database (www.otseeker.com) and OT-CATs website (www.otcats.com). Her research has investigated the effect of teaching health professionals how to search for and appraise evidence, the process of becoming an evidence-based practitioner and evidence indexed on OTseeker. Annie is currently investigating the implementation of evidence by community rehabilitation teams in Sydney, to help improve outcomes for people with stroke.

Ann McKibbon MLS, PhD

Associate Professor, Health Information Research Unit, Department of Clinical Epidemiology and Biostatistics, McMaster University, Ontario, Canada

Ann's background is information sciences and her PhD is in medical informatics, and she has been part of the evidence-based medicine movement for many years. She teaches in the Health Research Methodology program, although most of her recent effort has been to develop a new MSc in eHealth and an affiliated eHealth Research Network. Her research focuses on the use of information resources by health professionals, information retrieval and knowledge translation.

Angela Morgan BSpAud (Hons), PhD

Senior Research Fellow, Murdoch Children's Research Institute, Melbourne, Victoria, Australia; Speech Pathology Department, Royal Children's Hospital, Melbourne, Victoria, Australia; Department of Paediatrics, University of Melbourne, Victoria, Australia

Angela has 15 years of clinical and research experience in paediatric speech pathology in Australia and the UK. She gained an international view of evidence-based practice in paediatric speech pathology through her experience as a Research Lecturer in the UK from 2004 to 2006 (at the Institute of Child Health, University College London). Angela currently holds a National Health and Medical Research Council Career Development Award and her current program of research focuses on (1) understanding the neural and genetic bases of paediatric communication disorders; and (2) developing an evidence base for the management of these conditions.

Lisa Nissen BPharm, PhD, FPS, FHKAPh, FSHP

Professor (Head), School of Clinical Sciences, Queensland University of Technology; Honorary Professor, School of Pharmacy, The University of Queensland, Australia

Lisa's research focuses on improving the quality use of medicines in the wider community, with a focus on professional service development for pharmacists and the factors which influence prescribing of medicines. Her research and teaching activities are firmly centred around evidence-based practice. She is actively involved in the pharmacy profession and is the current Pharmaceutical Society of Australia (Queensland) Branch President and past national vice-president.

Denise O'Connor BAppScOT(Hons), PhD

Senior Research Fellow and NHMRC Public Health Fellow, School of Public Health and Preventive Medicine, Monash University, Melbourne, Victoria, Australia

Denise is an active Cochrane author, editor with the Cochrane Effective Practice and Organisation of Care (EPOC) Group and associate editor with *Implementation Science*. She contributes to several collaborative research projects which aim to increase the uptake of research into clinical practice by designing and evaluating interventions to change health professional behaviour. Previously she worked as a lecturer with the Australasian Cochrane Centre, where she coordinated training and support for Australasian Cochrane authors.

Alan Pearson AM, RN, ONC, DipNEd, MSc, PhD, FCN, FRCNA, FAAG, FRCN

Professor of Evidence-Based Healthcare and Executive Director, The Joanna Briggs Institute, The University of Adelaide, South Australia, Australia

Alan has extensive experience in clinical practice in the UK, the USA, Papua New Guinea and Australia. He is the Editor of the *International Journal of Nursing Practice* and is Director of the Cochrane Nursing Care Field.

Marie Pirotta MBBS, FRACGP, M Med, PhD

Associate Professor of General Practice, Primary Care Research Unit, Department of General Practice, University of Melbourne, Melbourne, Victoria, Australia

Marie is an academic general practitioner with a strong research interest in evaluating complementary therapies. She is the current chair of the Royal Australian College of General Practitioner's National Standing Committee—Research and a member of the Therapeutic Guidelines of Australia's advisory committee on complementary medicines. Her current research includes two National Health and Medical Research Council funded randomised controlled trials evaluating acupuncture.

Sheena Reilly BAppSc, PhD

Professor of Paediatric Speech Pathology, Department of Paediatrics, The University of Melbourne, Victoria, Australia; Professor-Director of Speech Pathology, The Royal Children's Hospital, Melbourne, Victoria, Australia; Associate Director, Clinical and Public Health Research, Murdoch Children's Research Institute, Melbourne, Victoria, Australia

Sheena holds a National Health and Medical Research Council practitioner fellowship; her research focuses on speech and language development, and the prevalence and predictors of communication and swallowing difficulties in children. Sheena has a strong interest in evidence-based practice, particularly the application of evidence-based practice to speech pathology. She is co-editor of the book *Evidence-Based Practice in Speech Pathology* and is on the editorial board of *Evidence-Based Communication Assessment and Intervention.*

Claire Rickard BN, RN, GradDip(CriticalCare), PhD, FRCNA

Professor, NHMRC Centre of Research Excellence in Nursing Interventions for Hospitalised Patients, Griffith Health Institute, Griffith University, Brisbane, Australia

Claire is a registered nurse with many years of experience in clinical research. Claire's primary focus is leading large-scale, multi-centre trials of interventions to reduce complications and promote evidence-based practice for patients with intravascular devices. In addition she is involved in a number of systematic reviews for the Cochrane Collaboration.

Sharon Sanders BSc(Pod), MPH

Centre for Research in Evidence-Based Practice, Bond University, Gold Coast, Australia

While working as a podiatrist in the public health service Sharon completed a Masters of Public Health and, for the last 12 years, she has been working at The University of Queensland and Bond University researching and teaching the skills of evidence-based practice to students and health professionals from a range of disciplines. Sharon is currently completing a PhD on the value, useability and use of clinical prediction rules for making diagnoses.

Michal Schneider-Kolsky BSc, DipEd, MRepSc, GradCertHealthProfEdu, PhD

Senior Lecturer, Department of Medical Imaging and Radiation Sciences, Monash University, Melbourne, Victoria, Australia

Michal trained as a scientist gaining a PhD in Obstetrics and Gynaecology and a masters in Reproductive Physiology. Since 2002, she has conducted research in diagnostic imaging and radiation therapy using both quantitative and qualitative research methods. She conducts lectures and workshops on evidence-based practice and research methodology to undergraduate and postgraduate students, and acts as a reviewer for several international journals.

Ian Scott FRACP, MHA, MEd

Director of Internal Medicine and Clinical Epidemiology, Princess Alexandra Hospital, Brisbane, Queensland, Australia

Ian is a consultant general physician with a long-standing interest in evidence-based medicine, quality improvement and health services research. He sits on the Queensland Health Patient Safety and Quality Executive Committee and the Quality Expert Advisory Group of the Royal Australasian College of Physicians. He is Associate Professor of Medicine at the University of Queensland and Adjunct Associate Professor of Medicine at Monash University in Melbourne.

Jemma Skeat BSpPath(Hons), PhD

National Advisor, Research and Policy, Speech Pathology Australia; Department of Paediatrics, University of Melbourne, Victoria, Australia

Jemma is a clinical speech pathologist and researcher, with a background in both qualitative and quantitative research. Jemma has an interest in evaluating qualitative evidence and speech pathologists' use of evidence in practice. She is co-editor of the book *Embedding Evidence-Based Practice in Speech and Language Therapy*.

Alan Spencer MPH, Grad Dip Diet, BSc(Hons)

Director of Nutrition Services, Gold Coast Health Service District, Queensland, Australia

Alan is a clinical dietitian for the Intensive Care Unit and parenteral nutrition services at the Gold Coast Hospital. He is also a teaching fellow for the School of Health Science at Bond University. He has a long-standing interest in evidence-based practice, is a member of the Gold Coast District evidence-based practice committee and is an active contributor to Bond University's evidence-based practice workshops.

Leigh Tooth BOccThy(Hons) PhD

Senior Research Fellow, Australian Longitudinal Study on Women's Health, School of Population Health, The University of Queensland, Brisbane, Australia

Leigh is a graduate in occupational therapy and has had both a clinical and a research career. She was previously a National Health and Medical Research Council Fellow with the Longitudinal Studies Unit in the School of Population Health, researching statistical methodology and teaching in the epidemiology program. Her current research interests include women's health, socio-economic determinants of health, outcome evaluation, longitudinal methods, quality of life, comorbidity and epidemiology. Leigh is one of the founding chief investigators of the OTseeker database.

Merrill Turpin BOccThy, Grad Dip Counsel, PhD

Senior Lecturer, Division of Occupational Therapy, School of Health and Rehabilitation Sciences, The University of Queensland, Brisbane, Australia

Merrill's professional areas of expertise include occupational therapy philosophy and professional issues and clinical/professional reasoning and evidence-based practice. She uses a range of qualitative research methods to understand diverse aspects of people's experiences as well as organisational culture and service development processes.

Nancy L Wilczynski MSc, PhD

Assistant Professor and Research Manager, Health Information Research Unit (HIRU), Department of Clinical Epidemiology and Biostatistics, McMaster University, Hamilton, Ontario, Canada
Nancy teaches in the Health Research Methodology Program in the Faculty of Sciences, which provides training at the MSc and PhD levels. She oversees the research conducted in the HIRU, which is focused on the field of health information science and is dedicated to the generation of new knowledge about the nature of health and clinical information problems, the development of new information resources to support evidence-based health care and the evaluation of various innovations in overcoming healthcare information problems.

Caroline Wright MSc, PGCE, BSC (Hons), DCR (T)

Senior Lecturer in Radiation Therapy, Department of Medical Imaging and Radiation Sciences, Monash University, Melbourne, Victoria, Australia
Caroline's current role is convening the graduate-entry masters in Radiation Therapy at Monash University. Her research interests include the assessment and regulation of fitness to practise in students and professionals, clinical assessment and advancing practice in the profession. She is a member of the Editorial Review Board for the *Journal of Radiotherapy in Practice* and a member of the Medical Radiations Practitioner Board of the Victoria Education Committee.

Reviewers

Heleen Blijlevens MHSc (Hons)

Lecturer/Programme Leader, Faculty of Health and Environmental Sciences, Department of Occupational Science and Therapy, AUT University, Auckland, New Zealand

Marina Ciccarelli BAppSc (OccThy), MSc, PhD

Associate Professor, School of Occupational Therapy and Social Work, Faculty of Health Sciences, Curtin University, Perth, Western Australia

Steven A Frost BN, MPH

Lecturer, School of Nursing and Midwifery, University of Western Sydney and Intensive Care, Liverpool Hospital, Sydney, Australia

Anne Howard BHSc (Nat), Adv Dip (Herb Med), Adv Dip (Nutritional Med)

Senior Lecturer, Naturopathy, Department of Occidental Medicine, Endeavour College of Natural Health, Melbourne, Australia

Debbie Howson AssDipMedrad (RT), MSc

Lecturer, Division of Health Sciences, School of Health Science, The University of South Australia, Adelaide, Australia

PhD Candidate, International Centre for Allied Health Evidence, The University of South Australia, Adelaide, Australia

Preface

When the publishers asked us to prepare a second edition, they asked us to respond to feedback that was in the form of popular demand: more examples for more health professionals, please. We are delighted to oblige. This edition of the book contains new material that is relevant to exercise physiologists and human movement specialists, pharmacists, paramedics, and complementary and alternative medicine practitioners, in addition to the 10 disciplines that were included in the first edition.

We have expanded our contributor team and as well as adding discipline experts, we have been joined by a host of international and national experts in numerous fields of evidence-based practice. We welcome our new contributors to the book and thank all of the authors for their valuable contributions.

The overwhelmingly positive reaction to the first edition, and the developments that evolved from it, delighted us. The field of evidence-based practice is sometimes naïvely and incorrectly viewed as a relatively slow-changing area. Yet, as we updated each of the chapters even we were surprised by the number of developments and progress since we prepared the first edition four years ago. For example, into Chapter 12 we have added information about qualitative evidence synthesis. We have also added a new chapter (Chapter 17—*Embedding evidence-based practice into routine clinical care*) which reflects on the importance of an organisational environment which promotes evidence-based practice and describes specific supportive strategies.

Finally, we hope that this book helps bring together health team members from different disciplines for a common purpose, in the same way that we have done so in producing this book—so that, quite apart from enjoying each other's company, we can deliver seamless, integrated and up-to-date evidence-based care to our patients.

Tammy Hoffmann, **Sally Bennett** and **Chris Del Mar**

Chapter 1

Introduction to evidence-based practice

Tammy Hoffmann, Sally Bennett and Chris Del Mar

LEARNING OBJECTIVES

After reading this chapter, you should be able to:

- Explain what is meant by the term evidence-based practice
- Understand the origins of evidence-based practice
- Explain why evidence-based practice is important
- Describe the scope of evidence-based health care
- List and briefly explain each of the five steps that make up the evidence-based practice process

WHAT IS EVIDENCE-BASED PRACTICE?

There is a famous definition by Professor David Sackett and some of his colleagues which declares evidence-based medicine to be explicit and conscientious attempts to find the best available research evidence to assist health professionals to make the best decisions for their patients.[1] Even though this definition was originally given with respect to evidence-based medicine, it is often extended beyond the medical profession and used as the definition of evidence-based practice as well. The definition may sound rather ambiguous, so let us pick its elements apart so that you can fully appreciate what is meant by the term *evidence-based practice*.

The purpose of evidence-based practice is to assist in clinical decision making. To make informed clinical decisions, we need to integrate lots of pieces of information. As health professionals, we are typically very good at seeking information from our patients and their families and from the settings in which we work; but, traditionally, we have not been as aware of the information that we can gain from research. When Sackett and his colleagues refer to 'evidence', they clarify it by specifying 'evidence from research'. So, although we need information from many sources, evidence-based practice shows how research can also play a role in informing clinical decisions. Let us sidetrack for a moment to look briefly at what research can offer us to enhance our clinical decision making.

We are familiar with the importance of research for testing theories and for providing us with the background information that forms part of our clinical knowledge. Knowledge about subjects such as anatomy, pathology, psychology and social structures that is essential to our work has been refined over many years through research. Our science-based training gives us models on which to base our clinical management of patients. Of course, having an understanding of the mechanisms is important—for example, we could never have made sense of heart failure or diabetes without understanding the basic mechanisms of these illnesses. Yet, focusing only on the mechanisms of illness can be misleading. Evidence-based practice encourages us to concentrate instead on testing the information directly. This is actually difficult for health professionals to do, because we have been trained to consider primarily the underlying mechanisms. Table 1.1 gives some clinical examples to illustrate how the two approaches differ.

Returning to exploring the elements of the definition of evidence-based practice, the definition very deliberately states that attempts to find evidence should be 'explicit' and 'conscientious'. There is a good

TABLE 1.1: EXAMPLES OF HOW FOCUSING ONLY ON THE MECHANISMS OF ILLNESS CAN BE MISLEADING		
Previous recommendation (based on a mechanism approach)	Rationale based on a mechanism approach	The empirical research that showed it was wrong
Put babies onto their fronts when they go to sleep	If they should vomit in their sleep, they might swallow the vomit into their lungs and develop pneumonia (Dr Spock in the 1950s)[2]	Observational data have shown that babies are more likely to die of sudden infant death syndrome (SIDS) if they lie on their fronts, rather than on their backs, when sleeping[3]
Bed rest after a heart attack (myocardial infarction)	The heart needs resting after an insult in which some of the heart muscle dies	Randomised controlled trials showed that bed rest makes thromboembolism (a dangerous condition in which a clot blocks the flow of blood through a blood vessel) much more likely[4]
Covering skin wounds after removal of skin cancer	To prevent bacteria gaining access and therefore causing infection	A randomised controlled trial showed that leaving the skin wounds open does not increase the infection rate[5]

reason for this. Prior to the advent of evidence-based practice, the way in which many health professionals accessed research was somewhat haphazard and their understanding of how to accurately interpret research results was often superficial. In other words, we may not have been making the best use of research to inform our clinical decision making. For example, simply using whatever research evidence you happen to obtain from reading the few journals that you subscribe to is not going to sufficiently meet your clinical information needs or keep you updated with new research.[6] Hence, the definition of evidence-based practice encourages us to be 'explicit' and 'conscientious' in our attempts at locating the best evidence from research.

That leads us to explore what is meant by the term *best* evidence from research. Understanding what the different study designs can and cannot help you with and, if you like, what their pros and cons are is important. Part of the skill of evidence-based practice is being able to locate the type of study design that is best suited to the particular type of information that you need in order to make a clinical decision. Further, as we explain in more detail later in this chapter, some studies have not been designed very well and this reduces the confidence that we have in their conclusions. We therefore need to attempt to find the best quality research that is available.

The beginning of the definition of evidence-based medicine according to Sackett and colleagues,[1] introduced at the beginning of this chapter, is well known and often quoted. However, the section that follows it is also important. It reads:

> The practice of evidence-based medicine means integrating individual clinical expertise with the best available external clinical evidence from systematic research. By individual clinical expertise we mean the proficiency and judgement that individual clinicians acquire through clinical experiences and clinical practice. Increased expertise is reflected in many ways, but especially in more effective and efficient diagnosis and in the more thoughtful identification and compassionate use of individual patients' predicaments, rights, and preferences in making clinical decisions about their care.[1]

This definition makes it clear that evidence-based practice also requires clinical expertise, which includes thoughtfulness and compassion as well as knowledge of effectiveness and efficiency. As this is a key aspect of evidence-based practice, we consider the concept of clinical expertise in more depth in Chapter 15.

A simple definition of evidence-based practice

Over time, the definition of evidence-based practice has been expanded upon and refined. Nowadays one of the most frequently used and widely known definitions of evidence-based practice acknowledges that it involves the integration of the best research evidence with clinical expertise and the patient's unique values and circumstances.[7] It also requires the health professional to take into account characteristics of the practice context in which they work. This is illustrated in Figure 1.1. As you read this book, keep this definition in mind. Evidence-based practice is *not* just about using research evidence, as some critics of it may suggest. It is also about valuing and using the education, skills and experience that you have as a health professional. Furthermore, it is also about considering the patient's situation and values when making a decision, as well as considering characteristics of the practice context (for example, the resources available) in which you are interacting with your patient. This requires judgment and artistry, as well as science and logic. The *process* that health professionals use to integrate all of this information is *clinical reasoning* (in Chapter 15, this process is discussed in more detail). When you take these four elements and combine them in a way that enables you to make decisions about the care of a patient, then you are engaging in evidence-based practice.

Before we continue, just a note about the language used throughout the book: we have chosen to use the word 'patient', although we acknowledge that different terms (such as 'client' or 'consumer') are used in different disciplines.

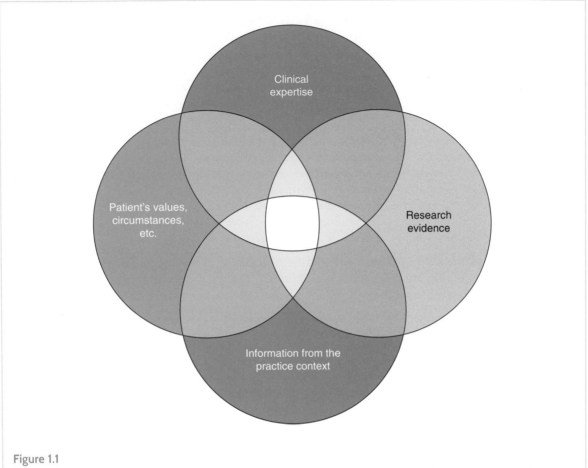

Figure 1.1

Evidence-based practice involves using clinical reasoning to integrate information from four sources: research evidence, clinical expertise, the patient's values and circumstances, and the practice context.

Where did evidence-based practice come from?

It came from a new medical school that started in the 1970s at McMaster University in Canada. The new medical program was unusual in several respects. One difference was that it was very short (only three years). This meant that its teachers realised that the notion of teaching medical students everything they needed to know was clearly impossible. All they could hope for was to teach them how to find for themselves what they needed to know. How could they do that? The answer was the birth of evidence-based medicine, and hence evidence-based practice.

What happened before evidence-based practice?

This is a good question, and one that patients often ask whenever we explain to them what evidence-based practice is all about. We often relied just on 'experience', on the expertise of colleagues who were older and 'better' and on what we were taught as students. Each of these sources of information can be flawed and there are good data to show this.[8] Experience is very subject to flaws of bias. We over-emphasise the mistakes of the recent past, and underestimate the rare mistakes. What we were taught as students is often woefully out of date.[9–11] The health professions are, by their nature, very conservative, and so relying on colleagues who are older and better (so-called 'eminence-based practice'[12]) as an information source will often provide us with information that is out of date, biased and, quite simply, often wrong.

This is not to say that clinical experience is not important. In fact, it is so important that it is a key feature in the definition of evidence-based practice. Clinical experience (discussed further in Chapter 15) is knowledge that is generated from practical experience and involves thoughtfulness and compassion as well as knowledge about the practices and activities that are specific to a discipline. However, rather than simply relying on clinical experience alone for decision making, we need to use our clinical experience *together* with other types of information. To help us make sense of all of the information that we have—from research, from clinical settings, from our patients and from clinical experience—we use clinical reasoning processes.

Is evidence-based practice the same as 'guidelines'?

No. As you will see in Chapter 13, guidelines are one way that evidence-based practice can help to get the best available evidence into clinical practice, but they are by no means the only way. Unfortunately, some documents that call themselves 'guidelines' are *not* evidence-based guidelines (for example, they may contain recommendations that are derived from a mixture of research evidence and expert opinion). When this is the case, they are worse than any evidence-based practice alternatives, because health professionals may mistakenly believe that the 'recommendations' are evidence-based when in fact they are opinion-based, with all the biases that accompany opinion.

Is evidence-based practice the same as randomised controlled trials?

No. As you will see in Chapter 4, it is certainly true that randomised controlled trials are the cornerstone of research investigating whether *interventions* ('treatments') work. However, questions about the effectiveness of interventions are not the only type of question that health professionals need good research information about. For example, health professionals also need good information about questions of: *aetiology* (what causes disease or makes it more likely); *frequency* (how common it is); *diagnosis* (how we know if the patient has the disease or condition of interest); *prognosis* (what happens to the condition over time); and what *patients' experiences and concerns* are in particular situations. In this book, we will primarily focus on how to answer four main types of questions—concerning the effects of interventions, diagnosis, prognosis and patients' experiences and concerns—as these questions are relevant to a range of health professionals and are asked commonly by them. Each question type requires a different type of research design (of which randomised controlled trials are just one example) to address it. Other research designs include *qualitative research, case-control studies, cross-sectional studies* and *cohort studies*. There are many others. They can all be examples of the best evidence for some research questions. This is explored in more depth in Chapter 2.

Can anyone practise evidence-based practice?

Yes. With the right training, practice and experience, any of us can learn how to do evidence-based practice competently. You do not have to be an expert in anything. Having access to the internet and databases (such as PubMed and the Cochrane Library) is good. And having some trustworthy colleagues to check your more surprising findings is also good.

Do health professionals have time for an activity like evidence-based practice?

Health professionals do not have to commit more time to evidence-based practice than they are comfortable with. Actually, if you are a practising health professional, you will probably find that you can replace a lot of what you currently do, such as (for example) reading journals, attending in-service training or other continuing professional development activities, with evidence-based practice. Simply reading a journal or attending a conference or in-service training session is not evidence-based practice—although, of course, these activities often form part of evidence-based practice. When they do, the process which is followed, and the way in which the 'answers' to the clinical questions are subsequently used, is different (as described in Chapter 17).

WHY IS EVIDENCE-BASED PRACTICE IMPORTANT?

Put simply, the main reason why evidence-based practice is important is because it aims to provide the most effective care that is available, with the aim of improving patient outcomes. However, there are many other reasons why it is important. When you seek health care for yourself from a health professional, do you expect that you will receive care that is based on the best available evidence? Of course you do. Likewise, our patients expect that we will provide them with the most effective care and the most accurate healthcare information that is available. As the internet plays such a large role in today's society, patients are now more aware of and educated about health conditions and issues such as intervention options and available tests. For example, it is not uncommon for patients to show their health professional information about a new intervention that they read about on the internet and ask to receive that intervention. As their treating health professional, we need to be able to assess the accuracy of this information, determine the suitability of the intervention for our patient and work with them to decide if this intervention is an appropriate and effective option for them.

Evidence-based practice promotes an attitude of inquiry in health professionals and gets us thinking about questions such as: Why am I doing this in this way? Is there evidence that can guide me to do this in a more effective way? As such, evidence-based practice has an important role in facilitating our professional accountability. By definition, we are *professionals* whose job is to provide health care to people who need it (hence the term 'health professionals'). As part of providing a professional service it is our responsibility, when it is possible, to ensure that our practice is informed by the best available evidence. When we integrate the best available evidence with information from our clinical knowledge, patients and practice context, the reasoning behind our clinical decisions becomes more apparent and this serves to reinforce both our professional accountability and our claim of being a health professional.

Evidence-based practice also has an important role to play in ensuring that health resources are used wisely and that relevant evidence is considered when decisions are made about funding health services. There are finite resources available to provide health care to people. As such, we need to be responsible in our use of healthcare resources. For example, if there is good quality evidence that a particular intervention is harmful or not effective and will not produce clinically meaningful improvement in our patients, we should not waste precious resources providing this intervention—even if it is one that has been provided for years. That is not to say, however, that if no research exists that clearly supports what we do, the interventions that we provide should not be funded. As discussed later in this book, absence of evidence and evidence of ineffectiveness (or evidence of harm) are quite different things.

SCOPE OF EVIDENCE-BASED HEALTH CARE

As mentioned earlier, evidence-based practice is a concept that emerged out of evidence-based medicine. Although this book will concentrate largely on the use of evidence-based practice in clinical settings, evidence-based concepts now permeate all of health care (and beyond). That is why you will hear, from time to time, terms such as 'evidence-based purchasing' (where purchasers are informed by research to make purchases of health and social care services and resources that are useful and safe), 'evidence-based policy' (where policy makers integrate research evidence into the formation of policy documents and decisions to address the needs of the population) or 'evidence-based management' (where managers integrate research findings into a range of management tasks). Evidence-based practice has had a significant impact in more than just the clinical domain, and its influence can be seen in many of the major health systems and government health policies across the world. In fact, if you are interested, you might like to do a quick internet search that will show that 'evidence-based' principles are now being applied in social care, criminology, education, conservation, engineering, sport and many other disciplines.

COMMON CRITICISMS OF EVIDENCE-BASED PRACTICE

Once you start reading widely in this area you will notice that many have criticised evidence-based practice.[13] Criticisms that have been raised are often due to lack of knowledge or misinformation, so we will have a look at some of them here.

Some authors criticise evidence-based practice for relying too heavily on quantitative research. Qualitative research is very important in helping us to understand more about how individuals and communities perceive health, manage their own health and make decisions related to health-service usage. There is growing appreciation of the value and contribution of qualitative research to evidence-based practice. This is partially reflected in the growth of mixed-methods research papers (those that use a combination of qualitative and quantitative approaches); both primary studies, such as those that are answering questions about intervention effectiveness, and systematic reviews that critically review the quality and synthesise the findings of individual studies.

Authors from a range of health professions have also highlighted the limitations of relying on research to provide the evidence on which to base practice. They point to limited available research, particularly in some areas of allied health. Similarly, questions have been raised as to whether it is possible to develop sufficient and appropriate research to support the complexity and rapidly changing nature of professional practice.[14] While we agree that there will never be enough research to provide answers to every possible clinical question, evidence-based practice emphasises using the best research evidence *available* and acknowledges the need to draw on expert opinion where research does not exist. Further, clinical experience, which is one of the key components of evidence-based practice, must be relied on even more where there is a lack of evidence or uncertainty.

Many authors have debated the nature of 'evidence', arguing that evidence comes from many sources other than research. While it is vital to incorporate information from many different sources, the term 'evidence' in evidence-based practice serves a specific purpose. Its purpose is to highlight the value of information from research which has so often been ignored. In fact, some have suggested that, instead of the term *evidence-based practice*, 'knowledge-based practice' or 'information-based practice' should be used. While these alternatives avoid the contentiousness about what evidence is and what it is not, it would be impossible to find a health professional who does not base their practice on knowledge or information. In other words, use of the term 'evidence' (where evidence is taken to mean evidence from research) helps to highlight a source of information that has been under-utilised. Use of the term 'evidence' to highlight the role of research in clinical decision making by no means discounts the importance of information and knowledge from patients and health professionals themselves, and this is something we hope to demonstrate throughout this book.

THE PROCESS OF EVIDENCE-BASED PRACTICE

Rather than being just a vague concept that is difficult to incorporate into everyday clinical practice, the process of evidence-based practice is actually quite structured. The process can be viewed as a number of steps that health professionals need to perform when an information need (that can be answered by research evidence) arises:[7]

1. Convert your information needs into an answerable clinical question.
2. Find the best evidence to answer your clinical question.

3. Critically appraise the evidence for its validity, impact and applicability.

4. Integrate the evidence with clinical expertise, the patient's values and circumstances, and information from the practice context.

5. Evaluate the effectiveness and efficiency with which steps 1–4 were carried out and think about ways to improve your performance of them next time.

Some people may prefer to remember these steps as the five **A**s:[15]

- **A**sk a question
- **A**ccess the information
- **A**ppraise the articles found
- **A**pply the information
- **A**udit.

Regardless of which list you prefer to use to remember the process of evidence-based practice, the basic steps are the same and they are explained in more detail below.

Step 1. Convert your information needs into an answerable clinical question

The process of evidence-based practice begins with the recognition that you, as a health professional, have a clinical information need. Some types of clinical information needs can be answered with the assistance of research evidence. Chapter 2 describes the different types of clinical information needs and which ones research evidence can help you to answer. An important step in the evidence-based practice process is turning this information need into an answerable clinical question, and there are some easy ways to do this which are demonstrated in Chapter 2.

You may have a question about:

- **intervention** (that is, treatment)—for example, in adults with rheumatoid arthritis, is education about joint protection techniques effective in reducing hand pain and improving function?
- **diagnosis**—for example, in adults admitted to a chest pain unit, which elements of serial diagnostic testing are the most sensitive and specific predictors of cardiac involvement?
- **prognosis**—for example, in people undergoing total knee replacement for osteoarthritis, what improvement in walking ability is expected after six weeks?
- **patients' experiences and concerns**—for example, what does the lived experience of older adults transitioning to residential aged-care facilities mean for their ability to integrate and find a sense of identity?

The type of question will determine the type of research that you need to look for in order to answer your question. This is explained further in Chapter 2.

Step 2. Find the best evidence to answer your clinical question

Once you have structured your clinical question appropriately and know what type of question you are asking and, therefore, what sort of research you need to look for, the next step is to find the research evidence to answer your question. It is important that you are aware of the many online evidence-based resources and which will be most appropriate for you to use to search for the evidence to answer your question. Being able to *efficiently* search the online evidence-based resources is a crucial skill for anyone who practises evidence-based practice. Chapter 3 contains information about the key online evidence-based resources and how to look for evidence efficiently.

Step 3. Critically appraise the evidence for its validity, impact and applicability

Upon finding the evidence, you will need to critically appraise it. That is, you need to examine the evidence closely to determine whether it is worthy of being used to inform your clinical practice.

Why do I need to critically appraise the evidence? Is not all published research of good quality?

Unfortunately, not all published research is of good quality. In fact, there are a number of studies that suggest that much of it is of poor quality (see, for example, references 16–25). There is a range of reasons why this is the case. Conducting a well-designed research study is hard work—there are many issues to consider during the design phase. Sometimes, even when researchers have designed a great study, things that they have no control over can happen—such as losing many of the participants to follow-up (despite their best attempts to avoid this happening), or an unexpected change in the type or number of patients who are eligible for recruitment into the study. There are many practical and ethical considerations that can also make it difficult to conduct a study that uses methods to avoid introducing bias into a trial. For example, as you will see in Chapters 2 and 4, lack of blinding can introduce bias in a study. However, in the overwhelming majority of randomised controlled trials that evaluate an allied health intervention, it is not possible to blind either the participants or the therapists who are providing the intervention as to whether the participants are in the intervention group or the control group. Too often, research is conducted by people who do not have a full awareness of the issues surrounding research design and, as a result, the studies that they conduct are flawed. The way in which some researchers report their studies also can be incomplete and, as readers, we are often left wondering about the details of some aspects of the study and unsure whether the researchers did or did not consider particular aspects of study design. Sadly, the people who peer-review the studies for journals are sometimes no more informed about all of the latest issues in study design than the researchers who conducted the studies are.

Fortunately, it appears that this situation is changing, with some emerging data showing that the quality of studies is improving over time as researchers increase their use of methods to minimise the risk of bias.[23,26-29] This is most likely because there is now a growing awareness of the importance of strong study design (thanks in part to the proliferation of evidence-based practice) on the part of authors of studies, reviewers of studies and journal editors. As you will see in various chapters throughout the book, guides for how certain types of studies should be reported have been developed (for example, in Chapter 4, you will learn about the CONSORT statement for randomised controlled trials). A list of the reporting guidelines for various study types is available at the website of the EQUATOR Network (www.equator-network.org). A growing number of journals now require authors of studies to carefully follow these guides if they wish their article to be considered for publication. All of this is good news for us (health professionals who wish to use evidence to inform their clinical decision making), as it has the potential to make interpreting research reports easier, but there is still a very long way to go to remedy the multitude of ways in which bias can creep in to the design and re-porting of research studies.

Because of this, before you can use the results of a research study to assist you in making a clinical decision, you need to determine whether the study methods are sound enough to provide you with potentially useful information or, alternatively, whether the methods are so flawed that they might potentially provide misleading results. Studies that are poorly designed may produce results that are distorted by bias (and, often, more than one type of bias). Some of the common types of bias are intro-duced in Chapter 2. The main types of bias that are relevant to each of the question types are explained in detail in the corresponding chapter that discusses how to appraise the evidence for each question type.

What is involved in critically appraising evidence?

There are three main aspects of the evidence (that is, each study) that you need to appraise (in the following order):

1. **Internal validity.** This refers to whether the evidence is trustworthy. That is, can you believe the results of the study? You evaluate the validity of the study by determining whether the study was carried out in a way that was methodologically sound. In this step, we are concerned with the study's *internal validity*—this is explained more fully in Chapter 2.

2. **Impact.** If you decide that the validity of the study is sufficient that you can believe the results, you then need to look closely at the results of the study. The main thing that you need to determine is the impact (that is, the clinical importance) of the evidence. For example, in a study that compared the effectiveness of a new intervention with an existing intervention, did the new intervention have a *large enough effect* on the clinical outcome(s) of interest that you would consider altering your practice and using the new intervention with your patient?

3. **Applicability.** If you have decided that the validity of the study is adequate and that the results are clinically important, the final step of critical appraisal is to evaluate whether you can apply the results of the study to your patient. Essentially you need to assess whether your patient is so different from the participants in the study that you cannot apply the results of the study to your patient. This step is concerned with assessing the *external validity* (or the 'generalisability' or 'applicability') of the study—this is explained more fully in Chapter 2.

Many chapters in this book (Chapters 4–12) are devoted to helping you learn how to critically appraise various types of evidence. There are plenty of appraisal checklists that you can use to help you critically appraise the evidence. Many of the checklists are freely available on the internet. Most of them contain more or less the same key items. The checklists that we have used in this book as a general guide for the appraisal of research are based on those developed by the UK National Health Service Public Health Resource Unit as part of the Critical Appraisal Skills Programme (CASP). In turn, these checklists were derived from the well-known *Journal of the American Medical Association (JAMA)* Users' Guides.[29] The CASP checklists are freely available at www.casp-uk.net. For the appraisal of qualitative research, we have also used the Qualitative Assessment and Review Instrument (QARI) developed by the Joanna Briggs Institute. The QARI can be accessed as part of a software package which you can download for free (once you have registered) at www.joannabriggs.edu.au. In addition, the CASP checklist for appraising qualitative studies is also described and the two approaches are compared in Chapter 10.

Each of the CASP checklists begins by asking two screening questions. These questions are designed to filter out studies of low methodological quality. This is so that you do not waste your time proceeding to appraise the validity, impact and applicability of a study that is going to be of too poor a quality for you to use in clinical decision making. In the worked examples in Chapters 5, 7, 9 and 11, you will notice that these screening questions are not included in the examples. This is because, prior to appraising their chosen article, the authors of each of the worked examples had already conducted a screening process when they decided which article was the best available evidence to use to answer their clinical question. When you are critically appraising research articles, keep in mind that no research is perfect and that it is important not to be overly critical of research articles. It just needs to be *good enough* to assist you to make a clinical decision.

Step 4. Integrate the evidence with clinical expertise, the patient's values and circumstances, and information from the practice context

The fourth step in the evidence-based practice process involves integrating the findings from the critical appraisal step with your clinical expertise, your patient's needs and the practice (clinical) context. As discussed earlier in this chapter and illustrated in Figure 1.1, these four elements form the definition of evidence-based practice. 'Clinical expertise' refers to a health professional's cumulative experience, education and clinical skills. As evidence-based practice is a problem-solving approach that initially stems from a patient's needs, any clinical decision that is made in relation to the patient should involve consideration of the unique needs, values, preferences, concerns and experiences that each patient brings to the situation. Many of the chapters of this book discuss the need for and process of integrating research evidence with clinical expertise and the patient's needs, with appropriate consideration also given to the practice context.

Step 5. Evaluate the effectiveness and efficiency with which steps 1–4 were carried out and think about ways to improve your performance of them next time

As evidence-based practice is a process that is intended for health professionals to incorporate into their routine clinical practice, it is important that you learn to do it as efficiently as possible so that it does not become a time-consuming or onerous task. Asking yourself self-reflection questions after you have completed steps 1 to 4 of the evidence-based practice process can be a useful way to identify which steps you are doing well and areas where you could improve. Box 1.1 contains some examples of self-reflection questions that you could ask when evaluating how well you performed steps 1 to 4 of the evidence-based practice process.

HOW THIS BOOK IS STRUCTURED

The process of evidence-based practice that was just described has been used as a structure for this book. In addition to the key steps that form the evidence-based practice process, there are other topics that are important for health professionals who wish to practise evidence-based practice to know. Topics such as how to implement evidence into practice and how to communicate with patients about evidence are also addressed in chapters of this book.

BOX 1.1

Examples of self-reflection questions when evaluating your performance of steps 1 to 4 of the evidence-based practice process

- Am I asking well-formulated clinical questions? (See Chapter 2)
- Am I aware of the best sources of evidence for the different types of clinical question? (See Chapter 3)
- Am I searching the databases efficiently? (See Chapter 3)
- Am I using the hierarchy of evidence for each type of clinical question as my guide for the type of evidence that I should be searching for? (See Chapter 2)
- Where possible, am I searching for and using information that is higher up in the pyramid of levels of organisation of evidence (for example, syntheses, synopses, summaries and pre-appraised original studies)? (See Chapter 3)
- Am I integrating the critical appraisal into my clinical practice? (See Chapters 4–13)
- Can I clearly explain what the evidence means to my patients and involve them in shared decision making where appropriate? (See Chapter 14)
- Am I proactively monitoring for newly emerging evidence in my field of practice?[30] (See Chapter 3)

Chapter 1—Introduction to evidence-based practice	This chapter addresses some of the background information about evidence-based practice, such as what it is, why it was developed, why it is important and the five key steps that underlie the process of evidence-based practice.
Chapter 2—Information needs, asking questions and some basics of research studies	Chapter 2 provides details about clinical information needs, how to convert them into an answerable question and how the type of research that you look for differs according to the type of question you are asking. This chapter also contains some of the background statistical information that you need to understand before being able to critically appraise the research evidence.
Chapter 3—Finding the evidence	Chapter 3 contains information about how to undertake the second step of the evidence-based practice process, which is searching for the evidence to answer your clinical question.
Chapter 4—Evidence about effects of interventions	This chapter explains what to do when you have a clinical question about the effects of an intervention, with the focus on how to perform the third and fourth steps of the evidence-based practice process. It gives details about how to assess the validity of the evidence, understand the results and use the evidence to inform clinical practice.
Chapter 5—Questions about the effects of interventions: examples of appraisals from different health professions	As the steps of evidence-based practice become easier with practice, this chapter provides you with a number of worked examples of questions about interventions so that you can see, step-by-step, for various clinical scenarios how questions are formulated and evidence is found, appraised and applied. In keeping with the multidisciplinary nature of this book, examples from a range of health professions are provided.
Chapter 6—Evidence about diagnosis	This chapter follows the same structure as Chapter 4, but the content is focused on how to appraise the evidence when your clinical question is about diagnosis.
Chapter 7—Questions about diagnosis: examples of appraisals from different health professions	Chapter 7 contains a number of worked examples of questions about diagnosis from a range of health professions that commonly have diagnostic/assessment informational needs.
Chapter 8—Evidence about prognosis	This chapter follows the same structure as Chapters 4 and 6, but the content is focused on how to appraise the evidence when your clinical question is about prognosis.
Chapter 9—Questions about prognosis: examples of appraisals from different health professions	Chapter 9 contains a number of worked examples of questions about prognosis from a range of health professions that commonly consider prognostic issues.

Chapter 10—Evidence about patients' experiences and concerns	This chapter follows the same structure as Chapters 4, 6 and 8, but the content is focused on how to appraise the evidence when your question is about patients' experiences and concerns and you are using qualitative research to answer the question.
Chapter 11—Questions about patients' experiences and concerns: examples of appraisals from different health professions	Chapter 11 contains a number of worked examples of questions about patients' experiences and concerns from a range of health professions.
Chapter 12—Appraising and understanding systematic reviews and meta-analyses	As discussed in Chapter 2, systematic reviews and meta-analyses are a very important research study type. They are so important that we have devoted an entire chapter to explaining how to appraise and make sense of them.
Chapter 13—Clinical guidelines	Clinical practice guidelines can be a useful tool in evidence-based practice. Chapter 13 provides you with information about what they are, how they are developed, where to find them and how to assess their quality to determine if you should use them in clinical practice.
Chapter 14—Talking with patients about evidence	Knowing how to talk with patients and explain, in a way that they can understand, what the evidence you have found means for them is an important skill for health professionals. Chapter 14 describes how to do this and how to involve your patients in the decision-making process.
Chapter 15—Clinical reasoning and evidence-based practice	Clinical reasoning is the process by which health professionals integrate information from many different sources. Having an understanding of clinical reasoning can clarify, and hopefully improve, our clinical decision making.
Chapter 16—Implementing evidence into practice	After finding and appraising the evidence, patient outcomes will only be altered if the evidence is then implemented into clinical practice. Chapter 16 describes the process for doing this, along with some of the barriers that may be encountered during the process, and strategies for overcoming them.
Chapter 17—Embedding evidence-based practice into routine clinical care	While individual health professionals will always be key in advancing evidence-based practice, an organisational environment which recognises the value of, and encourages, evidence-based practice is also important. Chapter 17 describes why organisations should promote evidence-based practice, characteristics of organisations that do this and specific strategies which organisations can use to support evidence-based practice.

SUMMARY POINTS OF THIS CHAPTER

- Evidence-based practice is a problem-based approach where research evidence is used to inform clinical decision making. It involves the integration of the best available research evidence with clinical expertise, each patient's values and circumstances, and consideration of the clinical (practice) context.

- Evidence-based practice is important because it aims to improve patient outcomes and it is what our patients expect. However, it also has a role in facilitating professional accountability and guiding decisions about the funding of health services.

- Evidence-based practice has extended to all areas of health care and is now used in areas such as policy formulation and implementation, purchasing and management.

- There are five main steps in the evidence-based practice process: (1) asking a question; (2) searching for evidence to answer it; (3) critically appraising the evidence; (4) integrating the evidence with your clinical expertise, the patient's values and information from the practice context; and (5) evaluating how well you performed steps 1–4 and how you can improve your performance the next time you complete this process.

- Not all research evidence is of sufficient quality that you can confidently use it to inform your clinical decision making. Therefore, you need to critically appraise it before deciding whether to use it. The three main aspects of the evidence that you need to critically appraise are its: (1) validity—can you trust it?, (2) impact—are the results clinically important? and (3) applicability—can you apply it to your patient?.

References

1. Sackett D, Rosenberg W, Gray J, et al. Evidence based medicine: what it is and what it isn't: it's about integrating individual clinical expertise and the best external evidence. BMJ 1996;312:71–2.
2. Spock B. Baby and child care. London: The Bodley Head; 1958.
3. Gilbert R, Salanti G, Harden M, et al. Infant sleeping position and the sudden infant death syndrome: systematic review of observational studies and historical review of recommendations from 1940 to 2002. Int J Epidemiol 2005;34:874–87.
4. Allen C, Glasziou P, Del Mar C. Bed rest: a potentially harmful treatment needing more careful evaluation. Lancet 1999;354:1229–33.
5. Heal C, Buettner P, Raasch B, et al. Can sutures get wet? Prospective randomised controlled trial of wound management in general practice. BMJ 2006;332:1053–6.
6. Hoffmann T, Erueti C, Thorning S, et al. The scatter of research: a cross-sectional comparison of randomised trials and systematic reviews across specialties. BMJ 2012;344:e3223. doi: 10.1136/bmj.e3223.
7. Straus S, Richardson W, Glasziou P, et al. Evidence-based medicine: how to practice and teach EBM. 4th ed. Edinburgh: Churchill Livingstone; 2011.
8. Oxman A, Guyatt G. The science of reviewing research. Ann N Y Acad Sci 1993;703:125–33, discussion 133–4.
9. Sibley J, Sackett D, Neufeld V, et al. A randomised trial of continuing medical education. N Engl J Med 1982;306:511–15.
10. Ramsey P, Carline J, Inui T, et al. Changes over time in the knowledge base of practising internists. JAMA 1991;266:1103–7.
11. Evans C, Haynes R, Birkett N, et al. Does a mailed continuing education program improve clinical performance? Results of a randomised trial in antihypertensive care. JAMA 1986;255:501–4.
12. Isaacs D, Fitzgerald D. Seven alternatives to evidence based medicine. BMJ 1999;319:1618.
13. Straus S, McAlister F. Evidence-based medicine: a commentary on common criticisms. Can Med Assoc J 2000;163:837–41.
14. Higgs J, Titchen A, editors. Practice knowledge and expertise in the health professions. Oxford: Butterworth–Heinemann; 2001.
15. Jackson R, Ameratunga S, Broad J, et al. The GATE frame: critical appraisal with pictures. ACP J Club 2006;144:2.

16. Anyanwu C, Treasure T. Surgical research revisited: clinical trials in the cardiothoracic surgical literature. Eur J Cardiothorac Surg 2004;25:299–303.

17. DeMauro S, Giaccone A, Kirpalani H, et al. Quality of reporting of neonatal and infant trials in high-impact journals. Pediatrics 2011;128:e639–44.

18. Sinha S, Sinha S, Ashby E, et al. Quality of reporting in randomised trials published in high-quality surgical journals. J Am Coll Surg 2009;209:565–71.

19. Kjaergard L, Frederiksen S, Gludd C. Validity of randomised clinical trials in gastroenterology from 1964–2000. Gastroenterology 2002;122:1157–60.

20. Dickinson K, Bunn F, Wentz R, et al. Size and quality of randomised controlled trials in head injury: review of published studies. BMJ 2000;320:1308–11.

21. Chan S, Bhandari M. The quality of reporting of orthopaedic randomised trials with use of a checklist for nonpharmacological therapies. J Bone Joint Surg Am 2007;89:1970–80.

22. Hoffmann T, McKenna K, Hadi T, et al. Quality and quantity of paediatric research: an analysis of the OTseeker database. Aust Occup Ther J 2007;54:113–23.

23. Hoffmann T, Bennett S, McKenna K, et al. Interventions for stroke rehabilitation: analysis of the research contained in the OTseeker evidence database. Top Stroke Rehabil 2008;15:341–50.

24. Bennett S, McKenna K, McCluskey A, et al. Evidence for occupational therapy interventions: effectiveness research indexed in the OTseeker database. Br J Occup Ther 2007;70:426–30.

25. McCluskey A, Lovarini M, Bennett S, et al. What evidence exists for work-related injury prevention and management? Analysis of an occupational therapy evidence database (OTseeker). Br J Occup Ther 2005;68:447–56.

26. Moseley A, Herbert R, Sherrington C, et al. Evidence for physiotherapy practice: a survey of the Physiotherapy Evidence database (PEDro). Aust J Physiother 2002;48:43–9.

27. Moseley A, Herbert R, Maher C, et al. Reported quality of randomized trials of physiotherapy interventions has improved over time. J Clin Epidemiol 2011;64:594–601.

28. Falagas M, Grigori T, Ioannidou E. A systematic review of trends in the methodological quality of randomised controlled trials in various research fields. J Clin Epidemiol 2009;62:227–31.

29. Guyatt G, Rennie D. Users' guides to the medical literature. JAMA 1993;270:2096–7.

30. Keister D, Tilson J. Proactively monitoring for newly emerging evidence: the lost step in EBP? Evid Based Med 2008;13:69.

Chapter 2

Information needs, asking questions, and some basics of research studies

Chris Del Mar, Tammy Hoffmann and Paul Glasziou

LEARNING OBJECTIVES

After reading this chapter, you should be able to:
- Describe the types of clinical information needs that can be answered using research
- Differentiate between 'just-in-case' information and 'just-in-time' information
- Convert your information needs into answerable, well-structured clinical questions, using the PICO format
- Describe the basic design of some of the common study types that are used in evidence-based practice
- Explain the hierarchy of evidence for questions about the effects of interventions, the hierarchy for diagnostic questions and the hierarchy for prognostic questions
- Explain what is meant by internal validity and external validity
- Describe some of the main types of bias that can occur in studies
- Differentiate between statistical significance and clinical significance and briefly explain how each of them is determined

This chapter provides background information that you need to know for understanding the details of the evidence-based practice process that follow in the subsequent chapters of this book. In that sense, this chapter is a somewhat diverse but important collection of topics. We start by describing the types of clinical information needs that health professionals commonly have and discuss some of the methods that health professionals use to obtain information to answer those needs. As we saw in Chapter 1, converting an information need into an answerable, well-structured question is the first step in the process of evidence-based practice and, in this chapter, we explain how to do this. We then explain the importance of matching the type of question asked with the most appropriate study design. As part of this, we will introduce and explain the concept of 'hierarchies of evidence' for each type of question. In the last sections of this chapter, we will explain some concepts that are fundamental to the critical appraisal of research evidence, which is the third step in the evidence-based practice process. The concepts that we will discuss include internal validity, chance, bias, confounding, statistical significance, clinical significance and power.

CLINICAL INFORMATION NEEDS

Health professionals need information all the time to help assess patients, make decisions, reassure patients, formulate treatment, make practical arrangements and so on. Some of the necessary information can be usefully assembled from existing research, and some cannot. Table 2.1 provides examples of some of the obvious types of information that can or cannot be gathered from research. This book will help you to learn how to deal with information needs that can be answered to some extent by research. Along the way we will also discuss the types of information that come from patients and the types of information that come from clinical experience. When we consider these together—information

TABLE 2.1: CLINICAL INFORMATION NEEDS–EXAMPLES OF QUESTIONS THAT CAN AND QUESTIONS THAT CANNOT BE ANSWERED BY EVIDENCE-BASED PRACTICE			
		Information	Examples
These questions typically *cannot* be answered by research	Local	Background information	Is this patient eligible for treatment subsidy? What are the regulations for the use of a type of treatment? Who can be referred to this service? What are the opening hours of the hospital outpatients' administration? Is there an organisation that runs a chronic disease self-management program in this community? What is a Colles' fracture?
These questions *can* usually be informed by research	General	Aetiology/frequency	Is this risk factor associated with that disease? How many people with those symptoms have this disease?
		Prognosis	What happens to this illness without treatment?
		Diagnosis	If I elicit this sign among people with these symptoms, how many have that disease? If this test is negative, how sure can I be that the patient does *not* have the disease?
		Treatment/ intervention	How much improvement can I expect from this intervention? How much harm is likely from the intervention? Is this intervention more effective than that intervention?
		Patients' experiences and concerns	What is the experience of patients concerning their condition or intervention? What is happening here and why is it happening?

from research, patients and experience—we are working within an evidence-based practice framework.

DEALING EFFECTIVELY WITH INFORMATION NEEDS

Having established that health professionals have many information needs, this section explains how you can effectively deal with these information needs. A simple overview of one way of doing this is as follows:

- Recognise when we have a question.
- Record the question—do not lose that moment!
- Attempt to find the answer.
- Record the answer so that it can be re-used later.
- Stop and reflect on what you have been looking up and dealing with. Is it helping you to answer your question?

The size of the problem

The clinical literature is big. Just how big is staggering. There are thousands of new studies published every week. For example, there are about 75 randomised controlled trials and 11 systematic reviews (this is where primary studies have been systematically located, appraised and synthesised) published per day.[1] That is about one trial published every 19 minutes! Worse than that, randomised controlled trials represent a small proportion (less than 5%) of the research that is indexed in PubMed, which, as you will see in Chapter 3, is just one of several databases available for you to search to find evidence. This means that the accumulated literature is a massive haystack to search for that elusive, yet important, needle of information you need. The information might mean the difference between effective or ineffective (or even harmful) care for your patient. One of the purposes of this book, then, is to help you find evidence needles in research haystacks.

Noting down your clinical question

It is important that we keep track of the questions we ask. If not, it is all too easy to lose track of them and then the opportunity evaporates. If you cannot remember what you wanted to know when in the midst of managing a patient, the chances are you will never go back to answering that question.

How should we do this? One way is to keep a little book in which to write them down in your pocket or handbag. Date and scribble. A more modern way is electronically, of course, using a smart-phone, iPad/tablet or computer (if simultaneously making patient records). Some health professionals tell the patient what they are doing:

> 'I'm just making a note of this to myself to look it up when I have a moment. Next time I see you, I will be able to let you know if we need to change anything.'

Or:

> 'Let's get online and look that up right now, because I want to make sure that we are using the latest research when we make decisions about your ...'

(This second strategy is risky until you have had a lot of practice with the first!)

In Chapter 1, we discussed the general process of looking up, appraising and applying the evidence that we find. Remember also to keep track of the information that you have found (in other words, write it down!), and how you evaluated and applied it. In the end, the information that is found might result in you changing (hopefully improving) your clinical practice. The way it does this is often un-coupled from the processes you undertook, so it takes some time to realise what led you to make the changes—often systematic—to the way you do things. In Chapter 17 there is more information about how this process can occur. Sometimes the research information just reassures us, the health professional, that we are on the right track, but this is important also.

DIFFERENT WAYS OF OBTAINING INFORMATION: PUSH OR PULL? JUST-IN-CASE OR JUST-IN-TIME?

Push: just-in-case information

In advertising jargon, the term *push* means that the information is sent out, or broadcast. This is the traditional means of disseminating information. This is basically the function of journals. After research has been undertaken it is either sent directly to you, or pre-digested in some way (perhaps as an editorial, review article, systematic review or guideline). 'Just-in-case' information is made available when it is generated, or when it is thought (by someone other than you, the health professional) that health professionals ought to hear about it.

Figure 2.1 shows some examples of information that can be *pushed*. Other sources of 'push' information include conferences, professional newsletters, textbooks and informal chats to colleagues and other people from other professional groups.

As can be seen, there are many ways in which a piece of research can percolate through to you as a health professional. The picture is actually more complex than this: what is picked up for review, systematic review and so on is determined by several factors, including which journals the primary data were first published in, how relevant readers think the research is and how well it fits into the policy being formulated or already in existence. There are, in fact, different sorts of information that we might consider accessing and this is explained in detail in Chapter 3 (see Figure 3.1). But this is only the start. All these methods rely on the information arriving at your place of work (or home, post box, email inbox, online blog, etc). Then it has to be managed before it is actually put into practice. How does this happen? There are a number of different stages that can be considered, and these are explained in Table 2.2.

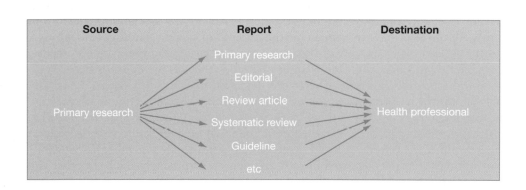

Figure 2.1
Ways in which research data get to you.

TABLE 2.2:
THE PROCESSES INVOLVED IN MAKING SURE THAT *JUST-IN-CASE* INFORMATION IS USED PROPERLY TO HELP PATIENTS

Task		Explanation
Read the title Read the abstract		Decide whether something is worth reading at all.
Read the full paper		We have obviously not tossed this paper aside (that means we have turned the page).
Decide whether it is …	(a) relevant	A lot of research is not aimed at health professionals who are looking for better information to manage their patients. Much of it is researcher-to-researcher information. Just some of it is information that we think might be useful, either now or in the future when this might become part of everyday practice.
	(b) believable	Methodologically sound. That means the information is not biased to the extent that we cannot believe the result. This is explained further later in this chapter and in Chapters 4–12.
Wonder whether the technique is available		A lot of research reports do not spell out the treatment, diagnostic procedure or definitional terms adequately so that we can simply put the research into practice–even if we believe it!
Store the paper so we can recall it when the right patient comes along		Different health professionals do this in different ways: • tear out the paper and file it • meticulously make out reference cards • store a copy electronically (through a reference manager) • just try to remember it. Most health professionals do the last. And then forget!
Ensure that we have the necessary resources to incorporate the research into our practice		There may be prerequisites, such as availability of resources and skills to carry it out or perhaps some policy needs to be instituted before this can happen.
Persuade the patient		… that this is the best management.

Clearly this is not an easy process—how do we get just the right article from the thousands published each week? We often feel overloaded by this, but as Clay Shirky has said: 'It's not information overload. It's filter failure.'[2] The filtering of research information has many steps where the flow can be distorted or interrupted. All the steps have to happen for the research to run the gauntlet through to the patient. One part of the solution is to use one of the good abstracting services (there are also many poor ones, so check their filtering process first). One example of a good service is the *Evidence Based Medicine* online journal (see ebm.bmj.com). This type of service is described in depth in Chapter 3 but, in a nutshell, such journals only provide abstractions of previous research (that is, they contain no primary research). Papers are abstracted only if they survive a rigorous selection process that begins with a careful methodological appraisal; and then, if the paper is found to be sufficiently free of bias, it is sent for appraisal by a worldwide network of health professionals who decide whether the research is relevant. The resultant number of papers reported in each discipline is surprisingly small. In other words, only a few papers are not too biased *and* also relevant!

A word of caution, though: most journal scanning services are insufficient for health professionals to use as a method for keeping up to date with research in their area of practice.[3] This is partly due to the problem of research scatter, where trials and systematic reviews are scattered across hundreds of specialty and general journals.[3] Personal journal subscriptions (and traditional habits such as scanning a few specialty journals) are insufficient for keeping up to date and need to be supplemented by other methods such as journal scanning systems.[3] However, few of the current journal scanning services or systems cover sufficient journals and filter for quality and relevance. Happily for health professionals, however, there is an alternative option to 'just-in-case' information.

Pull: just-in-time information

Pull is advertising jargon for information that potential customers look for (rather than simply waiting for it to be *pushed* to them). This is information that the health professional seeks in relation to a specific question arising from their clinical work, and so this gives it certain characteristics. This is illustrated in Table 2.3 using the five As that were introduced in Chapter 1 as a way of simply describing the steps in the evidence-based practice process.

If this looks familiar to you, well, this is the essential core of evidence-based practice. How feasible is it to incorporate this way of finding information 'just-in-time'? Again, there are several steps which are not easy—they all need mastering and practice (like almost everything in clinical care). For example, asking questions is difficult. It requires health professionals to be open to not knowing everything. Doctors are notorious for having trouble with this—perhaps because society has bestowed some god-like attributes on them that made it potentially too disappointing if they admitted not knowing stuff. The truth is that most people in modern times welcome the honesty that goes with questioning the management you are proposing to give them. It shows how we health professionals are taking extra and meticulous care.

How often do we ask questions? Is this something that we can aspire to realistically? Most health professionals are worried that they do not ask questions enough. Relax. You probably do. Studies have been undertaken in a number of settings (mostly to do with doctors, sadly) to show that they ask questions much more than they realised. For example, a study undertaken in Iowa, USA, examined what questions family doctors working in the community asked during the course of their work. Just over 100 doctors asked >1100 questions over 2.5 days, which is approximately 10 questions each, or 4 per person per day.[4]

A similar Spanish study to the one above found that doctors had a good chance (nearly 100%) of finding an answer if it took less than 2 minutes, but were much less likely to do so (<40%) if it took 30 minutes.[5] A study of doctors found that they are more likely to chase an answer if they believe that an answer exists, or if the information need is urgent.[6] Nurses working in a similar setting were more

TABLE 2.3: PROCESSES INVOLVED IN *JUST-IN-TIME* INFORMATION: THE FIVE AS	
Task	**Explanation**
Ask a question: re-format the question into an answerable one	This ensures relevance–by definition!
Access the information: searching	Decide whether to look now (in front of the patient) or later. Searching is a special skill, which is described in Chapter 3.
Appraise the papers found	We talk about this (in fact, we talk about this a lot) in Chapters 4–12.
Apply the information	This means with the patient who is in front of you.
Audit	Check whether the evidence-based practice processes that you are engaged in are working well.

likely to ask someone or look in a book in order to answer their questions.[7] Despite advances in electronic access, health professionals do not seem to be doing well at effectively seeking answers to clinical questions,[8] even though there is good (randomised controlled trial) evidence to show that getting information this way (that is, just-in-time) improved clinical decision-making.[9]

If we are not able in the hurly burly of daily clinical practice to look up questions immediately, it is important (as we mentioned earlier in the chapter) to write them down in a questions log book (paper or electronic).

HOW TO CONVERT YOUR INFORMATION NEEDS INTO AN ANSWERABLE CLINICAL QUESTION

We will now look at how you can take a clinical question and convert it into an *answerable* clinical question which you can then effectively search to find the answers to. Remember from Chapter 1 that forming an answerable clinical question is the first step of the evidence-based practice process. Asking a good question is central to successful evidence-based practice. Converting our clinical question into an 'answerable question' is necessary because it prevents the health professional from forgetting any of the important components of the clinical question. Typically there are four components,[10] which can be easily remembered using the PICO mnemonic:

P **P**atient or **p**roblem (or **p**opulation or **p**erson)

I **I**ntervention (or diagnostic test or prognostic factor or issue)

C **C**omparison

O **O**utcome(s).

A few questions are only 'PO's—population and outcome. For example, '*What is the chance that an elderly person who falls* (P) *will have a second fall within 12 months* (O)?' But most questions have three or four PICO elements, so we will now address each in turn.

Patient or problem (or population or person)

This component makes sure that you are clear *who* the question relates to. It may include information about the patient, their primary problem or disease, or coexisting conditions—for example, '*In children with autism …*' Sometimes we specify the sex and age of a patient if that is going to be relevant to the diagnosis, prognosis or intervention—for example, '*In elderly women who have osteoporosis …*'

Intervention (or diagnostic test or prognostic factor or issue)

The term 'intervention' is used here in a broad sense. It may refer to the intervention (that is, treatment) that you wish to use with your patient—for example, '*In people who have had a stroke, is home-based rehabilitation as effective as hospital-based rehabilitation in improving ability to perform self-care activities?*' In this case, home-based rehabilitation is the intervention that we are interested in. Or, if you have a diagnostic question, this component of the question may refer to which diagnostic test you are considering using with your patients—for example, '*Does the Mini-Mental State Examination accurately detect the presence of cognitive impairment in older community-living people?*' In this example, the Mini-Mental State Examination is the diagnostic test that we are interested in. A question about prognosis may specify a particular factor or issue that might influence the prognosis of your patient—for example, in the question '*What is the likelihood of hip fracture in women who have a family history of hip fracture?*', the family history of hip fracture is the particular factor that we are interested in. If you want to understand more about patients' perspectives, you may want to focus on a particular issue. For example, in the question '*How do adolescents who are being treated with chemotherapy feel about hospital environments?*', the issue of interest is adolescent perceptions of hospital environments.

Comparison

Your questions may not always include this component, but it is usually useful to consider. It is mainly questions about the effects of intervention (and sometimes diagnosis) that use this component. Add a comparison element to your question if you are interested in comparing the intervention component of your question with another intervention and wish to know if one intervention is more effective than another—which might include nothing. In the example we used above, '*In people who have had a stroke, is home-based rehabilitation as effective as hospital-based rehabilitation in improving ability to perform self-care activities?*', the comparison is hospital-based rehabilitation. Often, the comparison that you are interested in may be 'usual' (or standard) care. While intervention questions sometimes do not include this component, other types of questions that are less likely to include this component include:

- frequency questions (for example, '*How common is dementia in residents of nursing homes?*'—a 'PO' question)
- prognosis questions (for example, '*How long before a runner with an ankle sprain can return to training?*')
- qualitative questions (for example, '*How do adolescents who are being treated with chemotherapy feel about hospital environments?*').

Outcome(s)

This component of the question should clearly specify what outcome (or outcomes) you are interested in. For some outcomes you may also need to specify whether you are interested in increasing the outcome (such as the score on a functional assessment or chance of recovery) or decreasing it (such as the reduction of pain or the risk of relapse). In the stroke question example above, the outcome of interest was an improvement in the ability to perform self-care activities. As you will see in Chapter 14, shared decision making is an important component of evidence-based practice and it is important, where possible, to involve your patient in choosing the goals of intervention that are most important to them. As such, there will be many circumstances where the outcome component of your question will be guided by your patient's preferences.

The exact way that you structure your clinical question varies a little depending on the type of question. This is explained more in the relevant chapter—Chapter 4 for questions about the effects of intervention, Chapter 6 for diagnostic questions, Chapter 8 for prognostic questions and Chapter 10 for qualitative questions.

NOW THAT THE QUESTION IS FORMULATED, WHAT TYPES OF INFORMATION SHOULD BE LOOKED FOR?

Not all types of information are equally useful—some are much more useful than others. This is because useful pieces of information are:

1. more relevant

or

2. more believable

than others.

Relevant information

One problem when searching is that there is so much information that deciding what to download and use can be distorted by finding something that *nearly* answers what you asked, *but not quite*. It is all too easy to be distracted by interesting-looking (but sadly, not directly relevant) information. Information may be published as *researcher-to-researcher* communication. For example, research into the most valid and reliable instrument for measuring trial outcomes is unlikely to be directly useful to any question you need answered as a practising health professional.

Deciding how relevant information is can be partly achieved by using the PICO mnemonic explained above. This can help you decide in advance what you need to ask, and then ensure that you are thinking about the relevance of each of the components of your question.

Truthful information

Some information *appears* to answer your question, but either does not or, worse, cannot. Much published research is unhelpful to health professionals for several reasons:

1. The research (even if attempting to answer your question) used a design that cannot answer the question. This is often because the *wrong study type* (to provide the best type of evidence for the question being asked) was used. There are many different study designs, and the right one must be used to answer the question at hand. Using the wrong study design may mean either no direct answer or that there is too much bias to rely on the result.

2. The research (even though it does attempt to answer your question) had some flaws in its conduct that also leaves it vulnerable to bias, leaving too much uncertainty to answer the question securely. For example, the research may have failed in a large number of different ways so that we are unsure that the apparent 'result' is true.

3. There were insufficient numbers of participants or 'events' (that is, things of clinical importance that happen). This may mean that there is not enough *statistical power*.

We will now look at these reasons in detail.

WHAT ARE THE DIFFERENT STUDY TYPES?

First we need to understand some of the different study types that exist. They are briefly explained in Table 2.4, and illustrated in Figure 2.2.

There are some important things to notice about the study types listed in Table 2.4:

1. Only one study type is particularly good at addressing intervention questions—randomised controlled trials. Even better is a pooled analysis of several randomised controlled trials, something called a *meta-analysis* (a type of *systematic review* where the results from individual studies are combined). Systematic reviews and meta-analyses are discussed in detail in Chapter 12.

2. A subgroup of randomised controlled trials is the n-of-1 trial, described in Table 2.4. These may represent the best evidence for an individual patient, because they are undertaken in the same individual that the results will be applied to.

3. All the other study types are observational studies. They are not the best at answering questions about the effect of interventions (you will see in Chapter 4 why a randomised controlled trial is best primary study type for answering intervention questions), but they are good at answering *other* types of questions, including questions about prognosis, diagnosis, frequency and aetiology.

4. Different questions require different study designs; this is explained more fully in the next section. Although randomised controlled trials can sometimes answer questions about prognosis (for example), by examining just the control group (who did not receive any intervention) of a randomised controlled trial, this can be inefficient.

This means that there is no single 'hierarchy of evidence' (a rank order of study types from *good* to *bad*), as is sometimes claimed. However, hierarchies of evidence do exist for each question type.

TABLE 2.4:
SOME OF THE MAIN STUDY TYPES THAT YOU NEED TO KNOW ABOUT FOR EVIDENCE-BASED PRACTICE

Study type	How it works	The type of questions that it is good at answering
Randomised controlled trial	This is an experiment. Participants are randomised into two (or more) different groups and each group receives a different intervention. At the end of the trial, the effects of the different interventions are measured.	Questions about interventions, such as: *Is the intervention effective?* *Is one intervention more effective than another?*
n-of-1 randomised trial	This is a sub-group of a randomised controlled trial and is conducted on just *one* participant. Different time periods are randomised and the participant receives one treatment in one time period and a different treatment in another (and this can be repeated several times).[12] The average differences in clinical outcomes between the two time periods are compared.	Intervention questions–particularly those which address stable illnesses (such as chronic ones which cannot be 'cured'), so that the intervention can be tested over time.
Cohort	This is an observational study. It is a type of longitudinal study where participants are followed over time. Participants with specific characteristics are identified as a 'cohort', differences between them are measured and they are followed over time. Finally, differences in outcome are observed and related to the initial differences.	Several questions: Risks–*what risk factors predict disease?* Aetiology–*what factors cause these outcomes?* Prognosis–*what happens with this disease over time?* Diagnosis–*if the test is positive, what happens to the patient?*
Case-control	Observational study. Participants who have experienced an outcome already (such as developing a disease) are identified. They are then 'matched' with other participants who are similar– except they do *not* have the outcome (for example, the disease being studied). Differences in risk factors between the two groups of participants are then analysed.	Several questions: Risks–*what risk factors predict disease?* Prognosis–*what happens with this disease over time?* Diagnosis–*does this new test perform as well as the old 'gold standard'?*
Cross-sectional	These sample a population at a particular point in time and measure them to see who has the outcome. Often, associations between risk factors and a certain outcome are analysed. Or, comparisons between an established test ('gold standard') and a new candidate test are made.	Observational questions: Frequency–*how common is the outcome (disease, risk factor etc)?* Aetiology–*what risk factors are associated with these outcomes?* Diagnosis–*does the new test perform as well as the 'gold standard'?*
Qualitative	There are several kinds, including: • Interviews (asking people) • Focus groups (a representative group of people who will provide a wide spectrum of information) • Participant observation (the researcher joins the group to understand what is going on)	Observational questions: *Why do people ...?* *What are the possible reasons for ...?* *How do people feel about ...?*
Case series	Descriptions of a group of patients who are exposed to the factor (such as an intervention) that is being studied. They usually do not provide definitive evidence, but more usually are 'hypothesis-generating' (meaning they give rise to questions that need one of the higher level of study designs to answer).	*Should we research this question?* (which might be about intervention, prognosis, or diagnosis, etc)

Figure 2.2 illustrates the various types of questions that can arise from a particular clinical scenario and how different study types are most appropriate to answer each of the question types. The clinical scenario used in Figure 2.2 is patients with stroke. Starting on the left before the disease has become manifest, you might ask about risk factors that might lead to stroke (for example hypertension, diabetes and so on). There are two principal study types that can be used to answer these questions: a cohort study or a case-control study, and both have their own pros and cons (see Table 2.4).

Or you might ask about the prevalence of stroke—for example, *'How common is a history of stroke in nursing-home residents who are older than 70 years?'*. For this question, a simple cross-sectional survey would be the best way of providing the answer and the type of study you should look for. A similar cross-sectional study design may be best for answering diagnosis questions (although sometimes a cohort design is necessary). For example, *'Which depression screening instrument is as good at diagnosing post-stroke depression as the "gold standard" assessment of depression?'* Another method testing diagnostic alternatives is a cohort study, especially when there is no gold standard and the patient outcome (*'Did the patient become clinically depressed?'*) has to be the gold standard instead.

The right-hand side of the figure shows the two types of questions that often occur when looking to the future: (1) prognosis questions (*what will happen* questions—such as *'How likely is it that a stroke*

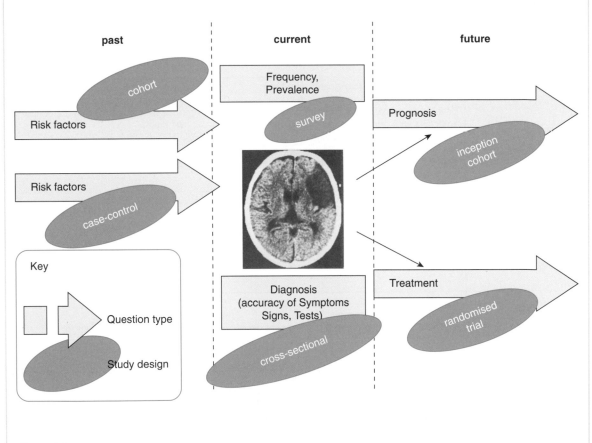

Figure 2.2
Example: how different question types (at different stages of the evolution of stroke) might be posed and the study types that might answer them.
CT scan reproduced with permission from Crawford MH et al. Cardiology, 3rd ed. Mosby; 2010, Fig. 11.1A.[11]

patient with expressive aphasia will experience full recovery of their speech?), which are best answered by an inception cohort study (see Table 2.4); and (2) intervention questions (such as '*Is mirror therapy effective at improving upper limb function in people who have had a stroke*'?), which are best answered by a randomised controlled trial.

HIERARCHIES OF EVIDENCE FOR EACH QUESTION TYPE

Hierarchies of evidence tell you what type of study provides the most robust (that is, the most free of bias) evidence, and therefore what you should first look for. There are different hierarchies for each question type. If there are no relevant studies of the type that are at the top of the hierarchy (for example systematic reviews of randomised controlled trials for an intervention question), proceed to search for the type of study next down the hierarchy (for example randomised controlled trials). This ensures that you select from the best available evidence. The higher up the hierarchy, the more likely a study can minimise the impact of bias on its results. We can also think of the hierarchy as representing a continuum of certainty (with higher levels of certainty at the top of the hierarchy). Consider, for example, the hierarchy of evidence for intervention questions—the continuum of certainty represents how certain we are that the effects found in the study are actually due to the intervention and not something else. This introduces two very important concepts in evidence-based practice, *bias* and *confounding*, which are explained in the next section of this chapter.

There are a number of published hierarchies of evidence assembled by different organisations. Although these are generally similar, they have subtle differences between them. So if you are a reading a document and it refers to a particular study as being (for example) *level III-1* evidence, it is a good idea to check which hierarchy of evidence the document followed, because level III-1 evidence in one hierarchy scheme may differ slightly from that in another. The hierarchies of evidence for the various types of questions shown in Table 2.5 are a simplified version of the hierarchies of evidence that have been developed by the National Health and Medical Research Council (NHMRC) of Australia.[13]

Most of the study types included in Table 2.5 have been explained already in this chapter. The intricate details of the main study types are explained in the relevant chapter that deals with how to appraise evidence for each of the question types. Here we briefly consider study types[12] additional to those in Table 2.5 and not already explained elsewhere in this chapter.

- A **non-randomised experimental trial** is essentially the same as a randomised controlled study except that there is no randomisation (hence it is lower down the hierarchy, as this opens it up to all kinds of bias). Participants are allocated to either an intervention or a control group and the outcomes from each group are compared.

- The basic premise of a **case-control study** was explained in Table 2.4, but not in relation to how it can be used to answer questions about the effects of intervention. When a case-control study has been used to answer a question about the effect of an intervention, 'cases' are participants who have been exposed to an intervention and 'controls' are participants who have not.

- **Interrupted time series** studies attempt to test interventions. Trends in an outcome are measured over multiple time-points *before* and *after* the intervention is provided to a group of participants, and these can then be compared with the outcomes at the same time-points for a control group of participants (who did not receive the same intervention). This type of study can also be conducted *without* a parallel control group being involved, comparing the *before* to the *after* data for just the one group, but this is a weaker design (and it lies lower down the hierarchy of evidence).

- In a **historical control study** the key word is *historical*, as the control group does not participate in the study at the same time as the intervention group. There are two main forms that this type of study can take. Data about outcomes are prospectively collected for a group of participants who received the intervention of interest. These data are compared with either:

TABLE 2.5:
HIERARCHIES AND LEVELS OF EVIDENCE FOR QUESTIONS ABOUT INTERVENTION, DIAGNOSIS AND PROGNOSIS (BASED ON NHMRC LEVELS OF EVIDENCE)[12]

Level	Intervention	Diagnosis	Prognosis
I	A systematic review of level II studies	A systematic review of level II studies	A systematic review of level II studies
II	Randomised controlled trial	A study of test accuracy with an independent, blinded comparison with a valid reference standard, among consecutive persons with a defined clinical presentation	Prospective cohort study
III-1	Pseudo-randomised controlled trial (that is, alternate allocation or some other method was used rather than true randomisation–see Chapter 4 for details about this)	As for level II, but a study that used *non-consecutive* participants	
III-2	Comparative study *with* concurrent controls: • non-randomised • experimental trial • cohort study • case-control study • interrupted time series with a control group	A comparison with a reference standard that does not meet the criteria required for level II or/and III-1 evidence	Analysis of the prognostic factors among the participants in one group of a randomised controlled trial
III-3	Comparative study *without* concurrent controls: • historical control study • two or more single arm study • interrupted time series without a parallel control group	Diagnostic case-control study	Retrospective cohort study
IV	Case series	Study of diagnostic yield (no reference standard)	Case series *or* Cohort study where participants are at different stages of the disease/condition

1. data about outcomes from a group of people who were treated at the same institution before the intervention of interest was introduced—this group is, in a sense, considered to be a control group who received standard care; or

2. data about outcomes from a group of people who received the control (or an alternative) intervention but the data comes from a previously published document.

- A **two or more single arm study** gathers the data from two or more studies and compares the outcomes of a single series of participants (in each study) who received the intervention of interest.

- A **case series** is simply a report on a series of patients (that is, 'cases') who have an outcome of interest (or received the intervention that is being studied). There is no control group involved.

- In a **diagnostic (test) accuracy study**, the outcomes from the test that is being evaluated (known as the *index test*) are compared with outcomes from a *reference standard test* to see how much agreement there is between the two tests. The outcomes are measured in people who are suspected of having the condition of interest. A reference standard test (often called the 'gold standard' test) is the test that is considered to be the best available method for establishing the presence or absence of the target condition of interest.

- In a **diagnostic case-control study**, the results from a reference standard test are used to create two groups of people—those who are known to have the condition of interest (the 'cases') and those who do not have it (the 'controls'). The index test results for the cases are then compared with the index test results for the controls.

- In a **study of diagnostic yield**, the index test is used to identify people who have the condition of interest. A reference standard test is not used to confirm the accuracy of the diagnosis and, therefore, this study design is at the bottom of the hierarchy of evidence for diagnostic questions.

- The basic idea of a **cohort study** was explained in Table 2.4, but there are two broad types of cohort studies that can be conducted and, as you can see in the prognosis column of Table 2.5, they sit at very different levels in the hierarchy of evidence for prognostic questions. The reasons for this are explained in Chapter 8, but for now we will just explain the main difference between them.

  - In a **prospective cohort study**, groups of participants are identified as a 'cohort' (based on whether they have or have not been exposed to a certain intervention or situation) and then followed prospectively over time to see what happens to them.

  - In a **retrospective cohort study**, the cohorts are defined from a previous point in time and the information is collected (for example, from past records) about the outcome(s) of interest. Participants are not followed up in the future to see what happens to them, as happens in a prospective cohort study.

Hierarchy of evidence for questions about patients' experiences and concerns

Questions about patients' experiences and concerns are answered using qualitative evidence. The various qualitative research methodologies are explained in depth in Chapter 10. There is currently no universally agreed-upon hierarchy of evidence for study types that seek to answer questions about patients' experiences and concerns.

INTERNAL VALIDITY: WHAT HAVE BIAS AND CONFOUNDING GOT TO DO WITH EVIDENCE-BASED PRACTICE?

Internal validity and external validity

As we saw in Chapter 1 when the process of evidence-based practice was explained, when reading a research study you need to know whether you can believe the results of the study. *Internal validity* refers to whether the evidence is trustworthy. That is, are the conclusions that the authors have stated for that particular study valid? Can we be sure that the association or effect found is not really due to some other factor? Three common alternative explanations that must be considered for the association or effect that is found in a study are: (1) chance, (2) bias and (3) confounding. We now look at each of these in turn. But first we need to briefly explain what external validity is so that you do not confuse it with internal validity. *External validity* refers to the generalisability of the results of a study. That is, to what extent can we apply the results of the study to people other than the participants of the study?

Chance

One possible explanation for a study's results is that any findings of differences between two groups are due to random variation. Random variation in data collected during research means that differences occur by chance alone. As we explain later in this chapter, determining whether findings are due to chance is a key feature of statistical analysis (hypothesis testing). Random variation is smaller when the sample size (that is, the number of participants or, more properly, the number of *events*) of the study is adequate. This is discussed in more detail later in the chapter.

Bias

Bias can be likened to the characteristic of lawn bowls which leads the bowl to roll in a curve. Although this characteristic of lawn bowls to 'not run true' (that is, not in a straight line) is useful in the game of bowls, it is a problem in study design. We use the term *bias* for any effect that prevents the study conclusions from running true. Whereas chance is caused by *random* variation, bias is caused by *systematic* variation. Bias is a systematic error in the way that participants are selected for a study, outcomes are measured or data are analysed which, in turn, leads to inaccurate results.

Biases can operate in either direction—to underestimate or overestimate an effect reported in a study. Consider an example of a randomised controlled trial of the effectiveness of a new intervention for back pain. If the participants allocated to the new intervention had more-severe symptoms (that is, had more back pain) at the start of the trial than the participants allocated to the control group, any differences at the end of the study might be the result of that initial difference rather than the effect of the new intervention. This bias is then called 'allocation bias'—the bias introduced by how participants were allocated to the two groups which creates initial differences that then undermine our confidence in any apparent effect.

There are dozens of other kinds of bias, and we need to be able to look for and recognise them. Table 2.6 briefly describes some of the common kinds of bias that can occur. Some are relevant to non-randomised studies and some to randomised studies. Chapter 4 discusses the biases that can occur in randomised controlled trials in more detail.

Assessing whether bias has occurred in a study is the main focus of the first step (*Is the evidence valid?*) in the three-step critical appraisal process that was described in Chapter 1. Being able to assess whether the evidence is valid is a key skill needed by those who wish to practise evidence-based practice. As such, this topic is given a lot of attention in this book, primarily in Chapters 4, 6, 8, 10 and 12.

Confounding

'Confound' comes from the Latin *confundere* [*com-* (together) + *fundere* (to pour)], meaning to confuse. Add another liquid to the pure initial one and it loses its purity. So it is with confounding factors. The factor of interest becomes confused with the confounding factor (the 'confounder'). In other words, confounding variables are generally variables that are causally associated with the outcome variable under investigation and non-causally associated with the explanatory variable of interest. Confounders do not cause error in *measurement*; rather, they involve error in the *interpretation* of what may be an accurate measurement.

In research study design, we want to minimise confounders. For randomised controlled trials, the easiest way of doing this is to randomly allocate participants to groups. The intention is to have confounders spread randomly—and hence evenly—between the groups and not stacked up in one group unfairly. Randomisation will ensure this, *provided* the sample is large enough (see below). In other study designs, a list of possible confounders is drawn up and either accounted for in the analysis (by stratification or statistical adjustment—'regression analysis'—methods) or restricted to subgroups. In fact, this is the method employed for observational studies (since there is no other option).

The problem with adjusting for confounders is *unknown* confounders—factors that we either cannot measure or do not even know about—that could influence the results. For example, participants' level of motivation to participate fully in an intervention (consider one that required people to perform certain exercises daily) is very difficult to measure accurately and could be a potential unknown confounder for a study that was examining the effectiveness of this intervention. Randomisation is the key, because the act of randomisation distributes all confounders, both known and unknown, fairly. A problem remains, though: what about the chance of an unequal distribution of confounders between groups? The answer to that is to do with two things: numbers and statistics.

TABLE 2.6:
SOME COMMON KINDS OF BIAS

Type	How it operates	How study design can prevent it	What to look for when critically appraising an article
Selection or sampling bias	Systematic differences between those who are selected for study and those who are not selected. This means that the results of the study may not be generalisable to the population from which the sample is drawn.	Good sampling ensures that the people who are participating are representative of the population you want to generalise to.	Check how the sampling was done. Look for any data that compare this sample with the population's characteristics.
Allocation bias	In experimental studies, allocation or selection bias can refer to intervention and control groups being systematically different.	Randomisation attempts to evenly distribute both known and unknown confounders. Assess differences between groups at baseline. Statistically control for differences in analysis.	Check the article for a comparison of the groups before an intervention to see if they look sufficiently similar (also known as *baseline similarity*).
Maturation bias	The effect might be due to changes that have occurred naturally over time, not because of any intervention.	Use a control group and random allocation to intervention or control group.	Check to see if a control group and random allocation were used.
Attrition bias	Participants who withdraw from studies may differ systematically from those who remain. Alternatively, there may be more participants lost from one group in the study than the other group.	Minimise loss to follow-up. Analyse the results by intention-to-treat.	Reject articles with a loss to follow-up of >15%. Check whether results were analysed by intention-to-treat.
Measurement bias in experimental studies	Errors in measuring exposure or outcome can lead to differential accuracy of information between groups. In other words, if the way that data are measured differs systematically between groups, this introduces bias. In experimental studies, this can be due to bias in the expectations of study participants, health professionals or researchers.	'Blinding' participants, health professionals or researchers will reduce this bias. Blinding is discussed further in Chapter 4.	Look to see if the study used methods to reduce the participants', health professionals' and/or researchers' awareness of a participant's group allocation (blinding).
Placebo effect	An improvement in the participants' condition may occur because they expect or believe that the intervention they are receiving will cause an improvement.	Have a control group of participants that receive approximately the same intervention (that is, raise no different expectations). 'Blinding' participants, health professionals or researchers will reduce this bias.	Check whether there is a suitable control group and look to see whether the study used methods to reduce the participants', health professionals' and/or researchers' awareness of a participant's group allocation (blinding).
Hawthorne effect	Participants may experience changes because of the attention that they are receiving from being a part of the research process.	Have a control group that is studied in the same way (except for the intervention)– that is, a randomised controlled trial.	Check whether there is a suitable control group to control for attention and whether the randomised controlled trial is designed properly.

STATISTICAL SIGNIFICANCE, CLINICAL SIGNIFICANCE, AND POWER

Statistical significance

The concern we identified above is that a randomised controlled trial could be biased because of a chance uneven distribution of confounders across the groups. The chance of this happening is reduced if the number of participants in the trial is increased (as the numbers get larger, the chance of unevenness decreases). However large the trial is designed to be, though, the chance of unevenness never decreases to zero. This means that there is always a chance of bias from confounders, so we have to tolerate some uncertainty; less so as the trial size gets larger, until the trial is sufficiently large that we can relax. The question is: how large? The answer comes from statistics, which is the science of dealing with this uncertainty and quantifying it. There are two main ways of deciding whether a difference in the summaries of two groups of participants is due to chance or to a real difference between them.

The *p* value

The *p* here is short for 'probability'. This test is based on one of the cornerstones of scientific philosophy: that we cannot ever prove anything, but rather can only *dis*prove it.[14] This means that we have to invert the test from the intuitive, which is:

> 'Are the measurements between the two groups different enough to assume that it is because of some factor other than chance?'

to

> 'Are the measurements between the two groups *similar* enough to assume that it is because of chance alone?'

If we can show that the latter statement is unlikely, then we can say that there must be some *other* factor responsible for the difference. In other words, the *p* value is estimated to establish 'how likely it is that the difference is because of chance alone'. Statisticians estimate a value of *p* that will be somewhere between 1.0 (absolutely sure that the difference is because of chance alone) and 0.0 (absolutely sure that the difference is *not* because of chance alone). Traditionally we set the arbitrary value of *p* as <0.05, at which point we assume that chance was so unlikely that we can rule it out as the cause of the difference. A value of 0.05 ($\frac{5}{100}$) is the same as 5% or 1:20. What we mean when we use this cut-off point for the *p* value is: 'We would have to repeat the study an average of 20 times for the result to happen once by chance alone.' When a study produces a result where the *p* value is <0.05, that result is considered to be 'statistically significant'.

Confidence intervals

Confidence intervals take a different approach, and instead estimate what range of values the true value lies within. *True value* refers to the population value, not just the estimate of a value that has come from the sample of one study (such as an estimate about how effective an intervention is)—this is explained in more depth in Chapter 4. The range of values is called the confidence interval, and is most commonly set at the same arbitrary level as *p* values (0.95, or 20:1), which is also called the 95% confidence interval. Another way to think of the value is graphically, as shown in Figure 2.3.

Figure 2.3 shows the range of possible values for an estimated measurement for two different studies, A and B. In each figure the two vertical lines indicate the two limits (or boundaries) of the confidence interval. The values in between these lines indicate the range of values within which we are 95% certain (or confident, hence the term confidence intervals) that the true value is likely to lie. The probability that the true value lies outside of this confidence interval is 0.05 (or 5%), with half of this value (2.5%)

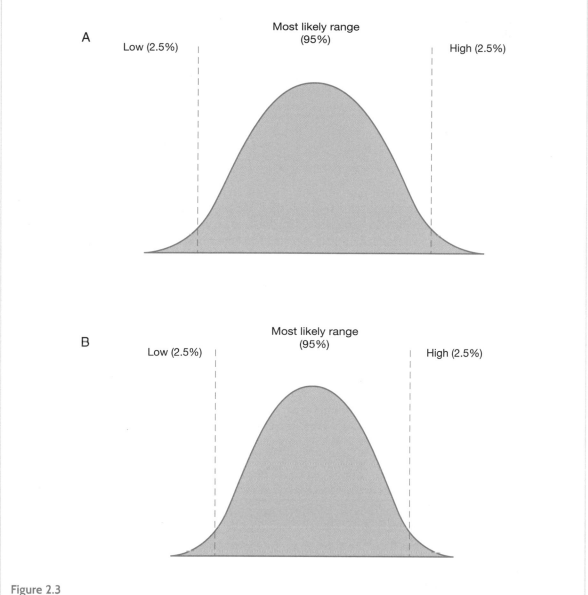

Figure 2.3
For two different studies, the range of possible values for an estimated measurement (with the 95% confidence interval) is shown. In the study represented by figure B, the 95% confidence interval is smaller (narrower) than the one in figure A. A smaller confidence interval can occur when the sample size of a study is larger.

lying in each tail of the curve. The most likely value is central and, in most cases, the distribution of possible values forms a normal distribution (that is, a bell-shaped curve). The spread of values will form a different shape according to different influences on the 95% confidence interval. For example, in the study that is represented by Figure 2.3B, the sample size is larger. This has the effect of narrowing the 95% confidence interval because the normal curve is more peaked. The same effect is achieved by samples that yield greater uniformity of the participants (that is, decreased variance of the sample). This is summarised in Table 2.7.

TABLE 2.7:
EFFECT OF SAMPLE SIZE AND VARIANCE ON A STUDY'S CONFIDENCE INTERVAL

Factor	Effect on the confidence interval
Sample size (the number of participants in the study)	The confidence interval narrows as the sample size increases–there is more certainty about the effect estimate. This is one of the reasons why it is important that studies have an adequate sample size. The importance of a smaller (narrower) confidence interval is explained in Chapter 4.
Variance (the amount of 'noise' or differences in values between participants in the sample)	The confidence interval widens as the variance increases–there is less certainty about the effect estimate.

Confidence intervals are an important concept to understand if you wish to use evidence-based practice, as they help you with the second step (*What is the impact of the evidence?*) of the three-step critical appraisal process described in Chapter 1. The role that confidence intervals play in helping you to determine the impact of the evidence is explained in more detail in Chapter 4.

Clinical versus statistical significance

There is one more essential consideration: how big a difference is worthwhile? Once we have established a difference that is unlikely to be attributable to chance (that is, it is statistically significant), how can we decide whether the difference is important? Clinical significance is defined as just that: the minimum difference that would be important to patients. (Because of this, some people use the term 'clinical importance' rather than 'clinical significance' to refer to this concept.)

We cannot use statistics to measure clinical significance because it is a judgment: we have to decide what difference would be important (meaning, would change clinical practice). This means choosing some difference based on what is clinically important. Such differences are called 'clinically significant'. For example, consider an intervention study where the outcome being measured was pain, using a visual analogue scale (a straight line with one end meaning 'no pain' and the other end meaning 'the most pain imaginable'). If the intervention had the effect of reducing participants' pain (on average) by 4 points on a 10-point visual analogue scale (where 1 = 'no pain' and 10 = 'the most pain imaginable'), we would probably judge a difference of this size to be clinically significant; whereas a reduction of 0.5 would probably not be considered clinically significant. Chapter 4 discusses in further detail the various approaches that can be used to help determine clinical significance.

Hopefully it is now clear that there are three main categories that the results of a study can fall into:

- a result that is not statistically significant—when this is the case, you do not need to bother deciding whether the result is clinically significant as you cannot even be very sure that the result was not due to chance.

- a result that is statistically significant but not *clinically* significant. This is, unfortunately, a common scenario and regrettably means that the difference is not large enough to be important (even though it is a 'real' not-by-chance difference).

- a result that is statistically significant *and* clinically significant—this is the type of result that is clear: there is a real and meaningful difference that can potentially inform our clinical practice and we can proceed to the third step in the three-step critical appraisal process—deciding whether you can apply the evidence to your patient.

Outcome measures–what you need to know about them

The issue of clinical significance raises another issue that is important when it comes to appraising articles—you need to know about the outcome measure that a study used, as this helps you to make a judgment about clinical significance. In our pain study example above, if the visual analogue scale that was used to measure pain was a 0–100 scale, then we would probably no longer consider a reduction in pain of 4 points (on a 100-point scale) to be clinically significant (although on a 10-point scale, we felt that it was). If you are lucky, the study that you are reading will include the scale range of the continuous outcome measures used in the study somewhere in the article (usually in the methods section or in a results table). If they do not, then you will need to find this information out for yourself. If it is an outcome measure that you are familiar with, great! If not, perhaps searching for it on the internet (even Google can be useful in this instance) may help you to find out more about it.

In addition to knowing about the actual measures used in a study to measure the outcomes, it is important that you consider whether the outcomes themselves are relevant, useful and important to your patient. An example is a patient who has had a stroke and, as a result, has difficulty using their arm to perform functional activities such as eating and getting dressed. The patient's goal is to return to doing these activities independently. You are considering using a physical rehabilitation technique on them to improve their ability to carry out these activities, primarily by working on the quality of the movement that they have in their affected arm. Let us suppose that when evaluating the evidence for the effectiveness of this intervention, there are two studies that you can use to inform your practice (for the sake of simplicity, we will assume that they both have a similar level of internal validity). The outcomes measured in one study (study A) are arm function and the ability to perform self-care activities, whereas the outcome measured in the other study (study B) is quality of arm movement. In this (very simplified!) example, if you choose study A to inform your clinical practice you will be able to communicate the results of the study to the patient and explain to them the estimated effect that the intervention may have on their ability to perform these activities. Remember that this is what your patient primarily wants to know. Although study B may provide you with information that is useful to you as a health professional, the effect that the intervention may have on the quality of arm movement may be of less interest to your patient than knowing how it may improve the function of their arm. Considering whether the outcomes measured by a study are useful to your patient is one way of considering the patient-centredness of the study. In Chapter 14, the concept of patient-centred care is explained and the importance of encouraging patients' involvement in decisions about their health care is discussed.

Putting it all together: thinking about power

As we mentioned earlier, we can have results that are statistically significant but not clinically significant. But statistical significance can be made more likely by increasing the size of the sample (or reducing the 'noise', more properly called 'variance'). If a study is large enough, its results will become statistically significant even though the differences are not important clinically—which is why we call on clinical significance to decide what is worthwhile. This means we can decide on the minimum size a study's sample has to be to give a definitive answer. This is important because it helps decide what would be wasteful (above the minimum is wasteful of research resources).

Estimating the minimum is called a 'power calculation'. A study has enough *power* (meaning that there is a large enough sample) if a statistically significant difference is found. In other words, the power of a study is the degree to which we are certain that, if we conclude that a difference does *not* exist, that it in fact does *not* exist. The accepted level of power is generally set at the arbitrary level of 80% (or 0.80).

What happens if the minimum sample size is not reached? Such a study is called 'underpowered', meaning that if a non-significant difference was found, it might nevertheless correspond to a truly clinically significant difference but this was something that was not detected because the sample was too small. In other words, a non-significant result might mean either that there is truly no difference or that the sample was too small to detect one. This state of affairs, where a study has incorrectly concluded that a difference does not exist, is also called a type-2 error. Because of the risk of this type of error occurring, when evaluating a study you need to decide whether the study had adequate power (that is, a large enough sample size). This can be determined by checking an article to see if the researchers did a power calculation. Researchers do a power analysis prior to conducting the study because it enables them to estimate how many participants they will need to recruit to be reasonably sure (to a given level of uncertainty) that they will detect an important difference if it really exists. You can then check if they actually did recruit at least as many participants as they estimated would be needed.

Can a study be too large? Surprisingly, the answer is yes. If a study is too large, then effort and money have been wasted in undertaking research unnecessarily. A more subtle reason is that a difference that is statistically significant can be found, but the difference may be so small that we judge its significance to not be meaningful. This can mean having a situation that we discussed earlier in this chapter, where a difference is *statistically* significant but *clinically* not significant.

SUMMARY POINTS OF THIS CHAPTER

- Questions about frequency, diagnosis, prognosis and the effects of interventions are among the types of clinical questions that can usually be answered using evidence-based practice.

- Converting your information needs into answerable clinical questions is the first step of the evidence-based practice process. A well-structured question can be achieved by using the PICO (Patient/Problem, Intervention, Comparison, Outcome[s]) format.

- Systematic reviews, randomised controlled trials, cohort studies, cross-sectional studies and case-control studies are some of the common study types that are used in evidence-based practice.

- For each type of question, there is a different hierarchy of evidence. The higher up the hierarchy that a study is, the more likely it is that the study can minimise the impact of bias on the results of the study. You should use the hierarchy of evidence that is appropriate to your question to guide your search for and selection of evidence to answer your question.

- For all question types, a systematic review of level II evidence is at the top of the hierarchy and you should always search for this type of evidence first. The study type that is level II evidence is different for each question type. For intervention questions, level II evidence is a randomised controlled trial; for prognostic questions, it is a prospective cohort study; and for diagnostic studies, it is a study of test accuracy that involved an independent, blinded comparison with a valid reference standard, among consecutive persons with a defined clinical presentation.

- Being able to recognise whether bias and/or confounding have occurred in a study is a crucial part of the critical appraisal process, as it enables you to determine the internal validity of the evidence. There are many types of bias and you need to be able to recognise them. Internal validity refers to how much we can trust the results of a study and is a reflection of the degree to which chance, bias and/or confounding are operating in a study.

- If the result of a study is statistically significant, it means that we are reasonably sure that the result (such as a difference in outcomes between two groups in a study) did not occur because of chance. Statistical significance can be indicated by p values or confidence intervals. In evidence-based practice, confidence intervals are much more useful than p values. If a result is statistically significant, you then need to consider if it is also clinically significant—that is, is the result important enough that you will use it in your clinical practice? Clinical significance is determined by judgment.

References

1. Bastian H, Glasziou P, Chalmers I. Seventy-five trials and eleven systematic reviews a day: how will we ever keep up? PLoS Med 2010;7:e1000326.

2. Shirky C. It's not information overload. It's filter failure. Title of talk, Web 2.0 Expo, New York, 2008.

3. Hoffmann T, Erueti C, Thorning S, et al. The scatter of research: a cross-sectional comparison of randomised trials and systematic reviews across specialties. BMJ 2012;e3223. doi: 10.1136/bmj.e3223.

4. Ely J, Osheroff J, Ebell M, et al. Analysis of questions asked by family doctors regarding patient care. BMJ 1999;319:358–61.

5. Gonzalez-Gonzalez A, Dawes M, Sanchez-Mateos J, et al. Information needs and information-seeking behaviour of primary care physicians. Ann Fam Med 2007;5:345–52.

6. Gorman P, Helfand M. Information seeking in primary care: how physicians choose which clinical questions to pursue and which to leave unanswered. Med Decis Making 1995;15:113–19.

7. Cogdill K. Information needs and information seeking in primary care: a study of nurse practitioners. J Med Libr Assoc 2003;91:203–15.

8. Coumou H, Meijman F. How do primary care physicians seek answers to clinical questions? A literature review. JAMA 2006;94:55–60.

9. McGowan J, Hogg W, Campbell C, et al. Just-in-time information improved decision-making in primary care: a randomised controlled trial. PLoS ONE 2008;3:e3785.

10. Straus S, Richardson W, Glasziou P, et al. Evidence-based medicine: how to practice and teach EBM. 4th ed. Edinburgh: Churchill Livingstone; 2011.

11. Crawford MH, DiMarco JP, Paulus WJ. Cardiology. 3rd ed. Philadelphia: Mosby; 2010.

12. Guyatt G, Keller J, Jaeschke R, et al. The n-of-1 randomised controlled trial: clinical usefulness. Our three-year experience. Ann Intern Med 1990;112:293–9.

13. National Health and Medical Research Council (NHMRC). NHMRC additional levels of evidence and grades for recommendations for developers of guidelines. Canberra: NHMRC; 2009. Online. Available: www.nhmrc.gov.au/_files_nhmrc/file/guidelines/developers/nhmrc_levels_grades_evidence_120423.pdf; 11 Mar 2012.

14. Hacking I. An introduction to probability and inductive logic. 1st ed. New York: Cambridge University Press; 2001.

Chapter 3

Finding the evidence

Nancy Wilczynski and Ann McKibbon

LEARNING OBJECTIVES

After reading this chapter, you should be able to:

- Describe the basic principles of efficient searching
- Understand how literature services are organised
- Be aware of the major online evidence-based resources and how they fit into the organisation of literature services
- Be aware of the discipline-specific online evidence-based resources
- Know which databases will be likely to have an answer when searching for evidence for each type of question (that is, intervention, diagnosis, prognosis and qualitative)
- Know how to search for evidence for each type of question

One of the most important and challenging aspects of implementing evidence-based practice can be finding the current best evidence relevant to your clinical question. The internet provides ready and free access to information, but the information explosion and the ever-increasing availability of online resources makes finding the current best evidence difficult. Many online resources falsely claim to be 'evidence-based', making it difficult for health professionals to navigate internet sites. In addition to discerning whether the information provided on the internet site is based on sound evidence, research shows that some of the obstacles that are most frequently encountered when attempting to find the answer to a clinical question are:

- the excessive amount of time required to find information
- difficulty in selecting an optimal filter to search for information
- failure of the selected resource to provide an answer.[1]

These barriers can be reduced by approaching the search for the current best evidence in a systematic way that harnesses the organisation of the literature to your advantage. In this chapter we will show you some of the main ways that you can do this. We will begin by describing the basics of searching, followed by a description of a model that outlines a categorisation of evidence-based information services and how this evidence is processed and presented. Within each category of this model, we will describe the types of evidence that are included and the resources that are available to find that type of evidence. We will concentrate on the resources which have the strongest evidence base, as these resources are the ones that are likely to be of most use to you in your clinical practice and are also typically the resources that are easier and faster to use. The chapter concludes with a number of clinical questions and examples of how you can find an answer to these questions using the model and the information resources described in the chapter.

THE BASICS OF SEARCHING

So that your search for evidence is as efficient as possible, it is a good idea to understand some of the basic principles of effective searching, which are:

1. Carefully define your clinical question.
2. Choose your key search terms.
3. Broaden your search if necessary, with synonyms, truncation and/or wildcards.
4. Use Boolean operators.

Carefully define your clinical question

Information about how to construct a well-formulated clinical question, using the PICO format, was provided in Chapter 2.

Choose your key search terms

Using the PICO format to structure your clinical question makes choosing key search terms relatively easy. Typically you would start your search using the 'P' (patients [or population]) and 'I' (intervention) terms or phrases from your question. For example, if your question was '*In people with chronic low back pain, is an operant–behavioural graded activity program more effective than physical training in improving functional ability?*' you would start your search with the phrases "chronic low back pain" ('P' terms) and "operant-behavioural graded activity" ('I' terms).

Broaden your search if necessary

Once you have identified key terms or phrases, you should consider broadening your search, particularly if your initial search yields no relevant articles.

- The first way to broaden your search is to consider using **synonyms and related terms**. For example, if you are searching for articles on patients with "rheumatoid arthritis" you can broaden your search by also searching with the terms "RA" and "rheumatologic disease". Several online resources list synonyms and related terms for many diseases and conditions, for example, eMedicine from WebMD (emedicine.medscape.com; choose a specialty and then a condition), eMedicineHealth from WebMD (www.emedicinehealth.com/script/main/hp.asp) and Genetics Home Reference from the US National Library of Medicine (ghr.nlm.nih.gov/glossary).

- Another way to widen your search is to use **truncation** and **wildcards**.

  - When using truncation in a search you enter the first part of a keyword, insert a symbol (usually an asterisk symbol*), and accept any variant spellings or word endings from the occurrence of the symbol onwards. For example, "disease*" would retrieve records with the word *disease*, as well as the words *diseases*, *diseased*, etc.

  - When using wildcards in a search you enter a wild card character (usually "?") within or at the end of a keyword to substitute for only one character. Wildcards are particularly useful when searching for some plural forms, such as "wom?n", which would retrieve records with the words *woman* and *women*. Wildcards are also very useful when searching for terms where there is a variation between the American and Australian spelling of words such as orthopaedic and paediatric. Searching with the term "orthop?edic" will find articles that use *orthopaedic* as well as *orthopedic*.

- Truncation symbols and wildcard characters vary between databases and database providers; for example, in PubMed the truncation symbol is an asterisk (*), whereas when searching MEDLINE in Ovid it is a colon (:) or dollar sign ($). Consult each database's online help section to determine which symbols or characters to use.

Use Boolean operators

Once you have determined the terms or phrases that you will include in your search, you should consider combining your search terms using the Boolean logical operators.

- The Boolean AND command is used when you want all search terms to be present in each article that is retrieved. For example, when searching using 'P' terms and 'I' terms you would combine these using the Boolean AND command as you would want to retrieve articles that have both your patient/population of interest *and* the intervention of interest. Using our back pain example above, your search filter would be "(chronic low back pain) AND (operant-behavioural graded activity)", thus narrowing your search.

- The Boolean OR command is used when you want *any* of the specified search terms to be present in the articles. When incorporating synonyms and related terms you would search using the Boolean OR command, for example "rheumatoid arthritis OR RA OR rheumatologic disease", thus broadening your search. When using this search you will retrieve articles that use any one of 'rheumatoid arthritis' *or* 'RA' *or* 'rheumatologic disease'. How search terms should be grouped together—that is, whether "double inverted commas" or brackets () should be used—varies between different databases, so it is useful to check this in the database's help section.

BASICS OF SEARCHING–AN EXAMPLE

To illustrate these basics of searching further, we will work through a step-by-step example.

You are a rehabilitation consultant who has recently seen a number of individuals with work-related neck muscle pain, especially pain from the descending part of the trapezius muscle. You know that physical exercise is generally recommended, but you do not know which type of training is more effective in relieving muscle pain–strength training of the painful muscle or general fitness training without direct involvement of the painful muscle.

STEP 1: IDENTIFY THE COMPONENTS OF YOUR QUESTION IN PICO FORMAT

P Patient population	I Intervention (therapy, diagnostic test, prognostic factor)	C Comparison	O Outcomes
Work-related neck muscle pain	Strength training of the painful muscle	General fitness training	Pain relief

STEP 2: COMPOSE YOUR CLINICAL QUESTION

Patients with work-related neck muscle pain	Patients
Strength training of the painful muscle	Intervention
General fitness training without direct involvement of the painful muscle	Comparison
Greater pain relief	Outcomes

STEP 3: CONSTRUCT THE FINAL CLINICAL QUESTION

'For patients with work-related neck muscle pain, does strength training of the painful muscle versus general fitness training without direct involvement of the painful muscle result in greater pain relief?'

STEP 4: RECORD KEYWORDS AND PHRASES

Keyword 1:	Keyword 2:	Keyword 3:	Keyword 4:
Neck muscle pain	Muscular strength training	General fitness	Pain relief

STEP 5: IDENTIFY SYNONYMS AND VARIANT WORDS

Keyword 1:	Keyword 2:	Keyword 3:	Keyword 4:
Neck strain Neck strains Neck strain injury Neck strain injuries Neck sprain Neck sprains Stiff neck Trapezius muscle pain	Strength training Muscle strengthening	Exercise	Pain

CLINICAL SCENARIO

You are a rehabilitation consultant who has recently seen a number of individuals with work-related neck muscle pain, especially pain from the descending part of the trapezius muscle. You know that physical exercise is generally recommended, but you do not know which type of training is more effective in relieving muscle pain—strength training of the painful muscle or general fitness training without direct involvement of the painful muscle.

STEP 6: USE TRUNCATION AND WILDCARDS WHERE APPROPRIATE AND BOOLEAN OPERATORS TO COMBINE TERMS

(Neck muscle pain OR Neck strain* OR Neck strain injur* OR Neck sprain* OR Stiff neck OR Trapezius muscle pain) AND (Strength training OR Muscle strengthening) AND (General fitness OR Exercise) AND (Pain*)

Note: The truncation symbol used in this example is for conducting a search in PubMed.

STEP 7: DECIDE WHICH ONLINE RESOURCE(S) TO SEARCH

The online resource that you decide to search in will depend on the type of question that you are asking (for example intervention, diagnostic, prognostic or qualitative question). As was explained in Chapter 2, for each type of question there is a hierarchy of evidence. This hierarchy should be used to guide your search so that you know what type of study design you are hoping to find when searching. The type of study design that you are looking for will, in turn, influence which online resource(s) you should search in.

For example, if your clinical question is a prognostic one related to rehabilitation, then you will be looking for a cohort study (or systematic review of cohort studies). Therefore, there is no point in searching the Cochrane Library, PEDro or OTseeker, as these resources do not contain cohort studies. The best resource for you to start your search in would probably be PubMed, using the Clinical Queries feature, or REHAB+ (see later in the chapter). All of these resources, and many others, are described in the following section and in the examples at the end of this chapter.

A MODEL OF EVIDENCE-BASED INFORMATION SERVICES

In this chapter we will use a six-level pyramid to discuss the organisation of evidence-based information services.[2] This '6S' model (see Figure 3.1) is hierarchical in nature and has:

- **original studies** (what was done in one study) at the base
- **synopses of studies** (what the evidence is in one study, along with an expert telling you its strengths and potential practice changes)—that is, succinct descriptions of original studies often accompanied by expert commentaries such as those found in evidence-based secondary journals like *ACP Journal Club*
- **syntheses** (what the evidence is across several studies on the same topic)—that is, systematic reviews of the literature
- **synopses of syntheses** (what the evidence is across several studies, along with an expert telling you its strengths and potential practice changes)—that is, succinct descriptions of systematic reviews, often accompanied by expert commentaries such as those found in evidence-based secondary journals like *ACP Journal Club*
- **summaries**—that is, management options for diseases or conditions arranged by clinical topics such as those that appear in the online resources *Physicians' Information and Education Resource (PIER)* and *Clinical Evidence* (quite like a textbook chapter with a broad-based summary of a content area)
- **systems**—that is, integrated decision support services which provide evidence plus 'actions' that should be taken in relation to a specific patient or situation.

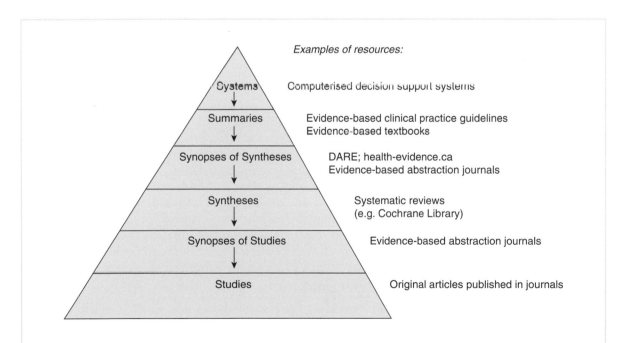

Figure 3.1
The 6S pyramid showing levels of organisation of evidence from healthcare research.

Reproduced with permission from DiCenso A, Bayley L, Haynes RB, Assessing preappraised evidence: fine-tuning the 5S model into a 6S model. American College of Physicians; 2009.[2]

As you are seeking the current best evidence, begin your search as high up in the pyramid as possible. The higher you go in the pyramid, the more the evidence has been collected, sifted and synthesised. As the synthesis and evaluation work has already been done by others, using evidence from the higher levels will save you time and labour and assist you to apply the best quality evidence that is currently available.

Deciding where to start on the pyramid depends largely on the question being asked and what resources are available to you. As explained earlier, you should be guided by the hierarchy of evidence for the type of question that you are asking. Additionally, you will also find that much of the content available at the higher levels of the pyramid is aimed at the medical profession, and that most of the evidence for nursing and allied health questions are found in levels one (bottom) and three of the pyramid and, at times, levels two and four. At each level of the '6S' pyramid, users of the evidence must appraise the quality of the evidence presented to ensure that the methods used to generate this evidence were sound. Detailed information about how to critically appraise evidence, once you have found it, is presented in Chapters 4–13 of this book. Each level of the pyramid will now be discussed further, starting at the top of the pyramid, where the best and most highly synthesised evidence can be found.

Systems–first layer (top) of the pyramid

Systems are found at the top of the '6S' pyramid. A system is an integrated clinical decision support service designed to improve clinical decision making. Such a system may be integrated into an electronic patient health record system or hospital clinical information system. Alternatively, the system may allow for entry of patient-specific characteristics, such as age, gender, renal function and allergy history. These computerised decision support systems reliably link patient characteristics with the current evidence-based guidelines for care. The system generates patient-specific recommendations (for example, lower the dose of insulin because of hypoglycaemic events or schedule a blood test because it is due next month). A key component of a clinical decision support service that differentiates it from other types of evidence-based information services is the integration of patient-specific variables.

Clinical decision support systems have been developed for various clinical issues, including the diagnosis of chest pain, the management of chronic disease (such as diabetes care) and the timely administration of preventive services (such as immunisations). Systematic reviews of the effects of computerised clinical decision support systems showed that some may improve health professionals' performance.[3–8] If you have such a system in your workplace, you are lucky as it is likely that you will not need to look further for the best evidence to answer your clinical question. However, most people will not be able to begin their search at the top of the pyramid because systems are relatively rare, existing for only a few diseases or conditions, and usually have a medical focus. Not all health professions have electronic patient medical records and, even if they do, many are not integrated with a decision support system that has an evidence-based guideline summarising the current best evidence on a topic of interest. Therefore, if you do not have access to a system that addresses your information needs, you will need to start your search for the current best evidence at the next level down in the pyramid.

Summaries–second layer of the pyramid

Summaries are information resources that provide regularly updated evidence, which is usually arranged by clinical topics. They are considered to be similar to traditional textbook chapters in form and content. Evidence-based clinical guidelines are also located at this level of the pyramid. Summaries provide guidance and/or recommendations for patient management and often provide links to other aspects of the disease or condition. Summaries can be found in disease-specific textbooks such as *Evidence-based endocrinology*[9] but, unless the textbook is accompanied by a website where the content can be regularly updated, the content in a print textbook quickly becomes outdated. Online textbooks that are regularly updated are becoming more common. Medicine has the most of these online textbooks, and some of these contain information which may be of interest to allied health professionals or nurses. All of the online textbooks listed as examples below are available on a subscription basis, but many workplaces, particularly academic and healthcare institutions, may have institutional subscriptions.

- *Clinical Evidence* (clinicalevidence.bmj.com/ceweb/index.jsp) is provided by the BMJ Publishing Group and summarises evidence on the benefits and harms of healthcare interventions for selected medical conditions. The evidence is drawn from systematic reviews and original studies. The content is presented in question format (for example, *What are the effects of interventions aimed at reducing relapse rates and disability in people with multiple sclerosis?*), with the levels of evidence used to answer the question and hyperlinks to the supporting evidence. A clinical guide (that is, a comment on how to use this information in clinical practice) is also presented.

- *Best Practice* (bestpractice.bmj.com/best-practice/welcome.html) is provided by the BMJ Evidence Centre (a division of the BMJ Group) and incorporates *Clinical Evidence*. The service combines the latest research evidence, guidelines and expert opinion regarding prevention, diagnosis, treatment and prognosis using a step-by-step approach (that is, presented for each medical condition/disease are highlights, basics, prevention, diagnosis, treatment and follow-up). Recommendations are supported with links to the evidence.

- *Physician's Information and Education Resource (PIER)* (pier.acponline.org/index.html), from the American College of Physicians (ACP), is an integrated summary service that provides evidence-based guidance and practice recommendations for health professionals. It is organised into seven topic types (diseases, screening and prevention, complementary and alternative medicine, ethical and legal issues, procedures, quality measures and drug resources), with each topic containing several modules. *PIER*'s authors are supported by an explicit evidence-based process, where current best evidence is provided to the authors of the chapters after comprehensive literature searches are conducted.

  PIER is available online to ACP members and can also be accessed through *STAT!Ref* (www.statref.com), an online healthcare reference that provides full-text access to key medical reference sources and textbooks, some of which are evidence-based resources. *STAT!Ref* is a subscription-based resource that is usually available in academic or hospital environments where institutional subscriptions exist. *PIER* is more directive than *Clinical Evidence*, as it contains recommendations rather than evidence summaries.

- *UpToDate* (www.uptodate.com) is an online textbook that is very comprehensive in its topic coverage. It is currently organised into 17 medical specialties (for example, adult primary care and internal medicine, cardiovascular medicine, endocrinology and diabetes, family medicine). *UpToDate* provides specific recommendations (guidelines) for health professionals for patient care and most, but not all, of these recommendations include an assessment of the quality of the evidence.

- *First Consult* (www.firstconsult.com/php/376749460-30/home.html) is part of *MD Consult*, from Elsevier, and is an evidence-based and continuously updated clinical information resource for primary care clinicians. Designed for use at point-of-care (for example at the bedside, in the clinic), information is arranged around the components of medical topics, differential diagnosis and procedures. Recommendations are made and the levels of evidence and links to supporting evidence accompany some recommendations.

- *DynaMed* (dynamed.ebscohost.com), from EBSCO Publishing, is a clinical reference tool for use at the point-of-care (for example at the bedside, in the clinic). It has clinically-organised summaries for more than 3200 topics. Recommendations are made and the levels of evidence and links to supporting evidence accompany some recommendations.

- *EBM Guidelines: Evidence-Based Medicine* (onlinelibrary.wiley.com/book/10.1002/0470057203), from Wiley Interscience, is a collection of clinical guidelines for primary care combined with the best available evidence. There are approximately 1000 primary care practice guidelines, which are continuously updated and cover a wide range of medical conditions. Both diagnosis and treatment are included.

Synopses of syntheses—third layer of the pyramid

If you do not find an answer to your clinical question in a summary, the next best place to search for an answer is in synopses of syntheses. Synopses of syntheses are structured abstracts or brief overviews of published systematic reviews that have been screened for methodological rigour. This means you do not have to do this step yourself! Synopses of syntheses can be found in the following online resources:

- *ACP Journal Club* (www.acpjc.org) is a pre-appraised secondary journal that is available online as well as in print within the *Annals of Internal Medicine*. To produce the content for this journal, research staff hand-search over 120 core healthcare journals and critically appraise the articles in each issue to identify high-quality primary studies and review articles that have potential for clinical application. From this pool of articles, practising health professionals rate the content for relevancy and newsworthiness. The studies and reviews that are considered to be the most clinically important are summarised in structured abstracts. A clinical expert comments on the methods and provides a clinical bottom line (that is, how to use the evidence in clinical practice).

  The focus of the content in *ACP Journal Club* is internal medicine, and it includes sections on therapy, diagnosis, prognosis, aetiology, quality improvement and continuing education, economics, clinical prediction guides and differential diagnosis. As well as being a subscription-based resource, *ACP Journal Club* is one of the databases available through Ovid (gateway.ovid.com), a company that designs search engines and makes several evidence-based databases available on a subscription basis. Many institutions such as libraries, hospitals and universities use Ovid and therefore have institutional subscriptions.

- **Evidence-Based Nursing** (http://ebn.bmj.com), **Evidence-Based Medicine** (http://ebm.bmj.com) and **Evidence-Based Mental Health** (http://ebmh.bmj.com) are all currently published by the BMJ Publishing Group. Articles and reviews that meet specified criteria for rigour and relevance to nursing, general medicine and mental health, respectively, are selected for inclusion. A commentary is provided that identifies the key findings and implications for clinical practice.

- **Database of Abstracts of Reviews of Effects (DARE)** (www.crd.york.ac.uk/crdweb) is produced by the Centre for Reviews and Dissemination (CRD) at the University of York in the United Kingdom and contains abstracts of quality-assessed non-Cochrane systematic reviews. Each abstract includes a summary of the review together with a critical commentary about the overall quality of the review. DARE covers a broad range of health-related interventions. At the time of writing, DARE included over 21,000 abstracts of systematic reviews. When searching on the CRD website, content is retrieved from DARE, NHS EED (National Institute for Health Research Economic Evaluation Database) and HTA (Health Technology Assessment Database) simultaneously. DARE, as well as NHS EED and HTA, are available free of charge.

- **Bandolier** (www.medicine.ox.ac.uk/bandolier) provides a summary service that covers selected medical topics. Information comes from systematic reviews, meta-analyses, randomised trials and high quality observational studies. The review of the clinical evidence is combined with a clinical commentary and a clinical bottom line. Bandolier's internet version is free of charge.

Several journals also have sections where they highlight critically appraised papers. They generally use similar principles and format to *ACP Journal Club*. Examples in the allied health professions are the *Journal of Physiotherapy, Australian Occupational Therapy Journal* and the Canadian Association of Occupational Therapists' *OT Now* publication.

A list of resources with hotlinks to pre-appraised resource journals (synopses) for various disciplines is maintained by The New York Academy of Medicine (www.nyam.org/fellows-members/ebhc/eb_publications.html).

Syntheses (systematic reviews)–fourth layer of the pyramid

When no synopses of syntheses can be found, the next best place to look for an answer to your clinical question is a systematic review. Systematic reviews provide syntheses of the highest quality evidence available for a specific clinical question. Information about how to appraise systematic reviews is presented in Chapter 12 of this book. Systematic reviews can be found in the following resources:

- **Cochrane Database of Systematic Reviews** (www.thecochranelibrary.com) is part of the Cochrane Library and is made up of several review groups that concentrate and synthesise the evidence in specific healthcare areas. For example, the focus of the Cochrane Musculoskeletal Group is synthesising the evidence from randomised controlled trials and controlled clinical trials of interventions that are concerned with the prevention, treatment and/or rehabilitation of musculoskeletal disorders.

  The focus of the Cochrane Database of Systematic Reviews was originally on healthcare interventions. However, from Issue 1, 2008, reviews on diagnostic test accuracy were introduced. At the time of writing (March 2012), there were over 7200 records available and most of these were completed reviews. Even with this many systematic reviews available, the Cochrane Collaboration contains less than a quarter of the world's supply of systematic reviews.

  The Cochrane Library, which houses the Cochrane Database of Systematic Reviews, is a subscription-based resource that is usually available in academic or hospital environments where institutional subscriptions exist. However, residents in a number of countries or regions can access The Cochrane Library online for free (for a list visit www.thecochranelibrary.com/view/0/FreeAccess.html). Cochrane systematic reviews are indexed in several large biomedical electronic databases such as MEDLINE, and are therefore also available through other vendors such as Ovid on a subscription basis and through PubMed (www.ncbi.nlm.nih.gov/sites/entrez?db=pubmed), which is free.

  There are a number of ways to search in the Cochrane Database of Systematic Reviews, such as Quick Search, Advanced Search and MeSH search (see Box 3.1 for an explanation of MeSH). As the Cochrane Library is such an important evidence-based practice resource, it is important that you know how to search in it efficiently. We highly recommend that you read the easy-to-read Cochrane Library User Guide (available for free at www.cochrane.org.au/libraryguide)

  Cochrane reviews are updated regularly, and previous versions of a review are archived on the Cochrane Library website under the 'Other versions' tab available on the article display page. Older versions of the review can only be retrieved via the 'Other versions' tab as they are not picked up by a Cochrane Library search. The Cochrane Library also includes DARE content.

- **Campbell Collaboration** (www.campbellcollaboration.org) conducts and maintains systematic reviews about the effects of interventions in the social, behavioural and educational arenas (for example social skills training). As of March 2012, the free searchable database contained more than 200 systematic reviews.

- **Various biomedical databases**—many systematic reviews are available in the large electronic biomedical databases such as MEDLINE and EMBASE. These databases are available through various providers such as Ovid (gateway.ovid.com) on a subscription basis. MEDLINE is also available free of charge through PubMed.

  It can be challenging to efficiently retrieve systematic reviews from these large databases because of the sheer volume of articles that they contain and because they also contain many other types of articles that are not useful for answering clinical questions. To assist with the retrieval of systematic

BOX 3.1

What are index terms and textwords?

INDEX TERMS

- These are somewhat like the index in a book. Index terms can be useful to search with, as they are designed to overcome the problem of different authors using different terms to describe the same concept. Index terms (usually between 10 and 20) are assigned to each article by staff at the electronic databases using a database-specific thesaurus. Of course, to keep users on their toes, different databases use different index terms! For example, MEDLINE uses MeSH (Medical Subject Headings), CINAHL uses CINAHL subject headings and EMBASE uses Emtree.

- Index terms are organised hierarchically, using a tree structure, with broader terms higher up in the 'tree'. This structure provides an effective way for users to make their search broader and narrower as needed. For example, part of the MeSH tree structure for 'stroke' is as follows:

> Nervous System Diseases
> > Central Nervous System Diseases
> > > Brain Diseases
> > > > Cerebrovascular Disorders
> > > > > Stroke
> > > > > > Brain Infarction
> > > > > > > Brain Stem Infarction
> > > > > > > > Cerebral Infarction

- For some topics that you want to search on, there may be no corresponding index terms. Sadly, this is the case for many of the interventions that are used by allied health professionals. When this occurs, you need to search using textwords.

- How do you know what MeSH to use? You can search the MeSH browser online (www.nlm.nih.gov/mesh/MBrowser.html); when searching MEDLINE via Ovid, you can choose to have your search automatically mapped to relevant MeSH; or you can look at relevant articles to see what MeSH have been assigned to those articles.

TEXTWORDS

You can also search using textwords. These are free-text words that are found in the title and abstract of the article and therefore are the words used by the authors of articles. The limitation of this method is that the authors may have used a different term (for example 'cerebrovascular accident') to the search term that you are using (for example 'stroke'). Although you are both describing the same thing, you may not retrieve their article in your search. The obvious way to overcome this is to use the relevant index term. However, if there is no corresponding index term, using synonyms and related terms (combining them with the Boolean operator OR) and truncation and wildcard symbols can help to broaden your search.

reviews, researchers have developed search filters for use in these large databases. The 'Clinical Queries' screen in PubMed (www.ncbi.nlm.nih.gov/pubmed/clinical or accessed by a link on the PubMed homepage) offers some assistance to efficient searching by providing a ready-to-use search filter for identifying systematic reviews. This feature is described in more detail later in this chapter when MEDLINE is discussed further.

- **Discipline-specific databases**—there are several discipline-specific databases which contain systematic reviews or index systematic reviews. For example:

  - **health-evidence.ca** (www.health-evidence.ca) is a free, searchable online registry of public health systematic reviews.

  - **EvidenceUpdates** (http://plus.mcmaster.ca/EvidenceUpdates) is a freely available resource. EvidenceUpdates is described in more detail in the following section on studies.

- **OBESITY+** (http://plus.mcmaster.ca/obesity/Default.aspx) provides access to a subset of the content found in EvidenceUpdates. The content focuses on obesity. OBESITY+ is described in more detail in the following section on studies.

- **REHAB+** (http://plus.mcmaster.ca/rehab/Default.aspx) provides access to the current best evidence about the causes, course, diagnosis, prevention, treatment and economics related to rehabilitation. REHAB+ is described in more detail in the following section on studies.

- **Nursing+** (http://plus.mcmaster.ca/NP) provides access to the current best evidence about the causes, course, diagnosis, prevention, treatment and economics related to nursing care. Nursing+ is described in more detail in the following section on studies.

- **OTseeker** (Occupational Therapy Systematic Evaluation of Evidence) is an occupational therapy evidence database and is freely available at www.otseeker.com. OTseeker is described in more detail in the following section on studies.

- **PEDro** is the Physiotherapy Evidence Database, from the Centre for Evidence-based Physiotherapy in Australia, and is freely available at www.pedro.org.au. PEDro is described in more detail in the following section on studies.

- **PsycBITE** (the Psychological Database for Brain Impairment Treatment Efficacy) is freely available at www.psycbite.com. PsycBITE is described in more detail in the following section on studies.

- **speechBITE** (Speech Pathology Database for Best Interventions and Treatment Efficacy) is freely available at www.speechbite.com and is described in more detail in the following section on studies.

- The Joanna Briggs Institute provides a library of systematic reviews that is available on a subscription basis (http://connect.jbiconnectplus.org). It contains reviews that are primarily of relevance to nursing.

Synopses of studies–fifth layer of the pyramid

When no syntheses can be found, the next best place to look for an answer to your clinical question is synopses of studies. Synopses of studies are structured abstracts or brief overviews of published individual studies that have been screened for methodological rigour. This means you do not have to do this step yourself. Synopses of studies are found in evidence-based abstraction journals, that is *ACP Journal Club* (www.acpjc.org), *Evidence-Based Nursing* (http://ebn.bmj.com), *Evidence-Based Medicine* (http://ebm.bmj.com) and *Evidence-Based Mental Health* (http://ebmh.bmj.com), as described in the section on synopses of syntheses.

Studies–sixth layer (bottom) of the pyramid

When none of the upper layers of the pyramid provide an answer to your clinical question, you must look for individual studies. There are millions of individual studies, which can make it difficult for you to efficiently find the evidence that you need to answer your clinical question. When searching for individual studies, you should start your search using databases that have screened many sources for you, include only the most important clinical studies and have pre-appraised the studies for you. Examples are:

- **EvidenceUpdates** (plus.mcmaster.ca/EvidenceUpdates) provides access to scientifically sound and clinically relevant systematic reviews and studies that have been published in over 120 premier healthcare journals. The content found in these 120 journals is critically appraised by research staff, and those studies and reviews that are scientifically sound are then rated for relevancy and newsworthiness by a worldwide panel of practising doctors. The content focuses on internal medicine and its subspecialties, general medical practice and nursing. Various types of articles are included, such as those concerned with therapy, diagnosis, prognosis, aetiology, quality improvement and continuing education, economics, clinical prediction guides and differential diagnosis. A searchable database is available for use after registering for this free service.

The following three databases are subsets of the content found in EvidenceUpdates. Their content is rated for relevancy and newsworthiness by a worldwide panel of practising health professionals who have a special interest in the area of interest of each database (for example, practising occupational therapists and physiotherapists provide the ratings for REHAB+). These databases are free to search after completing a quick registration process.

- **OBESITY+** (http://plus.mcmaster.ca/obesity/Default.aspx) provides access to the current best evidence about the causes, course, diagnosis, prevention, treatment and economics of obesity and its related metabolic and mechanical complications.

- **REHAB+** (http://plus.mcmaster.ca/rehab/Default.aspx) provides access to the current best evidence about the causes, course, diagnosis, prevention, treatment and economics related to rehabilitation.

- **Nursing+** (http://plus.mcmaster.ca/NP) provides access to the current best evidence about the causes, course, diagnosis, prevention, treatment and economics related to nursing care.

- **Cochrane Central Register of Controlled Trials** is part of the Cochrane Library and is the largest electronic registry of randomised controlled trials in existence (in September 2012, there were over 680,000 records). It is available as part of a subscription to the Cochrane Library and is also available through Ovid's Evidence-Based Medicine Reviews, which are packages of databases available on a subscription basis, as well as through several other services such as Wiley Interscience. This registry of individual controlled trials is a companion database to the Cochrane Database of Systematic Reviews, which was described earlier in the chapter. The articles in this registry are sourced from large databases including MEDLINE and EMBASE, hand-searches of major healthcare journals across many health disciplines and other sources that are utilised by the review groups within the Cochrane Collaboration.

- **OTseeker** (www.otseeker.com) is a discipline-specific database that contains abstracts of systematic reviews and randomised controlled trials relevant to occupational therapy (over 9000 as of November 2012). The trials included in this database have been critically appraised and rated to help you interpret the results and assess the validity of the findings. OTseeker is available free of charge.

- **PEDro** (www.pedro.org.au) is a discipline-specific database that contains abstracts of randomised controlled trials, systematic reviews and evidence-based clinical practice guidelines relevant to physiotherapy (over 22,000 as of November 2012). As with the articles on OTseeker, most trials in the database have been critically appraised and this assessment helps you to discriminate between trials which are likely to be valid and interpretable and those which are not. PEDro is available free of charge.

- **PsycBITE** (www.psycbite.com) catalogues studies (randomised and non-randomised controlled trials, case series and single subject design) and systematic reviews focusing on the cognitive, behavioural and other types of treatment for the psychological problems and issues that can occur as a result of acquired brain impairment. The methodological quality of most of the randomised trials, non-randomised controlled trials and case series has been rated.

- **speechBITE** (www.speechbite.com) is modelled on PsycBITE and contains treatment studies (systematic reviews, randomised and non-randomised controlled trials, case series and single subject design) across the scope of speech pathology practice. The randomised and non-randomised controlled trials have been critically appraised.

If you cannot find an answer to your clinical question using a pre-appraised service such as those outlined above, the next step is to use one or more of the large electronic bibliographic databases that are described in this section. When searching in the large electronic databases, it is often most effective if you search using a combination of index terms and textwords. These are explained in Box 3.1.

- **MEDLINE** is the largest biomedical database and currently has over 21 million citations. MEDLINE is produced by the US National Library of Medicine and is available for free through PubMed (www. ncbi.nlm.nih.gov/sites/entrez?db=pubmed). Searching efficiently in MEDLINE is important because of the large size of the database and also because many of the articles included in the database are not appropriate for use in evidence-based practice (for example literature reviews). MEDLINE is also available through providers, such as Ovid, on a subscription basis. When accessing MEDLINE via Ovid, content searches can also be limited by Clinical Queries for individual studies about therapy, diagnosis, prognosis, aetiology, clinical prediction guides, costs, economics and studies of a qualitative nature, as well as systematic reviews.

  - As mentioned previously in this chapter, the **Clinical Queries screen in PubMed** (www.ncbi.nlm. nih.gov/pubmed/clinical) can be a great tool to facilitate efficient clinical searching by providing ready-to-use search filters. These search strategies filter the retrieval of appropriate study types for the clinical categories of **therapy**, **diagnosis**, **aetiology**, **prognosis** and **clinical prediction**. For example, when searching for an article about therapy, the search filter attempts to restrict the retrieval to articles that report using a randomised controlled trial design.

  - Search strategies that filter the retrieval of appropriate study types for the clinical categories of **healthcare costs** and **healthcare quality** (and some **qualitative topics**) can be found on the **Health Services Research Queries** screen (www.nlm.nih.gov/nichsr/hedges/search.html) after clicking on the Special Queries link in PubMed.

When using the Clinical Queries or Health Services Research Queries interfaces, you only need to:

1. Enter basic content information (such as the keywords from your clinical question—try starting with the 'P' and 'I' keywords and then broaden or narrow your search as needed) and click on 'Search'.

2. Then, select the type of question that you are searching for an answer to (in Clinical Queries, you can choose from therapy, prognosis, diagnosis, aetiology or clinical prediction guides).

3. Decide if you want to conduct a broad (sensitive) or narrow (specific) search:

   a. A **sensitive (broad) search** increases the likelihood of retrieving every possible relevant study, which in PubMed can often result in an unmanageable number of search results.

   b. You may wish to begin by selecting a **specific (narrow) search**, which will minimise the number of irrelevant studies that are returned. If you get very few, or no, search results, you can then repeat the search and change the emphasis to sensitive.

That is all you have to do. Everything else, such as the methodological refining of the search filter, is done for you. The results will be presented in two columns: one containing primary studies (called 'clinical studies' by PubMed) and one containing systematic reviews (sometimes there can be some inaccuracies in this, with systematic reviews appearing in the primary study list and non-systematic reviews appearing in the systematic reviews list). There is also a third column called 'Medical Genetics', but the results in this column are unlikely to be of use for health professionals who are trying to answer a clinical question. A useful feature of Clinical Queries is that it also searches using the relevant MeSH terms (without you having to select them). Another handy feature of PubMed is the *Related Citations* feature—a list of related articles (as the name aptly suggests!) that appears on the right-hand margin of the search results screen. This can be a quick and easy way to locate some additional articles that are relevant to your search, or at least, some related terms to search with.

Figure 3.2 shows the search page of Clinical Queries and a basic search related to the clinical scenario that was outlined earlier in this chapter. Details of the search that Clinical Queries actually ran for you are shown in the 'search details' box on the right-hand side of the full search results page (once you click

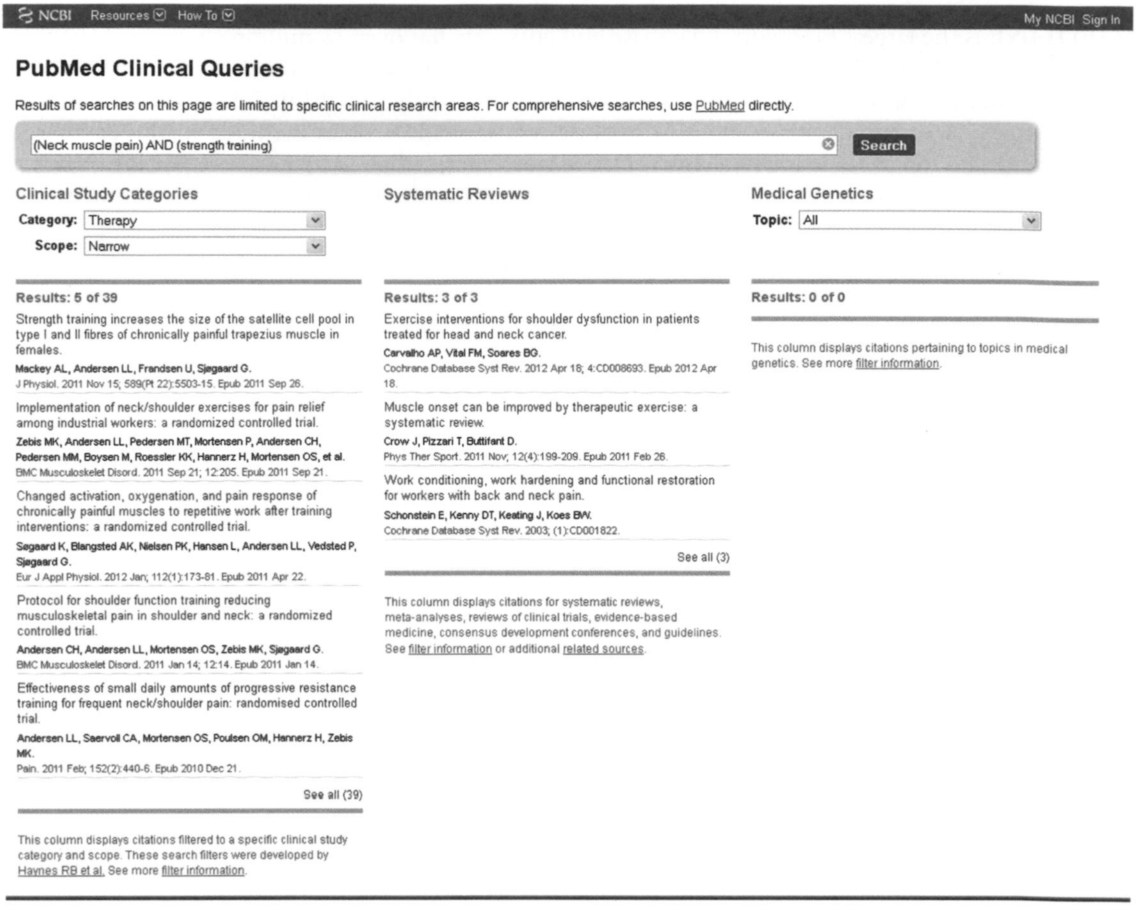

Figure 3.2
The Clinical Queries search page in PubMed.

Reproduced courtesy of National Center for Biotechnology Information/U.S. National Library of Medicine.

on 'see all' at the bottom of the first search results page that is displayed). In the example search that is shown in Figure 3.2, even though we only typed in *(Neck muscle pain) AND (strength training)*, this is what was actually searched for:

Therapy/Narrow[filter] AND ((("neck muscles"[MeSH Terms] OR ("neck"[All Fields] AND "muscles"[All Fields]) OR "neck muscles"[All Fields] OR ("neck"[All Fields] AND "muscle"[All Fields]) OR "neck muscle"[All Fields]) AND ("pain"[MeSH Terms] OR "pain"[All Fields])) AND ("resistance training"[MeSH Terms] OR ("resistance"[All Fields] AND "training"[All Fields]) OR "resistance training"[All Fields] OR ("strength"[All Fields] AND "training"[All Fields]) OR "strength training"[All Fields]))

Other large databases are:

- **EMBASE** is a large European database with over 20 million citations. EMBASE is similar to MEDLINE in scope and content, with an overlap in content between the two databases of about

30–50%. Compared with MEDLINE, EMBASE provides greater coverage of European and non-English-language publications and a broader coverage of topics concerned with pharmaceuticals, psychiatry, toxicology and alternative medicine. EMBASE is available through various providers, such as Ovid, on a subscription basis. Your hospital or academic institution library may have an institutional subscription to this resource. As in Ovid MEDLINE, Ovid EMBASE content searches can be limited by Clinical Queries for individual studies about therapy, diagnosis, prognosis, aetiology, economics and studies of a qualitative nature, as well as systematic reviews.

- **CINAHL** (Cumulative Index to Nursing and Allied Health Literature) is the premier nursing and allied health database, and contains over 2.3 million records. CINAHL is offered by the vendor EBSCOHost. As in Ovid MEDLINE and Ovid EMBASE, EBSCO CINAHL offers content searches that can be limited by Clinical Queries for individual studies about therapy, prognosis, aetiology and studies of a qualitative nature, as well as systematic reviews.

- **PsycINFO** is the comprehensive international bibliographic database of psychological literature from the 1800s to the present, and contains over 3 million records. As with the other large databases, multiple access routes are available and all require a subscription. In Ovid PsycINFO, Clinical Queries can be used to limit retrieval to individual studies about therapy and those of a qualitative nature, as well as systematic reviews.

When searching using the large electronic databases, it is important to use the help function that is found within each database so that you become familiar with how to search the database efficiently. The features and interfaces of databases change from time to time and, as mentioned earlier, there are some subtle differences across databases in terms of refining search techniques, such as the symbols for truncation and the use of double quotation marks instead of parentheses for combining terms.

Some tips for locating qualitative research

Finding qualitative research can be very difficult. One of the reasons is that it is indexed in a number of different ways. Using the term 'qualitative' as a search term is often not useful, as sometimes qualitative research is indexed by the specific method that was used to collect data (for example, focus group or in-depth interview) and other times it is indexed according to the methodology that was used (for example, phenomenology or grounded theory). Table 3.1 shows some empirically derived[10–13] search filters that can be used to locate qualitative studies in CINAHL, MEDLINE, EMBASE and PsycINFO. They are methodological search filters, meaning that they focus on the *methods of qualitative research* rather than the content. Combine these methodological search filters with your content terms, that is the keywords from your clinical question.

For example, to locate qualitative research about depression in women, you could try the following search string in Ovid MEDLINE:

depression.tw. AND wom*n.tw. AND [interview:.tw. OR px.fs OR exp health services administration]

The search filters shown in Table 3.1, except for the CINAHL filter, are in Ovid syntax (that is, Ovid language) so they will need translation if you are searching using another interface. The CINAHL filter provided is in EBSCO syntax, as CINAHL has only been available through this provider since 2009. The PubMed translation of the MEDLINE sensitive and specific search can be found on the Special Queries page of PubMed under Health Services Research Queries, which we described earlier in this chapter when MEDLINE was explained. As you can see in Table 3.1, there is a choice of three different search filters—'sensitive', 'specific' or 'best balance of sensitive and specific'.

- Use the sensitive search filter when you want a very broad search and do not want to risk missing any relevant articles.

TABLE 3.1:
SEARCH FILTERS FOR LOCATING QUALITATIVE RESEARCH IN MEDLINE, CINAHL, EMBASE AND PSYCINFO

Hedge	MEDLINE (Ovid syntax)	CINAHL (EBSCO syntax)	EMBASE (Ovid syntax)	PsycINFO (Ovid syntax)
Sensitive	interview:.tw. OR px.fs. OR exp health services administration	((MH "study design+" not MM "study design+") or MH "attitude" or (MH "interviews+" not MM "interviews+"))	interview:.tw. OR qualitative.tw. OR health care organization	experience:.mp. OR interview:.tw. OR qualitative:.tw.
Specific	qualitative.tw. OR themes.tw.	((MH "grounded theory" not MM "grounded theory") or (TI thematic analysis or AB thematic analysis or MW thematic analysis))	qualitative.tw. OR qualitative study.tw.	qualitative:.tw. OR themes.tw.
Best balance of sensitive and specific	interview:.mp. OR experience:. mp. OR qualitative.tw.	((TI interview or AB interview) or (MH "audiorecording" not MM "audiorecording") or (TI qualitative stud* or AB qualitative stud*))	interview:.tw. OR exp health care organization OR experiences.tw.	experiences.tw. OR interview:.tw. OR qualitative.tw.

Ovid syntax: colon (:) = truncation; exp = explosion; fs = floating subheading; mp = multiple posting, term found in title, abstract or index terms; px = psychology; tw = textword.

EBSCO syntax: + = explode; AB = abstract; MH = subject heading; MM = exact major subject heading; MW = subject heading word; TI = title.

- Use the specific search filter when you want to narrow your search and want to find just a few relevant articles.
- Use the 'best balance' search filters for a search that provides a good balance between sensitivity and specificity.

Alerting or updating services

Although it is not on the '6S' pyramid specifically, electronic communication (that is, email) can be a useful method of informing health professionals about newly published studies. Unlike all of the resources outlined above that require you to go and search for the evidence, alerting services bring the research literature to you in the form of email alerts or RSS (really simple syndication) feeds, which are simply a list of items that you sign up to receive. In Chapter 2, this was described as 'push' or 'just-in-case' information. Several alerting systems that target articles to individual health professionals have been developed. Some examples are:

- **EvidenceUpdates** (plus.mcmaster.ca/EvidenceUpdates) is a free service that alerts health professionals to newly published studies and systematic reviews from over 120 premier healthcare journals that are published in their discipline. It is the same process that the *ACP Journal Club* uses to select both clinically relevant and methodologically rigorous papers. If a paper is going to be clinically useful, it has a high probability of being selected in this database. Newly published studies and systematic reviews have been pre-appraised for methodological rigour, and clinical relevancy and newsworthiness. Users choose the frequency at which they wish to receive email notifications or RSS feeds and the disciplines in which they are interested (for example: general medicine practice, endocrinology) and set the score level for clinical relevance and newsworthiness to a level that is acceptable to them.

- **OBESITY+** (plus.mcmaster.ca/obesity/Default.aspx) offers a free alerting service that provides access to a subset of the content found in EvidenceUpdates. The content of OBESITY+ was described earlier in this chapter.

- **REHAB+** (plus.mcmaster.ca/rehab/Default.aspx) offers a free alerting service that provides access to a subset of the content found in EvidenceUpdates that is relevant to rehabilitation.

- **Nursing+** (plus.mcmaster.ca/NP) provides access to the current best evidence about the causes, course, diagnosis, prevention, treatment and economics related to nursing care and also has a free alerting service.

- **My NCBI** (www.ncbi.nlm.nih.gov/sites/myncbi) is an alerting service within PubMed that will email users with new citations from MEDLINE in the clinical areas that they have specified. Users set up a search that will automatically email them citations of newly published articles based on content (for example, asthma in adolescents) or journal titles. My NCBI is offered free of charge through PubMed. However, the newly published articles are not filtered by methodological rigour and you will need to critically appraise the articles that are sent to you before considering their use in clinical practice.

- **Journals** may enable you to register to have the table of contents emailed to you as each new issue of the journal is published. You may wish to do this for journals that you frequently consult. As with My NCBI, the newly published articles are not filtered by methodological rigour and you will need to critically appraise the articles that are sent to you before considering their use in clinical practice.

Other resources

Again, although not specifically on the '6S' pyramid, many search engines are available for use on the internet. When using these search engines (for example Google), you are not searching a defined database but are searching the internet in general. A major negative aspect of using these search engines is that evidence-based information may be difficult to find and much high quality clinical research (such as that located in databases) cannot be located at all in this way. On the other hand, positive aspects are that an internet search can be a quick way of tracking down a specific article and obtaining information about issues that keep changing, such as listings of country-specific vaccination rules for travellers. Examples of internet search engines are:

- **Google** (www.google.com), **Yahoo** (www.yahoo.com), **MSN** (www.msn.com) and **Ask** (www.ask.com). All four internet search engines are commonly used and freely accessible. Search Engine Watch (searchenginewatch.com/article/2048976/Major-Search-Engines-and-Directories) maintains a list of major search engines on the web and rates the usefulness of each. Note that when searching using Google, truncations or wild cards for letters of the alphabet are not an option. In Google, the use of wild cards is for words rather than letters. For example, typing *personal * records* would retrieve items that include *personal health records*, *personal medical records*, *personal records*, etc.

- **Google Scholar** (scholar.google.com) is a free service provided by Google that provides searching of the scholarly literature. From one site, you are able to search across many disciplines and sources such as peer-reviewed papers, theses, books, abstracts and articles that are from academic publishers, professional societies, preprint repositories, universities and other scholarly organisations. Google Scholar sorts articles by weighting the full text of the article, the author, the publication in which the article appears and how often the article has been cited in other scholarly literature. This sorting results in the most relevant articles being likely to appear on the first page.

- Search engines that retrieve and combine results from multiple search engines (meta-search engines) also exist.

Finally, you may be faced with a clinical question where you do not know which of the evidence-based resources may be best for answering your particular clinical problem. In these situations, 'federated search engines' provide a means to search many resources, with the retrieval of results organised according to the source of evidence. Examples are:

- **ACCESSSS** (plus.mcmaster.ca/accessss) is a free health-related meta-search engine that searches multiple databases with just one entry of your search term(s). ACCESSSS is designed to find the best evidence-based answer to your clinical questions by simultaneously searching the leading evidence-driven medical publications and high quality clinical literature. As of September 2011, sources included in ACCESSSS searches included *DynaMed, UpToDate, STAT!Ref PIER, Best Practice*, DARE, McMaster Premium Literature Service (PLUS), *ACP Journal Club*, PubMed Clinical Queries and PubMed. ACCESSSS searches and groups the results according to the '6S' pyramid. ACCESSSS is a product of the McMaster Health Knowledge Refinery (http://hiru.mcmaster.ca/hiru) which is a continuously updated resource for evidence-based clinical decisions. After registering for the service, alerts to new evidence tailored to your clinical/research needs are provided, as well as links to prescribing and patient information.

- **SUMSearch 2** (sumsearch.org) is a free health-related meta-search engine that simultaneously searches for original studies, systematic reviews and practice guidelines from multiple sources. You can focus (for example, *intervention*) and limit (for example, *age*) your search. By using SUMSearch 2, you can search multiple medical databases with one entry of search terms. For example, the entry of two words, 'spinal manipulation' in SUMSearch 2 provided links to 19 guidelines that are available through the US National Guidelines Clearinghouse, 4 guidelines in PubMed, 231 systematic reviews in PubMed and 51 original studies in PubMed. By contrast, when an internet search engine such as Google (www.google.com) was used to perform this search, it retrieved approximately 2.8 million entries for 'spinal manipulation' and the items were not grouped by source (for example PubMed) or type of evidence (for example systematic reviews).

- **TRIP** (Turning Research Into Practice, www.tripdatabase.com) is similar to SUMSearch 2 in that it searches multiple databases and other evidence-based resources with just one entry of your search term(s). TRIP groups the search results into evidence-based synopses, systematic reviews, guidelines (from Australia and New Zealand, Canada, UK, USA and other locations), clinical questions and answers, core primary research, e-textbooks and more. Any articles that are retrieved from MEDLINE are organised by purpose—therapy, diagnosis, systematic review, prognosis and aetiology. You can register for My TRIP and obtain access to extra features including alerts to new evidence.

SEARCH EXAMPLES

In this section we will use some of the resources described in this chapter to answer several different clinical questions—one from each of the four major question types that are covered in this book (effects of intervention, diagnosis, prognosis, and questions about patients' experiences and concerns).

Clinical question about the effects of intervention

You are a physiotherapist and currently have two patients who are pregnant and experiencing pelvic and back pain. You wonder:

> In pregnant women, is acupuncture more effective than standard treatment in relieving pregnancy-related pelvic and back pain?

Starting at the top of the '6S' pyramid, you confirm that there is nothing at the top three levels of the pyramid, which is often the case for allied health clinical questions. As your question is one about intervention effectiveness, you are ideally hoping to find a systematic review of randomised controlled trials. Therefore, your next step is to look for a systematic review (fourth level of the pyramid—syntheses) by searching in the Cochrane Database of Systematic Reviews, using the keywords from your clinical question (pregnan* AND acupuncture).

Your search retrieves one review[14] that summarises interventions for preventing and treating pelvic and back pain in pregnancy. As all but one study included in the review had moderate to high potential for bias (as stated by the authors of the review), you decide to look for other systematic reviews, ideally ones where acupuncture was the only intervention of focus.

Since PEDro contains systematic reviews and pre-appraised articles related to physiotherapy, you decide to search there next. On the advanced search page, you type in the terms 'pregnancy acupuncture', and select the body part 'lumbar spine, sacro-iliac joint and pelvis'. Note that in PEDro you do not need to type in Boolean operators; just tick the box at the bottom of the advanced search page indicating whether you want the search terms to be combined with AND or OR. Your search retrieves 13 records, and three of these are systematic reviews. One was the Cochrane review that you had already found. One focuses on transcutaneous electrical nerve stimulation (TENS) for pain relief with labour. The third review is a systematic review of acupuncture for pelvic and back pain in pregnancy,[15] which appears to be exactly what you are after.

Note that during this search you try the Cochrane Database of Systematic Reviews and the relevant discipline-specific database (PEDro in this case) before trying the large electronic databases such as MEDLINE, as it is typically much more efficient to locate evidence about an intervention question in these databases than in the large electronic databases.

Clinical question about diagnosis

You are an occupational therapist who works in a community health centre. The team that you work in is putting together an initial assessment form for newly referred patients, and they wish to include some screening questions that will provide useful information to various members of the team. You are interested in including a brief cognitive screening test, such as the Mini-Mental State Examination (MMSE), as part of this initial assessment but wonder how accurate this test is at predicting cognitive impairment in older people who live in the community. Your question is:

> Does the MMSE accurately detect the presence of cognitive impairment in older community-living people?

After confirming that there is nothing available at the top three levels of the pyramid, you proceed to the fourth level of the pyramid (syntheses). You conduct a search in the Cochrane Database of Systematic Reviews, but no search results are returned. Since the Cochrane database only recently started adding diagnostic reviews, you are not surprised that no relevant reviews are retrieved.

You then search using PubMed Clinical Queries (with 'diagnosis' selected as the category and a narrow search chosen) with the terms:

> (MMSE OR Mini-Mental State Examination) AND (cognitive impairment) AND (older OR elder*)

This produces 109 hits, which you decide is too many to look through. You add the word 'community' to your search string and this produces 30 articles, three of which are exactly what you are after.[16–18]

Clinical question about prognosis

You are a recently graduated speech pathologist who has just commenced working in a stroke rehabilitation unit. One of your patients is 2 months post-stroke and has severe dysphagia (difficulty swallowing). His wife asks you how likely it is that his swallowing will get better in the next few months and that he will be able to return to eating a normal diet. As you are new to this area of clinical practice and have little clinical experience to guide your answer, you form the following clinical question:

> In adults with dysphagia following stroke, what is the likelihood of recovery within 6 months of the stroke?

You search using PubMed Clinical Queries (with prognosis selected as the clinical category and a narrow search chosen) with the terms:

> (dysphag* OR swallow*) AND (stroke OR CVA) and (recover*)

This produces 23 hits, two of which are exactly what you are after.[19,20]

Clinical question about patients' experiences and concerns

You are a dietitian working with children who are obese. The children are having a very difficult time losing weight. You wonder why it is that children who are obese often find it so difficult to lose weight when the lifestyle factors that contribute to the condition are so widely recognised. Your question is:

> What are the barriers to losing weight from the child's perspective?

This question would best be answered by a qualitative research design. Currently, qualitative studies are most likely found on the bottom layer of the pyramid: studies. You start your search using CINAHL (through EBSCOhost), as this can be a useful database to search when looking for qualitative research. You search using the search string:

> barrier* AND weight loss AND child*

choosing the 'TX All Text' searching field. You also limit the search by using the Clinical Queries feature of CINAHL and select 'qualitative—best balance' as you only want to retrieve qualitative articles.

Your search produces 11 hits, one of which is directly on target.[21] You notice that one of the other hits is also very relevant, but when you look at the abstract of it you realise that it is actually a synopsis[22] of the original article that has been published in *Evidence-Based Nursing*, which is a synopsis journal— located on the third and fifth layer of the pyramid (synopses of syntheses and synopses of studies). This is great news for you, as it means that this original article has been pre-appraised for you and considered to be clinically important and that the synopsis will also contain a clinical bottom line that has been written by a clinical expert in this field!

Another approach for this search would be to use PubMed, using the Health Services Research Queries feature (accessed by clicking on the 'Topic-Specific Queries' link on the main PubMed page followed by the 'Health Services Research [HSR] Queries' link) that was described earlier in this chapter. One of the categories for searching on this page is qualitative research. You choose this category and 'Narrow, specific search' for the scope, and enter the same search terms as we used above in CINAHL. The search retrieves 13 citations. The eleventh article on the list of search results is the same primary article[21] that you found using CINAHL.

SUMMARY POINTS OF THIS CHAPTER

- Using the PICO format to structure your clinical question makes choosing key search terms easier.
- Combining search terms using the Boolean operators (AND, OR) helps to narrow or broaden your search as required, and wildcard and truncation symbols are also useful.
- Organising your literature search using the '6S' pyramid is an effective and efficient approach to finding the best evidence.
- Where to start your search on the '6S' pyramid depends largely on the type of question that is being asked and what resources are available to you.
- Although many online evidence-based resources require a subscription, other exellent resources are readily available on the internet free of charge.
- Many clinical questions can be answered by searching online for the best evidence.

References

1. Ely J, Osheroff J, Ebell M, et al. Obstacles to answering doctor's questions about patient care with evidence: qualitative study. BMJ 2002;324:710–16.
2. DiCenso A, Bayley L, Haynes RB. Assessing preappraised evidence: fine-tuning the 5S model into a 6S model. Ann Intern Med 2009;151:JC3-2–3.
3. Roshanov P, Misra S, Gertein H, et al. Computerised clinical decision support systems for chronic disease management: a decision-maker–researcher partnership systematic review. Implement Sci 2011;6:92.
4. Sahota N, Lloyd R, Ramakrishna A, et al. Computerised clinical decision support systems for acute care management: a decision-maker–researcher partnership systematic review of effects of process of care and patient outcomes. Implement Sci 2011;6:91.
5. Nieuwlatt R, Connolly S, MacKay J, et al. Computerised clinical decision support systems for therapeutic drug monitoring and dosing: a decision-maker–researcher partnership systematic review. Implement Sci 2011;6:90.
6. Hemens BJ, Holbrook A, Tonkin M, et al. Computerised clinical decision support systems for drug prescribing and management: a decision-maker–researcher partnership systematic review. Implement Sci 2011;6:89.
7. Roshanov P, You J, Dhaliwal J, et al. Can computerised clinical decision support systems improve practitioners' diagnostic test ordering? A decision-maker–researcher partnership systematic review. Implement Sci 2011;6:88.
8. Souza N, Sebaldt R, Mackay J, et al. Computerised clinical decision support systems for primary preventive care: a decision-maker–researcher partnership systematic review of effects on process of care and patient outcomes. Implement Sci 2011;6:89.
9. Montori VM. Evidence-based endocrinology. Totowa, NJ: Humana Press; 2005.
10. Wong S, Wilczynski N, Haynes RB, et al. Developing optimal search strategies for detecting clinically relevant qualitative studies in MEDLINE. Medinfo 2004;11:311–16.
11. Wilczynski N, Marks S, Haynes RB. Search strategies for identifying qualitative studies in CINAHL. Qual Health Res 2007;17:705–10.
12. Walters L, Wilczynski N, Haynes RB, et al. Developing optimal search strategies for retrieving clinically relevant qualitative studies in EMBASE. Qual Health Res 2006;16:162–8.
13. McKibbon KA, Wilczynski N, Haynes RB. Developing optimal search strategies for retrieving qualitative studies in PsycINFO. Eval Health Prof 2006;29:440–54.
14. Pennick VE, Young G. Interventions for treating and preventing pelvic and back pain in pregnancy. Cochrane Database Syst Rev 2007;2:CD001139. doi: 10.1002/14651858. CD001139.pub2.
15. Ee C, Manheimer E, Pirotta M, et al. Acupuncture for pelvic and back pain in pregnancy: a systematic review. Am J Obstet Gynecol 2008;198:254–9.
16. Gagnon M, Letenneur L, Dartigues J, et al. Validity of the Mini-Mental State examination as a screening instrument for cognitive impairment and dementia in French elderly community residents. Neuroepidemiology 1990;9:143–50.
17. Loewenstein D, Barker W, Harwood D, et al. Utility of a modified Mini-Mental State Examination with extended delayed recall in screening for mild cognitive impairment and dementia among community dwelling elders. Int J Geriatr Psychiatry 2000;15:434–40.

18. Scazufca M, Almeida O, Vallada H, et al. Limitations of the Mini-Mental State Examination for screening dementia in a community with low socioeconomic status: results from the Sao Paulo Ageing & Health Study. Eur Arch Psychiatry Clin Neurosci 2009;259:8–15.
19. Mann G, Hankey G, Cameron D. Swallowing function after stroke: prognosis and prognostic factors at 6 months. Stroke 1999;30:744–8.
20. Han T, Paik N, Park J, et al. The prediction of persistent dysphagia beyond six months after stroke. Dysphagia 2008;23:59–64.
21. Murtagh J, Dixey R, Rudolf M. A qualitative investigation into the levers and barriers to weight loss in children: opinions of obese children. Arch Dis Child 2006;91:920–3.
22. Macdonald M. Clinically obese children identified facilitators and barriers to initiating and maintaining the behaviours required for weight loss. Evid Based Nurs 2007;10:92.

Chapter 4

Evidence about effects of interventions

Sally Bennett and Tammy Hoffmann

LEARNING OBJECTIVES

After reading this chapter, you should be able to:

- Understand more about study designs appropriate for answering questions about effects of interventions
- Generate a structured clinical question about an intervention for a clinical scenario
- Appraise the validity of randomised controlled trials
- Understand how to interpret the results from randomised controlled trials and calculate additional results (such as confidence intervals) where possible
- Describe how evidence about the effects of intervention can be used to inform practice

This chapter focuses on research that can inform us about the effects of interventions. Let us first consider a clinical scenario that will be useful for illustrating the concepts that are the focus of this chapter.

CLINICAL SCENARIO

You are working in a community health centre and, during a regular team meeting, the general practitioner notes that there are a large number of older people attending the clinic who have had multiple falls. He questions whether there is a need for the delivery of a preventative program for this group. A number of staff have similar concerns and decide to form a small group to look for research regarding the effectiveness of falls prevention programs. In your experience working with people who have a history of falling, you are aware that many of them have low confidence in their ability (this is also known as self-efficacy) to prevent themselves from falling. You are therefore particularly interested in finding evidence about the effectiveness of falls prevention programs that have looked at improving participants' self-efficacy as well as reducing the number of falls that they experience.

This clinical scenario raises several questions about the interventions that might be effective for reducing falls in people who are at risk of falling. Is balance and strength training effective in reducing the risk of falls? Does providing advice about how to modify a person's home to make it safer prevent falls in people who are at risk of falling? Which of these interventions is most effective, or are both combined more effective than one intervention alone? How cost-effective are multifactorial falls prevention education programs? These are questions that health professionals might ask when making decisions about which interventions will be most effective and will optimise outcomes for their patients.

As we saw in Chapter 1, clinical decisions are made by integrating information from the best available research evidence with information from our patients, the practice context and our clinical experience. Given that one of the most common information needs in clinical practice relates to questions about the effects of interventions, this chapter will begin by reviewing the role of the study design that is used to test intervention effects, before moving on to explaining the process of finding and appraising research evidence about the effects of interventions.

STUDY DESIGNS THAT CAN BE USED FOR ANSWERING QUESTIONS ABOUT THE EFFECTS OF INTERVENTIONS

There are many different study designs that can provide information about the effects of interventions. Some are more convincing than others in terms of the degree of bias that might be in play given the methods used in the study. From Chapter 2, you will recall that *bias* is any systematic error in collecting and interpreting data. In Chapter 2, we also introduced the concept of *hierarchies of evidence*. The higher up the hierarchy that a study design is positioned, in the ideal world, the more likely it is that the study design can minimise the impact of bias on the results of the study. That is why randomised controlled trials (sitting second from the top of the hierarchy of evidence for questions about the effects of interventions) are so commonly recommended as the study design that best controls for bias when testing the effectiveness of interventions. Systematic reviews of randomised controlled trials are located above them (at the top of the hierarchy), because these can combine the results of multiple randomised controlled trials. This can potentially provide an even clearer picture about the effectiveness of interventions, providing they are undertaken rigorously. Systematic reviews are explained in more detail in Chapter 12.

One of the best methods for limiting bias in studies that test the effects of interventions is to have a control group.[1] A control group is a group of participants in the study who should be as similar in as many ways as possible to the intervention group except that they do not receive the intervention being studied. Let us first have a look at studies that do not use control groups and identify some of the problems that can occur.

Studies that do not use control groups

Uncontrolled studies are studies where the researchers describe what happens when participants are provided with an intervention, but the intervention is not compared with other interventions. Examples of uncontrolled study designs are case reports, case series and before and after studies. These study designs were explained in Chapter 2. The big problem with uncontrolled studies is that when participants are given an intervention and simply followed for a period of time with no comparison against another group, it is impossible to tell how much (if any) of the observed change is due to the effect of the intervention itself or is due to some other factor or explanation. There are some alternative explanations for effects seen in uncontrolled studies, and these need to be kept in mind if you use this type of study to guide your clinical decision making. Some of the forms of bias that commonly occur in uncontrolled studies are described below.

- **Volunteer bias.** People who volunteer to participate in a study are usually systematically different from those who do not volunteer. They tend to be more motivated and concerned about their health. If this is not controlled for, it is possible that the results can make the intervention appear more favourable (that is, more effective) than it really is. This type of bias can be controlled for by randomly allocating participants, as we shall see later in this chapter.

- **Maturation.** A participant may change between the time of pre-test (that is, before the intervention is given) and post-test (after the intervention has finished) as a result of maturation. For example, consider that you wanted to measure the improvement in fine motor skills that children in grade 2 of school experienced as a result of a fine-motor-skill intervention program. If you test them again in grade 3, you will not know if the improvements that occurred in fine motor skills happened because of natural development (maturation) or because of the intervention.

- **Natural progression.** Many diseases and health conditions will naturally improve over time. Improvements that occur in participants may or may not be due to the intervention that was being studied. The participants may have improved on their own with time, not because of the intervention.

- **Regression to the mean.** This is a statistical trend that occurs in repeated non-random experiments, where participants' results tend to move progressively towards the mean of the behaviour/outcome that is being measured. This does not occur due to maturation or improvement over time, but due to the statistical likelihood of someone with high scores not doing as well when a test is repeated or of someone with low scores being statistically likely to do better when the test is repeated. Suppose, for example, that you used a behavioural test to assess 200 children who had attention deficit hyperactivity disorder and scored their risk of having poor academic outcomes, and that you then provided the 30 children who had the poorest scores with an intensive behavioural regimen and medication. Even if the interventions were not effective, you would still expect to observe some improvement in the children's scores on the behavioural test when it is next given, due to regression to the mean. When outliers are repeatedly measured, subsequent values are less likely to be outliers (that is, they are expected to be closer to the mean value of the whole group). This always happens, and health professionals who do not expect this to occur often attribute any improvement that is observed to the intervention. The best way to deal with the problem of regression to the mean is to randomly allocate participants to either an experimental group or a control group. The regression to the mean effect can only be accounted for by using a control group (which will have the same regression to the mean if the randomisation succeeded and the two groups are similar). How to determine this is explained later in this chapter.

- **Placebo effect.** This is a well-known type of bias where an improvement in the participants' condition occurs because they expect or believe that the intervention they are receiving will cause an improvement (even though, in reality, the intervention may not be effective at all).

- **Hawthorne effect.** This is a type of bias that can occur when participants experience improvements not because of the intervention that is being studied, but because of the attention that participants are receiving from being a part of the research process.

- **Rosenthal effect.** This occurs when participants perform better because they are expected to and, in a sense, this expectation has a similar sort of effect as a self-fulfilling prophecy.

Controlled studies

It should now be clear that having a control group which can be compared with the intervention group in a study is the best way of making sure that bias and extraneous factors that can influence the results of a study are limited. However, it is not as simple as just having a control group as part of the study. The way in which the control group is created can make an enormous difference to how well the study design actually controls for bias.

Non-randomised controlled studies

You will recall from the hierarchy of evidence about the effects of interventions (in Chapter 2) that case-control and cohort studies are located above uncontrolled study designs. This is because they make use of control groups. Cohort studies follow a cohort that has been exposed to a situation or intervention and have a comparison group of people who have not been exposed to the situation of interest (for example, they have not received any intervention). However, because cohort studies are observational studies, the allocation of participants to the intervention and control groups is not under the control of the researcher. It is not possible to tell whether the participants in the intervention and the control groups are similar in terms of all the important factors and, therefore, it is unclear to what extent the exposure (that is, the intervention) might be the reason for the outcome rather than some other factor.

We saw in Chapter 2 that a case-control study is one in which participants with a given disease (or health condition) in a given population (or a representative sample) are identified and are compared with a control group of participants who do not have that disease (or health condition). When a case-control study has been used to answer a question about the effect of an intervention, the 'cases' are participants who have been exposed to an intervention and the 'controls' are participants who have not. As with cohort studies, because this is an observational study design, the researcher cannot control the assembly of the groups under study (that is, which participants go into which group). Although the controls that are assembled may be similar in many ways to the 'cases', it is unlikely that they will be similar with respect to both known and unknown confounders. Chapter 2 explained that confounders are factors that can become confused with the factor of interest (in this case, the intervention that is being studied) and obscure the true results.

In a non-randomised experimental study, the researchers can control the assembly of both experimental and control groups, but the groups are not assembled using random allocation. In non-randomised studies, participants may choose which group they want to be in, or they may be assigned to a group by the researchers. For example, in a non-randomised experimental study that is evaluating the effectiveness of a particular public health intervention (such as an intervention that encourages walking to work) in a community setting, a researcher may assign one town to the experimental condition and another town to the control condition. The difficulty with this approach is that the people in these towns may be systematically different to each other and so confounding factors, rather than the intervention that is being trialled, may be the reason for any difference that is found between the groups at the end of the study.

So not only are control groups essential, but in order to make valid comparisons between groups they must also be as similar as possible at the beginning of a study. This is so that we can say, with some certainty, that any differences found between groups at the end of the study are likely to be due to the factor under study (that is, the intervention), rather than because of bias or confounding. To maximise the similarity between groups at the start of a study, researchers need to control for both known and unknown variables that might influence the results. The best way to achieve this is through randomisation. Non-randomised studies are inherently biased in favour of the intervention that is being studied, which can lead researchers to reach the wrong conclusion about the effectiveness of the intervention.[2]

Randomised controlled trials

The key feature of randomised controlled trials is that the participants are randomly allocated to either an intervention (experimental) group or a control group. The outcome of interest is measured in participants in both groups before (known as pre-test) and again after (known as post-test) the intervention has been provided. Therefore, any changes that appear in the intervention group pre-test to post-test, but not in the control group, can reasonably be attributed to the intervention. Figure 4.1 shows the basic design of a randomised controlled trial.

You may notice that we keep referring to how randomised controlled trials can be used to evaluate the effectiveness of an intervention. It is worth noting that they can also be used to evaluate the efficacy of an intervention. *Efficacy* refers to interventions that are tested in ideal circumstances, such as where intervention protocols are very carefully supervised and participant selection is very particular. *Effectiveness* is an evaluation of an intervention in circumstances that are more like real life, such as where there is a broader range of participants included and a typical clinical level of intervention protocol supervision. In this sense, effectiveness trials are more pragmatic in nature (that is, they are accommodating of typical practices) than are efficacy trials.

There are a number of variations on the basic randomised controlled trial design, which partly depend on the type or combination of control groups used. There are many variations on what the participants in a control group in a randomised controlled trial actually receive. For example, participants may receive no intervention of any kind (a 'no intervention' control), or they may receive a placebo, some form of social control or a comparison intervention. In some randomised controlled trials, there are more than two groups. For example, in one study there might be two intervention groups and one control group or, in another study, there might be an intervention group, a placebo group and a 'no intervention' group. Randomised crossover studies are a type of randomised controlled trial in which all participants

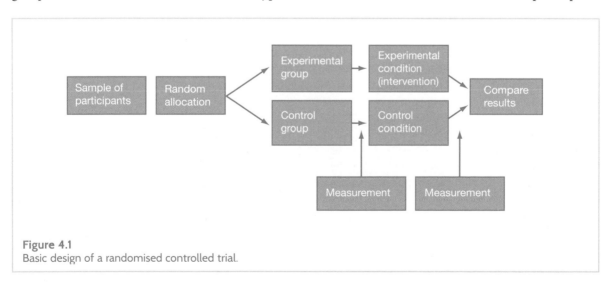

Figure 4.1
Basic design of a randomised controlled trial.

take part in both intervention and control groups, but in random order. For example, in a randomised crossover trial of transdermal fentanyl (a pain medication) and sustained-release oral morphine (another pain medication) for treating chronic non-cancer pain, participants were assigned to one of two intervention groups.[3] One group was randomised to four weeks of treatment with sustained-release oral morphine, followed by transdermal fentanyl for four weeks. The second group received the same treatments but in reverse order. A difficulty with crossover trials is that there needs to be a credible wash-out period. That is, the effects of the intervention provided in the first phase must no longer be evident prior to commencing the second phase. In the example we used here, the effect of oral morphine must be cleared prior to the fentanyl being provided.

As we have seen, the advantage of a randomised controlled trial is that any differences found between groups at the end of the study are likely to be due to the intervention rather than to extraneous factors. But the extent to which these differences can be attributed to the intervention is also dependent on some of the specific design features that were used in the trial, and these deserve close attention. The rest of this chapter will look at randomised controlled trials in more depth within the context of the clinical scenario that was presented at the beginning of this chapter. In this scenario you are a health professional who is working in a small group at a community health centre and you are looking for research regarding the effectiveness of falls prevention programs. To locate relevant research, you start by focusing on what it is that you specifically want to know about.

HOW TO STRUCTURE A QUESTION ABOUT THE EFFECT OF AN INTERVENTION

In Chapter 2, you learnt how to structure clinical questions using the PICO format: Patient/Problem/Population, Intervention/Issue, Comparison (if relevant) and Outcomes.

In our falls clinical scenario, the *population* that we are interested in is elderly people who live in the community who fall. We know from our clinical experience that people who have had falls in the past are at risk of falling again, so it makes sense to target our search for interventions aimed at people who are either 'at risk' of falling and/or have a history of falling.

The *intervention* that we think could most readily be delivered in our setting would be a falls prevention education group which targets multiple risk factors for falling and incorporates exercise. Are we interested in a *comparison* intervention? While we could compare the effectiveness of one type of intervention with another, for this scenario it is probably more useful to start by first thinking about whether the intervention is effective. To do this we would need to compare the intervention to either a placebo (a concept we will discuss later) or to usual care.

There are a number of *outcomes* that we could consider important for people who fall. The most obvious outcome of interest is a reduction in the number of falls. However, we could also look for interventions that consider the factors contributing to falls, such as balance problems or, in our scenario, a person's confidence (or self-efficacy) to undertake actions that will prevent them from falling.

CLINICAL SCENARIO (CONTINUED)
The question

While there are a number of questions about interventions that can be drawn from the scenario presented at the beginning of this chapter, you decide to form the following clinical question:

- In community-dwelling older people with a history of falling, are falls prevention group education and exercise programs effective in reducing falls and increasing self-efficacy compared with usual care?

HOW TO FIND EVIDENCE TO ANSWER QUESTIONS ABOUT THE EFFECTS OF AN INTERVENTION

Our clinical scenario question is a question about the effectiveness of an intervention to prevent falls and to improve self-efficacy. You can use the hierarchy of evidence for this type of question as your guide to know which type of study you are looking for and where to start searching. In this case, you are looking for a systematic review of randomised controlled trials. If there is no relevant systematic review, you should next look for a randomised controlled trial. If no relevant randomised controlled trials are available, you would then need to look for the next best available type of research, as indicated by the hierarchy of evidence for this question type shown in Chapter 2.

As we saw in Chapter 3, the best source of systematic reviews of randomised controlled trials is the Cochrane Database of Systematic Reviews, so this would be the logical place to start searching. The Cochrane Library also contains the Cochrane Central Register of Controlled Trials, which includes a large collection of citations of randomised controlled trials. If you are looking for randomised controlled trials specifically in the rehabilitation field, two other databases that you could consider searching for this topic are PEDro (www.pedro.org.au) or OTseeker (www.otseeker.com). These databases were explained in Chapter 3. One of their advantages is that they have already evaluated the risk of bias that might be of issue in the randomised controlled trials that they index.

Once you have found a research article that you are interested in, it is important to critically appraise it. That is, you need to examine the research closely to determine whether and how it might inform your clinical practice. As we saw in Chapter 1, to critically appraise research, there are three main aspects to consider: (1) its internal validity (in particular, the risk of bias); (2) its impact (the size and importance of any effect found); and (3) whether or how the evidence might be applicable to your patient or clinical practice.

CLINICAL SCENARIO (CONTINUED)
Finding evidence to answer your question

You search the Cochrane Database of Systematic Reviews, and there are three reviews concerning falls prevention.

One of these reviews evaluated the effect of interventions that were designed to reduce the incidence of falls in the elderly, but not just those who are community-living—it also included those in institutional care and hospital care. The second review focused on population-level interventions. The third review looks promising, as it focuses on falls prevention for community-living people. Although it reviewed over 100 studies, only a few were of groups which included both education and exercise.

You therefore decide to look at one of these studies in more detail (for the purpose of demonstrating how to appraise a randomised controlled trial in this chapter, we will choose just one to appraise).

The study you choose is a randomised controlled trial that has investigated the effectiveness of a program (called the 'Stepping On' program) for reducing the incidence of falls in the community-living elderly.[4] As you found this article indexed in a Cochrane review, it has also been evaluated with respect to risk of bias. You obtain the full text of the article in order to think about the effects of any bias more carefully, determine whether the trial measured self-efficacy as an outcome, specifically examine the results of the trial and determine whether the findings may be applicable to your clinical scenario.

CLINICAL SCENARIO (CONTINUED)

Structured abstract of our chosen article (the 'Stepping On' trial)

Citation: Clemson L, Cumming R, Kendig H, et al. The effectiveness of a community-based program for reducing the incidence of falls in the elderly: a randomised trial. J Am Geriatr Soc 2004; 52:1487–94. The structured abstract is adapted from this reference.

Design: Randomised controlled trial.

Setting: Community venues and follow-up home visits in New South Wales, Australia.

Participants: 310 community-living people aged 70 years and older (mean age 78.4 years, 74% female) with a history of falling in the past year or who were concerned about falling.

Intervention: A community-based small-group education program that aimed to help older people reduce falls and enhance their self-efficacy in fall-risk situations. Key content that was covered by the program included: lower limb balance and strength exercises, coping with visual impairment, medication management and home and community safety. One session also involved community mobility practice. A cognitive–behavioural approach was used, with practice and application of behaviours encouraged during and after groups. The program consisted of 2-hour group sessions (held weekly for 7 weeks), an individual home visit (held within 6 weeks of the last group session) and a 3-month group booster session. All intervention was provided by an experienced occupational therapist. Participants in the control group received one or two social home visits from a student.

Outcomes: The primary outcome measure was the occurrence of falls (for which a specific definition was used). There was also a range of secondary outcome measures used. Of particular interest to this clinical scenario, there were two self-efficacy outcome measures used. One was the Modified Falls Efficacy Scale, which assesses how confident a person is in their ability to avoid falls when performing basic activities of daily living. The other was the Mobility Efficacy Scale, which assesses how confident a person is in their ability to avoid falls when performing functional tasks that require a greater degree of postural challenge than the tasks assessed by the Modified Falls Efficacy Scale.

Follow-up period: Approximately 14 months (median 420 days).

Main results: The intervention group experienced a 31% reduction in falls relative to the control group.

Conclusion: Cognitive–behavioural learning in a small-group environment can reduce falls, and the Stepping On program is an option for effective falls prevention.

IS THIS EVIDENCE LIKELY TO BE BIASED?

In this chapter we will discuss six criteria that are commonly used for appraising the potential risk of bias in a randomised controlled trial. These six criteria are summarised in Box 4.1 and can be found in the *Users' guides to the medical literature*[5] and in many appraisal checklists such as the Critical Appraisal Skills Program (CASP) checklist and the PEDro scale.[6] A number of studies have demonstrated that estimates of treatment effects may be distorted in trials that do not adequately address these issues.[7,8] As you work through each of these criteria when appraising an article, it is important to consider the direction of the bias (that is, is it in favour of the intervention or the control group?) as well as its magnitude. As we pointed out in Chapter 1, all research has flaws. However, we do not just want to know what the flaws might be, but whether and how they might influence the results of a study.

BOX 4.1

Key questions to ask when appraising the validity (risk of bias) of a randomised controlled trial

1. Was the assignment of participants to groups randomised?
2. Was the allocation sequence concealed?
3. Were the groups similar at the baseline or start of the trial?
4. Were participants, health professionals and study personnel 'blind' to group allocation?
5. Were all participants who entered the trial properly accounted for at its conclusion, and how complete was follow-up?
6. Were participants analysed in the groups to which they were randomised using intention-to-treat analysis?

Was the assignment of participants to groups randomised?

Randomised controlled trials, by definition, randomise participants to either the experimental or the control condition. The basic principle of randomisation is that each participant has an equal chance of being assigned to any group, such that any difference between the groups at the beginning of the trial can be assumed to be due to chance. The main benefit of randomisation is related to the idea that, this way, both known and unknown participant characteristics should be evenly distributed between the intervention and control groups. Therefore, any differences between groups that are found at the end of the study are likely to be because of the intervention.[9]

Random allocation is best done using a random numbers table which can be computer-generated. Sometimes it is done by tossing a coin or 'pulling a number out of a hat'. Additionally, there are different randomisation designs that can be used and you should be aware of them. Researchers may choose to use some form of restriction, such as blocking or stratification, when allocating participants to groups in order to create a greater balance between the groups at baseline in known characteristics.[10] Different randomisation designs are summarised below.

- **Simple randomisation:** involves randomisation of individuals to the experimental or the control condition.
- **Cluster randomisation:** involves random allocation of intact *clusters* of individuals rather than individuals (for example, randomisation of schools, towns, clinics or general practices).
- **Stratified randomisation:** in this design, participants are matched and randomly allocated to groups. This method ensures that potentially confounding factors such as age, gender or disease severity are balanced between groups. For example, in a trial that involves people who have had a stroke, participants might be stratified according to their initial stroke severity as belonging to a 'mild', 'moderate' or 'severe' stratum. This way, when randomisation to study groups occurs researchers can ensure that, within each stratum, there are equal numbers of participants in the intervention and control groups.
- **Block randomisation:** in this design, participants who are similar are grouped into 'blocks' and are then assigned to the experimental or control conditions within each block. Block randomisation often uses stratification. An example of block randomisation can be seen in a randomised controlled study of a community-based parenting education intervention program designed to increase the use of preventive paediatric healthcare services among low-income, minority mothers.[11] Two hundred and eighty-six mother–infant dyads recruited from four different sites in Washington DC were assigned to either the standard social services (control) group or the intervention group. To ensure that there were comparable numbers within each group across the four sites, site-specific block randomisation

was used. By using block randomisation, selection bias due to demographic differences across the four sites was avoided.

CLINICAL SCENARIO (CONTINUED)

Was the assignment of participants to groups randomised?

In the Stepping On trial, it is explicitly stated that participants were randomised and that the randomisation was stratified in blocks of four, according to participants' gender and number of falls in the previous 12 months.

Was the allocation sequence concealed?

As we have seen, the big benefit of a randomised controlled trial over other study designs is the fact that participants are randomly allocated to the study groups. However, the benefits of randomisation can be undone if the allocation sequence is manipulated or interfered with in any way. As strange as this might seem, a health professional who wants their patient to receive the intervention being evaluated may swap their patient's group assignment so that their patient receives the intervention being studied. Similarly, if the person who recruits participants to a study knows which condition the participants are to be assigned to, this could influence their decision about whether or not to enrol them in the study. This is why assigning participants to study groups using alternation methods, such as every second person who comes into the clinic, or assigning participants by methods such as date of birth is problematic because the randomisation sequence is known to the people involved.[9]

Knowledge about which group a participant will be allocated to if they are recruited into a study can lead to the selective assignment of participants, and thus introduce bias into the trial. This knowledge can result in manipulation of either the sequence of groups that participants are to be allocated to or the sequence of participants to be enrolled. Either way, this is a problem. This problem can be dealt with by concealing the allocation sequence from the people who are responsible for enrolling patients into a trial or from those who assign participants to groups, until the moment of assignment.[12] Allocation can be concealed by having the randomisation sequence administered by someone who is 'off-site' or at a location away from where people are being enrolled into the study. Another way to conceal allocation is by having the group allocation placed in sealed, opaque envelopes. Opaque envelopes are used so that the group allocation cannot be seen if the envelope is held up to the light! The envelope is not to be opened until the patient has been enrolled into the trial (and is therefore now a participant in the study).

Hopefully, the article that you are appraising will clearly state that allocation was concealed, or that it was done by an independent or off-site person or that sealed opaque envelopes were used. Unfortunately, though, many studies do not give any indication about whether allocation was concealed,[13,14] so you are often left wondering about this, which is frustrating when you are trying to appraise a study. It is possible that some of these studies did use concealed allocation, but you cannot tell this from reading the article.

CLINICAL SCENARIO (CONTINUED)

Concealed allocation

In the Stepping On trial, allocation was concealed. The article states that the randomisation was conducted by a researcher who was not involved in participant screening or assessment.

Were the groups similar at the baseline or start of the trial?

One of the principal aims of randomisation is to ensure that the groups are similar at the start of the trial in all respects, except for whether they received the experimental condition (that is, the intervention of interest) or not. However, the use of randomisation does not guarantee that the groups will have similar known baseline characteristics. This is particularly the case if there is a small sample size. Authors of a research article will usually provide data in the article about the baseline characteristics of both groups. This allows readers to make up their own minds as to whether the balance between important prognostic factors (variables that have the potential for influencing outcomes) is sufficient at the start of the trial. Consider, for example, a study about the effectiveness of acupuncture for reducing pain from migraines compared with sham acupuncture. If the participants who were allocated to the acupuncture group had less severe or less chronic pain at the start of the study than the participants who were allocated to the sham acupuncture group, any differences in pain levels that were seen at the end of the study might be the result of that initial difference and not the acupuncture that was provided.

Differences between the groups that are present at baseline after randomisation have occurred due to chance and, therefore, determining whether these differences are statistically significant by using p values is not an appropriate way of assessing such differences.[15] That is, rather than using the p value that is often reported in studies, it is important to examine these differences by comparing means or proportions visually. The extent to which you might be concerned about a baseline difference between the groups depends on how large a difference it is and whether it is a key prognostic variable, both of which require some clinical judgment. The stronger the relationship between the characteristic and the outcome of interest, the more the differences between groups will weaken the strength of any inference about efficacy.[5] For example, consider a study that is investigating the effectiveness of group therapy in improving communication for people who have chronic aphasia following stroke compared with usual care. Typically, such a study would measure and report a wide range of variables at baseline (that is, prior to the intervention) such as participants' age, gender, education level, place of residence, time since stroke, severity of aphasia, side of stroke and so on. Some of these variables are more likely to influence communication outcomes than others. The key question to consider is: are any differences in key prognostic variables between the groups large enough that they may have influenced the outcome(s)? Hopefully, if differences are evident the researchers will have corrected for this in the data analysis process.

As a reader (and critical appraiser) of research articles, it is important that you are able to see data for key characteristics that may be of prognostic value in both groups. Many articles will present such data in a table, with the data for the intervention group presented in one column and the data for the control group in another. This enables you to easily compare how similar the groups are for these variables. As well as presenting baseline data about **key socio-demographic characteristics** (for example, age and gender), articles should *also* report data about important **measures of the severity of the condition** (if that is relevant to the study—most times it is) so that you can see whether the groups were also similar in this respect. For example, in a study that involves participants who have had a stroke, the article may present data about the initial stroke severity of participants, as this variable has the potential to influence how participants respond to an intervention. In most cases, socio-demographic variables alone are not sufficient to determine baseline similarity.

One other area of baseline data that articles should report is the **key outcome(s)** of the study (that is, the pre-test measurement(s)). Let us consider the example presented earlier of people receiving group communication treatment for aphasia to illustrate why this is important. Although such an article would typically provide information about socio-demographic variables and clinical variables (such as severity of aphasia, type of stroke and side of stroke), having information about participants' initial (that is, pre-test) scores on the communication outcome measure that the study used would be helpful for considering baseline similarity. This is because, logically, participants' pre-test scores on a communication measure are likely to be a key prognostic factor for the main outcome of the study, which is communication ability.

When appraising an article, if you do conclude that there are baseline differences between the groups that are likely to be big enough to be of concern, hopefully the researchers will have statistically adjusted for these in the analysis. If they have not, you will need to try to take this into account when interpreting the study.

CLINICAL SCENARIO (CONTINUED)
Baseline similarity

In the Stepping On trial, the baseline characteristics shown in Tables 1 and 2 of the article are similar between the study groups and include most of the likely confounders. The authors point out that there is a small difference (6% in the intervention group, 10% in the control group) in the number of participants with a previous hip fracture, but go on to report that there were no differences in the trial results when data were re-analysed after adjusting for history of hip fracture. The baseline scores of the outcome measures are also similar between the two groups.

Were participants, health professionals and study personnel 'blind' to group allocation?

People involved with a trial, whether they be the participants, the treating health professionals or the study personnel, usually have a belief or expectation about what effect the experimental condition will or will not have. This conscious or unconscious expectation can influence their behaviour, which in turn can affect the results of the study. This is particularly problematic if they know which condition (experimental or control) the participant is receiving. Blinding (also known as masking) is a technique that is used to prevent participants, health professionals and study personnel from knowing which group the participant was assigned to so that they will not be influenced by that knowledge.[10]

In many studies, it is difficult to achieve blinding. Blinding means more than just keeping the name of the intervention hidden. The experimental and control conditions need to be indistinguishable. This is because even if they are not informed about the nature of the experimental or control conditions (which, for ethical reasons, they usually are) when they sign informed consent forms, participants can often work out which group they are in. Whereas pharmaceutical trials can use placebo medication to prevent participants and health professionals from knowing who has received the active intervention, blinding of participants and the health professionals who are providing the intervention is very difficult (and often impossible) in many non-pharmaceutical trials. We will now look a little more closely at why it is important to blind participants, health professionals and study personnel to group allocation.

A **participant's** knowledge of their treatment status (that is, if they know whether they are receiving the intervention that is being evaluated or not) may consciously or unconsciously influence their performance during the intervention or their reporting of outcomes. For example, if a participant was keen to receive the intervention that was being studied and they were instead randomised to the control group, they may be disappointed and their feelings about this might be reflected in their outcome assessments, particularly if the outcomes being measured are subjective in nature (for example, pain, quality of life or satisfaction). Conversely, if a participant knows or suspects that they are in the intervention group, they may be more positive about their outcomes (such as exaggerating the level of improvement that they have experienced) when they report them, as they wish to be a 'polite patient' and are grateful for receiving the intervention.[16]

The **health professionals** who provide the intervention often have a view about the effectiveness of interventions, and this can influence the way they interact with the study participants and the way they deliver the intervention. This in turn can influence how committed they are to providing the intervention in a reliable and enthusiastic manner, affecting participants' compliance to the intervention and participants' responses on outcome measures. For example, if a health professional believes strongly in the value of the intervention that is being studied, they may be very enthusiastic and diligent in their delivery of the intervention, which may in turn influence how participants respond to this intervention. It is easy to see how a health professional's enthusiasm (or lack of) could influence outcomes. Obviously some interventions (such as medications) are not able to be influenced easily by the way in which they are provided, but for many other interventions (such as rehabilitation techniques provided by therapists), this can be an issue.

Study personnel who are responsible for measuring outcomes (the assessors) and who are aware of whether the participant is receiving the experimental or control condition may provide different interpretations of marginal findings or differential encouragement during performance tests, either of which can distort results. For example, if an assessor knows that a participant is in the intervention group, they might be a little more generous when scoring a participant's performance on a task than they would be if they thought that the participant was in the control group. Studies should aim to use blinded assessors to prevent measurement bias from occurring. This can be done by ensuring that the assessor who measures the outcomes at baseline and at follow-up is unaware of the participant's group assignment. Sometimes this is referred to as the use of an *independent assessor*. The more objective the outcome that is being assessed, the less critical this issue becomes. However, there are not many truly objective outcome measures, as even measures that appear to be reasonably objective (for example, measuring muscle strength manually or functional ability) have a subjective component and, as such, can be susceptible to measurement bias. Therefore, where it is at all possible, studies should try to ensure that the people who are assessing participants' outcomes are blinded. Ideally, studies should also check and report on the success of blinding assessors and, where this information is not provided, you may wish to reasonably speculate about whether or not the outcome assessor was actually blinded as claimed.

However, there is a common situation that occurs, particularly in many trials in which non-pharmaceutical interventions are being tested, that makes assessor blinding not possible to achieve. If the participant is aware of their group assignment, then the assessment cannot be considered to be blinded. For example, consider the outcome measure of pain that is assessed using a visual analogue scale. The participant has to complete the assessment themselves due to the subjective nature of the symptom experience. In this situation, the participant is really the assessor and, if the participant is not blind to which study group they are in, then the assessor is also not blind to group allocation. Research articles often state that the outcome assessors were blind to group allocation. Most articles measure more than one outcome and often a combination of objective and subjective outcome measures are used. So, while this statement may be true for objective outcomes, if the article involved outcomes that were assessed by participant self-report and the participants were not blinded, you cannot consider that these subjective outcomes were measured by a blinded assessor.

CLINICAL SCENARIO (CONTINUED)
Blinding

In the Stepping On trial, the primary outcome measure was the occurrence of falls and this was measured by participant self-report. Participants had to fill out a monthly postcard calendar, noting whether they did or did not fall on each day of the month, and post this to the researchers. Participants who reported falling received a telephone call to verify whether the fall met the definition of falling that was being used in the trial.

As the primary outcome measure was measured by participant self-report and participants were not blinded, technically the measurement of the primary outcome measure was not done by a blinded assessor. However, participant self-report is an appropriate, and widely used and accepted, measure of collecting data about falling in community-living people and there is not really any other feasible method that enables this type of data to be collected in a blinded manner.

All other outcome measures were assessed, at the 14-month follow-up assessment, by a research assistant who was blind to group allocation. Neither the participants nor the health professionals who provided the intervention were blind to group allocation. For this type of intervention, blinding is not possible for participants or those providing the intervention.

Were all participants who entered the trial properly accounted for at its conclusion, and how complete was follow-up?

In randomised controlled trials, it is common to have missing data at follow-up. There are many reasons why data may be missing. For example, some questionnaires may not have been fully completed by participants, some participants may have decided to leave the study or some participants may have moved house and cannot be located at the time of the follow-up assessment. How much of a problem this is for the study, with respect to the bias that is consequently introduced, depends on *why* participants left the study and *how many* left the study.

It is therefore helpful to know whether all the participants who entered the trial were properly accounted for. In other words, we want to know what happened to them. Could the reason that they dropped out of the study have affected the results? This may be the case, for example, if they left the study because the intervention was making them worse or causing adverse side effects. If this was the case, this might make the intervention look more effective than it really was. Did they leave the study simply because they changed jobs and moved away, or was the reason that they dropped out related to the study or to their health? For example, it may not be possible to obtain data from participants at follow-up measurement points because they became unwell, or maybe because they improved, and no longer wanted to participate. Hopefully, you can now see why it is important to know why there are missing data for some participants.

The more participants who are 'lost to follow-up', the more the trial may be at risk of bias because participants that leave the study are likely to have different prognoses from those who stay in the study. It has been suggested that 'readers can decide for themselves when the loss to follow-up is excessive by assuming, in positive trials (that is, trials that showed that the intervention was effective), that all participants lost from the treatment group did badly, and that all lost from the control group did well, and then recalculating the outcomes under these assumptions. If the conclusions of the trial do not change, then the loss to follow-up was not excessive. If the conclusions would change, the strength of inference is weakened (that is, less confidence can be placed in the study results)'.[5]

When large numbers of participants leave a study, the potential for bias is enhanced. Various authors suggest that *if more than 15–20% of participants leave the study* (with no data available for them), then the results should be considered with much greater caution.[16,17] Therefore, you are looking for a study to have a minimum follow-up rate of at least 80–85%. To calculate the loss to follow-up, you just need to divide the number of participants included in the analysis at the time point of interest (such as the 6-month follow-up) by the number of participants who were originally randomised into the study groups. This gives the percentage of participants who were followed up. In some articles it is straightforward to find the necessary data that you need to calculate this, particularly if the article has provided a flow diagram (see Figure 4.2). It is highly recommended that trials do this, and this is explained more

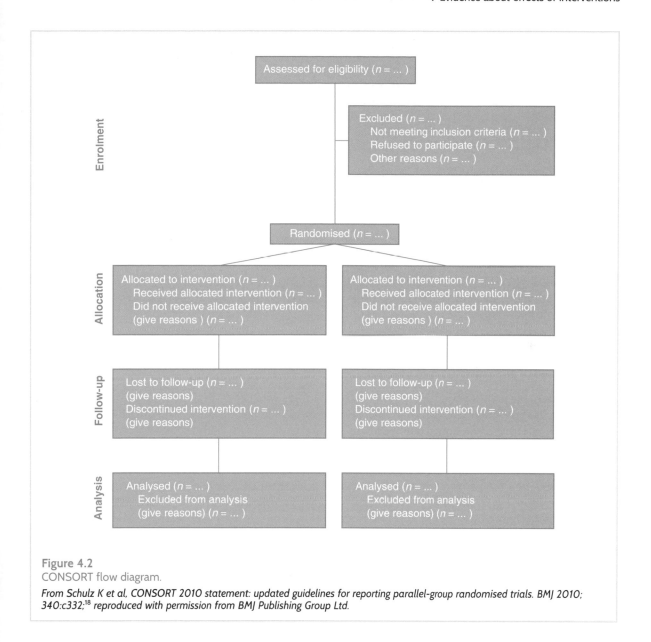

Figure 4.2
CONSORT flow diagram.

From Schulz K et al, CONSORT 2010 statement: updated guidelines for reporting parallel-group randomised trials. BMJ 2010; 340:c332;[18] *reproduced with permission from BMJ Publishing Group Ltd.*

fully later in the chapter when the recommended reporting of a randomised controlled trial is discussed. In other articles, this information can be obtained from the text, typically in the results section. In some articles, the only place to locate information about the number of participants who remain in the groups at a particular time point is from the column headers in a results table. And finally, in some articles, despite all of your best hunting efforts, there may be no information about the number of participants who were retained in the study. This may mean that there were no participants lost to follow-up (which is highly unlikely, as at least some participants are lost to follow-up in most studies) or the authors of the article did not report the loss of participants that occurred. Either way, as you cannot determine how complete the follow-up was, you should be suspicious of the study and consider the results to be potentially biased.

It is worth noting that where there is loss to follow-up in both the intervention and the control groups and the reasons for these losses are both *known* and *similar* between these groups, it is less likely that bias will be problematic.[19] When the reasons why participants leave the study are unknown, or when they are known to be different between the groups and potentially prognostically relevant, you should be more suspicious about the validity of the study. That is why it is important to consider the reasons for loss to follow-up and whether the number of participants lost to follow-up was approximately the same for both of the study groups, as well as the actual percentage of participants who were lost to follow-up.

> ### CLINICAL SCENARIO (CONTINUED)
> #### Follow-up of participants
>
> In the Stepping On trial, participants were followed from baseline to 14 months post-randomisation. The flow of participants through the trial is clearly provided in Figure 1 of the article. Loss to follow-up was minimal, with 8% of participants lost to follow-up before the 14-month assessment (therefore a 92% follow-up rate). Loss to follow-up for secondary outcome measures was higher (15.5%), but this is still around the 85% follow-up rate that is considered acceptable when evaluating a trial's internal validity.

Were participants analysed in the groups to which they were randomised using intention-to-treat analysis?

The final criterion for assessing risk of bias that we will address in this chapter is whether or not data from all participants were analysed in the groups to which participants were initially randomised, regardless of whether they ended up receiving the treatment. This analysis principle is referred to as *intention-to-treat analysis*. In other words, participants should be analysed in the group that corresponds to how they were *intended* to be treated, not how they were actually treated.

It is important that an intention-to-treat analysis is performed, because study participants may not always receive the intervention or control condition as it was allocated (that is, intended to be received). In general, participants may not receive the intervention (even though they were allocated to the intervention group) because they are either unwell or unmotivated, or for other reasons related to prognosis.[5] For example, in a study that is evaluating the effect of a medication, some participants in the intervention group may forget to take the medication and therefore do not actually receive the intervention as intended. In a study that is evaluating the effects of a home-based exercise program, some of the participants in the intervention group may not practise any of the exercises that are part of the intervention because they are not very motivated. Likewise, in a study that is evaluating a series of small-group education sessions for people who have had a heart attack, some participants in the intervention group may decide not to attend some or all education sessions because they feel unwell. From these examples, you can see that even though these participants were in the intervention group of these studies, they did not actually receive the intervention (either at all or only partly). It may be tempting for the researchers who are conducting these studies to analyse the data from these participants as if they were in the control group instead. However, doing this would increase the numbers in the control group who were either unmotivated or unwell. This would make the intervention appear more effective than it actually is because there would be a greater number of participants in the control group who were likely to have unfavourable outcomes. It may also be tempting for researchers to discard the results from participants who did not receive the intervention (or control condition) as was intended. This is also an unsuitable way of dealing with this issue, as these participants would then be considered as lost to follow-up and we saw in the previous criterion why it is important that as few participants as possible are lost to follow-up.

For the sake of completeness, it is important to point out that it is not only participants who are allocated to the intervention group but do not receive the intervention that we should think about. The opposite can also happen. Participants who are allocated to the control group can inadvertently end up receiving the intervention. Again, intention-to-treat analysis should be used and these participants should still be analysed as part of the control group.

The value of intention-to-treat analysis is that it preserves the value of randomisation. It helps to ensure that prognostic factors that we know about, and those that we do not know about, will still be, on average, equally distributed between the groups. Because of this, any effect that we see, such as improvement in participants' outcomes, is most likely to be because of the intervention rather than unrelated factors.

The difficulty in carrying out a true intention-to-treat analysis is that the data for *all* participants is needed. However, as we saw in the previous criterion about follow-up of participants, this is unrealistic to expect and most studies have missing data. There is currently no real agreement about the best way to deal with such missing data (probably because there is no ideal way), but researchers may sometimes estimate or impute data.[20] Data imputation is a statistical procedure that substitutes missing data in a data file with estimated data. Other studies may simply report that they have carried out an intention-to-treat analysis or that participants received the experimental or control conditions as allocated without providing details of what was actually done or how missing data were dealt with. In this case, as the reader of the article, you may choose to accept this at face value or to remain sceptical about how this issue was dealt with, depending on what other clues are available in the study report.

CLINICAL SCENARIO (CONTINUED)
Intention-to-treat analysis

In the Stepping On trial, it is stated that data were analysed using intention-to-treat; however, no details about how missing data were handled are provided.

The role of chance

So far in this chapter we have considered the potential for bias in randomised controlled trials. Another aspect that is important to consider is the possibility that the play of chance might be an alternative explanation for the findings. So, a further question that you may wish to consider when appraising a randomised controlled trial is: did the study report a power calculation that might indicate what sample size would be necessary for the study to detect an effect if the effect actually exists? As we saw in Chapter 2, having an adequate sample size is important so that the study can avoid a type II error occurring. You may remember that a type II error is the failure to find and report a relationship when a relationship actually exists.[21]

CLINICAL SCENARIO (CONTINUED)
Did the study have enough participants to minimise the play of chance?

In the Stepping On trial, 310 participants were recruited. A power calculation (with a power of 80% and an alpha of 5%) was performed, and it was estimated that 300 participants would be needed to detect a 40% relative reduction in fall rate. Therefore, it appears that an adequate number of participants were recruited into the trial.

COMPLETENESS OF REPORTING OF RANDOMISED CONTROLLED TRIALS

As we have seen in many places throughout this chapter, it can often be difficult for readers of research studies to know whether a study has or has not met some of the requirements to be considered a well-designed and well-conducted randomised controlled trial that is relatively free of bias. To help overcome this problem and aid in the critical appraisal and interpretation of trials, an evidence-based initiative known as the CONSORT (Consolidated Standards of Reporting Trials) statement[12,18] has been developed to guide authors in how to completely report the details of a randomised controlled trial. The CONSORT statement is considered an evolving document and, at the time of writing, it consisted of a 22-item checklist and a flow diagram (see Figure 4.2). Full details are available at www.consort-statement.org. The CONSORT statement is also used by reviewers of articles when the articles are being considered for publication, and many journals now insist that articles about randomised controlled trials follow the CONSORT statement. This is helping to improve the quality of reporting of trials but, as this is a recent requirement, many older articles do not contain all of the information that you need to know.

After determining that an article about the effects of an intervention that you have been appraising appears to be reasonably free of bias, you then proceed to looking at the importance of the results.

UNDERSTANDING RESULTS

One of the fundamental concepts that you need to keep in mind when trying to make sense of the results of a randomised controlled trial is that clinical trials provide us with an *estimate* of the *average* effects of an intervention. Not every participant in the intervention group of a randomised controlled trial is going to benefit from the intervention that is being studied—some may benefit a lot, some may benefit a little, some may experience no change and some may even be worse (a little or a lot) as a result of receiving the intervention. The results from all participants are combined and the *average* effect of the intervention is what is reported.

Before getting into the details about how to interpret the results of a randomised controlled trial, the first thing that you need to look at is whether you are dealing with continuous or dichotomous data:

- **Variables with continuous data** can take any value along a continuum within a defined range. Examples of continuous variables are age, range of motion in a joint, walking speed and score on a visual analogue scale.
- **Variables with dichotomous data** have only two possible values. For example, male/female, satisfied/not satisfied with treatment, and hip fracture/no hip fracture.

The way that you make sense of the results of a randomised controlled trial depends on whether you are dealing with outcomes that were continuous or dichotomous. We will look at continuous data first. However, regardless of whether the results of the study were measured using continuous or dichotomous outcomes, we will be looking at how to answer two main questions:

1. What is the **size** of the intervention effect?
2. What is the **precision** of the intervention effect?

Continuous outcomes—size of the intervention effect

When you are trying to work out how much of a difference the intervention made, you are trying to determine the size of the intervention effect. When you are dealing with continuous data, this is often quite a straightforward process.

> The best estimate for the size of the intervention effect is the **difference in means** (or medians if that is what is reported) **between the intervention and the control groups**.

Many articles will already have done this for you and will report the difference. In other articles, you will have to do this simple calculation yourself.

Let us consider an example. In a randomised controlled trial[22] that evaluated the efficacy of a self-management program for people with knee osteoarthritis in addition to usual care, compared with usual care, one of the main outcome measures was pain, which was measured using a 0–10 cm visual analogue scale with 0 representing 'no pain at all' and 10 representing 'the worst pain imaginable'. At the 3-month follow-up, the mean reduction in knee pain was 0.67 cm (standard deviation [SD] = 2.10) in the intervention group and 0.01 cm (SD = 2.00) in the control group. This difference was statistically significant ($p = 0.023$). You can calculate the intervention effect size (difference in mean change between the groups) as: 0.67 cm minus 0.01 cm = 0.66 cm.

Note that in this study, the authors reported the mean *improvement (reduction in pain) scores* at the 3-month follow-up (that is, the *change* in pain from baseline to the 3-month follow-up). Some studies report **change scores**; other studies report **end scores** (which are the scores at the end of the intervention period). Regardless of whether change scores or end scores are reported, the method of calculating the size of the intervention effect is the same. When dealing with change scores, it becomes the difference of the mean *change* between the intervention and control groups that you need.

Clinical significance

Once you know the size of the intervention effect, you need to decide whether this result is clinically significant. As we saw in Chapter 2, just because a study finds a statistically significant result it does not mean that the result is *clinically* significant. Deciding whether a result is clinically significant requires your judgment (and, ideally, your patient's, too) on whether the benefits of the intervention outweigh its costs. 'Costs' should be regarded in the broadest sense to be any inconveniences, discomforts or harms associated with the intervention, in addition to any monetary costs. To make decisions about clinical significance, it helps to determine what the smallest intervention effect is that you consider to be clinically worthwhile. Where possible, this decision is one which is reached in conjunction with the patient so that their preferences are considered.

To interpret the results of a study, the smallest clinically worthwhile difference (to warrant using a self-management program in addition to standard care) needs to be established. This might be decided directly by the health professional, by using guidelines established by research on the particular measure being used (if available), by consultation with the patient or by some combination of these approaches. Frequently, health professionals make a clinical judgment based on their experience with a particular measure and by discussion with the patient about their preferences in relation to the costs (including both financial costs and inconveniences) involved. Health professionals then need to consider how the smallest clinically worthwhile difference that was determined relates to the effect found in the study. This is handled in a number of different ways in the literature.

One of the earliest methods for deciding important differences using effect sizes was developed by Cohen.[23] Effect sizes (represented by the symbol *d*) were calculated by taking the difference between group average scores and dividing this by the average of the standard deviation for both groups. This effect size is then compared with ranges classified intuitively by Cohen: 0.2 being a small effect size, 0.5 a moderate effect size and 0.8 a large effect size. This general rule of thumb has consequently been used to determine whether a change or difference was important or not.

Norman and colleagues looked at effect sizes empirically (looking at a systematic review of 62 effect sizes from 38 studies of chronic disease that had calculated minimally important differences) and found that, in most circumstances, the smallest detectable difference was approximately half a standard deviation.[24] They thus recommend that, when no other information exists about the smallest clinically worthwhile difference, an intervention effect should be regarded as worthwhile if it exceeds half a standard deviation. However, the use of statistical standards for interpreting differences has been criticised because the between-patient variability, or number of standard deviation units, depends on the heterogeneity of the population (meaning whether the population is made up of different sorts of participants).[25]

A more direct approach is to simply compare the mean intervention effect with a nominated smallest clinically worthwhile difference. If the mean intervention effect lies below the smallest clinically worthwhile difference, we may consider it to be *not* clinically significant. For our knee osteoarthritis example, let us assume that in conjunction with our patient we nominate a 20% reduction of initial pain as the smallest difference that we would consider to be clinically worthwhile in order to add self-management to what the patient is already receiving. Our calculations show that a 20% reduction from the initial average pain of 4.05 cm experienced by participants in this study would be 0.8 cm. If the intervention has a greater effect than a 20% reduction in pain from baseline, we may consider that the benefits of it outweigh the costs and may therefore use it with our patient(s). In this study, the difference between groups in mean pain reduction (0.66 cm) is lower than 0.8 cm, so we might be tempted to conclude that the result may not be clinically significant for this patient.

An alternative approach that is sometimes used for considering the effect size relative to baseline values involves comparing the effect size to the scale range of the outcome measure. In this example we would simply compare the intervention effect size of 0.66 cm in relation to the overall possible score range of 0–10 cm, and see that this between-group difference is not very large and therefore conclude that the result is unlikely to be considered clinically significant.

Note, however, that as this is an *average* effect there may be some patients who do much better than this and, for them, the intervention is clinically significant. Of course, conversely, there may be some patients who do much worse. This depends on the distribution of changes that occur in the two groups. One way of dealing with this is to look for the proportion of patients in both groups who improved, stayed the same or got worse relative to the nominated smallest clinically worthwhile difference. However, these data are often elusive as they are often not reported in articles.

Another approach to determining clinical significance takes into account the uncertainty in measurement using the *confidence intervals* around the estimate. To understand this approach, we need to first look at confidence intervals in some detail.

Continuous outcomes–precision of the intervention effect

How are confidence intervals useful?

At the beginning of this results section we highlighted that the results of a study are only an *estimate* of the true effect of the intervention. The size of the intervention effect in a study approximates but **does not equal** the true size of the intervention effect in the population represented by the study sample. As each study only involves a small sample of participants (regardless of the actual sample size, it is still just a *sample* of all of the patients who meet the study's eligibility criteria and therefore is small in the grand scheme of things), the results of any study are just an estimate based on the sample of participants in that particular study. If we replicated the study with another sample of participants, we would (most likely) obtain a different estimate. As we saw in Chapter 2, the *true value* refers to the population value, not just the estimate of a value that has come from the sample of one study.

Confidence intervals are a way of describing how much uncertainty is associated with the estimate of the intervention effect (in other words, the precision or accuracy of the estimate). We saw in Chapter

2 how confidence intervals provide us with a range of values that the true value lies within. When dealing with 95% confidence intervals, what you are saying is that you are **95% certain that the true average intervention effect lies between the upper and the lower limits of the confidence interval**. In the knee osteoarthritis trial that we considered above, the 95% confidence interval for the difference of the mean change is 0.05 cm to 1.27 cm (see Box 4.2 for how this was calculated). So, we are 95% certain that the true average intervention effect (at 3 months follow-up) of the self-management program on knee pain in people with osteoarthritis lies between 0.05 cm and 1.27 cm.

How do I calculate a confidence interval?

Hopefully the study that you are appraising will have included confidence intervals with the results in the results section. Fortunately this is becoming increasingly common in research articles (probably because of the CONSORT statement and also growing awareness of the usefulness of confidence intervals). If not, you may be able to calculate the confidence interval if the study provides you with the right information to do so (see Box 4.2 for what you need). An easy way of calculating confidence intervals is to use an online calculator. There are plenty available, such as those found at

---

BOX 4.2

How to calculate the confidence interval (CI) for the difference between the means of two groups

A formula[26] that can be used is:

$$95\% \, CI \approx Difference + 3 \times SD/\sqrt{n_{av}}$$

where:

Difference = difference between the two means

SD = average of the two standard deviations

n_{av} = average of the group sizes

For the knee osteoarthritis study, Difference = 0.66; SD = (2.10 + 2.00) ÷ 2 = 2.05; and n_{av} = (95 + 107) ÷ 2 = 101.

Therefore:

$$95\% \, CI \approx 0.66 \pm 0.61$$
$$\approx 0.05 \, to \, 1.27$$

When you calculate confidence intervals yourself, they will vary slightly depending on whether you use this formula or an online calculator. This formula is an approximation of the complex equation that researchers use to calculate confidence intervals for their study results, but it is adequate for the purposes of health professionals who are considering using an intervention in clinical practice and wish to obtain information about the precision of the estimate of the intervention's effect.

Occasionally you might calculate a confidence interval that is at odds with the p value reported in the paper (that is, the confidence interval might indicate non-significance when in fact the p value in the paper is significant). This might occur because the test used by the researchers does not assume a normal distribution (as the 95% confidence interval does) or because the p value was close to 0.05 and the rough calculation of the confidence interval might end up including zero as it is a less precise calculation.

Note: if the study reports standard errors (SEs) instead of standard deviations, the formula to calculate the confidence interval is:

$$95\% \, CI = Difference \pm 3 \times SE$$

www.pedro.org.au/wp-content/uploads/CIcalculator.xls or www.graphpad.com/quickcalcs/index.cfm. If the internet is not handy, you can use a simple formula to calculate the confidence interval for the difference between the means of two groups. This is shown in Box 4.2.

Confidence intervals and statistical significance

Confidence intervals can also be used to determine whether a result is statistically significant. Consider a randomised controlled trial where two interventions were being evaluated and, at the end of the trial, it was found that, on average, participants in both groups improved by the same amount. If we were to calculate the size of the intervention effect for this trial it would be zero, as there would be no (0) difference between the means of the two groups. When referring to the difference between two groups with means, zero is considered a 'no effect' value. Therefore,

- if a confidence interval includes the 'no effect' value, the result is not statistically significant

and the opposite is also true:

- if the confidence interval does *not* include the 'no effect' value, the result *is* statistically significant.

In the knee osteoarthritis trial, we calculated the 95% confidence interval to be 0.05 cm to 1.27 cm. This interval does *not* include the 'no effect' value of zero, so we can therefore conclude that the result is statistically significant without needing to know the p value; although, in this case, the p value (0.023) was provided in the article and it also indicates a statistically significant result.

As an aside, if a result is *not* statistically significant, it is incorrect to refer to this as a 'negative' difference and imply that the study has shown no difference and conclude that the intervention was not effective. It has not done this at all. All that the study has shown is an absence of evidence of a difference.[27] A simple way to remember this is that non-significance does not mean no effect.

Confidence intervals and clinical significance

We now return to our previous discussion about clinical significance. Earlier we saw that there are a number of approaches that can be used to compare the effect estimate of a study to the smallest clinically worthwhile difference that is established by the health professional (and sometimes their patient as well). We will now explain a useful way of considering clinical significance that involves using confidence intervals to help make this decision.

Before we go on to explain the relationship between confidence intervals and clinical significance, you may find it easier to understand confidence intervals by viewing them on a **tree plot** (see Figure 4.3). A tree plot is a line along which varying intervention effects lie. The 'no effect' value is indicated in Figure 4.3 as the value 0. Effect estimates to the left of the no effect value may indicate harm. Also marked on Figure 4.3 is a dotted line that indicates the supposed smallest clinically worthwhile intervention effect. Anything to the left of this line but to the *right* of the no effect value estimate represents effects of the intervention that are too small to be worthwhile. On the contrary, anything to the right of this line indicates intervention effects that are clinically worthwhile.

In the situation where the **entire confidence interval is *below* the smallest clinically worthwhile effect**, this is a useful result. It is useful because at least we know with some certainty that the intervention is *not* likely to produce a clinically worthwhile effect. Similarly, when an **entire confidence interval is *above* the smallest clinically worthwhile effect**, this is a clear result, as we know with some certainty that the intervention is likely to produce a clinically worthwhile effect.

However, in the knee osteoarthritis trial, we calculated the 95% confidence interval to be 0.05 cm to 1.27 cm. The lower value is below 0.8 cm (20% of the initial pain level that we nominated as the smallest clinically worthwhile effect), but the upper value is above 0.8 cm. We can see this clearly if we

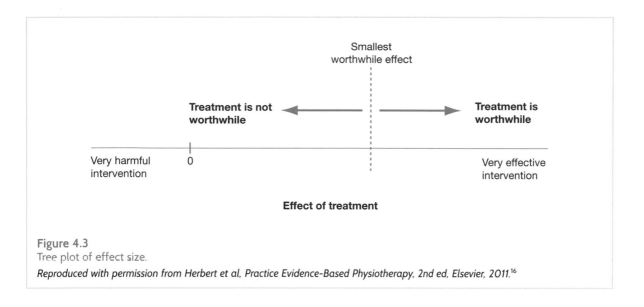

Figure 4.3
Tree plot of effect size.
Reproduced with permission from Herbert et al, Practice Evidence-Based Physiotherapy, 2nd ed, Elsevier, 2011.[16]

mark the confidence interval onto a tree plot (see Figure 4.4, tree plot A). This indicates that there is uncertainty about whether there is a clinically worthwhile effect occurring or not.

When the confidence interval *spans* the smallest clinically worthwhile effect, it is more difficult to interpret clinical significance. In this situation, the true effect of the intervention could lie either above the smallest clinically worthwhile effect or below it. In other words, there is a chance that the intervention may produce a clinically worthwhile effect, but there is also a chance that it may not. Another example of this is illustrated in tree plot B in Figure 4.4, using the data from a randomised controlled trial that investigated the efficacy of a guided self-management program for people with asthma compared with traditional asthma treatment.[28] One of the main outcome measures in this study was quality of life, which was measured using a section of the St George Respiratory Questionnaire. The total score for this outcome measure can range from −50 to +50, with positive scores indicating improvement and negative scores indicating deterioration in quality of life compared with one year ago. At the 12-month follow-up, the difference between the means of the two groups (that is, the intervention effect size) was 8 points (in favour of the self-management group), with a 95% confidence interval of 2 to 15. This difference was statistically significant ($p = 0.009$). Let us assume that we nominate a difference of 4 points to be the smallest clinically worthwhile effect for this example. In this example, the mean difference (8) is above what we have chosen as the smallest clinically worthwhile effect (4), but the confidence interval includes some values that are above the worthwhile effect and some values that are below it. If the true intervention effect was at the upper limit of the confidence interval (at 15), we would consider the intervention to be worthwhile, while if the true intervention effect was at the lower limit of the confidence interval (2), we may not. So, although we would probably conclude that the effect of this self-management intervention on quality of life was clinically significant, this conclusion would be made with a degree of uncertainty.

The situation of a confidence interval spanning the smallest clinically worthwhile effect is a common one, and there are two main reasons why it can occur. First, it can occur when a study has a small sample size and therefore low power. The concept of power was explained in Chapter 2. As we also saw in Chapter 2, the smaller the sample size of a study, the wider (that is, less precise) the confidence interval is, which makes it more likely that the confidence interval will span the worthwhile effect. Second, it can occur because many interventions only have fairly small intervention effects, meaning that their true effects are close to the smallest clinically worthwhile effect. As a consequence, they need to have very

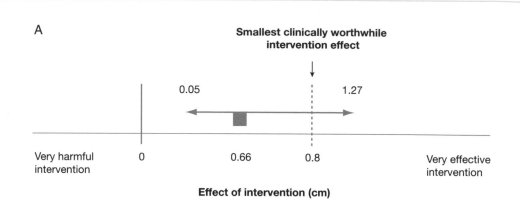

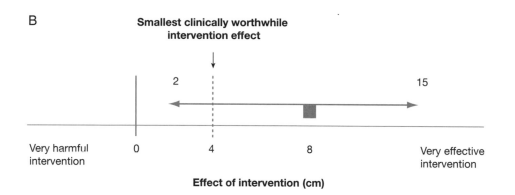

Figure 4.4
Tree plots showing the effect size, the smallest clinically worthwhile effect and the confidence interval associated with the effect size.

In tree plot A, the estimate of the intervention effect size (0.66 cm) sits below the smallest clinically worthwhile effect of 0.8 cm and the confidence interval (0.05 cm to 1.27 cm) spans the smallest clinically worthwhile effect of 0.8 cm. The estimate of the intervention effect size is indicated as a small square, the 95% confidence interval about this estimate is shown as a horizontal line and the dotted line indicates the supposed smallest clinically worthwhile intervention effect.

In tree plot B, the estimate of the intervention effect size (8) is above the smallest clinically worthwhile effect (4) and the confidence interval (2 to 15) spans the smallest clinically worthwhile effect.

narrow confidence intervals if the confidence interval is going to avoid spanning the smallest worthwhile effect.[16] As we just discussed, this typically means that a very large sample size is needed. In allied health studies in particular, this can be difficult to achieve.

There are two ways that you, as a health professional who is trying to decide whether to use an intervention with a patient, can deal with this uncertainty:[16]

- Accept the uncertainty and make your decision according to whether the difference between the group means is higher or lower than the smallest clinically worthwhile effect. However, keep the confidence interval in mind as it indicates the degree of doubt that you should have about this estimate.

- Try to increase the certainty by searching for similar studies and establishing whether the findings are replicated in other studies. This is one of the advantages of a systematic review, in particular a meta-analysis, as combining the results from multiple trials increases the sample size. The consequence of this is usually a more narrow (more precise) confidence interval which is less likely to span the smallest clinically worthwhile effect. Systematic reviews and meta-analyses are discussed in detail in Chapter 12.

CLINICAL SCENARIO (CONTINUED)

Main results–self-efficacy

In the Stepping On trial, the self-efficacy results are reported as change scores (follow-up score minus baseline score). For the Mobility Efficacy Scale, the mean difference (in the change score) between the two groups was 4.28 points (95% confidence interval = 8.40 to 0.54), which was statistically significant. Note that the confidence interval does not contain zero and therefore this result was statistically significant. We will assume for argument's sake that a 10% change in mobility efficacy would be considered clinically significant. A mean difference of 4.28 points compared with the initial average mobility efficacy baseline score of 66 points represents a change of only 6% (as $4.28/66 \times 100 = 6$). This mean difference in improvement of 4.28 (6% change) is smaller than the 10% we were hoping for, but for some patients it may still be clinically significant, depending on their values or preferences, as the confidence interval indicates that for some people the mean improvement achieved could be as high as 8.40 (or 12.7% change).

For the Modified Falls Efficacy Scale, the mean difference (in the change score) between the two groups was 1.74 (95% confidence interval = –6.14 to 2.67), which was not statistically significant. Note that the confidence interval does contain zero, as the result was not statistically significant. As the result for this outcome was not statistically significant, there is no need to consider the clinical significance of this result as we cannot be convinced that this result did not occur by chance.

Dichotomous outcomes–size of the treatment effect

Often the outcomes that are reported in a trial will be presented as dichotomous data. As we saw at the beginning of this results section, these are data for which there are only two possible values. It is worth being aware that data measured using a continuous scale can also be categorised, using a certain cut-off point on the scale, so that the data become dichotomised. For example, data on a 10-point visual analogue pain scale can be arbitrarily dichotomised around a cut-off point of 3 (or any point that the researchers choose), so that a pain score of 3 or less is categorised as mild pain and a score of above 3 is categorised as moderate/severe pain. By doing this, the researchers have converted continuous data into data that can be analysed as dichotomous data.

Health professionals and patients are often interested in *comparative* results—the outcome in one group relative to the outcome in the other group. This overall (comparative) consideration is one of risk. Before getting into the details, let us briefly review the concept of risk. *Risk* is simply the chance, or probability, of an event occurring. A probability can be described by numbers, ranging from 0 to 1, and is a proportion or ratio. Risks and probabilities are usually expressed as a decimal, such as 0.1667, which is the same as 16.67%. Risk can be expressed in various ways (but using the same data).[29] We will consider each of these in turn:

1. relative risk (or the flip side of this, which is referred to as relative benefit)
2. relative risk reduction (or relative benefit increase)
3. absolute risk reduction (or absolute benefit increase)
4. number needed to treat.

Risk and relative risk (or relative benefit)

Consider a hypothetical study that investigated the use of relaxation training to prevent the recurrence of migraines. The control group ($n = 100$) received no intervention and is compared with the intervention group ($n = 100$) who received the relaxation training. Suppose that at the end of the 1-month trial, 25 of the participants in the control group had had a migraine.

- The risk for recurrence of migraine in the control group can be calculated as 25/100, which can be expressed as 25%, or a risk of recurrence of 0.25. This is also known as the Control Event Rate (CER).
- If, in the relaxation group, only 5 participants had had a migraine, the risk of recurrence would be 5% (5/100) or 0.05. This is sometimes referred to as the experimental event rate (EER).

These data can be represented graphically, as in Figure 4.5.

We are interested in the comparison between groups. One way of doing this is to consider the **relative risk**—a ratio of the probability of the event occurring in the intervention group versus in the control group.[30] In other words, **relative risk is the risk or probability of the event in the intervention group divided by that in the control group**. The term *relative risk* is being increasingly replaced by use of the term *risk ratio*—this describes the same concept, but the term reflects that it is a ratio that is being referred to. In the migraine study, the relative risk (that is, the **risk ratio**) would be calculated by dividing the experimental event rate (EER) by the control event rate (CER):

$$0.05/0.25 = 0.20 \text{ (or 20\%)}$$

This can be expressed as: 'the risk of having a recurrence of migraine for those in the relaxation group is 20% of the risk in the control group'.

You may remember that when we were discussing continuous outcomes, the no effect value was zero (when referring to the difference between group means). When referring to relative risk, the no effect value (the value that indicates that there is no difference between groups) is 1. This is because if the risk is the same in both groups (for example, 0.25 in one group and 0.25 in the other group), there would be *no* difference and the relative risk (risk ratio) would be 0.25/0.25 = 1. Therefore, **a relative risk (risk ratio) of less than 1 indicates lower risk—that is, a benefit from the intervention**.[30]

If we are evaluating a study that aimed to improve an outcome (that is, make it more likely to occur) rather than reducing a risk, we might instead consider using the equivalent concept of

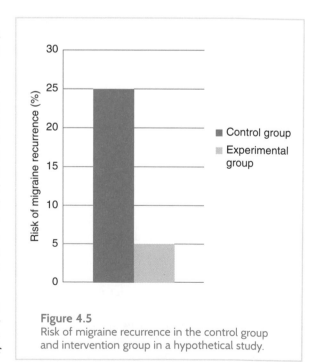

Figure 4.5
Risk of migraine recurrence in the control group and intervention group in a hypothetical study.

relative benefit. For example, in a study that evaluated the effectiveness of phonological training to increase reading accuracy among children with learning disabilities, we could calculate relative benefit as the study was about improving an outcome, not reducing the risk of it happening.

Sometimes a study will report an **odds ratio** instead of relative risk. It is similar, except that an odds ratio refers to a ratio of odds, rather than a ratio of risks. The odds ratio is the ratio of the odds of an event for those in the intervention group compared with the odds of an event in the control group. Odds are derived by dividing the event rate by the non-event rate for each group. The odds ratio is calculated by the following formula, where CER is the 'control event rate' and EER refers to the 'experimental event rate':

$$\text{Odds ratio (OR)} = [\text{EER}/(1 - \text{EER})] \div [\text{CER}/(1 - \text{CER})]$$

Also, some studies may report the intervention effect as a **hazard ratio**. This typically occurs when a survival analysis has been performed. A hazard ratio is broadly similar in concept to a risk ratio (relative risk) and so can be interpreted in a similar manner—that is, it describes how many times more (or less) likely a participant is to experience the event at a particular point in time if they were in the intervention group rather than the control group.

Relative risk reduction (or relative benefit increase)

Relative risk reduction is another way of expressing the difference between the two groups, and is simply the proportional reduction in an event of interest (for example, falls) in the intervention group compared with the control group, at a specified time point. Again, there is a flip side of this concept, which is known as relative benefit increase. When appraising an article and using this concept, you need to keep in mind whether you are considering negative or positive outcomes:

- Relative risk reduction (RRR) is used for expressing the reduction in risk of a negative outcome (such as falling).
- Relative benefit increase (RBI) is used for expressing an increase in the probability of a beneficial outcome (such as returning to work).

The formula that can be used for calculating relative risk reduction or relative benefit increase is:

$$(\text{CER} - \text{EER}) \div \text{CER} \times 100$$

Remember, we have said that the CER is the 'control event rate' and EER refers to the 'experimental event rate'.[29] The CER is simply the proportion of participants in the control group who experienced the event of interest. In our study of relaxation training to reduce migraines, this was 25% (or 0.25). Similarly, the EER is the proportion of participants in the intervention (experimental) group who experienced the event of interest. This was 5% (or 0.05) in the relaxation study.

Using our relaxation training study as an illustration, relative risk reduction can be calculated as: $(0.25 - 0.05) \div 0.25 = 0.80$. We could multiply this by 100 to get 80% and report that the relaxation training reduced the rate of migraines by 80%.

Alternatively, if you already know the relative risk, then the relative risk reduction can be calculated easily using the formula:

$$\text{RRR} = 1 - \text{RR}$$

In our example, where the relative risk (RR) is 0.20, the relative risk reduction is 0.80 or 80% (calculated as $1 - 0.20$).

The main difficulty in the use of relative risk reduction is that it does not reflect the baseline risk of the event.[31] This means that as a reader you are unable to discriminate between small intervention effects and large ones. **Baseline risk** has an important role to play. To understand this, you need to think about the risk in different populations. For example, in the general population the risk of migraine might be around 5–10% (depending on factors such as gender, age, and so on). Reducing the risk of migraine in a population that has a low risk to start with is very hard to achieve, and any risk reduction that is found would be fairly small (and as you will see in the next section, absolute risk reduction would be smaller still). However, in a population of people who commonly have migraines, the risk of recurrence is much higher and it would, therefore, be easier to achieve a larger relative risk reduction. Interventions that reduce the risk in populations who are at high risk of the event under consideration are likely to be clinically worthwhile.[32]

Another difficulty with the use of the relative risk reduction concept is that it can make results seem more impressive than they really are. Expressing the effects of an intervention in relative terms will result in larger percentages than when the same intervention is expressed in absolute terms. For example, suppose the use of a particular type of mattress reduced the risk of pressure sores from 0.05 to 0.025. In relative terms, the mattress reduces the risk by 50% (calculated by: 0.025 ÷ 0.05 = 0.5 or 50%), while in absolute terms it reduces the risk by 2.5% (calculated by: 0.05 – 0.025 = 0.025 or 2.5%). Similarly, in the hypothetical trial on relaxation training for reducing recurrence of migraines the *relative* risk reduction seems an impressive 80% but, as we will see later, the *absolute* difference in the rate of events between groups is only 20%. So we can see that the concept of relative risk reduction can inflate the appearance of intervention effectiveness.

You should also be aware that two studies might have the same relative risk reduction but there may be a large difference in the absolute risk reduction. As we saw in the example above about reducing the risk of pressure sores by using a particular type of mattress, a reduction in risk from 0.05 to 0.025 reduces the relative risk by 50%, while in absolute terms it reduces the risk by 2.5%. Let us say that another study found that the risk of pressure sores in a very-high-risk group of people was reduced from 0.8 to 0.4 because of the intervention (the mattress). In relative terms, although the mattress reduced the relative risk by 50% (calculated by: 0.8 ÷ 0.4 = 0.5 or 50%), the absolute risk reduction is 40%, which is a more clinically valuable result than the absolute risk reduction of 2.5% that the first study found.

Absolute risk reduction (or absolute benefit increase)

Another way of presenting information about dichotomous outcomes is by referring to the absolute risk reduction. The *absolute risk reduction* is simply the absolute arithmetic difference in event rates between the experimental (intervention) and the control groups.[33] This is shown graphically in Figure 4.6. Absolute values are simply the value of a number, regardless of its sign (positive or negative sign). The notation used for absolute values is vertical bars either side of the value, for example: |x|. The absolute arithmetic difference for risk reduction is calculated as: |EER – CER|. As with the previous methods of calculating risk that we

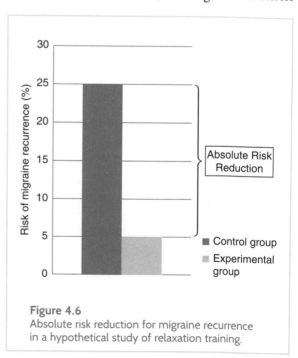

Figure 4.6
Absolute risk reduction for migraine recurrence in a hypothetical study of relaxation training.

have explained, there is a flip side to this concept. This is known as *absolute benefit increase* and is used when referring to a beneficial outcome (such as being discharged home instead of discharged to residential care).

In our hypothetical relaxation study for reducing recurrence of migraine, the absolute risk reduction would be 25% – 5% = 20%. This could be expressed as: 'the absolute risk of having a migraine recurrence was 20% less in the people who were in the relaxation group compared with those in the control group'.

A big absolute risk reduction indicates that the intervention is very effective, but how big is big enough to be considered clinically significant? A more meaningful measure, known as number needed to treat, can be used instead.

Number needed to treat

We saw that the absolute risk reduction of having migraine recurrence in the relaxation study was calculated as 20%, but is this clinically worthwhile? Number needed to treat (NNT) is a method of making the magnitude of the absolute risk reduction more explicit and is a more clinically useful concept.[30] The number needed to treat is simply the inverse of absolute risk reduction,[34] and is calculated as:

$$1 \div (EER - CER)$$

It tells you the number of people who would need to be treated to achieve the event of interest once. In the trial of relaxation training for preventing migraine recurrence, the number needed to treat is $1 \div (0.25 - 0.05) = 5$. So, in this example, you would have to treat 5 people for 1 month with the hypothetical relaxation intervention to prevent *one* (extra) person from having a recurrence of migraine (when compared with the control group). Obviously, a smaller number needed to treat is better than a large one. An intervention that has a smaller number needed to treat is more effective than an intervention that has a larger number needed to treat.

This concept of number needed to treat makes it easier to consider clinical significance, as you can more easily weigh up the benefits of preventing the event in one person against the costs and risks of providing the intervention. The size of the smallest clinically worthwhile effect (that is, the smallest worthwhile number needed to treat) will then depend on the seriousness of the event and the costs and risks of the intervention.

Another handy feature when using number needed to treat is that you can compare two different interventions (that are trying to achieve the same outcome) that have the same number needed to treat but have other features that are different. For example, one of the interventions may have a shorter intervention time and/or result in fewer side effects and/or be more convenient to patients and/or be less expensive. It is important to consider features such as these that a particular intervention has when making a decision about which intervention to use with a patient.

Applying results to your clinical situation

Most health professionals find it difficult to translate the results from studies to individual patients or to specific clinical situations, as studies usually only tell us about the *average* effects of the intervention. Further, the participants who took part in the study may be different to the patients that we see, and the intervention may differ to the intervention that we use. However, as a rough guide, if your patient is 'healthier' or the situation that you are considering is more optimistic than that in the study, the number needed to treat would be lower, the relative benefit increase would be higher, the mean difference would be larger, and so on. If, however, your patient is 'worse off' or the situation that you are considering is worse than that in the study, the number needed to treat would be higher, the relative benefit increase would be lower, the mean difference would be smaller, and so on. A solution to applying the results of a trial to patients with higher or lower levels of risk has been described by Straus and Sackett[35] and you may wish to read their article to learn more about this.

Dichotomous outcomes–precision of the treatment effect

Confidence intervals are also important to consider when examining dichotomous outcomes as, again, they indicate how much uncertainty is associated with the estimate of the intervention effect (in other words, the precision or accuracy of the estimate). The principles of confidence intervals associated with dichotomous data are similar to those for continuous data, but there is one very important difference to consider—what is the appropriate no effect value to use?

- For effect size estimates where **subtraction is involved**, such as mean differences (for continuous outcomes) and absolute risk reductions, the **no effect value is 0**.
- For effect sizes that involve **division**, such as risk ratios and odds ratios, the **no effect value is 1**.

Therefore, you can see that it is important to consider the *type* of effect measure you are interpreting in order to reliably interpret the confidence interval. The same general principle applies, though—a 95% confidence interval that does *not* include the no effect value indicates that the result is statistically significant. Table 4.1 presents a summary of the dichotomous effect measures, including what the no effect value is, that have been discussed in this section of the chapter.

As we could do with continuous outcomes, if the confidence interval has not been provided by the authors of the article it can be possible to calculate an approximate confidence interval. This is illustrated

TABLE 4.1: SUMMARY OF DICHOTOMOUS EFFECT MEASURES			
Type of measure	Definition	Formula	No effect value
Relative risk (RR) (also called risk ratio)	The ratio of the probability of the event occurring in the intervention group versus the control group. Expressed as either a decimal proportion or a percentage.	The risk of an event in the intervention group divided by the risk in the control group: EER ÷ CER	1
Relative risk reduction (RRR)	The proportion of the risk that is removed by the intervention. That is, the proportional reduction in an event of interest in the intervention group compared with the control group. Usually expressed as a percentage.	(CER – EER) ÷ CER x 100 *or* 1 – RR	0
Absolute risk reduction (ARR)	The absolute arithmetic difference in event rates between the experimental (intervention) and control groups. Usually expressed as a percentage.	|EER – CER|	0
Number needed to treat (NNT)	The number of people that would need to be treated for the event of interest to occur in 1 person.	1 ÷ ARR *or* 1 ÷ (EER – CER)	Infinity. Refer to article by Altman[36] for an explanation of why this is so.
Odds ratio (OR)	The odds of an event in the intervention group divided by the odds of an event in the control group. Usually expressed as a decimal proportion.	[EER/(1 – EER)] ÷ [CER/(1 – CER)]	1
CER = control event rate; EER = experimental event rate.			

BOX 4.3

How to calculate the confidence interval (CI) for absolute risk reduction

A formula[32] that can be used is:

$$95\% \text{ CI} \approx \text{Difference in risk} \pm 1/\sqrt{n_{av}}$$

where n_{av} = average of the group sizes.

For our study of relaxation training, the 95% confidence interval for the absolute risk reduction would be:

$$\approx (30\% - 5\%) \pm 1/\sqrt{100}$$

$$\approx 25\% \pm 0.1$$

$$\approx 25\% \pm 10\%$$

This tells us that the best estimate of the absolute risk reduction achieved from the relaxation training is 35% and that the 95% confidence interval extends from 15% to 35%.

in Box 4.3. Again, a simplified version of the more complex equation is used, but the confidence interval that is calculated is sufficient for use by health professionals who wish to use the information to assist in clinical decision making. Once you know the confidence interval for the absolute risk reduction, if you wish you could plot it, the effect estimate and the smallest clinically worthwhile effect on a tree plot in the same way that we did for continuous outcomes in Figure 4.4.

Calculating the confidence intervals for number needed to treat is fairly straightforward, as you just use the inverse of the numbers in the confidence interval of the absolute risk reduction.[30] However, understanding how to interpret the confidence intervals for number needed to treat can be complicated, and the article by Altman[36] is recommended to understand this in detail.

CLINICAL SCENARIO (CONTINUED)
Main results–falls

In the Stepping On trial, the **relative risk** (or **risk ratio**) was 0.69 (95% confidence interval = 0.50 to 0.96). As the relative risk is less than 1, it indicates that the intervention decreased the ratio of the risk (event rate) in the intervention group compared with the control group. Also note that the confidence interval does not extend across 1, indicating that this result was statistically significant.

The **relative risk reduction** was 31% (that is, the intervention group experienced a 31% reduction in falls relative to the control group). Unfortunately, no raw data (such as the number of events in each group) are reported in the article to enable calculation of the number needed to treat. It has been suggested in the literature that, for a falls intervention to be considered clinically significant, a reduction of at least 30% in the falls rate should be achieved.[37,38] This was achieved in this trial; therefore, the results can be considered clinically significant.

When making sense of the results of a randomised controlled trial, one further issue that you should be aware of is that trials usually report results from many different outcomes. With so much information to process it may be helpful, in some cases, for you to focus your attention on the main outcome(s) of the trial, the outcome(s) of interest to the question that you initially formed and/or the outcome that is of interest to your patient. If you have got to this point and determined that the article that you have been appraising not only appears to be reasonably free of bias but also contains some clinically important results, you then proceed to look at whether you can apply the results from the study to your patient or clinical situation. This is the third and final step of the critical appraisal process that we described in Chapter 1.

HOW CAN WE USE THIS EVIDENCE TO INFORM PRACTICE?

If you have decided that the validity of the study you are appraising is adequate and that the results are clinically important, the final step of the critical appraisal process is to consider the application of this information to the clinical situation that prompted your original clinical question. To do this, there are a few important questions which should be considered:

- Do the results apply to your patient or situation?
- Do the benefits found outweigh any harm, costs and/or inconveniences that are involved with the intervention?
- What other factors might need to be considered when applying this evidence?

Do the results apply to your patient or situation?

When considering whether the results apply to your patient or situation, you essentially need to assess whether your patient is so different from the participants in the study that you cannot apply the results of the study that you have been reading to your patient or situation. So, rather than just thinking about the study's eligibility criteria with respect to your patient, are the differences problematic enough that the results should not be applied? Further to this, results can sometimes be individualised to a particular patient by considering the individual benefit and harm for that patient. There is some complexity involved in doing so, which is beyond the scope of this book. If you wish to learn about this further, you are advised to read the article by Glasziou and Irwig[39] to understand how this may be done.

Do the benefits found outweigh any harm, costs and/or inconveniences that are involved with the intervention?

Understanding whether benefits outweigh harms or costs requires using information about benefits that is given in terms of the size of the intervention effect (e.g. mean differences, relative risk reduction, number needed to treat) and comparing this against possible harms or even inconveniences. When information about harm and cost is provided in the article, this is relatively straightforward. However, this type of information is often not provided and some estimate of the costs associated with the intervention might need to be made. Information about harm is obviously more difficult to estimate, and other sources might need to be consulted to get a sense of the potential harms involved. This is a grey area of practice in which clinical experience and discussion with patients about their preferences and values become very important.

What other factors might need to be considered when applying this evidence?

A further important question to consider is: what other factors might need to be considered when applying this evidence? When you are thinking about what other factors affect the delivery of an intervention, there are a few key questions that you can ask, such as:

- How much does it cost?
- How many sessions might be involved or how long would the patient need to stay in hospital?
- How far would the patient (or the health professional) need to travel?

- Are the resources (for example, any equipment that is needed) available to deliver the intervention?
- Do you or other health professionals working with you have the skills to provide the intervention?

A central component of applying research evidence to your patient is discussing the information with them. The success of many interventions is dependent on the health professional successfully providing the patient with appropriate information.

Involving the patient in the decision-making process is important, and this is discussed further in Chapter 14. In Chapter 1 we emphasised the need for integrating information from patients, clinical experience, research and the practice context. To do so is the art of evidence-based practice. Integrating so many pieces of information from many different sources is certainly an art form and one that requires clinical reasoning and judgment. The roles of clinical reasoning and judgment are discussed further in Chapter 15.

CLINICAL SCENARIO (CONTINUED)
Using the evidence to inform practice

So what can we conclude from our reading of the article about the Stepping On trial? You know, as a health professional, that falls are a major cause of accidental injury and death in the elderly, that they are costly in terms of loss of function and quality of life at both the individual and the community level, and that preventing falls is an important issue. In summary, the trial that evaluated the Stepping On program[4] was a well-constructed trial of a multifaceted educational and behavioural intervention for falls prevention. However, the trial design was unable to achieve blinding of participants, health professionals or study personnel, which leads you, as the reader, to be a bit cautious of results reported. For example, the falls data were collected by participant self-report which would not only be subject to error but also to differential bias (that is, there could be systematic differences in the self-reports of people in the intervention compared with those in the control group due to their knowledge about which group they were in). Participants in the intervention group received an individual home visit and a 3-month group booster session, whereas participants in the control group did not. This makes you wonder what part the attention (that intervention group participants received) might have played in influencing outcomes.

The intervention group experienced a 31% reduction in falls with sustained effect at 14 months and we could consider a result of this size to be clinically significant. Although the mean difference of 4.28 (95% confidence interval = –8.40 to –0.54) on the Mobility Efficacy Scale was statistically significant, you consider its clinical significance to be uncertain. However, participants' outcomes on the Modified Falls Efficacy Scale, which is an outcome that you were particularly interested in, were not statistically significant. As the reader of this article you need to contemplate how the biases present in this study might have affected these results. You then also need to consider how to apply these results in your situation.

DO THE RESULTS APPLY TO OUR PATIENT OR SITUATION?
The group of people that we were concerned about were community-living elderly people who had had multiple falls. The study that we looked at involved community-living men and women aged 70 years and older who had fallen in the previous year or were concerned about falling, but were not housebound and did not have cognitive impairment. It is likely that these results do apply to the group of people that we are concerned about; however, we would need to be aware that the results may not be as relevant for people who have cognitive impairment.

ARE THE BENEFITS WORTH THE HARMS AND COSTS?

There are no real 'harms' associated with this intervention. No details about costs of the intervention are provided in the article, but we do know that the intervention involved a group program (with approximately 12 participants per group) and a total of 15.5 hours of intervention. A very general idea of costs can be determined from this information. For individual patients, the 'cost' to them can be thought about in terms of the time commitment and travel involved in attending seven community-based sessions. Unfortunately data were not provided which enabled a number needed to treat to be calculated, which could have been valuable in helping us to interpret whether the benefits are worth the costs.

OTHER FACTORS TO CONSIDER

Other practical factors to consider are the availability of this type of comprehensive program in your clinical vicinity or, if you were to run it at the community health centre, the resources (such as staffing and space) and costs that would be involved. Data about the cost-effectiveness of this study would be valuable to further facilitate your team's decision making about whether to implement this intervention or not.

SUMMARY POINTS OF THIS CHAPTER

- The effects of intervention are best determined through rigorous randomised controlled trials (or better still, systematic reviews of randomised controlled trials), as their methods best reduce the risk of bias.
- Most randomised controlled trials are not free from bias. Key questions that should be asked when appraising the risk of bias in a randomised control trial are:
  - How were participants randomised to groups?
  - Was the allocation sequence concealed?
  - Were the groups similar at baseline?
  - Were participants, health professionals and study personnel blind to group allocation?
  - Was follow-up adequate?
  - Was intention-to-treat analysis used?
- Our understanding of the degree of bias that is present in a study is affected not just by the methods that the researchers used, but also by how well these are reported in the article that describes the study.
- Two factors to consider when making sense of the results of a randomised controlled trial are:
  - the size or magnitude of the intervention effect (this may be provided as continuous data or dichotomous data); and
  - the precision of the intervention effect (which can best be determined by inspecting the confidence interval for the intervention effect).
- Applying the results of the study requires thinking through whether the results apply to your patient or situation, whether benefits outweigh any harm, costs or inconveniences and a range of logistical factors that can affect the delivery of the intervention.

References

1. Portney L, Watkins M. Foundations of clinical research: applications to practice. Upper Saddle River, NJ: Prentice Hall Health; 2000.

2. Deeks J, Dinnes J, D'Amico R, et al. Evaluating non-randomised intervention studies. Health Technol Assess 2003;7:1–186.

3. Allan L, Hays H, Jensen N, et al. Randomised crossover trial of transdermal fentanyl and sustained release oral morphine for treating chronic non-cancer pain. BMJ 2001;322:1154–8.

4. Clemson L, Cumming R, Kendig H, et al. The effectiveness of a community-based program for reducing the incidence of falls in the elderly: a randomised trial. J Am Geriatr Soc 2004;52:1487–94.

5. Guyatt GH, Sackett DL, Cook DJ. Users' guides to the medical literature. II. How to use an article about therapy or prevention. JAMA 1993;270:2598–601.

6. Maher C, Sherrington C, Herbert R, et al. Reliability of the PEDro scale for rating quality of randomised controlled trials. Phys Ther 2003;83:713–21.

7. Shulz K, Chalmers I, Hayes R, et al. Empirical evidence of bias: dimensions of methodological quality associated with estimates of treatment effects in controlled trials. JAMA 1995;273:408–12.

8. Kunz R, Vist G, Oxman A. Randomisation to protect against selection bias in healthcare trials. Cochrane Database Syst Rev 2007;(2):MR000012. doi: 10.1002/14651858.MR000012.pub2.

9. Altman DG, Bland JM. Treatment allocation in controlled trials: why randomise? BMJ 1999;318:1209.

10. Hewitt C, Torgerson D. Is restricted randomisation necessary? BMJ 2006;332:1506–8.

11. El-Mohandes A, Katz K, El-Khorazaty M, et al. The effect of a parenting education program on the use of preventive paediatric health care services among low-income, minority mothers: a randomised, controlled study. Pediatrics 2003;111:1324–32.

12. Altman D, Schulz K, Moher D, et al. The revised CONSORT statement for reporting randomised trials: explanation and elaboration. Ann Intern Med 2001;134:663–94.

13. Pildal J, Chan AW, Hróbjartsson A, et al. Comparison of descriptions of allocation concealment in trial protocols and the published reports: cohort study. BMJ 2005;330:1049–54.

14. Bennett S, McKenna K, McCluskey A, et al. Evidence for occupational therapy interventions: status of effectiveness research indexed in the OTseeker database. Br J Occup Ther 2007;70:426–30.

15. Roberts C, Torgerson D. Understanding controlled trials: baseline imbalance in randomised controlled trials. BMJ 1999;319:185.

16. Herbert R, Jamtvedt G, Hagen K, et al. Practical evidence-based physiotherapy. 2nd ed. Edinburgh: Elsevier; 2011.

17. Dumville J, Torgerson D, Hewitt CE. Reporting attrition in randomised controlled trials. BMJ 2006;332:969–71.

18. Schulz K, Altman D, Moher D for the CONSORT Group. CONSORT 2010 statement: updated guidelines for reporting parallel-group randomised trials. BMJ 2010;340. doi: 10.1136/bmj.c332.

19. Higgins J, Altman D, Sterne J. Chapter 8: Assessing risk of bias in included studies. In: Higgins J, Green S, editors. Cochrane Handbook for Systematic Reviews of Interventions. Version 5.1.0 (updated March 2011). The Cochrane Collaboration; 2011. Online. Available: www.cochrane-handbook.org.

20. Hollis S, Campbell F. What is meant by intention to treat analysis? Survey of published randomised controlled trials. BMJ 1999;319:670–4.

21. Ottenbacher K, Maas F. How to detect effects: statistical power and evidence-based practice in occupational therapy research. Am J Occup Ther 1999;53:181–8.

22. Heuts P, de Bie R, Drietelaar M, et al. Self-management in osteoarthritis of hip or knee: a randomised clinical trial in a primary healthcare setting. J Rheumatol 2005;32:543–9.

23. Cohen J. Statistical power analysis for the behavioural sciences. 2nd ed. Hillsdale, NJ: Lawrence Erlbaum; 1988.

24. Norman G, Sloan J, Wyrwich K. Interpretation of changes in health-related quality of life: the remarkable universality of half a standard deviation. Med Care 2003;41:582–92.

25. Guyatt G. Making sense of quality-of-life data. Med Care 2000;39(II):175–9.

26. Herbert R. How to estimate treatment effects from reports of clinical trials. I: continuous outcomes. Aust J Physiother 2000;46:229–35.

27. Altman D, Bland J. Absence of evidence is not evidence of absence. BMJ 1995;311:485.

28. Lahdensuo A, Haahtela T, Herrala J, et al. Randomised comparison of guided self-management and traditional treatment of asthma over one year. BMJ 1996;312:748–52.

29. Guyatt G, Sackett D, Cook D. Users' guide to the medical literature: II. How to use an article about therapy or prevention: B. what were the results and will they help me in caring for my patients? JAMA 1994;271:59–63.

30. Cook R, Sackett D. The number needed to treat: a clinically useful measure of treatment effect. BMJ 1995;310:452–4.

31. Sackett D, Richardson W, Rosenberg W, et al. Evidence-based medicine. How to practice and teach EBM. New York: Churchill Livingstone; 1997.

32. Herbert R. How to estimate treatment effects from reports of clinical trials. II: Dichotomous outcomes. Aust J Physiother 2000;46:309–13.

33. Centre for Evidence-Based Medicine. Glossary. Oxford: University of Oxford. Online. Available: www.cebm.net/index.aspx?o=1116; 31 May 2012.

34. Laupacis A, Sackett D, Roberts R. An assessment of clinically useful measures of the consequences of treatment. N Engl J Med 1988;318:1728–33.

35. Straus S, Sackett D. Applying evidence to the individual patient. Ann Oncol 1999;10:29–32.

36. Altman D. Confidence intervals for the number needed to treat. BMJ 1998;317:1309–12.

37. Cumming R. Intervention strategies and risk-factor modification for falls prevention: a review of recent intervention studies. Clin Geriatr Med 2002;18:175–89.

38. Campbell A, Robertson M, Gardner M, et al. Falls prevention over 2 years: a randomised controlled trial in women 80 years and older. Age Ageing 1999;28:513–18.

39. Glasziou P, Irwig L. An evidence based approach to individualising treatment. BMJ 1995;311:1356–9.

Chapter 5

Questions about the effects of interventions: examples of appraisals from different health professions

Tammy Hoffmann, John W Bennett, Mal Boyle, Jeff Coombes, Mark R Elkins, Edzard Ernst, Angela Morgan, Lisa Nissen, Claire Rickard, Sharon Sanders, Alan Spencer and Caroline Wright

This chapter is an accompaniment to the previous chapter (Chapter 4) in which you learnt how to critically appraise evidence about the effects of interventions. In order to further illustrate the key points from Chapter 4, this chapter contains a number of worked examples of questions about the effects of interventions. As we mentioned in the preface of the book, we believe that it can be easier to learn the process of critical appraisal when you see some worked examples of how it is done, and it is even better when the examples are from your own health profession. Therefore, this chapter (and likewise Chapters 7, 9 and 11) contains examples from a range of health professions. Some of the clinical examples are relevant to more than one health profession. Each example is formatted in a similar manner and contains the following elements:

- a clinical scenario that explains the origins of the clinical question
- the clinical question
- the search terms and databases used to find evidence to answer the clinical question
- a brief description of the article chosen and the reason for its selection
- a structured abstract of the chosen article
- an appraisal of the risk of bias of the evidence
- a summary of the main results of the article that are relevant to the clinical question
- a brief discussion about how the evidence can be used to inform practice.

You will notice that in most of the examples the type of article chosen to be appraised is a randomised controlled trial. You may wonder why this is the case when Chapters 2 and 4 explained that systematic reviews of randomised controlled trials should be the first choice of study design to answer questions about the effects of an intervention. There is a good reason behind this. The authors of the examples contained in this chapter were asked to not choose (or indeed, specifically search for) systematic reviews if these were available to answer their question. Why? Because it is easier to learn how to appraise a systematic review of randomised controlled trials if you have first learnt how to appraise a randomised controlled trial. This chapter and Chapter 4 are designed to help you learn how to appraise a randomised controlled trial. Once you know how to do this, Chapter 12 will help you learn how to appraise a systematic review.

As you read through these examples, keep in mind that the suggestions that the authors of these worked examples have provided in the 'how might we use this evidence to inform practice' section have been drawn from only one individual study. In reality, additional studies would need to be located and appraised prior to drawing clear conclusions about what should be done in clinical practice.

When appraising an article, you need to obtain and carefully read the full text of the article. We have not included the full text of the articles that are appraised. However, for each of the examples in this chapter (and Chapters 7, 9 and 11), the authors of the examples have prepared a structured abstract that summarises the article. This has been done so that you have some basic information about each article. As we mentioned in Chapter 1, the more you practise doing the steps of evidence-based practice, the easier it will become. This is particularly true of the critical appraisal step. You may find it useful if you approach these worked examples as a self-assessment activity and try to obtain a copy of the article that is appraised in each of the examples (or just the ones that are relevant to your health profession if you feel more comfortable with that). You can then critically appraise the articles for yourself and check your answers with those that are presented in the worked examples.

One other thing to note about the examples in this chapter (and Chapters 7, 9 and 11) is that the appraisal of articles is not an exact science and sometimes there are no definite right or wrong answers. As with evidence-based practice in general, the health professional's clinical experience has an important role to play, particularly in deciding about issues such as baseline similarity (as we saw in Chapter 4) and clinical significance (as we saw in Chapters 2 and 4). Some of the examples may contain statements that you do not completely agree with and that you, as a health professional, would interpret a little differently. Also, the examples are provided to give you an overall sense of the general process of evidence-based practice. The content that is presented in the examples is not exhaustive (particularly in the 'how do we use this evidence to inform practice' section), and there may be other factors or issues that you, as a health professional, would suggest or consider if you were in that situation. That is OK.

OCCUPATIONAL THERAPY EXAMPLE

CLINICAL SCENARIO

You are an occupational therapist who works in a recently opened community adult health centre. In the last few weeks, you have received referrals for a number of patients who have been diagnosed with rheumatoid arthritis in the last 1 or 2 years. Most of these patients are female and middle-aged, and their arthritis is causing them considerable pain (particularly in the hand) and affecting their ability to perform self-care activities. You are considering running an education group about joint protection techniques and wonder if this will be effective in reducing your patients' pain and improving their function.

CLINICAL QUESTION

In adults with rheumatoid arthritis, is group education about joint protection techniques effective in reducing hand pain and improving function?

Search terms and databases used to find the evidence

Database: OTseeker.

Search terms: 'rheumatoid arthritis' AND 'joint protection'

This search retrieved 14 randomised controlled trials. Only four of these articles specifically evaluated the effectiveness of a joint protection program and the two most relevant articles were both based on the same study, with one describing the 6- and 12-month results and the other reporting the long-term (4-year) effects of the intervention. You choose to appraise the article that presents the long-term results to see if there is a sustained effect of joint protection education. As you discover that the full methodology of the trial is described in the earlier article (2001), you also obtain the full text of this article.

Articles chosen

Hammond A, Freeman K. The long-term outcomes from a randomized controlled trial of an educational–behavioural joint protection programme for people with rheumatoid arthritis. Clin Rehabil 2004;18:520–8.

Hammond A, Freeman K. One-year outcomes from a randomized controlled trial of an educational–behavioural joint protection programme for people with rheumatoid arthritis. Rheumatology 2001; 40:1044–51.

Structured abstract (adapted from the above)

Study design: Randomised controlled trial.

Setting: Outpatients from the occupational therapy departments of two hospitals in the UK.

Participants: 127 patients with rheumatoid arthritis; aged between 18 and 65 years (mean age 50.5 years, 76% female); diagnosed with rheumatoid arthritis within the last 5 years, a history of wrist or metacarpophalangeal joint pain and inflammation and experiencing hand pain during activity. Exclusion criteria included no other medical condition that affected hand function.

Intervention: Two small-group education interventions, both of 8 hours duration, were compared. One group attended a standard arthritis education program, which included 2.5 hours of joint protection education. Approximately 15–45 minutes was spent practising joint protection techniques. The other group attended a joint protection education program that used educational–behavioural teaching methods and aimed to enhance self-efficacy and motor learning. Participants in this program spent about two-thirds of their time practising and receiving feedback about hand joint protection methods.

Outcomes: *Primary measures:* hand pain experienced during a moderate activity (such as cooking or housework) within the last week (measured using a 100 mm visual analogue scale); adherence with joint protection. *Secondary measures:* functional status (measured using the Arthritis Impact Measurement Scales [AIMS2] with a range of 0–10 where 0 indicated better function), indicators of disease severity, hand status and psychological status.

Follow-up period: 4 years. Assessments were performed at baseline, 6 months, 12 months and 48 months.

Main results: At 4 years, compared with participants in the standard group, participants in the joint protection group had significantly better adherence to joint protection, less early-morning stiffness, higher AIMS2 activities of daily living (ADL) scores and fewer deformities in metacarpophalangeal and wrist joints.

Conclusion: Among those who attended the joint protection program, some of the significant improvements (in adherence and maintenance of functional ability) that were found at 1 year were maintained at 4 years, suggesting that an educational–behavioural joint protection program should be used in clinical practice.

Is the evidence likely to be biased?

- *Was the assignment of participants to groups randomised?*
  Yes. Participants were randomly allocated, using a four-block sequence.

- *Was the allocation sequence concealed?*
  Yes. Allocation occurred using sealed envelopes that had been prepared in advance.

- *Were the groups similar at the baseline or start of the trial?*
  Yes. The baseline characteristics were similar between the two study groups. There is a small difference between the two groups in terms of steroid use (6% of participants in the standard group and 20% of participants in the joint protection group), but this difference is probably not large enough to have affected the results. The baseline scores of the outcome measures were also similar between the two groups.

- *Were participants blind to which study group they were in?*
  No. For this trial, it was not possible for participants to be blinded to group allocation.

- *Were the health professionals who provided the intervention blind to participants' study group?*
  No. For this trial, it was not possible for the health professionals who provided the intervention to be blinded to group allocation.

- *Were the assessors blind to participants' study group?*
  Yes, for some measures. Assessments were conducted by independent assessors who were not informed of group allocation. The assessor was also asked to avoid discussing the education programs with the participants. However, for the outcomes that were measured by participant self-report (such as hand pain), the assessment of these outcomes was not blind as participants were not blinded to group allocation.

- *Were all participants who entered the trial properly accounted for at its conclusion, and how complete was follow-up?*
  Yes. The follow-up rate was 95.3% at 6 months and 96.8% at 12 months. By 4 years, the follow-up rate was 77%. Reasons are given as to why some participants were not able to be followed up, as well as which group they were in.
- *Was intention-to-treat analysis used?*
  Yes. The authors state that an intention-to-treat analysis was conducted.
- *Did the study have enough participants to minimise the play of chance?*
  Yes. Based on data from a previous study, the authors conducted a power analysis and determined that, with a power of 80% and a significance level of 0.05, 63 participants would be needed in each group.

What are the main results?

These are given in Table 5.1. For hand pain at 1 year, the effect size is 12.98, which is a statistically significant result. Both the *p* value (0.02) and confidence interval (CI), which does not include the no effect value of zero, show this. As hand pain was measured using a 100 mm visual analogue scale, an effect size (between groups) of 13 is probably large enough to also be considered clinically significant. However, the confidence interval is very wide, indicating some imprecision in the result. Thus, for some people the intervention effect may not be large enough to be considered clinically significant, whereas for other people the effect could be quite large and deemed clinically significant.

However, by 4 years, the between-group difference in hand pain is no longer statistically significant. Unfortunately, in the 4-year follow-up article the authors present results differently than they did in the 1-year article. Two of the problems with this are that: (1) as medians are used to present 4-year results, confidence intervals cannot easily be calculated; and (2) it is difficult to compare the results of the 1- and 4-year follow-up papers as the results are presented differently.

With respect to function, the ADL subscale of the AIMS2 was used to measure participants' ability to perform self-care and household activities. The effect size for the ADL subscale at 12 months was 0.8, which is statistically significant (confirmed by both the *p* value and the confidence interval). However, as the AIMS2 is scored on a scale of 0–10, an effect size of 0.8 is small and may not be

TABLE 5.1:
HAND PAIN AND FUNCTIONAL OUTCOME FOR INTERVENTION AND CONTROL GROUPS AT 1 YEAR AND 4 YEARS

Outcomes relevant to clinical question	Mean of joint protection group	Mean of standard group	Difference in mean	95% confidence interval[a]	*p* value
Hand pain at 1 year	33.63	46.61	12.98	1.98 to 23.98	0.02
AIMS2 ADL at 1 year	1.33	2.13	0.8	0.03 to 1.57	0.04
	Median of joint projection group	Median of standard group	Difference in medians	Confidence interval[b]	*p* value
Hand pain at 4 years	38	52.5	14.5	–	0.21
AIMS2 ADL at 4 years	1.25	1.87	0.62	–	0.04

[a]*Not provided by authors–calculated using data provided in the article. Confidence intervals may vary slightly depending on the formula used and the extent of the rounding.*
[b]*Not able to be calculated based on the information provided by authors in the article.*
ADL = activities of daily living; AIMS2 = Arthritis Impact Measurement Scales.

considered by many to be a clinically significant result. However, if we consider that the upper end of the confidence interval is 1.57, it is possible that the effect of this intervention could be clinically significant for some people. As explained in Chapter 4, the decision about clinical significance is a subjective one and depends on a number of factors such as the costs involved and preferences of the individual concerned.

At 4 years, the between-group difference remains statistically significant, but because the results are now presented in medians, it is difficult to compare the change from 1 year, not possible to calculate confidence intervals and difficult to consider clinical significance.

How might we use this evidence to inform practice?

As you are reasonably confident about the validity of the study's results and some of the results were of clinical importance, you proceed to assessing the applicability of this evidence to your clinical scenario. The patients with rheumatoid arthritis that you see are similar to the study participants in a number of ways such as age, gender (predominantly female) and disease duration. The majority of the participants in the study were assessed as having mild or moderate rheumatoid arthritis. You have yet to assess the disease severity in your recently referred patients. Once you do, you will check whether their disease severity is comparable to that of the study participants before making a decision about whether to implement a joint protection program.

Before making the decision, you will also need to consider whether you and the health centre where you work have the resources available to offer a joint protection program such as the one that was evaluated in the study. You will also need to obtain further, more detailed, information about the content of the program and the teaching strategies that were used. The article mentions that further details may be obtained in another published article, so you will start by obtaining that article and, if you have questions after reading that, you will contact the authors of the article for more information.

Although the study found a statistically and clinically significant effect of the intervention on hand pain at 1 year, this was not maintained by 4 years. The effect on the other outcome (self-care) that you were particularly interested in may not be conclusively clinically significant at either 1 year or 4 years. Although it is unlikely that the program would cause any harm and it appears to offer some benefits to participants, these mainly appear to be in the short term and there are considerable staffing resources associated with providing the program. Before making a decision about whether to implement the program at your workplace, you decide to search for other approaches to providing joint protection education and training to people with rheumatoid arthritis (and not necessarily education that is group-based or uses an educational–behavioural approach).

PHYSIOTHERAPY EXAMPLE

CLINICAL SCENARIO

As a physiotherapist on the cardiac surgery ward, you attend a conference and hear that some of your peers at another hospital are providing inspiratory muscle training to patients who are undergoing coronary artery bypass graft (CABG) surgery. The training is performed preoperatively in an attempt to reduce the likelihood of pulmonary complications occurring postoperatively. You are unaware of any research that has investigated the use of this intervention in patients undergoing cardiac surgery, and decide to search for evidence to decide whether this is something you should institute at the hospital where you work.

CLINICAL QUESTION

Does preoperative inspiratory muscle training in addition to standard care prevent postoperative pulmonary complications in patients who are undergoing CABG surgery?

Search terms and databases used to find the evidence

Database: PEDro (using the Advanced Search option).

Search terms: You decide that *inspiratory muscle training* is likely to be mentioned in the title of the article, although it may be described as *respiratory muscle training*. You therefore enter **spiratory muscle training* in the 'Title' field. You consider that the patient population might be broadly defined in the title using a phrase like *cardiac surgery*, but you expect that it would be defined using *coronary artery bypass graft* or *coronary artery bypass surgery* in the abstract. Therefore, you enter *coronary artery bypass* in the 'Abstract & Title' field. You want both of these terms to be present, so you select the option 'Match all search terms' when searching.

The search returns eight records, but this represents only three separate trials as some of these trials had multiple publications that were retrieved by the search. For the first trial, by Hulzebos et al, there is the main publication which is accompanied by a report of pilot data, an English translation of the primary Dutch publication, a consumer summary of the trial and an analysis of the feasibility of the intervention using data from the trial. For the second trial, there is the main publication and a Hebrew-to-English translation. The third trial has only one publication, but it is about postoperative respiratory muscle training, so it is not relevant to your question.

Although the first and second trials examine inspiratory muscle training for patients who are undergoing CABG surgery, several features of the first trial show that it probably provides less-biased evidence to answer your question. Unlike the second trial, it used concealed allocation, blinded outcome assessment and intention-to-treat analysis and fewer participants were lost to follow-up. In addition, the sample size of the trial was larger ($n = 279$ vs $n = 84$) and the trial was conducted more recently, so the surgical procedure and standard care in the postoperative period are more consistent with that offered at your hospital. Therefore, you decide on the first article.

Article chosen

Hulzebos E, Helders P, Favie N, et al. Preoperative intensive inspiratory muscle training to prevent postoperative pulmonary complications in high-risk patients undergoing CABG surgery: a randomized clinical trial. JAMA 2006;296:1851–7.

Structured abstract (adapted from the above)

Study design: Randomised controlled trial.

Setting: University medical centre in Utrecht, the Netherlands.

Participants: 279 patients (mean age 66.9 years; 77.9% male) undergoing CABG surgery at high risk of developing postoperative pulmonary complications, indicated by the presence of two or more of these criteria: age >70 years, productive cough, diabetes mellitus, smoking, chronic obstructive pulmonary disease and body mass index >27. Exclusion criteria included: surgery within 2 weeks of initial contact; a history of stroke; use of immunosuppressive medication for 30 days before surgery; and presence of a neuromuscular disorder, cardiovascular instability or an aneurysm.

Intervention: Participants were randomly assigned to receive either preoperative inspiratory muscle training ($n = 140$) or usual care ($n = 139$). The intervention group trained daily (20 minutes), 7 times a week (6 times without supervision), for at least 2 weeks before the surgery. Both groups received the same postoperative physical therapy and other standard care.

Outcomes: *Primary outcome:* the incidence of postoperative pulmonary complications, defined according to recognised criteria. *Secondary outcome:* duration of postoperative hospitalisation, in days.

Main results: Postoperative pulmonary complications occurred in 25 (18%) of the participants in the intervention group and 48 (35%) of the control group, odds ratio 0.52 (95% CI 0.30 to 0.92). Median duration of hospitalisation was 7 days (range 5–41) in the intervention group and 8 days (range 6–70) in the control group ($p = 0.02$).

Conclusion: Preoperative inspiratory muscle training reduced the incidence of pulmonary complications and the duration of postoperative hospitalisation in patients who were at high risk of developing a pulmonary complication after CABG surgery.

Is the evidence likely to be biased?

- *Was the assignment of participants to groups randomised?*
  Yes. Participants were appropriately randomised, using a computer-generated number list.

- *Was the allocation sequence concealed?*
  Yes. The number list was sealed in envelopes which were held by an external investigator.

- *Were the groups similar at the baseline or start of the trial?*
  Yes. The baseline characteristics were similar between the two study groups. Although in the table of baseline characteristics the authors of the article have reported a difference between the two groups in terms of median duration of mechanical ventilation (4 hours in the intervention group vs 5 hours in the control group), this is technically not a baseline characteristic as it was measured after the intervention had been provided. Additionally, it is unlikely that a difference of this size would be of clinical importance and have affected the results.

- *Were participants blind to which study group they were in?*
  No. For this trial, it was not possible for participants to be blinded to group allocation.

- *Were the health professionals who provided the intervention blind to participants' study group?*
  No. For this trial, it was not possible for the therapists who provided the intervention to be blinded to group allocation.

- *Were the assessors blind to participants' study group?*
  Yes. The investigators who assessed outcomes were blinded to participants' treatment group.

- *Were all participants who entered the trial properly accounted for at its conclusion, and how complete was follow-up?*
  Yes. Apart from three participants who died before surgery, all participants were followed up. This is a 98.9% follow-up rate.

- *Was intention-to-treat analysis used?*
  Yes. It is stated that an intention-to-treat analysis was conducted.

- *Did the study have enough participants to minimise the play of chance?*
  Yes. A power calculation was performed, but the trial was terminated before this number was reached because safety monitoring determined that statistically and clinically significant results had been achieved at the interim analysis.

What are the main results?

Pulmonary complication: The risk of pulmonary complications is presented appropriately, using an odds ratio with a 95% confidence interval (refer to Table 5.2). The reduction in risk is both statistically and clinically significant. The 95% confidence interval includes only clinically worthwhile reductions in risk. Therefore, the results are sufficiently precise to make clinical recommendations.

The data for the first outcome, pulmonary complications, can be used to estimate two useful statistics. First, let us calculate the absolute risk reduction (ARR), which is simply the risk in the control group minus the risk in the intervention group: 35% – 18% = 17%. Using the formula (95% confidence

TABLE 5.2: FREQUENCY OF PULMONARY COMPLICATIONS IN BOTH GROUPS				
Outcome	Intervention group	Control group	Odds ratio	95% confidence interval
Pulmonary complications	25/139 (18%)	48/137 (35%)	0.52	0.30 to 0.92

interval $\approx$ difference in risk $\pm 1 \sqrt{n_{av}}$) that was provided in Box 4.3 in Chapter 4, you also calculate the 95% confidence interval of the ARR to be 9% to 25%. The ARR statistic is useful in clinical practice because, if you decide to implement the intervention, you can use it to explain to patients the value that they can expect from undertaking the inspiratory muscle training regimen. After explaining what a pulmonary complication is and how it can delay recovery, many patients would consider the training program worthwhile to reduce their risk of such a complication from 35% to 18%.

An alternative statistic is the relative risk reduction (RRR). This is calculated by dividing the difference in risk between the two treatment groups by the risk in the control group:

$$RRR = (control\ group\ risk - treatment\ group\ risk) \div control\ group\ risk$$
$$= (35\% - 18\%) \div 35\% = 49\%$$

When an adverse outcome occurs fairly frequently in a study, the RRR is a useful statistic; but when the outcome is rare, a large RRR may still be found even though the ARR is very small, which can be misleading. Therefore you decide to use ARR instead of RRR.

You then use the ARR to calculate the number of people that need to be treated in order to prevent one pulmonary complication:

$$number\ needed\ to\ treat = 1 \div ARR$$
$$= 1/17$$
$$= 5.88\%$$

The 95% confidence interval of this number needed to treat is 4 to 12. This was calculated by using the inverse of the numbers in the confidence interval of the ARR that you calculated earlier (so 1/25% and 1/9%). Therefore, for every 6 high-risk patients that we treat, 1 pulmonary complication will be prevented that would have otherwise occurred with usual care. However, this number needed to treat could be as low as 4 or as high as 12.

Duration of hospitalisation: The median duration of postoperative hospitalisation was 7 days (range 5 to 41) in the treatment group and 8 days (range 6 to 70) in the control group, and this difference was statistically significant.

How might we use this evidence to inform practice?

You decide that the trial is valid and that the results are important. Pulmonary complications are dangerous and uncomfortable for the patient and they are expensive to treat. Therefore, the effect of this intervention on this outcome alone is clinically worthwhile, and the number needed to treat of 6 is useful in justifying the introduction of the service. Further justification of the clinical worth of this intervention comes from the other significant outcome, which was a reduction in the duration of hospitalisation. You plan to discuss the results of this study with your head of department as there are resource implications associated with introducing the service, particularly providing an intervention of the same intensity as was provided in the study. However, it is your recommendation that this intervention should be introduced.

PODIATRY EXAMPLE

You are a podiatrist who works in a private practice. In recent days, you have seen several patients with heel pain which you believe is plantar fasciitis. Your management of this condition often includes prescription of customised orthoses (devices made to a cast of the patient's foot with an individualised prescription). Because it takes several weeks for the orthotics to be manufactured, you wonder whether prefabricated orthotics (mass-produced devices made to fit a generic foot shape) which can be bought over the counter and started immediately are as effective. You decide to search for the evidence.

CLINICAL QUESTION

In people with plantar fasciitis, are prefabricated orthotic devices as effective as customised orthoses in reducing pain and improving foot function?

Search terms and databases used to find the evidence

Database: The Cochrane Library. A systematic review of randomised controlled trials or a randomised controlled trial would be the ideal study design to answer this question. Ideally the randomised controlled trial would have three arms, allowing comparison of the two types of orthotic devices with each other and a control group.

Search terms: You start by checking for MeSH terms related to the population and intervention of interest, and combine these with textword terms using the Boolean operator OR in the 'Search History' and 'Advanced Search' features of The Cochrane Library:

(Fasciitis, plantar (MeSH) OR plantar fasciitis OR (heel OR calcan* NEAR pain)) AND (orthotic devices (MeSH) OR orthotic* OR orthoses)

This search produced 30 hits, comprising 7 Cochrane Reviews, 3 other non-Cochrane systematic reviews, 19 trials and 1 economic evaluation. Two Cochrane reviews look as though they may answer your question. Unfortunately, the first one you look at, titled 'Interventions for the treatment of heel pain', has been withdrawn from the Library because it is out of date. The second review, titled 'Custom-made orthoses for the treatment of foot pain', examines the effect of customised orthoses on foot pain of any type or aetiology. As you read through the review, you find that it included six trials which assessed the effect of customised orthoses for plantar fasciitis, and in three of these, customised orthoses were compared with prefabricated devices. The review is very helpful as it not only describes, assesses the risk of bias and synthesises the results of studies which address your clinical question, but it also provides information on the comparative effectiveness of other interventions such as night splinting and stretching.

Of the three relevant trials, one is a three-arm trial which compares the effect of customised, prefabricated and sham orthoses in participants with plantar fasciitis. Measures of pain and function at 3 and 12 months are reported. The other trials also compare customised orthoses with a range of other interventions, including prefabricated orthoses and in-shoe devices; however, participants in these studies were only followed up for a maximum of 3 months. You decide that assessment of pain and function at 12 months is preferable, so you select the trial titled 'Effectiveness of foot orthoses to treat plantar fasciitis' for appraisal.

Article chosen

Landorf KB, Keenan A, Herbert RD. Effectiveness of foot orthoses to treat plantar fasciitis. Arch Intern Med 2006;6:1305–10.

Structured abstract (adapted from the above)

Study design: Randomised controlled trial.

Setting: A university podiatry clinic, Melbourne, Australia.

Participants: 136 participants, mean age 48 years, 67% female, with a clinical diagnosis of plantar fasciitis who had experienced symptoms for at least 4 weeks. People with a major orthopaedic or medical condition that may have influenced the condition were excluded.

Intervention: Participants were randomised to receive one of: (a) 'sham' orthoses which were made of soft foam moulded over an unmodified cast of the foot; (b) prefabricated orthoses made from a thicker, firmer-density foam moulded over the cast; or (c) customised foot orthoses made from semi-rigid polypropylene moulded over neutral-position plaster casts with a firm foam heel post.

Outcomes: The primary outcome of the trial was self-reported pain and function at 3 and 12 months, which were measured using the pain and function domains of the Foot Health Status Questionnaire (on a 0–100 measurement scale).

Follow-up period: 12 months.

Main results: This trial found that pain and function improved in all three groups over time. Participants receiving prefabricated and customised orthoses showed greater improvement in function than the sham group at 3 months (mean difference of 8.4 points on the function domain between prefabricated and sham orthoses, and mean difference of 7.5 points between customised and sham orthoses). Prefabricated and customised orthoses also reduced pain compared with sham orthoses at 3 months (8.7 points and 7.4 points respectively), although these differences were not statistically significant. At 12 months, there were no significant differences in pain and function between any of the three groups.

Conclusion: Both prefabricated and customised orthoses have similar small short-term benefits for people with plantar fasciitis and negligible long-term effects.

Is the evidence likely to be biased?

- *Was the assignment of participants to groups randomised?*
  Yes. The randomisation sequence was generated using an appropriate method (computer-generated randomisation sequence).

- *Was the allocation sequence concealed?*
  Yes. The allocation was concealed from participants and from the investigator enrolling participants in the trial. The allocation sequence appears to be held off-site and, once a participant was enrolled and baseline assessments were completed, the allocation sequence was obtained by telephone or email.

- *Were the groups similar at the baseline or start of the trial?*
  Table 1 in the article shows that study groups were balanced in terms of most of the baseline variables that were measured. One important exception is participant's weight, where the mean weight of participants in the prefabricated orthoses group was approximately 10 kg more than in the other two study groups. This is a clinically important difference that may influence the outcome. You notice that the results are not adjusted for this difference and keep this in mind. You also notice a considerable difference between the sham and prefabricated groups in the foot function score at baseline, but are satisfied that this has been adjusted for in the analysis.

- *Were participants blind to which study group they were in?*
  Cannot tell. Although the article states that it was a 'participant blinded' trial, you cannot tell this for sure. The investigators attempted to 'blind' participants to the orthoses they received by making the devices as similar as possible in terms of colour and shape. Participants were told they would receive soft, medium or hard orthoses. All participants had a cast of the foot taken. However, because the material used for the three devices was different (foam, polyethylene,

polypropylene), some participants may have been able to work out which device they had received. Because some participants may not have been blind to which study group they were in and because the study outcomes were measured by participant self-report, you cannot be sure that any treatment effect (or lack of effect) that is reported in this study is not biased. Evaluation of the success of participant blinding was not reported.

- *Were the health professionals who provided the intervention blind to participants' study group?*
  No. Due to the nature of the intervention, the podiatrist who assessed the participants and provided them with their orthoses was not blind to the intervention allocation.

- *Were the assessors blind to participants' study group?*
  Cannot tell. For the same reason that participants may not have been blind to study group allocation, the investigators who were in contact with participants during outcome measurement may also not have been blind to study group allocation. To prevent study investigators from biasing measures of outcome (and potentially influencing participants' responses), participants completed the Foot Health Status Questionnaire at the beginning of each appointment before they had any interaction with the investigator. However, as the Foot Health Status Questionnaire is a self-report outcome, if participants are not blind to their allocation then the assessment cannot be considered blind either.

- *Were all participants who entered the trial properly accounted for at its conclusion, and how complete was follow-up?*
  Yes. The flow of participants through this study is clearly reported in a flow diagram. Five of the 136 participants (4%) were lost to follow-up, three from the sham orthoses group (though one of these withdrew before any baseline measures were conducted or treatment was received) and one each from the prefabricated and customised orthoses groups. The article also reports the number of participants who crossed over to alternative orthoses. This was highest in the sham orthoses group, with two of the 44 participants using alternative orthoses at 3 months and seven (of the 43) at 12 months.

- *Was intention-to-treat analysis used?*
  Yes. The article states that an intention-to-treat analysis was conducted.

- *Did the study have enough participants to minimise the play of chance?*
  Yes. The authors report conducting a power calculation prior to commencing participant recruitment. They determined the number of participants required based on the significance level (risk of type 1 error 5%), statistical power (90%) and an estimated difference in effect between any of the study groups. According to the power calculation, 136 participants were required, which is how many were randomised.

What are the results?

As you are interested in the comparison between prefabricated orthoses and customised orthoses, you look for these results first. The results are presented in the article as the mean difference (and 95% confidence intervals) in pain and function scores between the groups at 3 and 12 months (adjusted for baseline scores). See Table 5.3 for a summary of these results.

Pain: At 3 months, the mean difference in pain between prefabricated and customised orthoses was 1.3 (95% CI –7.6 to 10.2) points on the Foot Health Status Questionnaire pain domain, and at 12 months, it was 2.3 points (95% CI –5.6 to 10.1).

Function: On the function domain, the mean difference between prefabricated and customised orthoses at 3 months was 0.9 points (95% CI –6.3 to 8.1), and at 12 months, it was 1.2 points (95% CI –6.1 to 8.5).

None of these results are statistically significant (as seen by the confidence intervals which all contain the no effect value of zero). You therefore do not need to consider the clinical significance

TABLE 5.3:
EFFECT OF INTERVENTION ON PAIN AND FOOT FUNCTION

Outcome	Mean difference (95% CI) in scores between prefabricated and customised orthoses (adjusted for baseline score)
Pain 3 months 12 months	1.3 (−7.6 to 10.2) 2.3 (−5.6 to 10.1)
Function 3 months 12 months	0.9 (−6.3 to 8.1) 1.2 (−6.1 to 8.5)

of these results. The results show that the effects of prefabricated and customised orthoses on pain and function are similar.

The study also presents the effects on foot function as a number needed to treat by dichotomising the data. In the dichotomisation, an improvement in function was considered to have occurred when function increased by more than one-third of the baseline value. The prefabricated foot orthoses produced one additional improved outcome for every six people treated for 3 months, and the customised foot orthoses produced one additional beneficial outcome for every four people treated for 3 months.

Other results show that pain and function improved in all study groups over time and that, at 12 months, differences in pain and function between all the groups were small and not statistically significant. However, at 3 months, the prefabricated and customised orthoses group showed greater improvement in pain and function than the sham group. The mean difference in function was statistically significant–a difference of 8.4 (95% CI 1.0 to 15.8) points for prefabricated orthoses vs sham orthoses, and a difference of 7.5 (95% CI 0.3 to 14.7) points for customised orthoses vs sham orthoses. Although the authors do not provide any guidance about the amount of difference on the 0–100 scale that would be needed for this to be considered a clinically significant difference, the upper ends of the confidence intervals indicate that these intervention effects may be considered clinically significant to some people, depending on their preferences. However, the lower ends of the confidence intervals suggest that it is also possible that some people may not find much benefit from this intervention.

How might we use this evidence to inform practice?

You decide that the trial is valid and that the results are important. Given the similarity in the effects of the prefabricated and the customised orthoses, it would be reasonable to prescribe a prefabricated device rather than a custom-made devices for your patients with plantar fasciitis. A major benefit you see in this approach is that the patient can start the treatment almost straight away, as opposed to the several weeks it takes for customised devices to be manufactured. However, you think there are other factors to consider. First, several of your patients have had symptoms for only a few weeks. You wonder if they would respond the same way as participants in the trial where the condition was more chronic (symptoms were experienced for a median of 12 months). You also wonder how the results might vary if you use different prefabricated orthoses or customised orthoses manufacturers to those that were used in the study.

The prefabricated orthoses used in the study are easily obtained for a cost of around AUD $40 to $70. This is considerably cheaper than customised orthoses, which can cost anywhere from AUD $250 to $400. However, prefabricated devices do not last as long as customised devices, which are usually made from more-durable polypropylene, and may need to be replaced a number of times depending on wear. If, as the results of this study suggest, most people recover from plantar fasciitis by 1 year, then two or three pairs of prefabricated devices over a 12-month period would still be cheaper than customised devices. You know from experience, though, that once people start to wear orthoses and feel they are beneficial, they often continue to use them long-term and, if this is the case, customised orthoses which last for several years may be more economical. Your experience also tells you that often patients also need to purchase footwear that can accommodate orthotic devices. This, together with the cost of the actual orthoses, can be an issue for some patients. You decide that it is important to discuss the results of this study with your patients, working with them to determine the best management option for each situation.

SPEECH PATHOLOGY EXAMPLE

CLINICAL SCENARIO

You are a speech pathologist working in a children's hospital. Ben, a 10-year-old boy, was admitted to hospital with severe traumatic brain injury following a horse-riding accident. He was intubated and ventilated at hospital admission due to difficulty breathing. Two weeks after admission, Ben was in a medically stable condition and had been weaned from the ventilator and extubated. He could understand basic commands and speak in two- to three-word phrases at this time, but had severe dysarthria due to persistent breathing difficulties and poor breath support for speech. At two months post-injury Ben was speaking in full sentences, but the dysarthric impairment was persistent. You have previously used an eclectic range of traditional behavioural approaches to treat this form of dysarthria (e.g. using a manometer tube and breathing tasks alongside speech drills). However, you recall hearing about instrumental biofeedback options for dysarthria at a recent conference. You remember that the biofeedback equipment sounded expensive, but wonder whether you should make a case to your manager for buying this equipment to pursue a biofeedback approach for Ben.

CLINICAL QUESTION

Are instrumental biofeedback treatment approaches more effective than traditional behavioural treatment approaches at improving acquired dysarthria associated with underlying respiratory support issues in children?

Search terms and databases used to find the evidence

Databases: PubMed and speechBITE.

Search terms: (dysarthria OR speech) AND (respiration OR breathing) AND ((brain injur* OR (traumatic brain injur*) OR (trauma) OR (acquired brain injur*)) AND (child* OR p?ediatric) AND (treatment or intervention)

Twenty-four articles were generated by the search (3 in speechBITE; 21 in PubMed). You reviewed the title and abstract of the articles and determined that only three seemed appropriate for the clinical question, and obtained the articles. The first article, a Cochrane review examining interventions for childhood-acquired dysarthria, indicated that a single-case study was the only relevant paper addressing the clinical question of interest. This same single-case study was also the second relevant paper identified from the search. The third article was inappropriate because it was a non-treatment-based review of speech aerodynamic behaviour. The chosen article was therefore the paper that was independently generated by the search and also identified in the Cochrane review. While the article is a single-case study and is classified low on the evidence hierarchy, at the time of searching it was the only article available that was most relevant to the clinical question.

Article chosen

Murdoch B, Pitt G, Theodoros D, et al. Real-time continuous visual biofeedback in the treatment of speech breathing disorders following childhood traumatic brain injury: report of one case. Paediatr Rehabil 1999;3:5–20.

Structured abstract (adapted from the above)

Study design: Quasi-experimental single-case A-B-A-B study design.

Study question: What is the efficacy of traditional (B1) versus instrumental biofeedback (B2) therapy for dysarthria associated with poor respiratory support for speech?

Participant and selection: The study participant was a 12-year-old male who had sustained left parietal lobe damage due to a motor vehicle accident as a cyclist, two and a half years prior to the study commencement. The participant had a chronic mixed spastic–ataxic–flaccid dysarthria, with severely impaired respiratory function being the predominant impairment. Inclusion and exclusion criteria were specified.

Assessment: The participant underwent a comprehensive battery of both instrumental and traditional behavioural assessments at baseline (A1), during a 10-week withdrawal phase between treatments (A2), and at the end of the second treatment period (A3). Further monitoring assessments were also conducted at several time points during both B1 and B2. Outcome measures included multiple physiological instrumental measures and perceptual measures across all levels of the speech sub-system (that is, respiration, laryngeal, velopharyngeal and articulatory). All were clinician-rated (that is, no parent or child report) and were impairment-based and focused on the isolated function level of speech production (such as vowel prolongation) or on the single word or sentence level of speech production (for example, the Assessment of Intelligibility of Dysarthric Speech).

Intervention: The main aims of each treatment were to: (1) increase the participant's control of inhalation and exhalation; and (2) improve the participant's coordination of phonation and exhalation. Both treatments used a bottom-up intervention approach, with the participant being required to progress along a hierarchy of speech and non-speech tasks. More specifically, traditional therapy involved eight 30- to 45-minute sessions across 2 weeks, and consisted of a range of tasks largely based on adult treatment approaches that were described in a previous article. These tasks included the use of the U-tube manometer to increase the participant's control of subglottal air pressure via a form of simple traditional visual feedback, and description and demonstration of an appropriate breathing pattern for speech. The therapist provided verbal feedback to the participant on issues such as the duration of tasks, depth and speed of inhalation and voice latency.

In relation to the instrumental visual biofeedback, inductance plethysmography (Respitrace system) was used to provide real-time continuous biofeedback of ribcage circumference to the participant during breathing. The participant received eight sessions over 2 weeks. Tasks involved trying to match a target trace provided at the top of the computer screen through the performance of various non-speech and speech tasks at certain levels. The specific computer feedback enabled the participant to visualise the exact point at which inspiration ended and expiration began, enabling him to try to coordinate phonation with this point. This biofeedback was augmented by the therapist explaining the visual feedback to the participant and instructing him to make adjustments to his breathing and voice onset coordination with expiration.

Main results: The continuous biofeedback treatment was not only effective, but superior to traditional therapy in the modification of speech breathing patterns for a child with persistent dysarthria following severe traumatic brain injury.

Conclusion: A physiological biofeedback treatment approach is potentially useful for the remediation of speech breathing impairment in the paediatric dysarthric population.

Is this evidence likely to be biased?

Given that this was a single-case study, it was not appropriate to appraise this article for risk of bias using the criteria that are typically applied to randomised controlled trials.

- Appropriate inclusion and exclusion criteria were applied in participant selection.
- The methodology was appropriate for addressing the research question and methodological strengths included explicit reporting of the baseline assessment characteristics and the reporting of missing data or data that were unable to be analysed.
- The treatment methods were outlined in extensive detail and would enable replication of most components of the study. More prescriptive detail could have been provided about the steps in the progression along the treatment hierarchy, including the number of items administered within each level of the hierarchy.
- A large number of assessment points and assessments were used during baseline assessments and for treatment monitoring. Some level of change in some measures was likely to be found when so many assessments were conducted, which potentially limits the conclusions about treatment efficacy.
- No direct statistical tests were performed to compare treatment outcomes from traditional versus instrumental biofeedback approaches. Rather, multiple quantitative descriptive results were reported for pre- and post-treatment changes that are difficult for the reader to interpret.
- All outcome measures were administered by the treating therapist. This may have introduced rater bias.

What are the main results?

Multiple perceptual and physiological measures were made; however, two key measures included voice onset latencies and phonation time.

- Following traditional treatment, the participant's voice onset latencies were reduced (mean = 1.14 seconds, range = 0.5 ± 2 seconds) and phonation time increased (mean = 2.57 seconds, range = 1.5 ± 4 seconds). The authors stated that both of these results were minimal, and not convincing evidence of improvement in the participant's control of his breath pattern for speech.
- Using visual biofeedback treatment of ribcage excursion, the participant was able to produce a reduced mean voice onset latency of 1 second (range = 0 ± 2 seconds) and to increase mean phonation time to 4.4 seconds (range = 3.5 ± 5 seconds).

How might we use this evidence to inform practice?

In the case of Ben, no firm conclusions are able to be drawn about which treatment method is optimal for dysarthria treatment. This is because the current treatment evidence in this field is limited to a single-case study. The participant in the chosen article was also a male and of similar age and aetiology (i.e. traumatic brain injury) to Ben. However, it is difficult to generalise the findings of one case study to other cases, regardless of these similarities. Further research and evidence is required in this field before any one treatment method can be definitively advocated for use in clinical practice. While the authors reported a slight improvement with the use of instrumental biofeedback methods, this approach requires the use of expensive equipment which is not currently available in many settings. The evidence is not strong enough for you, as Ben's speech pathologist, to present a case to your manager of the need to purchase this equipment for patient care. Thus, in the absence of the necessary instrumental equipment and the absence of strong evidence for applying a biofeedback approach, you decide that you will continue to use a typical traditional behavioural treatment approach with Ben.

Undertaking the above process of finding and appraising research evidence ensured that you were educated about current research in the field so that you could confidently discuss the treatment literature with Ben and his parents. Importantly, you were able to reassure Ben's parents that the intervention that was being applied was appropriate to continue using. Reading the treatment methodology outlined in the study also encouraged you to reflect upon the structure of Ben's treatment. The study provided a guide as to what may be an appropriate number of treatment sessions for Ben, what the duration of treatment sessions should be and what treatment targets may be useful, and suggested methods for how to progress the patient along treatment targets in an hierarchical fashion, moving towards functional speech outcomes.

MEDICINE EXAMPLE

CLINICAL SCENARIO

You are a general practitioner who provides travel medicine advice in Australia. Many of your patients seek advice about travel to destinations where traveller's diarrhoea is frequent. Sarah, aged 48, is going to travel to Thailand for 4 weeks and plans to include an extended stay in the northern border areas with one of the hill tribes. On a previous holiday Sarah experienced an episode of diarrhoea that 'ruined' her holiday. She asks what you might recommend to limit this risk on this holiday. Standard treatment is t o recommend loperamide (an anti-diarrhoeal medication) and an antibiotic. You are unsure of the benefits of taking these in combination, as compared with separately. You decide to research the effects of these medications taken together.

CLINICAL QUESTION

In travellers' diarrhoea, does the use of both loperamide and an antibiotic lessen the effects of traveller's diarrhoea, compared with a single agent?

Search terms and databases used to find the evidence

Database: PubMed–Clinical Queries (with 'therapy category' and 'narrow scope' selected).

Search terms: travel* diarrh* AND loperamide

This search retrieved six results. Five were randomised trials, but only one of these was a study that compared agents available in Australia and currently recommended for the treatment of travellers' diarrhoea.

Article chosen

Ericsson C, DuPont H, Okhuysen P, et al. Loperamide plus azithromycin more effectively treats travelers' diarrhea in Mexico than azithromycin alone. J Travel Med 2007;14:312–19.

Structured abstract (adapted from the above)

Study design: Randomised controlled trial.

Setting: USA students attending sessions in the University of Arizona, University of San Diego and Universidad Autonoma de Guadalajara summer programs.

Participants: 176 US adults who were recently arrivals in Guadalajara, Mexico during the summer of 2002 and 2003. Inclusion criteria: adults (over 18) who developed acute diarrhoea, which was defined as 'passage of three or more unformed (defined later) stools in the preceding 24 hours accompanied by one or more signs or symptoms of enteric infection.' Exclusion criteria: pregnancy, breastfeeding, an unstable medical condition, had taken two or more doses of an anti-diarrhoeal medication in the 24 hours or symptomatic therapy within 2 hours of enrolment, or receiving an antimicrobial drug aimed at enteric bacterial pathogens within 7 days prior to enrolment.

Intervention: Participants were randomised to one of three oral treatment groups:

1. azithromycin 1000 mg (single dose)
2. azithromycin 500 mg (single dose)
3. azithromycin 500 mg (single dose) plus loperamide as a 4 mg loading dose followed by 2 mg after each loose stool; not to exceed a total of 16 mg/day over 2 days.

Double dummies were used to blind the study.

Outcomes: Participants gave a pre- and post-treatment stool sample for analysis and maintained daily diaries of symptoms and passage of stools. Stool form was divided into three categories: 'formed' (stool retains its shape), 'soft' (stool takes the shape of a container) and 'watery' (stool can be poured).

Follow-up period: 4 days (96 hours).

Main results: The duration of diarrhoea was significantly ($p = 0.0002$) shorter after treatment with azithromycin and loperamide (11 hours) than with either dose of azithromycin alone (34 hours). In the first 24 hours, the average number of unformed stools passed was 3.4 (azithromycin alone) and 1.2 (combination) for a significant ($p < 0.0001$) difference of 2.2 unformed stools. This difference equated with 20% of azithromycin-treated subjects continuing to pass six or more unformed stools in the first 24 hours post-treatment compared with only 1.7% of combination-treated subjects.

Conclusion: For the treatment of travellers' diarrhoea in an *Escherichia coli* predominant region of the world, a single 500 mg dose of azithromycin appeared as effective as a 1000 mg dose. Loperamide plus azithromycin (500 mg) was safe and more effective than either dose of azithromycin alone. Loperamide should routinely be used in combination with an antimicrobial agent to treat travellers' diarrhoea.

Is the evidence likely to be biased?

- *Was the assignment of participants randomised?*
  Yes, participants were randomly allocated. Medications were randomised in blocks of 12 participants.

- *Was allocation concealed?*
  Cannot tell. It is not clear if concealed allocation occurred.

- *Were the groups similar at baseline or the start of the trial?*
  Yes. There were no clinically important differences in demographic characteristics or clinical features of illness between the three study groups at enrolment.

- *Were participants blind to which study group they were in?*
  Yes. The use of the double dummy technique should have ensured this occurred. This means that the medications could not be made to look identical, so an extra set was made. This meant that all participants took two types of tablets or capsules.

- *Were the health professionals who provided the intervention blind to participants' study group?*
  Cannot tell. The article does not explicitly state that the health professionals who provided the mediations were blind to participant group allocation. Although the methods section states that a double dummy technique was used and that the study was double-blind, it is not clear if the 'double' part of the blinding is referring to the health professionals or the assessors (as participants were one part of the 'double blind', as described above).

- *Were the assessors blind to participants' study group?*
  Yes. As the main outcomes were self-reported and participants were blind to group allocation, the participants were actually the assessors.

- *Were all participants who entered the trial properly accounted for at its conclusion, and how complete was follow-up?*

Yes. Only 14 participants dropped out, giving a follow-up rate of 91%. Reasons were given for loss to follow-up, as well as which group they were in.

- *Was intention-to-treat analysis used?*
  Yes. It is explicitly stated that an intention-to-treat analysis was conducted.
- *Did the study have enough participants to minimise the play of chance?*
  A power calculation was presented 'in which sample sizes permitted detection of diarrhea from over 24 hours to less than 12 hours in a three-way comparison at a power of 0.8'.

What are the main results?

The intention-to-treat analysis showed a statistically significant reduction in average number of hours taken for the diarrhoea to cease for the azithromycin/loperamide treated group (11 hours) over either group treated with azithromycin alone (34 hours). Confidence intervals are not provided, but the *p* value of 0.0002 confirms statistical significance of this between-group difference of 23 hours. This is also a clinically significant reduction, as this equates to one and a half days of diarrhoea with just antibiotics versus just on half a day with the combined treatment.

How might we use this evidence to inform practice?

Although this study is conducted only on young adults and in one region of Mexico, the strong methodological features mean that you are reasonably confident about the results. You discuss the results of this study with Sarah, who happily accepts the option of taking both loperamide (4 mg initially and 2 mg with each subsequent loose stool, up to a maximum of 16 mg/day for 2 days) and azithromycin (500 mg) should she suffer with diarrhoea during her upcoming holiday. After presenting this article to your practice-based journal club and discussing it with your colleagues, you also alter your practice handouts on travel medicine to reflect this new advice.

MIDWIFERY EXAMPLE

CLINICAL SCENARIO

You are a midwife who is newly employed in the postnatal unit of a tertiary hospital. You have noticed diversity of practice surrounding the provision of perineal ice-packs for pain relief in patients after spontaneous vaginal delivery. In addition to providing oral anti-inflammatories, some of your colleagues provide perineal ice-packs to these women in order to relieve perineal postpartum pain, while other nurses and midwives do not. You decide to find out about the effectiveness of an ice-pack applied during the immediate postpartum period in reducing perineal pain.

CLINICAL QUESTION

Following spontaneous vaginal delivery, does the application of an ice-pack to the perineal area reduce postpartum perineal pain?

Search terms and databases used to find the evidence

Database: PubMed–Clinical Queries (with 'therapy category' and 'narrow scope' selected).

Search terms: (perineal pain) AND ice

This search results in 5 articles. One matches your clinical question and you retrieve its full text.

Article chosen

Leventhal L, de Oliveira S, Nobre M, et al. Perineal analgesia with an ice pack after spontaneous vaginal birth: a randomised controlled trial. J Midwifery Women's Health 2011;56:141–6.

Structured abstract (adapted from the above)

Study design: Randomised controlled trial.

Setting: In-hospital birth centre averaging 900 births per month in São Paulo, Brazil.

Participants: 114 nulliparous women recovering from spontaneous vaginal deliveries, who experienced perineal pain ≥ 3 (0 = no pain to 10 = worst imaginable pain) within 2 and 48 hours following childbirth, regardless of perineal condition. Exclusion criteria included maternal, obstetric or clinical complications such as haemorrhoids, haematomas, newborn complications or instrumental births, multiple births, non-cephalic fetal presentation, postpartum fever treatment with antibiotics or had received a postpartum analgesic within 6 hours prior to inclusion into the study.

Intervention: The intervention group applied an ice-pack for a single instance for a 20-minute period in the perineal region between 2 and 48 hours postpartum. The placebo group applied a water-pack at room temperature for a single instance for a 20-minute period in the perineal region between 2 and 48 hours postpartum. The control group received no treatment in addition to routine care. All participants received routine care, consisting of 500 mg of metamizole, an anti-inflammatory agent which was administered orally every 8 hours. No other non-pharmacological treatment to alleviate perineal pain was provided.

Outcomes: The primary outcome measure was perineal pain, measured using a 0 (no pain) to 10 (worst imaginable pain) scale.

Follow-up period: Perineal pain was assessed prior to the intervention (baseline), immediately after the application of the pack (20 minutes), then 20 minutes later (40 minutes) and again 20 minutes later (60 minutes).

Main results: A comparison of the mean pain score at baseline and at 20 minutes showed a significant reduction of pain ($p < 0.001$) in all three groups. However, the intervention group had a lower average pain score at 20 minutes compared with the control group (1.6 versus 3.3, $p = 0.032$).

Conclusion: The use of ice-packs for 20 minutes was effective for the relief of perineal pain for women after spontaneous vaginal delivery.

Is this evidence likely to be biased?

- *Was the assignment of participants to groups randomised?*
  Yes. Participants were randomly allocated to intervention, placebo or control group in a 1:1:1 ratio by computer-generated randomisation. Blocks of six were used.
- *Was the allocation sequence concealed?*
  Yes. Allocation was concealed in an opaque, numbered sealed envelope which was opened by an individual not involved in the research.
- *Were the groups similar at the baseline or start of the trial?*
  Yes. The three groups had similar baseline mean pain scores and were similar on other characteristics such as socio-demographic characteristics, ambient, axillary and perineal temperatures and birth-related characteristics (for example, degree of perineal trauma).
- *Were participants blind to which study group they were in?*
  No. For this type of intervention it was not possible to blind participants.
- *Were the health professionals who provided the intervention blind to participants' study group?*
  No. Due to the nature of the intervention the research nurse who applied the intervention could not be blinded.

- *Were the assessors blind to participants' study group?*
  No. Even though the article states that there was an outcome assessor who was blinded and that participants were instructed not to inform the researcher which intervention they received, as the outcome was pain that was measured by participant self-report, the assessment of this was not blind as participants were not blinded to group allocation.
- *Were all participants who entered the trial properly accounted for at its conclusion, and how complete was the follow-up?*
  Yes. Although there is no figure showing participant flow through the trial, the article reports that no participants withdrew from the study (most likely to due to the short duration of the intervention and follow-up period) and that there was no migration of women among the groups.
- *Was intention-to-treat analysis used?*
  Cannot tell. The article does not specifically mention using intention-to-treat analysis, although it is likely that this is what occurred as there were no participants lost to follow-up or migration among groups.
- *Did the study have enough participants to minimise the play of chance?*
  Yes. The authors had undertaken a pilot study to inform sample size calculations and concluded that for a significance level of 5% and power level of 80%, a sample size of 38 patients per group was required. They adequately recruited to this sample size.

What are the main results?

The study reports the mean pain scores (and 95% confidence intervals) for all three groups at all time points (see Table 5.4). Although the article reports that all three groups had a statistically significant reduction in the mean pain score at 20 minutes compared with baseline, it is the between-group comparisons that you are interested in. The only statistically significant between-group difference was between the intervention (ice) group and control group at 20 minutes (a difference of 1.7). As standard deviations are not presented, a confidence interval for this effect size cannot be calculated.

The article also presents the data transformed into categories (pain worsened, improved <30%, improved 30–50%, improved >50%) at the end of the intervention (presumably 60 minutes); see Table 5.5. The authors nominate a decrease in pain of ≥30% as clinically significant. It is unclear whether the analysis by categorisation was planned a priori or an attempt to find significant results. If you use the authors' cut-off of ≥30% improvement and calculate the number of participants in each group who reported ≥30% improvement in pain, using the data in Table 5.5, this gives 20/38 (53%) in the control group, 31/38 (82%) in the placebo group, and 35/38 (92%) in the intervention group. You then calculate the following (using the formula for calculating 95% CI for absolute differences given in Box 4.3 in Chapter 4):

TABLE 5.4: MEAN PAIN (95% CI) AT FOUR TIME PERIODS FOR ALL GROUPS			
Time period	Mean (95% CI)		
	Control group (*n* = 38)	Placebo group (*n* = 38)	Intervention group (*n* = 38)
Baseline	4.5 (4.0 to 5.0)	4.6 (3.9 to 5.2)	4.6 (4.0 to 5.1)
20 minutes	3.3 (2.6 to 4.1)	2.1 (1.6 to 2.7)	1.6 (1.0 to 2.3)
40 minutes	3.3 (2.5 to 4.1)	1.8 (1.2 to 2.5)	1.5 (0.9 to 2.2)
60 minutes	3.1 (2.4 to 3.9)	1.8 (1.2 to 2.6)	1.5 (0.9 to 2.1)

TABLE 5.5:
NUMBER AND PERCENTAGE OF PARTICIPANTS IN EACH CATEGORY AT END OF INTERVENTION

Categorisation of pain	Control group (n = 38)	Placebo group (n = 38)	Intervention group (n = 38)
Worsened	3 (7.9)	1 (2.6)	0
Improved <30%	15 (39.5)	6 (15.8)	3 (7.9)
Improved 30–50%	12 (31.6)	15 (39.5)	13 (34.2)
Improved >50%	8 (21.1)	16 (42.1)	22 (57.9)

- Intervention group vs control group:

$$\text{Absolute benefit increase} = (92\% - 53\%) = 39\% \ (95\% \ CI \ 23\% \ to \ 55\%)$$
$$\text{Number needed to treat} = 1/39 = 3$$

- Intervention group vs placebo group:

$$\text{Absolute benefit increase} = (92\% - 82\%) = 10\% \ (95\% \ CI -6\% \ to \ 26\%)$$

As this effect is not statistically significant, there is no need to calculate number needed to treat.

- Placebo group vs control group:

$$\text{Absolute benefit increase} = (82\% - 53\%) = 29\% \ (95\% \ CI \ 13\% \ to \ 45\%)$$
$$\text{Number needed to treat} = 1/29 = 4$$

How might we use this evidence to inform practice?

You are reasonably confident of the results of this study. While there was no difference in pain outcomes between the intervention (ice-pack) and placebo (water-pack) groups, there was a difference between *any* pack (that is, either water-pack or ice-pack) and *no* pack. This difference may have been due to the placebo effect. In addition, all participants had a researcher remain at their side for 20 minutes providing guidance about postpartum care such as breastfeeding and postpartum bleeding, and this may have confounded the results. That is, the reduction in pain in all groups may be partially explained by the psychosocial support and distraction of having an experienced midwife's presence and support.

As there is unlikely to be any harm from using ice-packs (although it is advised that they should be removed after 20 minutes' use) and they are inexpensive, you decide that it may be worthwhile having ice-packs available to women as an option. Some women may not like using an ice-pack (in this study, 3 out of 117 declined to participate), so asking women if they wish to use this intervention will be important. Your ward already has the logistical issues associated with using ice-packs (such as a suitably-sized freezer that is accessible to staff, and appropriate infection control processes) in place.

NUTRITION THERAPY EXAMPLE

CLINICAL SCENARIO

As a clinical dietitian who works in the orthopaedic ward of a hospital, you are asked to review a 72-year-old woman admitted to the accident and emergency department 2 days ago with a fractured neck of femur. She went to theatre yesterday morning. Today, the orthopaedic team have commenced her on a full ward diet, but due to her thin and malnourished appearance they are concerned that she may develop a pressure ulcer. They have requested a dietitian consult for advice about whether supplementary nutritional support may reduce the risk of this occurring.

CLINICAL QUESTION

Does nutritional support prevent pressure ulcer development in people who have undergone surgery for a fractured neck of femur?

Search terms and databases used to find the evidence

Database: PubMed–Clinical Queries (with 'therapy category' and 'broad scope' selected).

Search terms: ((hip fracture*) OR (fractured neck of femur)) AND (nutritional support) AND (pressure ulcer*)

This search yielded three clinical studies and one systematic review. The systematic review relates to enteral nutrition and is therefore not relevant to the clinical question. Of the three clinical studies, only two relate to the clinical question; and as only one is a randomised controlled trial, this study is chosen.

Article chosen

Houwing R, Rozendaal M, Wouters-Wesseling W, et al. A randomised, double-blind assessment of the effect of nutritional supplementation on the prevention of pressure ulcers in hip-fracture patients. Clin Nutr 2003; 22:401–5.

Structured abstract (adapted from the above)

Study design: Randomised controlled trial.

Setting: Three medical centres in the Netherlands.

Participants: 103 participants who were post-surgery for a hip fracture and had a pressure ulcer risk score >8 according to the CBO risk-assessment tool. Exclusion criteria included: terminal care, metastatic hip fracture, insulin-dependent diabetes, renal disease (creatinine >176 mmol/L), hepatic disease, morbid obesity, need for a therapeutic diet incompatible with supplementation, and pregnancy or lactation.

Intervention: Participants in the intervention group (n = 51) received 400 mL daily of a nutritional supplement enriched with protein, arginine, zinc and antioxidants. Participants in the control group (n = 52) received a water-based placebo. The supplement and placebo were commenced postoperatively and continued for 4 weeks or until discharge. Participants in both groups also received a regular diet.

Outcomes: Pressure ulcer development (assessed using a four-stage classification); time of onset, size and location of any pressure ulcer(s) were also recorded.

Follow-up period: 4 weeks or until discharge. Participants were assessed daily by nursing staff.

Main results: There was no difference in the incidence of developing a pressure ulcer between the intervention (55%) and placebo (59%) groups; however, the supplemented group had a lower incidence of stage II ulcers and showed a trend towards later development of a pressure ulcer.

Conclusion: People with hip fracture are prone to developing pressure ulcers at an early postoperative stage. Initiating nutritional support at this stage may delay ulcer development and progression, but is unlikely to prevent this process occurring. The authors surmise that nutritional supplementation may be more effective if it is started earlier.

Is the evidence likely to be biased?

- *Was the assignment of participants to groups randomised?*
  Yes, participants were randomised to receive the study or placebo supplement in addition to their regular diet; however, the method of randomisation is not specified.

- *Was the allocation sequence concealed?*
  Cannot tell. The article does not describe how participants were allocated to groups.

- *Were the groups similar at the baseline or start of the trial?*
  The baseline characteristics of participants appear similar between the two study groups. There was also no difference in the median time between the start of supplementation and surgery or admission to hospital between the two study groups.

- *Were participants blind to which study group they were in?*
  Yes. Although participants may have been aware of what they were receiving due to the different taste and viscosity of the two drinks, it is unlikely that this was the case as there was no crossover of drinks between the study groups and participants would have been unlikely to know what each drink tasted like prior to the study.

- *Were the health professionals who provided the intervention blind to participants' study group?*
  Cannot tell. It is stated that nursing staff recorded each participant's daily intake of the supplement, but it is not clear who gave the supplements to the participants in between their regular meals each day.

- *Were the assessors blind to participants' study group?*
  Yes. The authors of the study acknowledge that, although each of the supplements (intervention supplement and placebo supplement) had a different look and taste, both supplements were provided in similar blinded packages to mask this difference. It is therefore unlikely that nursing staff would have been able to tell the difference between the two supplements. The presence of pressure ulcers was assessed daily by nursing staff according to a four-stage classification system based on the European Pressure Ulcer Advisory Panel Guidelines.

- *Were all participants who entered the trial properly accounted for at its conclusion, and how complete was follow-up?*
  No. The article does not state whether any participants were lost to follow-up or, if so, the reasons for this. However, based on the data provided in Table 4 of the article, it appears that two participants were lost from the intervention group and one from the control group. This would give a 97% follow-up rate.

- *Was intention-to-treat analysis used?*
  Cannot tell. The authors do not explicitly state that an intention-to-treat analysis was conducted; therefore, it is assumed that it was not. There was no mention of percentage error in drinks given, which may mean that there was no error; however, this should also have been stated in the article.

- *Did the study have enough participants to minimise the play of chance?*
  No. This study did not have enough participants to identify a significant difference in outcome between the two groups. A power calculation is described indicating that 350 participants were required in each group to detect a 25% decrease in pressure ulcer incidence. The study only recruited 14% of this required amount.

What are the main results?

As indicated by the confidence intervals and the p values, there were no statistically significant differences in any of the outcomes shown in Table 5.6. Based on the data that are provided in the article, you were able to calculate the absolute risk reduction (ARR), the 95% confidence interval associated with the ARR, and the number needed to treat. The development of one pressure ulcer would be prevented for every 27 people who receive the nutritional supplement and the development of one stage II pressure ulcer would be prevented for every 11 people who receive the nutritional supplement.

How might we use this evidence to inform practice?

There are a number of pieces of information which are relevant to this study but are not discussed in the article. For example, were participants using a pressure-ulcer relieving mattress prior to and/ or after the surgery? What was the immediacy of surgery and had participants been fasted a number of times preoperatively?

It may be difficult to generalise the results of this study to other populations as the sample in the study had specific characteristics, such as a pressure ulcer risk score of around 11, average age of 81 years, 81% of the group being female, a well-nourished population (average body mass index 23.5–24.5 kg/m^2) and a haemoglobin level of 7.1 g/L. These specific characteristics may partly explain the low number of participants who were able to be recruited into this study. The consequence of such specific characteristics is that the results can only be translated to patients who have similar characteristics. The patient in your clinical scenario differs from the study sample in a number of ways, and you do not feel confident that you can generalise the results to her. Additionally, the intervention was with a very specific supplement which was enriched with arginine, zinc and antioxidants (Cubitan®, from N.V. Nutricia in the Netherlands), and this product is not readily available in your region.

In conclusion, although this study had reasonably good internal validity, it does little to inform the dietitian about changing practices because it was severely underpowered and the sample population had a restricted profile. As such, nutritional practitioners should continue to provide nutritional support based on stronger data in the literature from different, yet related, patient populations. You are aware of good quality research studies that have demonstrated the positive effects of nutritional supplementation on pressure ulcer development in different clinical populations, for example malnourished patients or elderly people recovering from the acute phase of a critical illness, and so wonder if the lack of statistically significant results in this study was due to the fact that it was underpowered. Until a larger, sufficiently powered study is conducted with people with hip fractures, your practice will be guided by the research that has been conducted with other clinical populations.

TABLE 5.6: DEVELOPMENT OF PRESSURE ULCERS AFTER SUPPLEMENTATION OR PLACEBO						
Outcomes of interest to clinical question	Supplemented group ($n = 51$)	Placebo group ($n = 52$)	Difference (absolute risk reduction)	95% confidence interval for ARR	Number needed to treat	p value
Incidence of pressure ulcer (%)	55.1	58.8	58.8% − 55.1% = 3.7%	−10.2% to 17.6%	1/3.7 = 27	0.42
Incidence of stage II ulcer (%)	18.4	27.5	27.5% − 18.4% = 9.1%	−4.8% to 23%	1/9.1 = 10.99	0.34
ARR = absolute risk reduction.						

RADIATION THERAPY EXAMPLE

CLINICAL SCENARIO

You are a radiation therapist who is currently assisting at a radiation therapy clinic in preparation for your new advanced practice role in radiation therapy side-effect review. One of the clinic patients is Mr Jones who is 58 years old and has a glioblastoma (a brain tumour). He is being treated with palliative high-dose radiation therapy to 60 Gy in 30 fractions, over 6 weeks. Prior to starting his treatment, Mr Jones had surgery to de-bulk as much of the tumour as possible. When he attends the weekly radiation oncology review at the clinic with his wife, Mrs Jones says that they have been looking at the internet for other possible treatment options for her husband's terminal brain tumour. She mentions that they have seen some information which suggests that a drug named temozolomide is being used in conjunction with radiation therapy in other hospitals to improve survival and control of the disease. They ask why it is not being used in their case. You decide to look for evidence about the use of this drug, particularly its success with respect to survival post-treatment.

CLINICAL QUESTION

Does the use of concomitant and adjuvant temozolomide with radiation therapy improve survival for people with glioblastoma compared with high-dose palliative radiation therapy alone?

Search terms and databases used to find the evidence

Database: PubMed–Clinical Queries (with 'therapy category' and 'narrow scope' selected).

Search terms: (glioblastoma) AND (temozolomide) AND (radiotherapy OR radiation therapy) AND (survival)

The search resulted in 23 articles. Of these, three articles are relevant to your question and compare radiation therapy combined with temozolomide to radiation therapy alone. One of these is a Phase II randomised controlled trial with 130 participants. In this study, overall survival, progression-free survival and toxicity are the primary outcomes. The other publication (a 2005 article) is a Phase III international multi-centre randomised controlled trial with 573 participants. The primary outcome of this study is overall survival, with secondary outcomes being progression-free survival, safety and quality of life. You choose the second article to fully appraise, as it is the most relevant to your question and because it is a Phase III trial and had a larger sample size. The third article is a more recent (2009) article that reports the 5-year follow up results of the Phase III trial, and you decide to review both articles related to this study.

Articles chosen

Stupp R, Mason W, van den Bent M, et al. Radiotherapy plus concomitant and adjuvant temozolomide for glioblastoma. N Engl J Med 2005;352:987–96.

Stupp R, Hegi M, Mason WP, et al. Effects of radiotherapy with concomitant and adjuvant temozolomide versus radiotherapy alone on survival in glioblastoma in a randomised phase III study: 5-year analysis of the EORTC-NCIC trial. Lancet Oncol 2009;10:459–66.

Structured abstract (adapted from the above)

Study design: Phase III, multi-centre, randomised controlled trial.

Setting: Participants were recruited from 85 radiation oncology institutions in 15 countries throughout Europe and Canada.

Participants: 573 participants aged between 18 and 70 years (median age 56 years) with newly diagnosed histologically confirmed glioblastoma. Participants needed a World Health Organization performance status of 2 or less (indicating that they were relatively fit and self-caring). Additional specific inclusion criteria related to haematological, renal and hepatic function; serum creatinine and bilirubin levels.

Intervention: Participants in the control group ($n = 286$) received only radiation therapy (60 Gy, 30 fractions, 5 days a week for 6 weeks). Participants in the intervention group ($n = 287$) received radiation therapy (same dose and fractionation as the control group) and concomitant temozolomide (75 mg per square metre of body surface area per day, given 7 days a week from the first to the last day of radiation therapy, but for no longer than 49 days). Intervention group participants then had a 4-week break before receiving up to 6 cycles of adjuvant temozolomide (5-day schedule every 28 days) as well as prophylactic antibiotics due to increased chance of infection and prophylactic anti-emetics due to increased chance of nausea/vomiting.

Outcomes: The primary outcome was survival. Secondary outcomes were progression-free survival, safety (toxicity) and quality of life.

Follow-up period: Median follow-up was 51 months (in 2009 article). During radiation therapy, participants were seen every week. After the radiation therapy was completed, participants were seen 21–28 days after this, and every 3 months thereafter. Participants in the intervention group received a monthly clinical evaluation while receiving the adjuvant temozolomide therapy and a comprehensive assessment at the end of cycles 3 and 6.

Main results: During the 5 years of follow-up, 254 (89%) of the intervention group participants and 278 (97%) of the control group participants died. Overall survival was 27.2% (95% CI 22.2 to 32.5) at 2 years, 16.0% (12.0 to 20.6) at 3 years, 12.1% (8.5 to 16.4) at 4 years and 9.8% (6.4 to 14.0) at 5 years for the intervention group, compared with 10.9% (7.6 to 14.8), 4.4% (2.4 to 7.2), 3.0% (1.4 to 5.7) and 1.9% (0.6 to 4.4) in the control group (hazard ratio 0.6, 95% CI 0.5 to 0.7, $p < 0.0001$).

Conclusion: Benefits of temozolomide in addition to radiation therapy for people with newly diagnosed glioblastoma lasted throughout 5 years of follow-up.

Is the evidence likely to be biased?

- *Was the assignment of participants to groups randomised?*
  Yes. Participants were randomly allocated to either the intervention or the control group, although details of the exact method of randomisation are not provided. Participants were stratified according to performance status, previous surgery and treatment centre.

- *Was the allocation sequence concealed?*
  Yes. The article states that participants were centrally randomised over the phone or internet at the headquarters of a European research centre.

- *Were the groups similar at the baseline or start of the trial?*
  Yes. The article provides details about a large range of participant characteristics and the two groups appear to have been well balanced at baseline.

- *Were participants blind to which study group they were in?*
  No. For this trial, it was not possible for participants to be blinded to group allocation.

- *Were the health professionals who provided the intervention blind to participants' study group?*
  No. For this trial, it was not possible for the health professionals who provided the intervention to be blinded to group allocation.

- *Were the assessors blind to participants' study group?*
  No. Because of the nature and toxic effects of both treatments it was not possible to blind the assessors to the study group. The assessments were performed by qualified radiation oncologists.

- *Were all participants who entered the trial properly accounted for at its conclusion, and how complete was follow-up?*
  Yes. The article includes a flowchart showing participant flow throughout the trial. Of the 287 participants randomised to the intervention group, 3 did not start treatment, 14 discontinued the radiotherapy and 37 discontinued the temozolomide; 287 were included in the intention-to-treat analysis and 284 in the safety analysis. Of the 286 control group participants, 7 did not start treatment and 19 discontinued treatment; 286 were included in the intention-to-treat analysis and 279 in the safety analysis. Because of the population (palliative patients) and primary outcome of this study (survival), participants who died would not have been considered as lost to follow-up.
- *Was intention-to-treat analysis used?*
  Yes. The article stated that all analyses were conducted on an intention-to-treat basis, which is important as there were a number of reported deviations from the treatment allocation and treatment protocol.
- *Did the study have enough participants to minimise the play of chance?*
  Yes. This study had 80% power at a significance level of 0.05 to detect a 33% increase in median survival (hazard ratio for death, 0.75), assuming that 382 deaths occurred.

What are the main results?

Survival and disease progression: A total of 254 (89%) of the intervention group participants and 278 (97%) of the control group participants had died by the 5-year follow-up. The article reports that the hazard ratio for survival among participants in the intervention group compared with those in the control group was 0.6 (95% CI 0.5 to 0.7), which is statistically significant. Table 5.7 shows the overall survival according to group.

The median difference between the two groups in length of survival (that is, the median survival benefit) was 14.6 – 12.1 = 2.5 months. In the 2005 article it is reported that during the concomitant temozolomide therapy, 7% of participants had a grade 3 (severe adverse effect) or 4 (life-threatening effect) haematological effect. At the 5-year follow up, severe late toxicity was observed in 2 patients in the intervention group (visual disturbance and seizure) and in 1 patient in the control group (fatigue).

How do we use this evidence to inform practice?

You are satisfied with the validity of the study's results and consider the results to be important and, when you compare the demographic and clinical details of Mr Jones to the study participants, they compare well. Therefore, you decide to consider the side-effect profile of temozolomide (which includes fatigue and immunosuppression) before discussing this study with the radiation oncologist for consideration about the potential use of temozolomide in the clinic where you work.

The article does not provide data about the effects of the interventions on participants' quality of life. The article describes collecting data about quality of life as a secondary endpoint but does not report the data in this main article. As this is an important issue to consider, you will search for an article that contains the quality-of-life data.

TABLE 5.7: OVERALL SURVIVAL ACCORDING TO GROUP		
Outcome	Intervention group (*n* = 287)	Control group (*n* = 286)
Median overall survival - months (95% CI)	14.6 (13.2 to 16.8)	12.1 (11.2 to 13.0)
Overall survival at 5 years - % (95% CI)	9.8 (6.4 to 14.0)	1.9 (0.6 to 4.4)

There are also a number of resource issues related to the use of temozolomide which have to be evaluated in order to ensure that, if the decision is made to use this treatment, there is adequate funding for staff and equipment to support its use. If the clinic decides to implement the use of temozolomide, together with the radiation oncologist, you will make a time to explain the results of the study to Mr and Mrs Jones.

COMPLEMENTARY AND ALTERNATIVE MEDICINE EXAMPLE

CLINICAL SCENARIO

As an acupuncturist, you have had years of experience in treating people with drug addictions. In your experience, auricular acupuncture is particularly useful for reducing anxiety during drug withdrawal. You were invited to present your observations to clinicians at a local meeting. After your lecture, you were approached by a consultant who specialises in detoxification for drug dependency. He claimed that, as far as he was aware, the evidence for acupuncture was not convincing but said that he would invite you to join his team, if you could produce sound data demonstrating that acupuncture is, in fact, effective and practical for treating drug addictions.

CLINICAL QUESTION

Is auricular acupuncture effective at reducing anxiety in people with drug addictions who are undergoing withdrawal?

Search terms and databases used to find the evidence

Database: PubMed–Clinical Queries (with 'therapy category' and 'narrow scope' selected).

Search terms: (auricular acupuncture) AND (withdraw*) AND (anxiety)

This search retrieves two results. Of these, one article was directly relevant to the question.

Article chosen

Black S, Carey E, Webber A, et al. Determining the efficacy of auricular acupuncture for reducing anxiety in patients withdrawing from psychoactive drugs. J Subst Abuse Treat 2011;41:279–87.

Structured abstract (adapted from the above)

Study design: Randomised controlled trial.

Setting: Outpatient addiction service in Canada.

Participants: 140 patients were randomised. Patients aged 18 years or older were included if suffering from self-reported alcohol, cocaine, nicotine, cannabis, opioid, benzodiazepine or amphetamine dependency. Patients were excluded if they had received acupuncture during the last 3 months, were currently receiving anti-anxiety treatments or had a history of a bleeding disorder.

Intervention: Participants were randomised into three groups. The experimental group had needles inserted in both auricles at the 5 points specified by the National Acupuncture Detoxification Association protocol. Needles were inserted into the cartilage to a depth of 1–3 mm and left in situ for 45 minutes. The control group had 5 needles inserted into non-acupuncture points on the helix of both auricles; otherwise the procedure was identical. Participants in a second control group received no acupuncture, but the treatment setting (designed to encourage relaxation) and pre-needle procedure was the same as the other two groups. Three acupuncture sessions of 45 minutes duration were given to participants in groups A and B during a maximum of a 2-week period.

Outcomes: The primary outcome measure was participant state anxiety (measured using the Spielberger State–Trait Anxiety Inventory (STAI)). Secondary outcome measures were changes in heart rate and blood pressure.

Follow-up period: Assessments were performed on the day of recruitment and immediately pre and post each treatment.

Main results: 101 participants completed at least one, 71 completed two, and 49 completed all three treatment sessions. There were no significant between-group differences in dropout rates. Intention-to-treat analysis of the 101 participants who had at least one acupuncture session showed no significant effects on any outcome measure of real versus sham-acupuncture or of real versus no acupuncture. No adverse effects were noted.

Conclusion: Real acupuncture was not more effective than sham-acupuncture or no acupuncture in reducing anxiety of patients with mixed dependences during withdrawal.

Is the evidence likely to be biased?

- *Was the assignment of participants to groups randomised?*
  Yes. Participants were randomised using a computerised random-number generation procedure.

- *Was the allocation sequence concealed?*
  Cannot tell. It is not clear whether this was achieved. The article states that research staff did not have access to the master list which linked participants' study ID number to treatment allocation, but this may refer to assessor blinding rather than concealed allocation.

- *Were the groups similar at the baseline or start of the trial?*
  Yes. The demographic and clinical characteristics and pre-treatment anxiety scores appear to be similar across all three groups.

- *Were participants blind to which study group they were in?*
  Cannot tell. This is not clearly reported. It appears that there was some attempt to blind participants, as the article states that participants were not aware of the placebo condition during treatment. So, it is possible that there was participant blinding for acupuncture versus sham-acupuncture groups, but the success of patient-blinding was not tested. Therefore we do not know whether some patients managed to guess which group they had been allocated to.

- *Were the health professionals who provided the intervention blind to participants' study group?*
  No. This would be difficult (but not impossible) to achieve in acupuncture trials.

- *Were the assessors blind to participants' study group?*
  Yes, for some measures. The article states that the research staff who administered the outcome measures were blind to participants' treatment allocation, thus assessment of heart rate and blood pressure was blinded. However, as anxiety was assessed using a self-report measure, the assessment of this outcome was not blind as it is unlikely that participants were blinded to group allocation.

- *Were all participants who entered the trial properly accounted for at its conclusion, and how complete was follow-up?*
  No. There was a high proportion of dropouts (28% by session 1, 50% by session 2 and 65% by session 3), as one might expect in this type of setting and study. There was no significant difference in dropout rates between the groups. Reasons are not given for why participants were lost to follow-up, although the article states that no participant explicitly withdrew from the study or reported an adverse effect.

- *Was intention-to-treat analysis used?*
  Cannot tell. Although the authors do not explicitly state that an intention-to-treat analysis was conducted, the article does state that data from participants were used in the analysis regardless of the number of sessions that they attended; so it appears that an intention-to-treat analysis was possibly conducted.
- *Did the study have enough participants to minimise the play of chance?*
  Yes. Prior to the study, the authors calculated that they would need to recruit 22 participants per group to detect a significant difference ($p = 0.05$) with a power of 80%, and this number was recruited.

What are the main results?

There was a decrease in state anxiety scores from pre-treatment to post-treatment in all three groups. However, this change was very similar in all three groups and there were no statistically significant between-group differences. The same applies to the secondary endpoints of heart rate and blood pressure.

How might we use this evidence to inform practice?

There are a number of aspects of the methodology and conduct of this study that were poorly reported (which makes assessing internal validity difficult), and several other caveats of this study to consider. The reported findings relate to measurements taken before the first and immediately after the last treatment. We therefore cannot tell anything about medium- or long-term effects. We also are unable to say whether there are any effects on drug usage or other variables not quantified in this study. Similarly, we cannot be sure whether a different acupuncture protocol (for example, longer treatment periods) would have generated different effects; nor can we tell from this study that acupuncture has no effects on specific addictions (for example, exclusively cocaine dependence).

The research question posed by this study was fairly narrow. It may be tempting to extrapolate from these findings that acupuncture is ineffective for drug withdrawal. Strictly speaking, this would not be permissible on the basis of the results of this study. All we can say with a reasonable degree of certainty is that, for patients with mixed addictions, three sessions of an accepted auricular acupuncture protocol did not reduce anxiety immediately after treatment significantly more than sham acupuncture or a relaxation control. This conclusion is nevertheless meaningful in the present context. The acupuncturist did have the initial impression that acupuncture was highly effective in reducing withdrawal-induced anxiety. This research thus shows how wrong such clinical impressions can be.

HUMAN MOVEMENT EXAMPLE

CLINICAL SCENARIO

As a clinical exercise physiologist working in a health and fitness centre you have received a referral from a general practitioner for a 53-year-old male who underwent a prostatectomy 14 months ago and has been on androgen suppression therapy (AST) since the operation. You undertake a fitness appraisal and determine that the man has an average exercise capacity but has very low strength. He complains of feeling tired and weak and is now not strong enough to complete tasks around the home and activities such as lifting up his grandchildren. You wonder whether there are any benefits of resistance training in the context of AST.

CLINICAL QUESTION

Is resistance training effective at improving muscle strength in a man taking androgen suppression therapy?

Search terms and databases used to find the evidence

Database: PubMed–Clinical Queries (with 'therapy category' and 'narrow scope' selected).

Search terms: You are aware that the terms 'androgen suppression therapy' and 'androgen deprivation therapy' are used synonymously, therefore your search terms are: (androgen (suppression OR deprivation) therapy) AND (resistance training)

This search retrieved 5 results. A quick read of the abstracts showed that two were protocol papers, and one used resistance training only and looked at adherence. Another compared the effects of aerobic training, resistance training and a control group (three groups). The other trial (Galvão et al 2010) included 57 patients in a two-group design where the effects of a combined aerobic and resistance training program was compared with a control group. Given that you are considering giving your patient an exercise program that contains aerobic training, you choose the Galvão et al (2010) study to determine whether resistance training is able to improve strength alongside aerobic exercise.

Article chosen

Galvão D, Taaffe DR, Spry N, et al. Combined resistance and aerobic exercise program reverses muscle loss in men undergoing androgen suppression therapy for prostate cancer without bone metastases: a randomised controlled trial. J Clin Oncol 2010;28:340–7.

Structured abstract (adapted from the above)

Study design: Randomised controlled trial.

Setting: Participants were recruited from a hospital in Perth, Western Australia. The exercise training site locations were not supplied.

Participants: 57 participants directly referred by oncologists. Inclusion criteria: histologically documented prostate cancer, minimum prior exposure to AST longer than 2 months, without prostate-specific antigen evidence of disease activity, and anticipated to remain hypogonadal for the subsequent 6 months. Exclusion criteria: bone metastatic disease, musculoskeletal, cardiovascular or neurological disorders that could inhibit them from exercising, inability to walk 400 metres or undertake upper and lower limb exercise, and resistance training in the previous 3 months.

Intervention: Participants were randomly assigned to a program of resistance and aerobic exercise ($n = 29$) or usual care ($n = 28$) for 12 weeks. The resistance exercises included chest press, seated row, shoulder press, triceps extension, leg press, leg extension and leg curl, with abdominal crunches also performed. Sessions commenced and concluded with general flexibility exercises. The resistance exercise program was designed to progress from 12- to 6-repetition maximum (RM) for two to four sets per exercise. The aerobic component of the training program included 15 to 20 minutes of cardiovascular exercises (cycling and walking/jogging) at 65–80% maximum heart rate and perceived exertion at 11 to 13 (6 to 20 point, Borg scale). Sessions were conducted in small groups of one to five participants under direct supervision of an exercise physiologist.

Outcomes: *Primary outcomes:* whole-body and regional lean mass, fat mass and percentage fat. *Secondary outcomes:* muscle strength and endurance, functional performance, cardiorespiratory capacity balance, falls self-efficacy, blood biomarkers and quality of life.

Follow-up period: 12 weeks. Assessments were administered at baseline and at the end of the 12-week intervention.

Main results: Compared with usual care, participants in the intervention group had significant increases in lean mass for total body, upper limb and lower limb, increased muscle strength (chest press, seated row, leg press and leg extension) and 6-metre walk time, improvement in some aspects of quality of life (general health and less fatigue), and decreased levels of C-reactive protein.

Conclusion: Resistance exercise in combination with aerobic training improved muscle mass, strength, physical function and balance in hypogonadal men.

Is the evidence likely to be biased?

- *Was the assignment of participants to groups randomised?*
  Yes, Participants were randomly allocated using a computer random-assignment program.
- *Was the allocation sequence concealed?*
  Yes. The allocation sequence was concealed from the project coordinator and exercise physiologist involved in assigning participants to groups.
- *Were the groups similar at the baseline or start of the trial?*
  Yes. There were no significant differences between groups at baseline in regard to demographics, clinical characteristics or primary and secondary outcome measures.
- *Were participants blind to which study group they were in?*
  No. For this trial it was not possible for participants to be blinded to group allocation.
- *Were the health professionals who provided the intervention blind to participants' study group?*
  No. For this trial it was not possible for the exercise physiologists who provided the intervention to be blinded to group allocation.
- *Were the assessors blind to participants' study group?*
  Cannot tell. There is no mention in the article of whether the assessors were blinded to group allocation, so it is assumed that they were not.
- *Were all participants who entered the trial properly accounted for at its conclusion, and how complete was follow-up?*
  Yes. The study had a follow-up rate of 96.5%. One participant in the usual care group was lost to follow-up and one in the intervention group discontinued the intervention.
- *Was intention-to-treat analysis used?*
  Yes. The authors explicitly state that intention-to-treat analysis was used.
- *Did the study have enough participants to minimise the play of chance?*
  Yes. A power calculation was performed with change in whole-body lean mass used as the primary outcome measure. This found that 25 participants per group were needed to detect a mean difference in change of 1 kg (SD = 1.25) at the end of the 12 weeks (80% power and alpha = 0.05). The study recruited a total of 57 participants.

What are the main results?

The outcome measures relevant to the clinical question are shown in Table 5.8. In the article, the authors provide the mean scores (and their standard deviation) at baseline and at 12 weeks for both groups, along with the adjusted group difference in mean change over the 12 weeks and the 95% confidence interval for the mean change. For all of the strength outcome measures shown in the table, the between-group differences were statistically significant (note that none of the confidence intervals include the no effect value of 0).

How might we use this evidence to inform practice?

After critically appraising the internal validity of this trial, you believe that there is only a low likelihood that these results are biased. There was a statistically significant between-group difference, in favour of the intervention group, for the strength outcome measures. You discuss the results of the trial with your patient, the benefits and likely increase that he may experience in lean mass and strength and explain what the exercise program would involve. He decides that he would like to try it.

TABLE 5.8:
EFFECT OF INTERVENTION ON STRENGTH OUTCOMES

Outcomes of interest to clinical question	Adjusted group difference in mean change over 12 weeks (95% confidence interval)	p value
Total body lean mass (kg)	0.76 (0.01 to 1.5)	0.047
Upper limb lean mass (kg)	0.26 (0.11 to 0.42)	<0.001
Lower limb lean mass (kg)	0.54 (0.09 to 1.0)	0.019
Chest press strength (kg)	2.8 (0.5 to 5.1)	0.018
Seated row strength (kg)	5.1 (3.3 to 7.0)	<0.001
Leg press strength (kg)	30.8 (20.1 to 41.6)	<0.001
Leg extension strength (kg)	11.5 (7.2 to 15.8)	<0.001

PARAMEDICINE EXAMPLE

CLINICAL SCENARIO

You are a paramedic and, in your experience, adrenaline has been used as part of the standard care for the management of out-of-hospital cardiac arrest. You recently attended a paramedic conference and as part of a discussion with some paramedics from another country, you were interested to hear that they do not routinely use adrenaline as part of the management of out-of-hospital cardiac arrest. Given these contradictory practices, you wonder if there is any evidence of the effectiveness of adrenaline in improving the survival to hospital discharge of patients who have a cardiac arrest in an out-of-hospital setting.

CLINICAL QUESTION

For patients who have an out-of-hospital cardiac arrest, does the use of adrenaline, in addition to usual care, improve survival to hospital discharge?

Search terms and databases used to find the evidence

Database: PubMed–Clinical Queries (with 'therapy category' and 'narrow scope' selected).

Search terms: As you are aware that adrenaline is referred to as epinephrine in some countries, you use this as a synonym in your search terms: (cardiac arrest) AND (epinephrine OR adrenaline) AND (out-of-hospital)

The search identified 33 articles. Following review of the titles and abstract, you choose the article which most closely matched your clinical question for appraisal.

Article chosen

Jacobs I, Finn J, Jelinek G, et al. Effect of adrenaline on survival in out-of-hospital cardiac arrest: a randomised double-blind placebo-controlled trial. Resuscitation 2011;82:1138–43.

Structured abstract (adapted from the above)

Study design: Randomised controlled trial.

Setting: Out-of-hospital cardiac arrest patients attended by St John Ambulance Western Australia paramedics.

Participants: Patients ($n = 601$) who experienced an out-of-hospital cardiac arrest from any cause who were over 18 years of age, with resuscitation commenced by paramedics.

Intervention: The administration of either the intervention drug, adrenaline 1 mg in 1 mL (10 mL vial), or the control drug, placebo (normal saline) 1 mL (10 mL vial) intravenously at 3 minute intervals to a maximum of 10 mL of either drug, along with other normal resuscitation procedures (that is, defibrillation) when indicated.

Outcomes: The primary outcome was survival to hospital discharge. Secondary outcomes were pre-hospital return of spontaneous circulation and Cerebral Performance Category at hospital discharge.

Follow-up period: This was not specified in the article. However, as the outcome was survival to hospital discharge, the follow-up period would have had to have been at least until hospital separation. Outcome data were obtained from the Western Australian Emergency, Hospital Morbidity and Mortality Data system.

Main results: Pre-hospital return of spontaneous circulation occurred in 23.5% of adrenaline group participants and 8.4% of control group participants (odds ratio = 3.4; 95% CI 2.0 to 5.6). Survival to hospital discharge was 5 (1.9%) of the control group and 11 (4.0%) of the adrenaline group (odds ratio = 2.2; 95% CI 0.7 to 6.3).

Conclusion: Patients who received adrenaline during resuscitation for cardiac arrest had no significant improvement in survival to hospital discharge compared with the placebo group. However, there was a higher likelihood of achieving a return of spontaneous circulation in the pre-hospital setting following adrenaline administration.

Is the evidence likely to be biased?

- *Was the assignment of participants to groups randomised?*
  Yes. A computer-generated randomisation schedule was used.

- *Was the allocation sequence concealed?*
  Yes. The intervention and control vials were commercially prepared (independently of the researchers) in identical 10 mL vials with a tamperproof seal and were only identifiable by a randomisation number on the vial.

- *Were the groups similar at the baseline or start of the trial?*
  Yes. Participants in the groups were similar on most patient and arrest characteristics. The intervention group had a higher proportion of patients who were transported to hospital (88.6% compared with 82.1% in the control group). It is unclear whether this baseline difference may have had a confounding effect on the results.

- *Were participants blind to which study group they were in?*
  Yes. The patients were in cardiac arrest and blinded to the study group they were in and the contents of the vial that was administered.

- *Were the health professionals who provided the intervention blind to participants' study group?*
  Yes. The intervention and control vials were identical 10 mL vials with a tamperproof seal, the only difference being the randomisation number on the vial.

- *Were the assessors blind to participants' study group?*
  Yes. It appears that the assessors were blinded for at least some of the outcomes. Data for the outcome of Cerebral Performance Category were extracted from patient hospital records by a blinded assessor. Data about the primary outcome were extracted from the Emergency, Hospital Morbidity and Mortality data systems, so it is possible that the extraction of this data was performed in a blinded manner.

- *Were all participants who entered the trial properly accounted for at its conclusion, and how complete was follow-up?*
  Yes. The authors provide a flow diagram which shows that after randomisation of 601 participants, 67 were subsequently excluded as the randomisation number was lost or not recorded. This left 262 participants in the placebo group (of these, 6 did not receive the placebo) and 272 in the adrenaline group (of these, 8 did not receive the adrenaline). Reasons are provided for why these 14 participants did not receive the placebo or adrenaline as intended.
- *Was intention-to-treat analysis used?*
  Yes. The authors stated they used an intention-to-treat analysis.
- *Did the study have enough participants to minimise the play of chance?*
  No. The authors calculated that they needed to recruit 2213 patients per group; however, their actual recruitment was much lower than this ($n = 601$). The authors stated in the discussion that the study was underpowered to detect a significant effect in survival to hospital discharge. The lack of study participants was due to an unforeseen lack of participation by other Australian and New Zealand ambulance services after initial agreement to participate in the trial.

What are the main results?

The between-group difference for survival to hospital discharge was not statistically significant (4% in the intervention group vs 1.9% in the control group; odds ratio of 2.2, 95% CI 0.7 to 6.3). Because this confidence interval includes the no effect value (of 1), it indicates that the difference is not statistically significant. The study was underpowered (sample size of only 601 recruits out of the 2213 estimated by a statistical power calculation). This means that we cannot be sure whether the lack of statistical difference was the result of insufficient real effect–that is, the adrenaline does not contribute to survival–or too small a sample. There was a statistically significant difference between the groups for pre-hospital return of spontaneous circulation, in favour of the intervention group (odds ratio = 3.4; 95% CI 2.0 to 5.6).

How might we use this evidence to inform practice?

It is difficult to make use of this study in deciding intervention options for patients with out-of-hospital cardiac arrest. A naïve interpretation of the study's results would suggest that adrenaline does not produce benefit except in short-term outcomes (although a return of spontaneous circulation–if it does not lead to a better chance of leaving hospital alive–is probably not enough for most patients). However, because the study sample was (much) smaller than the estimated required minimum to achieve adequate power, we cannot know whether inadequate sample size rather than ineffectiveness of adrenaline caused the non-significant result. In other words, we still do not know whether adrenaline is effective or not. Accordingly, it is reasonable to either continue to use it (as you do in your service) or not (as other services do), until a repeat trial with adequate power is conducted.

PHARMACY EXAMPLE

CLINICAL SCENARIO

You are the professional services programs manager for a large group of community pharmacies. Your role is to oversee the programs offered by the pharmacies, including the development and implementation of new professional programs and services for delivery across the group. There are 20 pharmacies in the group, including medical centre, strip and shopping centre pharmacies in metropolitan and regional locations. Your pharmacies are very actively engaged with the wider community, currently offering professional services in the area of asthma, sleep, healthy eating (weight), wound care and baby care. Many of these services involve the integration of other health professionals within and outside of the pharmacy.

Although these current services are working well, patients with diabetes are becoming a key focus of the pharmacies you work with. Many of them already offer a variety of diabetes products, and links with National Diabetes Services and other local health professionals. Diabetes is a significant health issue in the wider community and the majority of the patients seen in the pharmacies have type 2 diabetes. The pharmacists within the group would like to provide a more structured and focused pharmacy-based service for patients with type 2 diabetes. They think this service should be centred on the monthly visits that patients make to collect their regular prescriptions, and strongly believe that this service would improve patients' clinical care. They have approached you as the professional services programs manager to investigate whether this type of program would be feasible for the group. You search the literature for evidence to support their assertions.

CLINICAL QUESTION

In adults with type 2 diabetes, can a focused, community-pharmacy-delivered education and management service improve clinical outcomes?

Search terms and databases used to find the evidence

Database: PubMed–Clinical Queries (with 'therapy category' and 'narrow scope' selected).

Search terms: community AND pharmac* AND education AND diabetes

This search resulted in 15 articles. Only two are relevant to your question, and you choose the one that most closely matches it.

Article chosen

Krass I, Armour C, Mitchell B, et al. The Pharmacy Diabetes Care Program: assessment of a community pharmacy diabetes service model in Australia. Diab Med 2007;24:677–83.

Structured abstract (adapted from the above)

Study design: Randomised controlled trial.

Setting: 56 randomly selected urban and rural Australian community pharmacies (28 intervention, 28 control).

Participants: 289 patients with type 2 diabetes (149 in intervention group and 140 in control group). Inclusion criteria were patients who had (1) $HbA_{1c} \geq 7.5\%$ and were taking at least one oral glucose-lowering medication or insulin; or (2) $HbA_{1c} \geq 7.0\%$ and were taking at least one oral glucose-lowering medication or insulin and who were on at least one anti-hypertensive, angina or lipid-lowering drug.

Intervention: Pharmacy-delivered diabetes service which comprised an ongoing cycle of assessment, management and review, provided at regular intervals (5 times) over 6 months. Services included support for self-monitoring of blood glucose, education, adherence support and reminders of checks for diabetes complications. Control pharmacists provided usual care (that is, no specialised diabetes service).

Outcomes: Primary outcome was change in HbA_{1c} (%); secondary outcomes were: blood pressure, lipid measures, body mass index and a quality-of-life measure (EQ-5D assessment tool).

Follow-up period: 6 months.

Main results: There was a significant improvement in glycaemic control in the intervention group compared with the control group: a reduction in HbA_{1c} in intervention group participants of −0.97% (95% CI −0.8 to −1.14) compared with −0.27% (95% CI −0.15 to −0.39) in control group participants. Improvements in blood pressure control and quality-of-life indicators were also seen in the intervention group.

Conclusion: The pharmacy-delivered diabetes service resulted in significant improvements in clinical and humanistic outcomes for type 2 diabetes patients.

Is the evidence likely to be biased?

- *Was the assignment of participants to groups randomised?*
  Yes. Pharmacies were randomly allocated to either the intervention or the control group (that is, this was a cluster trial), but no further details are given about the process.

- *Was the allocation sequence concealed?*
  Cannot tell. There is no mention in the article of concealed allocation.

- *Were the groups similar at the baseline or start of the trial?*
  Yes, for some characteristics. The article reports that the two groups were similar in terms of only very basic pharmacy (cluster) characteristics (number of staff, location), pharmacists (age, gender, position in pharmacy) and most participant characteristics (demographics, diabetes history and most clinical characteristics). However, there was a baseline difference in the primary outcome of HbA_{1c} (8.9% in intervention vs 8.3% in control group), which the authors adjusted for in the analyses.

- *Were participants blind to which study group they were in?*
  No. For this intervention, it was not possible to blind participants to group allocation.

- *Were the health professionals who provided the intervention blind to participants' study group?*
  No. For this intervention, it was not possible to blind the pharmacies to group allocation.

- *Were the assessors blind to participants' study group?*
  No for some measures, and cannot tell for other measures. Data for the outcomes of HbA_{1c}, blood pressure and lipids were obtained from participants' GPs. It is not described whether participants' GPs knew which group participants were in, but it is possible that at least some of them would have been aware of group allocation (if for no other reason than that they would have been involved in increased management of participants in the intervention group). For the primary outcome measure of HbA_{1c}, the uncertainty regarding blinding is not of concern as it is an objective outcome measure. However, for other measures such as quality of life, assessment was not blinded.

- *Were all participants who entered the trial properly accounted for at its conclusion, and how complete was follow-up?*
  Yes and no. The article provides a participant flowchart showing that 19 (12%) participants withdrew from the control group ($n = 159$ at baseline) and 27 (15%) from the intervention group ($n = 176$ at baseline). In addition, the article reports that final data from participants' GPs were unable to be obtained for 33 intervention and 39 control group participants (some who withdrew and some who did not), giving loss to follow-up of approximately 22%. However, as this is a cluster trial it would also have been useful to have information about whether any clusters withdrew, but this information is not provided.

- *Was intention-to-treat analysis used?*
  No. The article does not mention whether intention-to-treat analysis was conducted. There is no mention of any attempt to handle the data that were missing for some participants, and therefore it is assumed that intention-to-treat analysis was not done.

- *Did the study have enough participants to minimise the play of chance?*
  No. The article stated that to detect a 0.5% reduction in HbA_{1c} in the intervention group compared with the control group, with a power of 90% at the 5% significance level, at least 180 patients were required in each group. The study collected baseline data for 159 control group participants and 176 intervention group participants, which is less than the required amount.

TABLE 5.9: MEAN CHANGE SCORE (BASELINE TO 6 MONTHS) FOR THE INTERVENTION AND CONTROL GROUPS FOR OUTCOMES WITH A STATISTICALLY SIGNIFICANT BETWEEN-GROUP DIFFERENCE				
	Mean (95% CI) change score		Difference in mean change scores	p value
	Intervention group	Control group		
HbA$_{1c}$ (%)	−1.0 (−0.8 to −1.3)	−0.3 (−0.003 to −0.5)	−0.7	<0.01
Health state scale of the EQ-5D (range 0 to 100)	5.3 (1.7 to 8.8)	1.1 (−1.6 to 3.8)	4.2	0.02

EQ-5D is a standardised quality-of-life/health status assessment tool.

What are the main results?

Table 5.9 shows the outcomes for which there was a statistically significant between-group difference in the change scores at follow-up. The main benefit of the study results are the improvement of HbA$_{1c}$ scores by a mean change of 0.7%, which was statistically significant (unfortunately, confidence intervals for this cannot be calculated from the data the authors provide). We must now ask ourselves if this is large enough to be considered clinically significant and therefore enough to change practice. Questions about clinical significance are subjective. Ideally a 'minimally important clinical difference' in HbA$_{1c}$ would be set before the study was conducted (in fact, as a hypothesis). Since this did not happen, we must use our judgment. A reduction of a patient's HbA$_{1c}$ by between 0.5% and 1% is associated with a better outcome from diabetes, and so this *does* appear to be an important enough improvement. There were no significant between-group differences for body mass index, blood pressure, total cholesterol, triglycerides or the utility score of the quality-of-life measure.

How might we use this evidence to inform practice?

First of all, do we believe the results of the study? Our critical appraisal suggests that there are some threats to the internal validity of the study. Again, we have to exercise judgment to decide whether the study was robust enough to change clinical practice according to its results. Added to this concern is the issue of whether the right outcome measure was measured. We must remember that HbA$_{1c}$ is a 'surrogate measure'; it is not a direct measure of the patient's health status. Instead we are reliant on a series of assumptions about a lower HbA$_{1c}$ leading to better health, something that is actually somewhat controversial. Do we have sufficient well-established evidence that high HbA$_{1c}$ is a cause of diabetes complications, such that reducing it means that complications will be inevitably reduced? Not everyone believes that this is the case, and you are aware that some recent trials have found this may not be the case.

The intervention that was evaluated is a complex intervention that had lots of components. It is not clear which part of the intervention was effective. Was it the self-monitoring, the education, adherence support or reminders for diabetes checks, and in what combination? If we decided to implement this intervention, we would have to try to replicate the exact same intervention as in the study (which is not clearly outlined in the article). You decide that there is sufficient concern about the surrogate nature of the outcome measure (HbA$_{1c}$), which of the intervention components was effective and the risk of bias in the results that you will await further research before asking for additional funds to provide this extra service in your group of pharmacies.

Chapter 6

Evidence about diagnosis

Jenny Doust

LEARNING OBJECTIVES

After reading this chapter, you should be able to:

- Generate a structured clinical question about diagnosis for a clinical scenario
- Appraise the validity of diagnostic evidence
- Understand how to interpret the results from diagnostic studies and calculate additional results (such as positive and negative predictive values and likelihood ratios) where possible
- Describe how diagnostic evidence can be used to inform practice

Let us consider a clinical scenario that will be useful for illustrating the concepts of evidence about diagnosis that are the focus of this chapter.

CLINICAL SCENARIO

You are working in private practice as a physiotherapist. During your Monday clinic, you see a 24-year-old man who twisted his right knee while playing football the day before. He has been suffering with pain and swelling in the knee since the time of the injury, and is able to weight-bear but with difficulty. You examine his knee and wonder how well physical examination determines the cause of knee injury.

Diagnosis is essential in all areas of clinical practice and includes the history, physical examination, assessment tools, pathology and imaging tests that may be performed. Health professionals need to understand how each of these elements contributes to the final diagnosis, whether that be the diagnostic label that we use for patients or the various categories and stratifications within the diagnostic label that we use to assist with decisions about management. This chapter will address the process of using diagnostic evidence to assess the clinical examination of the knee. We will start by defining the components of a structured clinical question about diagnosis. Then we will see how to appraise the evidence to determine its likely validity. Subsequent sections of the chapter will review how to understand the results of a diagnostic study and how to use the evidence to inform practice.

Physical signs are a form of diagnostic test. They help health professionals to decide whether a client has a disease or not. Like all diagnostic tests, they can be measured against a 'gold-standard' test (a test that is known to be highly accurate for the disease being considered) to measure how well they rule in or rule out a diagnosis. Various measures may be used to estimate the accuracy of the test, such as the sensitivity and specificity or the positive and negative likelihood ratios. We will explain these measures later in the chapter.

STUDY DESIGNS THAT CAN BE USED FOR ANSWERING QUESTIONS ABOUT DIAGNOSIS

Studies of diagnostic tests generally measure how accurately a test can detect the presence or absence of a disease by comparing the test with a reference test or 'gold standard'. As we saw in Chapter 2, the best type of study to estimate diagnostic accuracy is a 'consecutive cohort study'. This is a study that compares the test of interest with a gold-standard test in every client who presents with a similar type of clinical problem in a particular setting over a particular time period. As we saw in Chapter 2, systematic reviews are even better than an individual study or trying to read all the studies that are available. Systematic reviews will be discussed further in Chapter 12.

Other study designs are also possible, such as a cross-sectional study of a convenience sample of patients who have had both the test of interest and the reference test, or studies that compare the test results of the index test and the reference test in patients who are known to have the disease of interest (cases) versus the test results in patients who are known not to have the disease of interest (controls). As these studies do not enrol patients with the whole spectrum of disease that may be seen in clinical practice (for example, they may only include patients who have a 'mild' form of the disease of interest), these study types can lead to biased estimates of diagnostic accuracy. Case-control studies, because they enrol patients who clearly have or do not have the disease, are known to overestimate the diagnostic accuracy of a test.[1]

Diagnostic accuracy studies are often more difficult to find than studies assessing the effectiveness of interventions. As yet, there is no publication type that specifically indexes this type of study in Medline or the other major databases, as there is for randomised controlled trials. A possible approach to searching for diagnostic studies is:

1. In PubMed Clinical Queries, choose the 'diagnosis' and 'narrow scope' options.
2. Type in the name of the test. If the test is used for more than one condition, you may also need to use the name of the target disorder in your search.
3. If you do not find a relevant study, try a sensitive search.
4. If you find too many studies, use the name of the target disorder or the 'gold-standard' test in your search.

CLINICAL SCENARIO (CONTINUED)
Structuring the clinical question

As with clinical questions about the effectiveness of interventions, we can define the clinical question for diagnostic questions using the PICO format that was outlined in Chapter 2. There are often several possible questions than can be asked, so it is worth spending a few minutes to consider the question you wish to ask more carefully.

In the case of the 24-year-old footballer described at the beginning of this chapter, you may be considering a meniscal injury, an injury to the anterior cruciate ligament or a soft-tissue injury. You may want to define the population in the question broadly, such as in 'all people', or more narrowly, such as in 'adults with a knee injury'. How narrowly you define the question may depend on whether you think that the test may perform differently in different sub-groups of patients.

The disorders of meniscal injuries and anterior cruciate ligament injuries are the possible outcomes for the diagnostic test, and in this example we will focus on the physical examination for determining the presence of an anterior cruciate ligament injury. For anterior cruciate injuries, tests include the anterior drawer test, Lachman's test and the pivot shift test[2] (see Figure 6.1). Each of these parts of the physical examination of the knee can be the index tests.

The comparator test should be the most accurate method of diagnosing these conditions. In general, the most accurate test for diagnosing intra-articular damage to the knee is arthroscopy. However, magnetic resonance imaging (MRI) is also a highly accurate test for meniscal and ligament injuries of the knee and may be used in some studies because it is less invasive than surgery. Unless patients have a reasonably high probability of the disease or are considering surgery, it is difficult to justify performing surgery in patients to verify the results of physical examination, so many studies will not have used the results of arthroscopy or will only have included patients who are being scheduled for surgery. For this clinical question, both forms of investigation can be considered as the gold-standard test.

You decide on the following question:

• In adults with a knee injury, how well does physical examination, compared with arthroscopy or MRI, determine the presence of anterior cruciate ligament injury?

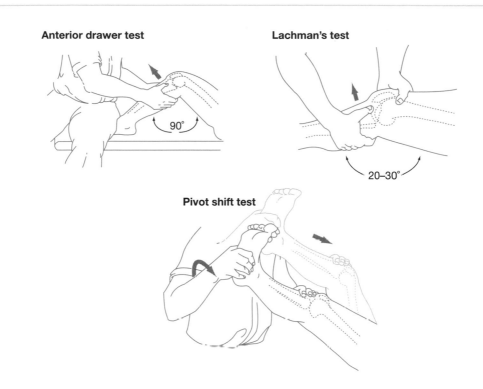

Figure 6.1
Description and illustration of the anterior drawer test, Lachman's test and the pivot shift test.

Anterior drawer test: Place patient supine, flex the hip to 45° and the knee to 90°. Sit on the dorsum of the foot, wrap your hands around the hamstrings (ensuring that these muscles are relaxed), then pull and push the proximal part of the leg, testing the movement of the tibia on the femur. Do these manoeuvres in three positions of tibial rotation: neutral, 30° externally and 30° internally rotated. A normal test result is no more than 6–8 mm of laxity.

Lachman's test: Place the patient supine on examining table, leg at the examiner's side, slightly externally rotated and flexed (20–30°). Stabilise the femur with one hand and apply pressure to the back of the knee with the other hand, with the thumb of the hand exerting pressure placed on the joint line. A positive test result is movement of the knee with a soft or mushy endpoint.

Pivot shift test: Fully extend the knee and rotate the foot internally. Apply a valgus stress while progressively flexing the knee, watching and feeling for translation of the tibia on the femur.

Adapted with permission from Jackson J et al, Evaluation of acute knee pain in primary care, Annals of Internal Medicine, 2003.[2]

CLINICAL SCENARIO (CONTINUED)

Finding the evidence to answer your question

As we saw in Chapter 3, one of the best options for finding diagnostic accuracy studies is PubMed Clinical Queries. If you are looking for studies on a particular test, you may type in the name of the test and select 'diagnosis' and 'narrow scope'. This may be enough to find what you want. If you do not find anything with a narrow search, you can then look for more studies by selecting 'broad scope'. If the test is used for diagnosing more than one disease, you will also need to type in the name of the disease to narrow the search to only the disease that you are considering (for example, ultrasound AND breast cancer).

In the current scenario, the test is the physical examination of the knee. You could type in the names of the different types of test (such as anterior drawer), but it would take quite a while to search for each separate test.

Using the search terms (knee injury AND physical examination) and with the 'diagnosis' and 'narrow scope' options selected in PubMed Clinical Queries, your search finds 91 articles. You find a systematic review of the diagnostic accuracy of physical examination to detect anterior cruciate injury.[3] As the purpose of this scenario is to demonstrate how to appraise a diagnostic study, one of the studies included in the systematic review, rather than the review itself, will be chosen for appraisal (and although this article is quite old, the format in which its results are presented makes it a suitable paper to use for explaining the various results which can be used in a diagnostic study). One of the larger and more recent studies included in the systematic review was an audit of 203 patients who were referred to orthopaedic clinics in Bristol, UK, by general practitioners or accident and emergency departments.[4]

CLINICAL SCENARIO (CONTINUED)

Structured abstract of the chosen article

Citation: Boeree N, Ackroyd C. Assessment of the menisci and cruciate ligaments: an audit of clinical practice. Injury 1991;22:291–4.[4] The structured abstract has been adapted from this reference.

Question: Can clinical assessment of the knee accurately target which patients need arthroscopy, without the need for alternative methods of investigation?

Design: The reliability of clinical assessment of the menisci and cruciate ligaments of the knee was evaluated by evaluating participants using magnetic resonance imaging (MRI).

Setting: Patients of orthopaedic clinics in Bristol, United Kingdom.

Participants: 203 patients (mean age 32.7 years, 76% male) who were seen during a 2-year period in orthopaedic clinics. Of these, 169 patients were referred by their general practitioner and 34 were from accident and emergency departments.

Test: Clinical assessment of the knee (included clinical symptoms and physical signs such as Lachman's test, the anterior drawer sign and the pivot shift test).

Diagnostic standard: MRI of the knee.

Main results: Physical signs proved insufficiently sensitive in detecting abnormalities. Overall, the accuracy of clinical diagnosis was 80.8% for the anterior cruciate ligament, 62.9% for the medial meniscus and 74.9% for the lateral meniscus.

Conclusions: Investigations that are accurate enable arthroscopy to be used for those who are likely to obtain therapeutic benefit. Use of clinical judgment alone would have resulted in an 89% increase in arthroscopic procedures. MRI or arthrography investigations appear to be cost-effective methods of avoiding unnecessary hospitalisation and morbidity.

IS THIS EVIDENCE LIKELY TO BE BIASED?

As we saw in Chapter 4, for studies about the effectiveness of interventions it is important to critically appraise the diagnostic test studies that you find to determine whether the study is adequate to inform your clinical practice. As with the other types of study designs, the main elements to consider are: (1) internal validity (in particular, the risk of bias); (2) the results (the estimates of diagnostic accuracy); and (3) whether or how the evidence might be applicable to your client or clinical practice.

We will use the Critical Appraisal Skills Program (CASP) checklist for appraising a diagnostic test study to explain how to assess the likelihood of bias in this type of study. The key questions to ask when appraising the validity of a diagnostic study are summarised in Box 6.1. The checklist begins with two simple screening criteria that, if not met, indicate that the article is unlikely to be helpful and that further assessment of potential bias is probably unwarranted. Also, you learnt in Chapter 4 that there is a standard for the reporting of randomised controlled trials (the CONSORT statement). There is also one for diagnostic accuracy studies. It is known as the STARD (STAndards for the Reporting of Diagnostic accuracy studies) statement. Further details are available at: www.STARD-statement.org.

BOX 6.1

Key questions to ask when appraising the validity (risk of bias) of a diagnostic study

1. Was there a clear question for the study to address?
2. Is the comparison with an appropriate reference standard?
3. Did all participants get the diagnostic test and the reference standard?
4. Could the results of the test of interest have been influenced by the results of the reference standard, or vice versa?
5. Was there a clear description of the disease status of the tested population?
6. Was there sufficient description of the methods for performing the test?

Was there a clear question for the study to address?

The first criterion on the checklist is whether there was a clear question for the study to address. For diagnostic evidence, the study should clearly define the population, the index and comparator tests, the setting and the outcomes considered.

CLINICAL SCENARIO (CONTINUED)

Did the study address a clearly focused issue?

The study examined the accuracy of the clinical examination of the knee in people who were referred to an orthopaedic outpatient clinic compared with the results of an MRI examination of the knee in determining injuries of the anterior cruciate ligament and the medial and lateral meniscus. This is slightly different to our clinical question, which concerned adults with a knee injury. Not all of the participants in the study had a knee injury. It is unclear from the article what proportion of participants had such an injury, although it appears that these data were recorded as part of the study.

It is important to think through the question clearly before searching for the answer so you can think how this might affect your interpretation of the results of the studies that you find.

Is the comparison with an appropriate reference standard?

The second criterion is whether there was a comparison with an appropriate reference standard. The reference standard should, in general, be the most accurate method available to diagnose the target disorder(s). If the reference test used in the study is not 100% accurate, the diagnostic accuracy of the index test may be either over- or underestimated.

Sometimes, the reference standard will be a combination of a number of tests. For example, a test for diagnosing heart failure may be tested against the combined results of clinical examination and echocardiography. If the index test is included in the reference standard (this is called incorporation bias), the diagnostic accuracy of the test is likely to be overestimated.

CLINICAL SCENARIO (CONTINUED)
Comparison with an appropriate reference standard

The most accurate method for diagnosing knee injuries is by arthroscopy. However, clearly this is too invasive a test to be used in all patients and it would be unethical to perform this test in patients where the clinical examination indicated no need for arthroscopy. The authors of the chosen study had previously demonstrated that MRI is a relatively accurate investigation for assessing the anterior cruciate ligament,[5] and therefore used MRI to assess the diagnostic accuracy of the clinical examination of the knee. Although MRI is slightly less accurate than arthroscopy, and is therefore not a perfect gold-standard test, it can be used for all the participants in the study; so for pragmatic and ethical reasons is used as the reference standard in this study.

Did all participants get the diagnostic test and the reference standard?

As we explained earlier in this chapter, the best type of study to estimate diagnostic accuracy is a 'consecutive cohort' of patients. That is, every client who presents with a similar type of clinical problem in a particular setting over a particular time period receives both tests and the results are compared. In some studies, not all those who receive the test that is being evaluated receive the reference test, or only those who receive both tests are included in the study. This is particularly common when the reference test is harmful or invasive. It results in a biased spectrum of patients. Receiving the gold-standard test generally overestimates the sensitivity and underestimates the specificity of the test. This type of bias is known as *verification bias*. Sensitivity and specificity will be explained in the results section of this chapter.

Sometimes verification bias is unavoidable. For example, in the clinical question we are considering (the diagnosis of anterior cruciate ligament tears), the gold-standard test is arthroscopy. However, as we explained earlier, it would be unethical to perform arthroscopy in patients where no abnormality is suspected after clinical examination (the index test). Therefore, it is not possible to perform the gold-standard test in all patients. In these cases, it may be necessary to use two gold standards, such as arthroscopy for patients with an abnormality on clinical testing and clinical follow-up for patients who initially show no abnormality on clinical testing.

A common form of verification bias occurs when the authors of a study use client records to select patients to include in the study who have had both the index test and the reference test. For example, in this study it appears that patients were included in the study if they attended an orthopaedic clinic and had both a physical examination and an MRI scan. Patients who had both a suspected anterior cruciate ligament injury and an MRI scan are likely to be a different spectrum of patients to all patients who present to an orthopaedic clinic with a suspected anterior cruciate ligament injury. When client records are used to select patients for a study, the study participants are likely to be different from the type of patients who present to a clinic with a particular clinical problem, and are therefore likely to give a biased estimate of the accuracy of the diagnostic test.

CLINICAL SCENARIO (CONTINUED)
Did all participants get the diagnostic test and the reference standard?

The study included 203 patients who had suspected meniscal or cruciate ligament injuries who had been further investigated with an MRI study. The study does not state how many patients were examined in clinics for the above conditions and not investigated with an MRI study. Therefore, there is the possibility of verification bias in this study.

Could the results of the test of interest have been influenced by the results of the reference standard, or vice versa?

The results of the index test and the reference test should each be decided without knowledge of the results of the other test. That is, the person who interprets the test should be blinded to the results of the other test. Knowledge of one test result may bias the reading of the other, particularly where the reading is subjective, such as physical examination or the interpretation of imaging results.

CLINICAL SCENARIO (CONTINUED)
Could the results of the test of interest have been influenced by the results of the reference standard, or vice versa?

Imaging tests are generally performed after the physical examination, so it is likely that the index tests were not influenced by the reference standard. However, it is not clear from the study report whether the clinical examination was performed independently of any previous investigation, such as X-ray reports. It is not reported in the study whether the MRI was performed independently of the physical examination. If the results of the physical examination were included on the radiological request forms, this could have resulted in a bias in the interpretation of the MRI results.

Was there a clear description of the disease status of the tested population?

The test should be investigated in a clinical setting that is as close as possible to the clinical setting in which it will be used. The spectrum of patients included in the study can affect the sensitivity or specificity or both, and therefore may affect the observed accuracy of the test. For example, if the study is conducted in a tertiary referral centre (as compared with a general practitioner's office, for example), patients may have more-severe symptoms and this may affect the sensitivity and/or the specificity of the physical examination.

CLINICAL SCENARIO (CONTINUED)
Clear description of the disease status of the tested population

The study describes the participants as patients who were referred to the orthopaedic clinic for suspected meniscal and anterior cruciate ligament injuries who had been investigated with MRI imaging. The internal validity of the study may be compromised if not all patients who were seen for these suspected disorders were investigated with an MRI. This is not reported in the study, so it is difficult to assess this from the information that is provided in the article.

Was there sufficient description of the methods for performing the test?

Both the index test and the reference standard test should be described in sufficient detail so that it is possible to: (1) reproduce the test; and (2) determine whether the test was performed adequately and is similar to the test being conducted in your own clinical setting.

CLINICAL SCENARIO (CONTINUED)
Sufficient description of the methods for performing the test

The study reports that 'in the examination of the anterior cruciate ligament, the physical signs that were studied included Lachman's test, the anterior drawer sign and the pivot shift (jerk) test.'[4] No further details of either the physical examination techniques or the methods for performing the MRI were given. The reader would need to consider whether these tests are standard enough that no further details are required.

If you have got to this point and determined that the article about diagnosis that you have been appraising is valid, you then proceed to looking at the importance and applicability of the results.

WHAT ARE THE RESULTS?

Sensitivity and specificity

There are a number of ways in which the results of diagnostic accuracy studies may be reported. Diagnostic studies often report sensitivity and specificity results. The most useful results for you as a health professional are the post-test probabilities of a positive and negative test, which we will explain in the next section. However, as many articles report sensitivity and specificity results it can be useful to have an understanding of them.

- The **sensitivity** of a test measures how well a test performs in detecting a disease in people who have the disease. It is the probability that a test is positive in people who have a disease (true positives ÷ [true positives + false negatives]). Using data from our clinical scenario article,[4] this is represented graphically in Figure 6.2.

- The **specificity** of a test measures how well a test performs in determining that disease is *not* present in people who do not have the disease. It is the probability that a test is negative in people who do not have the disease (true negatives ÷ [true negatives + false positives]). Using data from our clinical scenario article,[4] this is represented graphically in Figure 6.2.

Box 6.2 shows how to calculate sensitivity and specificity. It is difficult to convert sensitivity and specificity to the probability that the client does or does not have the disease. It is therefore difficult to apply these values clinically, which is why it is important to understand the concepts of positive and negative predictive values. These are explained in the following section.

Post-test probabilities of a positive and a negative test

These are the most useful way of interpreting results for you as a health professional:

- The **post-test probability of a positive test** (also known as **positive predictive value**) tells you the probability that a patient has disease if he or she has a positive test result. The closer that this number is to 100%, the better the test is at ruling in disease. Its calculation (true positives ÷ [true positives + false positives]) is represented graphically in Figure 6.3, using data from our clinical scenario article.[4]

- Conversely, the **post-test probability of a negative test** (which is the *complement* of the **negative predictive value**) tells you the probability that a client has the disease if he or she has a negative test result.

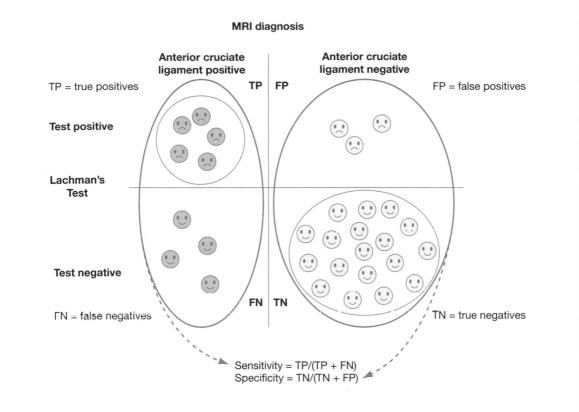

Figure 6.2
Graphical representation of sensitivity and specificity.

BOX 6.2

Measuring diagnostic accuracy: sensitivity and specificity

This box uses data (see Table 6.1) about the diagnostic accuracy of Lachman's test for detecting anterior cruciate ligament injuries of the knee from our clinical scenario article[4] as an example.

$$\text{The \textbf{sensitivity} of Lachman's test} = \frac{\text{true positives}}{\text{true positives} + \text{false negatives}}$$

$$= \frac{37}{37+22}$$

$$= \frac{37}{59}$$

$$= 63\%$$

$$\text{The \textbf{specificity} of Lachman's test} = \frac{\text{true negatives}}{\text{true negatives} + \text{false positives}}$$

$$= \frac{130}{130+14}$$

$$= \frac{130}{144}$$

$$= 90\%$$

TABLE 6.1: THE SENSITIVITY AND SPECIFICITY OF LACHMAN'S TEST FOR DETECTING ANTERIOR CRUCIATE LIGAMENT INJURY AS REPORTED BY BOEREE AND ACKROYD[4]			
	Anterior cruciate ligament injury present	Anterior cruciate ligament injury not present	Total
Lachman's test positive	True positives 37	False positives 14	51
Lachman's test negative	False negatives 22	True negatives 130	152
Total	59	144	203

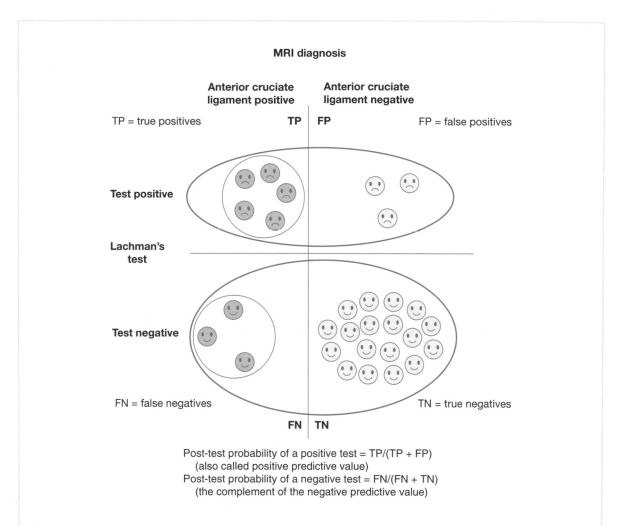

Figure 6.3
Graphical representation of post-test probabilities of positive and negative tests.

The closer that this number is to 0%, the better the test is at ruling out disease. Its calculation (false negatives ÷ [false negatives + true negatives]) is represented graphically in Figure 6.3, using data from our clinical scenario article.[4] The closer that a *negative predictive value* approaches 100%, the better the test is at ruling out disease. Its calculation is true negatives ÷ (false negatives + true negatives).

The difficulty with post-test probabilities (positive and negative predictive values) is that you need to know the pre-test probability of disease (that is, the likelihood of having the disease before having the test) in order to be able to calculate them. This is different to sensitivity and specificity results, which do not change with the pre-test probability (prevalence) of disease. When the percentage of people in the sample who have the disease increases, the post-test probability of both positive and negative tests will increase.[6] So, if you use post-test probabilities to guide your decision about whether to use a diagnostic test or not, this means it is particularly important that you check the spectrum of patients that were included in the diagnostic accuracy study to ensure that they match the sort of patients that you see in your practice. Box 6.3 explains how to calculate post-test probabilities of positive and negative test results, as well as the pre-test probability of disease.

Positive and negative likelihood ratios

Another pair of values that can be used to report results is the **positive/negative likelihood ratios**. Box 6.4 shows how likelihood ratios can be calculated. These results have the advantage of being relatively stable across different clinical settings, but also give an indication of how well the test rules in or rules out disease (refer to Box 6.4).

CLINICAL SCENARIO (CONTINUED)
What are the results?

A summary of the pooled results for each of the physical examination tests in our chosen article is presented in Table 6.2 (see Box 6.4 for how to interpret these results). Using the positive likelihood ratios, we can see that all three of the physical examination tests for anterior cruciate ligament injury are moderately good at detecting an injury if present. Looking at the negative likelihood ratios, we can see that if Lachman's test or the anterior drawer sign is negative, it is moderately helpful for ruling an anterior cruciate ligament injury out, but a negative pivot shift test does not rule out this injury.

TABLE 6.2:
ESTIMATES OF THE DIAGNOSTIC ACCURACY OF THE ANTERIOR DRAWER TEST, LACHMAN'S TEST AND PIVOT SHIFT TEST FOR THE DIAGNOSIS OF ANTERIOR CRUCIATE LIGAMENT INJURIES[4]

	Sensitivity	Specificity	Positive likelihood ratio	Negative likelihood ratio
Anterior drawer test	56%	92%	6.7	0.48
Lachman's test	63%	90%	6.4	0.41
Pivot shift test	30%	96%	8.8	0.72

How changes in the cut-off affect test performance

For many diseases, there is no clear threshold between the presence and absence of a disease. For example, blood pressure and blood glucose levels exist on a spectrum, and the cut-offs that have been chosen to define hypertension or diabetes are, to some extent, arbitrary. In cases where the cut-off for normal/abnormal levels can be raised or lowered, this will affect the test characteristics, and the choice of cut-off

Measuring diagnostic accuracy: post-test probabilities of a positive and a negative test result

As a health professional, what you want to know is that if you receive a positive or a negative test result for a client, what is the probability that he or she has the disease? These values are the post-test probabilities of a positive and a negative test. However, most diagnostic accuracy studies report the sensitivity and the specificity of a diagnostic test. The probability of a disease after a positive or a negative test result requires further calculation, and also needs us to consider the *prevalence* (also called the pre-test probability) of the disease.

Using some of the data from our clinical scenario article[4] as an example:

Lachman's test had a sensitivity of 63% and a specificity of 90%. The study reports that 59 of the 203 participants included in the study had an anterior cruciate ligament injury. The **prevalence or pre-test probability** in this study is therefore $59 \div 203 = 29\%$.

$$\text{The } \textbf{post-test probability of a positive test} = \text{the probability of having an anterior cruciate}$$
$$\text{ligament injury with a positive Lachman's test}$$
$$= \frac{\text{true positives}}{\text{true positives} + \text{false positives}}$$
$$= \frac{37}{37 + 14}$$
$$= \frac{37}{51}$$
$$= 73\%$$

$$\text{The } \textbf{post-test probability of a negative test} = \text{the probability of having an anterior cruciate}$$
$$\text{ligament injury given a negative test result}$$
$$= \frac{\text{false negatives}}{\text{false negatives} + \text{true negatives}}$$
$$= \frac{22}{22 + 130}$$
$$= \frac{22}{152}$$
$$= 14\%$$

To help people remember whether tests rule in or rule out disease, the following mnemonics may be helpful:

- **SpPIn** (Specificity-Positive-In) = if a test has a high specificity and the result is positive, it rules the disease in.
- **SnNOut** (Sensitivity-Negative-Out) = if a test has a high sensitivity and the result is negative, it rules the disease out.

Note that this is a generalisation, and that the post-test probability depends on both sensitivity and specificity and on the prevalence of the disease.[7] Even though Lachman's test has a relatively high specificity, it is not a good example of a SpPIn. A positive test result is only a moderate predictor of the disease being present.

Note: When the pre-test probability is low, for example in screening programs, even tests with high sensitivity and specificity will have a low positive predictive value; that is, most positive test results will be false positives.

BOX 6.4

Measuring diagnostic accuracy: positive and negative likelihood ratios

The *positive likelihood ratio* is the probability that a test is positive in people with the disease divided by the probability that the test is positive in people without the disease.

The *negative likelihood ratio* is the probability that a test is negative in people with the disease divided by the probability that the test is negative in people without the disease.

Using some of the data from our chosen article[4] as an example:

$$\text{The positive likelihood ratio for Lachman's test} = \frac{(\text{true positives/people who have the disease})}{(\text{false positives/people who do not have the disease})}$$

$$= \frac{(37/59)}{(14/144)}$$

$$= 6.4$$

$$\text{The negative likelihood ratio for the Lachman's test} = \frac{(\text{false negatives/people who have the disease})}{(\text{true negatives/people who do not have the disease})}$$

$$= \frac{(22/59)}{(130/144)}$$

$$= 0.41$$

If the article only reports the sensitivity and specificity of the tests, another way to calculate likelihood ratios is:

$$\text{Positive likelihood ratio (LR+)} = \text{sensitivity}/(100 - \text{specificity})$$

$$\text{Negative likelihood ratio (LR−)} = (100 - \text{sensitivity})/\text{specificity}$$

When interpreting likelihood ratios, as a rough guide:

- A positive likelihood ratio > 2 indicates a test that helps rule in disease.
- A positive likelihood ratio > 10 is an extremely good test for ruling in disease.
- A negative likelihood ratio of < 0.5 indicates a test that helps rule out disease.
- A negative likelihood ratio of < 0.1 is an extremely good test for ruling out disease.

will involve a trade-off between the sensitivity and the specificity of the test. If higher values indicate more-abnormal test results, as the cut-off is raised then the sensitivity will increase and the specificity will decrease. A receiver operating characteristic (ROC) curve (see Figure 6.4) plots this trade-off between sensitivity and specificity with changes in the cut-off. The curve demonstrates the trade-off between sensitivity and specificity of a test as the cut-off point changes.

How can we use this evidence to inform practice?

As part of our judgment about whether to use the results of this study in our own practice, we need to think about how likely it is that the test performs in a similar way in our own clinical setting to the diagnostic accuracy in this study.[8] We need to consider:

1. Is the spectrum of patients in the diagnostic study similar to the spectrum of patients in the clinical setting in which you are working?
2. Is the prevalence of disease in the diagnostic study similar to the prevalence in the clinical setting in which you are working?

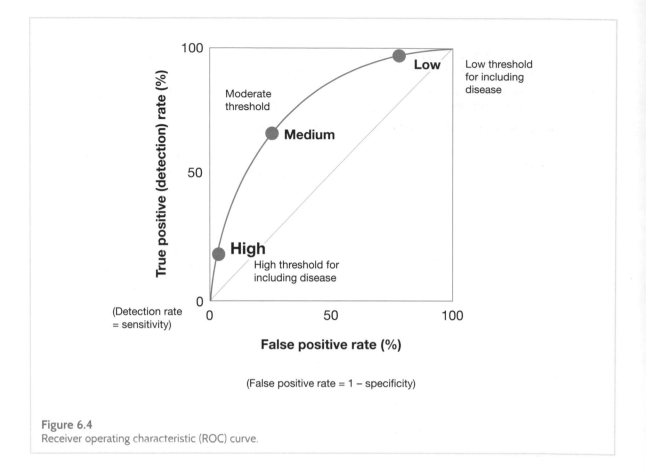

Figure 6.4
Receiver operating characteristic (ROC) curve.

3. Is the method for using the index test similar in the diagnostic study and the clinical setting in which you are working? This includes both the method for performing the index test and the person performing the test. In the clinical scenario chosen, the physical examination was performed by orthopaedic consultants and registrars. Will this alter the diagnostic accuracy of the physical examination?

4. Is the method for using the reference test similar in the diagnostic study and the clinical setting in which you are working?

5. Is the study defining the target disorder in the same way as in your own clinical setting?

CLINICAL SCENARIO (CONTINUED)
Using the evidence to inform practice

Our chosen study shows that the anterior drawer sign, Lachman's test and the pivot shift test are all moderately good at ruling in an anterior cruciate ligament injury, and Lachman's test and the anterior drawer sign are moderately good at ruling such an injury out.

COULD THE QUALITY OF THE STUDY HAVE BIASED THE RESULTS?
There are some reasons why we may doubt the results of this study. It seems likely that not all patients with a normal physical examination received the MRI reference test (the exclusion of

patients with normal physical examination will overestimate sensitivity and underestimate specificity). It is also possible that the MRI test was interpreted without blinding to the results of the physical examination test results. Because of these possible biases, it is likely that these signs are even less accurate than estimated by this study.

COULD OTHER FACTORS HAVE AFFECTED THE RESULTS, FOR EXAMPLE THE SETTING OF THE STUDY?

The study was conducted in an outpatient orthopaedic clinic, and many of the patients had been referred to the clinic by a primary care doctor. This may also affect the sensitivity and specificity of the results seen in this study. There is also a limitation with the external validity of the study. External validity was explained in Chapter 2 and refers to the generalisability of the results of a study. The study assessed the diagnostic accuracy of the physical examination in patients who were referred to an orthopaedic clinic and examined by orthopaedic consultants and registrars. This may not be an accurate estimate of the same tests performed in another clinical setting.

SHOULD I USE THESE TESTS?

Even though these tests have only a moderate discriminatory value, the alternative diagnostic tests (arthroscopy or MRI) are more expensive and have potential harmful effects. Establishing the diagnosis will be of importance primarily in cases where surgery is being considered. If the client is someone for whom the consequences of the injury may be high (such as an elite athlete) or the client has particularly severe symptoms and may benefit from surgery, he or she may benefit from further investigation, such as an MRI. Patients with low demands, however, may be treated conservatively, whatever the findings of the clinical examination. If there is no resolution of symptoms within a reasonable timeframe, the client may then require further investigation.

OTHER TYPES OF TEST STUDIES

So far, we have considered diagnostic test accuracy. These results measure how valid a test is. Not all test studies measure diagnostic accuracy. Some studies measure the *reliability* of a test; that is, whether you get the same test result when the test is done by different health professionals or by the same health professional at different times. The first are usually called *studies of inter-observer reliability* and the latter *studies of intra-observer reliability.*[9] The agreement between different operators of the test (or different groups of operators) can be assessed using measures of agreement such as Cohen's kappa scores. These scores measure the agreement that is seen beyond that expected by chance.

Other clinical tests are used for assessing or monitoring patients. For example, assessments of ability to perform self-care skills, assessments of pain, or haemoglobin A_{1c} (HbA_{1c}) for monitoring glycaemic control in patients with diabetes. These types of tests can be used for many reasons, such as assessing a patient's progress, predicting the likelihood of needing further treatment and/or monitoring a patient's response to intervention and whether adjustments to intervention are needed.

Tests that are used for monitoring need to be reliable, and they are evaluated using measures of reliability such as those described above or the coefficient of variation. Sometimes in clinical practice we use the *average* of several measures in order to improve the reliability of a test. For example, by taking an average of several blood pressure measurements, we reduce the random error that would be seen in a single measurement. When tests are used to monitor a patient, the most appropriate study design is a randomised controlled trial. In these clinical settings, the test is being used as part of a strategy to intervene in the patient's clinical course. Therefore, these tests should be evaluated in the same way as other interventions (see Chapter 4), and preferably by considering studies that used outcomes that are clinically relevant to the patient.[10]

SUMMARY POINTS OF THIS CHAPTER

- The diagnostic accuracy of a test (whether that be part of the clinical history, physical examination or a pathological or radiological investigation) is best assessed by a study of the test against a 'gold-standard' reference test in a consecutive series of patients presenting with a clinical problem.

- Some of the main risks of bias in a diagnostic accuracy study are: (1) only a selected portion of the patients get both the index test and the reference test; and (2) the results of the two tests are not interpreted independently to the other test or blinded to the results of the other test.

- The most common methods for reporting the results of a diagnostic accuracy study are the sensitivity and the specificity of a test. However, the most useful results for a health professional are the post-test probabilities of a positive and a negative test, or the positive and negative likelihood ratios.

- Along with the assessment of the risk of bias in a diagnostic accuracy test, it is also necessary to think how the results may be affected by the setting of the study and the types of patients included in the study.

- Using the results of a diagnostic accuracy study can help you decide whether the test is useful at ruling in or ruling out the diagnosis, or both.

- Tests are also used for assessing and/or monitoring patients, and studies reporting about tests used for this purpose should also be critically appraised.

References

1. Rutjes A, Reitsma J, Di Nisio M, et al. Evidence of bias and variation in diagnostic accuracy studies. CMAJ 2006;1744:469–76.
2. Jackson J, O'Malley P, Kroenke K. Evaluation of acute knee pain in primary care. Ann Intern Med 2003;139:575–88.
3. Scholten R, Opstelten W, van der Plas C, et al. Accuracy of physical diagnostic tests for assessing ruptures of the anterior cruciate ligament: a meta-analysis. J Fam Pract 2003;52:689–94.
4. Boeree N, Ackroyd C. Assessment of the menisci and cruciate ligaments: an audit of clinical practice. Injury 1991;22:291–4.
5. Boeree N, Watkinson A, Ackroyd C, et al. Magnetic resonance imaging of meniscal and cruciate injuries of the knee. J Bone Joint Surg Br 1991;73:452–7.
6. Peat J, Barton B, Elliott E. Statistics workbook for evidence-based healthcare. Chichester: Wiley-Blackwell; 2008.
7. Pewsner D, Battaglia M, Minder C, et al. Ruling a diagnosis in or out with 'SpPIn' and 'SnNOut': a note of caution. BMJ 2004;329:209–13.
8. Deeks J. Using evaluations of diagnostic tests: understanding their limitations and making the most of available evidence. Ann Oncol 1999;10:761–8.
9. Byrt T, Bishop J, Carlin J. Bias, prevalence and kappa. J Clin Epidemiol 1993;46:423–9.
10. Glasziou P, Irwig L, Mant D. Monitoring in chronic disease: a rational approach. BMJ 2005;330(7492):644–8.

Chapter 7

Questions about diagnosis: examples of appraisals from different health professions

Chris Del Mar, Sally Bennett, Mal Boyle, Jeff Coombes, Mark R Elkins, Angela Morgan, Lisa Nissen, Claire Rickard, Sharon Sanders, Michal Schneider-Kolsky and Jemma Skeat

This chapter accompanies the previous chapter (Chapter 6) where the steps involved in answering a clinical question about diagnosis or assessment were explained. In order to further help you learn how to appraise the evidence for this type of question, this chapter contains a number of worked examples of questions about diagnosis from a range of health professions. These worked examples follow the same format as those in Chapter 5. As with the worked examples that are in Chapter 5, the authors of the worked examples in this chapter were also asked not to choose a systematic review, but to instead find and use the next best available level of evidence to answer the clinical question that is in the worked example. This is because it is easier to learn how to appraise a systematic review of test accuracy studies if you have first learnt how to appraise a study about test accuracy. Chapter 12 will help you to learn how to appraise a systematic review.

OCCUPATIONAL THERAPY EXAMPLE

CLINICAL SCENARIO

You are a paediatric occupational therapist who works in private practice. You often work in local schools with children who have a range of developmental disorders. You frequently use the Bruininks–Oseretsky Test of Motor Proficiency to identify children who may have developmental coordination disorder. The busy nature of your practice, and the time it takes to administer the Bruininks–Oseretsky (often 45–60 minutes), means you would like to know more about a test that you have recently heard about called the Motor Performance Checklist because it is only a 12-item measure and was designed for identifying children with motor performance difficulties such as developmental coordination disorder.

CLINICAL QUESTION

Among children with motor performance problems, is the Motor Performance Checklist as accurate as the Bruininks–Oseretsky Test of Motor Proficiency for identifying developmental coordination disorder?

Search terms and databases used to find the evidence

Database: PubMed—Clinical Queries (with 'diagnosis category' and 'narrow scope' selected).

Search terms: (The Motor Performance Checklist)

The PubMed Clinical Queries diagnosis 'narrow scope' filter automatically combines this phrase with the term 'specificity' in the title or abstract. An alternative search approach would have been to enter this phrase in the CINAHL database and combine it with the term 'specificity'.

This search retrieves four titles. The second title is obviously relevant, so you obtain the full text of the article.

Article chosen

Gwynne K, Blick B. Motor performance checklist for 5-year-olds: a tool for identifying children at risk of developmental co-ordination disorder. J Paediatr Child Health 2004;40:369–73.

Structured abstract (adapted from the above)

Study design: This study used a cross-sectional design to compare a new measure of motor performance with a 'gold standard' test for identifying children with developmental coordination disorder.

Setting: The study was conducted in schools in Sydney, Australia.

Participants: All 5-year-old children in a random sample of seven schools from 59 primary schools in the northern beaches sector of Sydney were invited to participate. Of the total population of children in the participating schools, 141 (60%) participated in the study (mean age 5 years and 5 months; 54% male). The prevalence of developmental coordination disorder in the study population was 4.2%.

Description of test: The Motor Performance Checklist is a 12-item instrument for identifying children at risk of developmental coordination disorder.

Diagnostic standard: The Bruininks–Oseretsky Test of Motor Proficiency Long Form. A composite standard score of 40 (1 standard deviation below the mean) was used as the Bruininks–Oseretsky Test of Motor Proficiency Long Form cut-off/failure point to direct children to occupational therapy.

Main results: The Motor Performance Checklist was found to have a sensitivity of 83% and a specificity of 98%. The post-test probability of a positive test was 72% and of a negative test 1% at the cut-off score of 4.

Conclusion: The Motor Performance Checklist has the potential to aid in identifying children who are in need of referral to community occupational therapy services.

Is the evidence likely to be biased?

- *Did all participants get the diagnostic test and the reference standard?*
  Yes. The study report states that all children were tested using both measures. The reference standard used for this study was the Bruininks–Oseretsky Test of Motor Proficiency Long Form. It is a well-validated and frequently used measure for assessing motor performance difficulties in children.

- *Could the results of the test of interest have been influenced by the results of the reference standard, or vice versa?*
  No. A nurse was trained to administer the Motor Performance Checklist, and an occupational therapist blinded to the Motor Performance Checklist results administered the Bruininks–Oseretsky Test of Motor Proficiency.

- *Is the disease status of the tested population clearly described?*
  Yes. The study included children from a random sample of seven out of 59 primary schools in a district of Sydney, Australia. The article states that the population from which the sample was drawn was fairly homogenous with 11% from non-English-speaking backgrounds. Twenty per cent of this population had a tertiary education. There was an approximately even distribution between male (54%) and female (46%) children who participated in the study.

- *Were the methods for performing the test described in sufficient detail?*
  No. Nurses who administered the Motor Performance Checklist were trained in its use for the purpose of this study and a reference to an article that describes the test procedure in detail is provided. However, the actual testing conditions were not clearly described. As the Bruininks–Oseretsky Test of Motor Proficiency is a standardised test, it would have to have been carried out as per the standardised instructions.

What are the main results?

In this study, 6 (4.2%) children were identified by the Bruininks–Oseretsky Test of Motor Proficiency as having developmental coordination disorder. This study presents the sensitivity, specificity, post-test probabilities and likelihood ratios for identifying developmental coordination disorder using the Motor Performance Checklist (see Table 7.1) and compares this with the Bruininks–Oseretsky Test of Motor Proficiency Long Form using a cut-off score of 40 points.

The Motor Performance Checklist has high specificity (98%), which means that there would be very few false positives. The sensitivity of 83% is also reasonably high, meaning that not many children who had developmental coordination disorder would be missed (few false negatives).

TABLE 7.1: ASCERTAINING DEVELOPMENTAL COORDINATION DISORDER						
Assessment	Sensitivity	Specificity	Post-test probability for a:		Positive likelihood ratio	Negative likelihood ratio
			positive test	negative test		
The Motor Performance Checklist	83%	98%	72%	1%	41.5	0.17

The post-test probability of a positive test looks at the data in a different way. A post-test probability of 72% means that the chance of a child actually having developmental coordination disorder if they have a positive Motor Performance Checklist result (using the cut-off score of 4) is 72%. Similarly, using the post-test probability of a negative test, the chance of a child having the disorder with a negative test is 1%.

As you saw in Chapter 6, two things contribute to the post-test probabilities: the *quality of the test* (how well it performs as described by the sensitivity and specificity) and the *prevalence of the disorder*. In this example, only about 4% of children had the condition. This means that we can only generalise the post-test probabilities to other populations that have a similar prevalence.

Another way to deal with this is to look at likelihood ratios, which use a clever algebraic approach enabling us to not have to rely on prevalence to describe the usefulness of a test, yet also employ both sensitivity and specificity. The positive likelihood ratio is the likelihood of a positive test result in a child with the condition compared with the same likelihood in one without the condition. In this study, the positive likelihood ratio is 41.5 [calculated as sensitivity ÷ (100 – specificity)]. Using the approximate guide values that were presented in Chapter 6, a positive likelihood ratio over 10 indicates that the test is extremely good for ruling in the presence of developmental coordination disorder if it is present. The negative likelihood ratio was 0.17 [calculated as (100 – sensitivity) ÷ specificity] which, again using the values presented in Chapter 6, indicates that it is a test that can also help rule out the presence of developmental coordination disorder.

How might we use this evidence to inform practice?

Although this study may be prone to some types of bias that are common in cross-sectional studies, it was otherwise well-designed and you are reasonably confident about the results. There are three factors about this study to think about, though. First, the ability of the Motor Performance Checklist to identify children with developmental coordination disorder was restricted in this study to children who were 5 years old. Testing this measure with children from 4 to 10 years is needed, as this is the age range that this assessment was designed to be used with. Second, the study reports a low prevalence of developmental coordination disorder, and the authors state that this is lower than reported in the literature. This means that, in populations with a higher prevalence of developmental coordination disorder, the post-test probability of a positive test (the chance of the test being correct) will be greater than reported in this study. Finally, the brevity of this measure is appealing and the article also reports on the concurrent validity and reliability of this measure, which are other psychometric test properties that must be considered when considering using an assessment with patients.

You think back to your original dilemma. Can you use the Motor Performance Checklist for identifying children with developmental coordination disorder? The study was limited to children aged 5 years, so you are just a little uncertain whether the study can be applied to those older and younger, although this is likely.

PHYSIOTHERAPY EXAMPLE

CLINICAL SCENARIO

A 25-year-old male cricketer presents to your physiotherapy outpatient clinic with right shoulder pain. The pain began without any acute injury and is aggravated by repetitive throwing and catching. The location of the pain and your standard physical examination make you suspect, among other possible diagnoses, that he may have a lesion of the posteroinferior portion of the labrum of his shoulder. You are only aware of manual tests to diagnose superior labral lesions, and wonder if there is a formal test for posteroinferior lesions. Also, you have recently read a systematic review that examined a range of widely used manual tests for shoulder pathology.[1] The review indicated that several of the tests have limited diagnostic accuracy compared with the 'gold standard' of seeing the pathology during surgery. You decide to search for a study of the diagnostic accuracy of any test for posteroinferior labral lesions.

CLINICAL QUESTION

In athletes with shoulder pain, is there a manual test for diagnosing posteroinferior lesions of the labrum, and what is its diagnostic utility?

Search terms and databases used to find the evidence

Database: PubMed–Clinical Queries (with 'diagnosis category' and 'narrow scope' selected).

Search terms: posteroinferior (labral OR labrum)

The search returns five records. One of these articles seems very promising: a comparison of the ability of two manual tests to diagnose posteroinferior labral tears, with surgical observation as the gold standard. It looks highly relevant, but you are concerned that your search is too narrow. You repeat the search, selecting the 'broad, sensitive search' option. This returns 20 records, but none of these is as relevant as the original article you found.

Article chosen

Kim S, Park J, Jeong W, et al. The Kim test: a novel test for posteroinferior labral lesion of the shoulder–a comparison to the jerk test. Am J Sports Med 2005;33:1188–92.

Structured abstract (adapted from the above)

Study design: Cohort study.

Setting: Department of Orthopaedic Surgery at a hospital in Korea.

Participants: 172 adults awaiting arthroscopic examination for undiagnosed shoulder pain. Exclusion criteria were septic arthritis, fracture of the greater tuberosity, arthroscopic capsular release due to frozen shoulder, frozen shoulder, and previous surgery.

Description of tests: For the Kim test, the patient sits with the trunk against a backrest and the arm abducted to 90°. The examiner applies axial force along the humerus at the elbow to compress the glenohumeral joint and elevates the arm by 45°. With the other hand, the examiner applies downward and backward force to the upper arm. Sudden onset of pain indicates a positive test. For the jerk test, the patient sits with the arm abducted to 90° and internally rotated 90°. The examiner stands behind and supports the scapula with one hand. With the other hand, axial force is applied at the elbow and maintained while the arm is horizontally adducted. Sharp pain indicates a positive test. Each test was performed by two independent examiners.

Diagnostic standard: Arthroscopic examination of the glenohumeral joint and subacromial space.

Main results: Thirty (17%) of the 172 participants had a posteroinferior labral lesion. The Kim test had sensitivity of 80% and specificity of 94%. The positive predictive value of the Kim test was 0.73 and the negative predictive value was 0.96. The jerk test had sensitivity of 73% and specificity of 98%. The positive predictive value of the jerk test was 0.88 and the negative predictive value was 0.95. The sensitivity in detecting a posteroinferior lesion increased to 97% when the two tests were combined.

Conclusion: The two tests, particularly in combination, have worthwhile clinical utility in the diagnosis of posteroinferior labral lesions.

Is the evidence likely to be biased?

- *Did all participants get the diagnostic test and the reference standard?*
  Yes. All participants received the diagnostic tests of interest and the reference standard.

- *Could the results of the test of interest have been influenced by the results of the reference standard, or vice versa?*
  No. The manual tests were performed before the arthroscopy (so the arthroscopic examination could not have influenced them). And the results of the arthroscopy could not have been influenced by the results of the manual tests because the surgeon was blinded.

- *Is the disease status of the tested population clearly described?*
  Yes. The description of the study population is reassuring: eligible patients were recruited consecutively from an orthopaedic surgical clinic. All participants entered the study with preliminary clinical diagnoses that were potentially consistent but not definitive of the diagnosis of interest.

- *Were the methods for performing the test described in sufficient detail?*
  Yes. The diagnostic tests of interest are described in sufficient detail for you to replicate them in your clinical practice.

What are the main results?

Thirty (17%) of the 172 participants had a posteroinferior labral lesion. The article presents the sensitivity, specificity, positive predictive value and negative predictive value of the two tests. You also use these results to calculate the positive and negative likelihood ratios (see Table 7.2).

The post-test probability of the Kim test indicates that, on average, 73% of people with a positive test result actually have a posteroinferior labral lesion. The post-test probability of the jerk test indicates that, on average, 88% of people with a positive result actually have a posteroinferior labral lesion. Using the approximate guide values that were presented in Chapter 6, as both of the positive likelihood ratios are over 10 this indicates that these tests are very helpful for ruling in a posteroinferior labral lesion if it is present. Also, as the negative likelihood ratios are <0.5, this suggests that these tests are moderately helpful in ruling out a posteroinferior labral lesion.

Test	Sensitivity	Specificity	Post-test probability for a:		Positive likelihood ratio	Negative likelihood ratio
			positive test	negative test		
Kim test	80%	94%	0.73	0.04	13.3	0.21
Jerk test	73%	98%	0.88	0.05	36.5	0.28

TABLE 7.2:
RESULTS OF THE KIM TEST AND JERK TEST

How might we use this evidence to inform practice?

You are satisfied that the study is valid and the results are clinically useful. The study population was reasonably similar to the patient to whom you are considering applying the tests; although in your practice not all patients are severe enough to be scheduled for arthroscopy, so the prevalence of posteroinferior labral lesions is likely to be lower. The tests can be performed quickly and without requiring specialised equipment. However, before applying these tests, you should consider other diagnoses. The patient's description of the location of the pain suggests that the posteroinferior labrum is involved. Furthermore, the following tests are negative: the apprehension test (for detecting anterior shoulder instability), the impingement test (for detecting rotator cuff inflammation or impingement), the horizontal adduction test (for assessing acromioclavicular joint impingement) and tests for superior labral lesions as mentioned in the clinical scenario. In doing this, you confirm that a posteroinferior labral lesion is the diagnosis that you primarily suspect. You decide to apply the Kim test and the jerk test to your patient and use the results of these tests to guide the diagnosis and subsequent management of your patient.

PODIATRY EXAMPLE

CLINICAL SCENARIO

You are a podiatrist working in a community health centre, and you have just seen a 28-year-old male plumber with a diffuse scaling rash which covers most of his instep area, extending towards the digits of his right foot. It has been present for about 8 weeks, is itchy and there are some vesicles in the instep area. Several weeks ago he tried a topical steroid cream bought from the pharmacy. According to the patient, the rash did not really improve and he stopped applying the cream after a few days. You suspect a fungal infection, suggest an antifungal cream that is available over the counter and discuss foot hygiene with him. You wonder how accurate the diagnosis of tinea pedis (a fungal foot infection) is, based on clinical presentation.

CLINICAL QUESTION

In a person with suspected tinea pedis, how accurate is clinical examination compared with a 'gold standard' of microbiological confirmation in making a diagnosis?

Search terms and databases used to find the evidence

Database: PubMed–Clinical Queries (with 'diagnosis category' and 'narrow scope' selected).

Search terms: tinea OR (athletes foot)

This search retrieves 34 titles. Several studies look promising but, on reading through their abstracts, they are either comparing different laboratory methods for diagnosing mycoses or are case-control studies. You know that case-control studies can overestimate the accuracy of diagnostic tests, so you reject these. There is only one study that, on the basis of the abstract, appears to compare the clinical diagnosis of tinea pedis with laboratory methods, although the operating characteristics of the tests are not reported. This study investigated the diagnostic value of signs and symptoms compared with culture for diagnosing dermatomycosis in general practice. You consider whether this study, which appears to have looked at the diagnosis of fungal infection on any hairless part of the body, could be relevant to your clinical situation. As there do not appear to be any studies that have looked specifically at the clinical diagnosis of tinea pedis, you obtain the full text of this study.

Article chosen

Lousbergh D, Buntinx F, Piérard G. Diagnosing dermatomycosis in general practice. Fam Pract 1999;16:611–15.

Structured abstract (adapted from the above)

Design: This study compared clinical examination, microscopy of a potassium hydroxide preparation and cyanoacrylate surface skin scraping (CSSS) for detecting fungal infection of the skin, with culture as the reference standard.

Setting: General practices in Belgium.

Participants: 148 consecutive general practice patients with red scaly lesions of the glabrous (smooth, hairless) skin. Participants whose lesions had already been treated with antifungal therapy were excluded.

Description of tests: Scales were collected from the border of the lesion for microscopic testing using a potassium hydroxide preparation (KOH test) and culture. A strip biopsy (CSSS) was also made from the same site. Each participant's general practitioner also noted their diagnosis, based on each participant's characteristics, and local signs and symptoms.

Diagnostic standard: Culture of scales collected from the border of the lesion.

Main results: 18% of participants had a positive fungal culture. The sensitivity of the clinical diagnosis was 81% (95% confidence interval [CI] 60% to 93%) and the specificity was 45% (95% CI 36% to 54%). The likelihood ratio of clinical examination was 1.47 (95% CI 1.15 to 1.88) for a positive test result and 0.43 (95% CI 0.19 to 0.96) for a negative test result. The most accurate diagnostic method was CSSS, which had a likelihood ratio of 5.17 for a positive test result and 0.43 for a negative test result.

Conclusion: In people with red scaly (erythrosquamous skin) lesions, clinical diagnosis has low diagnostic accuracy for detecting dermatomycosis.

Is this evidence likely to be biased?

- *Did all participants get the diagnostic test and the reference standard?*
  Yes. It appears that all participants received the index tests and the reference standard test. Culture of skin scrapings is the reference test used in this study.

- *Could the results of the test of interest have been influenced by the results of the reference standard, or vice versa?*
  Cannot tell. The article does not clearly state that the index test results were interpreted blind to the results of the reference standard test. You think it is likely, however, that direct microscopy of the scales collected using the traditional method and the strip biopsy would have been performed before the results of the reference standard became available (cultures were examined after 4 weeks incubation) and that interpretation of the results of the KOH and CSSS tests would be without knowledge of the results of the culture. It also appears that signs and symptoms and general practitioner diagnosis were obtained before the results of the culture would have been available from the laboratory. You are also not sure whether the results of the culture were interpreted without knowledge of the results of the index tests.

- *Is the disease status of the tested population clearly described?*
  No. There is no information that you can use to judge whether the spectrum of participants included in this study is similar to those you see in your practice. There is no information about the severity or the duration of the lesions or their location. Demographic and clinical features of the participants in this study are also not reported.

- *Were the methods for performing the test described in sufficient detail?*
  Yes. The microscopy and culture of the samples was done by a laboratory which would need to adhere to testing standards. There is a reasonable description of how the CSSS was performed, but you think that more information about how the skin samples for the KOH test and culture were collected would be helpful. For example, what was used to collect the sample, how was it stored and was the lesion cleaned with alcohol before collection?

What are the main results?

In this study, 26 cultures (18%) were considered positive. Table 7.3 presents the sensitivity, specificity, post-test probabilities and likelihood ratios for the clinical diagnosis of dermatomycosis. Table 7.3 shows that clinical examination has moderate sensitivity and low specificity for diagnosing dermatomycosis in general practice. The positive likelihood ratio of 1.47 is of little diagnostic value, suggesting only a minimal increase in the likelihood of dermatomycosis with a positive clinical diagnosis. The likelihood ratio for a negative test (0.42) suggests that it is of some value in ruling out fungal infection, representing a small decrease in the likelihood of disease when a negative clinical diagnosis is made.

How might we use this evidence to inform practice?

This study suggests that a positive clinical diagnosis of fungal infection is of little help in determining that a person has dermatomycosis. You have some doubts about the validity of the study, as the methods of the study were not reported in sufficient detail for you to accurately judge the level of bias that may be present. Your general reading in the area has also led you to question the validity of the gold-standard test (culture of skin scrapings) used in this study. For numerous reasons, including sampling error and errors in the culture process, fungal culture may not be the best method for establishing the presence or absence of dermatophyte infection. Use of an 'imperfect' reference standard may lead to the over- or underestimation of the diagnostic accuracy of clinical judgment.

You also have some concerns about how generalisable the study is to your situation, but you have been unable to find any other studies which answer your question. As this study was carried out in general practices, you think that the population is more likely to be similar to yours than if the study had recruited people from dermatology specialist clinics; however, with the limited information that is provided in the article, it is difficult to be sure about this. You reflect on your management of your patient and wonder if you should have referred him for further testing. Further testing would mean extra costs for the patient. The study that you just reviewed found that the KOH test and the CSSS test provide additional diagnostic value if a positive clinical diagnosis (from clinical examination) is made. You think that the probability that your patient has tinea is quite high and that suggesting antifungal treatment without further testing was a reasonable approach. The antifungal treatments that are available are reasonably cheap, easy to obtain and use and generally well tolerated. You advise your patient to see his general practitioner for further testing if the rash does not clear.

TABLE 7.3:
USING CLINICAL EXAMINATION TO DIAGNOSE DERMATOMYCOSIS

Test	Sensitivity (95% CI)	Specificity (95% CI)	Post-test probability (with 95% CI) for a:		Positive likelihood ratio (95% CI)	Negative likelihood ratio (95% CI)
			positive test	negative test		
Clinical examination	81% (60% to 93%)	45% (36% to 54%)	24% (16% to 34%)	92% (81% to 97%)	1.47 (1.15 to 1.88)	0.42 (0.19 to 0.96)

SPEECH PATHOLOGY EXAMPLE

CLINICAL SCENARIO

You are a junior speech pathologist working in a rotational position at a tertiary adult hospital. Mr Pitt, a 33-year-old man with Friedrich's ataxia (a neurodegenerative genetic disorder), has been referred to you with recurrent aspiration. He was first diagnosed with the disorder at the age of 16 and had relatively good health until his motor function deteriorated, leaving him wheelchair-dependent with moderate dysarthric speech. Despite this, he is a bright and witty young man with intact language skills. He has just completed a university degree in art history. Recently he developed severe swallowing difficulties and has had two successive admissions to hospital with aspiration pneumonia in the last 9 months. On his first admission, he was referred to speech pathology for a swallowing assessment by videofluoroscopy (VFS). This demonstrated aspiration on thin fluids. The previous therapist recommended a modified diet of nectar-thick fluids only, using a chin-tuck posture.

However, the problem has not resolved when you see him during his second hospital admission. You wonder what investigations you should use this time and into the future, as many more will probably be needed as he deteriorates. VFS involves large X-ray doses. You consider using fibre-optic endoscopic evaluation of swallowing (FEES), which does not have this problem, but you are not sure if it is sensitive enough.

CLINICAL QUESTION

How do VFS and FEES compare for detecting aspiration in adults with dysphagia?

Search terms and databases used to find the evidence

Database: PubMed–Clinical Queries (with 'diagnosis category' and 'narrow scope' selected).

Search terms: (fiberoptic endoscop*) AND aspiration AND dysphagia AND (videofluoroscop*)

This search results in 0 hits. You repeat it, this time selecting the 'broad' scope, and it still results in no hits. You repeat the search using the main PubMed search function (rather than Clinical Queries), and this results in 14 hits. There are four studies which compared VFS and FEES; one of these was a study in children. Of the remaining three, two studies compared the two procedures and provided primary data. However, the FEES and VFS procedures in both studies were conducted on separate days in one paper and within a 2-week period in the second paper, rather than being conducted simultaneously (which is a weaker method, more open to bias than if the procedures are conducted at the same time). The remaining article is more recent and appears to be the most appropriate to answer your clinical question, as it directly compares VFS and FEES which were conducted simultaneously for each participant.

Article chosen

Kelly A, Drinnan M, Leslie P. Assessing penetration and aspiration: how do videofluoroscopy and fiberoptic endoscopic evaluation of swallowing compare? Laryngoscope 2007;117:1723–7.

Structured abstract (adapted from the above)

Study design: Prospective single-blind comparative study.

Study question: Does the type of instrumental evaluation (VFS vs FEES) influence the speech-language pathologist's rating of penetration and aspiration?

Participants: *Participants with dysphagia*–15 consecutive participants referred to speech–language pathology for dysphagia assessment at one UK hospital. They presented with a wide range of primary diagnoses (such as bilateral vocal-fold palsy, previous stroke and skull-base tumour, cervical spine degeneration, base of tongue carcinoma). Participants were excluded if they were nil by mouth or judged to be at high risk of aspiration of all oral intake. *Speech-language pathologist raters*–20 therapists were invited to participate, 17 consented and the ratings of 15 were included in the final analyses. All were experienced in performing and interpreting FEES and VFS (with a mean of 6 years of experience for VFS, based on performing and interpreting approximately once per week each year, and a mean of 4.9 years for FEES).

Data collection: *Dysphagia assessments*–All participants underwent both FEES and VFS simultaneously on one occasion. Two therapists, one radiologist and one radiographer performed the examinations. Each participant swallowed two test boluses: 5 mL liquid from a cup and 15 mL yoghurt from a standard dessert spoon. Both boluses were dyed with 1 mL of blue food dye to enable clear visualisation of the bolus. All participants swallowed the boluses in the same order. Thirty recording clips (15 VFS and 15 FEES) were recorded in random order onto two compact discs, with the order randomly changed for the second. *Rating*–Each rater used the Penetration–Aspiration Scale to rate all swallows for both procedures (the scale ranges from 1 = material does not enter the airway to 8 = material enters the airway, passes below the vocal folds and no effort is made to eject). Each 'clip' was to be viewed no more than twice. The 30 clips on one disc were rated first, and the clips on the second disc were rated 1 week later.

Main results: The Penetration–Aspiration Scale scores were significantly higher (mean difference in scores was 1.15 points) for the FEES recordings than for the VFS recordings.

Conclusion: Penetration aspiration is perceived to be greater (more severe) from FEES than from VFS images.

Is this evidence likely to be biased?

This study does not compare a new test with a gold-standard test and, therefore, is not designed to determine test accuracy as is the case in many of the other examples in this chapter. Therefore, the same criteria for considering validity are not used here. Instead, more-general questions for determining the potential for bias are used in this example. The focus is on the examination of bias in the participants and raters, methods and analysis.

- **Participants.** *People with dysphagia:* minimal inclusion and exclusion criteria were applied in participant selection, and the 15 participants recruited to the study were extremely heterogeneous in age, diagnosis, treatment history and severity of swallowing difficulty. This makes it difficult to generalise the findings of this study to any particular population with dysphagia. *Speech-language pathology raters:* raters' experience in performing and rating FEES/VSF was only quantified for 14 of the 17 original participants. While the mean years of experience appears high (6 for VSF and 4.9 for FEES), the standard deviation (4.5 for VSF and 4.3 for FEES) shows that there was wide variation in the actual experience level of these 14 raters.
- **Methods.** Strengths include all participants undergoing VFS and FEES simultaneously, the use of a well-validated and commonly used aspiration-penetration rating tool, the randomisation of VFS versus FEES procedures, the use of a large number of raters from a number of different institutions (15 raters from 12 different institutions), the use of a week-long period between ratings of both discs to minimise recall bias, blinding raters to participants' age and aetiology and to the other raters' responses, and the inclusion of both inter- and intra-rater reliability ratings.
- **Replicability.** The assessment methods were well detailed and would enable replication of the study. For example, details were provided about the FEES and VFS procedure, including specific information about the ratio of food/fluid to barium in the bolus administered and the exact type of barium used.

- **Statistical analyses.** Both five-way analysis of variance (ANOVA) and logistic regression were used to examine the variables that had the greatest impact on ratings of aspiration–penetration. The variables investigated were: the *examination* (FEES vs VFS), *bolus type* (liquid or yoghurt), *rating order* (first or second), *rater* and *participant*. The analyses were limited by the small number of participants and the heterogeneity of the participant sample. The total number of swallows rated across the group was high ($n = 1800$) and the number of raters used was considerable ($n = 15$). However, given that the same 15 individuals were producing each of the swallows, the swallows were all highly related and were therefore not independent data points, potentially reducing the statistical power of the study. The small and diverse participant sample also limits the ability to directly generalise these findings to any particular population with dysphagia.

What are the main results?

Both penetration and aspiration in patients with dysphagia were rated more severely by experienced health professionals using FEES than using VFS. The authors concluded that FEES and VSF should not be used interchangeably in clinical practice, as they do not lead to equivalent interpretations of swallowing function/dysfunction.

How might we use this evidence to inform practice?

After appraising the article, you come to a number of conclusions. First, you realise that although the Penetration–Aspiration Scale scores were higher for the FEES than for the VFS recordings, the article does not provide information about the sensitivity or specificity of the results in relation to a gold standard for detecting aspiration, and you decide to look for further research in this area. Second, FEES and VSF are not interchangeable and swapping between them for a single patient may provide a misleading view of the patient's changes over time. However, since FEES is more appropriate for repeated use for a patient like Mr Pitt, and this is only his second instrumental swallowing assessment, you will consider using FEES from this point onwards, in order to ensure a homogenous interpretation of Mr Pitt's swallowing over time. Third, it is not clear which test is best at predicting aspiration pneumonia. Finally, you do not know whether Mr Pitt's type of dysphagia (neurological degenerative) is best predicted by the FEES test, as any sub-group analysis was limited by the small sample of widely differing types of dysphagia.

MEDICINE EXAMPLE

CLINICAL SCENARIO

You are a general practitioner working with a primary care team. One of the issues for the team is dealing with the standard way of screening for renal disease (albuminuria) in diabetes of pregnancy, which is becoming a more frequent problem. The standard method is a 24-hour collection of urine from which the lab estimates the albumin excreted. However, this method is a problem because it is very inconvenient for women, who dislike having to collect it (especially a problem if they have to urinate while out of the home) and bring a large, bulky container to the clinic. Yet the information is important, as the presence of microalbuminuria predicts the rate of pre-eclampsia well in women with diabetes of pregnancy. The nurses in the practice consider that adherence to the 24-hour urine collections is not good, with missing urines leading to underestimates of albuminuria. At a staff meeting, one of the nurses asks 'Isn't the usual screening, which is just measuring the urine albumin-to-creatinine ratio, as we do for pregnant women without diabetes, just as good?'

CLINICAL QUESTION

In women with diabetes of pregnancy, how accurate is the urine albumin-to-creatinine ratio compared with the 'gold standard' of 24-hour excretion of albumin when screening for albuminuria?

Search terms and databases used to find the evidence

Database: PubMed–Clinical Queries (with 'diagnosis category' and 'broad scope' selected).

Search terms: albuminuria diabetes pregnancy

This search retrieved 40 titles. The 14th article listed was the most relevant to the question. The full text is available at: http://care.diabetesjournals.org/cgi/reprint/29/4/924

Article chosen

Justesen T, Petersen J, Ekbom P, et al. Albumin-to-creatinine ratio in random urine samples might replace 24-h urine collections in screening for micro- and macroalbuminuria in pregnant woman with type 1 diabetes. Diabetes Care 2006; 29:924–5.

Structured abstract (adapted from the above)

Study design and participants: All women with diabetes in pregnancy who were admitted to the hospital's obstetrics department before 14 weeks of gestation were invited to participate, and 119 were enrolled in the study. The urine samples were collected between gestational weeks 7 and 22.

Setting: A university hospital in Denmark.

Description of test: Two random samples of urine collected at different times were used to estimate the albumin-to-creatinine ratio. The cut-off point was >2.5 mg albumin/mmol of creatinine.

Diagnostic 'gold standard': 24-hour urine collections were tested for albumin. The cut-off point was >30 mg albumin/24 hours.

Main results: The albumin-to-creatinine ratio had a sensitivity of 94% and a specificity of 100%. Its post-test probability for a positive test was 100% and the post-test probability for a negative test was 1%.

Conclusion: The simpler and more convenient test (two samples of urine rather than the 24-hour collection) performs well.

Is the evidence likely to be biased?

- *Did all participants get the diagnostic test and the reference standard?*
  Yes. The article describes that all eligible women used both tests.
- *Could the results of the test of interest have been influenced by the results of the reference standard, or vice versa?*
  No. The tests were analysed by the laboratory and were presumably automated, so that one result could not have influenced the other.
- *Is the disease status of the tested population clearly described?*
  Yes. The women were clearly defined. Their mean age was 30 ($\pm$4) years; they had had diabetes for a mean of 16 ($\pm$7) years; and their HbA$_{1c}$ (glycated haemoglobin level) was 7.6% ($\pm$1%).
- *Were the methods for performing the test described in sufficient detail?*
  Yes. The cut-off points are described. Details of the biochemical tests are described in detail and this will enable people to replicate them.

What are the main results?

Table 7.4 shows how the 119 women tested for both tests, and Table 7.5 shows a summary of the test accuracy for the test that used two random urine samples. These results show that testing for albuminuria had a high specificity, which means that there would be very few false positives. There were none in this sample, but the numbers were small enough to lend some uncertainty, which is expressed by the 95% confidence interval's lower value being less than 100%, that is, 94%. The sensitivity was also high at 94%, suggesting that few women with albuminuria would be missed–that is, few false negatives. In this study, there was only one. The post-test probability of the positive test refers to the chance of a woman having albuminuria after having two random samples of urine test positive, and is 100%. Similarly, the post-test probability of a negative urine test means the chance of a woman having albuminuria after a negative test is 1%.

The positive likelihood ratio is the ratio of the probability of the test being positive among women with albuminuria divided by that of those who do not have albuminuria. The negative likelihood ratio is the ratio of the probability of the test being negative among women who do not have albuminuria divided by that of those who do. In this study, the positive likelihood ratio is ∞, because dividing the sensitivity of 94% by [100 – specificity (100%)] would give an infinitely large number. In other words, the test is extremely good for ruling in the presence of albuminuria if it is present. Using the values presented in Chapter 6, the negative likelihood ratio of 0.06 indicates that it is a test that is extremely good for ruling out the presence of albuminuria.

How might we use this evidence to inform practice?

The simpler test seems to perform so well that your team decides to use it at the practice instead of the slightly more accurate one, judging that the extra convenience of the two random urine samples is much more likely to be adhered to than the cumbersome, embarrassing and inconvenient 24-hour urine collection gold standard.

TABLE 7.4:
RESULTS FOR 24-HOUR URINE COLLECTION AND TWO RANDOM URINE SAMPLES FOR ALL PARTICIPANTS

		Albuminuria >30 mg/24 hours (by 24-hour urinary collection)		Total
		positive	negative	
(Mean of two) random urine samples' albumin:creatinine ratio >2.5 mg/mmol	positive	15	0	15
	negative	1	103	104
Total		16	103	119

TABLE 7.5:
SUMMARY OF THE TEST ACCURACY FOR THE TEST THAT USED TWO RANDOM URINE SAMPLES

Diagnosis	Sensitivity (95% CI)	Specificity (95% CI)	Post-test probability for a:		Positive likelihood ratio	Negative likelihood ratio
			positive test	negative test		
Albuminuria	94% (70% to 100%)	100% (94% to 100%)	100%	1%	∞	0.06

∞ = an infinitely large number.

NURSING EXAMPLE

CLINICAL SCENARIO

You are a nurse who works in a medical ward in a large tertiary hospital. Many of the patients you care for are elderly people with a variety of health conditions. You regularly conduct assessments using the STRATIFY falls screening tool to gauge your patients' risk of falling. It is a five-item checklist, assessing previous falls, agitation, visual impairment, toileting frequency and transfer/mobility problems. Each item is scored 1 for 'yes' or 0 for 'no'. A score of 2 or greater determines a high risk of falling. You wonder whether the STRATIFY falls scoring tool accurately predicts which patients are at risk of falling.

CLINICAL QUESTION

Among elderly hospitalised patients, is the STRATIFY falls screening tool an accurate predictor of falls risk?

Search terms and databases used to find the evidence

Database: PubMed–Clinical Queries (with 'diagnosis category' and 'narrow scope' selected).

Search terms: (STRATIFY tool) AND fall* AND hospital*

This search yields 14 hits. A number of the articles involve the STRATIFY tool and you choose the article that most closely matches your clinical question.

Article chosen

Webster J, Courtney M, Marsh N, et al. The STRATIFY tool and clinical judgment were poor predictors of falling in an acute hospital setting. J Clin Epidemiol 2010;63:109-13.

Structured abstract (adapted from the above)

Design: Prospective cohort study.

Setting: Large tertiary teaching hospital in Australia.

Participants: 788 patients over 65 years of age who were admitted to any hospital unit.

Description of test: The STRATIFY tool was used by researcher officers on all patients within 48 hours of admission.

Diagnostic 'gold standard': Information about occurrence of falls was extracted from weekly reports from the Patient Incident Reports database and/or a review of participants' medical chart on discharge.

Main results: 788 patients were screened, and the STRATIFY tool classified 335 (43%) as at risk of falling. Of these, 59 (18%) patients fell (sensitivity = 0.82, specificity = 0.61, positive predictive value = 0.18, negative predictive value = 0.96).

Conclusion: The STRATIFY tool is not useful for fall screening in acute hospital settings.

Is this evidence likely to be biased?

- *Did all participants get the diagnostic test and the reference standard?*
  Yes. All patients who were recruited (consecutively) were assessed for falls risk using STRATIFY, and   it was checked (by medical chart review at discharge and examination of weekly reports from the hospital's incidence database) whether a fall occurred for each participant.

- *Could the results of the test of interest have been influenced by the results of the reference standard, or vice versa?*
  Cannot tell. It is possible that health professionals who recorded the falls may have known the results of the STRATIFY screening and this may have influenced their reporting of a fall. Although it is possible this might have happened in some cases, the presence or absence of a fall was probably usually unequivocal.
- *Is the disease status of the tested population clearly described?*
  Yes. Participants are described by treating specialty, age group, length of stay and the ward they were in—surgical (41.5%), medical (41.2%), oncology (7%), extended-stay or geriatric assessment and rehabilitation unit (5.6%) and mental health unit (4.7%).
- *Were the methods for performing the test described in sufficient detail?*
  Yes. The 5 items of the STRATIFY tool and the scoring of these are listed. Information was gathered from either patient notes or the nurse caring for the participant. The study reports that research officers were trained in the use of the tool, but no details about this training are provided.

What are the main results?

Table 7.6 shows the actual numbers of participants who fell, and the number who were 'at risk' of falling (a score of ≥2) and those who were not according to the STRATIFY tool. The authors provide the sensitivity of the tool as 0.82. Using the data in Table 7.6, you can see how this was calculated using the formula: true positives/(true positives + false negatives) = 59/(59 + 13) = 0.82. The article provides a specificity of 0.61. This can be calculated as: true negatives/(true negatives + false positives) = 440/(440 + 276) = 0.61.

The sensitivity (0.82) is greater than the specificity (0.61). This means that a negative (or 'not at risk of falling') STRATIFY score (a score <2) will be reasonable at ruling out a fall (see the SnNOUT mnemonic, 'if a test has a high sensitivity and the result is negative, it rules the disease out', Chapter 6). Unfortunately, because of the low specificity, an 'at risk' STRATIFY score (that is, ≥2) will be poor at predicting a fall (see the SpPIN mnemonic—'if a test has a high specificity and the result is positive, it rules the disease in').

The post-test probability of a positive ('at risk') score predicting a fall was 0.18. This can be calculated as: true positives/(true positives + false positives) = 59/335 = 0.18 (or 18%). This means that for every 100 patients who were classified as 'at risk' of falling on the STRATIFY tool, only 18 actually did fall. The post-test probability for a negative ('not at risk') score was 0.03. This can be calculated as: false negatives/(true negatives + false negatives) = 13/453 = 0.03 (or 3%). This means that 3% of participants who were correctly classified as 'not at risk'—that is, 3 out of every 100 who scored as not at risk on the STRATIFY tool—actually fell.

How might we use this evidence to inform practice?

A high falls risk score on a tool such as the STRATIFY is designed to prompt staff to utilise additional resources to prevent patient falls. Unfortunately, it is the post-test probability that is central to the

TABLE 7.6: NUMBER OF PATIENTS WHO SCORED AT RISK OF FALLING ACCORDING TO THE STRATIFY TOOL, AND WHETHER PATIENTS ACTUALLY FELL			
	Fell	Did not fall	Total
'At risk' score on STRATIFY tool	59	276	335
'Not at risk' score on STRATIFY tool	13	440	453
Total	72	716	788

decision to employ extra staff and resources to look after patients who might fall (we rarely wonder whether to reduce them because a patient is unlikely to fall!). It is difficult to see how we can use the STRATIFY tool usefully in acute hospital settings to accurately predict falls. Perhaps being aware of which patients have known modifiable falls risk factors such as poor mobility, certain medications (such as sedatives), continence problems and confusion and designing an intervention plan that is tailored for each patient is a more appropriate option than just calculating a score on screening tool. You decide to present the results of this appraisal at the next ward journal club so that your ward's approach to falls prevention can be discussed.

MEDICAL IMAGING EXAMPLE

CLINICAL SCENARIO

As the newly appointed chief radiographer of a metropolitan public hospital which has a large gastroenterology unit, you are relieved to learn that the department has recently upgraded much of its medical imaging equipment and now offers a full digital imaging service including a 64-slice computed tomography (CT) scanner. As you review the range of CT examinations that have been performed since its installation, you are surprised at the small number of referrals for CT colonography. This was in contrast to what occurred in your previous hospital, where some selected symptomatic and screening patients were offered CT colonography instead of colonoscopy. Your Director of Medical Imaging is sympathetic with your interest in ensuring that referring clinicians are made aware of the full diagnostic capabilities of the imaging modalities available to them. However, first he asks you to tell him what research evidence supports the broader use of CT colonography in preference to colonoscopy.

CLINICAL QUESTION

What are the sensitivity and specificity of CT colonography, compared with colonoscopy, in the detection of small polyps and lesions in symptomatic people?

Search terms and databases used to find the evidence

Database: PubMed–Clinical Queries (with 'diagnosis category' and 'narrow scope' selected).

Search terms: (computed tomography colonography) AND (polyps OR lesions) AND symptomatic

The search yields 13 articles. Based on the abstracts, three articles appear to be potentially relevant and one of these used a similar patient population to the one in your clinic, so you retrieve the full text of this article.

Article chosen

Roberts-Thomson IC, Tucker GR, Hewett PJ, et al. Single-center study comparing computed tomography colonography with conventional colonoscopy. World J Gastroenterol 2008;14:469–73. The article is available at: www.wjgnet.com/1007-9327/14/469.asp

Structured abstract (adapted from the above)

Design: A cohort study comparing sensitivity and specificity of CT colonography with colonoscopy.

Setting: A metropolitan teaching hospital in Australia.

Participants: 227 patients (mean age 60 years; 51% male) presenting with appropriate indications for colonoscopy. Exclusion criteria included inflammatory bowel disease and major coexisting medical disorders.

Description of tests: CT colonography was performed with a multi-slice helical CT scanner with 2 mm collimation that was reconstructed into intervals of 1.0–1.5 mm. Colonic distension was achieved by insufflation of carbon dioxide and the use of intravenous Buscopan (butylscopolamine). Participants were scanned in both supine and prone positions during a single breath-hold. Images were read in two-dimensional format with the use of a targeted three-dimensional format when necessary.

Diagnostic standard: Colonoscopy.

Main results: The sensitivity of CT colonography was 71% (95% CI 52% to 85%) for polyps ≥6 mm in size. Specificity was 67% (95% CI 56% to 76%) for polyps ≥6 mm in size.

Conclusion: CT colonography is well accepted by patients and carries a low risk of adverse effects. However, it is not sensitive enough for widespread application in symptomatic patients.

Is this evidence likely to be biased?

- *Did all participants get the diagnostic test and the reference standard?*
  Yes. All participants received the CT colonography and the colonoscopy. Both tests were performed on the same day. Of the 227 patients recruited, 202 were successfully evaluated with both procedures. Twenty-five (11%) of participants were excluded from analysis participation due to incomplete colonoscopy or poor bowel preparation, both of which are factors that cannot be predicted.

- *Could the results of the test of interest have been influenced by the results of the reference standard, or vice versa?*
  No. Colonoscopists were blinded to the CT colonography results prior to the colonoscopy but were segmentally unblinded during the procedure (that is, CT colonography results of the right colon were made available after the colonoscopy of the right colon had been done, and then the same occurred for the left colon). This ensured that all findings reported by CT colonography could be verified during the colonoscopy in real time and any discrepancies clarified by the colonoscopy while the participant was sedated.

- *Is the disease status of the tested population clearly described?*
  Yes. The article states that participants were symptomatic patients with appropriate indications for colonoscopy such as rectal bleeding, abdominal pain and/or change in bowel habits. Some participants also had a family history of colorectal cancer, previous colonic polyps or recent positive faecal occult blood test.

- *Were the methods for performing the test described in sufficient detail?*
  Partially. The procedure for each of the tests was described in reasonable detail. The type of bowel preparation for the CT colonography was not standardised and was determined by the colonoscopist, with little detail provided about this.

What are the main results?

Table 7.7 shows the sensitivity, specificity and positive and negative likelihood ratios of CT colonography when analysed according to polyp size. These results show that CT colonography had low to moderate sensitivity and specificity, although this improved when the polyps were larger (≥6 mm). According to the positive likelihood ratio, only when polyps are ≥6 mm is CT colonography likely to be of some diagnostic value, suggesting a minimal increase in the likelihood of ruling in the presence of polyps if positive. Similarly, the negative likelihood ratios indicate that only when polyps are ≥6 mm is CT colonography likely to be able to help rule out polyps when negative.

TABLE 7.7:
SENSITIVITY, SPECIFICITY AND POSITIVE AND NEGATIVE LIKELIHOOD RATIOS OF CT COLONOGRAPHY WHEN ANALYSED ACCORDING TO POLYP SIZE

Polyp size	Sensitivity (95% CI)	Specificity (95% CI)	Positive likelihood ratio	Negative likelihood ratio
<6 mm	42% (30% to 55%)	63% (52% to 73%)	1.13	0.92
≥6 mm	71% (52% to 85%)	67% (56% to 76%)	2.15	0.43

How might we use this evidence to inform practice?

The study participants were selected from patients who were referred for a colonoscopy on the basis of symptoms suggestive of colonic pathology, and are well matched with the types of patients that you encounter in your clinic in terms of age and indications for colonoscopy. Patients in which CT colonography might be indicated include elderly people who are contraindicated for colonoscopy and those with known bowel obstruction, which it would overcome. However, the results are dependent on polyp size, which limits the usefulness of CT colonography as a screening tool for patients with small (<6 mm) lesions. Given that the sensitivity and specificity of CT colonography are not yet sufficient to implement it on a routine basis, you propose to recommend its use only among suitable patients who could benefit from this procedure. Relative costs and complications of the procedures must also be considered.

HUMAN MOVEMENT EXAMPLE

CLINICAL SCENARIO

You have been employed to facilitate increased physical activity in a retirement village. You know that some residents are active, but you want to identify those who are not, because focusing on them may help to prevent the development of chronic diseases. You wonder if there is a simple validated questionnaire that tests the physical activity of older-aged community-based people.

CLINICAL QUESTION

In a population of older community-based people, is there a validated instrument for assessing physical activity levels?

Search terms and databases used to find the evidence

Database: PubMed–Clinical Queries (with 'diagnosis category' and 'narrow scope' selected).

Search terms: (Physical activity) AND (assessment) AND (sensitivity and specificity) AND (old*)

This search retrieved 23 results, and you choose the one that most closely matched your clinical question.

Article chosen

Topolski T, LoGerfo J, Patrick D, et al. The Rapid Assessment of Physical Activity (RAPA) among older adults. Prev Chronic Dis 2006;3:A118. Full test available free at www.ncbi.nlm.nih.gov/pmc/articles/PMC1779282/pdf/PCD34A118.pdf

Structured abstract (adapted from the above)

Study design: Cross-sectional study.

Setting: Community settings in the Seattle area, USA.

Participants: 115 non-institutionalised men and women (mean age 73.3 years, range 51–92 years, 72% female).

Description of tests: All participants completed three short questionnaires: (1) a new tool called the Rapid Assessment of Physical Activity (RAPA) consisting of nine yes/no questions; (2) the Patient-centred Assessment and Counselling for Exercise (PACE) tool; and (3) the activity measure on the Behavioural Risk Factor Surveillance System. (The last two measures are not the focus of this clinical question, so their results are not reported.)

Diagnostic standard: The Community Healthy Activities Model Program for Seniors (CHAMPS) questionnaire–a research instrument which has been previously validated against an objective measure of physical activity.

Main results: The RAPA had a sensitivity of 81%, positive predictive value of 77% and negative predictive value of 75%.

Conclusion: The RAPA is an easy-to-use valid instrument for measuring physical activity in older people.

Is this evidence likely to be biased?

- *Did all the participants get the diagnostic test and the reference standard?*
  Cannot tell. It is implied, although not clearly stated, that all participants completed both the RAPA and the CHAMPS.

- *Could the results of the test of interest have been influenced by the results of the reference standard, or vice versa?*
  Cannot tell. The article does not detail whether the two tests were administered blinded to the results from each other, so it is possible that the results of one may have influenced the results of the other.

- *Is the disease status of the tested population clearly described?*
  Yes. Although in this study, it is the physical activity status (rather than disease status) that is described; 55% of the participants were described as being physically active by exercising regularly, which provides us with a crude prevalence.

- *Were the methods for performing the test described in sufficient detail?*
  Yes. Required information regarding the administration of the questionnaires is provided and a website for obtaining a copy of the questionnaire is provided.

What are the main results?

The article provides the sensitivity (81%), specificity (69%) and post-test probability for a positive test (77%) for the RAPA compared with the longer CHAMPS questionnaire. The article provides the negative predictive value (75%), which can be converted into the more useful post-test probability of a negative test (25%) by subtracting the negative predictive value from 100%. This tells you that the RAPA would lead to incorrectly classifying people who are non-exercisers as 'exercisers' 25% of the time.

How might we use this evidence to inform practice?

It appears from this study that the RAPA was able to discriminate well between older adults who did and did not engage in regular moderate physical activity and is short and easy-to-use. As the study is not very well reported and you have some concerns about its validity, you decide to search to see whether other studies have evaluated the RAPA before deciding whether this is the best assessment tool for you to be using with the retirement village residents.

PARAMEDICINE EXAMPLE

CLINICAL SCENARIO

You are a paramedic at a planning meeting of your Emergency Medical Service. There is a recurring issue on the agenda: do we have to immobilise the cervical spines of all patients–even those who do not have neck pain, are reasonably conscious, do not have distracting injuries and are not intoxicated–with severe trauma where there is a possible mechanism for spinal injury? Your impression is that large numbers of patients are immobilised although very few ever have a fractured cervical spine, which potentially delays the patient getting to a hospital emergency department. Computed tomography (CT) scans have replaced plain X-rays for detecting cervical spine fractures, as they have better sensitivity. You know that some pre-hospital Emergency Medical Services use a decision-rule based on the National Emergency X-Radiography Utilisation Study (NEXUS) criteria to decide whether trauma patients should be spinally immobilised prior to transport.

CLINICAL QUESTION

Can patients with blunt trauma meeting trauma team activation criteria have cervical spine fracture excluded by using NEXUS criteria, against CT scan as a gold standard?

Search terms and databases used to find the evidence

Database: PubMed–Clinical Queries (with 'diagnosis category' and 'narrow scope' selected).

Search terms: (cervical spine rule) AND ((computed tomography) OR CT) AND (blunt trauma)

The search identified 34 articles. Following a review of the titles and abstracts, one was considered most relevant to the clinical question and chosen for appraisal.

Article chosen

Duane T, Mayglothling J, Wilson S, et al. National Emergency X-Radiography Utilization Study criteria is inadequate to rule out fracture after significant blunt trauma compared with computed tomography. J Trauma 2011;70(4):829–31.

Structured abstract (adapted from the above)

Study design: Prospective cohort study.

Setting: Trauma patients transported to a single Level 1 trauma centre in Richmond, Virginia, USA.

Participants: Patients (>16 years of age) who suffered blunt trauma.

Description of test: The NEXUS criteria assessment of the patient is: (1) conscious and alert (Glasgow Coma Scale [GCS] of 15); (2) no evidence of intoxication; (3) no clinically distracting injury (that is, pain from another injury site); (4) no mid-line cervical spine tenderness or pain; and (5) no neurological deficits.

Diagnostic standard: Routine CT scan (2-mm-thick axial cuts at 2 mm increments with sagittal multi-planar reformatted images, from the base of the skull to the level of the third thoracic vertebra).

Main results: Out of 1361 eligible patients, 64 had a cervical spine fracture on CT scanning. Patients in the fracture group were more likely to be older, white, involved in a motor vehicle accident and initially have a lower GCS and blood pressure. For patients who had a GCS of 15, no other distracting injury and were not intoxicated, the NEXUS criteria had a sensitivity of 59%, specificity 80%, positive predictive value of 13% and negative predictive value of 97.5%. (The article presents results for other subsets of patients, but these subsets are not relevant to your scenario.)

Conclusion: The NEXUS criteria are inaccurate at diagnosing cervical spine fractures in patients who meet trauma team activation criteria, and CT scans are necessary.

Is this evidence likely to be biased?

- *Did all participants get the diagnostic test and the reference standard?*
  Yes. All participants received the diagnostic test (NEXUS) and the reference standard (CT scan).
- *Could the results of the test of interest have been influenced by the results of the reference standard, or vice versa?*
  No. First, the NEXUS test (diagnostic test) was conducted prior to the reference standard (CT scan); and second, it seems unlikely that the CT imaging and interpretation would have been influenced by the NEXUS result.
- *Is the disease status of the tested population clearly described?*
  Yes. Patients who had sustained blunt trauma and met the trauma team activation criteria were assessed on arrival at the emergency department of one Level 1 trauma centre. The number who had a fractured cervical vertebra is also reported.
- *Were the methods for performing the test described in sufficient detail?*
  Yes. The NEXUS criteria were stated clearly. However, there is an assumption that we know how to establish a patient's conscious state (using the Glasgow Coma Scale) and assess whether the patient has any neurological deficit, although this is reasonable.

What are the main results?

The study reported the sensitivity, specificity and negative and positive predictive values (see above in structured abstract) for the subset of patients who match the ones that triggered your clinical question. Table 7.8 shows the number of patients who met the NEXUS criteria and their results following a CT scan. It shows that 26 patients (out of 64) with cervical fractures were missed by NEXUS criteria screening. Of these, most (19; 73%) required intervention.

The post-test probability of a positive test (that is, a cervical spine fracture if there is a positive clinical examination based on the NEXUS criteria) was 0.125 (or 0.13 if rounded). This can be calculated as: true positives/(true positives + false positives) = 38/(38 + 266) = 0.13 (or 13%). This means that for every 100 patients who met the NEXUS criteria, 13 actually had a cervical spine fracture. The post-test probability for a negative test (that is, not meeting the NEXUS criteria to have only clinical examination) was 0.02. This can be calculated as: false negatives/(true negatives + false negatives) = 26/1057 = 0.02 (or 2%). This means that 2 out of every 100 patients who did not meet the NEXUS criteria had a cervical spine fracture.

TABLE 7.8:
OUTCOMES OF PATIENTS ACCORDING TO THE NEXUS CRITERIA AND CT SCAN RESULTS

NEXUS criteria	CT positive (for cervical spine fracture)	CT negative	Total
Positive	38	266	304
Negative	26	1031	1057
Total	64	1297	1361

How might we use this evidence to inform practice?

This study suggests that the NEXUS test is not sensitive enough to rule out cervical spine factures, and therefore cannot be used in this setting to avoid immobilising cervical spines. At your Emergency Service meeting, you decide that you must continue the current procedure of immobilising the cervical spine of patients who have sustained blunt trauma which might have resulted in a fracture, even if the patient has no pain in the neck, is alert, is not intoxicated and does not have a distracting injury.

PHARMACY EXAMPLE

CLINICAL SCENARIO

You are the pharmacy manager of a busy local medical centre pharmacy. The pharmacy is part of a group of five pharmacies in the area. Your pharmacy group implemented a new dispensing software system 1 year ago which included a modified drug-interaction alert tool as part of a dispensary management system upgrade. Overall you have been reasonably happy with the new software; however, at a recent manager's meeting, one of the other store managers reported that they have had a number of situations where the new software failed to pick up expected drug–drug interactions during the dispensing process. This prompted a discussion about the reliability of the software package.

CLINICAL QUESTION

How accurate are commercial pharmacy dispensing software packages at detecting drug–drug interactions?

Search terms and databases used to find the evidence

Database: PubMed Clinical Queries (with 'diagnosis category' and 'narrow scope' selected).

Search terms: pharmac* AND software AND (drug interaction*)

This gives 11 hits. You choose the one that most closely matches your clinical question.

Article chosen

Saverno K, Hines L, Warholak T, et al. Ability of pharmacy clinical decision-support software to alert users about clinically important drug–drug interactions. J Am Med Inform Assoc 2011;18:32–7. Free text available at http://jamia.bmj.com/content/18/1/32

Structured abstract*

Design: Cross-sectional study.

Setting: 64 pharmacies (40 community pharmacies, 14 inpatient hospital pharmacies and 10 others, such as long-term care) using a range of clinical decision-support and drug-interaction software embedded in their dispensing systems, in one state in the USA.

Description of tests: Each pharmacy system was presented, for a fictitious patient, with 18 different prescriptions which included 19 drug pairs: 6 non-interacting drug pairs and 13 potentially interacting pairs (generated from a list of common and important drug interactions generated from the literature).

*Reproduced and adapted from the above reference with permission from BMJ Publishing Group Ltd.

Main results: The median percentage of correct drug–drug interaction responses was 89% (range 47% to 100%). The median sensitivity to detect well-established interactions was 0.85 (range 0.23 to 1.0); median specificity was 1.0 (range 0.83 to 1.0); median positive predictive value was 1.0 (range 0.88 to 1.0) and median negative predictive value was 0.75 (range 0.38 to 1.0).

Conclusion: Many pharmacy clinical decision-support software systems perform less than optimally with respect to identifying well-known, clinically relevant interactions.

Is this evidence likely to be biased?

- *Did all participants get the diagnostic test and the reference standard?*
  Yes. All prescriptions were analysed by the software, except in four pharmacies which did not stock at least one of the medications. In about 40% of cases, the pharmacies had turned off the alerts for at least some of the interactions. This means that the failure rate of detection of drug–drug interactions may be an over-estimate of the usual experience.

- *Could the results of the test of interest have been influenced by the results of the reference standard, or vice versa?*
  No. The 'gold standard' was the drug–drug interactions which were derived from appropriate evidence-based summaries.

- *Is the disease status of the tested population clearly described?*
  In this study, this refers to the type of drug–drug interactions chosen. This was done from an analysis of the literature—choosing common and important interactions, but based on fictitious prescriptions. These may not be representative of the prescriptions normally presented to the pharmacies.

- *Were the methods for performing the test described in sufficient detail?*
  Yes. The 'test' itself of giving the fictitious orders to the systems was simple. However, it is not clear where the pharmacy dispensing systems sourced their drug information data from.

What are the main results?

As reported in the abstract above, the study reported the sensitivity, specificity and positive and negative predictive values for each of the pharmacy systems. The software was better at detecting no drug interactions (89–100% of the time) than detecting drug–drug interactions (as low as 45% for one pair, and up to 90% for the best-detected pair of interactions). Only 27/60 (45%) (missing data for four) pharmacies correctly identified one of the drug-pair interactions (digoxin and itraconazole), while the best was 90% (for simvastatin and itraconazole), with a median percentage of correct drug–drug interactions of 89%.

How might we use this evidence to inform practice?

Commonly used pharmacy information systems are poor at automatically detecting drug–drug interactions, although better at detecting no interaction. This study highlights the need for a high level of vigilance around drug–drug interactions in the pharmacy, particularly for important interactions. Interaction software cannot be relied on to alert pharmacists of all drug–drug interactions, and therefore should never replace good clinical practice.

Reference

1. Hegedus E, Goode A, Campbell S, et al. Physical examination tests of the shoulder: a systematic review with meta-analysis of individual tests. Br J Sports Med 2008;42:80–92.

Chapter 8

Evidence about prognosis

Mark R Elkins

LEARNING OBJECTIVES

After reading this chapter, you should be able to:

- Generate a structured clinical question about prognosis for a clinical scenario
- Appraise the validity of prognostic evidence
- Understand how to interpret the results from prognostic studies and calculate additional results (such as confidence intervals) where possible
- Describe how prognostic evidence can be used to inform practice
- Clearly explain prognostic information to a patient

Let us consider a clinical scenario that will be useful for illustrating the concepts of evidence about prognosis that are the focus of this chapter.

CLINICAL SCENARIO

Mrs Wilson is a 68-year-old woman with osteoarthritis affecting her knees and left hip. Her local doctor has referred her to an orthopaedic surgeon regarding her right knee. The pain in her right knee has been worsening for the past 6 months, making it difficult to manage stairs. The surgeon has recommended a total knee arthroplasty (knee replacement). Mrs Wilson also has mild chronic obstructive pulmonary disease. She takes no medication for this and has not smoked for almost 30 years. Mrs Wilson cares for her husband who has Parkinson's disease. He recently fractured his arm in a fall at home, but has recovered well. Mrs Wilson has not decided whether to proceed with the total knee arthroplasty.

The clinical scenario above raises several questions about the future of the patient's condition. What change in pain and mobility can Mrs Wilson expect if she chooses not to undergo the surgery? If she decides not to have the operation now, for how long will she remain a suitable candidate for surgery? Assuming the surgery is performed, many more questions are raised. How long will it take for the immediate symptoms associated with the surgery to resolve? Will complications occur? How much improvement in mobility can she expect after the surgery? How long will it take to achieve this level of mobility? Will surgical revision of the joint replacement become necessary and, if so, when? These types of questions will be the focus of this chapter on prognosis.

Prognosis is about predicting the future—the future of a patient's condition. While it is impossible for anyone to predict the future with absolute certainty, we can use evidence from the past to make informed and sensible predictions about the future. These evidence-based predictions about the future can be useful in many ways. They can help reassure patients by removing some doubt about the future, especially if their expectations are unjustifiably pessimistic. Predictions about natural recovery can help you and your patient to jointly decide whether interventions need to be considered at all. Sometimes an intervention is chosen that is typically applied only once, as with joint replacement or organ transplant. In such cases, the optimal time to apply the intervention can be determined by predictions about the rate of deterioration before it and the rate of recovery after it. Predictions about the average course of a particular condition can also be adjusted for individual patients. This adjustment is possible when other features about a patient or the patient's health or management, besides the primary diagnosis, have been shown to affect outcomes.

This chapter will address the process of using prognostic evidence to make these predictions and incorporating them into clinical practice. We will start by defining the components of a structured clinical question about prognosis. Then we will see how to appraise the evidence to determine its likely validity. Subsequent sections of the chapter will review how to understand the results of a prognostic study, how to use the evidence to inform practice and how to explain prognostic information clearly to patients.

HOW TO STRUCTURE A PROGNOSTIC QUESTION

You will recall from Chapter 2 that clinical questions can be structured using the PICO format: Patient/Problem, Intervention/Issue, Comparison (if relevant) and Outcomes. When our question was about the effect of an intervention, the comparison was an important component. The effect of an intervention was always estimated by comparison against this component, even if it was a 'no-intervention' or usual care control. Questions about prognosis, instead, are questions about expected outcomes, not questions about what has caused those outcomes. Therefore, the comparison component is not used in questions about prognosis. Let us look at each of the remaining components in more detail.

Patient/problem

The patient/problem component can simply be specified as previously described, for example: '*In patients with coronary heart disease …*', '*Among children with epilepsy …*' or, from our scenario, '*In adults with osteoarthritis of the knee …*'. Sometimes, the prognosis for typical patients with the condition is quite different to the prognosis for patients with some extra characteristic. For example, the prognosis for patients with cystic fibrosis who become infected with the bacteria *Burkholderia cepacia* is worse than for those who do not.[1] Characteristics that influence outcomes are known as **prognostic factors**. If you suspect that some characteristic of your patient might be a prognostic factor, this can be incorporated into the patient/problem component. Let us assume for a moment that Mrs Wilson, the patient in our scenario at the beginning of this chapter, is mildly obese. This may be a prognostic factor, so we could incorporate this into our clinical question: '*In adults with osteoarthritis of the knee who are obese …*' In addition to comorbidities like obesity, prognostic factors can also relate to the severity of the condition, for example: '*In patients with coronary heart disease (New York Heart Association Functional Class IV) …*'. The New York Heart Association functional classification is a simple way of describing the extent of heart disease. It places patients in one of four categories based on the severity of their symptoms and how much they are limited during exercise. The history of the condition can also be a prognostic factor, for example: '*Among children who have had their first epileptic seizure …*'.

Intervention/issue

The next component of the question is the intervention/issue. If you are interested in the natural course of a condition, then you can simply add the term 'untreated' to your clinical question, for example: '*In children with untreated nocturnal enuresis …*'. This will remind you when you search for evidence that you are interested in prognostic evidence about untreated patients. It is logical to assume that a patient's prognosis may be affected by receiving an intervention, especially if the intervention has been shown to be effective. Therefore, a clinical question about prognosis should specify what intervention a patient has received or is receiving for their condition. In fact, some questions are only relevant to a population that has received an intervention, such as in these two examples:

> *In patients undergoing surgical skin grafts for major burns, what is the risk of postoperative complications?*

and

> *Among patients who no longer stutter at the end of a course of intensive therapy, what is the probability that their stuttering will relapse in the next year?*

Outcomes

The last component of a clinical question about prognosis is outcomes. It is important to consider outcomes that will have the greatest impact on the patient's goals and priorities. The prognosis can also change over time. For example, among alcoholic women who are able to stop drinking alcohol and remain abstained from it, the average improvements in memory and psychomotor speed at 1 year are minimal, while by 4 years they have usually returned to within the normal range.[2] Therefore, it is sometimes worthwhile adding a timeframe to the outcome component of your clinical question.

CLINICAL SCENARIO (CONTINUED)

Structuring the clinical question

There are many prognostic questions that can be drawn from our scenario. Let us assume that Mrs Wilson has had further discussions with her orthopaedic surgeon and has now decided to go ahead with the surgery. Her primary concern is arranging care for her husband while she is incapacitated by the surgery. Mrs Wilson is keen to know how long it will take for her to regain the function in her knee, particularly her ability to walk independently. Mrs Wilson is eligible for 2 weeks of respite care and the Wilsons' son is able to take 4 weeks off work to assist with the care of his father. From this scenario, a suitable prognostic question would be:

- In patients undergoing total knee arthroplasty for osteoarthritis, what improvement in walking ability would be expected after 6 weeks?

CLINICAL SCENARIO (CONTINUED)

Finding the evidence to answer your question

You start by looking for a prospective cohort study in PubMed Clinical Queries, filtering your search with the 'prognosis' and 'narrow' options selected and using the search terms *osteoarthritis AND (total knee) AND walking*. You have included 'total knee' in your search terms, rather than 'total knee arthroplasty', as you are aware that it is sometimes referred to as total knee replacement and you wanted to find articles which had used either term. This search results in 15 articles. A quick scan of the titles confirms that several of the articles are probably relevant. One of these is very close to what we require, but the earliest point at which outcomes are measured is 6 months after the surgery. Another appears to be exactly what we require, as it provides data about mean walking ability from 1 week to 1 year after the surgery.[3] Throughout the rest of this chapter, we will refer to this study as the 'knee arthroplasty study'.

The results of your search—only 15 articles with a substantial proportion seeming relevant—suggests that the search may be too narrow. Using the 'broad' search option (this gives 82 results) or adjusting the search terms may help. A third strategy is to click on the 'Related Articles' link next to the most relevant article we have retrieved. This triggers a search in which PubMed seeks the most similar articles it can find to the one you have indicated. In this instance, 147 articles are retrieved. A scan of the titles, and of the abstracts for the most promising titles, identifies very similar types of articles but nothing more suitable than the best article that you chose from the original search.

CLINICAL SCENARIO (CONTINUED)

Structured abstract of our chosen article

Citation: Kennedy D, Stratford P, Riddle D, et al. Assessing recovery and establishing prognosis following total knee arthroplasty. Phys Ther 2008;88:22–32. The structured abstract has been adapted from this reference.

Question: In patients undergoing a primary knee replacement for osteoarthritis, what is the pattern of improvement in lower limb function and walking ability from 1 week to 1 year after surgery?

Design: Inception cohort followed prospectively for 1 year.

Setting: Tertiary care orthopaedic facility in Toronto, Canada.

Participants: Eighty-four patients with osteoarthritis (mean age 66 years, 52% female) undergoing primary total knee arthroplasty. Participants needed to be able to communicate in written and spoken English. Exclusion criteria were any neurological, cardiac or psychiatric disorders or other medical conditions that would substantially compromise physical function.

Prognostic factors: Gender, preoperative lower limb function and preoperative 6-Minute Walk Test distance.

Outcomes: Lower Extremity Functional Scale–a self-reported, 20-item scale of lower extremity function that includes activity limitation and participation restriction concepts and is scored from 0 (lowest function) to 80 (highest function). 6-Minute Walk Test–a submaximal exercise test in which participants walk the greatest distance they can in 6 minutes on flat ground with standard encouragement.

Main results: In general, there was a deterioration in both scores at the immediate postoperative measurement. From this point, there was rapid improvement in both scores initially, with progressively slower gains in improvement with increasing time postsurgery. Gender and preoperative function were prognostic factors for each outcome. For the Lower Extremity Functional Scale, assuming the average preoperative function of the cohort, females had scores of 18 at 1 week, 38 at 6 weeks and 53 at 6 months. Males had scores of 25 at 1 week, 43 at 6 weeks and 60 at 6 months. For the 6-Minute Walk Test, assuming the average preoperative function of the cohort, females achieved 200 m at 1 week, 330 m at 6 weeks and 470 m at 6 months. Males achieved 250 m at 1 week, 440 m at 6 weeks and 580 m at 6 months. All the 6-month values were maintained to 1 year.

Conclusions: For both outcomes, the rate of improvement was greatest immediately following surgery. Roughly half of the postoperative improvement was observed in the first 6 weeks. This brought patients to an adequate level of function for typical daily activities. Almost all of the remaining improvement had occurred by 6 months, with both outcomes then being maintained until the end of the year.

IS THIS EVIDENCE LIKELY TO BE BIASED?

We will use questions drawn from the Critical Appraisal Skills Program (CASP) and associated checklists for appraising a cohort study to explain how to assess the likelihood of bias in a prognostic study. Note, however, that the checklist for cohort studies is intended not only for use with longitudinal single-group studies, but also with other study designs such as case-control studies. Therefore, not all the questions that are raised in the checklist will be explained in this chapter. The key questions to ask when appraising the validity of a prognostic study are summarised in Box 8.1. The checklist begins with two simple screening criteria that, if not met, indicate that the article is unlikely to be helpful and that further assessment of potential bias is probably unwarranted.

As you saw in Chapters 4 and 6, there are standards for reporting of randomised controlled trials (CONSORT statement) and diagnostic accuracy studies (STARD statement). The reporting standard for observational studies in epidemiological studies is known as the STROBE statement, and there is a particular checklist for cohort studies (and checklists for other study designs such as case-control studies and cross-sectional studies). Further details are available at www.strobe-statement.org.

Key questions to ask when appraising the validity (risk of bias) of a prognostic study

1. Was there a representative and well-defined sample?
2. Was there an inception cohort?
3. Was exposure determined accurately?
4. Were the outcomes measured accurately?
5. Were important prognostic factors considered and adjusted for?
6. Was the follow-up of participants sufficiently long and complete?

Did the study address a clearly focused issue?

The first criterion on the CASP checklist is whether the study addressed a clearly focused issue. For prognostic evidence, the article should clearly define the population, potential prognostic factors and the outcomes considered.

CLINICAL SCENARIO (CONTINUED)

Did the study address a clearly focused issue?

The knee arthroplasty study meets this criterion, as shown in the question it seeks to answer: *In patients undergoing a primary knee replacement for osteoarthritis, what is the pattern of improvement in lower limb function and walking ability from 1 week to 1 year after surgery?*

Appropriate study type

The second criterion is that the method used was appropriate to answer the question posed by the authors. In Chapter 2, we saw that longitudinal studies, particularly prospective cohort studies, provide the best evidence about prognosis. Even better than that is a systematic review of prospective cohort studies. However, currently there are so few systematic reviews of prognostic studies in this area that it is probably not realistic for you to expect to find one.

Although prospective cohort studies are typically the study type that you should use to answer prognostic questions, you should be aware that prognostic information can also be generated by other study designs. For example, if you are interested in the natural history of a condition, then the outcomes of an untreated control group in a randomised controlled trial can provide this information. Conversely, case-control studies or case series, where all cases receive a particular treatment, give prognostic information about a treated cohort.

CLINICAL SCENARIO (CONTINUED)

Appropriate study type

The researchers in the knee arthroplasty study wanted to find prognostic data and they used the ideal study design for this: a prospective, longitudinal study of an inception cohort of patients undergoing primary total knee arthroplasty. Therefore, we can move on to the more detailed criteria on the CASP checklist.

Was there a representative and well-defined sample of participants?

The next criterion on the checklist is whether the cohort was recruited in a way that ensured it was representative of the larger population of interest. This criterion is important, as a study's estimate of prognosis will be biased if the study's sample is systematically different from (and therefore not representative of) the larger population of interest. It is important that a study clearly defines its inclusion and exclusion criteria, as this can help in recruiting a representative sample. Clearly defined criteria help make it clear to everyone (researchers, participants, you) just what the target population of the study was. A representative sample is also more likely to be obtained if the study recruits all of the eligible patients who presented at the recruitment site into the study. When appraising a study, look for a statement in the article that describes either recruiting 'all patients' or recruiting 'consecutive cases'. Recruiting all eligible patients prevents bias in the data that could arise if some eligible patients avoided recruitment and these patients differ in some systematic way from those who were recruited. The greater the proportion of eligible patients that are recruited into the study, the more representative of the target population the sample is likely to be.

CLINICAL SCENARIO (CONTINUED)
Representative and well-defined sample

In the knee arthroplasty study, the researchers were unable to achieve consecutive recruitment because of an outbreak of severe acute respiratory syndrome (SARS) in Toronto during their data collection period. However, we are not too concerned about this as it is unlikely to have caused recruitment of an unrepresentative sample. Additionally, the inclusion and exclusion criteria of the study are clearly defined. We conclude that the cohort is likely to be representative of the target population.

The problem with retrospective studies

As we saw in Chapter 2, cohort studies can either be prospective or retrospective, with retrospective studies being lower down the hierarchy of evidence for prognostic questions. The reason for this is that studies that identify patients retrospectively are more likely to have recruitment bias. This is because it is relatively common for patients with a particular characteristic to be systematically missed. As an extreme example, one retrospective study examined 81 patients with infections after total knee arthroplasty.[4] Clearly, we cannot use this cohort to determine the likelihood of joint infection, because this cohort was selected to ensure that 100% of patients had an infection. It is also inappropriate to use the cohort to determine, for example, the likelihood of independent mobility 1 year after total knee arthroplasty, as the mobility of individuals with infections may differ from that of all individuals who undergo knee arthroplasty. In other retrospective studies, the cohort is selected because they presented for treatment. For example, another study examined 1012 patients who presented for treatment of knee complaints after any previous knee injury.[5] The severity of the changes in bone and cartilage were compared with details in their health records to identify prognostic factors for the progression of osteoarthritis. Note that this study does not capture people who sustain a knee injury but do not present for treatment of knee complaints later, such as those who develop very mild or no osteoarthritis. The data from this study could therefore lead to excessively pessimistic predictions about the likely severity of osteoarthritis after knee injury. Instead, what is needed is a study in which patients are identified at the time of knee injury and followed for decades to assess the development of osteoarthritis.[6]

Was there an inception cohort?

Although it is not explicitly mentioned on the CASP checklist (but rather is covered by the question 'Was the cohort recruited in an acceptable way?' on the checklist), one of the things that will help you to determine whether the cohort was recruited in an acceptable way—a key issue that affects the validity of a cohort study (by minimising selection bias)—is whether there was an inception cohort. In other words, were participants recruited at a similar well-described point in the course of the disease? It is important that this was done because a group of people with the same condition may vary in their prognoses because of how long they have had the condition. Consider the scenario of a disease that is sometimes fatal, with the deaths that do occur usually being within 2 years of its onset. If we consider the prognosis for short-term mortality, it is likely to be worse in newly diagnosed patients than in those who have had the disease for 5 years. This is because the 5-year survivors have survived the 'danger period' and now have a short-term mortality that is similar to people without the disease. This means that, in a cohort study that recruited people with this disease, the average prognosis could be greatly affected by the proportions of participants who are newly diagnosed and participants who are chronic (that is, diagnosed some time ago) that are recruited. Some studies recruit from sources, such as patient support groups, that can bias recruitment towards these survivors, which makes any prognostic estimate favourable when this is really not an accurate estimate for this disease.

Avoiding this bias is solved by recruiting participants at a consistent and defined point in their disease. When this point is very early in the disease process, the cohort is called an 'inception' cohort. Some studies recruit participants at diagnosis. However, the point of diagnosis is not always at an early or a uniform point in the disease process. This is particularly the case for chronic conditions, for example rheumatoid arthritis or low back pain. You must therefore consider carefully whether a true inception cohort has been identified when recruitment occurs at diagnosis.

CLINICAL SCENARIO (CONTINUED)
Inception cohort

In the knee arthroplasty study, the participants were not recruited at the inception of their osteoarthritis, but we still have an inception cohort. They were recruited at their inception into our target population of patients undergoing total knee arthroplasty for osteoarthritis.

Was exposure determined accurately?

The next criterion on the checklist is whether exposure was determined accurately. The term 'exposure' can be confusing when referring to a simple prognostic cohort study, as it is more commonly considered in case-control studies. For a simple prognostic cohort study, we can think of it as whether we have accurately determined eligibility criteria (that is, the main condition or disease or event that we are interested in determining the prognosis of). In the knee arthroplasty study, the criterion amounts to whether we have accurately determined whether our patients have undergone a total knee arthroplasty for osteoarthritis. While there is probably little chance of confusion about whether someone has undergone this procedure, the diagnosis of osteoarthritis may be more prone to error. This is relevant given that other prognostic studies have shown that some outcomes after total knee arthroplasty is performed because of *rheumatoid* arthritis differ markedly from those outcomes that occur when the total knee arthroplasty is performed because of osteoarthritis.[7]

Determination of exposure

The knee arthroplasty article states that the study was conducted at a Centre of Excellence for knee replacement that is one of the largest centres in Canada that performs this procedure. While we cannot be completely certain, we can probably expect that the diagnoses were made correctly.

Were the outcomes measured accurately?

Accuracy is important not only in the application of eligibility criteria, but also in the measurement of outcomes. Researchers should specify and clearly define their outcomes at the start of the study. We must consider whether the outcome measures have been **validated**—that is, do they measure what they claim to measure? The article that you are appraising should provide details about the validity of the outcome measures that were used. The CASP checklist also suggests that we consider whether the outcomes are *objective* (for example, a fall) or *subjective* (for example, pain). Although it is not always possible, outcomes should be measured using **objective criteria** where possible. As the subjectivity of the outcome measures increases, the risk of bias increases. In this situation, where the outcomes are subjective and require a degree of judgment on the part of the person who is doing the assessing of the outcome, it becomes important that the **assessor is blinded to the prognostic factors** that each patient has. However, it can be difficult to blind assessors to certain prognostic factors of each patient, such as age and gender. Prognostic factors are explained in more detail in the following section.

When prognostic studies report dichotomous outcomes, the criterion of accuracy is that the events have been clearly defined and a reliable system for identifying them has been implemented. Otherwise, some events might have occurred but not been recorded. For example, consider a cohort study of patients who commenced non-invasive ventilation for acute respiratory failure which reported the number of patients that died during that hospital admission. As this study involved hospitalised patients, the death of a patient would have been recorded in the patient's medical record, so we could be confident about the accuracy of this outcome. Now consider a cohort study that followed up elderly patients who had received an intervention (such as home assessment and modification) to prevent falls and evaluated whether the patients sustained a musculoskeletal injury in the year following the intervention. This dichotomous outcome (did or did not sustain musculoskeletal injury) is more difficult to measure accurately than the outcome of death in the above cohort study. Even if musculoskeletal injuries were well defined and explained to patients, such injuries may not have been reported if a patient mis-judged whether the injury was musculoskeletal or forgot that it occurred.

Measurement of outcomes

The knee arthroplasty article cites supportive data regarding the reliability, validity and ability to detect change for the Lower Extremity Functional Scale and the 6-Minute Walk Test. In terms of subjective versus objective outcomes, it is reassuring that there is one subjective continuous outcome measure and one objective continuous outcome measure that each measures the same concept–walking ability. It is even more reassuring that the results of the two measures are in agreement. The article does not mention whether assessors were blind to participants' prognostic factors, so we will assume that they were not.

Confounding factors and prognostic factors

We saw in Chapter 2 how confounding factors are anything that can become confused with the outcome of interest and bias the results. Although the CASP checklist only refers to confounding factors, it can also be useful to consider a reasonable range of possible prognostic factors that may influence the outcome of interest in the study and check whether the study has considered (and also measured) these factors. A *prognostic factor* is any characteristic that can influence the outcome of interest and is associated strongly enough with the outcome that it can accurately predict the eventual development of the outcome. Note that this does not necessarily mean that the prognostic factor causes the outcome. Prognostic factors can include demographic characteristics (such as age), disease-specific characteristics (for example severity of a head injury) or whether the patient has any comorbid conditions (that is, other conditions, for example hypertension or diabetes).

Many prognostic studies will report results for various subgroups of participants who differ because of the presence of a certain prognostic factor (or factors), and the prognosis that is reported for each subgroup will probably be different. When a study reports subgroup results like this, you need to check whether the researchers did an adjusted analysis. By this we mean: did they check that these subgroup differences and predictions are not the result of another important prognostic factor? Information about any adjusted analysis that was done is usually presented in the data analysis section of an article. It is beyond the scope of this book to explain the statistical methods that are involved with adjusted analysis. If you are interested in understanding this, we suggest that you consult an additional statistical resource.

Was the follow-up of participants sufficiently long and complete?

There are two elements to this criterion, and you should assess whether the study meets both elements. You must use your knowledge about the condition of interest to judge whether the follow-up period was long enough for clinically important changes or events to occur. Consider a cohort study to determine the proportion of tracheotomised patients who can manage a speaking valve as soon as ventilatory support is weaned. The outcome from each participant can be determined within minutes. Therefore, a very short follow-up period is sufficient in this situation. Conversely, a cohort study of very low birth-weight infants may need to follow participants for a decade or more to accurately assess the extent of neurodevelopmental delay.

As we saw with randomised controlled trials in Chapter 4, the greater the loss to follow-up, the greater the opportunity for bias in the results, especially if there is something systematic about those who drop out. Some experts suggest using the '5 and 20' rule: a loss to follow-up of less than 5% is unlikely to influence the results much, while a loss greater than 20% starts to seriously threaten a study's validity.[8] Using the same rule-of-thumb guide (where a study that has at least 80–85% follow-up is unlikely to be seriously biased) that we discussed in Chapter 4 when explaining how to evaluate the adequacy of follow-up in a randomised controlled trial is another simple way to determine whether follow-up in a prognostic study was sufficiently complete. As with randomised controlled trials, a study should also state the reasons why participants were lost to follow-up. It can also be helpful if a study provides a comparison of prognostic factors for participants who were lost to follow-up and those who were not. This information can help you to determine whether there were certain types of participants who were selectively lost to follow-up.

Follow-up of participants

In the knee arthroplasty study, there was so little change in the outcomes in the second 6 months of the follow-up period that it appears that a 1-year follow-up in total was long enough for all clinically important postoperative improvement to be captured. For data on a long-term dichotomous outcome (such as the time to revision of the total knee arthroplasty) to be collected, a follow-up period of 15 or 20 years would be required.[9] A potential complication following total knee arthroplasty is deep vein thrombosis, but the greatest risk of this occurring is during the period of reduced mobility postoperatively.[10] Therefore, the follow-up period of 1 year was adequate to detect this outcome if it were to occur (which it did in one participant). The period of follow-up is inadequate to pick up long-term surgical revisions due to prosthetic wear, but it will identify early revisions due to postoperative complications such as infection.

There are no data provided in the article about the number of participants who were lost to follow-up, so you are unable to assess the adequacy of follow-up.

If you have got to this point and determined that the article about prognosis that you have been appraising is reasonably valid, you then proceed to look at the importance and applicability of the results.

WHAT ARE THE RESULTS?

Prognostic data can be presented in several ways, and the results of the study may have been measured using continuous or dichotomous outcomes. In a similar manner to the way in which we approached understanding the results of a randomised controlled trial in Chapter 4, when understanding prognostic results we will be looking at how to answer two main questions:

1. How **likely** are the outcomes over time?
2. How **precise** are the estimates of likelihood?

Likelihood of the outcomes over time

Regardless of the way the outcome was measured, the prognosis often changes over time. Thus, prognostic data are usually only relevant to a particular time period. For continuous outcomes, the expected value (usually the mean value) of the outcome at a certain point in time is what is usually reported. For example, men with aphasia after their first stroke showed an average improvement of 12.3 on the Aphasia Quotient 1 year after the stroke.[11] The Aphasia Quotient is a measure of the severity of aphasia, rated from 0 (worst) to 100 (best). Scores above 93.8 are considered normal (non-aphasic). Where the pattern of change in the outcome is of interest, the outcome may be graphed over time (see Figures 8.2 and 8.3, later in the chapter, for graphs related to the knee arthroplasty clinical scenario).

Dichotomous outcomes can be reported as the proportion of patients who experienced the event at a particular time (that is, the risk of the event). For example, among women who develop postnatal depression, 62% are likely to still have depression 3 months later.[12] Alternatively, the same information can be reported as the risk for an individual patient: for a woman who develops postnatal depression, the risk of having depression 3 months later is 62%. Where the change in risk over time is of interest, this may be graphed as a survival curve.

Survival curves are often used to present prognostic data, and they show how the likelihood of an event changes over time. Figure 8.1 shows a survival curve from a study that examined the long-term

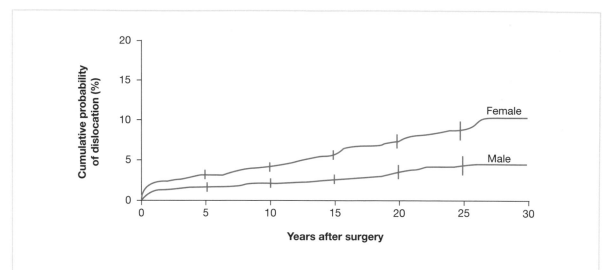

Figure 8.1
Cumulative probability of a first-time hip dislocation for female and male patients.

Reproduced with permission from Berry DJ, von Knoch M, Schleck CD, Harmsen WS, The cumulative long-term risk of dislocation after primary Charnley total hip arthroplasty, The Journal of Bone and Joint Surgery, Inc.[13]

risk of dislocation following total hip arthroplasty (replacement).[13] In this particular survival curve, the cumulative risk of hip dislocation following hip replacement is presented separately for females and males. You can see that at 25 years the risk of dislocation for females was 8.9% (the authors also provide the 95% confidence interval for this, 7.7% to 10.2%), whereas the risk for males was 4.5% (95% confidence interval 3.3% to 5.8%). You can also see, by looking at the slope of the curve, that female participants had both a higher early risk of dislocation as well as a higher late risk than male participants.

Precision of the estimates of likelihood

To properly interpret a prognostic study, it is necessary to know how much uncertainty is associated with its results. Just as we saw with estimates of the effect of an intervention in Chapter 4, a 95% confidence interval indicates the precision of the estimate of prognosis. As with the confidence intervals for randomised controlled trials, the larger the size of the prognostic study, the narrower (and more precise) the confidence interval will be. Confidence intervals can often be calculated if the authors of an article have not provided them.

Calculating a confidence interval for continuous outcomes

For continuous outcomes, the 95% confidence interval (CI) provides the range of average values within which we are 95% certain that the true average value lies. The confidence interval can be calculated approximately using the formula:

$$95\% \text{ CI} = \text{mean} \pm (3 \times \text{standard deviation} \div \sqrt{2n})$$

where n is the number of patients. Let us assume in our example of aphasia in men after their first stroke that the mean improvement of 12.3 on the Aphasia Quotient had a standard deviation of 18 and was determined using data from 83 patients:

$$95\% \text{ CI} = \text{mean} \pm (3 \times \text{standard deviation} \div \sqrt{2n})$$
$$= 12.3 \pm [(3 \times 18) \div \sqrt{(2 \times 83)}]$$
$$= 12.3 \pm 4.2$$
$$= 8.1 \text{ to } 16.5$$

Therefore, we could expect that, in men with aphasia after their first stroke, the average level of improvement would be between 8 and 16 on the Aphasia Quotient 1 year after their stroke.

Calculating a confidence interval for dichotomous outcomes

For dichotomous outcomes, which are reported as the risk of an event, the 95% confidence interval provides the range of risks within which we are 95% certain that the true risk lies. The confidence interval can be calculated approximately using the formula:

$$95\% \text{ CI} = \text{risk} \pm (1 \div \sqrt{2n})$$

where n is the number of patients. Let us assume, in our example of postnatal depression in women, that the 62% risk of still having depression 3 months later was determined using data from 24 patients:

$$95\% \text{ CI} = \text{risk} \pm (1 \div \sqrt{2n})$$
$$= 62\% \pm [1 \div \sqrt{(2 \times 24)}]$$
$$= 62\% \pm 14\%$$
$$= 48\% \text{ to } 76\%$$

Therefore, we could assume that the risk of postnatal depression persisting for 3 months is between 48% and 76%.

Identification and analysis of prognostic factors

In prognostic studies, data about the likelihood of the outcome are typically presented first, and then an analysis of prognostic factors is presented if the study conducts such an analysis. Such data may be presented simply by reporting the prognosis for various subgroups of participants, where each subgroup has a certain prognostic factor (or if dealing with a continuous variable, varying degrees of the factor). Data about prognostic factors may also be presented in a more complex way using multivariate predictive models which assess how each prognostic factor is associated with each other prognostic factor and the overall prognosis. Explanation about multivariate analysis techniques is beyond the scope of this book.

An example of how a prognostic factor can be reported in a way that treats it as continuous data comes from a study about risk factors for hip fracture in women.[14] In this study, increasing age was reported as a risk factor for hip fracture in women over 65 years of age. For every 5-year increment in age, the risk of a hip fracture increased 1.5 times. This study also treated other risk factors dichotomously. For example, having a maternal history of hip fracture was found to double a woman's risk of hip fracture.

What are the results?

In the knee arthroplasty article, the average pattern of postoperative improvement in the Lower Extremity Functional Scale is presented in a graph—see the middle curve in Figure 8.2. Note that these data are for females only. The authors elected to analyse the data for males and females separately because gender has previously been shown to influence functional mobility after total knee arthroplasty.[15,16] Females had average scores of 27 preoperatively, 18 at 1 week, 38 at 6 weeks and 53 at 6 months. The 6-month value was then maintained until 12 months.

A similar pattern of improvement was seen on the 6-Minute Walk Test. Females achieved an average distance of 353 m preoperatively, 200 m at 1 week, 330 m at 6 weeks and 470 m at 6 months. The 6-month value was again maintained until 12 months. For a graph of the average pattern of improvement, see the middle curve in Figure 8.3.

In addition to gender, there is another prognostic factor for functional mobility in the postoperative period: preoperative functional mobility. The higher a patient's Lower Extremity Functional Scale score was preoperatively, the higher their postoperative Lower Extremity Functional Scale score was throughout the following year. For a graph of the average effect of preoperative Lower Extremity Functional Scale score on postoperative recovery, see the top and bottom curves in Figure 8.2.

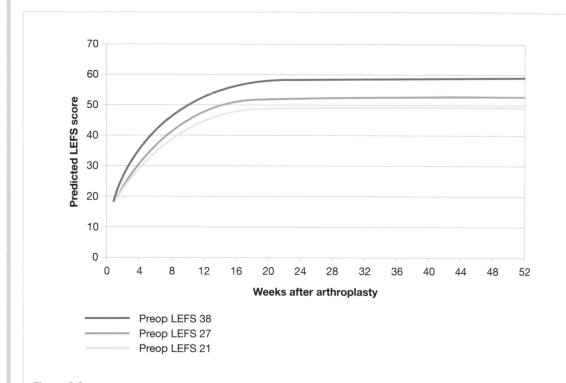

Figure 8.2

Change in average Lower Extremity Functional Scale (LEFS) scores for females (middle curve), with adjustment for higher (top curve) and lower (bottom curve) preoperative LEFS scores.

Reproduced with permission from Kennedy D et al, Assessing recovery and establishing prognosis following total knee arthroplasty, American Physical Therapy Association, 2008, Fig 2b.[3] This material is copyrighted, and any further reproduction or distribution requires written permission from APTA.

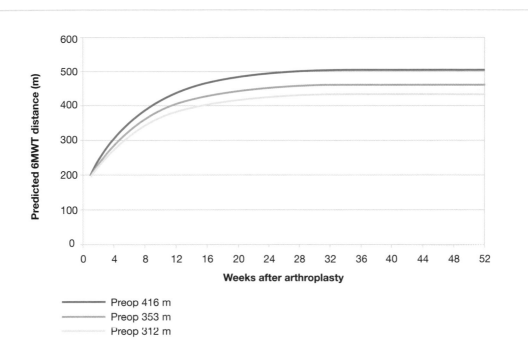

Figure 8.3

Change in average 6-Minute Walk Test: distances for females (middle curve), with adjustment for longer (top curve) and shorter (bottom curve) preoperative 6-Minute Walk Test distances.

Reproduced with permission from Kennedy D et al, Assessing recovery and establishing prognosis following total knee arthroplasty; American Physical Therapy Association 2008, Fig 3b.[3] This material is copyrighted, and any further reproduction or distribution requires written permission from APTA.

Similarly, a patient's preoperative 6-Minute Walk Test distance influenced the postoperative value—see the top and bottom curves in Figure 8.3.

For simplicity, let us assume that Mrs Wilson has average preoperative Lower Extremity Functional Scale and 6-Minute Walk Test results. It is important to remember that there is still a degree of uncertainty in using the average results for females as prognostic estimates for Mrs Wilson. For example, we have determined that her likely 6-Minute Walk Test distance at 1 year will be 470 m. The article tells us that the standard deviation around this estimate was 84.7 m and that this was determined with data from 44 female patients. Therefore, we can calculate a 95% confidence interval around that estimate.

$$95\% \ CI = mean \pm (3 \times standard \ deviation \div \sqrt{2n})$$
$$= 470\,m \pm [(3 \times 84.7) \div \sqrt{(2 \times 44)}]$$
$$= 470\,m \pm 27$$
$$= 443\,m \ to \ 497\,m$$

This is a reasonably precise estimate. We can be confident when discussing our estimate with Mrs Wilson, knowing that it is a good approximation of the true value that we are seeking to estimate. However, we should acknowledge and explain to her that the true average prognosis of the 6-Minute Walk Test may be a little higher or lower than our best estimate of 470 m.

HOW CAN WE USE THIS EVIDENCE TO INFORM PRACTICE?

As we saw in Chapter 4 in the section on using evidence about interventions, before applying the evidence about interventions from a study, you need to consider whether your patient is similar to the participants in the study. The same consideration needs to occur before applying the results from a prognostic study to your patient.

Prognostic information has several uses in clinical practice. Having information about the likely clinical course of a condition can help you to determine whether intervention needs to be considered for the condition. If the prognosis for natural recovery is very good, there may be little point in starting any intervention. Similarly, if the prognosis for a cohort treated with a particular intervention is very good, then alternative or additional interventions may not need to be considered for patients who can be managed successfully with that intervention. In such cases, using the information to counsel patients and provide them with explanation and reassurance may be all that is necessary.

However, if the prognosis for the condition may be able to be improved by intervention and there are available interventions that are likely to make a clinically important difference, the information that you have about prognosis can form the starting point for a discussion with your patient. In addition to explaining what is likely to occur in the future with respect to the condition, you also need to discuss the various intervention options (if there are more than one) with your patient and engage them in the decision-making process. Shared decision making is an important component of evidence-based practice (and indeed, clinical practice in general) and further information about this and strategies to facilitate shared decision making are discussed in Chapter 14.

Central to facilitating patient involvement in decision making is communicating with patients effectively. Again, Chapter 14 provides you with a number of practical strategies that you can use to ensure that you are communicating effectively with your patients. When explaining prognostic information to a patient, it is important to do so in a manner that the patient can understand and make it relevant to the patient's goals and priorities. It is therefore good to focus on the outcomes and timeframes that matter most to the patient. In addition, if the patient has prognostic factors that affect the prognosis, it is reasonable to consider explaining their influence, especially if any of them are modifiable (for example, being overweight).

CLINICAL SCENARIO (CONTINUED)
Using the evidence to inform practice

After reading about the characteristics of the study participants, you decide that Mrs Wilson is similar enough to the study participants that the results could apply to her. To explain Mrs Wilson's prognosis for the return of functional mobility, we could begin by explaining her predicted status at some key time-points: immediately after surgery, 6 weeks after surgery (when her support people are due to leave) and 6 months after surgery (when her maximum function is likely to be achieved). Remember that one purpose of generating this prognostic information was to help Mrs Wilson decide on arrangements for her husband's care after her surgery. Simply telling her the predicted Lower Extremity Functional Scale score and 6-Minute Walk Test distance at 6 weeks may not be very helpful in determining whether she will need assistance to care for her husband. Let us look at ways we can help Mrs Wilson to interpret these predicted results.

Mrs Wilson's Lower Extremity Functional Scale score is predicted to be 38 at 6 weeks. To link this overall score of 38 to ratings of difficulty with functional activities, we can draw upon further prognostic research[17] that provides data for 20 activities. For each activity, the average total Lower Extremity Functional Scale score is scored by participants who report the difficulty that they have doing the activity as: 0 (extreme difficulty), 1 (quite a bit of difficulty), 2 (moderate difficulty), 3 (a little bit of difficulty) or 4 (no difficulty). For the activity of walking between rooms, participants who had extreme difficulty had an average overall Lower Extremity Functional Scale score of 4; those who had quite a bit of difficulty had an average score of 15; those who had moderate difficulty had an average score of 22; those who had a little bit of difficulty had an average score of 36; and those who had no difficulty had an average score of 57. With her predicted score of 38 at 6 weeks after surgery, Mrs Wilson could expect to have little difficulty walking to her husband in another room by the time her support people are due to leave.

The meaning of the 6-Minute Walk Test result that Mrs Wilson is predicted to have at 6 weeks is much easier to understand. The distance that an individual is likely to be able to walk in 6 minutes is a simple concept. However, we can still help Mrs Wilson to interpret the distance. One way would be to compare it with normative data from healthy participants. Normative data[18] show that healthy 60- to 69-year-old women walk an average of 505 m in 6 minutes. Mrs Wilson's 330 m prognosis at 6 weeks represents 65% of the distance predicted for a healthy woman of her age (330 m/505 m = 65%). Viewed as a fraction of normative data, this percentage may be discouragingly low. Given that she is currently able to care for her husband, we could encourage her to compare it with her preoperative 6-Minute Walk Test distance instead. Her predicted result, 330 m, represents less than a 7% reduction in her current ability, 353 m, on the test.

Another approach is to compare it with distances that she must tackle in one session of walking, for example:

- back room of the house to the front door: 40 m
- kitchen to the letterbox and return: 60 m
- front door to neighbour's house and return: 180 m
- front door to nearby convenience store: 320 m

She should be able to manage all of these distances in 6 minutes. It is worth remembering that the 6-Minute Walk Test allows the participant to sit and rest as required. If she currently rests at all during her 6-Minute Walk Test and if there are no seats between her home and the nearby convenience store, she may have to consider organising assistance with shopping. She should also consider how quickly she recovered from her 6-Minute Walk Test and whether she could continue with shopping and then walk home again carrying it.

SUMMARY POINTS OF THIS CHAPTER

- Evidence about prognosis is often found in prospective cohort studies, although it may also be present in control-group data from a randomised controlled trial or in a systematic review of prognostic data from several studies.
- When searching for prognostic studies, include terms for the patient's problem, the intervention they receive (unless you are interested in the prognosis of the untreated condition) and the outcomes that are most important to the patient.

- The most valid prognostic evidence comes from studies in which the participants were identified at an early and uniform point in their disease (known as an 'inception cohort'). The participants included in the study should be representative of the population from which they were sampled and their condition should have been accurately diagnosed. Their outcomes should have been accurately measured with an appropriate and valid tool. Follow-up of the participants in the study needed to be sufficiently long and complete.

- The two main questions that you need to ask when determining if the results of a prognostic study are important are: (1) how likely are the outcomes over time? and (2) how precise are the estimates of likelihood?

- The average prognostic estimate for patients in the study can often be tailored to your particular patient by adjusting for the effect of certain characteristics which are known as prognostic factors.

- Most patients will require help to interpret prognostic estimates. This can sometimes be done by relating predicted values to threshold values, such as the patient's current value, the average value for healthy people and the values required for functional activities.

References

1. Liou T, Adler S, FitzSimmons B, et al. Predictive 5-year survivorship model of cystic fibrosis. Am J Epidemiol 2001;153:345–52.
2. Roseribloom M, Pfefferbaum A, Sullivan E. Recovery of short-term memory and psychomotor speed but not postural stability with long-term sobriety in alcoholic women. Neuropsychology 2004;18:589–97.
3. Kennedy D, Stratford P, Riddle D, et al. Assessing recovery and establishing prognosis following total knee arthroplasty. Phys Ther 2008;88:22–32.
4. Segawa H, Tsukayama D, Kyle R, et al. Infection after total knee arthroplasty. A retrospective study of the treatment of eighty-one infections. J Bone Joint Surg Am 1999;81:1434–45.
5. Roos H, Adalberth T, Dahlberg L, et al. Osteoarthritis of the knee after injury to the anterior cruciate ligament or meniscus: the influence of time and age. Osteoarthritis Cartilage 1995;3:261–7.
6. Gelber A, Hochberg M, Mead L, et al. Joint injury in young adults and risk for subsequent knee and hip osteoarthritis. Ann Intern Med 2000;133:321–8.
7. Bullens P, van Loon C, de Waal Malefit M, et al. Patient satisfaction after total knee arthroplasty. J Arthroplasty 2001;16:740–7.
8. Straus S, Richardson W, Glasziou P, et al. Evidence-based medicine: how to practice and teach EBM. 4th ed. Edinburgh: Elsevier Churchill Livingstone; 2011.
9. Robertsson O, Knutson K, Lewold S, et al. The Swedish Knee Arthroplasty Register 1975–1997. Acta Orthop Scand 2001;72:503–13.
10. White R, Romano P, Zhou H, et al. Incidence and time course of thromboembolic outcomes following total hip or knee arthroplasty. Arch Intern Med 1998;158:1525–31.
11. Pedersen P, Vinter K, Olsen T. Aphasia after stroke: type, severity and prognosis. Cerebrovasc Dis 2004;17:35–43.
12. Holden J, Sagovsky R, Cox J. Counselling in a general practice setting: controlled study of health visitor intervention in treatment of postnatal depression. BMJ 1989;298:223–6.
13. Berry J, Von Knoch M, Schleck C, et al. The cumulative long-term risk of dislocation after primary Charnley total hip arthroplasty. J Bone Joint Surg Am 2004;86:9–14.
14. Cummings S, Nevitt M, Browner W, et al. Risk factors for hip fracture in white women. N Engl J Med 1995;332:767–74.
15. Kennedy D, Stratford P, Pagura S, et al. Comparison of gender and group differences in self-report and physical performance measures in total hip and knee arthroplasty candidates. J Arthroplasty 2002;17:70–7.
16. Kennedy D, Hanna S, Stratford P, et al. Preoperative function and gender predict pattern of functional recovery after hip and knee arthroplasty. J Arthroplasty 2006;21:559–66.
17. Stratford P, Hart D, Binkley J, et al. Interpreting Lower Extremity Functional Status score. Physiotherapy Canada 2005;57:154–62.
18. Bohannon R. Six-minute Walk Test: a meta-analysis of data from apparently healthy elders. Topics Geriatric Rehabil 2007;23:155–60.

Chapter 9

Questions about prognosis: examples of appraisals from different health professions

Tammy Hoffmann, Marilyn Baird, John W Bennett, Mal Boyle, Jeff Coombes, Mark R Elkins, Lisa Nissen, Sheena Reilly, Claire Rickard and Sharon Sanders

This chapter is an accompaniment to the previous chapter (Chapter 8) where the steps involved in answering a clinical question about prognosis were explained. In order to further help you learn how to deal with prognostic clinical questions when they arise and appraise the evidence, this chapter contains a number of worked examples of questions about prognosis from a range of health professions. The worked examples in this chapter follow the same format as the examples in Chapter 5. In addition, as with the worked examples that were written for Chapter 5, the authors of the worked examples in this chapter were asked not to choose a systematic review (for the reason that was explained in Chapter 5), but instead to find the next best available level of evidence to answer the prognostic question that was generated from the clinical scenario.

OCCUPATIONAL THERAPY EXAMPLE

CLINICAL SCENARIO

You are an occupational therapist who has recently rotated into the outpatient department of a brain injury rehabilitation unit. After patients are discharged as inpatients and return home to live, they return to the hospital to receive outpatient therapy. One of your patients is Mary, a 21-year-old who sustained a mild traumatic brain injury in a motor vehicle accident 8 weeks ago. Her Glasgow Coma Scale was 14 on admission to hospital. Prior to the accident Mary worked full-time as an apprentice chef. She has been working in this job for 2 years and started after finishing high school. After discharge from hospital, Mary returned home to live with her parents and has been able to do simple tasks around the home and shopping with assistance from her mother.

Your initial outpatient assessment of Mary revealed that her current difficulties are poor endurance, poor memory and planning problems. Mary is already 2 months post-injury and her employer has just advised her that he is only able to keep her position in the apprenticeship scheme reserved for her for another 4 months. Mary has asked you how likely it is that she will be able to return to her job within that timeframe. As you are new to working in this area of clinical practice, you decide to search the literature to help you answer this question.

CLINICAL QUESTION

In adults with mild traumatic brain injury, what is the likelihood of returning to work within 6 months of the injury occurring?

Search terms and databases used to find the evidence

Database: PubMed–Clinical Queries (with 'prognosis category' and 'narrow scope' selected).

Search terms: (mild traumatic brain injury) AND (return to work*)

This search retrieves 10 results. After reading through the titles and abstracts of these articles, three appear to be relevant to your clinical question. One is primarily focused on the application of a particular outcome measure. Of the other two, you choose the article with the largest sample size and obtain its full text so that you can do a critical appraisal.

Article chosen

Stulemeijer M, van der Werf S, Borm G, et al. Early prediction of favourable recovery 6 months after mild traumatic brain injury. *J Neurol Neurosurg Psychiatry* 2008;79:936–42.

Structured abstract*

Study design: Prospective cohort study.

Setting: Level 1 trauma centre of a university medical centre in The Netherlands.

Participants: 452 patients with mild traumatic brain injury who were admitted to the emergency department and aged between 18 and 60 years (mean age 35.6 years, 78% female) were sent a questionnaire to complete (the 6-month questionnaire was returned by 201 patients). Other eligibility criteria were: able to speak and write in Dutch and did not have premorbid mental retardation or dementia.

Outcomes: Postconcussional symptoms (measured using Rivermead Post-Concussion Questionnaire) and return to work (without any negative change in work situation because of the injury).

Prognostic factors studied: *Pre-injury* (age, gender, education, premorbid emotional problems, physical comorbidities and prior head injury); *peri-injury* (Glasgow Coma Scale score; presence and duration of loss of consciousness; post-traumatic amnesia duration; brain computed tomography characteristics; dizziness, nausea/vomiting or headache in the emergency department; additional extracranial injuries); and *early post-injury* (postconcussional symptoms, post-traumatic stress, fatigue, pain and self-efficacy).

Follow-up period: 6 months (mean = 6.5 months, range 5.5 to 10 months).

Main results: At follow-up, 153 (76%) of the participating patients reported full return to work and 64% reported full recovery. Patients with more than 11 years of education, without nausea or vomiting on admission, with no additional extracranial injuries and only low levels of pain early after injury had a 90% chance of full return to work.

Conclusion: Early identification of patients with mild traumatic brain injury who are likely to have good 6-month recovery was feasible based on relatively simple prognostic models.

Is the evidence likely to be biased?

• *Was there a representative and well-defined sample?*
  Yes. There was a reasonably well-defined population and representative sampling. The article states that consecutive patients who were admitted to the trauma centre with a mild traumatic brain injury were eligible to participate in the study. A definition of what was considered a mild traumatic brain injury is provided. There were only a few inclusion criteria (between 18 and 60 years of age, able to speak and write in Dutch and no premorbid intellectual disability or dementia), although it is not detailed how these latter criteria were assessed. No specific exclusion criteria are provided. The exclusion of people who could not read or write may limit the generalisability of the study results.

• *Was there an inception cohort?*
  Yes. Participants were recruited at a similar well-described point, namely after they were admitted to hospital after the traumatic brain injury occurred.

• *Was exposure determined accurately?*
  Yes. In this study, it would have been very unlikely that an error was made in recruiting participants who had suffered a mild traumatic brain injury as a result of a motor vehicle accident, as this exposure (or in this case, eligibility criteria) can be easily determined. The authors also explain how the severity of participants' traumatic brain injury was determined (mild traumatic brain injury was defined as having a Glasgow Coma Scale admission score of 13–15, with or without a loss of consciousness of less than 30 minutes and with or without post-traumatic amnesia).

*Reproduced and adapted from the above reference with permission from BMJ Publishing Group Ltd.

- *Were the outcomes measured accurately?*
  Yes. The outcomes were postconcussional symptoms and return to work. *Postconcussional symptoms* were measured using the Rivermead Post-Concussion Questionnaire and the definition of a 'favourable' outcome using this measure is provided. *Return to work status:* participants were considered to have full return to work when they were not on sick leave at the time of follow-up or reported no change in working status (such as to part-time or a lower level) because of their injury. There are no details provided about what is meant by a lower level of working status and whether this included modified duties, which have been useful to know about.

  Participants provided the outcome measure information in a self-completed questionnaire at 6 months after recruitment to the study. It was not possible to measure outcomes in a blind fashion, as it was based on participant self-report. It was not possible to blind outcome assessors about participants' status on the prognostic factors, as the measures were based on participant self-report where the participant was technically the outcome assessor.

- *Were important prognostic factors considered?*
  Yes. The authors appear to have identified the major factors that could influence return to work. The study examined three main categories of possible prognostic factors (refer to the structured abstract).

- *Was the follow-up of participants sufficiently long and complete?*
  No, not sufficiently complete. The study identified 529 patients who met the inclusion criteria and of these, 452 were sent the early questionnaire (with most of the 77 missed due to logistical reasons). Complete questionnaires were returned by 280 patients and the follow-up questionnaire returned by 201 patients (which is 44% of those who were sent the early questionnaire and 72% of those who completed the first questionnaire). Compared with the total cohort, the group of participants that completed the follow-up questionnaire contained fewer men and were younger (mean difference of 2.6 years). With regards to length, the mean length of follow-up time was 6.5 months (range 5.5 to 10 months), which matches our clinical question. However, many studies that look at return to work after head injury follow participants for 12 months. Although only participants with mild traumatic brain injury were included in this study, they may have experienced impairments (physical, psychological and/or cognitive impairments) that could continue to have impacts on their ability to return to work beyond this amount of time post-injury.

What are the main results?

Return to work: Of the 201 participants who were able to be followed up, 153 (76%) reported full return to work by the time of the follow-up assessment. You calculate the 95% confidence interval (CI) to be 71% to 81% (using the formula that was provided in Chapter 8, where 95% CI = risk $\pm$ [1 $\div \sqrt{2n}$]). In other words, the likelihood of having returned to work by approximately 6.5 months after mild traumatic brain injury could be as low as 71% or as high as 81%.

Significant predictors of full return to work at 6 months: More than 11 years of education (odds ratio 6.4; 95% CI 2.3 to 18.3), without nausea or vomiting on admission (odds ratio 5.1, 95% CI 1.8 to 14.3), with no additional extracranial injuries (odds ratio 3.4, 95% CI 1.6 to 7.3) and only low levels of pain early after injury (odds ratio 2.3, 95% CI 0.9 to 5.9).

How might we use this evidence to inform practice?

As you have determined the internal validity of this study to be reasonably strong (although you keep in mind the bias from the incomplete follow-up) and the results useful, you proceed to assessing the applicability of the evidence by comparing your patient with the participants in the study, before deciding whether you can use the evidence to help inform your practice. Mary's mechanism and severity of injury is similar to the majority of the study participants. She is younger than the mean age of study participants, but meets the eligibility criterion for age and all of the other eligibility criteria of the study. In terms of the prognostic factors that were identified in this study, Mary has >11 years of education; did not have nausea, vomiting or extracranial injuries on admission; and had only low levels of pain early after injury. All of these factors were positively related to return to work, so this may increase the likelihood of her returning to work.

You explain to Mary that you think there is a reasonable chance that she will be able to return to her usual job by 6 months post-injury. As part of your treatment planning, you will arrange a time for Mary and yourself to meet with her employer to discuss the option of her returning to work in a modified capacity (such as shorter hours, different duties, graded return to work, etc) if this is necessary. During this meeting, you also plan to obtain more-detailed information about Mary's duties at work and then use this, in conjunction with Mary, to set her rehabilitation program and goals.

PHYSIOTHERAPY EXAMPLE

CLINICAL SCENARIO

A 32-year-old baker presents to your private physiotherapy practice 2 days after the onset of his first episode of acute low back pain. His pain is localised to his lumbar spine and is not accompanied by signs of more-serious pathology such as weight loss, weakness or paraesthesia. However, it is currently preventing him from working and he urgently needs to arrange a replacement until he is able to work again. He is therefore primarily interested in any advice you can give him with regard to when he can expect to improve enough to return to work. He is also interested to know how quickly his pain is likely to improve with usual intervention.

CLINICAL QUESTION

In adults with acute low back pain, what is the average time to return to work and to resolution of pain?

Search terms and databases used to find the evidence

Database: PubMed–Clinical Queries (with 'prognosis category' and 'narrow scope' selected).

Search terms: (acute OR recent) AND (low back pain) AND (return to work*)

The search returns 36 records. You scan the titles of the articles and read the abstracts of four studies that seem like they could be relevant. Of these, one is highly relevant as it is an inception cohort study of acute low back pain, it was conducted in the same healthcare setting as your work, it followed a large cohort and it measured the outcomes that are of primary concern to your patient.

Article chosen

Henschke N, Maher C, Refshauge K, et al. Prognosis in patients with recent onset low back pain in Australian primary care: inception cohort study. BMJ 2008;377:a171.

Structured abstract (adapted from the above)

Study design: Inception cohort study.

Setting: Medical, physiotherapy and chiropractic practices in Sydney, Australia. Participants: 973 participants (mean age 43.3 years; 54.8% male) aged at least 14 years with non-specific low back pain of less than 2 weeks' duration. Exclusion criteria included radiculopathy, cancer, spinal fracture, spinal infection and inflammatory arthritis.

Outcomes: Time to return to work (determined by self-report of returning to previous work status), time to complete resolution of pain and return to function.

Prognostic factors studied: Age, gender, intensity of low back pain and level of interference with function at baseline, plus individual variables grouped into seven factors—current history, past history, features of serious spinal pathology, sociodemographics, general health, psychological health and work.

Follow-up period: 1 year (with assessments also at baseline, 6 weeks and 3 months).

Main results: Median time to return to work was 14 days (95% confidence interval [CI] 11 to 17 days). Resolution of pain was much slower, at a median of 58 days (95% CI 52 to 63 days). A reasonable proportion of patients still had unresolved problems at 1 year. The cumulative probability of having returned to previous work status at 1 year was 89% and the cumulative probability of being pain-free at 1 year was 72%.

Conclusion: Prognosis of participants was not as favourable as is claimed in clinical guidelines. Most participants experienced slow recovery and almost one-third had not recovered from the presenting episode by the 12-month follow-up.

Is the evidence likely to be biased?

- *Was there a representative and well-defined sample?*
  Yes. The article states that consecutive participants who presented to primary care with recent-onset low back pain were invited to participate. Also, the target population is well-defined, as clear inclusion and exclusion criteria are provided.
- *Was there an inception cohort?*
  Yes. Participants were recruited within 2 weeks of onset of their condition, which minimises possible bias due to variable disease duration within the cohort.
- *Was exposure determined accurately?*
  Yes. Eligibility was determined by doctors, physiotherapists and chiropractors, so misclassification is unlikely unless participants misreported their symptoms.
- *Were the outcomes measured accurately?*
  Cannot tell. The outcomes (pain intensity, disability and work status) were based on participant self-report. Therefore, it was not possible to measure the outcomes in a blind fashion. Also, there is little indication of psychometric validation of any of the outcome measures, which may be one source of potential bias.
- *Were important prognostic factors considered?*
  Yes. The researchers identified an extensive range of prognostic factors (refer to the structured abstract).
- *Was the follow-up of participants sufficiently long and complete?*
  Yes. The follow-up rate was excellent (97%) and the length of follow-up appears to have been sufficient for the outcomes that were measured.

What are the results?

Return to work: The median time to return to work (to previous work hours and duties) was 14 days (95% CI 11 to 17 days). The cumulative probability of having returned to previous work status was 74.6% at 6 weeks, 83.2% at 12 weeks and 89.5% at 1 year.

Resolution of pain: The median time to resolution of pain was 58 days (95% CI 53 to 63 days). The cumulative probability of being pain-free was 39.9% at 6 weeks, 58.2% at 12 weeks and 72.5% at 1 year.

Complete recovery: This was measured by recovery on all three dimensions (return to work, no disability and no pain). The cumulative probability of being fully recovered was 39.0% at 6 weeks, 57.4% at 12 weeks and 71.8% at 1 year.

Prognostic factors: Factors associated with a longer time to recovery included older age, compensation cases, higher pain intensity, longer duration of low back pain before consultation, more days of reduced activity because of lower back pain before consultation, feelings of depression and a perceived risk of persistence.

How might we use this evidence to inform practice?

You compare your patient's characteristics with those of the participants in the sample, and decide that he is similar enough that you can apply this evidence to him and his situation. As this prognostic evidence has little risk of potential bias and the confidence interval extends only a few days either side of the estimate of median time to return to work, you can confidently reassure your patient that about 50% of people with acute low back pain return to work at about 2 weeks. Resolution of his pain is likely to take substantially longer, with 50% of people being pain-free by about 8 weeks. However, you also explain to your patient that there is a small risk that the condition will not have fully resolved by 1 year, with 28% of the study participants not considered as fully recovered by 1 year. Because he is young, self-employed and has only had the pain for 2 days, however, he does not have several of the prognostic factors that were found to predict a longer time to recovery. Therefore, it is likely that he may have a better than average prognosis for recovery. You clearly explain all of these findings to your patient.

PODIATRY EXAMPLE

CLINICAL SCENARIO

You are a podiatry student on clinical placement in a hospital podiatry department. You have just seen a 62-year-old man who attended with his wife. He has been referred by the diabetes educator for foot screening, education and management. He has had type 2 diabetes for approximately 10 years and, according to the patient, his control has been good.

Your examination indicates that neuropathy is present, vascular assessment is satisfactory, there is some foot deformity and there are active pressure lesions present plantar to the first metatarsal head bilaterally. Debridement of the callosity on the right foot reveals an ulcer. Together with your supervisor, you conduct a detailed ulcer assessment. The ulceration has white, macerated margins, the base is clean and pink to red and there is no exudate. The ulcer is round, 6 mm across and 4 mm deep. There do not appear to be any sinuses and you cannot probe to bone.

While discussing an intervention plan with your patient, his wife, who appears visibly worried, asks if he will end up losing his leg. You know that this is a possibility but are not sure of the actual risk, so your supervisor suggests you conduct a search to see if you can find some evidence to guide your answer to the question. You tell your patient and his wife that you will endeavour to answer her question more accurately when you see them again in a few days' time.

CLINICAL QUESTION

In a person with a first neuropathic foot ulcer, what is the risk of amputation?

Search terms and databases used to find the evidence

Database: PubMed–Clinical Queries (with 'prognosis category' and 'narrow scope' selected).

Search terms: (ulcer* AND (diabetic OR neuropathic)) AND amputat*

This search returns 77 systematic reviews and 116 studies. You quickly scan the titles of the first few systematic reviews, as a review of prognostic studies addressing your question would be more useful than a single study. In doing so, you notice a warning at the top of the page stating that 'the wildcard search for "ulcer" used only the first 600 variations'. To understand what this means, you click on 'details' to see how PubMed has dealt with your search terms. The 'Query Translation' box, which displays how the search was run, shows that the first 600 variations include the term 'ulcer' but not 'ulcers'. You think this term should also be searched, so go back and re-enter your search terms as:

((ulcer OR ulcers) AND (diabetic OR neuropathic) AND amputation*)

This slightly increases the number of studies retrieved, to 121. You decide this is too many abstracts to scan through, so you try to refine your search by adding the term 'first'. This retrieves a more reasonable 24 studies. You scan the titles and choose the following article which most closely matches your clinical question.

Article chosen

Winkley K, Stahl D, Chalder T, et al. Risk factors associated with adverse outcomes in a population-based prospective cohort study of people with their first diabetic foot ulcer. J Diabetes Complications 2007;21:341–9.

Structured abstract (adapted from the above)

Study design: Prospective cohort study.

Setting: Community and hospital foot clinics in London, UK.

Participants: 253 people (mean age 62.0 years; 63.6% male) with diabetes (type 1 or type 2) and their first foot ulcer. Exclusion criteria included not being fluent in English, a current independent comorbid medical condition, severe mental illness (such as psychosis or dementia), duration of foot ulcer greater than 1 year, or severely ischaemic feet (ankle brachial pressure index <0.5).

Outcomes: Death, amputation and recurrence of ulceration and the time taken for each outcome to occur.

Prognostic factors studied: Age, sex, smoking status, ulcer site (dorsal or plantar), size and severity of ulcer, severity of neuropathy, ischaemia, glycosylated haemoglobin, presence of micro- and macrovascular complications, and depression.

Follow-up period: 18 months (with assessments also at baseline, 6 months and 12 months).

Main results: At 18 months, 15.5% of participants had had an amputation, 15.8% had died and 43.2% had experienced ulcer recurrence. The severity of the ulcer at baseline was significantly associated with amputation (hazard ratio [HR] 3.18, 95% CI 1.53 to 6.59). Being older, having lower glycosylated haemoglobin, moderate ischaemia and depression were associated with mortality. Microvascular complications were associated with recurrent ulceration.

Is the evidence likely to be biased?

- *Was there a representative and well-defined sample?*
  Yes. It is likely that the sample was representative, as the article states that the records of each participating clinic were checked fortnightly so that eligible patients could be identified (using a standardised checklist of case definition and exclusion criteria) from all of the current and new patients that were being seen by the clinics. Also, there was a very high proportion of eligible patients that were recruited into the study (of the 260 people who were eligible, 253 were recruited), which helps to ensure the representativeness of the sample. The target population is well-defined, with clear inclusion and exclusion criteria described in the article.

- *Was there an inception cohort?*
  No. Although the range of time over which the ulcers had been present is not reported (mean duration was 3.1 months with a standard deviation of 3.6 months), it appears that the participants may have had the ulcers for as little as a few weeks or for as long as a year, and only participants

with an ulcer duration of greater than 1 year were excluded. As participants were not recruited at a similar point in the course of this condition, possible bias due to variable disease duration within the cohort may have been introduced into the study.

- *Was exposure determined accurately?*
  Yes. The article states that a clinically significant case definition of *diabetic foot ulcer* was used and go on to provide details about what this definition was. Also, participants were assessed by podiatrists at community and hospital foot clinics. Therefore it is likely that it was accurately determined whether participants had a foot ulcer or not.

- *Were the outcomes measured accurately?*
  Yes. The outcomes of death and amputation are valid, and objective and specific criteria were established to define the outcome of ulcer recurrence. The methods used to identify the occurrence of the outcomes of interest appear reliable. It is not clear whether the outcome assessors were blind to clinical characteristics or prognostic factors, although it does state in the discussion that they were blind to depression status. Given the objectivity of the outcome measures, the issue of blinding is not likely to be of great importance.

- *Were important prognostic factors considered?*
  Yes. The researchers identified an extensive range of factors that could have potential prognostic value.

- *Was the follow-up of participants sufficiently long and complete?*
  Yes. Follow-up was both sufficiently long and complete. Eighteen months is an adequate length of time to observe amputation and ulcer recurrence. You wonder if it is long enough to observe mortality, but notice that quite a number of participants (15%) had experienced this outcome during the follow-up period. The rate of follow-up was 100% for the death outcome, 92% for the amputation outcome and 90.5% for the recurrence outcome. While the loss to follow-up in this study is reasonably small (that is, <10%), there were some differences in baseline characteristics between the participants who were lost to follow-up and those that remained in the cohort. Participants with missing information had a shorter duration of diabetes and fewer microvascular problems. It is unclear whether this constitutes a certain type of participant who was selectively lost to follow-up.

What are the main results?

Amputation: By 18 months, 15.5% ($n = 36$) of the study population had undergone an amputation. Of the amputations, 10 were considered a major amputation (above the ankle) and the remainder were below the ankle (mainly of the toes). Using the data provided in the article, you calculate the 95% confidence interval for this 15.5% estimated risk of having an amputation to be 11.5% to 19.5%. In other words, the risk of amputation for a diabetic foot ulcer (at approximately 18 months after first seeking medical attention for the ulcer) is between 11.5% and 19.5%.

In a multivariate analysis, the severity of the ulcer was significantly associated with amputation (HR 3.34; 95% CI 1.53 to 6.59). The presence of an ulcer categorised as 'deep' according to the University of Texas Diabetic Wound Classification System increased the risk of amputation three-fold. As the confidence interval for the ratio does not contain 1 (the 'no effect' value), this result is statistically significant.

Recurrence of ulcer: By 18 months, 43% of participants developed another ulcer at the same or different site to the first ulcer. Microvascular complications (such as neuropathy) were associated with recurrent ulceration (HR 3.34; 95% CI 1.53 to 6.59).

Death: Being older (HR 1.07; 95% CI 1.04 to 1.11) and having moderate ischaemia (HR 2.74; 95% CI 1.46 to 5.14) and depression (HR 2.51; 95% CI 1.33 to 4.73) increased the risk of mortality. Better glycaemic control reduced mortality risk (HR 0.73; 95% CI 0.56 to 0.96).

How might we use this evidence to inform practice?

You consider the results of the study to be relatively free of bias, and your patient appears to be similar to the study participants in many respects including age, type and duration of diabetes and other clinical characteristics. You have not previously seen the wound classification system used in this study to assess the severity of the ulcers. The reference provided in the study report indicates that it is a validated instrument. In the study, the ulcers were categorised as either superficial (wound extended through the epidermis or dermis only) or deep (wound penetrates tendon, joint capsule, bone or joint). Using this categorisation, your patient's ulcer would be considered superficial. Given this, you feel that you can reassure the patient and his wife that he is at a lower risk of amputation than if the ulcer had penetrated to tendon, bone or joint. You will emphasise the importance of continued good control of his diabetes, as this may reduce the risk of death. However, due to the presence of peripheral neuropathy (a microvascular complication), your patient is at increased risk of recurrent ulceration. In conjunction with your supervisor, you discuss the findings of the study with your patient and his wife and also suggest that they schedule regular follow-up assessments to check frequently for ulcer recurrence and initiate prompt intervention if/when they recur to prevent them from progressing to deep ulcers.

SPEECH PATHOLOGY EXAMPLE

CLINICAL SCENARIO

You are a speech pathologist who works in a community child health centre. Mrs Overato brings her daughter Martha, aged 23 months, to see you. She is concerned that Martha has recently begun to stutter. Martha has a (dizygotic) twin brother, Steve, who does not stutter. There is no family history of stuttering. Mrs Overato reported that Martha first stuttered when she was about 18 months old, but this only lasted a few weeks and then stopped. She reports that the most recent bout of stuttering seemed to commence after Martha was frightened by their neighbour's dog.

Martha repeats words and initial sounds, but there is no blocking or prolongation occurring. She is reported to be as chatty as ever and appears unconcerned about her stuttering. There are no other concerns about Martha's development; she has a large vocabulary and she speaks in phrases and short sentences. Martha's speech development is normal and she is able to articulate words very clearly for her age. Mrs Overato is very anxious as Martha and Steve will soon be beginning day-care and, on a recent visit, the care staff remarked on her stuttering. She wonders if she should be seeking any intervention for Martha's stuttering. She has also heard that Martha is likely to grow out of her stuttering anyway. You decide to search the literature to obtain information about this issue.

CLINICAL QUESTION

When stuttering develops in infancy and early childhood in a twin, how likely is it that recovery will occur naturally and are there any indications about which children are most likely to recover?

Search terms and databases used to find the evidence

Database: PubMed–Clinical Queries (with 'prognosis category' and 'narrow scope' selected).

Search terms: (stutter* OR stammer*) AND (child*) AND (twin*) AND (recover*)

This search retrieves no articles. You repeat the search, this time with 'broad' scope selected. This retrieves one article and it is relevant to your clinical question.

Article chosen

Dworzynski K, Remington A, Rijsdijk F, et al. Genetic etiology in cases of recovered and persistent stuttering in an unselected, longitudinal sample of young twins. Am J Speech Lang Pathol 2007;16:169–78.

Structured abstract (adapted from the above)

Study design: Prospective, longitudinal twin study (in the UK).

Study question: What is the recovery rate from developmental stuttering in childhood and are there factors which predict recovery and persistence?

Participants: Participants were 12,892 twins recruited at 18 months of age.

Outcomes: Recovery of stuttering.

Follow-up period: Parent reports of the children's stuttering were obtained at 2, 3, 4 and 7 years of age.

Main results: Of the 12,892 children with at least two ratings, 950 children had recovered and 135 had a persistent stutter. Ratings of stuttering at 2 years of age were not predictive of later stuttering (at 7 years), but ratings at 3 and 4 years of age were. At 3, 4 and 7 years, the liability to stuttering was highly heritable.

Conclusion: Stuttering is a disorder that appears to have high heritability and little shared environment effect in early childhood and for recovered and persistent groups of children up to 7 years of age.

Is this evidence likely to be biased?

- *Was there a representative and well-defined sample?*
  Yes. This is one of the largest and most methodologically rigorous twin studies about stuttering that has been undertaken. Its strength lies in the fact that the study of stuttering was embedded within a larger study of twin development. The prospective and longitudinal nature of the study was ideal for addressing the research question. The families of all twins that were born in the UK between 1994 and 1996 were invited to participate in the larger study about twin development. Appropriate exclusion criteria were applied in participant selection, namely that children with a specific medical condition (such as a chromosomal anomaly) were excluded, as were cases where zygosity data were unavailable.

- *Was there an inception cohort?*
  No. Although the children in this study were recruited at a similar age (18 months), it is unlikely that they would have all been at a similar point with respect to the development/onset of stuttering.

- *Was exposure determined accurately?*
  No. Stuttering at ages 2, 3 and 4 years was used to predict stuttering at age 7 years. A parent questionnaire pack was sent to parents at each assessment point. Each questionnaire contained at least one question that specifically asked about stuttering/stammering. A weakness is that the study relied on parental report of the presence of stuttering and there was no clinical verification of the report. The authors argue that, in their studies of child language, clinical face-to-face assessments have verified parental report. However, this has not been tested satisfactorily in stuttering to date and the validity of using parent report alone to verify presence or absence of stuttering remains unknown.

- *Were the outcomes measured accurately?*
  No. A parent questionnaire pack was sent to parents at age 7 years (as was done for the measurement of exposure at ages 2, 3 and 4 years). The same issues that were discussed above with respect to the determination/measurement of exposure (that is, early stuttering) apply to the measurement of the outcome (that is, stuttering at 7 years).

- *Were important prognostic factors considered?*
  Yes. The researchers considered the effect of gender and genetic and environmental influences on stuttering outcomes.

- *Was the follow-up of participants sufficiently long and complete?*
  In terms of the length and completeness of follow-up, the overall length of follow-up (until children were 7 years old) is appropriate and one of the longest studies published to date. However, as the assessments were conducted when the participants were 2, 3, 4 and 7 years old, there were lengthy gaps (for example, 12 months) between the reports, so many short-lived bursts of stuttering may have been missed and data about onset prior to 2 years of age were not captured. The follow-up rate was 59% at 2 years of age, 64.8% at 3 years of age, 65% at 4 years of age and 62.4% at 7 years of age.

What are the main results?

Incidence of stuttering: The incidence was 1.1% (82/7164) at 2 years of age, 2.4% (180/7616) at 3 years and 2.5% (262/10,514) at 4 years of age. At 2 and 3 years, for every girl who stuttered there were 1.6 boys who stuttered; whereas at 4 and 7 years, there were 1.8 boys for every girl who stuttered.

Recovery and persistence rates: Of the children whose parents had provided at least two ratings across the ages, 970 (7%) were classified as recovered (comprised of 429 girls [45%] and 521 boys [55%]). In the 135 (1%) children in which stuttering persisted, 35 (26%) were girls and 100 (74%) were boys. These figures can be expressed as: for every girl who continued to stutter, there were 2.9 boys who continued to stutter. Of the 82 children who were reported to be stuttering at 2 years of age, 81 had recovered by 7 years of age. Recovery rates at 3 and 4 years were reported to be 79% and 53%, respectively. Not only are fewer girls than boys affected by stuttering, but this holds for each age as well as for the recovered and persistent groups.

Prediction of later stuttering: Using logistic regression, the authors explored whether reports of stuttering at early ages were predictive of stuttering at 7 years. Ratings of stuttering at 2 years of age were not predictive of later stuttering, but ratings at 3 and 4 years of age were.

Twin analyses: Monozygotic concordance rates were higher than dizygotic rates, which suggests that there is substantial genetic influence operating and little evidence of shared environmental influence. This was verified in formal statistical twin modelling. The authors examined recovery and persistence patterns where one child had been affected by stuttering and the other had not. Most often the other twin was not affected, with this pattern being more apparent in dizygotic pairs compared with monozygotic pairs. The data presented did not suggest gender differences in pairs where both twins stuttered, nor were there different recovery and persistence rates. The authors concluded that the factors that increase liability to stuttering do not seem to be different for male or female children.

How might we use this evidence to inform practice?

In the case of Martha, we can draw a number of conclusions based on the results of this study. First, reports of stuttering obtained close to 2 years of age are not predictive of stuttering later in childhood, for example at 7 years. In this study 81 of the 82 children who were reported to be stuttering at 2 years did not stutter at 7 years. Second, Martha's mother can be reassured that the factors that increase liability to stuttering do not seem to be different for male or female children. Third, because there is a large genetic component to stuttering and little evidence of shared environmental influences, it is unlikely that the traumatic incident that Martha experienced with the neighbour's dog is implicated in the onset of stuttering, especially as this was the second bout of stuttering. Fourth, Martha's mother can also be reassured of the likelihood of a favourable outcome as there is no family history of stuttering and the data suggest that girls are more likely to recover than boys.

Based on the evidence from this well-conducted study, we can infer that Martha's stuttering is less likely to persist because there is no family history of stuttering. Intervention therefore could be delayed and stuttering observed and monitored for up to 12 months after onset. There is limited research to suggest that Martha's dizygotic twin brother will start to stutter. It is unlikely that the stuttering onset can be linked to environmental influences such as Martha's experience with the neighbour's dog.

MEDICINE EXAMPLE

CLINICAL SCENARIO

As a general practitioner you regularly see a 48-year-old man who smokes about 25 cigarettes per day but is otherwise well. He is resistant to public health messages about smoking cessation, partly because he feels no immediate negative consequences from smoking. You thought it might be useful to provide him with current information about the effect of smoking on mortality and quality of life.

CLINICAL QUESTION

In people who are heavy smokers, what is the long-term effect on their quality of life and survival?

Search terms and databases used to find the evidence

Database: PubMed–Clinical Queries (with 'prognosis category' and 'narrow scope' selected).

Search terms: smok* AND (quality of life) AND (mortality OR survival) AND (long-term)

This search returned 45 studies. The first article listed in this search was the most current, most relevant and appeared from the abstract to have sound methods, so you obtain the full text of it so that you can appraise it in detail.

Article chosen

Strandberg A, Strandberg T, Pitkälä K, et al. The effect of smoking in midlife on health-related quality of life in old age: a 26-year prospective study. Arch Intern Med 2008;168:1968–74.

Structured abstract (adapted from the above)

Study design: Prospective cohort study.

Setting: Helsinki, Finland.

Participants: 1658 white men (born 1919–1934) of similar socioeconomic status who were participating in the Helsinki Businessmen Study. All were healthy at baseline (year 1974), when cardiovascular risk factors and smoking habits were assessed.

Outcomes: Health-related quality of life was measured with the RAND 36-Item Health Survey. Total mortality up to the year 2000 was determined from Finnish national registers.

Prognostic factors studied: Baseline smoking status.

Follow-up period: 26-year follow-up (from 1974 to 2000).

Main results: Those who had never smoked ($n = 614$) lived a mean of 10 years longer than heavy smokers (>20 cigarettes daily; $n = 188$). Those who had never smoked also had the best scores on all the RAND 36-Item Health Survey scales of survivors in 2000 ($n = 1131$). The largest differences were found between never-smokers and heavy smokers, ranging from 4 points on the scale of social functioning to 14 points on the physical functioning scale. The physical component summary score of the RAND decreased as the number of cigarettes that were smoked daily increased ($p = 0.01$).

Conclusion: Health-related quality of life deteriorated with an increase in daily cigarettes smoked in a dose-dependent manner. Never-smokers survived longer than heavy smokers and they had better quality of life.

Is the evidence likely to be biased?

- *Was there a representative and well-defined sample?*
  Yes. This was a well-defined sample with clear inclusion and exclusion criteria. Participants were healthy, professionally active in positions of responsibility and did not take regular medication or have signs of chronic diseases (including diabetes mellitus, cardiovascular disease, malignant neoplasms, psychiatric disorders or alcoholism). The participants were aged between 40 and 55 years at baseline. At baseline in 1974, data about detailed smoking status were available for 2464 men. However, only the data for 1658 men who were healthy were included. While these data are relevant for the particular patient that you are seeing (a 48-year-old, otherwise healthy male), extrapolation of the results of this study to the general population and to women must be done cautiously.

- *Was there an inception cohort?*
  No. 'Inception cohort' refers to cohorts that are assembled at a similar well-described point in the course of a disease. The participants in this particular study were all healthy at baseline, showed no signs of cardiovascular disease or other serious diseases, were taking no medications permanently and were professionally active.

- *Was exposure determined accurately?*
  No. Smoking status was assessed with a questionnaire. Participants were classified into five groups according to their self-reported smoking status in 1974: (1) never-smoked ($n = 614$), defined as men who had never smoked regularly and were not currently smoking; (2) ex-smokers ($n = 650$), defined as those who had previously been smokers but had quit smoking by 1974; and participants who smoked (3) 1 to 10 cigarettes per day ($n = 87$), (4) 11 to 20 cigarettes per day ($n = 119$) or (5) more than 20 cigarettes per day ($n = 188$). Information about the duration of the smoking habit during the study period was not available. Misclassification is possible as participants may have misreported their smoking status. However, as people who smoke may be more likely to under-report rather than over-report smoking, this would only strengthen the association if the people who smoked did not correctly identify their smoking status.

- *Were the outcomes measured accurately?*
  Partially. Health-related quality of life was measured using the RAND 36-Item Health Survey questionnaire—that is, it used participant self-report. Therefore, it was not possible to measure this outcome in a blind fashion. Total mortality of the study population was retrieved from the National Population Information System of the Finnish Population Register Centre, which includes data from all Finnish citizens. It is unclear whether the assessors who extracted this data were blind to participants' clinical characteristics or prognostic factors.

- *Were important prognostic factors considered?*
  Partially. Data about a range of factors such as alcohol consumption and cardiovascular risk factors were available from baseline to enable important prognostic factors to be adjusted for with respect to the mortality outcome. However, limited data were available for important

prognostic factors for health-related quality of life at baseline. Only participants' self-rating of health and physical fitness on a 5-point scale (very good, good, fair, poor or very poor) was available, as the RAND 36-Item Health Survey 1.0 questionnaire did not exist in 1974 (at baseline).

- *Was the follow-up of participants sufficiently long and complete?*
  Yes. The length of follow-up is the strength of this study. Mortality information was available for all participants. The total follow-up time was as long as 26 years, which generated 40,261 person-years of follow-up. Smoking status and health-related quality-of-life data were measured with a questionnaire that was mailed in the year 2000 to 1286 survivors and 1131 (87.9%) responded.

What are the results?

Mortality: Participants who had never smoked ($n = 614$) lived a mean of 10 years longer than heavy smokers (>20 cigarettes daily; $n = 188$).

Health-related quality of life: Among survivors in 2000 ($n = 1131$), the never-smokers had the best scores on all of the RAND 36-Item Health Survey scales. The largest differences were found between never-smokers and heavy smokers, ranging from 4 points on the scale of social functioning to 14 points on the physical functioning scale. The physical component summary score of the RAND decreased as the number of cigarettes that were smoked daily ($p = 0.01$) increased.

How might we use this evidence to inform practice?

This article clearly demonstrates that people who are heavy smokers are not only likely to live 10 years less than people who are non-smokers, but also that the more they smoke, the worse their physical functioning is likely to be in later years. The data provide further support for the already substantial evidence that warns about the negative risks of smoking. You consider the results of the study to be relatively free of bias. The data are directly relevant to your patient (a 48-year-old, otherwise healthy male). The editorial comment about this article from the same journal issue suggests that:

> It is not just that the heavy smoker loses 10 years of life expectancy but rather that at any given age, the functional capacities of the heavy smoker are equivalent to those of non-smokers who are 10 years older. The clear message is that smoking makes you old before your time, and this reality may be far less attractive to younger smokers than the macho image of dying young while still strong and active.[1]

You discuss the findings of the study with your patient and discuss methods that may support him as he quits smoking. As a starting point, you make a time to follow up with him about one of these methods, specifically nicotine replacement therapy.

NURSING EXAMPLE

CLINICAL SCENARIO

As the charge nurse in a nursing home, you frequently provide education on pressure-ulcer prevention to your nursing staff. One of the nurses points out that many patients have red areas that do not blanch (representing grade 1 ulcers) and wonders how many develop pressure ulcers (grade 2–4). You additionally wonder what factors may predict the development of pressure ulcers in these patients. You have a fairly clear idea of the most likely causes of pressure ulcer development, but want to ensure that your information is up-to-date before including this information in the in-service program. You advise the nurse that you will search for evidence and get back to him at next week's meeting.

CLINICAL QUESTION

In nursing-home patients with non-blanchable erythema, what factors are associated with the development of pressure ulcers?

Search terms and databases used to find the evidence

Database: PubMed–Clinical Queries (with 'prognosis category' and 'narrow scope' selected).

Search terms: ((nursing home) OR (care facility*)) AND ((pressure ulcer) AND (grade 1) OR (non-blanchable erythema))

The search returns two records. Of these, one is very relevant to your clinical question.

Article chosen

Vanderwee K, Grypdonck M, DeBacquer D, et al. The identification of older nursing home residents vulnerable for deterioration of grade 1 pressure ulcers. J Clin Nurs 2009;18:3050–8.

Structured abstract (adapted from the above)

Study design: Secondary analysis of data from a randomised controlled trial.

Setting: Eighty-four wards of 16 nursing homes in Belgium.

Participants: 235 participants (mean age 87 years, 16.6% male) with a grade 1 pressure ulcer, able to be repositioned, and with an expected length of stay in the nursing home greater than 3 days. Exclusion criteria included pressure ulcer grade 2–4 as defined by the European Pressure Ulcer Advisory Panel.

Outcomes: Incidence of a pressure ulcer lesion grade 2–4.

Prognostic factors studied: Age, body mass index, diabetes mellitus, history of cerebrovascular accident, urinary incontinence, faecal incontinence, dual incontinence, sleeping medication or tranquillisers, contractures, temperature, hypertension (systolic blood pressure ≥140 mmHg or diastolic blood pressure ≥90 mmHg), hypotension (systolic blood pressure <90 mmHg or diastolic blood pressure <60 mmHg), sensory perception, moisture, activity, mobility, nutrition, friction and shear.

Follow-up period: Patients were followed until they developed a pressure ulcer grade 2 or worse or until they were discharged or died. Mean follow-up period was 15 days.

Main results: A total of 44 (18.7%) participants developed a pressure ulcer grade 2–4. Predictive factors for developing a pressure ulcer were: hypotension (relative risk [RR] 3.42, 95% CI 1.6 to 7.5), history of stroke (RR 1.9, 95% CI 1.1 to 3.7), and contractures (RR 2.0, 95% CI 1.0 to 3.9). Urinary incontinence decreased the risk of developing a pressure ulcer by 76%.

Conclusion: Nursing-home residents with grade 1 pressure ulcers, hypotension, history of stroke, and/or contractures are at higher risk for the development of pressure-ulcer lesions.

Is the evidence likely to be biased?

- *Was there a representative and well-defined sample?* Yes–well-defined; no–representative. Data were collected as part of a randomised trial which examined the effect of turning residents with unequal time intervals on pressure ulcer lesions. Of 379 patients who were eligible for the study (because they had developed a grade 1 pressure ulcer and were from the total population of 2663 residents), only 235 gave informed consent and were included. Of these, all were Caucasian, the majority (83.4%) were women, and the median age was 87 years (with half aged ≥90 years). So although the target population is well-defined, with clear inclusion and exclusion criteria, the sample is not particularly representative of nursing-home residents in general.

- *Was there an inception cohort?*
  Yes. One of the eligibility criterion was that participants did not have a grade 2–4 pressure ulcer, but had to have a grade 1 pressure ulcer.
- *Was exposure determined accurately?*
  Yes. Exposure in this study refers to whether participants had a grade 1 pressure ulcer (non-blanchable erythema) at a pressure point on the skin. This was an eligibility criterion for the randomised controlled trial and the procedure for determining this is described in the article with the results of the trial.
- *Were the outcomes measured accurately?*
  Yes. Participants' skin was checked daily. Definitions were provided for each of the grades of pressure ulcer. All staff nurses received training in the observation of pressure ulcers using the European Pressure Ulcer Advisory Panel pressure ulcer classification educational program. Inter-rater reliability of the skin observations was carried out by the researcher and a study nurse who carried out unannounced weekly skin inspections of a random sample of participants.
- *Were important prognostic factors considered?*
  Yes. The study included a range of prognostic factors (refer to structured abstract) and these were selected based on a review of the literature.
- *Was the follow-up of participants sufficiently long and complete?*
  Yes. The follow-up period was quite short (mean of 15 days, interquartile range of 7 to 26 days); however, follow-up continued until participants developed a pressure ulcer grade 2–4, were discharged or died. The article does not mention if any participants were lost to follow-up; however, for this sample of participants (who were nursing-home residents) it is assumed that this did not occur (although it is possible that participants could have withdrawn from the study).

What are the main results?

A grade 2–4 pressure ulcer developed in 44 (18.7%) participants, with an incidence rate of 12.7 per 1000 days (95% CI 0.9 to 1.6). The majority of the participants developed a grade 2 pressure ulcer (*n* = 39). From a multivariate analysis, independent predictive factors which increased the risk of developing a pressure ulcer were: hypotension (relative risk [RR] 3.4, 95% CI 1.6 to 7.5), history of stroke (RR 1.9, 95% CI 1.1 to 3.7), and contractures (RR 2.0, 95% CI 1.0 to 3.9). Urinary incontinence decreased the risk of developing a pressure ulcer (RR 0.2, 95% CI 0.09 to 0.64). The authors hypothesise that this may be due to more-frequent position changes, to check incontinence materials, in these participants.

How might we use this evidence to inform practice?

You are reasonably satisfied with the validity of the results of this study, although aware that the sample may not be representative of typical nursing-home residents. The study found three significant risk factors for the progression of grade 1 pressure ulcers into grade 2–4 lesions. At next week's meeting you plan to discuss with your team what additional preventive nursing measures can be used with residents with these risk factors to reduce the occurrence of pressure ulcers. At the meeting you also plan to develop a clinical question that will lead to a review of the latest evidence of the most effective interventions for preventing pressure-ulcer development in nursing-home residents.

MEDICAL IMAGING EXAMPLE

CLINICAL SCENARIO

You are a radiographer with 5 years post-qualification experience. The large public teaching hospital where you have just started a new job has women's health as one of its specialties. In the course of your rotation through the breast unit, you become aware of the role played by the nurses in supporting the women who attend for the various breast-imaging examinations. It becomes clear to you that the women rely very much upon these nurses for information about the efficacy of the various imaging modalities in diagnosing cancer of the breast. One nurse in particular is keen to know whether it is possible for any of the imaging modalities (such as magnetic resonance [MR] imaging) to accurately predict which patients might survive breast cancer. She recently had some very anxious patients who asked her about their long-term chances of survival. You offer to do some searching and let the nurse know the answer later that week.

CLINICAL QUESTION

Can MR imaging be used to predict survival in women with breast cancer?

Search terms and databases used to find the evidence

Database: PubMed–Clinical Queries (with 'prognosis category' and 'narrow scope' selected).

Search terms: (MR imaging) AND (breast cancer) AND (survival)

This search results in 17 articles. You scan the titles, and one article is relevant to your clinical question.

Article chosen

Bone B, Szabo B, Perbeck L, et al. Can contrast enhanced MR imaging predict survival in breast cancer? Acta Radiol 2003;4:373–8.

Structured abstract (adapted from the above)

Study design: A longitudinal cohort study. This study followed up a cohort of participants who had previously been recruited for an earlier study that examined MR imaging in women with breast cancer.

Setting: Hospital in Sweden.

Participants: The initial study consisted of 50 consecutive breast-cancer patients (mean age at diagnosis = 59 years) who had undergone a preoperative contrast-enhanced MR imaging (CE-MRI) examination between September 1992 and December 1993. Inclusion criteria for the initial study were a histopathologically verified primary breast malignancy and a detectable abnormality at MR imaging (lesion visible on at least three consecutive images).

Outcomes: Disease-free survival and overall survival.

Prognostic factors studied: A range of established classical and molecular prognostic markers were analysed, such as age, lymph node status, tumour size and proliferating cell nuclear antigen index.

Follow-up period: Median follow-up was 95 months (range 23–111 months).

Main results: The cumulative 5-year and 7-year survival rates for the whole cohort were 63% and 59% for disease-free and 81% and 77% for overall survival, respectively. Local recurrence or metastasis of the primary disease developed in 20 (40%) patients. Independent and significant predictors of disease-free survival were tumour size and the signal enhancement ratio. Independent and significant predictors of overall survival were age, lymph node status, tumour size and proliferating cell nuclear antigen index.

Conclusion: CE-MRI is useful in predicting the disease-free survival of women with breast cancer.

Is the evidence likely to be biased?

- *Was there a representative and well-defined sample?*
  Cannot tell. When the cohort was gathered for the initial study, the article states that participants were consecutively investigated breast-cancer patients, which may indicate that the cohort was likely to be representative. However, it is not clear what is meant by 'investigated', as this could imply that only patients who had undergone a CE-MRI investigation were included and, if this was the situation, it is possible that these patients may have systematically differed in some way to the patients who did not undergo this investigation. The sample was reasonably well-defined, as clear inclusion criteria are provided; however, no exclusion criteria are stated.

- *Was there an inception cohort?*
  Cannot tell. The article does not provide any clear details about whether participants were in a similar stage in the disease process when they were recruited. Although it is likely that participants were recruited shortly after the time of diagnosis as they were patients who had undergone a CE-MRI examination preoperatively, no further details about this are provided.

- *Was the exposure determined accurately?*
  Yes. One of the inclusion criteria was that participants needed to have a histopathologically verified primary breast malignancy. In addition, all imaging and other clinical predictive markers were correlated and confirmed with the histopathological description of the biopsied tumour samples.

- *Were the outcomes measured accurately?*
  Yes. Data about the outcomes of overall survival and disease-free survival were obtained from the hospital medical records. Disease-free survival and overall survival are objective outcomes that were defined and the article states that participants who died from causes other than breast cancer were censored.

- *Were important prognostic factors considered?*
  No. The researchers identified some prognostic factors, but not all potentially important ones. For example, there was a mix of tumour types in this cohort and this may have affected the results, especially in such a small group. Ideally, results should have been stratified according to tumour type and grade, but this would require a much larger cohort.

- *Was the follow-up of participants sufficiently long and complete?*
  No. A major weakness of the study is that the follow-up was conducted retrospectively via hospital medical records. This implied that participants continued to be cared for by the same hospital throughout the study period, which may not have been the case. No information is provided as to whether all participants were able to be followed up (in this case, whether current medical records were available for all participants from the initial study). A prospective follow-up of patients would have strengthened the study. Additionally, the follow-up of participants was not long enough. Although the median follow-up time was appropriate at 95 months, the range was very large (23 to 111 months) and the reason for this large variation in the follow-up period is not explained.

What are the main results?

Predictors of disease-free survival: In a multivariate analysis, only the signal enhancement ratio obtained during the CE-MRI ($p = 0.014$) and tumour size at excision ($p = 0.001$) were significant and independent prognostic factors for disease-free survival.

Predictors of overall survival: In a multivariate analysis, age ($p = 0.003$), lymph node status ($p = 0.014$), tumour size ($p = 0.039$) and the proliferating cell nuclear antigen index ($p = 0.053$) were found to be significant and independent prognostic factors for overall survival.

How might we use this evidence to inform practice?

Because the study had a number of flaws which cast doubt on the validity of the results, you decide that the results should be treated with caution. You decide to tell the nurse that, although the results of this study seem to indicate a possible role for CE-MRI in predicting survival in breast cancer, the evidence is currently not adequate for it to be used to replace biological markers as predictors of survival in women with breast cancer.

HUMAN MOVEMENTS EXAMPLE

CLINICAL SCENARIO

Mr Roberts has been referred to you by his general practitioner. He is 47 years old with hypertension, high cholesterol, obesity and impaired glucose tolerance. You undertake a fitness assessment and determine that he has a low exercise capacity (lowest 20th percentile for his age). He is very worried about developing type 2 diabetes and wants to know if improving his fitness will make him less likely to develop diabetes. You want to give Mr Roberts evidence-based advice about this issue, and look for recent evidence to guide your discussion with him.

CLINICAL QUESTION

In a man with impaired glucose tolerance, does a high level of fitness lower the risk of developing type 2 diabetes?

Search terms and databases used to find the evidence

Database: PubMed–Clinical Queries (with 'prognosis category' and 'narrow scope' selected).

Search terms: (impaired glucose tolerance) AND fitness AND diabetes

This search results in nine articles, two which appear relevant from the abstracts. You obtain the full-text of each and find that both papers are describing the same cohort. You decide to use the 2009 article as it is based on more-recent data/analyses.

Article chosen

Lee D, Sui X, Church T, et al. Associations of cardiorespiratory fitness and obesity with risks of impaired fasting glucose and type 2 diabetes in men. Diabetes Care 2009;32:257–62.

Structured abstract (adapted from the above)

Study design: A prospective cohort study.

Setting: A medical clinic in Texas, USA.

Participants: 14,006 men in a larger study about diabetes; and of these, 7795 who had normal baseline glucose and were considered to be in an impaired fasting glucose group. Inclusion criteria were: men aged 20–79 years who had undergone at least two medical examinations at the clinic between 1974 and 2006. Exclusion criteria were: body mass index <18.5 kg/m²; abnormal resting or exercise electrocardiogram; history of heart attack, stroke, cancer or diabetes at baseline; or did not achieve at least 85% of their age-predicted maximal heart rate during the treadmill test.

Outcomes: Primary outcomes: development of impaired fasting glucose or type 2 diabetes.

Prognostic factors studied: Baseline age, examination year, waist girth, percent body fat, parental diabetes, current smoking, alcohol consumption, blood pressure, total cholesterol, baseline impaired fasting glucose, body mass index and exercise capacity (treadmill time for a maximal exercise test). Exercise was divided into fifths of treadmill time in each age group. The lowest 20% were classified as having fitness level 1, and in continuing increments of 20%, participants were classified as fitness levels 2 through 5.

Follow-up period: From baseline to first follow-up event (impaired fasting glucose or type 2 diabetes) or to the last follow-up in 2006 in participants who did not develop either condition.

Main results: 3612 men developed impaired fasting glucose and 477 men developed diabetes. Men in the highest fitness level (most fit 20%) showed a 52% lower risk of developing type 2 diabetes and a 14% lower risk of impaired glucose fasting compared with those in the lowest (least 20% fit) fitness level after accounting for body mass index.

Conclusion: Low fitness and obesity increased the risk of impaired glucose fasting and diabetes.

Is the evidence likely to be biased?

- *Was there a representative and well-defined sample?*
  Yes. The sample was recruited from all patients who received two medical examinations at the recruiting clinic, and clear inclusion and exclusion criteria are provided in the article.

- *Was there an inception cohort?*
  Yes. Participants in the study who had diabetes at baseline, a history of diabetes or were currently taking insulin were excluded from the study, thus leaving an inception cohort of participants without impaired fasting glucose or diabetes.

- *Was the exposure determined accurately?*
  Yes. Fitness was determined using total duration of a treadmill test which is highly correlated ($r = 0.92$) with the gold-standard measure (maximal oxygen uptake). It is not clear from the study how fitness was determined on an ongoing basis. The limitations section of the paper mentions that participants revisited the clinic every 1.5 years, on average, and that fasting glucose tests were done then, but it is not clear whether that is when the fitness tests were also done.

- *Were the outcomes measured accurately?*
  Yes. Impaired fasting glucose and diabetes were diagnosed according to the American Diabetes Association criteria.

- *Were important prognostic factors considered?*
  Yes. Important known risk factors for developing diabetes were measured and considered in the statistical analyses.

- *Was the follow-up of participants sufficiently long and complete?*
  Cannot tell. Participants were followed until they developed diabetes or impaired fasting glucose, or until the study ceased recruiting. The mean follow-up period was 5.1 years for the 7795 men with normal baseline glucose and 7.2 years for the entire cohort. The article does not provide any details about loss to follow-up of participants from the study. We know that some were lost to follow-up, as there is a brief mention in the limitations about comparing the main variables for men who were lost to follow-up and those who were not, but no further information is given.

What are the main results?

Men with a body mass index ≥ 30.0 kg/m², waist girth >102 cm or percent body fat $\geq 25\%$ had 2.7, 1.9 and 1.3 fold higher risks for type 2 diabetes, compared with those for non-obese men. Table 9.1 shows the relative risk of developing diabetes for each fitness level category. For example, men in the highest

TABLE 9.1:
ADJUSTED RELATIVE RISK OF DEVELOPING TYPE 2 DIABETES ACCORDING TO FITNESS LEVEL

	Fitness levels (divided into fifths)				
	1 (least fit 20%)	2	3	4	5 (most fit 20%)
Baseline mean treadmill time (minutes) ± SD	12.0 ± 2.2	15.2 ± 1.9	17.4 ± 2.0	20.2 ± 2.1	24.6 ± 2.9
Rate of developing diabetes[a]	12.4	5.6	4.5	3.5	2.4
Adjusted relative risk[b] (95% CI)	1.00 (referent)	0.65 (0.49 to 0.86)	0.53 (0.40 to 0.71)	0.43 (0.32 to 0.58)	0.30 (0.22 to 0.41)
Adjusted relative risk[c] (95% CI)	1.00 (referent)	0.80 (0.60 to 1.08)	0.71 (0.52 to 0.96)	0.62 (0.45 to 0.85)	0.48 (0.34 to 0.68)

[a]Per 1000 person-years adjusted for age and examination year.
[b]Model 1 = Adjusted for age, examination year, parental diabetes, current smoking, alcohol consumption, systolic and diastolic blood pressure, total cholesterol, and impaired fasting glucose.
[c]Model 2 = Adjusted for model 1 plus body mass index.
CI = confidence interval; SD = standard deviation.

fitness level (most fit 20%) showed a 52% lower risk of developing type 2 diabetes compared with those in the lowest (least 20% fit) fitness level after accounting for body mass index. As fitness improved, there was a lower risk of developing diabetes. The addition of body mass index into model 2 shows that the associations between fitness levels and the risks of developing diabetes were still significant irrespective of whether body weight was changed. The dose–response relationship between fitness and onset of diabetes remained in all multivariate-adjusted models.

How might we use this evidence to inform practice?

You are reasonably confident of the validity of this study, although a little cautious given that details regarding the completeness of follow-up are not reported in this article (although possibly are in other articles related to this cohort of patients). This study provides evidence to support your response to Mr Roberts that he could decrease his risk of developing diabetes if he increased his fitness level, even without a change in his body weight. Mr Roberts decides that he would like to increase his fitness level and you plan to design a training program to achieve this goal, taking into account his comorbidities, medications, limitations and personal preferences.

PARAMEDICINE EXAMPLE

CLINICAL SCENARIO

You are a paramedic who is at a social function when a friend asks what to do if a stranger collapses with a heart attack. 'I couldn't bring myself to do mouth-to-mouth on a total stranger,' he says. 'Well, the good news is that you don't have to. It has been shown that chest compression-only resuscitation can be used instead,' you reply. 'Yeah, maybe, but what's the point–aren't they all pretty much in a coma afterwards? I doubt any make a good recovery' is the reply. You decide to look up the evidence so that you can provide your friend with a research-based answer to his query.

CLINICAL QUESTION

For patients who have an out-of-hospital cardiac arrest and receive chest compression only, how many people survive to hospital discharge with reasonable neurological function?

Search terms and databases used to find the evidence

Database: PubMed–Clinical Queries (with 'prognosis category' and 'narrow scope' selected).

Search terms: (cardiac arrest) AND (chest compression only) AND surviv*

This resulted in nine articles, two of which match your clinical question. They both used a similar study design, so you choose the largest and most recent study to appraise.

Article chosen

Bobrow B, Spaite D, Berg R, et al. Chest compression–only CPR by lay rescuers and survival from out-of-hospital cardiac arrest. JAMA 2010;304:1447–54.

Structured abstract (adapted from the above)

Study design: Prospective cohort study.

Setting: Arizona, USA (and occurred following a state-wide multifaceted promotion of chest-compression-only cardiopulmonary resuscitation).

Participants: Patients ($n = 4415$) ≥18 years of age who experienced an out-of-hospital cardiac arrest of a presumed cardiac origin which was not witnessed by Emergency Medical Services (EMS) personnel which occurred between 2005 and 2009.

Outcomes: The primary outcome was survival to hospital discharge. Additional outcomes were Cerebral Performance Category (CPC) on hospital discharge and the frequency and type of bystander cardiopulmonary resuscitation (CPR).

Prognostic factors studied: Age, sex, witnessed arrest, shockable rhythm, bystander CPR provision and type, location of arrest, EMS response interval, type of EMS resuscitation protocol (minimally interrupted cardiac resuscitation vs conventional basic life support/advanced cardiac life support), use of post-arrest therapeutic hypothermia and year.

Follow-up period: The patients were followed up until hospital discharge.

Main results: Of the 4415 patients, 2900 received no bystander CPR, 666 received standard CPR by a bystander, and 849 received chest compression only CPR by a bystander. Rates of survival to hospital discharge and good neurological outcome were 5.2% and 2.1% for no bystander CPR, 7.8% and 3.8% for standard CPR, and 13.3% and 6.5% for chest-compression-only CPR, respectively.

Conclusion: For patients with out-of-hospital cardiac arrest of presumed cardiac aetiology, bystander chest compression only was associated with increased survival to hospital discharge compared with conventional CPR and no bystander CPR.

Is the evidence likely to be biased?

- *Was there a representative and well-defined sample?*
  Cannot tell, but probably. The study investigated all patients ≥18 years of age who suffered an out-of-hospital cardiac arrest, of cardiac origin, not witnessed by emergency medical service (EMS) staff, over a 5-year period for the whole state of Arizona, USA. Although it is probably implied by the authors of the article, we do not how many people were not included in this sample (that is, was it the entire state of Arizona that was potentially eligible?). However, it is hard to imagine a systematic bias towards patients with any better, or worse, prognosis.

- *Was there an inception cohort?*
  Yes. Patients were included in the study following arrival of the ambulance.
- *Was the exposure determined accurately?*
  Yes. All patients were assumed to be in cardiac arrest, unless they had obvious alternative explanations (such as drowning or trauma). Exposure to CPR was determined by the paramedics either by observation on their arrival or by questioning bystanders during the ongoing resuscitation attempt. Although there is some possibility of bias during collection of these data (such as misclassification of type of CPR that was performed), attempts were made to minimise this by training EMS staff in how to document the presence and type of bystander CPR.
- *Were the outcomes measured accurately?*
  Yes. Patient survival to hospital discharge was determined by review of hospital records and the state health database. Neurological outcome was categorised, according to neurological status at discharge, using a 5-level Cerebral Performance Category (good cerebral performance, moderate cerebral disability, severe cerebral disability, coma or vegetative state and death).
- *Were important prognostic factors considered?*
  Yes. Important prognostic factors were accounted for (see list in structured abstract).
- *Was the follow-up of participants sufficiently long and complete?*
  Yes. Data was collected on participants until hospital discharge (which was the primary outcome measure) and few participants were lost to follow-up, mainly due to missing data (1.4% in the 'no resuscitation' group; 1.6% in the conventional CPR group; and 0.5% in the chest-compression-only CPR group).

What are the main results?

Patients in each of the three groups were similar in age and gender, with the same response time for the EMS. Table 9.2 shows that patients who have a witnessed cardiac arrest and who receive some form of CPR are more likely to survive to hospital discharge with a good neurological outcome (scored 1 in the Cerebral Performance Category).

How might we use this evidence to inform practice?

This was a well-conducted study that suggests that the outcomes of patients who are given chest-compression-only CPR by bystanders is not hopeless, with about 13% surviving to hospital discharge and of those, about 6–7% with good neurological outcomes. The question about whether chest-compression-only CPR is better than conventional CPR is suggested by these results, but this is really a question that should be answered by a randomised controlled trial (if this were possible). However, you do feel empowered to tell your friend that there is reasonable evidence, from a large state-wide study, that chest-compression-only CPR from a lay person results in about 1 person in 15 surviving with a good outcome.

TABLE 9.2:
OUTCOMES ACCORDING TO TYPE OF BYSTANDER CPR

	No CPR ($n = 2900$)	Standard CPR ($n = 666$)	Chest-compression-only CPR ($n = 849$)
Survival to hospital discharge, n (%)	150 (5.2)	52 (7.8)	113 (13.3)
Good neurological outcome, n (%)	60 (2.1)	25 (3.8)	53 (6.5)

PHARMACY EXAMPLE

CLINICAL SCENARIO

You are a pharmacist working in a community pharmacy. One of your regular customers has just returned from her general practitioner (GP) after seeing him for worsening hip and knee pain. She has a history of osteoarthritis in these areas and until now has used regular paracetamol to manage the pain. Her GP suggested that she try taking a non-steroidal anti-inflammatory drug (NSAID) for a few weeks to see if that helps with the pain, as she is showing some signs of inflammation. Today she has a prescription for diclofenac 50 mg tablets, 1–2 tablets twice a day. However, after leaving the GP, she realised that she forgot to ask him whether taking a NSAID will give her a stomach ulcer and anxiously asks you if that is the case.

CLINICAL QUESTION

For primary-care patients who need to take NSAIDs, what is the likelihood of a gastric ulcer developing?

Search terms and databases used to find the evidence

Database: PubMed–Clinical Queries (with 'prognosis category' and 'narrow scope' selected).

Search terms: (primary care) and (ulcer*) and (NSAID)

This resulted in 14 articles, one of which matched your clinical question.

Article chosen

Hollenz M, Stolte M, Leodolter A, et al. NSAID-associated dyspepsia and ulcers: a prospective cohort study in primary care. Dig Dis 2006;24:189–94.

Structured abstract (adapted from the above)

Study design: Prospective cohort study.

Setting: A single primary-care practice in Germany.

Participants: 104 patients (mean age 53 years, 88% female) who were >18 years, not currently being treated for dyspepsia and starting treatment with an NSAID that was estimated by the GP to be needed for at least 2 weeks.

Outcomes: Development of upper gastrointestinal tract ulcers and/or troublesome dyspepsia.

Prognostic factors studied: Age, gender, smoking, regular consumption of alcohol, history of upper gastrointestinal tract disease and concomitant medication.

Follow-up period: After at least 2 weeks of NSAID treatment.

Main results: 16% of patients experienced an ulcer, 35% developed dyspepsia that required treatment and 44% developed ulcer and/or dyspepsia. 41% of the patients with an ulcer had no dyspepsia.

Conclusion: Primary-care patients frequently develop treatment-requiring dyspeptic symptoms and ulcers while on NSAIDs; the latter were not identifiable from symptoms or risk factors.

Is the evidence likely to be biased?
- *Was there a representative and well-defined sample?*
  Partially. This was a typical cohort of patients being treated with NSAIDs in primary care, for typical reasons (most for pain from degenerative spinal column and joint disease). There was a preponderance of females (88%), which weakens the generalisability of the study results.

Participants were consecutively recruited; however, we do not know what the refusal rates were. Although the paper mentions that two patients were excluded after recruitment because they refused the gastroscopy, we do not know if this was a supplement to a larger number who declined before recruitment. The article describes clear inclusion and exclusion criteria.

- *Was there an inception cohort?*
  Cannot tell. Although patients were recruited prior to beginning NSAID treatment, we do not know much about participants' prior history of upper gastrointestinal tract disease.

- *Was the exposure determined accurately?*
  Partially. The exposure was prescription of NSAIDs. However, it is possible that not all patients adhered to treatment and this was not measured explicitly.

- *Were the outcomes measured accurately?*
  Yes. Dyspeptic symptoms were measured using a structured questionnaire. Although it is not mentioned whether this was a validated instrument, this may not be critical because whether or not patients are experiencing symptoms is a direct and simple construct. Additionally, participants had an abdominal examination and a gastroscopy (with removal of two biopsies), which was probably objective.

- *Were important prognostic factors considered?*
  Yes. There was measurement of known confounders such as smoking, alcohol consumption and previous history of upper gastrointestinal disease and all of these existed in credibly typical rates in the cohort.

- *Was the follow-up of participants sufficiently long and complete?*
  No. Participants were followed up after at least 2 weeks of NSAID treatment, which may be considered to be a rather short duration of follow-up. No justification for choosing this minimum duration was provided. Actual follow-up was treatment of <1 month duration in 64%, 1–3 months in 16% and >3 months in 19%. It is possible that the results might have been more striking with a longer follow-up. The article reports that data were analysed for 100 (of the 104 participants), as 2 refused gastroscopy and 2 had had a partial gastrectomy. No other details about follow-up completeness are provided.

What are the main results?

An ulcer was diagnosed in 17 patients, giving an ulcer prevalence of 16%. These patients were not identifiable on the basis of their symptoms. Predictors for the development of an ulcer were smoking (odds ratio [OR] 5.1, 95% CI 1.6 to 16.5), regular use of alcohol (OR 4.5, 95% CI 1.3 to 15.1) and duration of treatment <1 month (OR 4.9, 95% CI 1.1 to 23.1).

How might we use this evidence to inform practice?

You have some concerns about the validity of this study's results, but it appears to be the best available evidence to answer this question at this time. The ulcer prevalence of 16% seems quite high and begs the question of what the figure would have been had the patients *not* been using NSAIDs, which we can only guess at (and would be difficult to answer; not least because of the ethical considerations of performing a gastroscopy on otherwise healthy people). We could mention to our concerned lady that there is a reasonable chance that she will suffer either dyspeptic symptoms (sometimes called 'indigestion') or even an ulcer following starting the NSAID diclofenac. However, it is not clear how much these adverse outcomes are actually *caused* by the diclofenac (which would require a randomised controlled trial).

Reference

1. Burns D. Live fast, die young, leave a good-looking corpse. Arch Intern Med 2008;168:1946–7.

Chapter 10

Evidence about patients' experiences and concerns

Alan Pearson and Karin Hannes

LEARNING OBJECTIVES

After reading this chapter, you should be able to:

- Appreciate the role of qualitative research in providing information about patients' experiences and concerns
- Describe the basic assumptions that underpin the common qualitative research methodologies of phenomenology, grounded theory, ethnography, action research, feminist research, and discourse analysis
- Develop a qualitative clinical question
- Have a basic understanding of how to search for qualitative research
- Critically appraise qualitative research articles
- Have a basic understanding of how to interpret the findings of qualitative research articles
- Discuss how the findings of qualitative research may be used in practice

A team of general practitioners, nurses, physiotherapists, occupational therapists, dietitians and medical receptionists working in a government-funded health centre have invested a great deal of energy and resources to develop a team-based approach to patient care. Overall, they are pleased with the progress made and are anxious to consider the degree to which their efforts relate to improving patients' experiences. They have agreed that, given the growing size of the team and the increase in the number of different members of the team interacting with patients with chronic illnesses, their most urgent need is to find out what, from the patients' perspective, *continuity* really means.

This chapter focuses on questions that relate to the experiences of patients and health professionals and the meaning that patients and health professionals associate with these experiences. In general terms, evidence-based health care has tended to focus on the search for objective evidence to establish the degree to which a particular intervention or activity results in defined outcomes. The importance of basing practice on the best available evidence is now well accepted, and ways of finding, appraising and applying evidence related to diagnosis, prognosis, the effects of an intervention and experiences and perceptions from those involved in health care are becoming increasingly well understood. Thus, evidence-based practice is generally conceptualised as searching for, appraising and synthesising the results of high quality research and transferring the findings to practice and policy domains to improve health outcomes.

Health professionals seek evidence to substantiate the worth of a very wide range of activities and interventions, and thus the type of evidence needed depends on the nature of the activity and its purpose. Pearson and colleagues[1] have described a model of evidence-based health care in which they assert that, if evidence is needed to address the multiple questions, concerns or interests of health professionals or the users of health services, it must come from a wide range of research traditions. Evidence that arises out of qualitative inquiry is frequently sought and utilised in clinical practice.[2] Qualitative research seeks to make sense of phenomena in terms of the meanings that people bring to them.[3] Evidence from qualitative studies that explore the experience of patients and health professionals has an important role in ensuring that the particularities associated with individual patients, families and communities are just as important as information that arises out of quantitative research.

Qualitative researchers attempt to increase our understandings of:

- how individuals and communities perceive health, manage their own health and make decisions related to health service usage
- the culture of communities and of organisations in relation to implementing change and overcoming barriers to the use of new knowledge and techniques
- how patients experience health, illness and the health system
- the usefulness, or otherwise, of components and activities of health services that cannot be measured in quantitative outcomes (such as health promotion and community development)
- the behaviours/experiences of health professionals, contexts of health care and why we behave/experience things in certain ways.

Qualitative research can generate evidence that informs clinical decision making on matters related to the feasibility, appropriateness or meaningfulness of a certain intervention or activity. Pearson et al.[2] describe feasibility as the extent to which an activity is practical and practicable. *Clinical feasibility* is about whether or not an activity or intervention is physically, culturally or financially practical or possible within a given context. They define *appropriateness* as the extent to which an intervention or activity fits with or is apt in a situation. *Clinical appropriateness* is about how an activity or intervention relates to the context in which care is given. *Meaningfulness* refers to how an intervention or activity is experienced by the patient. It relates to the personal experience, opinions, values, thoughts, beliefs and interpretations of patients. Evidence-based practice in its fullest sense is about making decisions about the feasibility, appropriateness, meaningfulness and effectiveness of interventions—and quantitative and qualitative evidence are often of equal importance in this endeavour. Qualitative research does not always involve the evaluation of an intervention. It may also seek to understand how patients try to cope with their disease, or how they experience illness in a broader social–cultural context. Apart from focusing on an intervention, qualitative research can also focus on a certain phenomenon of interest.

This chapter explores the value of different qualitative methodologies that can be used in qualitative research to address patients' experiences and concerns. It also presents a stepwise approach to developing qualitative clinical questions and searching for, appraising and applying qualitative evidence. Clinical scenarios and relevant qualitative articles are used to illustrate these processes.

QUALITATIVE RESEARCH: THE VALUE OF DIFFERENT PHILOSOPHICAL PERSPECTIVES AND METHODOLOGIES IN RESEARCHING PATIENTS' EXPERIENCES AND CONCERNS

Qualitative research that focuses on patients' (and health professionals') experiences and concerns assists people to tell their stories about what it is like to be a certain person, living in a particular time and place, in relation to a set of circumstances, and analyses the data generated to describe human experience and meaning. Qualitative researchers collect and analyse words, pictures, drawings, photos and other non-numerical data because these are the media through which people express themselves and their relationships to other people and their world. This means that if researchers want to know what the experience of care is like, they will ask the people receiving that care to describe or visualise their experience in order to capture the rich meaning. Through these approaches, the enduring realities of people's experiences are not over-simplified and subsumed into a number or a statistic.

All research has underlying philosophical positions or assumptions. In qualitative research, two common philosophical perspectives are the *interpretive* and *critical* perspectives. Interpretive research is undertaken with the assumption that reality is socially constructed through the use of language and shared meanings. Therefore, interpretive researchers attempt to *understand* phenomena through listening to people or watching what they do in order to interpret their meanings.[4] From the critical perspective, knowledge is considered to be value-laden and shaped by historical, social, political, gender and economic conditions. This in turn is thought to shape social structures and assumptions that, if they remain unquestioned, may serve to oppress particular groups.[5] Critical approaches in qualitative research ask not just what is happening, but why, and seek to generate theory and knowledge in order to help people bring about *change*.

Different qualitative methodologies may be used depending on the underlying philosophical perspective. For example, phenomenology, grounded theory and ethnography as commonly used 'interpretive' methodological approaches to research because they all aim to describe and understand phenomena. Critical researchers, on the other hand, seek to generate change by bringing problems or injustices forward for conscious debate and consideration, and therefore may choose methodological approaches such as action research, feminism and discourse analysis. Although these six methodologies are discussed separately in this chapter, qualitative researchers often combine elements from different methodologies when undertaking their research. Different qualitative research approaches set out to achieve different things and when differing perspectives are put together, they provide a multifaceted view of the subject of inquiry that deepens our understanding of it. In this sense they are not substitutes for each other due to some essential superiority of one method over another, but rather they represent a theoretical 'tool kit' of devices. Depending on the task at hand, one methodology on one occasion may be a more useful tool than another. We will describe these six commonly used methodologies below.

QUALITATIVE METHODOLOGIES USED IN HEALTH RESEARCH
Interpretive approaches to research
Phenomenology

A phenomenological research approach values human perception and subjectivity and seeks to explore what an experience is like for the individual concerned.[6] The basis of this approach is a concept called 'lived experience', which means that people who are living presently, or have lived an experience previously, are in the best position to speak of it, to inform others of what the experience is like or what it means to them. Phenomenology is concerned with discovering the 'essence' of experience. It usually draws on a very small sample of 3 to 10 research subjects, asking the question: '*What was it like to have that experience?*' Large sample sizes such as those found in quantitative research are not required in qualitative research, as the aim is to gather detailed information to understand the depth and nature of experiences. Data are collected using a focused, but non-structured, interview technique to elicit descriptions of the participant's experiences. This style of interview supports the role of the researcher as one who does not presume to know what the important aspects of the experience to be revealed are. Several steps are involved in thematic data analysis.[6] The interviews are transcribed verbatim and read by researchers who attempt to totally submerge themselves in the text in order to identify the implicit or essential themes of the experience, thus seeking the fundamental meaning of the experience.

The strength of the phenomenological method is that it seeks to derive meaning and knowledge from the phenomena themselves and, although it is generally conceded that unmediated access to a phenomenon is never a possibility (that is, the exclusion of all prior perceptions and research bias), the emphasis on the experience of the participants ensures that this model represents as closely as possible the participants' perspective.[7,8] In this sense the perspectives that arise from the phenomenological approach help to shape the categories of concern in terms of the issues that the participants themselves identify. Through the phenomenological method, participants contribute substantially to informing and describing the field of inquiry that future policy needs to address.

CLINICAL SCENARIO (CONTINUED)
Potential contribution of evidence from phenomenological research

The findings of phenomenological research studies could usefully provide evidence to the primary healthcare team related to the lived experience of being a patient and the meanings that patients associate with this experience.

Grounded theory

Grounded theory is a methodology developed by sociologists Glaser and Strauss[9] to express their ideas of generating theory from the 'ground' to explain data collected during the study, using an 'iterative' (or cyclical/circular) approach whereby data are gathered using an ongoing collection process from a variety of sources. Grounded theorists use a theoretical sample of people that are most likely to be the best informants to deliver the building blocks for the theory to be developed. Theoretical samples work towards a saturation point. That is, the point in which no new themes or issues emerge from the data. Glaser and Strauss developed this approach in their ground-breaking work on death and dying in hospitals.[9] Strauss and Corbin[10] have developed an approach that begins with open coding of data and requires the researcher to take the data apart. The approach distinguishes itself from phenomenology in putting a heavy emphasis on understanding the parts from a text to construct the overall picture of *'What is going on here?'*

CLINICAL SCENARIO (CONTINUED)

Potential contribution of evidence from grounded theory research

The findings of grounded theory research studies could usefully provide evidence to the primary healthcare team related to the development of a new, theoretical understanding of what being a person receiving primary health care means, grounded or based on the experience of patients themselves.

Ethnography

The term *ethnography* was used originally to describe a research technique that was used to study groups of people who: shared social and cultural characteristics; thought of themselves as a group; and shared common language, geographical locale and identity. Classic ethnographies portray cultures, providing 'a portrait of the people' (the literal meaning of the term ethnography), and move beyond descriptions of what is said and done in order to understand 'shared systems of meanings that we call culture'.[11] An ethnographer comes to understand the social world of the group in an attempt to develop an inside view while recognising that it will emerge from an outside perspective. In this sense the researcher attempts to experience the world of the 'other' (euphemistically referred to as 'going native'), while appreciating that the experience emerges through the 'self' of the researcher. Ethnography involves participant observation, the recording of field notes and interviewing key informants. The identifying feature of participant observation is the attempt to reconstruct a representation of a culture that closely reflects 'the native's point of view'.

CLINICAL SCENARIO (CONTINUED)

Potential contribution of evidence from ethnography

The findings of ethnographic research studies could usefully provide evidence to the primary healthcare team related to the norms, patterns and group meanings of patients who are receiving primary health care, based on observation and the accounts of members of the group.

Critical approaches to research

Action research

Action research is the pursuit of knowledge through working collaboratively on describing the social world and acting on it in order to change it. Through acting on the world this way, critical theory and understandings are generated. Action research asks the question, *'What is happening here and how could it be different?'* It involves reflecting on the world in order to change it and then entering into a cyclical process of reflection, change and evaluation. Data collected in action research include transcripts of group discussions as well as quantitative and qualitative data suggested by the participative group. Both of these types of data are analysed concurrently. Themes, issues and concerns are extracted and discussed by both the research team and the participative group. Action research provides a potential means for overcoming the frequent failure of externally generated research to be embraced by research consumers, who often regard this form of research as unrelated to and not associated with their practice.

CLINICAL SCENARIO (CONTINUED)

Potential contribution of evidence from action research studies

The findings of action research studies could usefully provide evidence to the primary healthcare team related to outcomes of involving patients themselves in critiquing the care they receive and in developing and implementing action to change those things that they identify as inappropriate or as barriers to optimal living.

Discourse analysis

Discourse analysis has its roots in postmodern thinking and emerged in a number of academic disciplines in the last two or so decades of the 20th century. It has played an important role in creating new ways of developing ideas in the arts, science and culture. At its simplest (and it is far from simple!), postmodernism is a response to modernity—the period when science was trusted and represented progress—and essentially focuses on questioning the centrality of both science and established principles, disciplines and institutions to achieving progress. The nature of 'truth' is a recurring concern to postmodernists, who generally claim that there are no truths but instead there are multiple realities and that understanding of the human condition is dynamic and diverse. The notion that no one view, theory or understanding should be privileged over another is a belief of postmodernist critique and analysis. The scrutiny and breakdown of ideas that are associated with postmodernism are most frequently applied through the discursive analysis of texts. Discourse is defined as to 'talk, converse; hold forth in speech or writing on a subject; give forth'.[12] Thus, discourse analysis essentially refers to the capturing of public, professional, political and even private discourses and deconstructing these 'messages'. Discursive analysis aims at revealing what is being said, thought and done in relation to a specific topic or issue.

CLINICAL SCENARIO (CONTINUED)

Potential contribution of evidence from discursive studies

The findings of discursive studies could usefully provide evidence to the primary healthcare team that arises out of deconstructing what patients and health professionals say; the origins of existing, dominant views; and the way in which strongly held, powerful discourses may 'silence' or 'marginalise' the voices of patients.

Hopefully by now you will have realised that qualitative research evidence is an important source of knowledge related to the 'culture, practices, and discourses of health and illness'.[13,14] The value of such research and its methodologies lies in its ability to systematically examine questions about issues such as experiences, opinions and reasons for behaviours that are unable to be answered by means of quantitative research that often uses frequencies and associations.

USING QUALITATIVE EVIDENCE: A STEPWISE APPROACH

Structuring a qualitative question

The team that was described in the clinical scenario at the beginning of this chapter want to find out what receiving care from a large primary healthcare team is like for people who have a chronic illness.

The PICO format that was described in Chapter 2 does not do justice to the variety of qualitative questions that can emerge within different methodologies; however, it is a helpful tool to structure qualitative questions. Generally there is no 'comparison' in a qualitative question, and the 'I' refers to 'interest' or 'issue' rather than intervention. And sometimes you may wish to add the term 'evaluation', as this is more appropriate than outcome ('*What are we evaluating in the study?*').

CLINICAL SCENARIO (CONTINUED)
Structuring the question

From this scenario, a suitable qualitative question would be:

- In adults with any chronic illness that requires frequent primary health care (*Population*), what are patients' perceptions and experiences of continuity and of receiving that care from different members of the primary healthcare team (*Issue*)?

Searching for qualitative evidence

Because the question for our clinical scenario explicitly seeks *qualitative* information, the team will clearly need to search for qualitative research articles. It may be clear from the previous section that using the term 'qualitative research' is, however, in itself problematic. The word 'qualitative' is frequently used to describe a singular, specific methodology (for example, 'in this study a qualitative methodology was pursued'), when in its broadest sense it is an umbrella term that encompasses a wide range of methodologies stemming from a number of diverse traditions.

Finding qualitative research papers through database searches is often difficult.[15] It has been claimed that finding quantitative studies is much easier because the progress that has been made in indexing specific quantitative designs has not been paralleled in the qualitative domain. In Chapter 3, we provided you with some search strategies for locating qualitative research in MEDLINE, CINAHL, Embase and PsycINFO (refer to Table 3.1 in Chapter 3). For example, you may remember that, in MEDLINE, the best multiple-term strategy that minimised the difference between a sensitive and a specific search[16] was to combine the content terms with the following methodological terms: *interview:.mp. OR experience:. mp. OR qualitative.tw*. However, if you wish to look for a particular method, relevant terms such as *phenomenology* or *grounded theory* will need to be used.

CLINICAL SCENARIO (CONTINUED)
Finding the evidence to answer the question

One possible search strategy that the primary healthcare team could use is to search in PubMed using the Health Services Research Queries feature (see Chapter 3) with the following search terms:

(primary health care) AND (chronic illness) AND (patient perceptions) AND continuity

Using the narrow search scope does not retrieve any relevant articles. You repeat the search using the broad search scope. This particular search, conducted in January 2012, resulted in 34 articles. One of these articles seemed to directly address patient experiences of continuity of care in a chronic illness. It specifically explores continuity of care in a group of people with diabetes.

CLINICAL SCENARIO (CONTINUED)

Structured abstract of the chosen article

Citation: Naithani S, Gulliford M, Morgan M. Patients' perceptions and experiences of 'continuity of care' in diabetes. Health Expect 2006;9:118–29. The structured abstract has been adapted from this reference.

Study design: This is a 'qualitative' study.

Study question: The study explored patients' experiences and values with respect to continuity in diabetes care.

Context: Participants lived in relatively deprived inner-city areas of London that have young, mobile and ethnically diverse populations.

Participants: Participants were 25 people with type 2 diabetes from 14 general practices in two inner London boroughs. Participants were purposively sampled to include main ethnic minority groups.

Data collection method: In-depth semi-structured interviews.

Analysis: Analysis initially involved coding segments of transcripts that described patients' views and experiences of their diabetes care. These were then mapped to the dimensions of continuity of Freeman et al,[17] which are further described in the article. This model was selected as forming the product of a synthesis of previous approaches to continuity of care and emphasising the primary–secondary interface.

Key findings: Patients' accounts identified four dimensions of experienced continuity of care. These were: (1) receiving regular reviews with clinical testing and provision of advice over time (longitudinal continuity); (2) having a relationship with a usual care provider who knew and understood them (relational continuity); (3) flexibility of service provision in response to changing needs or situations (flexible continuity); (4) consistency and coordination between different members of staff and settings (team and cross-boundary continuity). Lack of continuity occurred largely at transitions between sites of care, between providers or with significant changes in patients' needs.

Conclusion: The study offers a patient-based framework for determining continuity of care in chronic disease management. It also identifies problematic aspects of continuity related to key transition points. The authors suggest that it is important that service design for chronic disease management take patients' experience of continuity of care into account.

Critically appraising qualitative evidence—is the evidence likely to be biased?

Qualitative approaches are located in diverse understandings of knowledge; they do not distance the researcher from the researched; and the data analysis is legitimately influenced by the researcher when they interpret the data. This poses considerable challenges in appraising the quality of qualitative research. Dixon-Woods, Agarwal and Smith[18] suggest that 'there are now over 100 sets of proposals on quality in qualitative research' and it seems to be unlikely that the international research community will come to an agreement on which particular instrument to put forward as the standard for quality appraisal in qualitative research, at least in the short term. A useful point to start the process of quality appraisal is to read the chapter on critical appraisal of qualitative research written by the Cochrane Qualitative Research Methods Group and available as supplemental guidance to the *Cochrane Handbook of Systematic Reviews of Interventions*.[19] Although it focuses on qualitative evidence appraisal in the context of systematic reviews, it lists the core concepts to be considered in quality appraisal of qualitative research and a selection of instruments that are available for quality appraisal. It also provides some guidance on the phases that need to be considered in critical appraisal and on how to deal with the outcome of a critical appraisal exercise.[20]

In the rest of this chapter we will cross-compare the quality criteria and discuss some of the strengths and weaknesses of two commonly used critical appraisal tools: the QARI (Qualitative Assessment and Review Instrument)[21] critical appraisal instrument and the CASP (Critical Appraisal Skills Programme)[22] instrument. Both instruments contain 10 quality criteria.

In this comparison we will emphasise the extent to which both instruments facilitate the assessment of validity in qualitative research. In earlier chapters of this book you have seen that assessing the risk of bias of a study is also a major aim when critically appraising quantitative data. Validity in quantitative research is assessed by establishing the extent to which the design and conduct of a study address potential sources of bias. This focus on limiting bias to establish validity does not fit with the philosophical foundations of qualitative approaches to inquiry. There is no emerging consensus on what the actual focus of quality appraisal in qualitative research should consist of. Some argue that the focus should be on the *rigour* of the research design as well as on the quality of reporting. Others argue that quality of reporting is only a facilitator of appraising qualitative research papers and that the main focus should be on evaluating validity, referring to the kinds of understanding we have of the phenomena under study (accounts identified by researchers) and whether or not these are subject to potential flaws. Potential flaws can occur, for example, in the translation from statements of study participants into researcher statements or from study findings into a conclusion.

We tend to adopt the latter approach, emphasising that statements need to be grounded in research evidence, that we need to know whether statements from a researcher accurately reflect the ideas participants intended to reveal, and that the set of arguments or the conclusion derived from a study necessarily follows from the premises. To facilitate comparison between the QARI and the CASP, we took the 11 main headings (left column of Table 10.1) reported in Hannes et al[23] and adapted the original table for the purpose of this comparison.

Earlier we indicated that the philosophical stance one takes influences the research methodology one uses for research. In the same way, the methodological position chosen influences the way in which data are collected.[4] One feature of the QARI tool, that is not present in the CASP tool, is to check the congruence between these aspects of a study. QARI also focuses on the extent to which the influence of the researcher is acknowledged, and that what participants said is represented in the findings and form the basis of any conclusions drawn.

The CASP checklist, with its pragmatic focus on the different phases in a research project, does not engage with the theoretical and paradigmatic level for which one needs to be an experienced qualitative researcher. As a consequence it is more friendly to novice researchers. Overall, CASP does a better job than QARI in capturing the audit trail of individual studies and, as such, enables reviewers to evaluate whether a study has been conducted according to the 'state of the art' for a particular method. Specifically, the CASP tool reminds the reader to think about the idea of *rigour* (whether thorough and appropriate approaches have been applied to key research methods in the study); *credibility* (whether the findings are well presented and meaningful); and *relevance* (how useful the findings are to you and your organisation). Within the qualitative research tradition, there are specific strategies that the researcher can use to improve the credibility of the research, and these are indicated in the CASP tool

TABLE 10.1:
COMPARISON OF APPRAISAL CRITERIA IN THE QARI INSTRUMENT AND THE CASP CHECKLIST

Main heading	QARI instrument appraisal criteria (original criterion numbering)	CASP checklist instrument appraisal criteria (original criterion numbering)
	There is congruity between:	Screening questions: (1) Was there a clear statement of the aims of the research? *Consider what the goal of the research was, why it is important, its relevance.* (2) Is a qualitative methodology appropriate? *Consider whether the research seeks to interpret or illuminate the actions and/or subjective experiences of research participants.*
Theoretical framework	(1) The stated philosophical perspective and the research methodology. *Consider whether the article clearly states the philosophical or theoretical premises on which the study is based. Does the article clearly state the methodological approach on which the study is based? Is there congruence between the two? For example:* • *an article may state that the study adopted a critical perspective and a participatory action research methodology was followed. There is congruence between a critical view (focusing on knowledge arising out of critique, action and reflection) and action research (an approach that focuses on working with groups to reflect on issues or practices and to consider how they could be different, on acting to change and on identifying new knowledge arising out of the action taken).* • *an article states that the study adopted an interpretive perspective and that a survey methodology was followed. In this example, there is incongruence between an interpretive view (focusing on knowledge arising out of studying what phenomena mean to individuals or groups) and surveys (an approach that focuses on asking standard questions to a defined study population).* • *an article may state that the study was qualitative or used qualitative methodology (such statements do not demonstrate rigour in design) or make no statement about the philosophical orientation or methodology.*	
Appropriateness of research design	(2) The research methodology and the research question or objectives *This question seeks to establish whether the study methodology is appropriate for addressing the research question. For example:* • *a report may state that the research question was to seek understandings of the meaning of pain in a group of people with rheumatoid arthritis and that a phenomenological approach was taken. Here, there is congruity between this question and the methodology. However, a report which states that the research question was designed to establish the effects of counselling on the severity of pain experience and that an ethnographic approach was pursued lacks congruity. This is because cause-and-effect cannot be addressed using an ethnographic approach.*	(3) Was the research design appropriate to address the aims of the research? *Consider whether the researcher has justified the research design (for example, have they discussed how they decided which methods to use?)*

TABLE 10.1:
COMPARISON OF APPRAISAL CRITERIA IN THE QARI INSTRUMENT AND THE CASP CHECKLIST–CONT'D

Main heading	QARI instrument appraisal criteria (original criterion numbering)	CASP checklist instrument appraisal criteria (original criterion numbering)
Data collection	(3) The research methodology and the methods used to collect data. *This question guides reviewers to consider whether the data collection methods are appropriate to the stated methodology.* *For example:* • *an article may state that the study pursued a phenomenological approach and that data were collected through phenomenological interviews. In this instance there is congruence between the methodology and data collection.* • *an article stated that the study pursued a phenomenological approach and that data were collected through a postal questionnaire. This would indicate incongruence between the methodology and data collection. This is because phenomenology seeks to elicit rich descriptions of the experience of a phenomenon that cannot be achieved through seeking written responses to standardised questions.*	(4) Was the recruitment strategy appropriate to the aims of the research? *Consider whether the researcher has explained how the participants were selected, explained why the participants they selected were the most appropriate to provide access to the type of knowledge sought by the study and whether there are any discussions around recruitment (for example, why some people chose not to take part).* (5) Were the data collected in a way that addressed the research issue? *Consider whether the setting for data collection was justified. it is clear how data were collected (e.g. focus group, semi-structured interview, etc), the researcher has justified the methods chosen, the researcher has made the methods explicit (for example, for interview method, is there an indication of how interviews were conducted, did they use a topic guide?), methods were modified during the study (if so, has the researcher explained how and why?), the form of data is clear (for example, tape recordings, video material, notes, etc), the researcher has discussed saturation of data.*
Data analysis	(4) The research methodology and the representation and analysis of data. *Are the data analysed and represented in ways that are congruent with the stated methodological position?* *For example:* • *an article may state that the study pursued a phenomenological approach to explore people's experience of grief by asking participants to describe their experiences of grief. If the text generated from asking these questions is searched to establish the meaning of grief to participants and the meanings of all participants are included in the report findings, then this represents congruity.* • *an article might focus only on the meanings that were common to all participants and discard single reported meanings, which would not be appropriate in phenomenological work.*	(8) Was the data analysis sufficiently rigorous? *Consider whether there is an in-depth description of the analysis process, thematic analysis is used (if so, is it clear how the categories/themes were derived from the data?), whether the researcher explains how the data presented were selected from the original sample to demonstrate the analysis process, whether sufficient data are presented to support the findings, to what extent contradictory data are taken into account, whether the researcher critically examined their own role, potential bias and influence during analysis and selection of data for presentation.*

Continued

231

Main heading	QARI instrument appraisal criteria (original criterion numbering)	CASP checklist instrument appraisal criteria (original criterion numbering)
TABLE 10.1: COMPARISON OF APPRAISAL CRITERIA IN THE QARI INSTRUMENT AND THE CASP CHECKLIST–CONT'D		
Findings	(5) The research methodology and the interpretation of results. *Are the results interpreted in ways that are appropriate to the methodology?* *For example:* • *an article may state that a study pursued a phenomenological approach to explore people's experience of facial disfigurement and these results are used to inform health professionals about accommodating individual differences in care. In this example, there is congruence between the methodology and this approach to interpretation.* • *an article states that the study pursued a phenomenological approach to explore people's experience of facial disfigurement and the results are used to generate practice checklists for assessment. In this case, there is incongruence between the methodology and this approach to interpretation, as phenomenology seeks to understand the meaning of a phenomenon for the study participants and cannot be interpreted to suggest that this can be generalised to total populations to a degree where standardised assessments will have relevance across a population.*	(9) Is there a clear statement of findings? *Consider whether the findings are explicit, there is adequate discussion of the evidence both for and against the researcher's arguments, the researcher has discussed the credibility of their findings (for example, triangulation, respondent validation, more than one analyst) and whether the findings are discussed in relation to the original research questions.*
Context	(6) There is a statement locating the researcher culturally. *Are the beliefs and values and their potential influences on the study declared? The researcher plays a substantial role in the qualitative research process, and it is important when appraising evidence that is generated in this way to know the researcher's cultural and theoretical orientation. A high quality report will include a statement that clarifies this.*	
Impact of investigator	(7) The influence of the researcher on the research and vice versa is clear. *Are the potential for the researcher to influence the study and the potential of the research process itself to influence the researcher and the interpretations acknowledged and addressed?* *For example: Is the relationship between the researcher and the study participants addressed? Does the researcher critically examine their own role and potential influence during data collection? Is it reported how the researcher responded to events that arose during the study?*	(6) Has the relationship between researchers and participants been adequately considered? *Consider whether it is clear that the researcher critically examined their own role, potential bias and influence during formulation of research questions, data collection, including sample recruitment and choice of location, how the researcher responded to events during the study and whether they considered the implications of any changes in the research design.*
Believability	(8) Participants, and their voices, are heard. *Generally, articles should provide illustrations from the data (such as quotes from participants) to show the basis of their conclusions and to ensure that participants are represented in the article.*	

TABLE 10.1:
COMPARISON OF APPRAISAL CRITERIA IN THE QARI INSTRUMENT AND THE CASP CHECKLIST–CONT'D

Main heading	QARI instrument appraisal criteria (original criterion numbering)	CASP checklist instrument appraisal criteria (original criterion numbering)
Ethics	(9) The research is ethical according to current criteria or, for recent studies, there is evidence of ethical approval by an appropriate body. *An ethics committee approved the project proposal.*	(7) Have ethical issues been taken into consideration? *Consider whether there are sufficient details of how the research was explained to participants for the reader to assess whether ethical standards were maintained, the researcher has discussed issues raised by the study (for example, issues around informed consent or confidentiality or how they have handled the effects of the study on the participants during and after the study).*
Evaluation/ Outcome	(10) Conclusions drawn in the research report do appear to flow from the analysis, or interpretation, of the data. *This criterion concerns the relationship between the findings reported and the views or words of study participants. In appraising an article, appraisers seek to satisfy themselves that the conclusions drawn by the research are based on the data collected–the data being the text that is generated through observation, interviews or other processes.*	
Value and implications of research		(10) How valuable is the research? *Consider whether the researcher discusses the contribution the study makes to existing knowledge or understanding (for example, do they consider the findings in relation to current practice or policy, or relevant research-based literature?), they identify new areas where research is necessary. the researchers have discussed whether or how the findings can be transferred to other populations or considered other ways the research may be used.*

as a prompt for the reader to consider them. For example, the researcher may make use of triangulation and respondent validation. To explain further: *triangulation* occurs when data are collected and considered from a number of different sources, which may help to confirm the findings or to increase the completeness of data collected.[24] *Respondent validation* (also known as member checking) is where the researcher seeks confirmation and clarification from the participants that the data accurately reflect what they meant or wanted to say.

Another important feature of qualitative research is that the researcher is integral to the research process. It is therefore important that their role is considered and explained in the research report. The CASP tool prompts the reader to ask whether the researcher critically examined their own role, potential bias and influence during analysis and selection of data for presentation. One of the strengths of the QARI tool is that it suggests that the reader evaluate whether or not the researchers have reflected on their cultural and theoretical background and provided a rationale for the methodological choices made to control their impact on the research. However, it goes even further—also evaluating whether researchers have invested in an epistemological type of reflexivity. Thinking about how the choice of method might have influenced the findings is equally as important as thinking about what the potential impact of the researcher has been.

To illustrate the critical appraisal process, we will evaluate the clinical scenario using the 10 QARI criteria. Additional insights generated by using the CASP tool are added at the end of each of the QARI comments.

CLINICAL SCENARIO (CONTINUED)
Critical appraisal of the chosen article

1. CONGRUITY BETWEEN THE STATED PHILOSOPHICAL PERSPECTIVE AND THE RESEARCH METHODOLOGY
The study sought to understand patients' experience (interpretation) and used what it describes as 'a qualitative' approach. This is a somewhat meaningless description that offers little when trying to address this criterion. However, it appears that the researchers were taking an interpretive position and used a constructivist methodology, but they do not explicitly describe the methodology. Thus, when evaluating this criterion, it appears that there is insufficient information to make a judgment.

The CASP checklist does not evaluate this criterion.

2. CONGRUITY BETWEEN THE RESEARCH METHODOLOGY AND THE RESEARCH QUESTION OR OBJECTIVES
Given that the aim was to understand patient/patient experiences, this criterion appears to be met.

Additional comment from the CASP checklist: The study design or methodology was not mentioned, so it is not possible to evaluate whether it was appropriate to address the aims of the research.

3. CONGRUITY BETWEEN THE RESEARCH METHODOLOGY AND THE METHODS USED TO COLLECT DATA
The method used was in-depth semi-structured interviews with 25 people with type 2 diabetes. This method is consistent with the overall design of the study.

Additional comment from the CASP checklist: A clear audit trail of how participants have been recruited is included in the study; however, a rationale for the choice of the people or the reasons for drop-out at the level of recruitment have not been described. The authors do well in making their methods explicit. They mention the topics addressed in their interview guide and describe how (e.g. 30 to 120 minutes, tape-recorded, the use of probing strategies) and where (home setting) the interviews were conducted. It remains unclear who has conducted the interviews and what the characteristics of the interviewer are. Saturation of data is not discussed; however, this is not a prerequisite as the study does not aim to build theory.

4. CONGRUITY BETWEEN THE RESEARCH METHODOLOGY AND THE REPRESENTATION AND ANALYSIS OF DATA
Interviews were transcribed and responses analysed thematically and grouped into dimensions of continuity of care. This is congruous with the overall approach.

Additional comment from the CASP checklist: The thematic analysis is justified through the use of a deductive approach to analysis, using an existing framework to classify data. The author provides the reader with some indications on the profile of the participants from whom the excerpts (or illustrations) are selected (such as GP, hospital or shared care setting); however, there is no attempt to differentiate for these settings in the findings or discussion section.

5. CONGRUENCE BETWEEN THE RESEARCH METHODOLOGY AND THE INTERPRETATION OF RESULTS

The results were interpreted as patients valuing four dimensions of continuity of care. These were: receiving regular reviews with clinical testing and provision of advice over time (longitudinal continuity); having a relationship with a usual care provider who knew and understood them, was concerned and interested and took time to listen and explain (relational continuity); flexibility of service provision in response to changing needs or situations (flexible continuity); and consistency and coordination between different members of staff and between hospital and general practice or community settings (team and cross-boundary continuity). Problems of a lack of experience of continuity mainly occurred at transitions between sites of care, between providers or with major changes in patients' needs.

Additional comment from the CASP checklist: The analysis seems rigorous. The findings are explicit and the empirical data collected are generally well mapped onto an existing scheme of continuity of care developed. The authors clearly discuss the limitations of trying to map their data to this model (for example, in stating that this particular process of categorisation risks losing data).

6. LOCATING THE RESEARCHER CULTURALLY OR THEORETICALLY

The researchers do not describe this.

The CASP checklist does not specifically address whether the researcher has declared their cultural or theoretical position.

7. INFLUENCE OF THE RESEARCHER ON THE RESEARCH, AND VICE VERSA, IS ADDRESSED

The researchers do not describe this.

Additional comment from the CASP checklist: There are no traces of a thorough critical examination of the researcher's own role, potential bias and influence in this paper. The authors do state that the analysis has been conducted by at least two different researchers, which improves the credibility of the findings and limits the risk of bias resulting from the researcher's personal perspective. The authors also describe the difficulties reaching consensus between researchers and how they dealt with this.

8. REPRESENTATION OF PARTICIPANTS AND THEIR VOICES

The article illustrates each of the themes by presenting excerpts from the patient interview transcripts and therefore demonstrates compliance with this criterion.

Additional comment from the CASP checklist: This item is a ddressed as part of the representation of the findings (item 4).

9. ETHICAL APPROVAL BY AN APPROPRIATE BODY

An ethics committee approved the project proposal.

Additional comment from the CASP checklist: The authors outline the procedure of how participants were approached by stating that they developed letters, an information sheet explaining what the study was about, and indicated that all interviewees gave written informed consent.

10. RELATIONSHIP OF CONCLUSIONS TO ANALYSIS OR INTERPRETATION OF THE DATA

The study develops a patient-based framework for assessing continuity of care in chronic disease management and identifies key transition points with problems of lack of continuity. It concludes that it is important that service redesign and developments in vertically integrated services for chronic disease management take account of impacts on the patient's experience of continuity of care.

Additional comment from the CASP checklist: The authors stress the importance of the identified aspects of the patient's experiences and hence identify new areas where research is necessary.

Further comments comparing the QARI and CASP approaches to critical appraisal

Before finishing off this section on critical appraisal, we will highlight some of the interesting topics we came across when evaluating this particular study with the quality criteria of both the QARI tool and the CASP checklist. The most important issue is that the influence of the researcher on the research, or vice versa, is hardly addressed in this study and neither is the cultural or theoretical background of the researchers. The lack of sensitivity to these issues can be problematic, because most qualitative research is largely inductive. Researchers typically look at reality and try to develop a theory from the information derived from the field. The philosophical position of the researcher towards the research project determines not only the choice of an appropriate method, but also the window through which he or she will be looking at the data. It has a direct impact on the way the findings will be interpreted and presented. Therefore, a research project that does not reveal what view of reality the researcher holds can be called highly mechanistic.[23]

We have highlighted the fact that there are several methodologies which could be considered in qualitative research. If you decide to go down one particular path, you need to understand and articulate how the knowledge tradition you opt for, together with its claims to understanding, influence your data collection, analysis and conclusion. Clarifying and justifying the window that determines your view will allow an experienced reviewer to judge the impact of your theoretical and methodological choices.

There are some other interesting differences between the instruments compared, as reported by Hannes et al.[23] The QARI tool does not include an item about relevance or transferability (which the CASP checklist addresses in item 10). Whether or not 'relevance' is an issue that needs to be evaluated in the context of a critical appraisal exercise is debatable. Like ethics, the 'relevance' criterion most likely has its roots in the idea that research should address the concerns of health professionals rather than be the product of individual academic interest. This also raises the important question of whether or not an ethics approval has direct implications on the methodological quality of a study. To conclude our comments about these two approaches for appraising qualitative research, both instruments can assist us in evaluating methodological quality of studies; however, their approach to appraising qualitative research is somewhat different.

How, then, do we make sense of the appraisal as a whole? Pearson[21] offers the following categorisation of judgment about a qualitative article. Overall the article may be considered:

- *Unequivocal:* the evidence is beyond reasonable doubt and includes findings that are factual, directly reported/observed and not open to challenge.
- *Credible:* the evidence, while interpretative, is plausible in light of the data and theoretical framework. Conclusions can be logically inferred from the data but because the findings are essentially interpretative, these conclusions are open to challenge.
- *Unsupported:* findings are not supported by the data and none of the other level descriptors apply.

The next issue to consider is how we might use the findings in practice.

Applying qualitative evidence

Research from qualitative studies can inform health professionals' thinking about similar situations/populations that they are working with. However, the way in which findings from qualitative evidence might be used in practice differs from quantitative research. Quantitative research findings are reported in terms of the probability (for example) of an outcome occurring when a particular intervention is implemented, in the same way, for a defined patient group. This therefore requires health professionals to accept a generalisation that the research findings can be applied to patients similar to those participating in the study. In quantitative research, this concept is referred to as *generalisability*. There are objections to the application of qualitative findings in practice because of the theoretical underpinnings of many qualitative methodologies. Principally this relates to the idea that 'truth' is contextual, or for certain methodologies 'in the moment', and therefore only representative of a particular person or group at *that* time and within *that* context. Therefore it is argued that the findings of a qualitative study of one group of people in a single study cannot be extrapolated to other people, groups or contexts. Researchers who follow this line of argument claim that the pooling and/or application of qualitative findings is, in effect, an attempt to formulate a result that can be generalised across a population and, as such, is an inappropriate use of qualitative findings.

Other researchers have developed a strong opposing view and suggest that the term *generalisability* is being misinterpreted. Sandelowski and colleagues[25] have put forward that the argument against the pooling or application of qualitative findings is founded on a 'narrowly conceived' view of what constitutes generalisability—that is, a view that sees it in relation to the representativeness (in terms of size and randomisation) of a sample and of statistical significance. They argue that qualitative research has the capacity to produce generalisations—but they are suggestive or naturalistic (or realistic) in nature rather than generalisations that are predictive, as is the case in quantitative research.[25] The CASP checklist adds the criterion of relevance or transferability of findings as an important issue to be evaluated when reading a research paper and, depending on the type of qualitative design used, it seems reasonable to do so. There is little reason to believe that a theoretical or conceptual model that is based on a theoretical sample that used a maximum variation strategy (sampling to maximise diversity of participants represented), reached a point of saturation and was tested in different settings (for example, as grounded theory approaches do) could not be considered generalisable or relevant to other settings. However, bear in mind that many qualitative researchers aim to just understand a phenomenon, rather than to generalise the findings to other settings.

Applying qualitative evidence to the clinical scenario

A strategy for applying the findings of qualitative research within the primary healthcare team could include:

- Raising awareness of the patient's experiences within the team in relation to longitudinal continuity, relational continuity, flexible continuity and team and cross-boundary continuity.

- Conducting a clinical audit of care-giving to people with a chronic illness and assessing the degree to which these four areas of continuity are achieved.

- Involving the multidisciplinary team in reviewing the way in which people with a chronic disease are cared for in relation to longitudinal continuity, relational continuity, flexible continuity, and team and cross-boundary continuity.

- Engaging the multidisciplinary team in service redesign and the development of services for chronic disease management that include:
  - offering patients regular reviews
  - identifying a 'usual care provider' for all patients with a chronic condition
  - a degree of flexibility of service provision in response to changing needs or situations
  - consistency and coordination between different members of staff and between hospital and general practice or community settings.

- Evaluating the effects of the changes implemented on the patient experience by eliciting and analysing patient feedback.

SUMMARY POINTS OF THIS CHAPTER

- The experiences of patients are a rich source of evidence for practice and can increase our understandings of how individuals and communities perceive health, manage their own health and make decisions related to health service usage.

- High quality qualitative research uses rigorous processes to elicit and analyse data related to patient experience and perceptions.

- There are a number of well-established qualitative research methodologies including (but not limited to) phenomenology, grounded theory, ethnography, action research, feminist research, and discourse analysis. These methods are adaptive and may be used in conjunction with each other.

- Appraising qualitative evidence requires an assessment of the quality of the research in relation to the research methodology, methods and analyses used and the interpretation of data. Critical appraisal instruments may help us in evaluating whether studies are methodologically sound. However, as with appraisal instruments for quantitative research, appraisal checklists only capture what has been reported.

References

1. Pearson A, Wiechula R, Court A, et al. The JBI model of evidence-based healthcare. Int J Evidence-based Healthcare 2005;3:207–15.
2. Pearson A, Field J, Jordan Z. Evidence-based clinical practice in nursing and health care. Oxford: Blackwell Publishing; 2007.
3. Denzin NK. The art and politics of interpretation. In: Denzin N, Lincoln Y, editors. Handbook of qualitative research. Thousand Oaks, CA: Sage; 1994. pp. 500–15.
4. The Joanna Briggs Institute. CSR Study Guide Module 4. The systematic review of evidence generated by qualitative research, narrative and text. Adelaide, South Australia, Australia: The Joanna Briggs Institute; 2012. Online. Available: www.joannabriggs.edu.au/documents/train-the-trainer/module4/ttt_m4_studyguide.pdf; 15 Jul 2012.
5. Berman H, Ford-Gilboe M, Campbell JC. Combining stories and numbers: a methodologic approach for a critical nursing science. Adv Nurs Sci 1998;21(1):1–15.
6. van Manen M. Researching lived experience: human science for an action sensitive pedagogy. Toronto: Althouse Press; 1997.
7. Koch T. Establishing rigour in qualitative research: the decision trail. J Adv Nurs 1993;19:976–86.
8. Koch T. Implementation of a hermeneutic inquiry in nursing: philosophy, rigour and representation. J Adv Nurs 1996;24:174–84.
9. Glaser B, Strauss A. The discovery of grounded theory: strategies for qualitative research. New York: Aldine de Gruyter; 1967.
10. Strauss A, Corbin J. Basics of qualitative research: grounded theory procedures and techniques. London: Sage; 1990.
11. Boyle J. Styles of ethnography. In: Morse J, editor. Critical issues in qualitative research methods. Thousand Oaks, CA: Sage; 1994. pp. 159 85.
12. Concise Oxford English Dictionary. Oxford: Oxford University Press; 1964.
13. McCormick J, Rodney P, Varcoe C. Reinterpretations across studies: an approach to meta-analysis. Qual Health Res 2003;13:933–44.
14. Green J, Britten N. Qualitative research and evidence based medicine. BMJ 1998;316:1230–2.
15. Shaw R, Booth A, Sutton A, et al. Finding qualitative research: an evaluation of search strategies. BMC Med Res Methodol 2004;4:5.
16. Wong S, Wilczynski N, Haynes RB, et al. Developing optimal search strategies for detecting clinically relevant qualitative studies in MEDLINE. Medinfo 2004;11:311–16.
17. Freeman G, Shepperd S, Robinson I, et al. Report of a scoping exercise for the National Co-ordinating Centre for NHS Service Delivery and Organisation R&D (NCCSDO). London: NCCSDO; 2000. Online. Available: www.netscc.ac.uk/hsdr/files/project/SDO_ES_08-1009-002_V01.pdf; 19 Nov 2012.
18. Dixon-Woods M, Shaw R, Agarwal S, et al. The problem of appraising qualitative research. Qual Saf Health Care 2004;13:223–5.
19. Higgins JPT, Green S, editors. Cochrane Handbook for Systematic Reviews of Interventions Version 5.1.0 [updated March 2011]. The Cochrane Collaboration; 2011. Online. Available: www.cochrane-handbook.org; 8 Nov 2012.
20. Hannes K. Chapter 4: Critical appraisal of qualitative research. In: Noyes J, Booth A, Hannes K, et al, editors. Supplementary guidance for inclusion of qualitative research in Cochrane systematic reviews of interventions. Version 1 [updated August 2011]. Cochrane Collaboration Qualitative Methods Group; 2011. Online. Available: cqrmg.cochrane.org/supplemental-handbook-guidance; 8 Nov 2012.
21. Pearson A. Balancing the evidence: incorporating the synthesis of qualitative data into systematic reviews. JBI Reports 2004;2:45–64.
22. Critical Appraisal Skills Programme (CASP). 10 questions to help you make sense of qualitative research. England: Public Health Resource Unit; 2006. Online. Available: www.casp-uk.net/wp-content/uploads/2011/11/CASP_Qualitative_Appraisal_Checklist_14oct10.pdf; 14 Nov 2012.
23. Hannes K, Lockwood C, Pearson A. A comparative analysis of three online appraisal instruments' ability to assess validity in qualitative research. Qual Health Research 2010;20:1736–43.
24. Shih F. Triangulation in nursing research: issues of conceptual clarity and purpose. J Adv Nurs 1998;28(3):631–41.
25. Sandelowski M, Docherty S, Emden C. Focus on qualitative methods. Qualitative metasynthesis: issues and techniques. Res Nurs Health 1997;20:365–71.

Chapter 11

Questions about patients' experiences and concerns: examples of appraisals from different health professions

Sally Bennett, John Bennett, Mal Boyle, Jeff Coombes, Craig Lockwood, Lisa Nissen, Marie Pirotta, Sharon Sanders and Jemma Skeat

This chapter is an accompaniment to the previous chapter (Chapter 10) where the steps involved in answering a clinical question about patients' experiences and concerns were explained. In order to further help you learn how to appraise the evidence for this type of question, this chapter contains a number of worked examples of questions about patients' experiences and concerns.

The Critical Appraisal Skills Program (CASP) qualitative checklist[1] for critically appraising qualitative research has been used as a guide in each of the examples that follow, with additional comments added from the QARI instrument at the end of each example.

The CASP checklist is lengthy, and so for the purpose of brevity we have omitted the two screening items at the beginning of the checklist that ask: '*Was there a clear statement of the aims?*' and '*Is a qualitative methodology appropriate?*'. The authors who contributed examples to this chapter had already screened their chosen articles, and therefore we have not provided comments on these two items and you will see that each appraisal begins with item 3 of the checklist.

It is important to understand that the CASP checklist for qualitative research provides a technical/ pragmatic appraisal rather than a theoretical appraisal (as the QARI instrument does). The CASP tools were developed from guides produced by the Evidence-Based Medicine Working Group and published in the *Journal of the American Medical Association*.[2] One of the guides addresses qualitative research.[3] This guide does not consider theoretical perspectives of qualitative research, but asks the reader to judge the methodological rigour of the report by critically appraising the research/study design and analysis. You will note that the third item in the CASP checklist also asks about *research design*, and this needs clarification as it is subject to interpretation. Specifically it asks: '*Was the research design appropriate to address the aims of the research?*' It also prompts the reader to consider whether '*the researcher has justified the research design (for example, have they discussed how they decided which methods to use?)*'. There are no specific guidelines about what the CASP tool means by 'research design' or 'methods to use'. One could interpret this as meaning 'identify which research methodology was used', e.g. phenomenology, grounded theory, discourse analysis and so on. However, the perspective taken from the *User's guide*[3] is that 'research design' is about the practicalities of how the research was carried out, not which type of qualitative research methodology was used. In the examples that follow, we have therefore taken both approaches where relevant information was reported. As the CASP checklist does not ask about the philosophical perspectives of the researcher, we have added relevant comments from the QARI tool at the end of each worked example.

Although there are other checklists available for appraising qualitative evidence that have a slightly different focus, there is no consensus about the ideal approach that should be used. An explanation and comparison of the features of the QARI tool and the CASP checklist was provided in Chapter 10.

OCCUPATIONAL THERAPY AND PHYSIOTHERAPY EXAMPLE

CLINICAL SCENARIO

You have been working as a therapy manager in the multidisciplinary rehabilitation unit of a major metropolitan hospital for people with acquired brain injury, and want to understand the experience of patients of the inpatient rehabilitation setting as you think this might help inform ongoing refinements and developments within the rehabilitation unit. You are planning to meet with all staff on a rolling basis about how things might be improved in the unit, and decide to find studies that have specifically sought patients' views.

CLINICAL QUESTION

How do people who have had an acquired brain injury and their family members perceive the inpatient rehabilitation experience?

Search terms and databases used to find the evidence

Database: PubMed—Health Services Research Queries (with 'qualitative research' category and 'narrow scope' selected), which is accessed through the 'Topic-specific queries' link on PubMed.

Search terms: (brain injury) AND rehabilitation AND inpatient

This search strategy retrieved 10 articles. Two very recent articles focused on inpatient rehabilitation for people who have an acquired brain injury. One article considered a residential rehabilitation unit and the other considered the experience of an inpatient rehabilitation unit from the perspective of patients and their family members. This is the article that you choose to appraise.

Article chosen

Fleming J, Sampson J, Cornwell P, et al. Brain injury rehabilitation: the lived experience of inpatients and their family caregivers. Scand J Occup Ther 2012;19:184–93.

Structured abstract (adapted from the above)

Study design: This study was part of a larger qualitative research study about transitions from hospital to home for people with acquired brain injuries. This study reports on a subset of questions from this larger study, pertaining to their experiences of the rehabilitation unit, using a phenomenological approach.

Study question: To describe and interpret the inpatient brain injury rehabilitation experience from the perspective of patients and their carers.

Context: The inpatient rehabilitation ward was a secured ward in a large metropolitan hospital in Australia. It was a 26-bed ward with shared and single rooms, and had a dining room, recreational space, physiotherapy gym and outdoor courtyards. The multidisciplinary rehabilitation team included medical and nursing staff, occupational therapists, physiotherapists, speech pathologists, a social worker and a neuropsychologist.

Participants: Criterion-based purposeful sampling was used until data saturation was reached, resulting in a sample size of 20 patients and 18 nominated family carers.

Data collection method: Semi-structured interviews using an interview guide were conducted separately with participants and their nominated carers in a quiet room in the final week prior to discharge from the rehabilitation unit. The interview questions informing this study were the initial questions from the larger study intended for building rapport and obtaining background information regarding rehabilitation received up to the point of hospital discharge.

Analysis: Analysis of the interviews was conducted using a 'manifest content analytic' approach. The transcribed interview data were approached with the question: *'How do patients and family perceive the inpatient brain injury rehabilitation unit?'* Analysis occurred as follows. Two researchers independently extracted content related to the question from one interview transcription. Once accuracy of extraction was confirmed, one author extracted relevant data from the remaining transcripts. Data was organised by two researchers independently into core meanings (meaning units), which were then grouped and condensed into representative codes. Codes were then used to identify themes and categories, and all researchers met to establish a framework of themes and categories. This framework was then used by one author to code the remaining interviews. Emerging themes and codes were discussed if they arose.

Key findings: Three themes were identified: 'rehabilitation context/environment', 'activity/occupation' and 'support and adjustment'. The *rehabilitation context/environment* theme encompassed concerns about the limitations/restrictions of the physical environment and positive and negative perceptions related to organisational factors and staff attitudes. The theme of *activity/occupation* reflected the perceived importance of activities related to therapy sessions and other structured activities contrasting with the boredom experienced by some participants during unstructured time regardless of unstructured activities being available to them. The *support/adjustment* theme emphasised the pivotal role played by family members and friends in providing support to patients that was unable to be provided by staff, carers' need for information, and barriers experienced by carers in terms of communication and difficulty accessing staff.

Conclusion: This study improves understanding of rehabilitation from the patient's and family members' perspective and can assist rehabilitation teams to better meet the needs of people with acquired brain injury. Specifically highlighted was the need for a more therapeutic environment, meaningful occupations, and family-centredness in inpatient settings.

Is the evidence rigorous and sufficiently reported?

Detailed questions from CASP

3. Was the research design appropriate to address the aims of the research?

Consider:

• *Whether the researcher has justified the research design (for example, have they discussed how they decided which method to use?).*
   The authors clearly indicate that a phenomenological methodology was used and the justification for this was provided in the article. This study utilised semi-structured interviews with patients and nominated family carers in the week prior to patients being discharged from rehabilitation. The design and methods used for this study were clearly justified by the authors and addressed the study aims ('to describe and interpret the inpatient brain injury rehabilitation experience from the perspective of patients and their caregivers').

4. Was the recruitment strategy appropriate to the aims of the research?

Consider:

• *Whether the researcher has explained how the participants were selected.*
   Criterion-based purposeful sampling was used to select 'information-rich' participants who met a predetermined set of criteria, from whom comprehensive and detailed data regarding the rehabilitation experience were collected. Participants were recruited from a brain injury rehabilitation unit at a large metropolitan hospital in Australia.

• *Whether they explained why the participants they selected were the most appropriate to provide access to the type of knowledge sought by the study.*
   Some information is available about this through the eligibility criteria (for example, they needed to be current inpatients in a brain injury rehabilitation unit and able to communicate satisfactorily); it is also clear that those selected were appropriate for providing information with respect to the aims of this study.

5. Were the data collected in a way that addressed the research issue?

Consider:

• *Whether the setting for data collection was justified.*
   Participants were interviewed in the week prior to discharge home from the brain injury rehabilitation unit. Interviews were undertaken in the occupational therapy department and thus data was collected in a way that could address the research issue.

- *Whether it is clear how data were collected (for example, focus group, semi-structured interview etc).*
  Data were collected using semi-structured interviews separately with patients and a nominated family member.
- *Whether the researcher has justified the methods chosen.*
  Authors indicate that they used interviews in an attempt to gain a deep understanding of the phenomena.
- *Whether the researcher has made the methods explicit (for example, for interview method, is there an indication of how interviews were conducted, or did they use a topic guide?)*
  Although the authors explained the data collection process clearly, this study was part of a larger study and so it was not clear what specific questions were asked of the participants relevant to this component. The authors just state that this article was based on: 'a set of initial questions based around participants' experiences in the rehabilitation unit'. Referring to earlier articles did not improve the clarity of this issue.
- *Whether methods were modified during the study. If so, has the researcher explained how and why?*
  There is no mention that the research methods were changed during the study period.
- *Whether the form of data is clear (for example, tape recordings, video material, notes, etc).*
  It is clearly stated that interviews were tape-recorded and field notes taken.
- *Whether the researcher has discussed saturation of data*
  The saturation principle was used to determine the sample size of the study. Saturation was identified as the point at which no new information (that is, major themes) was emerging from the data-collection process, and this was determined through collaborative discussion between members of the research team.

6. Has the relationship between researcher and participants been adequately considered?

Consider:
- *Whether the researcher critically examined their own role, potential bias and influence during:*
  - *Formulation of the research questions.*
    There is no comment about this in the article.
  - *Data collection, including sample recruitment and choice of location.*
    The authors only state that 'recruitment and data collection were completed by an occupational therapist who had experience at the rehabilitation unit, but was not employed by the hospital'. However, there is no actual examination of her role beyond this statement.
- *How the researcher responded to events during the study and whether they considered the implications of any changes in the research design.*
  No changes occurred. The authors note that the injuries of participants may have affected their ability to clearly articulate and reflect upon their experiences as required during the interview process. However, they also note that triangulation with family carer interviews reduced the impact of bias that this might have introduced.

7. Have ethical issues been taken into consideration?

Consider:
- *Whether there are sufficient details of how the research was explained to participants for the reader to assess whether ethical standards were maintained.*
  All participants in the study signed a written consent statement.
- *Whether the researcher has discussed issues raised by the study (for example, issues around informed consent or confidentiality or how they have handled the effects of the study on the participants during and after the study).*

This is an important issue for a population who have sustained brain injuries and have related cognitive impairments. However, the ability of the participants to provide informed consent was determined by the patient's treating occupational therapist. Patients were excluded from the study if there was evidence of a premorbid psychiatric illness or cognitive impairment that impeded their ability to provide informed consent.

- *Whether approval has been sought from the ethics committee.*
  Approval from an ethics committee was provided.

8. Was the data analysis sufficiently rigorous?

Consider:

- *Whether there is an in-depth description of the analysis process. Whether thematic analysis is used. If so, is it clear how the categories/themes were derived from the data?*
  This is very clearly explained in the paper. Analysis of the interviews was conducted using a 'manifest content analytic' approach.

- *Whether the researcher explains how the data presented were selected from the original sample, to demonstrate the analysis process.*
  This was not clearly explained; however, representative quotes were given in table format for each of the themes and categories.

- *Whether sufficient data are presented to support the findings. To what extent contradictory data are taken into account.*
  Sufficient data were presented and both positive and negative perspectives were reported.

- *Whether the researcher critically examined their own role, potential bias and influence during analysis and selection of data for presentation.*
  The researcher did not critically examine their own role or potential biases and influence during analysis and selection of data.

9. Is there a clear statement of findings?

Consider:

- *Whether the findings are explicit. Whether there is adequate discussion of the evidence both for and against the researcher's arguments.*
  The authors presented a balanced discussion of the issues derived from participants' statements, reflecting both their positive and their negative perceptions.

- *Whether the researcher has discussed the credibility of their findings (for example, triangulation, respondent validation, more than one analyst).*
  The authors report features that improve the credibility of their findings, including triangulation of data from family members and patients, using respondent validation and involving more than one analyst in at least a few aspects of data analysis.

- *Whether the findings are discussed in relation to the original research question.*
  The findings were very clearly discussed in relation to the original objective of the research.

10. How valuable is the research?

Consider:

- *Whether the researcher discusses the contribution the study makes to existing knowledge or understanding (for example, do they consider the findings in relation to current practice or policy, or relevant research-based literature?).*
  The authors discuss the implications of this research and how it might inform rehabilitation team members, managers, and those designing rehabilitation units of this type. They also consider their findings in the light of contemporary research findings.

- *Whether they identify new areas where research is necessary.*
  The authors indicate that further research may address the impact of secured wards in brain injury rehabilitation, time use during inpatient rehabilitation settings and the associated issues of boredom and the psychosocial adjustment of individuals during post-acute rehabilitation.
- *Whether they identify new areas where research is necessary. Whether the researchers have discussed whether or how the findings can be transferred to other populations or considered other ways the research may be used.*
  The authors suggest that further research might be necessary to confirm whether these findings are common across brain injury rehabilitation units or specific to the unit in this study. However, the principles of considering environmental design, occupation and family-centred practice are relevant across many different settings.

Additional comments from the QARI instrument

In addition to the CASP criteria, it would also be helpful to consider congruity between the philosophical position adopted in the study, study methodology, representation of the data and interpretation of the results as outlined in QARI. While the study does not explicitly state that an interpretive perspective is taken when trying to understand the experiences and views of people who have received inpatient rehabilitation for acquired brain injuries and their family carers, the authors do state clearly that a phenomenological perspective was taken and this is an appropriate methodology for an interpretive philosophy. The objectives of the study are congruent with this methodology, as are the methods used to collect and analyse the data.

What are the main findings?

People who receive inpatient rehabilitation following brain injury and their family members perceive the rehabilitation environment as restrictive and that patients' motivation was influenced by both positive and negative organisational factors and staff attitudes. Therapy sessions and related activities were valued as contributing towards recovery, but boredom was experienced by participants during unstructured time, contributing to a feeling of frustration. It was clear that family members and friends provided pivotal support to patients that was unable to be provided by staff. Carers identified a need for information about brain injury, the process of rehabilitation and discharge, specific treatment goals and outcomes, and available community services. However, they experienced a number of barriers in terms of communication during the inpatient rehabilitation time, and difficulty accessing staff.

How might we use this evidence to inform practice?

As the authors indicate, this study improves our understanding of rehabilitation from the patient and family member's perspective and can assist rehabilitation teams to better meet the needs of people with acquired brain injury. Specific issues to consider in future developments of the rehabilitation unit in our clinical scenario (and perhaps other rehabilitation units that might be of a similar nature to that described in this study) are how the physical environment might be enhanced to reduce the sense of restriction while maintaining safety standards, considering how to provide more meaningful and structured activities and occupations during inpatient stays and the importance of enacting a family-centred approach in inpatient settings with systematic processes to support clear and consistent communication between all.

PODIATRY EXAMPLE

CLINICAL SCENARIO

You are a member of a recently established multidisciplinary team of health professionals who are involved in the management of patients with diabetic foot complications. During a case conference, you begin a discussion about a patient who has developed a new ulcer on the plantar surface of her foot after a recent digital amputation. While the patient has a pair of therapeutic shoes that can accommodate pressure-deflective devices, she does not wear them. Recognising that many of the patients who are seen by the team do not appear to wear their prescribed footwear or well-fitting, protective non-prescription shoes as advised, the endocrinologist asks whether you have any suggestions about how to tackle this problem. Before coming up with any strategies, you say that first you would like to gain an understanding of people's attitudes to, beliefs about and experiences with prescribed footwear. You think this understanding may help you come up with strategies that might improve patients' concordance with footwear advice. You agree to present your findings at the next case conference.

CLINICAL QUESTION

What are people's experience with prescribed footwear, and what factors determine whether they will follow footwear advice?

Search terms and databases used to find the evidence

Database: PubMed and CINAHL.

Search terms: (footwear OR shoe*) AND (perspective* OR attitude* OR view* OR experience*) in the study title.

This search retrieves 20 articles in PubMed and 17 in CINAHL. Looking through the titles, there are several studies that have examined people's experiences with prescribed footwear or have investigated factors associated with a person's decision to follow footwear advice. You think it will be important that you review them all for your presentation. To begin with, you select the following study which gives the views of patients with diabetes and of health professionals caring for people with diabetes-related foot complications on the use of therapeutic footwear.

Article chosen

Johnson M, Newton P, Goyder E. Patient and professional perspectives on prescribed therapeutic footwear for people with diabetes: a vignette study. Pat Educ Couns 2006;64:167–72.

Structured abstract (adapted from the above)

Study design: Qualitative analysis of semi-structured interviews using the framework approach.

Study question: To explore the experiences and views of people involved in prescribing and wearing footwear designed to reduce diabetes-related complications.

Context: Diabetes foot clinics, North Sheffield, UK.

Participants: 15 health professionals with experience in delivering care to people with diabetes-related foot complications and 15 patients from two diabetes foot clinics who had been prescribed footwear designed to reduce diabetes-related complications.

Data collection method: Participants were interviewed using a vignette depicting the experiences of a fictitious patient with diabetes-related foot complications. Prompts were used after each vignette section to explore participant views.

Analysis: Interviews were taped and analysed using the framework approach.

Key findings: There was incongruence between patients and health professionals in terms of the expectations and reality of preventive behaviour. Health professionals, while advocating preventive measures in order to limit morbidity, are aware of how difficult this can be for patients. For patients, the reality of wearing prescribed footwear conflicted with personal and social norms. Both patients and health professionals expressed concerns about shoe fit when foot shape, size and structure are constantly changing.

Is the evidence rigorous and sufficiently reported?

Detailed questions from CASP

3. Was the research design appropriate to address the aims of the research?

Consider:

- *Whether the researcher has justified the research design.*
  There was no clear statement of the chosen research methodology. This study aimed to explore issues identified by health professionals and patients of diabetic foot care clinics that have impacts on the use of therapeutic footwear. The arrangement of conditions for collecting and analysing data in this study is congruent with the aims of the research.

4. Was the recruitment strategy appropriate to the aims of the research?

Consider:

- *Whether the researcher has explained how the participants were selected.*
  A purposive sampling strategy was used to identify health professionals from a range of disciplines and patients of varying ages from a range of socio-economic circumstances who may or may not have used prescribed footwear. In addition, health professionals identified a purposive sample of patients from the two diabetes foot clinics.

- *Whether they explained why the participants they selected were the most appropriate to provide access to the type of knowledge sought by the study.*
  The researchers explain that these participants provided a broad spectrum of beliefs and attitudes to therapeutic footwear. The recruitment strategy is appropriate to the aims of the research, although whether (and why) any invited participants declined to participate in the study is not discussed.

5. Were the data collected in a way that addressed the research issue?

Consider:

- *Whether the setting for data collection was justified.*
  The setting for data collection was described: health professionals were interviewed in one of two hospital sites or in primary care, and patients were interviewed at their home or at one of the hospital-based diabetes foot clinics; however, the justification for this was not provided. One could assume that these locations were selected for convenience.

- *Whether it is clear how data were collected.*
  In this study, individual interviews were conducted with patients and health professionals using a vignette depicting the experience of a fictitious patient with diabetes-related complications.

- *Whether the researcher has justified the methods chosen.*
  The researchers believe that this approach facilitated the expression of opinions, beliefs and attitudes in a less personal and non-threatening way. The researchers also justified their use of individual interviews as opposed to focus groups.

- *Whether the researcher has made the methods explicit.*
  Individual interviews with health professionals and patients were conducted using a vignette. Prompts were used after each vignette section to explore participant views. Responses were then followed up as necessary to increase the clarity and depth of information.

- *Whether methods were modified during the study. If so, has the researcher explained how and why?*
  There is no mention that the research methods were changed during the study period.
- *Whether the form of data is clear.*
  Yes. It is stated that interviews were tape-recorded.
- *Whether the researcher has discussed saturation of data.*
  This was not reported.

6. Has the relationship between researcher and participants been adequately considered?

Consider:

- *Whether the researcher critically examined their own role, potential bias and influence during:*
  - *Formulation of the research questions.*
    There is no comment about this issue.
  - *Data collection, including sample recruitment and choice of location.*
    The article does not specify who conducted the interviews with study participants, nor the possible professional or personal relationships between the researcher and participants; and how this may have influenced recruitment and data collection is not considered.
- *How the researcher responded to events during the study and whether they considered the implications of any changes in the research design.*
  No changes were reported to have occurred during the study.

7. Have ethical issues been taken into consideration?

Consider:

- *Whether there are sufficient details of how the research was explained to participants for the reader to assess whether ethical standards were maintained.*
  Details were not provided in this article but are provided in an earlier article by these authors.
- *Whether the researcher has discussed issues raised by the study.*
  Not reported.
- *Whether approval has been sought from the ethics committee.*
  Approval from an ethics committee was provided.

8. Was the data analysis sufficiently rigorous?

Consider:

- *Whether there is an in-depth description of the analysis process. Whether thematic analysis is used. If so, is it clear how the categories/themes were derived from the data?*
  A detailed description of the process of analysis was provided and the researchers adequately described how the study findings emerged from the data. The interviews were analysed using the framework approach. In this method, after becoming familiar with the data, investigators classified the data according to key themes and concepts. In this study, two researchers carried out this process with a sample of transcripts before applying the framework to the remaining data.
- *Whether the researcher explains how the data presented were selected from the original sample, to demonstrate the analysis process.*
  The researchers drew on quotes from different participants to validate the identified themes; however, the validity of the interpretations does not appear to have been examined.
- *Whether sufficient data are presented to support the findings.*
  The extent to which contradictory data are taken into account is not clear. Sufficient data were provided to support the findings, but there were no clear examples of contradictory data presented.
- *Whether the researcher critically examined their own role, potential bias and influence during analysis and selection of data for presentation.*

The beliefs and values of researchers are not described and the potential influence of these on data analysis is not known.

9. Is there a clear statement of findings?

Consider:

- *Whether the findings are explicit. Whether there is adequate discussion of the evidence both for and against the researcher's arguments.*
  Yes. The study concluded that patient perspectives need to be taken into account in shoe provision. The researchers' conclusions are clearly drawn from the key themes they identified and inform the people prescribing footwear designed to reduce diabetes-related complications.
- *Whether the researcher has discussed the credibility of their findings.*
  Two researchers developed the thematic framework from which to classify or 'code' the data and applied it to the data. No report of respondent validation or triangulation was noted.
- *Whether the findings are discussed in relation to the original research question.*
  Yes. The findings were very clearly discussed in relation to the original objective of the research.

10. How valuable is the research?

Consider:

- *Whether the researcher discusses the contribution the study makes to existing knowledge or understanding.*
  This study makes a useful contribution to the limited body of research which has explored the experiences and views of health professionals and patients regarding therapeutic footwear. The researchers discussed how these findings relate to existing research and current practice.
- *Whether they identify new areas where research is necessary.*
  The authors recommend that further research, as part of research with larger samples, explore the issues involved for patients with diabetes who receive self-care advice.
- *Whether the researchers have discussed whether or how the findings can be transferred to other populations or considered other ways the research may be used.*
  The researchers do mention transferability of the findings, suggesting that the small sample in this study prevents generalisation to a larger population of people with foot complications. However, they stated that the issues raised are transferable to similar settings.

You reflect on your appraisal of this study and, while the design and methods of data collection were generally appropriate, there was inadequate detail within this report to make clear judgments on the relationship of the researchers to participants and how this may have influenced recruitment, data collection and analysis.

Additional comments from the QARI instrument

While the study does not clearly state the philosophical or theoretical premises on which it is based, it appears to take an interpretive perspective in trying to understand the experiences and views of people involved in prescribing and wearing footwear that is designed to reduce diabetes-related complications. It would be suited to phenomenological methodology, although this was not stated as such. The objectives of the study are congruent with this methodology, as are the methods used to collect and analyse the data.

What are the main findings?

The researchers present two themes which summarise issues relating to prescribed footwear that are important to patients and health professionals. The first theme relates to prescribed versus routine behaviour. There is incongruence between health professional recommendations regarding footwear and patients' behaviour, with patients finding it difficult to carry out advice that does not fit in with usual behaviour or with that of others. The second theme explores issues related to the fitting of footwear when foot shape, size and structure may be constantly changing. This was problematic for prescribers and patients. The researchers concluded that the insensitiveness of prescribed shoes to the varying contexts in which they are to be used, or the varying shapes of the patient's foot, may be the reason for low levels of use of prescribed footwear.

How might we use this evidence to inform practice?

The researchers discuss how the results of this study might be used in practice and suggest that negotiating the extent of use of prescribed footwear, providing varied styles of therapeutic footwear for different contexts, and more-detailed evaluation of shoe fit may improve the acceptance of prescribed footwear. Furthermore, involving patients in footwear design and obtaining views about the acceptability of the recommendations may help in developing more-realistic aims that are relevant to the patient.

There is limited information provided by which you can compare your setting with the study setting. However, the demographic details of the study sample seem similar to those of your patients in terms of their age, duration of diabetes and the type of intervention being received. There is no further detail on the types of footwear that participants in this study had been prescribed.

You reflect on discussions that you have had with patients about their footwear. Some of the experiences described in the study seem consistent with what your patients have talked about. Many patients with prescribed therapeutic shoes (shoes that have features such as extra depth, broad sole, deep toe box) comment negatively on the appearance and many complain that the shoes are not suitable for the hot climate in which they live. They also report difficulty being able to put the shoes on. Before moving on to the next study, you draw up a table which you will use to summarise the methods and results of the studies that you have found. You plan to present this at the next case conference, using it to stimulate discussion on possible strategies to improve concordance with footwear advice.

SPEECH PATHOLOGY EXAMPLE

CLINICAL SCENARIO

Mr Fallon, a 34-year-old man with a moderate to severe stutter, has previously attended your clinic and has returned today for advice. He has previously received individual speech therapy for 6 months, but was disappointed when this did not 'cure' his fluency difficulties. He would like to discuss some other options for therapy, particularly a 'prolonged speech'/'smooth speech' group program which he has heard about. From this program, he wants to see a difference for himself, is concerned at being able to maintain and transfer the techniques in everyday life after the program, and wants to 'sound normal'. You wonder what the evidence is for patient-perceived benefit from prolonged-speech approaches to therapy for dysfluency.

CLINICAL QUESTION

How do adults with moderate to severe chronic dysfluency experience the outcomes of prolonged-speech approaches?

Search terms and databases used to find the evidence

Database: PubMed (although CINAHL or Embase would also be appropriate to search).

Search terms: 'stutter*' AND (prolonged speech) AND 'experience*'

This returns three articles, one of which was relevant to the question. This article was chosen because a scan of the title and abstract revealed that it was potentially the most appropriate to the question, as it investigated the experiences of adults who had undergone prolonged speech therapy.

Article chosen

Cream A, Onslow M, Packman A, et al. Protection from harm: the experience of adults after therapy with prolonged-speech. Int J Lang Communi Disord 2003;38:379–95.

Structured abstract (adapted from the above)

Study design: Qualitative investigation using phenomenology as the method of inquiry.

Study question: What are the experiences of adults who use prolonged speech to control stuttering?

Context: Sydney, Australia. Therapy based on prolonged speech had been available through the speech pathology departments of public hospitals in Sydney for some time.

Participants: 10 adults (aged 24–54 years; 9 male) who had received prolonged-speech treatment. Participants were purposively sampled, on the basis of representing different viewpoints or experience. However, all had objectively experienced success with the prolonged-speech treatment, as a criterion for inclusion was that 'they had experienced zero stuttering at the end of treatment'.

Data collection method: Face-to-face interviews and informal discussions (face-to-face or over the telephone) were held with participants over a 2-year period. At the end of the study, participants attended group interviews for further discussion. Interviews were 'conversational' in nature, with an open-ended rather than a structured format. A total of 34 interviews/discussions were included in the data.

Analysis: Content analysis was used to determine emerging themes. Transcripts were analysed using, consecutively, a line-by-line approach (to identify all emergent themes), a holistic approach (to understand the overall meaning of the interviews/discussions) and a selective approach (aiming to discover the primary themes). Additional data were sought and analysed to gain further understanding of experiences of people who have undertaken prolonged speech treatment. Analysis occurred concurrently to data collection and emerging themes were discussed with participants.

Key findings and conclusion: Even after prolonged-speech treatment, there is an ongoing risk of stuttering occurring. Although patients may have experience of being able to control stuttering, they also continue to feel different from people who do not stutter and these feelings may be exacerbated after treatment. The maximum benefits of prolonged speech are achieved when patients use a strategic approach to control stuttering and everyday communication.

Is the evidence rigorous and sufficiently reported?

Detailed questions from CASP

3. Was the research design appropriate to address the aims of the research?

Consider:

- *Whether the researcher has justified the research design.*
  The authors have used phenomenology as the methodology for the research. The methods used for this study were clearly justified by the authors and addressed the study aims. The authors collected data over a period of 2 years, which supports their understanding of how patients' experiences with prolonged speech change over time.

4. Was the recruitment strategy appropriate to the aims of the research?

Consider:

- *Whether the researcher has explained how the participants were selected.*
  The article has clear detail about the purposive sampling methods in which each participant was recruited because of their potential representation of different viewpoints.

- *Whether they explained why the participants they selected were the most appropriate to provide access to the type of knowledge sought by the study.*
  The article contains a list of reasons for selecting participants (for example, having had therapy experience outside of the research centre, or having had experience of a non-intensive model of therapy). Recruitment decisions were based on the need to explore themes more fully.

5. Were the data collected in a way that addressed the research issue?

Consider:

- *Whether the setting for data collection was justified.*
  Participants were recruited in the context of ongoing treatment and participation in support groups in Sydney, but justification of the setting is not provided.
- *Whether it is clear how data were collected.*
  The study used formal and informal individual interviews, as well as group interviews, and the authors describe and justify the interview format (a 'conversational' approach). Authors explain the strategies used within the interviews (for example, encouraging patients to reflect on their own experiences rather than generalising by suggesting what 'people who stutter' might feel).
- *Whether the researcher has justified the methods chosen.*
  The authors explained the importance of helping participants focus on specific experiences for phenomenological research so that their own experiences are captured.
- *Whether the researcher has made the methods explicit.*
  A conversational approach was used, in which the interviewer followed the participant's lead. Hermeneutic interviewing was used, in which analysis occurred concurrently with interviews and emerging themes were discussed with participants.
- *Whether methods were modified during the study. If so, has the researcher explained how and why?*
  There is no mention that the research methods were changed during the study period.
- *Whether the form of data is clear.*
  It is clearly stated that interviews were tape-recorded.
- *Whether the researcher has discussed saturation of data.*
  This is not reported in this study.

6. Has the relationship between researcher and participants been adequately considered?

Consider:

- *Whether the researcher critically examined their own role, potential bias and influence during:*
  - *Formulation of the research questions.*
    This is not clearly reported.
  - *Data collection, including sample recruitment and choice of location.*
    The article states that the 'interviewer (the first author) attempted to bracket assumptions about therapy that were based on clinical experience as a speech pathologist, professional reading and contact with persons who stutter'.
- *How the researcher responded to events during the study and whether they considered the implications of any changes in the research design.*
  No changes were reported.

7. Have ethical issues been taken into consideration?

Consider:

- *Whether there are sufficient details of how the research was explained to participants for the reader to assess whether ethical standards were maintained.*
  There was only one comment in the article referring to maintaining ethical standards, indicating the voluntary nature of the interviews and ability to withdraw data: 'Participants were able to turn off the tape recorder at any time or request some parts to be omitted.'

- *Whether the researcher has discussed issues raised by the study.*
  This was not reported.
- *Whether approval has been sought from the ethics committee.*
  Approval from an ethics committee was not reported. However, it is unlikely that this did not occur given that this paper was published in 2003. It is more likely to be a reporting omission.

8. Was the data analysis sufficiently rigorous?

Consider:

- *Whether there is an in-depth description of the analysis process. Whether thematic analysis is used. If so, is it clear how the categories/themes were derived from the data?*
  There is a clear description of data analysis. To identify themes, three approaches were used: transcripts were analysed line-by-line and by 'holistic' and 'selective' approaches.
- *Whether the researcher explains how the data presented were selected from the original sample, to demonstrate the analysis process.*
  This is not clearly explained.
- *Whether sufficient data are presented to support the findings.*
  Sufficient data are provided to illustrate the themes. There were no contradictory data as such, but it was clear that participants had positive and negative perspectives on the use of prolonged speech that were described in the findings.
- *Whether the researcher critically examined their own role, potential bias and influence during analysis and selection of data for presentation.*
  This was not done explicitly for this aspect of the study; however, evidence of reflexivity in earlier phases of this study (through bracketing) may potentially have carried over to the analysis phase.

9. Is there a clear statement of findings?

Consider:

- *Whether the findings are explicit. Whether there is adequate discussion of the evidence both for and against the researcher's arguments.*
  A balanced discussion of the findings for and against therapy with prolonged speech is evident.
- *Whether the researcher has discussed the credibility of their findings*
  The study incorporated member checking/discussion of interpretations with participants, prolonged engagement with the participants and triangulation of data with other data sources (such as websites). For example, the authors stated that they tested their developing insights against 'descriptions of the period after PS contained in the newsletters of the Speak Easy Association and the Internet Stuttering Home Page'.
- *Whether the findings are discussed in relation to the original research question.*
  The findings were very clearly discussed in relation to the original objective of the research.

10. How valuable is the research?

Consider:

- *Whether the researcher discusses the contribution the study makes to existing knowledge or understanding.*
  The study discusses the findings in relation to informing prospective patients of the experiential consequences of prolonged speech, selecting patients who might benefit and in terms of assisting patients to achieve optimal benefits from it. They also consider these findings in relation to existing research.
- *Whether they identify new areas where research is necessary.*
  The authors also consider implications of the research in relation to the structure of prolonged-speech treatments overall, as well as in relation to future prolonged-speech outcome research.

- *Whether the researchers have discussed whether or how the findings can be transferred to other populations or considered other ways the research may be used.*
  The researchers raise the need to study this same issue in other age groups to see whether similar perspectives are evident. No further discussion of transferability is provided, but researchers do suggest that this research might inform existing and future developments in prolonged-speech approaches overall.

Additional comments from the QARI instrument

The authors have used a constructivist paradigm for their research, a theoretical standpoint where reality and truth are understood to be 'constructed' differently by every individual, rather than something 'objective' that can be described or understood (and generalised). The authors have used phenomenology as the methodology for the research. Phenomenology is appropriate to discovering what makes up others' experiences, and attempting to get to the 'essence' of these experiences. The research aims, methodology, data collection and analysis are all congruent with the philosophical approach selected and chosen methodology.

What are the main findings?

The themes that emerged describe interwoven experiences of adults after prolonged-speech therapy. As prolonged-speech therapy does not 'cure' stuttering, participants reported that their feelings about their stuttering, and the need to 'protect themselves' from the negative consequences that they associate with stuttering, does not diminish even after success with prolonged-speech therapy. Being fluent speakers 'has a price' for participants, as prolonged speech feels unnatural to produce and may also sound unnatural. Thus, participants were bound to be 'different' whether they used prolonged speech or stuttered. Prolonged speech became a 'tool' that participants could apply, along with their own existing resources, to protect themselves from harm.

The authors concluded that successful use of prolonged speech from a patient's perspective is the strategic application of the technique in order to reduce harm from stuttering. In some situations, patients may choose the risk of sounding different by stuttering rather than the risk of sounding different through prolonged speech. The findings suggest that practising the technique (either in therapy or in booster/maintenance programs) is not likely to increase use of the technique in the long term. Clinical programs to teach prolonged speech should focus not just on the behavioural changes, but also on the integration of the technique alongside existing resources that the patient has for reducing harm. Clinicians should consider whether patients have the resources to benefit from prolonged speech. For example, patients who are already considerably anxious about being different may not be suitable for this type of treatment.

How might we use this evidence to inform practice?

In the case of Mr Fallon, caution should be used in recommending a prolonged-speech therapy course to him, given his existing anxiety about 'sounding normal' and his emphasis on maintaining any therapy technique that he tries. Mr Fallon should be counselled about the realistic benefits that he might perceive from using prolonged speech. For example, although he might be able to use the technique well, he may find it unnatural and will have to weigh up the benefits of applying the technique versus stuttering. It should be emphasised that prolonged speech is not a 'cure' for stuttering. If Mr Fallon does choose to begin prolonged-speech therapy, he should be directed towards groups/clinicians who emphasise integration of prolonged speech in everyday life, rather than simply 'teaching' patients how to be good users of the technique.

MEDICINE EXAMPLE

CLINICAL SCENARIO

As a new general practitioner working in a practice with a largely elderly demographic, you have seen a number of older people with chronic back pain whose pain has not been adequately controlled. One lady in her 80s concerns you in particular. She has a 3-year history of non-malignant lower back pain and evidence of spinal stenosis, has received physiotherapy and has been on extended-release paracetamol and paracetamol/codeine tablets for this period of time with little benefit. You want to reduce her pain, as she reports great difficulty carrying out even basic daily activities, has to receive a lot of assistance from her family and her pain is interfering with her sleep. This is confirmed by her daughter who attends the appointment with her. Knowing that anti-inflammatories have disagreed with her in the past, you wonder about the potential for opioid use with this lady but also decide to consider the prescribing experiences of other doctors in this patient group.

CLINICAL QUESTION

What are the experiences of prescribing opioids for elderly people with non-malignant chronic pain?

Search terms and databases used to find the evidence

Database: PubMed–Health Services Research Queries (with 'qualitative research' category and 'narrow scope' selected), which is accessed through the 'Topic-specific queries' link on PubMed.

Search terms: opioid* AND (elderly or "older adult") AND ("primary care" OR "general practice")

This search returned seven articles. One looked directly relevant to the question, so you obtain the full text to look at in detail.

Article chosen

Spitz A, Moore A, Papaleontiou M, et al. Primary care providers' perspective on prescribing opioids to older adults with chronic non-cancer pain: a qualitative study. BMC Geriatr 2011;11:35.

Structured abstract (adapted from the above)

Study design: The authors described this as a 'qualitative cross-sectional study'.

Study question: To describe primary care providers' experiences and attitudes towards prescribing opioids for older adults with chronic pain, and to identify perceived barriers and facilitators to their prescription.

Context: Doctors and nurse practitioners were recruited from two academically affiliated primary care practices with patient populations that are older (mean age in the mid-80s) and predominantly female. They were selected because providers had substantial experience caring for older adults. Additionally, providers were recruited from three community health centres that serve predominantly Latino patients. All settings were located in New York City.

Data collection method: Six focus groups were conducted with a total of 23 doctors and three nurse practitioners.

Analysis: Focus groups were audiotape-recorded and transcribed. The data were analysed using directed content analysis. These were generated from the data and in reference to related literature.

Key findings: Most participants (96%) employed opioids as therapy for some of their older patients with chronic pain, although not as first-line therapy. Providers identified the main barriers to prescribing opioids were fear of causing harm, the subjectivity of pain, stigma, patient/family member reluctance to try opioids and lack of knowledge.

Conclusion: Providers use opioids cautiously and perceive multiple barriers to prescribing them for older adults with chronic pain. There is a need to establish the long-term safety and efficacy of these medications, develop and implement provider and patient education about their prescription and understand more about communicating with patients about opioids in order to improve the management of chronic pain for older adults.

Is the evidence rigorous and sufficiently reported?

Detailed questions from CASP

3. Was the research design appropriate to address the aims of the research?

Consider:

- *Whether the researcher has justified the research design.*
  The authors simply state that this study was a 'qualitative, cross-sectional study that employed focus groups to generate discussions'. The specific research methodology used was not evident. Their sampling choices supported the research aims of the study. There was no explanation provided about their choice of using focus groups.

4. Was the recruitment strategy appropriate to the aims of the research?

Consider:

- *Whether the researcher has explained how the participants were selected.*
  All doctors and nurse practitioners at the identified centres were invited to participate and were simply recruited based upon their interest and availability (that is, convenience sampling) to attend one of the focus group sessions.

- *Whether they explained why the participants they selected were the most appropriate to provide access to the type of knowledge sought by the study.*
  The only information offered regarding this was that providers at two of the settings had substantial experience caring for older adults.

5. Were the data collected in a way that addressed the research issue?

Consider:

- *Whether the setting for data collection was justified.*
  The settings were justified. The study states that 'Focus groups were conducted at the Columbia Presbyterian Allen Pavilion Division of Geriatrics and the New York-Presbyterian (NYP) Wright Center on Aging. In addition one focus group was also conducted with 'providers from three community health centers within the NYP Ambulatory Care Network that serve predominantly Latino patients'. The first two settings were selected because 'they include providers with substantial experience caring for older adults'. The ambulatory-care settings were selected to increase the diversity of study sites.

- *Whether it is clear how data were collected.*
  Six focus groups were conducted with a total of 23 doctors and three nurse practitioners.

- *Whether the researcher has justified the methods chosen.*
  No justification was provided for the use of focus groups.

- *Whether the researcher has made the methods explicit.*
  One researcher moderated the semi-structured focus group discussion, using open-ended questions and probes developed following a review of the literature and pilot testing. The specific questions that were asked during the focus groups are provided.

- *Whether methods were modified during the study. If so, has the researcher explained how and why?*
  There is no mention that the research methods were changed during the study period.
- *Whether the form of data is clear.*
  It is stated that interviews were tape-recorded.
- *Whether the researcher has discussed saturation of data.*
  The authors indicate that focus groups were conducted until researchers agreed that no new themes were emerging.

6. Has the relationship between researcher and participants been adequately considered?

Consider:

- *Whether the researcher critically examined their own role, potential bias and influence during:*
  - *Formulation of the research questions.*
    There is no comment about this issue.
  - *Data collection, including sample recruitment and choice of location.*
    There is no comment about this issue.
- *How the researcher responded to events during the study and whether they considered the implications of any changes in the research design.*
  No changes were reported to have occurred.

7. Have ethical issues been taken into consideration?

Consider:

- *Whether there are sufficient details of how the research was explained to participants for the reader to assess whether ethical standards were maintained.*
  No details are provided other than the study was passed by an ethics review board.
- *Whether the researcher has discussed issues raised by the study.*
  The authors acknowledge that the focus groups may not have accurately captured the full extent of participants' views on this topic, as participants were colleagues. One can speculate here that the concern may be about revealing true attitudes, beliefs or practices about prescribing opioids. Concerns about legal/regulatory sanctions were not frequently raised in this study, but it is unknown whether this is due to lower likelihood of local administrative sanctions in this setting or to confidentiality concerns between participants.
- *Whether approval has been sought from the ethics committee.*
  Approval from an ethics committee was provided.

8. Was the data analysis sufficiently rigorous?

Consider:

- *Whether there is an in-depth description of the analysis process. Whether thematic analysis is used. If so, is it clear how the categories/themes were derived from the data?*
  Data were analysed via directed content analysis. Transcripts were read and preliminary themes generated. Interestingly, this process took into consideration themes (such as barriers to opioid prescribing) that have been identified in previous studies. It is possible, therefore, that some themes presented were not uniquely derived from the data.
- *Whether the researcher explains how the data presented were selected from the original sample, to demonstrate the analysis process.*
  This was done in a very basic, limited manner with one specific example provided in the paper.
- *Whether sufficient data are presented to support the findings. To what extent contradictory data are taken into account.*
  Perspectives on both barriers and facilitators to opioid prescription were ascertained during focus groups, and there was some indication of differing perspectives arising among focus group participants on a few issues (for example, misuse of opioids).

- *Whether the researcher critically examined their own role, potential bias and influence during analysis and selection of data for presentation.*
  This was not reported in the article.

9. Is there a clear statement of findings?

Consider:

- *Whether the findings are explicit. Whether there is adequate discussion of the evidence both for and against the researchers' arguments.*
  This was a descriptive study seeking to describe perceived barriers and facilitators to prescribing opioids and, as such, the author did not have any stated position. Findings were clearly presented.

- *Whether the researcher has discussed the credibility of their findings.*
  Triangulation of themes evident in related research was used and data were analysed independently by more than one researcher. There was no description of respondent validation.

- *Whether the findings are discussed in relation to the original research question.*
  Yes. The findings were very clearly discussed in relation to the original objective of the research.

10. How valuable is the research?

Consider:

- *Whether the researcher discusses the contribution the study makes to existing knowledge or understanding:*
  Yes. The authors discuss the clinical implications of the findings in relation to provider training, communication with patients and development of risk assessment tools and guidelines.

- *Whether they identify new areas where research is necessary:*
  This study identified the need for research about the long-term safety and efficacy of opioids in different subgroups of older patients and how they respond to varying opioid medication regimens.

- *Whether the researchers have discussed whether or how the findings can be transferred to other populations or considered other ways the research may be used.*
  The authors emphasise that most providers cared for predominantly older adults of white or Hispanic origin, and indicate that the findings may not be transferable to other race/ethnicity groups or non-elderly populations.

Additional comments from the QARI instrument

In this study there is no statement regarding the philosophical position taken or the specific research methodology selected, so it is not possible to determine congruence between the underlying philosophical perspective and research methodology of the study. This study aimed to describe primary care providers' experiences and attitudes towards prescribing opioids for older adults with chronic pain, and thus most likely would be considered within the 'interpretive' paradigm and would be suited to phenomenological methods, although this was not stated as such.

What are the main findings?

Opioids were prescribed by most participants for some of their older patients with chronic pain, but not as first-line therapy. This study found that primary care providers use opioids cautiously with the elderly due to a number of different barriers. These included the older patient and/or their family member being reluctant to take an opioid; fear of causing harm; the subjective nature of pain and the associated difficulty of accurately determining pain severity; stigma; and the possibility of opioid abuse by carers (such as family members and home attendants). Facilitators were provider education, specialist support, evidence-based guidelines, and studies demonstrating long-term benefit.

How might we use this evidence to inform practice?

This study broadened your understanding of the barriers (and facilitators) to prescribing opioids in the older adult population. In relation to your specific patient, you weigh up the risks associated with opioids (such as increased risk of fracture, hospitalisations and all-cause mortality) against the fact that your patient has an identifiable cause of the pain, has very restricted participation in everyday activities and is distressed by the pain. You decide to discuss the option of a careful trial of opioids with your patient and her daughter who brings her to see you, to ascertain their perspectives about trialling opioids.

NURSING EXAMPLE

CLINICAL SCENARIO

As an experienced nurse who works in a wound clinic with an emphasis on treating chronic vascular ulcers, you have noticed that treatment seems to concentrate on the application of therapies such as compression bandaging. Yet you are aware that some of the patients who are treated in the clinic have had their leg ulcer for a long time, have experienced significant pain, lifestyle alteration and discomfort and are reluctant participants in their therapy. The reasons for low concordance with wearing compression bandages, exercising and elevating their leg are unclear. You suspect that improved concordance could be achieved if the treating team had greater insight into the experiences of patients, particularly patients with ulcers of vascular origins, as many of their wounds on initial presentation are very large and poorly self-managed.

CLINICAL QUESTION

What is the lived experience of a person with chronic venous leg ulcers trying to adhere to advice during the transition to healing?

Search terms and databases used to find the evidence

Database: PubMed–Health Services Research Queries (with 'qualitative research' category and 'narrow scope' selected), which is accessed through the 'Topic-specific queries' link on PubMed.

Search terms: (leg ulcer*) AND adher*

This search returned 26 hits. You choose the one which appears to most closely match your question and scenario as it explores the issues of adherence to recommendations.

Article chosen

Van Hecke A, Grypdonck M, Beele H, et al. Adherence to leg ulcer lifestyle advice: qualitative and quantitative outcomes associated with a nurse-led intervention. J Clin Nurs 2011;20:429–43.

Structured abstract*

Study design: A qualitative evaluation approach and pre-/post-test design were used.

Participants: 26 patients with venous ulcers in a community care setting.

Data collection method: Interviews and participant observation. Frequency and duration of wearing compression, leg exercising and leg elevation, activity level, pain and ulcer size were registered at baseline, after the end of the intervention and 3 months later.

*Reproduced and adapted from Van Hecke A et al. 2011.

Analysis: Inductive content analysis (for the qualitative data).

Key findings: Knowledge about leg ulcer advice increased. The education contributed to patients more consciously following the advice. The rationale of the advice and its association with healing or recurrence often remained unclear. More patients performed exercises after the intervention and at follow-up. Patients often looked out onto a 'new' perspective where enhancement of quality of life and even healing might be attainable. Some patients regained independence after learning how to apply and remove compression garments themselves. No significant changes were reported on hours wearing compression.

Conclusions: The perceived changes suggest that the intervention holds promise for current home care. Combining qualitative and quantitative research assisted in determining the possible effects of the intervention, increasing the potential for a meaningful randomised trial in the future.

Is the evidence rigorous and sufficiently reported?

Detailed questions from CASP

3. Was the research design appropriate to address the aims of the research?

Consider:

- *Whether the researcher has justified the research design.*
  In this study, the authors describe using a qualitative evaluation approach (combined with a pre- and post-test design; however, we are focused on the qualitative evaluation for this scenario). The authors gave a limited description of collecting qualitative data using a semi-structured interview process.

4. Was the recruitment strategy appropriate to the aims of the research?

Consider:

- *Whether the researcher has explained how the participants were selected.*
  The study described inclusion criteria. They chose patients with known non-adherence with limited comorbidities. Purposive selection is a typical approach for qualitative research, as it ensures that the participants are able to participate more fully in responding to the research questions.

- *Whether they explained why the participants they selected were the most appropriate to provide access to the type of knowledge sought by the study.*
  Purposive sampling was used to recruit people for the intervention (and thus also for the qualitative component of the study), to include patients with different characteristics (age, gender, education level, duration of leg ulcer, recurrence rate, pain) and in a different context (amount of social support, living alone versus cohabiting), although the authors did not explicitly explain why.

5. Were the data collected in a way that addressed the research issue?

Consider:

- *Whether the setting for data collection was justified.*
  Interviews took place in the participant's home environment (in which they may have felt more comfortable).

- *Whether it is clear how data were collected.*
  25 semi-structured interviews (with some open-ended questions) were conducted.

- *Whether the researcher has justified the methods chosen.*
  This is not clearly reported, although the questions started with an open-ended question in order to 'encourage patients to tell their experiences and perceptions'.

- *Whether the researcher has made the methods explicit.*
  A topic guide was used with open-ended questions. The questions were derived from themes established in previous studies. To encourage patients to relate their experiences and perceptions,

the interview started with a general and open-ended question ('*What was it like for you to receive the intervention?*'). Questions regarding the depth of the open-ended questions are unresolved, as there was a lack of description other than this one question.

- *Whether methods were modified during the study. If so, has the researcher explained how and why?*
  There is no mention that the research methods were changed during the study period.
- *Whether the form of data is clear.*
  Yes. It is clearly stated that interviews were tape-recorded. Interview durations ranged between 18 and 81 minutes and were audiotaped, then transcribed verbatim.
- *Whether the researcher has discussed saturation of data.*
  There was no mention of data saturation in this study, and it must be highlighted that while 18 minutes is very short for a qualitative interview, 81 minutes is almost too long, and participants may have been too fatigued to give full and detailed answers by the late stage of the interview.

6. Has the relationship between researcher and participants been adequately considered?

Consider:

- *Whether the researcher critically examined their own role, potential bias and influence during:*
  - *Formulation of the research questions.*
    No information is provided.
  - *Data collection, including sample recruitment and choice of location.*
    The authors indicate that the researcher was in contact with the patients for a considerable period of time and that this could have increased the positive nature of the qualitative findings, as patients could feel an obligation to help the researcher. However, no other features of the relationship are considered and so we are unable to draw many conclusions as to the extent, nature and context of the influence.
- *How the researcher responded to events during the study and whether they considered the implications of any changes in the research design.*
  No changes were reported.

7. Have ethical issues been taken into consideration?

Consider:

- *Whether there are sufficient details of how the research was explained to participants for the reader to assess whether ethical standards were maintained.*
  While this study was scant on detail regarding the issues behind informed consent and data protection, there was clear reference to approval by an ethics committee.
- *Whether the researcher has discussed issues raised by the study.*
  This was not reported.
- *Whether approval has been sought from the ethics committee.*
  Yes. It is reported that approval from an ethics committee was provided.

8. Was the data analysis sufficiently rigorous?

Consider:

- *Whether there is an in-depth description of the analysis process. Whether thematic analysis is used. If so, is it clear how the categories/themes were derived from the data?*
  The qualitative component of this article included a clear and detailed description of how data analysis was managed (using specified software). The authors reported using a three-step approach to thematic analysis of coding, categorisation and higher-order theme generation. Researcher triangulation was described as the method for establishing trustworthiness of the resultant themes. Emerging themes were confirmed against the transcripts to ensure that the emerging findings were congruent with the participants' voices.

- *Whether the researcher explains how the data presented were selected from the original sample, to demonstrate the analysis process.*
  Quotes from participants were used to inform and illustrate the themes. The level of description about this process was substantive, and gives a clear indication of a detailed and robust process for the methods by which data analysis was undertaken.
- *Whether sufficient data are presented to support the findings. To what extent contradictory data are taken into account.*
  While there are sufficient data to support the findings, only very limited accounts of contradictory findings are presented.
- *Whether the researcher critically examined their own role, potential bias and influence during analysis and selection of data for presentation.*
  This is not reported.

9. Is there a clear statement of findings?

Consider:

- *Whether the findings are explicit. Whether there is adequate discussion of the evidence both for and against the researcher's arguments.*
  Discussion of findings from the qualitative component of the study is extremely limited and insufficient. The authors did note, however, that findings from the qualitative component of the study helped to explain why the intervention in the quantitative component of the study did not seem to have an effect for some participants.
- *Whether the researcher has discussed the credibility of their findings*
  The authors reported using researcher triangulation. To verify the findings against the data, two researchers who were not involved in the analysis read a random selection of transcripts. No respondent validation was reported.
- *Whether the findings are discussed in relation to the original research question.*
  The findings were only briefly discussed in relation to the original objective of the research.

10. How valuable is the research?

Consider:

- *Whether the researcher discusses the contribution the study makes to existing knowledge or understanding.*
  The authors highlighted that the purpose of the study was to use a qualitative, evaluative approach to enhance adherence to leg ulcer treatment. They report a lack of research from the qualitative perspective on home-based interventions. The qualitative data were reported separately to the quantitative data, which segregated the results rather than bringing them together. The findings of the qualitative arm of the study did provide better understanding of the cognitive, behavioural, emotional and physical changes associated with improved adherence.
- *Whether they identify new areas where research is necessary.*
  The authors recommend use of complementary methodologies to evaluate complex nursing interventions and to evaluate how complex nursing interventions influence patients.
- *Whether the researchers have discussed whether or how the findings can be transferred to other populations or considered other ways the research may be used.*
  The main recommendations from the discussion of the qualitative component is for future research to use both qualitative and quantitative methods.

Comments from the QARI instrument

The authors describe using a qualitative evaluation approach, but unfortunately they did not go on to describe a particular qualitative methodology (such as phenomenology or grounded theory) or identify a philosophical perspective. Instead, they gave a limited description of the collection of qualitative data using a semi-structured interview process. This makes it difficult to consider congruence between research methodology and other aspects of the research such as representation of data or interpretation of results. This problem is compounded by the limited interpretation of results provided.

What are the main findings?

The primary findings of the qualitative component of this study were based around four domains: cognitive changes, behavioural changes, emotional changes, and physical changes. Cognitively, participants variously described the importance of knowing both what to do and why to do it. Behavioural changes were found in the creative strategies implemented by participants to form good habits that would assist them to adopt lifestyle advice into their routine behaviours. Emotional changes were reported as relating to feelings of hope, a sense of independence gained and a return to a quality of life previously thought lost. The authors posit that understanding which outcomes and what aspects of care patients valued would enable nursing staff to match their care interventions to particular patient values.

How might we use this evidence to inform practice?

Qualitative evidence can be used to inform evidence from a range of perspectives. By itself, qualitative evidence informs experiential domains that are not amendable to experimental research, it opens a window into the perspectives, values and meanings that people identify with and may also have an impact on how they participate in their care. Qualitative evidence can also facilitate a deeper understanding of healthcare interventions and the circumstances in which they work or do not work for particular people; or, as this study found, qualitative research may also illuminate a more complete picture of clinical care.

Specifically, this study found that concordance with therapy was not static and that patients varied in how closely they adhered to recommendations and lifestyle changes. This indicates that typifying patients based on whether they are perceived to be 'compliant' or 'non-compliant' is not useful and may disadvantage patients when the labels are applied. In addition to avoiding labelling patients based on brief contacts, this study indicates that patients can be assisted to better know why there are preferred approaches to how a therapy such as compression should be worn. We know that patients with a chronic venous leg ulcer are used to self-managing at home, and therefore education which explains *why* a particular intervention will help was found to be as important as indicating which interventions were effective. From this, we can conclude that patients, as autonomous individuals, are better motivated to participate in their care and demonstrate concordance if knowledge transfer is based on their felt needs and values.

COMPLEMENTARY AND ALTERNATIVE MEDICINE EXAMPLE

CLINICAL SCENARIO

You are a general practitioner. Occasionally patients ask you whether acupuncture might be useful for their unresolved health issues. You are aware that acupuncturists who practise in Australia may be medical doctors or therapists trained in traditional Chinese medicine. There has been an increase in the number of practitioners of Western-style acupuncture, but you are unaware of patient experiences of this. You wonder if there is any research into patients' perceptions of receiving Western-style acupuncture for medical problems.

CLINICAL QUESTION

What are the perceptions and experiences of patients who have received treatment with Western-style acupuncture?

Search terms and databases used to find the evidence

Database: PubMed–Health Services Research Queries (with 'qualitative research' category and 'narrow scope' selected), which is accessed through the 'Topic-specific queries' link on PubMed.

Search terms: acupuncture AND experience AND western

The search with narrow scope selected returns only one article, and it is not relevant. You repeat the search with 'broad scope' selected. This gives 30 articles; you exclude quite a few as they involve acupuncture that was done in the context of a research study to evaluate acupuncture effectiveness or were conducted in Thailand, China or Vietnam. Of the remaining articles, you choose the one that most closely matches your question.

Article chosen

Paterson C. Patients' experiences of Western-style acupuncture: the influence of acupuncture 'dose', self-care strategies and integration. J Health Serv Res Pol 2007;Suppl 1:S1-39–45.

Structured abstract (adapted from the above)

Study design: Qualitative research design with participants being interviewed twice over a 4-month period.

Study question: To investigate patients' perspectives of the process and outcome of Western-style acupuncture for chronic health problems.

Context: This study was undertaken with people who lived in urban and rural areas of the UK. Participants received treatment in a range of different settings: pain clinics, outpatient clinics and community-based practices.

Participants: A purposive sample of 19 patients who were having Western-style acupuncture for the first time for a health problem of at least 3 months' duration.

Data analysis: Analysis involved a constant comparative method. Data were analysed across cases and within cases over time.

Key findings: Participants complained of chronic pain and moderate or severe disability which was resistant to conventional treatment. Their experience of acupuncture was diverse and varied according to the 'dosage' of acupuncture received, the inclusion of self-care strategies and their relationship with the practitioner. These three factors were interlinked and constituted individual styles of practice for each practitioner. The majority of patients benefited in terms of complete or partial relief of pain and disability, and reduction in conventional medication. However, some patients were disappointed by the treatment, and distressed about 'wasting people's time' and about the lack of continuity of care. Patients showed discerning judgment regarding the 'dosage' of acupuncture they required, and combined acupuncture with exercises to good effect.

Conclusions: Publicly funded health services should provide an acupuncture service that provides the optimal 'dosage' and uses pain relief to promote self-care.

Is the evidence rigorous and sufficiently reported?

Detailed questions from CASP

3. Was the research design appropriate to address the aims of the research?

Consider:

- *Whether the researcher has justified the research design.*
  The research aimed to investigate the experiences of people with long-standing health problems who receive Western-style acupuncture. The specific research methodology was not clear. The research methods involved recruitment of acupuncture practitioners who provided Western-style acupuncture and, through them, invitations to their new participants to take part in data-gathering interviews. For this aim, this design was appropriate.

4. Was the recruitment strategy appropriate to the aims of the research?

Consider:

- *Whether the researcher has explained how the participants were selected.*
  The author aimed to use maximum variation sampling. There were two stages of recruitment in this study, as described previously. The method of practitioner recruitment was not described. Six practitioners from a range of backgrounds (general practitioner, hospital and 'other' doctors, physiotherapists) and practice settings (hospital/outpatients/general practice, public/private, general/specialist services, city/town/rural) were recruited. These six practitioners were then asked to invite all new patients who met the inclusion criteria to contact the researcher if they were interested in participating in the study. No data were presented about whether consecutive patients were invited or how many potential participants declined participation. However, once volunteers met the inclusion criteria, all were included in the study.

- *Whether they explained why the participants they selected were the most appropriate to provide access to the type of knowledge sought by the study.*
  This was not explained, but one might assume that as they were patients of practitioners of Western-style acupuncture and had just begun acupuncture within the last 3 weeks that they might have relevant experiences to discuss.

5. Were the data collected in a way that addressed the research issue?

Consider:

- *Whether the setting for data collection was justified.*
  Interviews were conducted in participants' homes, which is appropriate to address the research aims of exploring people's experiences.

- *Whether it is clear how data were collected.*
  Two semi-structured interviews were carried out: the first within 4 weeks of commencing acupuncture and the second approximately 4 months later.

- *Whether the researcher has justified the methods chosen.*
  Yes. The interviews sought to understand descriptions, views and feelings of the treatment within the wider context of people's lives and experiences of illness across repeated interviews.

- *Whether the researcher has made the methods explicit.*
  The information underpinning the interview schedule, the way the interviews were conducted (such as opening questions for the first and second interviews) and what type of information was sought is well described.

- *Whether methods were modified during the study. If so, has the researcher explained how and why?*
  There is no mention that the research methods were changed during the study period.

- *Whether the form of data is clear.*
  It is stated that interviews were tape-recorded.

- *Whether the researcher has discussed saturation of data.*
  This was not reported.

6. Has the relationship between researcher and participants been adequately considered?

Consider:

- *Whether the researcher critically examined their own role, potential bias and influence during:*
  - *Formulation of the research questions.*
    This was not reported.
  - *Data collection, including sample recruitment and choice of location.*
    Yes. The author specifically stated that she kept reflexive notes about the role of her personal and social identities within the data collection and analysis phases. However, no further information is provided as to whether her relationship with the participants had any impact on her results.
- *How the researcher responded to events during the study and whether they considered the implications of any changes in the research design.*
  No changes were reported.

7. Have ethical issues been taken into consideration?

Consider:

- *Whether there are sufficient details of how the research was explained to participants for the reader to assess whether ethical standards were maintained.*
  There are several ethical issues to consider in this study design. The issue of the dependency relationship between practitioner and patient and the possibility of coercion was addressed by ensuring that the patient was free to contact (or not) the researcher without knowledge of the treating practitioner. All participants were required to provide written informed consent prior to the first interview.
- *Whether the researcher has discussed issues raised by the study.*
  Participants were informed that their practitioner would have no access to their interview data, thereby encouraging participants to feel free to be truthful regarding their experiences.
- *Whether approval has been sought from the ethics committee.*
  Approval from an ethics committee was provided.

8. Was the data analysis sufficiently rigorous?

Consider:

- *Whether there is an in-depth description of the analysis process. Whether thematic analysis is used. If so, is it clear how the categories/themes were derived from the data?*
  The method of data analysis is well described. A constant comparative method was used, whereby data collection and analysis occurred side-by-side, each informing the other. The researcher describes her method of thinking about the data over time, making notes on her thinking, and questions in memos. Data coded over the two interviews for each person were summarised into a story and this became the basis for the thematic analysis.
- *Whether the researcher explains how the data presented were selected from the original sample, to demonstrate the analysis process.*
  This was not explained.
- *Whether sufficient data are presented to support the findings. To what extent contradictory data are taken into account.*
  The author sought negative cases to challenge her developing ideas. Contradictory cases were taken into account. For example: 'While some patients benefited rapidly from small amounts of treatment, others felt short-changed.'
- *Whether the researcher critically examined their own role, potential bias and influence during analysis and selection of data for presentation.*
  Yes. The author specifically stated that she kept reflexive notes about the role of her personal and social identities within the data collection and analysis phases.

9. Is there a clear statement of findings?

Consider:

- *Whether the findings are explicit. Whether there is adequate discussion of the evidence both for and against the researcher's arguments.*
  The main three findings were clearly described as factors that have an impact on patients' satisfaction, namely acupuncture 'dosage', integration of the acupuncture with patients' conventional treatment, and the extent to which patients learnt self-help strategies to maintain the improvements in their symptoms.

- *Whether the researcher has discussed the credibility of their findings.*
  This study interviewed each person twice, which provided a longer period of engagement than single interviews. The study would have been strengthened by having a second investigator independently code the data and develop themes and using respondent validation.

- *Whether the findings are discussed in relation to the original research question.*
  Yes. The findings were clearly discussed in relation to the original objective of the research.

10. How valuable is the research?

Consider:

- *Whether the researcher discusses the contribution the study makes to existing knowledge or understanding.*
  The value of the research relates mainly to assisting in the improvement of the provision of acupuncture services by the National Health Service in the UK.

- *Whether they identify new areas where research is necessary.*
  The author indicates that further cross-cultural studies are required.

- *Whether the researchers have discussed whether or how the findings can be transferred to other populations or considered other ways the research may be used.*
  Participants in this study were mainly female, mean age was 59 years, and they were being treated for musculoskeletal problems such as back or neck pain. The author suggests that having 19 participants who encompassed a range of experiences and settings increased the ability to transfer these findings. Readers need to consider whether the setting and type of participants in this study are similar enough to their own patients when considering using these findings.

Comments from the QARI instrument

The author briefly describes the philosophical perspectives underpinning this research as drawing on the theoretical and empirical findings of medical sociology and using a subtle realist position for the analysis. This position assumes that we can only know reality from our own perspective of it and acknowledges multiple perspectives but not multiple realities.

What are the main findings?

The main finding was that most participants experienced an improvement in their symptoms with Western-style acupuncture and would recommend it to others and use it again themselves. However, participants' experiences with Western-style acupuncture in the UK were quite diverse and largely dependent on the practitioner who treated them. Unlike traditional Chinese medicine practitioners who take a holistic approach and incorporate acupuncture into the treatment of most health problems, most participants in this study were having acupuncture as a stand-alone treatment for one chronic health problem, most commonly some type of musculoskeletal pain. The dose of acupuncture and number, frequency and length of appointments was important to participants, but often severely constrained by the health system. Improvement in symptoms was not infrequently short-lived due to inordinately long periods of time between appointments or too few treatment sessions (as compared with what is used by traditional Chinese medicine practitioners).

Participants were much more likely to be satisfied with their acupuncture if their practitioner involved them in self-care strategies, treated more than just the one main symptom, or if a positive relationship developed with the practitioner. Participants treated with one or two needles for a few minutes by a practitioner running several consultation rooms concurrently were less likely to be satisfied by their treatment. Participants were generally not demanding, but expressed a desire for acupuncture treatment to continue until symptoms had resolved or had improved to the point that people could live with them, and a clear strategy to manage symptoms into the future was achieved.

How might we use this evidence to inform practice?

It is suggested by this small qualitative study that Western-style acupuncture is better suited to treat one-off problems in patients, rather than patients with multiple health problems.

Experiences of Western acupuncture varied with some participants reporting benefit and others not. While some participants were satisfied, others were concerned about 'wasting people's time', and the lack of continuity of care. The diversity in experiences was related to three main factors: dose; the extent to which acupuncture was integrated with their other conventional care and was appropriate in terms of their overall health; and the extent to which they also learnt self-care strategies to maintain improvements gained through acupuncture. Most participants felt they would recommend it to others and use it again themselves. Having read this article, you understand more about the range of issues involved and may consider it for patients who do not have complex health conditions. However, you decide to first look for randomised controlled trials (and systematic reviews) that have explored the effectiveness of acupuncture so that you understand this body of evidence also.

EXERCISE PHYSIOLOGY EXAMPLE

CLINICAL SCENARIO

You have been employed in a cardiac rehabilitation unit attached to a public hospital. The unit has been staffed by nurses and you will be the first clinical exercise physiologist who works in the team. The manager has stated that one of your first goals is to improve adherence to the Phase 2 (supervised ambulatory outpatient) program. You wish to understand the research that has examined reasons for non-adherence in cardiac rehabilitation programs. This may also provide guidance to develop an approach to investigate this in your unit's own patients.

CLINICAL QUESTION

What reasons are given by patients for non-adherence to a hospital-based cardiac rehabilitation program?

Search terms and databases used to find the evidence

Database: PubMed–Health Services Research Queries (with 'qualitative research' category and 'narrow scope' selected), which is accessed through the 'Topic-specific queries' link on PubMed.

Search terms: (cardiac rehabilitation) AND (adherence OR non-adherence)

This search retrieved 26 results. By reading the titles it could be seen that three were specific to heart failure, one to angina and one to transplant recipients. One was a review article and others investigated service delivery, provision and/or implementation or had very specific populations. One study appears to address non-adherence to cardiac rehabilitation and you retrieve the full text of this one.

Article chosen

Jones M, Jolly K, Raftery J, et al. 'DNA' may not mean 'did not participate': a qualitative study of reasons for non-adherence at home- and centre-based cardiac rehabilitation. Fam Pract 2007;v24:343–57. Available at: fampra.oxfordjournals.org/content/24/4/343.long

Structured abstract (adapted from the above)

Study design: Qualitative study with individual semi-structured interviews.

Study question: To explore patients' reasons for non-participation in or non-adherence to a home- or hospital-based cardiac rehabilitation program.

Context: Patients participating in the Birmingham Rehabilitation Uptake Maximisation study in the UK. This is a randomised controlled trial of home- versus hospital-based cardiac rehabilitation. This article describes results from a qualitative sub-study. The authors state that they were particularly interested in women, elderly patients and people from ethnic minority groups.

Participants: 49 participants who had not completed their cardiac rehabilitation program. Of the 49 patients, 21 (43%) had been in the home arm and 28 (57%) in the hospital arm.

Data collection method: Sampling was purposive and patients were invited for interview until at least 10 had been interviewed from each of the categories: female, elderly (aged $\geq$70 years), ethnic minority group and middle-aged males. The semi-structured interviews covered topics related to the patients' cardiac event, including expectations and experience of their rehabilitation program and lifestyle changes. All 49 interviews were conducted in the patient's home by one interviewer.

Analysis: Interview transcripts were analysed using the technique of charting. Transcripts were read independently by three of the authors, and the main themes and subthemes were identified and agreed. The reasons for non-adherence were grouped into categories and repeated reading of the transcripts and field notes enabled the identification of a 'critical' reason. The reasons were grouped into four main categories: (1) alternative exercise and activities; (2) other health problems; (3) personal reasons; and (4) program-related reasons.

Key findings: Reasons for not adhering to their program spanned all the categories, with no one overall reason emerging across all patients as a major factor. There were only minor trends by ethnicity, gender, cardiac event or age of the participants. Several patients changed to their own preferred exercise program, but these patients would be labelled as non-adherers. Current methods used to measure adherence to a rehabilitation program may not reflect what people actually do.

Conclusion: Reasons for non-adherence were generally multifactorial and individualistic.

Is the evidence rigorous and sufficiently reported?

Detailed questions from CASP

3. Was the research design appropriate to address the aims of the research?

Consider:

• *Whether the researcher has justified the research design.*
This study was a part of a large randomised trial of a home- or hospital-based cardiac rehabilitation program. The qualitative study attached to this trial involved semi-structured interviews with 49 participants who had not adhered to the cardiac rehabilitation program. Although the specific choice of methodology is not explicitly justified by the authors, the methods used (such as interviews) were appropriate for the aims of exploring patients' reasons for non-participation in or non-adherence to a home- or hospital-based cardiac rehabilitation program.

4. Was the recruitment strategy appropriate to the aims of the research?

Consider:

- *Whether the researcher has explained how the participants were selected.*
  Participants were recruited from patients taking part in the larger trial. The trial nurses provided the names of patients who had not adhered to a program. Sampling was then purposive and patients were invited for interview until at least 10 had been interviewed from each of the categories: female, elderly (aged ≥70 years), ethnic minority group and middle-aged males. The authors explained numbers who were recruited and why some did not participate as follows: 'Of the 131 trial patients who did not attend/adhere to their programme, 73 (56%) were approached: of these, 49 patients agreed to be interviewed, 1 had died, 16 could not be contacted and 7 refused.'
- *Whether they explained why the participants they selected were the most appropriate to provide access to the type of knowledge sought by the study.*
  No explanation was provided about why they purposively selected these participants; however, all had not adhered to the rehabilitation program and so would be able to provide information relevant to the aims of the study.

5. Were the data collected in a way that addressed the research issue?

Consider:

- *Whether the setting for data collection was justified.*
  Interviews took place in participants' homes. No specific reason was provided for this choice of setting, but it could be assumed that it might be due to convenience for participants.
- *Whether it is clear how data were collected.*
  Semi-structured interviews were used.
- *Whether the researcher has justified the methods chosen.*
  No specific justification was provided.
- *Whether the researcher has made the methods explicit.*
  The interview schedule was developed to address issues identified from previous studies in the literature and from an earlier study in the same locality of ethnic minority patients. Topics related to the patients' cardiac event, expectations and experience of their rehabilitation program and lifestyle changes.
- *Whether methods were modified during the study. If so, has the researcher explained how and why?*
  There is no mention that any changes occurred to the research methods.
- *Whether the form of data is clear.*
  Yes. It is clearly stated that interviews were tape-recorded.
- *Whether the researcher has discussed saturation of data.*
  This is not reported.

6. Has the relationship between researcher and participants been adequately considered?

Consider:

- *Whether the researcher critically examined their own role, potential bias and influence during:*
  - *Formulation of the research questions or data collection, including sample recruitment and choice of location.*
    There is no comment about this.
- *How the researcher responded to events during the study and whether they considered the implications of any changes in the research design.*
  No changes were reported as occurring.

7. Have ethical issues been taken into consideration?

Consider:

- *Whether there are sufficient details of how the research was explained to participants for the reader to assess whether ethical standards were maintained.*
  This was not described; however, the study was approved by an ethics committee.
- *Whether the researcher has discussed issues raised by the study.*
  This was not reported.
- *Whether approval has been sought from the ethics committee.*
  Yes. Approval from an ethics committee was provided.

8. Was the data analysis sufficiently rigorous?

Consider:

- *Whether there is an in-depth description of the analysis process. Whether thematic analysis is used. If so, is it clear how the categories/themes were derived from the data?*
  A detailed description of the analysis is provided. The authors used a technique called charting. Transcripts were read independently by three authors, and the main themes and subthemes were identified. The reasons for non-adherence were grouped into categories and identification of a crucial or 'critical' reason among those patients who had given more than one reason for non-adherence confirmed by re-reading transcripts and field notes.
- *Whether the researcher explains how the data presented were selected from the original sample, to demonstrate the analysis process.*
  A worked example from one participant is provided to demonstrate how the authors arrived at the main reason that participants did not adhere to rehabilitation. Examples of quotes from participants are provided to illustrate each of the four categories. Tables which list the main reason provided by each participant for not adhering to the cardiac rehabilitation program are also provided.
- *Whether sufficient data are presented to support the findings. To what extent contradictory data are taken into account.*
  Extensive examples of participant quotes are provided in the article. The research question does not particularly lend itself to considering contradictory data. There were diverse reasons provided for non-adherence, but they could generally be subsumed into the four categories. The reasons for non-adherence were compared by home and hospital, cardiac event, age, gender and ethnicity.
- *Whether the researcher critically examined their own role, potential bias and influence during analysis and selection of data for presentation.*
  This was not reported.

9. Is there a clear statement of findings?

Consider:

- *Whether the findings are explicit. Whether there is adequate discussion of the evidence both for and against the researcher's arguments.*
  The findings are very clearly presented and unexpected findings noted. For example, it was noted that many who had not 'adhered' to cardiac rehabilitation exercise had actually sought out exercise themselves in other ways.
- *Whether the researcher has discussed the credibility of their findings (e.g. triangulation, respondent validation, more than one analyst).*
  Transcripts were read independently by three of the authors and very simple triangulation between interview multiple readings and field notes was used. However, there was no report of respondent validation or further triangulation.
- *Whether the findings are discussed in relation to the original research question.*
  Yes. The findings were clearly discussed in relation to the original objective of the research.

10. How valuable is the research?

Consider:

- *Whether the researcher discusses the contribution the study makes to existing knowledge or understanding.*
  This study recommends that social characteristics, individual patient needs and preferences, and location of rehabilitation programs need to be considered when designing rehabilitation programs.

- *Whether they identify new areas where research is necessary.*
  The authors do not specifically recommend other research, but suggest that measurement of adherence needs to be reconsidered. This study noted that the way in which adherence is measured (by number of sessions attended) may not be accurate as individuals may find other ways to exercise.

- *Whether the researchers have discussed whether or how the findings can be transferred to other populations or considered other ways the research may be used.*
  The authors acknowledge that the sample was limited to those originally enrolled in a trial and who did not have a choice in the program they were randomised to. Motivations for people not enrolled in a trial might be quite different, so findings should be considered with this in mind.

Additional comments from the QARI instrument

There was no statement regarding either a philosophical perspective or a qualitative research methodology that guided this study. Therefore it is hard to comment on the congruence between these and the representation of the data and interpretation of results, for instance. As the authors indicate that they aimed to explore participants 'views and experiences' of cardiac rehabilitation and reasons for non-participation, this could be considered from an interpretivist perspective.

What are the main findings?

Participants' reasons for not attending varied and were grouped into four categories: (1) undertaking alternative exercise programs or activities; (2) other health problems which interfered with exercise; (3) personal reasons; and (4) factors associated with the individual programs. Overall there were no clear consistent reasons why patients were not adhering to their cardiac rehabilitation program. Patients in the home program cited problems with motivation, and those assigned to the hospital had more issues with communication and access. Individualised approaches need to consider social characteristics, individuals' needs and preferences, and the location of the programs when attempting to maximise participation.

How might we use this evidence to inform practice?

As the exercise physiologist in a cardiac rehabilitation unit, you note that this study highlights the importance of individualising approaches to cardiac rehabilitation. The various reasons given by participants for non-adherence were diverse, and a one-size-fits-all approach would not be conducive to a high level of participation. It was also evident that many participants were willing and able to adopt self-care behaviours to their rehabilitation, with some changing their programs to suit their needs. This also has implications for the way that adherence is measured, with a suggestion that measuring the 'total number of sessions' that patients complete may not be appropriate. Indeed, measuring clinical outcomes more objectively may be a more appropriate way of measuring adherence. You decide to look into how to measure adherence and outcomes more thoroughly and to consider ways to provide a more individualised approach to the cardiac rehabilitation that is offered.

PARAMEDICINE EXAMPLE

CLINICAL SCENARIO

Hospital adverse events can have negative impacts on patients, extending their hospital stay, and may even lead to death. In the pre-hospital environment, except for death, it is difficult to accurately measure the clinical effects or determine the overall cost of an adverse event. Clinical audit processes are performed in most emergency medical services to determine compliance with practice guidelines. The emergency medical services patient care record audit system does not necessarily examine all patient care records, which means that some substantial errors may go unnoticed. This patient care audit system focuses on the documentation of the patient's management; however, it misses errors that were not documented. This type of adverse event identification fails to detect actual or potential adverse events that may occur at any time while the patient is under the care of the pre-hospital care provider.

There are many negative attitudes towards the reporting of incidents and near-misses in the pre-hospital setting, especially in Australia. As a senior manager in a regional health district, you wonder whether an anonymous incident reporting system as part of a blameless culture might improve patient safety outcomes in the pre-hospital setting.

CLINICAL QUESTION

What are the barriers to the reporting of critical incidents in the pre-hospital setting?

Search terms and databases used to find the evidence

Database: PubMed—Health Services Research Queries (with 'qualitative research' category and 'narrow scope' selected), which is accessed through the 'Topic-specific queries' link on PubMed.

Search terms: ("emergency medical" or prehospital OR ambulance*) AND ("critical incident*" OR adverse)

The search identified 35 articles. Following review of the title and abstract, there was one article that was relevant to your question and specifically focused on barriers.

Article chosen

Jennings P, Stella J. Barriers to incident notification in a regional prehospital setting. Emerg Med J 2011; 28:526–9.

Structured abstract*

Study design: A qualitative approach involving the triangulation of a number of ethnographic methodologies; unscripted focus groups, informal interviews and qualitative aspects of surveys.

Setting: A regional area of Victoria, Australia.

Participants: All operational ambulance personnel and management staff of Ambulance Victoria.

Analysis: Data analysis involved identification of categories and themes.

Key findings: Barriers were identified and categorised into seven themes: burden of reporting, fear of disciplinary action, fear of potential litigation, fear of breaches of confidentiality and fear of embarrassment, concern that 'nothing would change' even if the incident was reported, lack of familiarity with process and impact of 'blame culture' within the ambulance service.

*Reproduced and adapted from the above reference with permission from BMJ Publishing Group Ltd.

Conclusion: There are numerous barriers to reporting critical incidents in the pre-hospital setting. One of the main approaches may be shifting to a systems-based patient safety focus rather than an individual 'shame and blame' approach.

Is the evidence rigorous and sufficiently reported?

Detailed questions from CASP

3. Was the research design appropriate to address the aims of the research?

Consider:

- *Whether the researcher has justified the research design.*
  This study reports on a small section of a larger study designed to describe the nature and incidence of errors in pre-hospital trauma management in order to design processes to reduce errors. This study specifically indicates taking an ethnographic methodology for this study. As part of this larger study, methods used included interviews, focus groups and open-ended questions within a survey. This article reports on the barriers to critical incident reporting that were reported in the interviews, focus groups and survey. The researchers did not justify the use of these methods in this article, but did briefly explain who the different methods were used with and at what time point in the study they were used.

4. Was the recruitment strategy appropriate to the aims of the research?

Consider:

- *Whether the researcher has explained how the participants were selected.*
  Yes. A purposive sampling was used to recruit pre-hospital ambulance personnel and management staff. All operational staff within the Barwon region of Ambulance Victoria were eligible to participate in the study.

- *Whether they explained why the participants they selected were the most appropriate to provide access to the type of knowledge sought by the study.*
  This is implied, as they were investigating why paramedics did not report critical incidents.

5. Were the data collected in a way that addressed the research issue?

Consider:

- *Whether the setting for data collection was justified.*
  No. There is no comment about the data collection setting.

- *Whether it is clear how data were collected.*
  Yes. Focus groups, informal interviews and open-ended questions in surveys.

- *Whether the researcher has justified the methods chosen.*
  No. There is no explicit reason for the methods chosen.

- *Whether the researcher has made the methods explicit.*
  No. The research has stated that focus groups, interviews and surveys were conducted but not how they were conducted.

- *Whether methods were modified during the study. If so, has the researcher explained how and why?*
  There is no mention that the data collection methods were changed during the study period.

- *Whether the form of data is clear.*
  No. There is no clear statement about the format of the data (for example, whether focus groups were recorded and then transcribed), whether the survey was paper-based or electronic or whether the interviews were recorded and transcribed.

- *Whether the researcher has discussed saturation of data.*
  There is no comment about data saturation.

6. Has the relationship between researcher and participants been adequately considered?

Consider:

- *Whether the researcher critically examined their own role, potential bias and influence during:*
  - *Formulation of the research questions.*
    There is no comment about this issue.
  - *Data collection, including sample recruitment and choice of location.*
    There is no comment about this issue.
- *How the researcher responded to events during the study and whether they considered the implications of any changes in the research design:*
  Yes. The authors managed the issue of potential for litigation by de-identifying retained data for the project.

7. Have ethical issues been taken into consideration?

Consider:

- *Whether there are sufficient details of how the research was explained to participants for the reader to assess whether ethical standards were maintained.*
  Yes. All participants in the study signed a written consent statement.
- *Whether the researcher has discussed issues raised by the study.*
  The issue of potential for litigation was resolved by the systematic de-identification of all retained data for the project so that no possible link to a specific patient or specific paramedic was possible.
- *Whether approval has been sought from the ethics committee.*
  Yes. Ethics committee approval was reported to have been provided.

8. Was the data analysis sufficiently rigorous?

Consider:

- *Whether there is an in-depth description of the analysis process. Whether thematic analysis is used. If so, is it clear how the categories/themes were derived from the data?*
  No. Thematic analysis was conducted; however, there is no description of how this process was undertaken or how the themes were arrived at.
- *Whether the researcher explains how the data presented were selected from the original sample to demonstrate the analysis process.*
  No. There is no comment about this process.
- *Whether sufficient data are presented to support the findings. To what extent contradictory data are taken into account.*
  The themes are reported with only very limited supporting information, in the form of participant comments.
- *Whether the researcher critically examined their own role, potential bias and influence during analysis and selection of data for presentation.*
  There was no report that the researchers critically examined their own role, potential biases and influence during analysis and selection of data.

9. Is there a clear statement of findings?

Consider:

- *Whether the findings are explicit. Whether there is adequate discussion of the evidence both for and against the researcher's arguments.*
  There is some comment about the findings and the issues associated with them. There is also reference made to other professions and studies to highlight these points.
- *Whether the researcher has discussed the credibility of their finding.:*
  Respondent validation occurred. Themes were fed back to participants during focus groups to validate the themes and further explore perceptions about this research issue. The authors report

that triangulation of data from three methods were used: (1) unstructured discursive focus groups utilising senior, management and operational Rural Ambulance Victoria personnel and senior emergency department staff; (2) informal interviews with operational Rural Ambulance Victoria personnel; and (3) qualitative portions of surveys were examined to elucidate interest, knowledge and free commentary on incident reporting and any perceived barriers.

- *Whether the findings are discussed in relation to the original research question.*
  This part of the larger study was designed to report on barriers to the reporting of critical incidents, and the findings are clearly discussed in relation to this aim.

10. How valuable is the research?

Consider:

- *Whether the researcher discusses the contribution the study makes to existing knowledge or understanding.*
  There is some comment about how this study adds to current knowledge and how it may change policy.
- *Whether they identify new areas where research is necessary.*
  No. This is not discussed.
- *Whether the researchers have discussed whether or how the findings can be transferred to other populations or considered other ways the research may be used.*
  The issue of transferability was not considered. One of the main conclusions was to consider approaches to how to shift to a 'systems-based focus' rather than an individual 'shame and blame' approach.

Additional comment from the QARI instrument

This study specifically indicates taking an ethnographic methodology for this study and, in this sense, the use of multiple sources and methods (interviews, focus groups, information from surveys) is congruent with this methodology. However, there is no specific statement of the underlying philosophical perspective. Overall, there is very limited representation of the data or interpretation of the results, and therefore the ability of the reader to understand, interpret and appraise this paper or use these findings is significantly hampered.

What are the main results?

Barriers for reporting critical incidents were identified and were categorised into the following themes:

- Burden of reporting: the need for a process that allowed reporting of incidents in a timely fashion which is quick and simple to complete, and is readily available in a range of locations (that is, ambulance stations and hospital emergency departments).
- Fear of disciplinary action was a significant barrier to reporting.
- Fear of potential litigation: issues surrounding indemnity from prosecution needed to be clarified; concerns about liability if personnel admitted to an incident which may have contributed to an adverse outcome for a patient in their care.
- Fear of breaches of confidentiality and fear of embarrassment: participants were sceptical about the ability of the 'system' to maintain their confidentiality; being linked to certain types of critical incidents could be embarrassing within their peer group.
- Concern that 'nothing would change' even if the incident was reported: repeated reporting of issues to management with no positive outcome would seem to reinforce this belief.
- Lack of familiarity with process: some participants stated that they had not reported a critical incident as they 'only started recently and didn't know I could'.
- Impact of 'blame culture': paramedics were frustrated that hospital staff were encouraged to submit reports on critical incidents involving paramedics, while paramedics were not encouraged to report on in-hospital incidents as this was not within the scope of the project.

How might we use this evidence to inform practice?

Despite the very limited methodological information in this article, some information might be drawn from it. The perception of paramedics that the ambulance manager culture of assigning 'blame' to someone for an incident or error needs to be changed for the success of an incident monitoring system to be fully realised. For an incident reporting system to be fully functional and effective, the organisation's direction must focus on patient safety, from the upper and middle management to the paramedics. It is not possible to eliminate all pre-hospital errors, even those that cause risk, harm or death to a patient. However, improvements can be assisted by designing systems and tasks so that incidents are minimised. The system as a whole needs to be analysed to determine which components have not met the standard to achieve a good or positive outcome, and this was one of the major recommendations in this article. As a whole, this article has some very useful observations, but you decide to look for additional studies to confirm its findings.

PHARMACY EXAMPLE

CLINICAL SCENARIO

You are a pharmacist working in primary care where you are accredited to undertake community-based medication reviews in the domiciliary setting. The service is free to patients and is aimed at maximising the benefits of their medications and preventing drug-related problems. The reviews are undertaken in collaboration with patients' general practitioners. During the medication review consultation you interview the patient, preferably in their own home although the interview may also be conducted in another setting (such as the medical practice) based on patient preference. You then provide the patient's general practitioner with a report which outlines the drug-related problems that were identified during the consultation and recommendations for potential solutions.

Although the clinical benefits of medication review services have been recognised nationally and internationally, you note that a number of patients have declined to proceed with the review when you have contacted them to set up a consultation time. You are also aware that the national uptake of the funded program has remained below projected targets, despite showing success in identification of drug-related problems and patient outcomes. There is significant advertising of the program to healthcare providers and specific facilitation activities to increase identification of patients who would benefit from the service. However, you wonder why consumers who would benefit from the service would not want to participate in something that could potentially improve their health, and whether there is something you or the general practitioners could be doing to improve the uptake of this service.

CLINICAL QUESTION

What factors affect consumer participation in a home medication review program?

Search terms and databases used to find the evidence

Database: PubMed–Health Services Research Queries (with 'qualitative research' category and 'narrow scope' selected), which is accessed through the 'Topic-specific queries' link on PubMed.

Search terms: (consumer) AND (home medication review)

Your initial search using the narrow scope does not provide any results. You change to the 'broad scope', which gives eight hits—one of which is relevant to your question.

Article chosen

White L, Klinner C, Carter S. Consumer perspectives of the Australian Home Medicines Review Program: benefits and barriers. Res Social Adm Pharm 2012;8:4–16.

Structured abstract (adapted from the above)

Study design: Qualitative, with semi-structured focus group interviews.

Research question: Investigation of the perceived benefits and barriers of the home medication review service by individuals who had used the service and by those who were eligible for it but had not used it.

Participants: 87 patients and carers (55% were female; age range 33–91 years) who were eligible for the home medication review (split into 14 focus groups held across four Australian states) were recruited through participating pharmacies or via a local carer support group.

Data collection: Semi-structured focus group discussions were used. Participants were separated into groups of those who had and had not experienced the review service before the study. Topics covered included: details of the home medication review program, expectations/apprehensions with the service process, influences the service may have on their medications or relationships with healthcare providers, safety concerns, and whether they would actively ask their general practitioner for a home medication review referral.

Analysis: Thematic analysis of interviews using a three-step process: (1) eight codes were generated and collated into tentative themes; (2) codes were connected into categories and subcategories and relationships established between categories to find themes; and (3) themes were mapped and defined and names for each theme generated.

Key findings: The major benefits reported were acquisition of medicine information, reassurance, feeling valued and cared for, and willingness to advocate medication changes to the general practitioner. Perceived barriers were concerns regarding upsetting the general practitioner, pride and independence, confidence issues with an unknown pharmacist, privacy and safety concerns regarding the home visit, and lack of information about the program. Participants agreed that the potential benefits of the service outweighed its potential barriers.

Conclusion: It is expected that direct-to-consumer promotion of home medication reviews would increase the uptake of them. It would be necessary to ensure that the process and benefits of the service are communicated clearly and sensitively to eligible patients and their carers, to remove common consumer misconceptions and/or barriers regarding the home medication review service.

Is the evidence rigorous and sufficiently reported?

Detailed questions from CASP

3. Was the research design appropriate to address the aims of the research?

Consider:

- *Whether the researcher has justified the research design.*
  This study does not use specific qualitative research methodology. The methods include use of semi-structured interviews. The study investigated the perceived benefits and barriers of the patients regarding the home medication review service. The authors discuss the benefits of using focus group methods for ascertaining participants' views.

4. Was the recruitment strategy appropriate to the aims of the research?

Consider:

- *Whether the researcher has explained how the participants were selected.*
  Participants were recruited through voluntarily participating pharmacists throughout Australia. The pharmacists approached potential participants either while dispensing medicines for them

or on the occasion of a home medication review visit. In addition, carers were recruited from a support group for family carers.

- *Whether they explained why the participants they selected were the most appropriate to provide access to the type of knowledge sought by the study.*
  The authors sought representation from patients who had had a home medication review in the past 6 months and from those who had never had a home medication review but were eligible for the service, in order to obtain views from these two perspectives. They also sought involvement from carers of people with a disability, mental health problem, chronic condition or who are frail aged.

5. Were the data collected in a way that addressed the research issue?

Consider:

- *Whether the setting for data collection was justified.*
  The place/s in which the interviews were carried out was not identified.
- *Whether it is clear how data were collected.*
  Fourteen focus groups were used with a semi-structured format.
- *Whether the researcher has justified the methods chosen.*
  The authors clearly justify their chosen method.
- *Whether the researcher has made the methods explicit.*
  A semi-structured interview guide was used. The topics discussed were clearly outlined in the article.
- *Whether methods were modified during the study. If so, has the researcher explained how and why?*
  There is no mention that the research methods were changed during the study period.
- *Whether the form of data is clear.*
  Yes. It is clearly stated that interviews were tape-recorded.
- *Whether the researcher has discussed saturation of data.*
  This was not reported.

6. Has the relationship between researcher and participants been adequately considered?

Consider:

- *Whether the researcher critically examined their own role, potential bias and influence during:*
  - *Formulation of the research questions.*
    There is no comment about this in the article.
  - *Data collection, including sample recruitment and choice of location.*
    There is no comment about this in the article.
- *How the researcher responded to events during the study and whether they considered the implications of any changes in the research design.*
  No changes were reported.

7. Have ethical issues been taken into consideration?

Consider:

- *Whether there are sufficient details of how the research was explained to participants for the reader to assess whether ethical standards were maintained.*
  All participants provided written consent to the research content and process, including audiotaping of the focus groups. Assurances were given regarding anonymity and confidentiality.
- *Whether the researcher has discussed issues raised by the study.*
  The only information provided about this issue is that assurances were given regarding anonymity and confidentiality.
- *Whether approval has been sought from the ethics committee.*
  Yes. Approval from an ethics committee was provided.

8. Was the data analysis sufficiently rigorous?

Consider:

- *Whether there is an in-depth description of the analysis process. Whether thematic analysis is used. If so, is it clear how the categories/themes were derived from the data?*
  A detailed description of the analysis is provided and a clear explanation provided as to how the categories and themes were derived.

- *Whether the researcher explains how the data presented were selected from the original sample to demonstrate the analysis process.*
  This was not explicitly explained; however, it can be seen that data presented were used to illustrate the themes and to represent data from both carers and patients.

- *Whether sufficient data are presented to support the findings. To what extent contradictory data are taken into account.*
  There is sufficient data to illustrate the findings. The authors sought to identify common themes and disparate perceptions.

- *Whether the researcher critically examined their own role, potential bias and influence during analysis and selection of data for presentation.*
  This was not reported.

9. Is there a clear statement of findings?

Consider:

- *Whether the findings are explicit. Whether there is adequate discussion of the evidence both for and against the researcher's arguments.*
  The findings are very clearly reported. The author aimed to improve understanding of the barriers and benefits to home medication review and, as such, presented a balanced and detailed discussion of these perspectives and their implications.

- *Whether the researcher has discussed the credibility of their findings.*
  There was a brief attempt to validate responses with participants. The focus groups were debriefed by one of the researchers, and agreement or contradicting ideas discussed. It is not stated when this debriefing occurred, but we assume it was probably at the end of the focus group session. If this was the case, then participants were not provided time to carefully reflect on the full discussion prior to commenting. No clear evidence of triangulation or use of independent analysts was provided, although discrepancies in analysis were reported to have been resolved by discussions amongst the research team.

- *Whether the findings are discussed in relation to the original research question.*
  Yes. The findings were clearly discussed in relation to the original objective of the research.

10. How valuable is the research?

Consider:

- *Whether the researcher discusses the contribution the study makes to existing knowledge or understanding.*
  The authors concluded that direct-to-consumer promotion of home medication review services would increase service uptake, and identified a number of issues to consider when communicating the availability of this service.

- *Whether they identify new areas where research is necessary.*
  The authors recommend that quantitative research should be used to confirm the findings of this study with respect to the perceived barriers and benefits.

- *Whether the researchers have discussed whether or how the findings can be transferred to other populations or considered other ways the research may be used.*
  The authors discuss restrictions on the transferability of the data in relation to carers, patients who were offered but refused to have a medication review, and those who were housebound and unable to attend a focus group.

Additional comments from the QARI instrument

This article simply states that semi-structured focus groups were undertaken by people with experience in qualitative research, and does not describe either a philosophical perspective or a specific qualitative research methodology. However, it appears that the authors were taking an interpretivist position, and phenomenological methodology could have been reasonable given that they aimed to understand the 'perceived benefits and barriers' of the patients regarding home medication reviews. The interview questions make it clear that the study sought participants' concerns, attitudes and experiences through focus groups and would thus be congruent with phenomenological methodology.

What were the main findings?

This study identified high consumer satisfaction levels with the home medication review. The major benefits reported were acquisition of medicine information, reassurance, feeling valued and cared for, and willingness to advocate medication changes to their general practitioner. However, specific problems that patients and carers perceived with respect to accepting or asking for a home medication review were identified. In brief, these included concerns regarding upsetting their general practitioner, pride and independence, confidence issues with an unknown pharmacist, privacy and safety concerns regarding the home visit, and lack of information about the program.

How might we use this evidence to inform practice?

These findings indicate that a more thorough explanation of the process of a home medication review is needed for patients, both at the general practitioner level and at the pharmacist level. This might include addressing concerns they may have about 'upsetting the GP' and fear they might have of an 'unknown pharmacist'.

References

1. Critical Appraisal Skills Program (CASP). 10 questions to help you make sense of qualitative research. Oxford: CASP; 2010. Online. Available www.casp-uk.net/wp-content/uploads/2011/11/CASP_Qualitative_Appraisal_Checklist_14oct10.pdf; 20 Nov 2012.
2. National Collaborating Centre for Methods and Tools. Critical appraisal tools to make sense of evidence. Hamilton, ON: McMaster University; 2011. Online. Available: www.nccmt.ca/registry/view/eng/87.html; 31 May 2012.
3. Giacomini M, Cook D for the Evidence-Based Medicine Working Group. Users' guides to the medical literature, XXIII: qualitative research in health care. Are the results of the study valid? JAMA 2000;284:357–62.

Chapter 12

Appraising and understanding systematic reviews of quantitative and qualitative evidence

Sally Bennett, Denise O'Connor, Karin Hannes and Susan Doyle

LEARNING OBJECTIVES

After reading this chapter, you should be able to:

- Understand what systematic reviews are
- Know where to look for systematic reviews
- Understand how systematic reviews are carried out
- Critically appraise a systematic review
- Understand how to interpret the results from systematic reviews
- Understand how systematic reviews can be used to inform practice

A systematic review is a method for systematically locating, appraising and synthesising research from primary studies and is an important means of condensing the research evidence from many primary studies. This chapter will describe systematic reviews of quantitative and qualitative evidence, discuss their advantages and disadvantages and briefly illustrate the use of systematic reviews for different types of clinical questions. The methods for carrying out systematic reviews will be described, and key factors that can introduce bias into reviews will be explained. Using worked examples, we will also demonstrate how to critically appraise a systematic review and how it can be used to guide decision making in practice.

WHAT ARE SYSTEMATIC REVIEWS?

Due to the massive increase in the volume of health research over the last 50 years or so, it was recognised that some system of synthesising this information was essential. The health literature has a long tradition of using literature or narrative reviews to help readers grasp the breadth of a particular topic. These literature reviews typically provide a reasonably thorough description of a particular topic and refer to many articles that have been published in that particular area. Nearly all students are required to do at least one literature review as part of their studies, so you probably know what literature reviews are all about.

More recently, **systematic reviews** have been embraced as a more comprehensive and trustworthy means of synthesising the literature.[1] Systematic reviews differ from literature reviews in that they are prepared using transparent, explicit and pre-defined methods that are designed to limit bias.[2] In contrast to literature reviews, systematic reviews:

- involve a clear definition of eligibility criteria
- incorporate a comprehensive search to identify *all* potentially relevant studies (although there are qualitative reviewers that opt for a purposeful sample of papers deemed relevant for generating theory)
- use explicit, reproducible and uniformly applied criteria in the selection of studies for the review
- rigorously appraise the risk of bias within individual studies, and
- systematically synthesise the results of included studies.[2]

Systematic reviews may summarise the results from quantitative studies, qualitative studies or a combination of quantitative and qualitative studies, depending on the clinical question and the methods used to conduct the review. In a *quantitative review* the results from two or more individual quantitative studies are typically summarised using a measure of effect, which enables each study's effect size to be statistically combined and compared in what is called a **meta-analysis**.[2] Meta-analyses generally provide a better overall estimate of a clinical effect than looking at the results from individual studies. However, sometimes it is not possible to combine the results of individual studies in a meta-analysis because the interventions or outcomes used in the different studies may be too diverse for it to be sensible to combine them. In these instances the results from these studies have to be synthesised narratively.

It may help you to think about these different types of reviews visually. As you can see in Figure 12.1, literature reviews make up the vast majority of reviews that are found in the overall health literature. Systematic reviews can be considered a subset of literature reviews, and meta-analyses are a smaller set again. Note that the circle representing meta-analyses overlaps both systematic and literature reviews. This is because not all meta-analyses are carried out systematically. For example, it is technically possible for someone to take a collection of articles that report randomised controlled trials from their desk and undertake a meta-analysis of these articles. This would not be considered systematic, as methods were not used to ensure that a systematic search for all relevant articles was conducted. Sometimes the terms 'systematic review' and 'meta-analysis' are used interchangeably, but in this chapter they are conceptualised as different entities. A systematic review does not need to incorporate a meta-analysis, but a

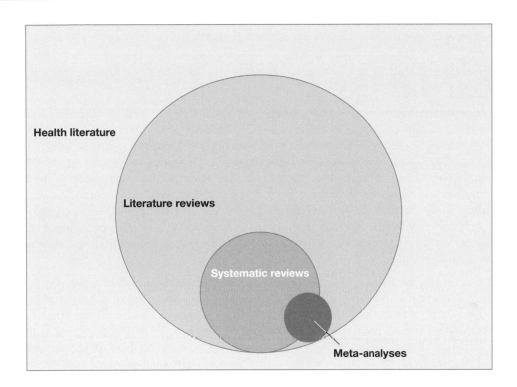

Figure 12.1
The relationships between the health literature, literature reviews, systematic reviews, and meta-analyses.

meta-analysis should only be done within the context of a systematic review (although occasionally it is not).

A *review of qualitative studies* (also known as qualitative evidence synthesis, QES) aggregates or integrates findings from individual qualitative basic research studies into categories or metaphors in order to generate new theory or advance our understanding of particular phenomena to advise professional practice or policy. In a *mixed-methods review*, both quantitative and qualitative studies are used in parallel or sequentially.[3]

ADVANTAGES AND DISADVANTAGES OF SYSTEMATIC REVIEWS

By combining the results of similar studies, a well-conducted systematic review can:

- improve the dissemination of evidence[2]
- hasten the assimilation of research into practice[3]
- assist in clarifying the heterogeneity of conflicting results between studies[4]
- establish generalisability of the overall findings[2]
- improve the understanding of a particular phenomenon or situation, and
- guide decision making.

Systematic reviews are important for health professionals and consumers of health care who are seeking answers to clinical questions, for researchers who are identifying gaps in research and defining future research agendas and for administrators and purchasers who are developing policies and guidelines.[2] Although systematic reviews have many advantages, as with any other study type they may be subject to bias, which will be discussed in detail later in this chapter.

SYSTEMATIC REVIEWS FOR DIFFERENT TYPES OF CLINICAL QUESTIONS

Systematic reviews synthesise studies using different study designs to address different research questions.[5] As we saw in Chapter 2 when we examined the hierarchies of evidence for various question types, systematic reviews are at the top of the hierarchy of evidence for questions about the effects of intervention, diagnosis and prognosis. For example, a well-conducted systematic review of randomised controlled trials is generally considered to be the best study design for assessing the effectiveness of an *intervention* because it identifies and examines all of the evidence about the intervention from randomised controlled trials (providing these are rigorous themselves) that meet pre-determined inclusion criteria.[6] This type of systematic review is by far the most common type of systematic review available. However, systematic reviews of quantitative studies may be carried out to address other types of questions, such as questions about *diagnosis* and *prognosis*.

Systematic reviews that focus on questions of prognosis or prediction best undertake a *synthesis of cohort studies*. Consider the following example in which a systematic review of cohort studies of patients in the subacute phase of ischaemic or haemorrhagic stroke was conducted with the aim of identifying prognostic factors for future place of residence at 6 to 12 months post-stroke.[7] The authors searched MEDLINE, EMBASE, CINAHL, Current Contents, Cochrane Database of Systematic Reviews, PsycLIT and Sociological Abstracts as well as reference lists, personal archives and consultations of experts in the field and guidelines to locate relevant cohort studies. They then assessed the internal, statistical and external validity of the 10 studies that they had selected for inclusion. Although the review found many factors that were predictive of a patient's future place of residence (for example, low initial functioning in activities of daily living, advanced age, cognitive disturbance, paresis of arm and leg), the authors concluded that there was insufficient evidence concerning possible predictors in the subacute stage of stroke with respect to place of future residence.

Systematic reviews of diagnostic test studies are carried out to determine estimates of test performance and consider variation between studies. This type of systematic review uses different methods to assess study quality and combine results than those used for systematic reviews of randomised controlled trials.[8] An example of this type of review is one that used meta-analytic procedures in a review of the accuracy of the Mini-Mental State Examination in the detection of dementia and mild cognitive impairment.[9] Thirty-four dementia studies and five mild cognitive impairment studies were included in the meta-analysis. It was concluded that the Mini-Mental State Examination offers modest accuracy with best value for ruling out a diagnosis of dementia in community and primary care.

Systematic reviews of qualitative studies allow us to have a more comprehensive understanding, for example, of patients' experience in relation to a particular issue. Noyes and colleagues[10] state that syntheses of evidence from qualitative research:

> explore questions such as how do people experience illness, why does an intervention work (or not), for whom and in what circumstances … what are the barriers and facilitators to accessing health care, or what impact do specific barriers and facilitators have on people, their experiences and behavior? … [Qualitative evidence syntheses] can aid understanding of the way in which an intervention is experienced by all of those involved in developing, delivering or receiving it; what aspect of the intervention they value, or not; and why this is so … [it] can provide insight into factors that are external to an intervention including, for example, the impact of other policy developments, factors which facilitate or hinder successful implementation of a programme, service, or treatment and how a particular intervention may need to be adapted for large-scale roll-out.

Systematic reviews of qualitative studies, often referred to as **qualitative evidence syntheses**, combine evidence from primary qualitative studies to create new understanding by comparing and analysing concepts and findings from different sources of evidence with a focus on the same topic of interest.[10] Qualitative evidence syntheses have gained significant recognition in the field of health care, both as a stand-alone product and as a scientific contribution able to inform, extend, enhance or supplement systematic reviews of effectiveness. Discussion among researchers about how systematic reviews of qualitative research should best be conducted continues. There is even ongoing debate about whether a synthesis of qualitative studies is appropriate and whether it is acceptable to combine studies that use a variety of different methods.[11]

There are at least 20 different approaches to the synthesis of qualitative studies that have been developed and identified by researchers, including the commonly used meta-ethnographic approach to synthesis, meta-study, thematic synthesis, narrative synthesis, content analysis, cross-study analysis, grounded theory, and framework synthesis.[12] Most of these approaches are interpretive in nature. They seek to increase the understanding of events based on the perspectives and experiences of the people studied by combining results of individual studies.

An alternative approach to qualitative evidence synthesis that is rapidly gaining recognition in the field is the *meta-aggregative approach to synthesis*. It is unique in taking an explicit integrative method to synthesis, as opposed to the more commonly accepted interpretive approach. This has been designed to model the Cochrane Collaboration's process of performing systematic reviews which summarise the results of quantitative studies, while being sensitive to the nature of qualitative research and its traditions.[13] In this chapter we will focus on this meta-aggregative approach, as the process and procedure will appeal to most health professionals who are familiar with effectiveness reviews. An interesting illustrative example of this approach can be found in a synthesis of studies on barriers to the implementation of evidence-based practice in health care.[14]

Methods for combining results from both quantitative and qualitative studies within a single review are generally referred to as *mixed-methods reviews*. Examples of mixed-method protocols can now be found in the Cochrane Library. An interesting example is a systematic review that examined older people's views, perceptions and experiences of falls prevention interventions.[15] The authors of the review searched eight databases using a broad search strategy in order to locate relevant qualitative and quantitative studies. The systematic review contained 24 studies, which consisted of 10 qualitative studies, 1 systematic review, 3 narrative reviews, 3 randomised controlled trials, 3 before/after studies and 4 cross-sectional observational studies. Synthesis of the *quantitative* studies in this review identified factors that encouraged older people's participation in falls prevention interventions, while the findings from the 10 *qualitative* studies demonstrated the importance of considering older people's views about falls interventions to ensure that these interventions are properly targeted.

So, contrary to common misconception, systematic reviews are not just limited to syntheses of quantitative studies such as randomised controlled trials. They are a methodology that can be used for many different study designs and research questions. Having pointed this out, the remainder of this chapter will outline the procedure for both an effectiveness review and a qualitative evidence synthesis using the meta-aggregative approach.

LOCATING SYSTEMATIC REVIEWS

It has been mentioned a number of times already in this book that a substantial difficulty in locating research evidence is the overwhelming quantity of information that is available and the diverse range of journals in which information is published. Unfortunately, systematic reviews are not immune to this problem either. As you saw in Chapter 3, the premier source for systematic reviews of quantitative studies answering clinical questions about intervention effectiveness is the Cochrane Database of Systematic

Reviews. These reviews are written by volunteer researchers who work with one of many review groups that are coordinated by The Cochrane Collaboration (www.cochrane.org). Each review group has an editorial team which oversees the preparation and maintenance of the reviews, as well as the application of rigorous quality standards. The Cochrane Collaboration has recently changed its policy towards including qualitative evidence in systematic reviews, with some versions of mixed-method reviews having already been published in the Library. It is expected that the number of these types of reviews will continue to increase.

Another source of reliable information contained within the Cochrane Library is the Database of Abstracts of Reviews (DARE). This contains abstracts of systematic reviews that have been quality-assessed. Each abstract includes a summary of the review together with a critical commentary about the overall quality. Chapter 3 provided the details of other resources that can be used to locate systematic reviews. These include the Joanna Briggs Institute, PEDro, OTseeker, PsycBITE, speechBITE and the large biomedical databases such as CINAHL and MEDLINE/PubMed (the latter contains a search strategy specifically for locating systematic reviews on the PubMed Clinical Queries screen).

HOW ARE SYSTEMATIC REVIEWS CONDUCTED?

We believe that it is easier to learn how to appraise a systematic review if you first have an understanding of what is involved in performing a systematic review. Undertaking a systematic review requires a significant time commitment, with estimates varying depending on the number of citations/abstracts involved. Obviously, for some topics there is very little research that has been done, whereas for other topics there is a huge amount of research to find and sort through. To give you an idea, one estimation is that it takes approximately 1139 hours or the equivalent of 6 months full-time work to complete a systematic review.[16]

We will now explain the basic steps involved in undertaking a systematic review, which are:

1. Define the research question and plan the methods for undertaking the review.
2. Determine the eligibility criteria for studies to be included.
3. Search for potentially eligible studies.
4. Apply eligibility criteria to select studies.
5. Assess the risk of bias in included studies.
6. Extract data from the included studies.
7. Synthesise the data.
8. Interpret and report the results.
9. Update the review at an appropriate time point in the future.

Define the research question and plan the methods for undertaking the systematic review

As with any research study, when conducting a systematic review the first place to start is planning the overall project. Planning also ensures that all aspects important to the scientific rigour of a review are undertaken to reduce the risk of bias. Each stage of the review needs to be thoroughly understood prior to moving on to plan the next stage.

The question needs to be clearly focused, as too broad a question will not produce a useful review. The question should also make sense clinically. Involving consumers, at both the health professional and the patient levels, may also be helpful when developing a plan, as this will ensure that areas of concern such as the types of interventions or outcomes that might not otherwise be considered are addressed.[17]

Planning a review also requires decisions to be made about the methods for searching, screening, appraisal and synthesis. These decisions should be made before commencing the review itself and ideally written up as a protocol, as this will help to make the whole process systematic and more transparent for all involved.

Determine the eligibility criteria for studies to be included in the review

The use of explicit, pre-defined criteria for including and excluding studies (eligibility criteria) is an important feature of systematic reviews. The eligibility criteria to be defined for, and applied in, a systematic review will depend on the type of review question (for example, whether the review is about effects of intervention or about diagnostic tests or patient experiences) and the population of interest.

Traditionally, eligibility criteria for systematic reviews of the effects of interventions have focused on defining *types of participants* (that is, people and populations), *types of interventions and comparisons* and *types of studies* (that is, the study designs most suitable for answering the review question). Although systematic reviews of the effects of interventions also typically pre-specify *types of outcomes* (the outcome measures that are important to answer the review question), these usually are not used to include or exclude studies but rather to guide how the findings from the included studies are reported. Generally, systematic reviews of the effects of interventions primarily focus on randomised controlled trials or quasi-randomised controlled trials. However, there are many reviews which include both randomised and non-randomised studies. While these reviews can provide a comprehensive overall picture of the available research, they require the reader to be particularly careful when interpreting the conclusions and to take into account the study types (and their associated strengths/weaknesses) that may have been used to contribute to the conclusion of the review.

Qualitative evidence syntheses generally include all sorts of qualitative study designs, including, for example, phenomenological studies, case studies, grounded theory designs and action research designs. Some review authors opt for the exclusion of opinion papers and editorials and papers without a clear methods and findings section. To date, there is little guidance on how to search for, critically appraise or extract data from these reports, or how to use them in a cross-comparison between papers.[10]

Search for potentially eligible studies

The search methodology needs to be developed prior to commencing the review and to be clearly explained and reproducible. All components of the question of the review (such as the participants, interventions, comparisons and outcomes) should be considered when developing the search strategy of the review. Synonyms and relevant Medical Subject Heading (MeSH) terms for key components of the search (for example, participants and interventions) should also be incorporated.[18] The search should not be limited by publication date, publication format or language unless there is a good reason for doing so (such as an intervention only being available after a certain point in time). Searching should occur across multiple databases, as it has been found that search strategies that are limited to one database do not identify all of the relevant studies.[18] The review authors should also ideally contact authors in the field in an attempt to locate other studies that have not already been identified and ongoing or planned studies in the area, and to ask about and obtain written copies of unpublished studies.[19] The reason for doing this is to limit a problem called '**publication bias**' that can occur due to study authors being more likely to submit studies with statistically significant results and journals being more likely to publish studies with positive results than those with negative outcomes.

As an illustration of how important it is that review authors use a comprehensive search strategy, one study found that 35% of all appropriate randomised controlled trials were not located by computerised searching[20] and another reported that 10% of suitable trials for systematic reviews were missed when only electronic searching was conducted.[21] Greenhalgh and Peacock[22] evaluated the appropriateness of standard searching procedures for the retrieval of qualitative research papers and found that only 30% were retrieved through databases and hand-searching. The rest were identified through a snowball procedure of following up on the references of relevant papers and by personal contacts. Hand-searching journals has been identified as important to conducting a high quality systematic review,[23] as not all journals are indexed in electronic databases or may be missed by the search strategy used. It is suggested[24] that authors of systematic reviews may perform hand-searching of the major journals that publish in the area relevant to the review question, to increase the comprehensiveness of their search strategy. Citation tracking or use of the references from the studies found may also help the reviewer to locate further studies on the topic and increase comprehensiveness of the search. Attempts could also be made to obtain unpublished studies (including masters and doctoral research and conference proceedings) by searching the CENTRAL database in the Cochrane Library and databases of grey literature (e.g. OpenSIGLE, Open System for Information on Grey Literature, www.opensigle.inist.fr). The same applies for reviewers who are conducting a qualitative evidence synthesis, although, as far as we are aware, specialised registers for qualitative research currently do not exist.

Apply eligibility criteria to select studies

Once the search has been completed and potentially relevant studies identified, the next task is to decide which of the studies should be included in the systematic review. Not all articles that are located during the search will be directly relevant to the review question. Eligibility criteria are established to guide the selection of studies to be included in the review. The criteria specify the studies, participants, interventions and outcomes that are to be included. The selection process should then be carried out by two or more authors independently to minimise bias. Titles and abstracts are screened for relevance and eligibility. At this point some citations will be excluded as it will be clear from the title and abstract that they do not meet the review eligibility criteria. For other citations, the decision on whether to include or exclude will be unclear due to insufficient information in the title and abstract. The full text of these potentially relevant studies is then retrieved so that a more detailed evaluation can be done. A final evaluation of the full-text articles is conducted and a decision is made whether to include or exclude the studies. If the review authors are conducting a Cochrane systematic review, studies that are excluded at this stage of the review process are listed in the review along with the reason why they were excluded.[24] A flow diagram summarising the study selection processes may also be appended to the review.

Assess the risk of bias in included studies

The next step is to evaluate the validity of the studies that have been included in the review. Assessing the validity, or 'risk of bias', of the results from the individual studies is vital to conducting a high quality systematic review. Including studies with a high risk of bias can serve to magnify the impact of that bias, and thus may raise doubts about the reliability of the systematic review's results and conclusions.[25] Where such studies are included in the review, it is important that the risk of bias is clearly communicated for the reader. To guard against errors and increase the reliability of the validity assessment, it is recommended that more than one person independently extract data and assess the risk of bias of the included studies.[26] Determining the potential for bias in individual studies can be done in a number of different ways, such as using the approach to appraising randomised controlled trials that was explained in Chapter 4 of this book. From the beginning of 2008, systematic reviews that are carried out through The Cochrane Collaboration have to use the 'risk of bias' tool.[26] The risk of bias tool includes seven different domains which are shown in Table 12.1, along with a definition of each of these criteria. Implementation of this tool requires two steps:

1. extracting information from the original study report about each criterion to describe what was reported to have happened in the study (see description column in Table 12.1); and then

TABLE 12.1:
THE COCHRANE COLLABORATION'S TOOL FOR ASSESSING RISK OF BIAS IN INDIVIDUAL STUDIES[26]

Domain	Description	Review authors' judgment*
Random sequence generation	Describe the method used to generate the allocation sequence in sufficient detail to allow an assessment of whether it should produce comparable groups.	Selection bias (biased allocation to interventions) due to inadequate generation of a randomised sequence.
Allocation concealment	Describe the method used to conceal the allocation sequence in sufficient detail to determine whether intervention allocations could have been foreseen in advance of, or during, enrolment.	Selection bias (biased allocation to interventions) due to inadequate concealment of allocations prior to assignment.
Blinding of participants and personnel Assessments should be made for each main outcome (or class of outcomes)	Describe all measures used, if any, to blind study participants and personnel from knowledge of which intervention a participant received. Provide any information relating to whether the intended blinding was effective.	Performance bias due to knowledge of the allocated interventions by participants and personnel during the study.
Blinding of outcome assessment Assessments should be made for each main outcome (or class of outcomes)	Describe all measures used, if any, to blind outcome assessors from knowledge of which intervention a participant received. Provide any information relating to whether the intended blinding was effective.	Detection bias due to knowledge of the allocated interventions by outcome assessors.
Incomplete outcome data Assessments should be made for each main outcome (or class of outcomes)	Describe the completeness of outcome data for each main outcome, including attrition and exclusions from the analysis. State whether attrition and exclusions were reported, the numbers in each intervention group (compared with total randomised participants), reasons for attrition/exclusions where reported and any re-inclusions in analyses performed by the review authors.	Attrition bias due to amount, nature or handling of incomplete outcome data.
Selective reporting	State how the possibility of selective outcome reporting was examined by the review authors and what was found.	Reporting bias due to selective outcome reporting.
Other sources of bias	State any important concerns about bias not addressed in the other domains in the tool.	Bias due to problems not covered elsewhere in the table.

* Judgment for each domain: 'Low risk' of bias, 'High risk' of bias, or 'Unclear risk' of bias.

Higgins JPT, Altman DG, Sterne JAC, editors. Chapter 8: Assessing risk of bias in included studies. In: Higgins JPT, Green S, editors. Cochrane Handbook for Systematic Reviews of Interventions. Version 5.1.0 [updated March 2011]. The Cochrane Collaboration; 2011. Online. Available: http://handbook .cochrane.org/

2. making a judgment about the likely risk of bias in relation to each criterion (rated as 'Low risk' of bias, 'High risk' of bias or 'Unclear risk' of bias) (see Review authors' judgment column in Table 12.1).

For the critical appraisal of qualitative studies, a number of different checklists and frameworks have been developed. Among them is the commonly used CASP checklist and QARI tool that were discussed and used in Chapters 10 and 11. The meta-aggregative approach encourages qualitative evidence synthesis review authors to assign an overall judgment to findings in an original article.[13] This allows the reviewer to decide which insights are valid enough to be considered for inclusion. These judgments are:

- *unequivocal* if the evidence is beyond reasonable doubt and includes findings that are factual, directly reported/observed and not open to challenge;

- *credible* if the evidence, while interpretative, is plausible in light of the data and theoretical framework; or

- *unsupported,* in case the findings are not supported by the data and none of the other level descriptors apply.

Extract data from the included studies

Generally, the data that are collected from quantitative research papers concern participant details, intervention details, outcome measures used, results of the study and the study methodology.[24] For qualitative research studies, the data to be extracted include setting, participant details, methodology and methods used, phenomenon of interest, cultural and geographical information, and findings of the study (such as the themes, metaphors or categories reported). Standardised data collection tools or processes are typically established regardless of the type of review so that the data are collected in a consistent manner and are relevant to the research question.

Synthesise the data

Before we explain what review authors do at this stage of the process, you first need to understand the principles of meta-analysis and meta-aggregation in more detail. We will deal with both issues, starting with the principles for conducting a meta-analysis. As we mentioned at the beginning of this chapter, a meta-analysis pools the data obtained from all studies answering the same clinical question included in a systematic review and produces an overall summary effect. The rationale behind a meta-analysis is that, as you are combining the samples of individual studies, the overall sample size is increased, which improves the power of the analysis as well as the precision of the estimates of the effects of the intervention.[18]

When review authors plan a systematic review, the process by which they will conduct the meta-analysis should be clearly outlined. It has been suggested that the process should include the following steps:[27]

1. The analysis strategy should clearly match the goals of the review.
2. Decide what types of study designs should be included in the meta-analysis.
3. Establish the criteria that would be used to decide whether or not to complete a meta-analysis (see when not to complete a meta-analysis, below).
4. Identify what types of outcome data are likely to be found in the studies and outline how each will be managed.
5. Identify in advance what effects measures will be used.
6. Decide the type of meta-analysis that will be used (random effects, fixed effects, or both).
7. Decide how clinical and methodological diversity will be managed, what characteristics would define the heterogeneity and if and how this will be incorporated into the analysis.
8. Decide how risk of bias in included studies will be assessed and addressed in the analysis.
9. Decide on how missing data will be managed.
10. Decide how publication and reporting bias will be managed.

There are two stages to doing a meta-analysis. First, the intervention effect, including the confidence intervals, for each of the studies is calculated. The statistics used will depend on the type of outcome data found in the studies, with commonly used statistics including odds ratios, risk ratios (also known as relative risks) and mean differences.[18] As we saw in Chapter 4 when learning how to interpret the results of randomised controlled trials, if the outcome is dichotomous then odds ratios or risk ratios may be used. For continuous outcomes, mean differences may be used.

TABLE 12.2: EXAMPLES OF STATISTICAL MEASURES OF INTERVENTION EFFECT THAT CAN BE USED IN A META-ANALYSIS	
Type of outcome data	Measures of intervention effect
Dichotomous or binary (one of two categories)	Risk ratio (RR) (also called relative risk) Odds ratio (OR) Risk difference (RD) Number needed to treat (NNT)
Continuous (numerical)	Mean difference
Ordinal (including measurement scales)	Proportional odds ratio Recalculated as binary data
Counts and rates (for example, number of events)	Rate ratio
Time to event (survival data)	Hazard ratio

Table 12.2 lists some of the statistical measures of intervention effect that can be used in a meta-analysis based on the outcome data type as outlined in the *Cochrane Handbook for Systematic Reviews of Interventions.*[27]

The second stage in a meta-analysis is calculating the overall intervention effect. This is generally an average of the summary statistics from the individual studies, each weighted to adjust for its sample size and variance. This is described in more detail later in this chapter.

The procedure of meta-aggregation used in qualitative evidence synthesis involves three steps: (1) assembling the findings of studies (variously reported as themes, metaphors, categories); (2) pooling them through further aggregation based on similarity in meaning, to (3) arrive at a set of synthesised statements presented as 'lines of action' for practice and policy.[12] In extracting the themes (step 1) identified by the authors of original studies, the reviewer takes the literal descriptions presented in the results sections of original articles into account and maintains representativeness with the primary literature. Similarity of meaning on the level of categories (step 2) is contingent on the reviewer's knowledge and understanding of the included studies. Having read and re-read the articles and extracted the findings from each included study, the reviewer looks for commonality in the themes and metaphors across all studies. Similarity may be *conceptual* (where a particular theme, metaphor or part thereof is identified across multiple papers) or *descriptive* (where the terminology associated with a theme or metaphor is consistent across studies). The actual move from findings to categories is similar to the procedures used in primary qualitative research methods (such as constant comparative analysis and thematic analysis). However, in a primary qualitative research project, the end result is a particular framework, matrix or conceptual model. In a meta-aggregation, it is declamatory statements or 'lines of action' (step 3) that are arrived at.[12] An adapted version of the process of meta-aggregation[28] is illustrated in Figure 12.2.

Interpret and report the results

The results of a systematic review are presented in the text, while the results of a meta-analysis are also displayed visually using a forest plot. Forest plots are made up of tree plots (explained in Chapter 4 and in Figure 4.3) represented in one figure. They display both the information from the individual studies included in the review (such as the intervention effect and the associated confidence interval) *and* an estimate of the overall effect (see Figure 12.4 later in the chapter). In some systematic reviews it is not proper to statistically combine data (because of *heterogeneity*, meaning the studies are not similar enough

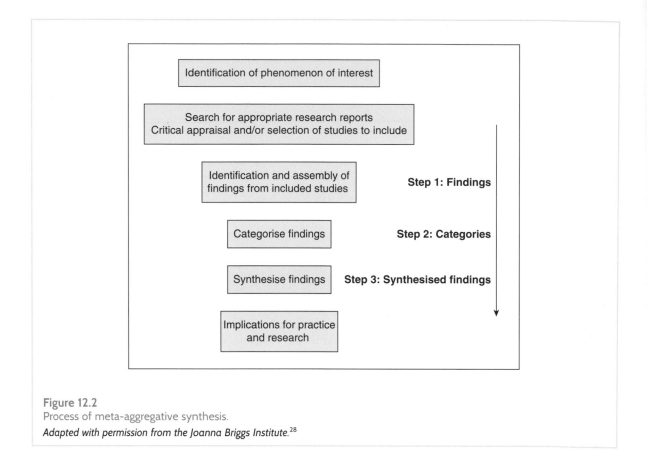

Figure 12.2
Process of meta-aggregative synthesis.
Adapted with permission from the Joanna Briggs Institute.[28]

in one or more respects); forest plots may still be presented but without an overall estimate (summary statistic). Forest plots are useful, as they allow readers to visually assess the amount of variation among the studies that are included in the review.[18]

How do you interpret a forest plot?

There was a previous convention that risk ratios and odds ratios less than 1 indicated that the experimental intervention was more effective than the control. When looking at the forest plot, this would mean that effect estimates to the left of the vertical line (the line of no effect) implied that the intervention was beneficial. This convention is no longer used, as the position of the effect estimates on the forest plot is influenced by the nature of the outcome (that is, outcome of benefit or harm). Instead, when interpreting a forest plot you should look for descriptors on the horizontal axis of the plot to indicate which side of the line of no effect is associated with benefit from the intervention.[29] We will take a closer look at interpreting a forest plot towards the end of this chapter when we look at the results from a specific systematic review.

Not all systematic reviews can undertake a meta-analysis, particularly when there is excessive heterogeneity. This means that the studies are not similar enough to allow them to be combined—for example because the interventions or outcomes were too different. For example, in a systematic review of family therapy for depression, three trials were found but the results were not combined as the studies were very heterogeneous in terms of the interventions, participants and measurement instruments that were involved.[30] These differences mean that pooling results is not appropriate. When this occurs, review authors describe the results of each study separately in a narrative way.

Conclusions that may be reached in systematic reviews include:

1. The results from a review consistently show positive (or negative) effects of an intervention. In this case a review might state that the results (that is, the evidence) are convincing.
2. Where there are conflicting results from studies within the review, the authors might state that the evidence is inconclusive.
3. A number of reviews find only a few studies (or sometimes none) that meet their eligibility criteria and conclude that there is insufficient evidence about that particular intervention.

As a reader of systematic reviews it is important that you do not confuse the concept of 'no evidence' (or 'no evidence of an effect') with 'evidence of no effect'. In other words, when there is inconclusive evidence, it is incorrect to state that the results of the review show that an intervention has 'no effect' or is 'no different' from the control intervention.[25]

For qualitative evidence syntheses, supporting tools such as the System for the Unified Management, Assessment and Review of Information (SUMARI) software and the Qualitative Assessment and Review Instrument (QARI) have been developed. These can be used to assist reviewers who are conducting a meta-aggregative approach in documenting each step of their decision process and linking synthesised statements to the findings retrieved from original studies.[31]

The outcome of a meta-aggregation generally looks like a chart such as the one presented in Figure 12.3.[32]

In meta-synthesis approaches that are interpretive in nature, research findings are more often presented as a web of ideas, theory or conceptual model. Their graphical display is less linear than the meta-aggregative type of presentation of findings that leads to particular lines of action. Two different formulations of a synthesised statement have been proposed that indicate direct action: an if-then structure or a declamatory form.[12] Both forms help authors of evidence syntheses to formulate suggestions to health professionals and policy makers on how to move forward with the results of the review.

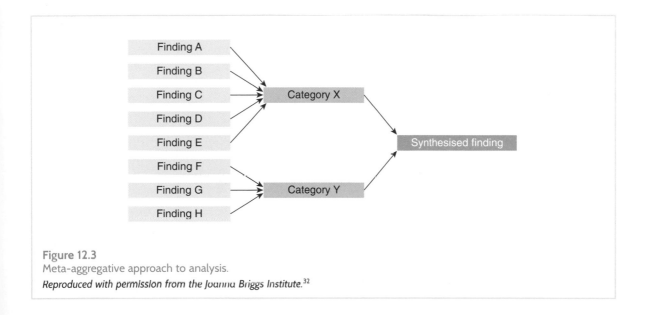

Figure 12.3
Meta-aggregative approach to analysis.
Reproduced with permission from the Joanna Briggs Institute.[32]

Two examples of the final syntheses derived from already published meta-aggregations are provided below:

- *Using the 'if-then' structure:* a review of caregivers' experiences of providing home-based care for people with HIV in Africa concluded that '*if* formal and informal support structures are available to caregivers providing home-based care to persons with HIV/AIDS, *then* the challenges and burdens they face may be lessened'.[33]

- *Using the declamatory form:* a review that explored the experiences of overseas-trained registered nurses working in Australia suggested that 'the clash of cultures between overseas nurses and the dominant Australian culture should be addressed in a transition program'.[34]

These forms emphasise the probability of the claim and lead directly to an operational prediction. In these cases, the 'line of action' is for putting in place formal and informal support structures, respectively, for 'inclusion of cultural awareness training in transition programs'. In practice, the synthesised statements are often accompanied by a short narrative summary.[35]

CRITICAL APPRAISAL OF SYSTEMATIC REVIEWS

Now that you have an understanding of what is involved in undertaking a systematic review of quantitative or qualitative studies, let us move on to looking at how to critically appraise systematic reviews. As with other types of studies, not all systematic reviews are carried out using rigorous methods and, therefore, bias may be introduced into the final results and conclusions of the review. A review of 300 systematic reviews found that not all systematic reviews were equally reliable and that their reporting could be improved if widely agreed reporting standards were adhered to by authors and journals.[36] Just because the evidence that you have found to answer your clinical question is a systematic review, this does not mean that you can automatically trust the results of that review. It is important that you critically appraise systematic reviews and determine whether you can trust their results and conclusions.

Using the three-step critical appraisal process that we have used elsewhere in this book to appraise other types of studies, the three key elements to be considered when appraising a systematic review are: (1) the validity of the review methodology; (2) the magnitude and precision of the intervention effect (or the trustworthiness of the findings for qualitative evidence syntheses); and (3) the applicability of the review to your specific patient or patient population.

There are a number of checklists or tools that can be used to critically appraise systematic reviews, many of which are based on the early Overview of Quality Assessment Questionnaire[37] and the article on overviews in the users' guide to evidence-based medicine.[38] Three commonly used appraisal checklists are the CASP checklist for appraising reviews (casp-uk.net); the Assessment of Multiple Systematic Reviews (AMSTAR)—an 11-item tool for that has good agreement, reliability, construct validity and feasibility;[39] and the criteria proposed by Greenhalgh and Donald.[40] Checklists or frameworks for appraising reviews of qualitative as well as quantitative studies are also available.[41]

Box 12.1 lists key questions that you can ask when critically appraising a systematic review. These questions are adapted from the appraisal criteria suggested by Greenhalgh and Donald.[40]

CRITICAL APPRAISAL OF SYSTEMATIC REVIEWS– A WORKED EXAMPLE

To help you further understand how to critically appraise and use systematic reviews to inform clinical decisions, we will consider an extended clinical scenario (with two parts), formulate relevant clinical questions, locate a systematic review of quantitative studies *and* a review of qualitative studies that might address those questions and then critically appraise the reviews. The box describes the clinical scenario that we will use.

Key questions to ask when critically appraising a systematic review

A. WERE THE METHODS USED IN THE REVIEW VALID?

1. Did the review address a clearly focused question with clearly defined eligibility criteria? The question should be focused in terms of the:
   a. Participants
   b. Intervention(s) and comparison(s)
   c. Outcome(s)

2. Did the review include high quality, relevant studies?
   a. Of robust study design (for example, randomised controlled trials)?
   b. That addressed relevant questions?
   c. Selected by more than one independent assessor?

3. Is it unlikely that the review missed important, relevant studies?
   a. Is the search strategy reproducible?
   b. Did the search strategy include synonyms for all terms?
   c. Is the search strategy sufficiently comprehensive? (Consider what sources were searched—for example, bibliographic databases, trial registers, unpublished literature, hand-searching, reference lists, correspondence with experts, unpublished data.)

4. Did the review include an assessment of the risk of bias of included studies and was this assessment incorporated into the review findings?
   a. Is the method for assessing risk of bias reproducible?
   b. Is the method for assessing risk of bias adequate?
   c. Was the risk of bias assessment conducted by more than one independent assessor?
   d. Was the risk of bias assessment incorporated into the review findings? For example, were results analysed for different sets of studies according to level of bias evident (sometimes referred to as *sensitivity analyses*) where possible?

5. Did the review combine the results from studies and, if so, was it reasonable to do so?
   a. Were the results similar from study to study (was an examination of heterogeneity undertaken)? In systematic reviews this might be tested statistically using the I^2 statistic or by looking at the degree of overlap between the studies' confidence intervals.
   b. Were reasons for variations in results discussed?

B. WHAT ARE THE RESULTS OF THE REVIEW?

1. What are the overall results of the review?
2. How precise are the results?

C. HOW RELEVANT ARE THE RESULTS TO ME?

1. Were all important outcomes considered (from the points of view of individuals/patients, policy makers, healthcare professionals, family/carers, the wider community)?
2. Can the results be applied to my patient/s? Consider how well your patient(s) and practice setting compare with the review population—for example, participant characteristics and disease/impairment characteristics, intervention(s) and outcomes(s).

CLINICAL SCENARIO (PART 1)

Clinical question and finding the evidence to answer the question

James, Samantha and Louise are a physiotherapist, occupational therapist and speech language pathologist who have been working in the acute care wards of a large regional hospital. They have been involved in an ongoing debate with the administration of the hospital about stroke patients who continue to be triaged to various medical wards on admission rather than consistently admitted to the stroke unit. They are concerned that patients who are sent to regular medical wards may not receive the optimal care and therapy that is needed to achieve the best outcomes after stroke. The administrator argues that patients still have access to all of the therapies in the regular medical wards.

To assist with clarifying their thoughts and developing an argument in preparation for a meeting that will be taking place the following week, the therapists decide to do a search of the literature to see whether there is any evidence to inform the debate. They know that the hospital administration is worried about the costs involved and the decreased flexibility to manage the overall hospital and feels that the benefits do not outweigh the costs. The team formed the clinical question:

- For people with acute stroke who are admitted to hospital, do patients cared for in stroke units have greater improvements in independence compared with patients who are cared for in general medical wards?

They searched using the phrase "stroke unit*'" in the search box on the home page of the Cochrane Library and located a systematic review[42] in the *Cochrane Database of Systematic Reviews* that appears relevant to their question.

CLINICAL SCENARIO (CONTINUED)

Structured abstract of chosen quantitative article

Citation: Stroke Unit Trialists' Collaboration. Organised inpatient (stroke unit) care for stroke. *Cochrane Database of Systematic Reviews* 2007;(4):CD000197. doi:10.1002/14651858.CD000197. pub2. The structured abstract has been adapted from this reference.

Objectives: The aim of this systematic review was to compare the effectiveness of care received in stroke units with other types of care.

Search strategy: The authors searched the Cochrane Stroke Group trials register and the reference lists of studies found through the initial search, and contacted researchers who were working in this area. The search was not limited by date or language.

Selection criteria: Individual studies that were included in the review were randomised controlled clinical trials that compared organised inpatient stroke unit care with an alternative form of care.

Data collection and analysis: The eligibility and quality of randomised controlled trials were assessed by two reviewers.

Main results: The review included 31 trials and found that more-organised care was associated with improved outcomes. In 26 trials, care in general wards was compared with care in stroke units. Stroke-unit care showed reductions in the odds of death at 1 year follow-up (odds ratio [OR] 0.86; 95% confidence interval [CI] 0.76 to 0.98), the odds of death or institutionalised care (OR 0.82; 95% CI 0.73 to 0.92) and death or dependency (OR 0.82; 95% CI 0.73 to 0.92). Organised stroke-unit care did not increase the length of hospital stay.

Authors' conclusions: People who had a stroke were more likely to have better outcomes in terms of survival, independence and avoiding institutional care when they received care in an organised inpatient stroke unit compared with those who did not receive care in a stroke unit.

Finding qualitative evidence relevant to the scenario

James, Samantha, and Louise are happy with the information they found. However, it is their general feeling that in order to present a stronger case at next week's meeting, it would be better to present additional information on the experiences of patients recovering from stroke. It is their opinion that health professionals may lack understanding of what patients think is important in the process of recovering from stroke, and how patients interpret and manage recovery after stroke. They search in PubMed, using the Health Services Research Queries (which is accessed through the 'Topic-specific queries' link on PubMed) and with 'qualitative research' category and 'narrow scope' selected and the search terms:

recover* AND stroke AND review

This resulted in 23 articles and they chose what appeared to be the most relevant review: a systematic review of qualitative studies which explored the psychosocial and spiritual experiences of elderly people recovering from stroke.[43] Despite the fact that the target group within this review somewhat differs from the general population addressed in the Cochrane systematic review of randomised controlled trials that the team had previously located, they decide to give it a closer look.

Structured abstract of chosen qualitative article

Citation: Lamb M, Buchanan D, Godfrey C, et al. The psychosocial spiritual experience of elderly individuals recovering from stroke: a systematic review. *International Journal of Evidence-Based Healthcare* 2008;6:173–205. Structured abstract reproduced with permission.

Objectives: To appraise and synthesise the best available evidence on the psychosocial, spiritual experience of elderly individuals recovering from stroke.

Selection criteria: Qualitative studies whose participants were adults, 65 years and older, and who had experienced at least one stroke. Studies were included that described the participant's own experience of recovering from stroke.

Search strategy: The review search strategy sought to find both published and unpublished studies and was not limited to English-language studies. An initial limited search of MEDLINE and CINAHL was undertaken, followed by an analysis of textwords contained in the title and abstract and of index terms used to describe the article. A second extensive search was then undertaken using all identified key words and index terms.

Methodological quality: Each study was assessed by two independent reviewers for methodological quality prior to inclusion in the review, using the Qualitative Assessment and Review Instrument (QARI). Disagreements were resolved through consultation with a third reviewer.

Data collection: Information was extracted from each study independently by two reviewers using the QARI data extraction tool. Disagreements were resolved through consultation with a third reviewer.

Data synthesis: Data synthesis aimed to portray an accurate interpretation and synthesis of concepts arising from the selected population's experience during their recovery from stroke. The process of meta-synthesis using this program involved categorising findings and developing synthesised topics from the categories.

Results: A total of 35 studies were identified and of those, 27 studies were included in the review. Four syntheses were developed related to the perceptions and experiences of stroke survivors: sudden unexpected event, connectedness, reconstruction of life and life-altering event.

Conclusion: The onset and early period following a stroke is a confusing and terrifying experience. The period of recovery involves considerable psychological and physical work for elderly individuals to reconstruct their lives. For those with a spiritual tradition, connectedness to others and spiritual connection is important during recovery. The experience of stroke is a life-altering one for most elderly individuals, involving profound changes in functioning and sense of self.

Using the questions that are outlined in Box 12.1, we will now step you through a critical appraisal of both the quantitative and the qualitative systematic reviews, alternating between each review for each item.

A. Were the methods used in the review valid?

1. Did the review address a clearly focused question with clearly defined eligibility criteria?

Review of quantitative studies

Yes. The research question for this review is concisely and clearly spelt out in the abstract. 'Objective: To assess the effect of stroke unit care compared with alternative forms of care for patients following a stroke.' The question is elaborated on further in the study, but is still clearly defined prior to the review being completed.

a. *Participants:*

Yes. The review stated that 'Any patients admitted to hospital who had suffered a stroke were eligible. We recorded the delay between stroke onset and hospital admission but did not use this as an exclusion criterion. We used a clinical definition of stroke: focal neurological deficit due to cerebrovascular disease, excluding subarachnoid haemorrhage and subdural haematoma.'

b. *Intervention(s) and comparison(s):*

Yes. The intervention under consideration in this review included stroke wards, acute stroke units which accept patients acutely but discharge early, rehabilitation stroke units and comprehensive stroke units (that is, combined acute and rehabilitation care). Each of these interventions was clearly defined in the review. The comparisons included mixed rehabilitation wards, mobile stroke teams or general medical wards.

c. *Outcome(s):*

Yes. As stated in this review, 'The primary analysis examined death, dependency and the requirement for institutional care at the end of scheduled follow-up of the original trial (two trials subsequently extended follow-up). Dependency was categorised into two groups where "independent" was taken to mean that an individual did not require physical assistance for transfers, mobility, dressing, feeding or toileting. Individuals who failed any of these criteria were considered "dependent." The criteria for independence were approximately equivalent to a modified Rankin score of 0 to 2, a Barthel Index of more than 18 out of 20, or an Activity Index (AI) of more than 83. The requirement for long-term institutional care was taken to mean care in a residential home, nursing home, or hospital at the end of scheduled follow-up. Secondary outcome measures included patient quality of life, patient and carer satisfaction, and duration of stay in hospital or institution or both.'

Review of qualitative studies (meta-aggregation)

No. The authors have not formulated a particular research question to be answered. However, the objective of the review is clear and it is stipulated as 'to appraise and synthesise the best available evidence on the psychosocial and spiritual experience of elderly individuals recovering from stroke.'

a. *Participants:*

Yes. This review included studies whose participants were adults, 65 years or older, in any setting, who had experienced a minimum of one stroke.

b. *Where relevant: Intervention(s) and comparison(s):*

Yes. Some qualitative evidence syntheses will evaluate experiences or opinions related to particular interventions. However, this should not be considered a standard approach to qualitative synthesis. Authors of reviews of qualitative studies should specify their particular research interest instead. This review indicates that the interest was both in experiences of recovering from stroke in relation to particular interventions, and in including descriptions of patients' experiences where intervention was not the focus.

c. *Evaluation (Outcomes):*

Yes. The authors list a couple of issues they intended to evaluate, more specifically the participant's experience through self-report. Reports from family and caregivers were excluded. Types of outcomes included sense of hope, hopelessness, connection and disconnection with others, disruptions in the sense of self and experience of time, loss, independence/dependence, discontinuity with previous way of life and sense of control.

2. Did the review include high quality, relevant studies?

Review of quantitative studies

a *Of robust study design?*

Yes. The review authors stated that they 'included all prospective trials that used some form of random allocation of stroke patients to an organised system of inpatient (stroke unit) care or an alternative form of inpatient care. Trials were included if treatment allocation was carried out on a strictly random basis or with a quasi-random procedure (such as bed availability or date of admission).'

b. *That addressed relevant questions?*

Yes. Refer to previous point.

c. *Selected by more than one independent assessor?*

Yes. The review stated that two review authors assessed the eligibility and methodological quality of published trials.

Review of qualitative studies (meta-aggregation)

a. *Of robust study design?*

Yes. The authors included all relevant, qualitative research papers that met the quality criteria according to their critical appraisal exercise using QARI. It is unclear, however, what their definition of a qualitative research paper is. They mention a few research designs, but also state that opinion papers, editorials or descriptive papers without a clear methods and findings section were excluded from their study.

b. *That addressed relevant questions?*

While this review had no specific research question, the studies selected seem to address the objective of the review.

c. *Selected by more than one independent assessor?*

No. There is no indication that the retrieved studies were screened for relevance by two different researchers. However, once selected, they were assessed for methodological validity by two independent reviewers prior to inclusion in the review.

3. Is it unlikely that the review missed important, relevant studies?

Review of quantitative studies

a. *Is the search strategy reproducible?*

Yes. The full search strategy used in this review is not documented within the review itself, but the authors provide a link to the Cochrane Stroke Group methods used in reviews, which provides the full search strategy.

b. *Did the search strategy include synonyms for all terms?*

Yes. The search strategy that was used (listed in the Cochrane Stroke Group) provides synonyms for all relevant terms.

c. *Is the search strategy sufficiently comprehensive?*
Yes, given that all trials in most databases (such as CINAHL, EMBASE) had been located and entered into the Cochrane Stroke Group Trials Register (see Cochrane Stroke Group Methods). The review authors stated that they 'searched the Cochrane Stroke Group Trials Register, which was last searched by the Review Group Coordinator in April 2006. In an effort to identify further published, unpublished and ongoing trials, we scanned the reference lists of relevant articles, contacted colleagues and researchers and publicised our preliminary findings at stroke conferences in the UK, Scandinavia, Germany, Netherlands, Switzerland, Spain, Canada, South America, Australia, Belgium, USA and Hong Kong. The search was not restricted by date, language or any other criteria to the best of our knowledge.'

Review of qualitative studies (meta-aggregation)

a. *Is the search strategy reproducible?*
No. The authors did not include a comprehensive list of key terms that were used to conduct the searches. They used a two-step search approach in scoping the literature, followed by an analysis of the keywords in title and abstract. The keywords and index terms from this analysis were then used to search various electronic databases.

b. *Did the search strategy include synonyms for all terms?*
No. The authors did not include a comprehensive list of key terms so it is hard to determine whether sufficient synonyms were used.

c. *Is the search strategy sufficiently comprehensive?*
No. The authors claim to have searched for published and unpublished studies. They list a variety of databases that were searched and report that reference lists of relevant studies were checked. However, these strategies would not identify unpublished studies. It is also unclear whether the search was comprehensive regarding locating non-English-language studies. Information on the dates of the search is also not provided.

4. Did the review include an assessment of the risk of bias of included studies and was this assessment incorporated into the review findings?

Review of quantitative studies

a. *Is the method for assessing risk of bias reproducible?*
Yes. The review authors stated that they 'did not use a formal scoring system to record methodological quality but recorded the method of allocation concealment, completeness of follow-up, presence of an intention-to-treat analysis and the presence of a blinded assessment of outcome.'

b. *Is the method for assessing risk of bias adequate?*
Yes, as above.

c. *Was the risk of bias assessment conducted by more than one independent assessor?*
Yes. The review stated that two review authors assessed the eligibility and methodological quality of published trials.

d *Was the risk of bias assessment incorporated into the review findings (for example, were sensitivity analyses used where possible)?*
Yes. The review stated: 'In view of the variety of trial methodologies described we carried out a sensitivity analysis based only on those trials with a low risk of bias: (1) secure randomisation procedures; (2) unequivocally blinded outcome assessment; (3) a fixed one-year period of follow-up. Seven trials are known to have met all of these criteria.'

Review of qualitative studies (meta-aggregation)

a. *Is the method for assessing risk of bias reproducible?*
Yes. The authors include the QARI tool that was used to appraise the qualitative studies and formulate a cut-off point of 6/10 to pass the quality appraisal. They explain the exclusion of eight studies in an appendix.

b. *Is the method for assessing risk of bias adequate?*
Yes. The QARI tool has been compared with other instruments and has been found adequate to evaluate the validity and overall quality of studies.[44] The cut-off point of 6/10 is, however, not explained by the authors.

c. *Was the risk of bias assessment conducted by more than one independent assessor?*
Yes. The review stated that two review authors assessed the methodological quality of the studies.

d. *Was the risk of bias assessment incorporated into the review findings (for example, were sensitivity analyses used where possible)?*
No. A sensitivity analysis has not been conducted. However, only the findings from the 27 studies that passed the cut-off point are combined in the overall synthesis. Reasons for excluding eight studies are provided in an appendix to the article.

5. Did the review combine the results from studies and, if so, was it reasonable to do so?

Review of quantitative studies

a. *Were the results similar from study to study (was an examination of heterogeneity undertaken)?*
Yes. Tests of heterogeneity were undertaken for all pooled outcomes. For the outcomes of 'death', 'death or institutional care' and 'death or dependency', there was no evidence of substantial heterogeneity in any of the comparisons, indicating that the results were similar from study to study for these outcomes. However, the outcome of 'length of stay (days) in a hospital or institution or both' had considerable heterogeneity.

b. *Were reasons for variations in results discussed?*
Somewhat. Some attempt at explaining variations in results for the outcome 'length of stay (days) in a hospital or institution or both' was made by the authors. They argued that length of stay was calculated in different ways, some trials recorded median rather than mean data and some trials did not provide measures of variability for effect estimates. They concluded: 'The analysis of length of stay is complicated by the different methods of reporting results, the widely varying baseline lengths of stay and the statistically significant heterogeneity between different trials.'

Review of qualitative studies (meta-aggregation)

a. *Were the results similar from study to study (was an examination of heterogeneity undertaken)?*
No. The results were not similar. However, this is not a prerequisite to conducting a meta-aggregation. The authors clearly indicate which finding is retrieved from which study and repeat these findings under the themes that have been derived from the analysis.

b. *Were reasons for variations in results discussed?*
No. However, the authors do attempt to discuss the experiences of stroke survivors with sensitivity to individual differences. One such example is the statement that those with comorbidities see discontinuity after the recovery of stroke as one particular event in their lifetime and those without comorbidities perceive the event as a discontinuity in their lives in general.

The importance of reporting in systematic reviews

Determining the methodological quality or risk of bias of a systematic review depends on how well the details of how the systematic review was conducted are reported. Based on studies which found that systematic reviews were generally poorly reported,[45] an international group developed a reporting guideline for reporting details of meta-analyses of randomised controlled trials called the QUOROM Statement (QUality Of Reporting Of Meta-analyses).[46] In 2009, the guideline was updated to encompass all types of systematic reviews about the effects of interventions, not just those using meta-analyses of randomised controlled trials. This reporting statement is called the Preferred Reporting Items for Systematic Reviews and Meta-Analyses, or the PRISMA statement.[47] Reporting statements improve the quality of *reporting* of studies[48] and therefore it is now recommended, or often insisted on, by an increasing number of journals that review authors use the PRISMA statement when writing their reviews.[49]

B. What are the results of the review?

In the stroke unit systematic quantitative review, you can see that the authors were dealing with dichotomous outcomes and therefore used odds ratios to calculate effect measures. The review authors state that they 'analysed dichotomous outcomes as the odds ratio (OR) with 95% confidence interval (CI) of an adverse outcome' and explained the statistical models used to do so. They went on to elaborate that 'subgroup analyses involved a re-analysis stratified by patient or service subgroup using tabular subgroup data provided by the trialists. We analysed data on length of stay in a hospital or institution using standardised mean difference ...'

In the meta-aggregation review, the authors strictly followed the three-step approach that was outlined earlier in this chapter. They indicate that where textual pooling was not possible, a narrative form was used.

1. What are the overall results of the review?

Review of quantitative studies

When organised stroke-unit care was compared with an alternative service, it was found that 'Case fatality recorded at the end of scheduled follow-up (median follow-up 12 months; range six weeks to 12 months) was lower in the organised (stroke unit) care in 22 of the 31 trial comparisons. The overall estimate gave an odds ratio of 0.82 (95% CI 0.73 to 0.92; $p = 0.001$), which was not complicated by statistically significant heterogeneity between trials.'

When reporting the second outcome, which was the odds of death or requiring institutional care at the end of scheduled follow-up, the review found a highly statistically significant result (OR 0.81; 95% CI 0.74 to 0.90; $p < 0.0001$) and no statistically significant heterogeneity between the trials.

The third outcome that was analysed was the combined adverse outcome of being dead or dependent in activities of daily living at the end of the scheduled follow-up. The authors report that 'the summary odds ratio for being dead or dependent if receiving organised (stroke unit) care rather than alternative (less organised) services was 0.79 (95% CI 0.71 to 0.88; $p < 0.0001$), indicating a significant reduction in odds of death or dependency in the organised (stroke unit) care group. There was no statistically significant heterogeneity between trials.'

Review of qualitative studies (meta-aggregation)

Meta-synthesis of included studies generated four synthesised findings. These synthesised findings were derived from 165 study findings that were subsequently aggregated into 20 categories. These categories were then analysed to identify four synthesised statements:

1. *Connectedness*–elderly individuals who have experienced stroke identify the importance of connectedness in their process of recovery.
2. *Reconstructing life*–elderly individuals describe the recovery process as reconstructing their lives following stroke. They are engaged in the recovery.
3. *Life-altering event*–individuals perceive the stroke as having life-altering consequences.
4. *Sudden unexpected event*–stroke survivors perceive the stroke experience as having a sudden onset, generating shock, fear and confusion.

2. How precise are the results?

Review of quantitative studies

The precision of the summary effect-size estimates that are reported in the previous results section is relatively high, as the confidence intervals are quite narrow.

Earlier in this chapter we introduced the idea of forest plots as a way of visually representing the results from multiple studies within a systematic review. Let us look at the first forest plot from the stroke unit systematic review,[42] shown in Figure 12.4, in a bit more detail. We find that the forest plot is labelled to show that effect measures to the *left* of the vertical line favour the intervention and those to the *right* of the line favour the control (comparison intervention).

The top of each forest plot is labelled to tell you what the **comparisons** are. The first forest plot that is included in the systematic review (and shown in Figure 12.4) is titled 'Organised stroke unit care versus alternative service' and has several subgroup analyses involved, with the first comparison being stroke ward versus general medical ward. The **outcome** of interest to each forest plot is also identified at the top of the forest plot. The outcome being reported in this forest plot is 'death by the end of scheduled follow-up'.

Each forest plot consists of a number of **horizontal lines**, with each horizontal line representing one of the individual studies that is included in the review. The length of the horizontal line represents the precision of the result or the confidence interval of the result of the study. In the forest plot in Figure 12.4, the first subgroup analysis involved 16 studies. There is a **square** on each of the lines which represents the intervention effect estimate from each of the individual studies. The **diamond** at the bottom of the plot represents the pooled quantitative result from the meta-analysis of the first subgroup.

At the bottom of the forest plot there is a line that tells you the *scale* for the intervention effect that you are measuring and at the top of the vertical line the type of effect (for example, odds ratio) is identified. In this example forest plot, it is the odds ratio. The **vertical line** in the middle of the plot is the line of no effect where the treatment and the placebo have the same effect on the risk of death in the follow-up period after stroke. To the left of the line, where the odds ratio is less than 1, the interpretation is that the intervention (organised stroke unit care) made death during follow-up less likely. Results to the right of the vertical line, where the odds ratio is greater than 1, mean the intervention made the risk of death during the follow-up period more likely.

The second and third columns in the forest plot are headed 'Treatment n/N' and 'Control n/N'. The 'n' represents the number of deaths in the group (treatment or control) and the 'N' represents the total number of participants in the group. The weight column (the fifth column in this forest plot) is the percentage weight given to each of the individual studies in the pooled meta-analysis. The weight used is a function of the sample size and its variance. The size of the square on each of the horizontal lines is proportional to the percentage of weight that is given to the study in the meta-analysis.

If the horizontal line for a study crosses the vertical line, it means that the study found no significant difference between the two groups. In our example forest plot, all of the studies except two (Athens and Orpington 1995)[50,51] cross the vertical line. The study given the largest weight is the second study in the analysis (author is Athens). The squares positioned to the left of the vertical line show that those studies found that the stroke unit was beneficial compared with the general ward. The squares positioned to the right of the vertical line show that the studies found that the general ward was beneficial compared with the stroke unit.

As mentioned earlier in this chapter, the middle of the diamond is the pooled treatment effect calculated in the meta-analysis. The **width of the diamond** is the certainty of the result, generally the 95% confidence interval.[52] In the first subgroup analysis shown in the forest plot, the intervention effect is significant. That is, the stroke ward was more effective than the general ward in reducing the number of deaths in the follow-up period after stroke. If the confidence interval crosses the vertical line, as is the case in the second subgroup analysis in our example forest plot, this indicates that there was no significant difference between the effectiveness of a mixed rehabilitation ward versus a general medical ward.

Review of qualitative studies (meta-aggregation)

Precision of results is not particularly relevant to a qualitative evidence synthesis. One should evaluate the richness of the findings instead. The authors have provided the reader with a very rich description of the experiences of elderly individuals recovering from stroke. Statements from the researcher are consequently informed by interview excerpts from the raw data. The authors' conclusion matches the outline of the findings as presented in Figure 12.5.[53]

Analysis 1.1. Comparison 1 Organised stroke unit care versus alternative service, Outcome 1 Death by the end of scheduled follow up.

Review: Organised inpatient (stroke unit) care for stroke

Comparison: 1 Organised stroke unit care versus alternative service

Outcome: 1 Death by the end of scheduled follow up

Study or sub group	Treatment n/N	Control n/N	Peto Odds Ratio Peto.Fixed. 95% CI	Weight	Peto Odds Ratio Peto.Fixed. 95% CI
1. Stroke ward versus general medical ward					
Akershus	61/271	70/279		13.8%	0.87 [0.59, 1.28]
Athens	103/302	127/302		19.7%	0.71 [0.51, 0.99]
Beijing	12/195	19/197		4.0%	0.62 [0.30, 1.29]
Dover (GMW)	34/98	35/89		6.0%	0.82 [0.45, 1.48]
Edinburgh	48/155	55/156		9.5%	0.82 [0.51, 1.32]
Goteborg-Ostra	16/215	12/202		3.6%	1.27 [0.59, 2.73]
Goteborg-Sahlgren	45/166	19/83		5.9%	1.25 [0.68, 2.27]
Joinville	9/35	12/39		2.1%	0.78 [0.29, 2.14]
Nottingham (GMW)	14/98	10/76		2.8%	1.10 [0.46, 2.61]
Orpington 1993 (GMW)	3/53	6/48		1.1%	0.43 [0.11, 1.70]
Orpington 1995	7/34	17/37		2.2%	0.33 [0.12, 0.87]
Perth	4/29	6/30		1.2%	0.65 [0.17, 2.50]
Stockholm	49/269	45/225		10.4%	0.89 [0.57, 1.40]
Svendborg	14/31	12/34		2.2%	1.50 [0.56, 4.02]
Trondheim	27/110	36/110		6.2%	0.67 [0.37, 1.20]
Umea	43/110	75/183		9.2%	0.92 [0.57, 1.50]
Subtotal (95% CI)	**2171**	**2090**		**100%**	**0.83 [0.71, 0.96]**

Total events: 489 (Treatment), 556 (Control)

Heterogeneity: Chi2 = 11.47, df = 15 (p = 0.72); I² = 0.0%

Test for overall effect: z = 2.57 (P = 0.010)

2. Mixed rehabilitation ward versus general medical ward					
Birmingham	4/29	2/23		6.9%	1.63 [0.30, 8.90]
Helsinki	26/121	27/122		54.1%	0.96 [0.52, 1.77]
Illinois	0/56	0/35		0.0%	0.0 [0.0, 0.0]
Kuopio	8/50	10/45		19.1%	0.84 [0.31, 2.28]
New York	0/42	0/40		0.0%	0.0 [0.0, 0.0]
Newcastle	11/34	12/33		19.9%	0.84 [0.31, 2.28]
Subtotal (95% CI)	**332**	**298**		**100%**	**0.91 [0.58, 1.42]**

Total events: 49 (Treatment), 51 (Control)

Heterogeneity: Chi2 = 0.86, df = 3 (p = 0.84); I² = 0.0%

Test for overall effect: z = 0.43 (P = 0.67)

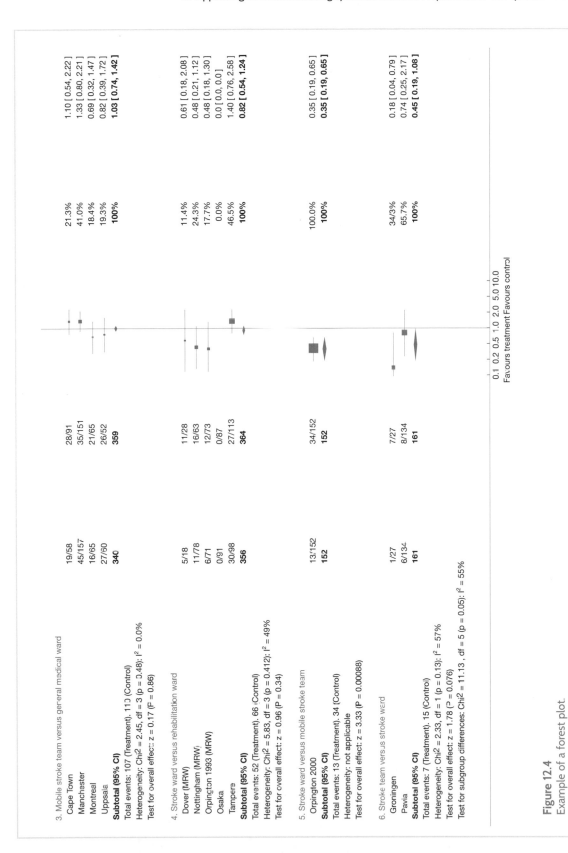

Figure 12.4
Example of a forest plot.

Stroke Unit Trialists' Collaboration, Organised inpatient (stroke unit) care for stroke, Issue 4, 2007.[42] Copyright The Cochrane Collaboration, reproduced with permission.

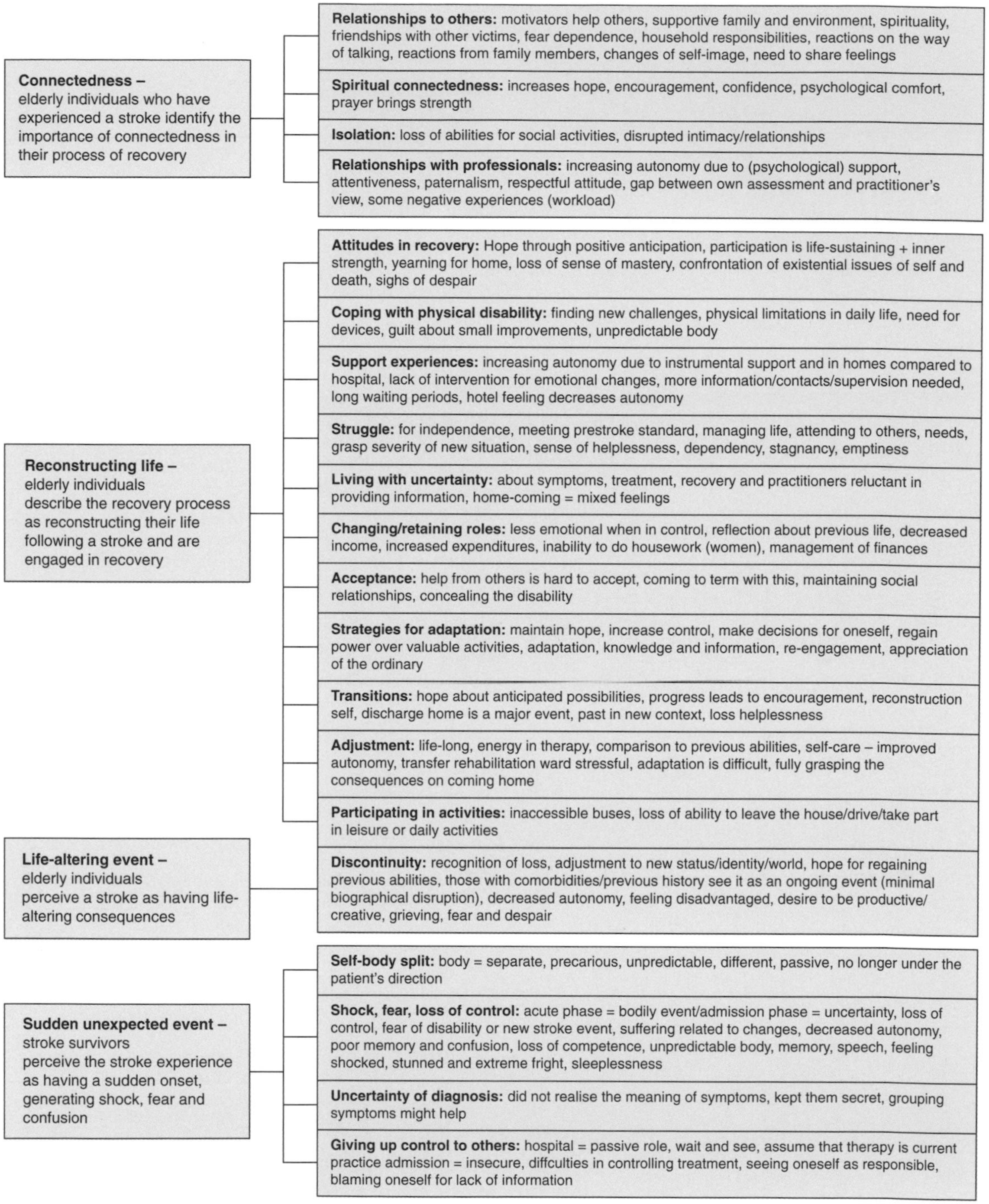

Connectedness – elderly individuals who have experienced a stroke identify the importance of connectedness in their process of recovery

Relationships to others: motivators help others, supportive family and environment, spirituality, friendships with other victims, fear dependence, household responsibilities, reactions on the way of talking, reactions from family members, changes of self-image, need to share feelings

Spiritual connectedness: increases hope, encouragement, confidence, psychological comfort, prayer brings strength

Isolation: loss of abilities for social activities, disrupted intimacy/relationships

Relationships with professionals: increasing autonomy due to (psychological) support, attentiveness, paternalism, respectful attitude, gap between own assessment and practitioner's view, some negative experiences (workload)

Reconstructing life – elderly individuals describe the recovery process as reconstructing their life following a stroke and are engaged in recovery

Attitudes in recovery: Hope through positive anticipation, participation is life-sustaining + inner strength, yearning for home, loss of sense of mastery, confrontation of existential issues of self and death, sighs of despair

Coping with physical disability: finding new challenges, physical limitations in daily life, need for devices, guilt about small improvements, unpredictable body

Support experiences: increasing autonomy due to instrumental support and in homes compared to hospital, lack of intervention for emotional changes, more information/contacts/supervision needed, long waiting periods, hotel feeling decreases autonomy

Struggle: for independence, meeting prestroke standard, managing life, attending to others, needs, grasp severity of new situation, sense of helplessness, dependency, stagnancy, emptiness

Living with uncertainty: about symptoms, treatment, recovery and practitioners reluctant in providing information, home-coming = mixed feelings

Changing/retaining roles: less emotional when in control, reflection about previous life, decreased income, increased expenditures, inability to do housework (women), management of finances

Acceptance: help from others is hard to accept, coming to term with this, maintaining social relationships, concealing the disability

Strategies for adaptation: maintain hope, increase control, make decisions for oneself, regain power over valuable activities, adaptation, knowledge and information, re-engagement, appreciation of the ordinary

Transitions: hope about anticipated possibilities, progress leads to encouragement, reconstruction self, discharge home is a major event, past in new context, loss helplessness

Adjustment: life-long, energy in therapy, comparison to previous abilities, self-care – improved autonomy, transfer rehabilitation ward stressful, adaptation is difficult, fully grasping the consequences on coming home

Participating in activities: inaccessible buses, loss of ability to leave the house/drive/take part in leisure or daily activities

Life-altering event – elderly individuals perceive a stroke as having life-altering consequences

Discontinuity: recognition of loss, adjustment to new status/identity/world, hope for regaining previous abilities, those with comorbidities/previous history see it as an ongoing event (minimal biographical disruption), decreased autonomy, feeling disadvantaged, desire to be productive/creative, grieving, fear and despair

Sudden unexpected event – stroke survivors perceive the stroke experience as having a sudden onset, generating shock, fear and confusion

Self-body split: body = separate, precarious, unpredictable, different, passive, no longer under the patient's direction

Shock, fear, loss of control: acute phase = bodily event/admission phase = uncertainty, loss of control, fear of disability or new stroke event, suffering related to changes, decreased autonomy, poor memory and confusion, loss of competence, unpredictable body, memory, speech, feeling shocked, stunned and extreme fright, sleeplessness

Uncertainty of diagnosis: did not realise the meaning of symptoms, kept them secret, grouping symptoms might help

Giving up control to others: hospital = passive role, wait and see, assume that therapy is current practice admission = insecure, diffculties in controlling treatment, seeing oneself as responsible, blaming oneself for lack of information

Figure 12.5
Meta-synthesis and related categories regarding experience of elderly individuals recovering from stroke.
Reproduced with permission from the Joanna Briggs Institute.[53]

C. How relevant are the results to me?

1. Were all important outcomes considered?

(From the points of view of individuals/patients, policy makers, healthcare professionals, family/carers, and the wider community.)

Review of quantitative studies

For people who have had a stroke, the important outcomes of death, dependency, requirement of institutional care, patient satisfaction and quality of life were considered by the review authors, and results for these outcomes were analysed where available. Other outcomes which may be of interest to policy makers and health professionals are the costs of providing organised stroke-unit care in comparison to general care. The review authors also point out that the results do not explain why stroke units may result in improved patient outcomes. They suggest that this may be the result of a number of factors such as better diagnostic procedures, better nursing care, early mobilisation, the prevention of complications or more effective rehabilitation procedures. These variables may be important to measure in future trials.

Review of qualitative studies (meta-aggregation)

Whether or not the findings from this meta-aggregation are relevant links into the question about whether or not the findings add to the theoretical and practical knowledge base regarding stroke and stroke units. The initial objective to appraise and synthesise the best available evidence on experiences of elderly individuals recovering from stroke has been met. From the findings, a number of implications for healthcare practice are drawn, such as: be sensitive to and acknowledge the overwhelming sense of terror and fear experienced in the early period; facilitate all aspects of connection with family and friends as well as spiritual connection and be alert to signs of isolation in the recovery period; recognise the huge amount of work, both psychological and physical, that is involved in reconstruction of a life and consider a plan of care; consider ways in which the health system, healthcare routines and practices support or do not support elderly persons who are recovering from a stroke; and provide opportunities for elderly persons recovering from a stroke to discuss their perceptions of improvement/progress and how their life has changed. The authors do not provide advice for other potential relevant stakeholders, such as family members, the wider community or policy makers.

2. Can the results be applied to my patient(s)?

Review of quantitative studies

Based on the large number of trials and participants (31 trials, involving a total of 6936 participants) and the subgroup analysis findings that outcomes were independent of patient age, sex or stroke severity, it can be suggested that the results can be extrapolated from the review population to other people who have had a stroke and receive organised stroke-unit care. If we go back to our clinical scenario that we raised at the beginning of this worked example, we see that the health professionals in the scenario are working in an acute hospital setting and with patients who have had a stroke. The question that they raised was: *'For people with acute stroke admitted to hospital, do stroke units have greater improvements in independence compared with general medical wards?'* This is directly addressed by this systematic review. The scenario does not provide us with details about the characteristics of the stroke patients that they see but, given that the therapists work in a general hospital setting and the studies included in the review were conducted in general hospital settings in various locations throughout the world, it is likely that the characteristics of the patients would be similar.

Review of qualitative studies (meta-aggregation)

The review authors provide a table which outlines the characteristics of the sample from each original study that was included in the synthesis. Whether or not this is sufficient to make a translation of the findings to a particular individual patient that one is working with is difficult to evaluate. Given the broad range of profiles included in the synthesis, it may be that the findings are applicable to the broader population of people who have had a stroke, not just the elderly. Extrapolating these findings to other people in other age categories who are recovering from stroke should be done very cautiously.

RESOLUTION OF CLINICAL SCENARIO

The review of quantitative studies that we have just appraised indicates that stroke units can result in improved outcomes in terms of survival, independence and avoiding institutional care when compared with care that is provided in alternative services. The outcome data from this review, particularly the data that compared stroke-unit care with care in medical wards, could be used by the therapists in our scenario when they are discussing hospital policy with the administrator to argue that people who have had a stroke should be cared for in the stroke unit. Data about the costs involved were not provided in the review; however, the review did find that there was no increase in the length of stay for participants who received care in stroke units. This is only a proxy for cost, and in future studies it would be important to ascertain full details of the costs involved. Discussions with the administrator about the feasibility of implementing a plan to ensure that all people who are admitted to hospital with a stroke are admitted to the stroke unit as soon as possible would also be needed.

From the meta-aggregation, a few important issues can be highlighted that would extend the discussion regarding stroke-unit care to include aspects of appropriateness and meaningfulness of stroke-unit care. The team members should consider how stroke-unit care could optimally support elderly persons who are in the process of recovering from stroke, given that they are often experiencing fear, feelings of disconnection with friends and family and while in hospital and following discharge will be required to do a huge amount of work, both physically and psychologically. Discussion about ways of providing opportunities for patients to discuss their perceptions of improvement and progress may also be warranted.

SUMMARY POINTS OF THIS CHAPTER

- Systematic reviews differ from literature reviews because they are prepared using explicit, transparent and pre-specified strategies that limit bias. They involve a comprehensive search of *all* potentially relevant articles; use explicit, reproducible and uniformly applied criteria in the selection of articles for the review; rigorously appraise the risk of bias within individual studies; and systematically synthesise the results of included studies.

- Systematic reviews synthesise the findings from different study designs depending on the research question of interest.

- A well-conducted systematic review can improve the dissemination of evidence and hasten the assimilation of research into practice. A review of quantitative studies can assist in clarifying the heterogeneity of conflicting results between studies and establish generalisability of the overall findings. A review of qualitative studies can deepen the understanding of a particular phenomenon or situation.

- Because systematic reviews vary in quality, you should know how to appraise them and recognise the key features that introduce bias into systematic reviews. When examining whether the review used valid methods, key questions that need to be asked are whether the review: (1) addressed a clearly focused question with clearly defined eligibility criteria; (2) included high quality, relevant studies; (3) is unlikely to have missed important, relevant studies; (4) included an assessment of the risk of bias of the included studies and incorporated this assessment into the review findings; and (5) combined the results from studies and, if so, was it reasonable to do so?

- Other key questions that you need to ask when examining the results of a systematic review are: (1) What are the overall results?; (2) How precise or rich are the results?; (3) Did the review consider all the important outcomes or evaluation measures?; and (4) Can the results be applied to your patients?

References

1. Mulrow C, Cook D, Davidoff F. Systematic reviews: critical links in the great chain of evidence. Ann Intern Med 1997;126:389–91.
2. Cook D, Mulrow C, Haynes RB. Systematic reviews: synthesis of best evidence for clinical decisions. Ann Intern Med 1997;126:376–80.
3. Hannes K, Van den Noortgate W. Master thesis projects in the field of education: who says we need more basic research? Educational Research 2012;3:340–4.
4. Greenhalgh T. How to read a paper: papers that summarise other papers (systematic reviews and meta-analyses). BMJ 1997;315:672–5.
5. Phillips B, Ball C, Sackett D, et al. Levels of evidence. Oxford: Centre for Evidence-based Medicine; 2009. Online. Available: www.cebm.net/index.aspx?o=1025; 31 May 2012.
6. National Health and Medical Research Council (NHMRC). NHMRC additional levels of evidence and grades for recommendations for developers of guidelines. Canberra: NHMRC; 2009. Online. Available: www.nhmrc.gov. au/_files_nhmrc/file/guidelines/developers/nhmrc_levels_grades_evidence_120423.pdf; 31 May 2012.
7. Meijer R, Ihnenfeldt D, van Limbeek J, et al. Prognostic factors in the subacute phase after stroke for the future residence after six months to one year. A systematic review of the literature. Clin Rehab 2003;17: 512–20.
8. Irwig L, Tosteson A, Gatsonis C, et al. Guidelines for meta-analyses evaluating diagnostic tests. Ann Intern Med 1994;120:667–76.
9. Mitchell A. A meta-analysis of the accuracy of the mini-mental state examination in the detection of dementia and mild cognitive impairment. J Psychiatr Res 2009;43:411–31.
10. Noyes J, Popay J, Pearson A, et al. Chapter 20: Qualitative research and Cochrane reviews. In: Higgins JPT, Green S, editors, Cochrane Handbook for Systematic Reviews of Interventions. Version 5.1.0 [updated March 2011]. The Cochrane Collaboration; 2011. Available from www.cochrane-handbook.org.
11. Goldsmith M, Bankhead C, Austoker J. Synthesising quantitative and qualitative research in evidence-based patient information. J Epidemiol Community Health 2007;61:262–70.
12. Hannes K, Lockwood C. Pragmatism as the philosophical underpinning of the Joanna Briggs meta-aggregative approach to qualitative evidence synthesis. J Adv Nurs 2011;67:1632–42.
13. Pearson, A. Balancing the evidence: incorporating the synthesis of qualitative data into systematic reviews. JBI Reports 2004;2:45–64.
14. Hannes K, Aertgeerts B, Goedhuys J. Obstacles to implementing evidence-based practice in Belgium: a context-specific qualitative evidence synthesis including findings from different health care disciplines. Acta Clinica Belgica 2012;67:99–107.
15 McInnes E, Askie L. Evidence review on older people's views and experiences of falls prevention strategies. World Views Evid Based Nurs 2004;1:20–37.
16. Allen IJ, Okin I. Estimating the time to conduct a meta-analysis from number of citations retrieved. JAMA 1999;282:634–5.
17. Jackson N, Waters E. Criteria for the systematic review of health promotion and public health interventions. Health Promot Int 2005;20:367–74.
18. Akobeng AK. Understanding systematic reviews and meta-analysis. Arch Dis Child 2005;90:845–8.
19. Bhandari M, Guyatt G, Montori V, et al. Current concepts review. Users guide to orthopedic literature: how to use a systematic review. J Bone Joint Surg 2002;84A:1672–82.
20. Hopewell S, Clarke M, Lefebvre C, et al. Handsearching versus electronic searching to identify reports of randomised trials. Cochrane Database Syst Rev 2007;(2):MR000001. doi: 10.1002/14651858.MR000001.pub2.
21. Kennedy G, Rutherford G. Identifying randomised controlled trials in the journal. Cape Town, South Africa: Presentation at the Eighth International Cochrane Colloquium; 2000.
22. Greenhalgh T, Peacock R. Effectiveness and efficiency of search methods in systematic reviews of complex evidence: audit of primary sources. BMJ 2005;331:1064–5.
23. Armstrong R, Jackson N, Doyle J, et al. It's in your hands: the value of handsearching in conducting systematic reviews. J Pub Health 2005;27:388–91.
24. Lefebvre C, Manheimer E, Glanville J. Chapter 6: Searching for studies. In: Higgins J, Green S, editors. Cochrane Handbook for Systematic Reviews of Interventions. Version 5.1.0 [updated March 2011]. The Cochrane Collaboration; 2011. Online. Available: http://handbook.cochrane.org/.
25. Juni P, Altman D, Egger M. Systematic reviews in health care: assessing the quality of controlled clinical trials. BMJ 2001;323:42–6.
26. Higgins JPT, Altman DG, Sterne JAC, editors. Chapter 8: Assessing risk of bias in included studies. In: Higgins JPT, Green S, editors. Cochrane Handbook for Systematic Reviews of Interventions. Version 5.1.0 [updated March 2011]. The Cochrane Collaboration; 2011. Online. Available: http://handbook.cochrane.org/.

27. Deeks JJ, Higgins JPT, Altman DG. Chapter 9: Analysing data and undertaking meta-analyses. In: Higgins JPT, Green S, editors. Cochrane Handbook for Systematic Reviews of Interventions. Version 5.1.0 [updated March 2011]. The Cochrane Collaboration, 2011. Available from www.cochrane-handbook.org.

28. The Joanna Briggs Institute. Joanna Briggs Institute Reviewers' Manual. Adelaide: Joanna Briggs Institute; 2008.

29. Schünemann H, Oxman A, Higgins J, et al. Chapter 11: Presenting results and 'Summary of findings' tables. In: Higgins J, Green S, editors. Cochrane Handbook for Systematic Reviews of Interventions. Version 5.1.0 [updated March 2011]. The Cochrane Collaboration, 2011. Available from www.cochrane-handbook.org.

30. Henken H, Huibers M, Churchill R, et al. Family therapy for depression. Cochrane Database Syst Rev 2007;(3):CD006728. doi: 10.1002/14651858.CD006728.

31. Joanna Briggs Institute. SUMARI. User's Manual Version 5.0. System for the unified management, assessment and review of information. Adelaide: Joanna Briggs Institute. Online. Available: www.joannabriggs.edu.au/documents/sumari/SUMARI%20V5%20User%20guide.pdf; 3 Jun 2012.

32. The Joanna Briggs Institute. Comprehensive Systematic Review Study Guide Module 4. Adelaide: The Joanna Briggs Institute; 2012.

33. McInerney P, Brysiewicz P. A systematic review of the experiences of caregivers in providing home-based care to persons with HIV/AIDS in Africa. JBI Library of Systematic Reviews 2009;7:130–53.

34. Konno R. Support for overseas qualified nurses in adjusting to Australian nursing practice: a systematic review. Int J Evid Based Healthc 2006;4:83–100.

35. McInnes E, Wimpenny P. Using qualitative assessment and review instrument software to synthesise studies on older people's views and experiences of falls prevention. Int J Evid Based Healthc 2008;6:337–44.

36. Moher D, Tetzlaff J, Tricco A, et al. Epidemiology and reporting characteristics of systematic reviews. PLoS Med 2007;4:e78. doi:10.1371/journal.pmed.0040078

37. Oxman A, Guyatt G. Validation of an index of the quality of review articles. J Clin Epidemiol 1991;44:1271–8.

38. Oxman A, Cook D, Guyatt G. Users' guides to the medical literature: VI. How to use an overview. JAMA 1994;272:1367–71.

39. Shea B, Hamel C, Wells G, et al. AMSTAR is a reliable and valid measurement tool to assess the methodological quality of systematic reviews. J Clin Epidemiol 2009;62:1013–20.

40. Greenhalgh T, Donald A. Evidence-based health care workbook: understanding research: for individual and group learning. London: BMJ Publishing Group; 2000.

41. Pope C, Mays N, Popay J. Synthesising qualitative and quantitative health research: a guide to methods. Maidenhead (UK): Open University Press; 2007.

42. Stroke Unit Trialists' Collaboration. Organised inpatient (stroke unit) care for stroke. Cochrane Database Syst Rev 2007;(4):CD000197. doi: 10.1002/14651858.CD000197.pub2.

43. Lamb M, Buchanan D, Godfrey C, et al. The psychosocial spiritual experience of elderly individuals recovering from stroke: a systematic review. Int J Evid Based Healthc 2008;6:173–205.

44. Hannes K, Lockwood C, Pearson A. A comparative analysis of three online appraisal instruments' ability to assess validity in qualitative research. Qual Health Res 2010;20:1736–43.

45. Sacks HS, Reitman D, Pagano D, et al. Meta-analysis: an update. Mt Sinai J Med 1996;63:216–24.

46. Moher D, Cook D, Eastwood S, et al, for the QUOROM group. Improving the quality of reporting of meta-analysis of randomised controlled trials: the QUOROM statement. Lancet 1999;354:1896–900.

47. Liberati A, Altman D, Tetzlaff J, et al. The PRISMA statement for reporting systematic reviews and meta-analyses of studies that evaluate health care interventions: explanation and elaboration. PLoS Med 2009;6:e1000100.

48. Simera I, Moher D, Hirst A, et al. Transparent and accurate reporting increases reliability, utility, and impact of your research: reporting guidelines and the EQUATOR Network. BMC Med 2010;26(8):24.

49. Tao K, Li X, Zhou Q, et al. From QUOROM to PRISMA: a survey of high-impact medical journals' instructions to authors and a review of systematic reviews in anesthesia literature. PLoS One 2011;6:e27611.

50. Kalra L, Eade J. Role of stroke rehabilitation units in managing severe disability after stroke. Stroke 1995;26:2031–4.

51. Vemmos K, Takis K, Madelos D, et al. Stroke unit treatment versus general medical wards: long term survival. Cerebrovasc Dis 2001;11:8.

52. Leonardi-Bee J. Presenting and interpreting meta-analyses. RLO, School of Nursing and Academic Division of Midwifery, University of Nottingham; 2007. Online. Available: www.nottingham.ac.uk/nursing/sonet/rlos/ebp/meta-analysis2/index.html; 31 May 2012.

53. Hannes K. The Joanna Briggs Institute Best Practice Information Sheet: the psychosocial and spiritual experiences of elderly individuals recovering from a stroke. Nurs Health Sci 2010;12:515–18.

Chapter 13

Clinical practice guidelines

Tammy Hoffmann and Heather Buchan

LEARNING OBJECTIVES

After reading this chapter, you should be able to:

- Describe what clinical practice guidelines are, their uses and their limitations
- Be aware of the major online resources for locating clinical practice guidelines
- Explain the major steps that are involved in the development of guidelines
- Appraise the quality of a clinical practice guideline to determine whether you should trust the recommendations that it contains
- Describe some of the issues related to using a clinical practice guideline
- Be aware of some of the legal issues associated with the use of guidelines

There are various forms of clinical guidance that recommend how to manage specific clinical conditions. This guidance is developed in different ways and can range from consensus-based documents compiled by an individual health agency to high quality evidence-based clinical practice guidelines which have undergone a much more rigorous development and review process. The latter is the type that we are interested in and will focus on in this chapter. However, we will also discuss how to assess the quality of a clinical practice guideline, as it is likely that you will come across many types of guidelines during your clinical practice.

In this chapter we will look at what clinical practice guidelines are, why they are used, where to search for guidelines, the steps involved in developing a guideline and how to appraise the quality of a guideline. We will also discuss some of the issues involved with using guidelines in clinical practice, including legal issues surrounding their use.

WHAT ARE CLINICAL GUIDELINES?

Until recently, the internationally accepted standard definition was that proposed by the United States Institute of Medicine (IOM) in 1992: clinical practice guidelines were:

> systematically developed statements to assist health professional and patient decisions about appropriate health care for specific circumstances.[1]

In 2011 a subsequent report by the IOM proposed a new definition aimed at better reflecting the consensus developed over the past 20 years. The new definition is:

> Clinical practice guidelines are statements that include recommendations intended to optimize patient care that are informed by a systematic review of evidence and an assessment of the benefits and harms of alternative care options.[2]

According to this definition, a well-developed, trustworthy guideline contains rigorously compiled information and recommended actions to guide practice. It should be developed by a knowledgeable, multidisciplinary panel of experts and representatives from key stakeholder groups, and be based on a systematic review of existing evidence, using an explicit and transparent process that minimises bias. It should consider important subgroups and patient preferences, clearly explain the relationship between alternative care options and health outcomes and provide ratings of both the quality of the evidence and the strength of the recommendations. Finally, it should be revised when important new evidence becomes available.[2]

Guidelines are designed to help health professionals and their patients reach decisions about the most appropriate ways to prevent, diagnose and treat the patient's presenting symptoms. For example, occupational therapists, physiotherapists, speech pathologists, doctors, nurses or other health professionals who work with people who are recovering from a stroke should find the National Stroke Foundation's 'Clinical Guidelines for Stroke Management 2010' useful for informing practice (available from www.strokefoundation.com.au/clinical-guidelines).

WHY USE GUIDELINES?

As we saw in Chapter 2, health professionals are continually exposed to an overwhelming amount of health research and there are thousands of new studies published each year. Keeping abreast of this enormous volume of information is not possible for busy health professionals, and the development of healthcare guidelines is one way in which information overload is being addressed. Guidelines are a useful tool for evidence-based practice as they help us to translate evidence into practice recommendations, which can then be applied to clinical situations.

Guidelines aim to help health professionals and patients make better decisions about health care. They aim to reduce variations in practice across health professionals for the same condition and improve patient outcomes. The *development* of guidelines—the act of amassing and scrutinising the relevant research about a specific topic and making research accessible to health professionals and patients—is part of evidence-based practice at the organisational level. The subsequent *translation and use* of guidelines in the clinical setting is more about evidence-based individual decision making, as well as the implementation of evidence into practice.

The number of clinical practice guidelines being produced has increased substantially over the last several years. A survey in 1993 identified 34 Australian clinical practice guidelines.[3] A more extensive search in 2007 found over 300 clinical practice guidelines that had been produced for use in Australia in the previous five years,[4] and many thousands of guidelines are now published in international guideline libraries.

Guidelines dealing with the same clinical condition may have differing recommendations about the care that should be provided. Sometimes this reflects a difference in quality of production, with some guidelines undergoing more-rigorous development processes than others. Differing recommendations may also arise because the guidelines have been developed for use in different settings, or with different population groups, or because of different views or approaches to valuing care outcomes.

Clinical guidelines are increasingly being used by health professionals. It is anticipated that their use will continue to become more common. The direct applicability to contemporary clinical practice is what makes a clinical guideline useful. As with other types of evidence, care needs to be taken to ensure that guidelines are of high quality, that the evidence that they use is relevant for the setting and population where they will be used, and that they are implemented effectively. Guidelines will not address all the uncertainties of current clinical practice and should be seen as only one strategy that can help improve the quality of patient care.[5]

Guidelines: the pros and cons

Guidelines have a number of benefits. High quality guidelines differ from systematic reviews in that they provide recommendations for care based on a combination of scientific research evidence, clinical expertise and patient values. They often provide an overview of the prevention, diagnosis and management of a condition or the use of an intervention, and so have a broader scope than systematic reviews, which tend to focus on a single clinical question. Use of guidelines can save time, improve decisions about health care and produce better health outcomes.[6–9]

Guideline development is not easy and involves large amounts of time, money, expertise and effort. As the development process can be lengthy, there is a possibility that the evidence used in a guideline may not be the most current evidence by the time the guideline is finally published. Many guidelines do not provide clear information about conflicts of interest within the guideline development group and how these were handled during the guideline development process.

When considering using a guideline, the key word to remember is 'guide'. Rigorously developed guidelines are the result of a comprehensive and systematic examination of the literature by a panel of experts with consumer input. This group considers how research findings should be applied in practice and aims to develop a useful, practical resource that can assist in the prevention, diagnosis and treatment of health conditions. However, guideline recommendations are *not* fixed protocols that must be followed. As with evidence-based practice in general, responsible and informed clinical judgment about the management of individual patients remains important. You need to work together with your patient to develop an intervention plan that is tailored to their specific needs and circumstances, and that is achievable, affordable and realistic.[10]

One of the potentially limiting factors about guidelines is that they generally tend to deal with a specific condition in isolation. However, in practice, patients often present with a range of comorbid conditions. Even when a patient presents without comorbidities, translating a guideline in practice still needs to take into account factors such as:

- individual patient preferences and desired outcomes
- the likelihood of adherence
- the patient's readiness to change behaviours
- the likely harms and benefits of alternative courses of action
- the availability and affordability of any services, medications or other interventions that are recommended in the guidelines.

Patient factors will be discussed in more detail later in this chapter when we discuss using a clinical guideline in practice.

HOW GUIDELINES FIT WITH OTHER EVIDENCE-BASED PRACTICE PRODUCTS

As well as clinical guidelines, there are other evidence-based practice products or aids that can help health professionals and patients to make decisions about care. Examples of these products include:

- 'handbooks', of which there are many and which differ from country to country. Some examples, primarily Australian ones, include:
  - The *Australian Medicines Handbook* (https://shop.amh.net.au)
  - The *Asthma Management Handbook* (www.nationalasthma.org.au/cms/index.php)
  - *Therapeutic Guidelines* (www.tg.org.au)—covers over 3000 topics, which will mostly be of relevance to medical practitioners. Some of the guidelines are available through the Clinical Guidelines Portal which is described in the 'Guideline-specific databases' section of this chapter. The topics are also produced electronically (known as eTG) for either a computer or a handheld device.
- Decision support tools for health care (sometimes these are available for both patients and health professionals). More detail about decision aids is provided in Chapter 14.
- Practice software and smart-phones/handheld computers which incorporate, or have links to, evidence-based guidelines.
- Educational modules and information packs which are sent out to health professionals by national and state health departments.
- Online resources that have been developed to help clinicians find evidence-based information relevant to their needs (in addition to those that were mentioned in Chapter 3), such as:
  - Some sites provide interactive topic-based information. For example, NICE Pathways brings together all related products from the United Kingdom's National Institute for Health and Clinical Excellence (NICE) so that users can quickly see all of NICE's recommendations on a specific clinical or health topic (pathways.nice.org.uk).
  - Other sites provide information in response to specific clinical questions e.g. BestBETS (www.bestbets.org) are Best Evidence Topics (BETs), developed in the Emergency Department of Manchester Royal Infirmary, UK. These provide evidence-based answers to real-life clinical questions.
  - EvidenceUpdates (plus.mcmaster.ca/EvidenceUpdates) is a free service arising from collaboration between the BMJ Group and McMaster University's Health Information Research Unit. This service scans over 120 clinical journals and carefully selects high quality papers. These are then

rated for clinical relevance and newsworthiness by an international panel of practising doctors. There is a searchable database and an email alerting system (that can be filtered by specialty/discipline).

Guidelines can complement these other products when the information contained in them is aligned and consistent. Some of these products may contain guidelines and sometimes the products may share the same evidence base as the relevant guidelines. However, there is not always consistency across products. Situations can arise where there are discrepancies in the recommendations made in various products. When discrepancies occur, you need to decide which resource to use. Later in this chapter, we discuss how to evaluate the quality of guidelines so that you can choose the one with the highest quality that will be of the most use to your particular clinical situation.

WHERE AND HOW TO FIND GUIDELINES

It is probably clear to you by now that there are thousands of clinical guidelines across the health professions. The obvious question is: *Where and how should you look for guidelines relevant to your patient/clinical situation?* In general, there are two main electronic sources that can be used to locate clinical guidelines:

- large bibliographic databases (such as PubMed, Embase, CINAHL)
- guideline-specific databases (such as the Australian Clinical Practice Guidelines Portal, National Guideline Clearinghouse and the Guidelines International Network library).

Bibliographic databases

Although the large bibliographic databases do contain some clinical guidelines, the problem is that only a small proportion of guidelines are published in journals. As a result, only a small proportion is indexed in the traditional databases. In addition, none of these bibliographic databases appraise the quality of guidelines, and it may be difficult to access more than just the abstract from their sites. However, if you decide to search the large bibliographic databases to locate guidelines, here are a few tips:

- PubMed: When searching for clinical guidelines in PubMed, you can select the limit 'practice guideline' under publication type.
- MEDLINE: Methodological search strategies for retrieving guidelines in MEDLINE (via Ovid) have been created[11] and are summarised in Table 13.1, showing strategies that are aimed at locating all

TABLE 13.1:
SEARCH STRATEGIES (HEDGES) FOR LOCATING PRACTICE GUIDELINES IN MEDLINE (VIA OVID)[11]

Hedge	All classified guidelines	Methodologically sound guidelines
Best sensitivity	exp health services administration OR tu.xs. OR management.tw.	guideline:.tw. OR exp data collection OR recommend:.tw. guidelines.tw. OR practice guidelines.sh. OR recommend:.tw.
Best specificity	guideline:.tw.	guideline adherence.sh. OR physician's practice patterns.sh. practice guidelines.tw. OR practice guidelines.sh.
Best optimisation of sensitivity and specificity	guide:.tw. OR recommend:. tw. OR exp risk	exp "quality assurance (health care)" OR recommend:.tw. OR guideline adherence.sh.

+ = explode; colon (:) = truncation; exp = explosion; sh = subject heading; tu = therapeutic use; tw = textword; xs = exploded subheading.

articles classified as a guideline and strategies that are aimed at locating methodologically sound guidelines. In the study that developed these search filters, all articles retrieved that met the definition of a clinical practice guideline were evaluated for methodological quality according to the following criteria if they were concerned with the *development* of a guideline:

1. the article contained an explicit statement that described the process of developing the guideline, including methods of evidence assembly, method of review of studies and at least one of (a) the organisations and the individuals involved, (b) the methods of formulating guidelines and (c) the methods of reaching agreement or consensus; and

2. evidence was cited in support of at least one of the recommendations contained in the guideline.

If the article related to the *application* (as opposed to development) of a clinical guideline, the following criterion was used to evaluate the article's scientific merit: at least one of the exact guidelines was provided in a table, figure or text of the article.

Combine the methodological search strategies in Table 13.1 with your content terms (such as the keywords from your clinical question) when searching for clinical guidelines in MEDLINE.

- Embase: Embase has a thesaurus term 'practice guideline' which you can use as part of your search strategy; however, be aware that the term refers to more than just clinical practice guidelines.

- CINAHL: You can select the limit 'practice guideline' under publication type when searching in CINAHL.

Chapter 3 provides further details about these databases, as well as advice about how to use search strategies such as those shown in Table 13.1 when looking for evidence to answer a clinical question.

Guideline-specific databases

One of the best ways to find a clinical guideline can be by searching a guideline-specific database. Details about some of the major guideline-specific databases where guidelines can be found are provided below.

- **Clinical Practice Guidelines Portal (Australia)** (www.clinicalguidelines.gov.au)

  This portal is maintained by the National Institute of Clinical Studies (NICS), an institute of the National Health and Medical Research Council (NHMRC). It provides links to clinical practice guidelines developed for use in Australian healthcare settings. To be included on the portal site, guidelines must have been produced within the last 5 years. At present the portal includes both guidelines that have been developed using systematic review processes and guidelines that do not use (or have documentation of) systematic literature reviews. A summary of key features of each guideline notes whether the guidelines are 'evidence-documented'. The browsing function supports looking for guidelines by topic as well as by developer. The portal also links to a register of guidelines in development.

- **National Guideline Clearinghouse (USA)** (www.guideline.gov)

  This database is maintained as a public resource by the Agency for Healthcare Research and Quality, USA Department of Health and Human Services. It contains guidelines from both USA-based and non-USA-based organisations, including guidelines from well-known guideline databases such as the Scottish Intercollegiate Guidelines Network (SIGN) and the New Zealand Guidelines Group. You can find guidelines by entering the topic you are interested in (using the National Library of Medicine's Medical Subject Headings (MeSH); www.nlm.nih.gov/mesh/2011/mesh_browser/MBrowser.html; see Box 3.1 in Chapter 3 for an explanation of MeSH) or by entering the name of the organisation or guideline developer. Guidelines must have been developed using a systematic literature search and review process and have been produced or reviewed within the past 5 years in order to be included on this site. The National Guideline Clearinghouse provides structured summaries of the guidelines, including information about availability and links to the developers' website. An interesting feature is the Guideline Comparison Utility, which gives users the ability to generate side-by-side comparisons of a combination of two or more guidelines. The Clearinghouse staff also prepare syntheses of selected guidelines that cover similar topic areas. In these syntheses, there is often a comparison of guidelines developed in different countries. This tool may assist health professionals by providing insight into the commonalities and differences in international health practices.

- **National Health Service (NHS) Evidence (UK)** (www.evidence.nhs.uk)

This database is managed by the UK's National Institute for Health and Clinical Excellence (NICE) and contains a large number of evidence resources, including guidelines. While some parts of the site are only available to people working within the NHS, most of the resources can be accessed by anyone and guidelines can be searched for by topic. An accreditation logo next to a guideline on the NHS Evidence site shows that the processes used by the organisation producing the guideline have been assessed as meeting NICE quality standards. Registering on the site enables you to save searches and results and be sent email updates of new evidence in your area of interest. All published NICE guidance is indexed by NHS Evidence and there are also guidelines from a variety of other sources. The guidelines on this site are also available at the website of the National Clinical Guideline Centre (www.ncgc.ac.uk), which is an easier site to search if it is primarily guidelines that you are looking for.

- **Guidelines International Network (G-I-N)** (www.g-i-n.net)

This is a global network with both organisational and individual members that aims to support collaboration on guideline development, adaptation and implementation. The Network has an International Guideline Library that contains more than 7500 guidelines, evidence reports and related documents, developed or endorsed by G-I-N member organisations. Anyone can access the library, but only network members can access the detailed information, save their searches, combine their searches or export the references to EndNote or RefMan.

- **Turning Research Into Practice (TRIP)** (www.tripdatabase.com)

The TRIP database was discussed in detail in Chapter 3. It is a search engine that searches a number of databases and thousands of sites for evidence relevant to clinical questions. The search results are grouped according to the type of evidence (for example, guideline). For guidelines, the search can be filtered further by choosing from Australia and New Zealand, Canada, UK, USA or 'other'.

For some specialties and geographical regions, there are other smaller databases which collate guidelines. These include:

- **Physiotherapy** (PEDro—the Physiotherapy Evidence Database; www.pedro.org.au): contains evidence-based clinical guidelines of relevance to physiotherapy. Some guidelines are also of relevance to other health professions. PEDro was described in more detail in Chapter 3.
- **Clinical Practice Rehabilitation Guidelines** (www.health.uottawa.ca/rehabguidelines/en/login.php): contains web-based guidelines of relevance to rehabilitation health professionals.
- **Canadian Medical Association Infobase—Clinical Practice Guidelines** (www.cma.ca/cpgs): contains more than 1200 guidelines that were developed or endorsed by an authoritative medical or health organisation in Canada.
- **Speech Pathology and Audiology** (www.asha.org/members/ebp/compendium): the American Speech-Language-Hearing Association have collated guidelines of relevance to these professions.
- **Oncology** (www.nccn.org/index.asp): contains guidelines produced by the National Comprehensive Cancer Network.

HOW ARE GUIDELINES DEVELOPED?

The steps involved in developing an *evidence-based* clinical guideline typically consist of:

1. Identifying the scope of a guideline—providing an outline of the aspects of care within the designated topic area that the guideline will cover.
2. Forming a guideline development group—usually made up of health professionals with expertise in the clinical area, representatives of patients and carers and people who have technical expertise in guideline development methods and in systematic literature reviewing.
3. Gaining agreement about the specific clinical questions or problems that will be addressed by the guideline and that will guide the search for evidence.
4. Searching systematically for evidence and appraising its quality.
5. Discussing and agreeing the implications of the evidence for clinical practice.
6. Formulating draft recommendations.
7. Obtaining external review and feedback of the guideline.
8. Ongoing review and update of the guideline to ensure it remains based on the most current best available evidence—a timeframe of 3 years is often used.

What gives rise to the variable quality of guidelines is that differences occur in this development process, typically in the following areas:

- the specific clinical questions that guide the search for evidence
- the comprehensiveness of the search used to locate evidence (it should be a systematic search)
- the quality of the evidence reviewed
- the rigour of the processes used to assess/grade the evidence
- the mix of people reviewing the evidence
- the way in which conflicts of interest are identified and managed throughout the guideline development process
- decisions that are made about the desirability of different clinical outcomes
- assessments of the likelihood of harms and benefits of interventions and where the balance should fall
- the processes used to develop agreement on the final guideline recommendations
- the strength of guideline recommendations and the extent to which they are linked to evidence
- the process for obtaining review and feedback on the guideline and the modifications made to the guideline as a result.

Guides to guideline development have been published by a number of international guideline development groups, including the NICE and the SIGN[12,13]—refer to the websites that are provided in the reference list for this chapter.

CAN I TRUST THE RECOMMENDATIONS IN A CLINICAL GUIDELINE?

With such a large number of clinical guidelines of varying quality available, you may be left wondering which guidelines you should, or should not, use in your clinical practice. You need to ask yourself the same question that we asked when appraising various study designs in earlier chapters of this book—'*Are the results of this study valid?*' When appraising clinical guidelines, the 'results' are the recommendations, so you are trying to determine whether you can trust the recommendations in a clinical guideline. As with the other types of evidence discussed in other chapters, it is important that you know how to appraise clinical guidelines and recognise the key features that discriminate high quality guidelines that can be used to guide practice from low quality clinical guidelines that should be used with caution. High quality guidelines can improve health care, but the adoption of low quality guidelines can lead to the use of ineffective interventions, the inefficient use of scarce resources and, most importantly, possible harm to patients.[14,15]

The AGREE II instrument

A number of instruments have been developed to help assess the quality of clinical practice guidelines.[16] The most widely used of these has been the AGREE instrument. The original AGREE instrument[17] was developed by an international group of guideline developers and researchers, the Appraisal of Guidelines Research and Evaluation (AGREE) collaboration. The Collaboration defined *quality of guidelines* as 'the confidence that the potential biases of guideline development have been addressed adequately and that the recommendations are both internally and externally valid, and are feasible for practice'.

The original AGREE Instrument was published in 2003 but has now been further refined to strengthen its measurement properties and improve its useability. The new AGREE II instrument[18] and instructions for its use can be downloaded for free from the AGREE Research Trust website (www.agreetrust.org). The AGREE II tool appraises guidelines based on how they score on 23 items, which are grouped into six major domains, followed by two global-rating overall assessment items. It is recommended that each guideline is assessed by at least two people (and preferably four) to increase the reliability of the assessment. Box 13.1 lists the domains and items of the AGREE II instrument. Each of the AGREE II items is rated on a 7-point scale (from 1 = strongly disagree to 7 = strongly agree) regarding the extent to which the guideline meets the particular item.

A quality score can then be calculated for each of the six AGREE II domains. Domain scores are calculated by summing up all the scores of the individual items in a domain and by scaling the total as a percentage of the maximum possible score for that domain. The six domain scores are independent and should not be aggregated into a single quality score. AGREE II asks for the assessor to make two overall assessments of the guideline—first, a judgment of the overall quality which takes into account the criteria considered in the assessment process; and second, a statement about whether the assessor would recommend use of the guideline.

Grading quality of evidence and strength of recommendations

Appraising the quality of the evidence that underpins the recommendations within a clinical practice guideline is a key part of the guideline development process. Some guideline recommendations are based on high quality evidence, while others are based on lower quality evidence that is more susceptible to bias, so it is important that users of guidelines are able to understand the strength of the evidence that supports any particular recommendation.[19] Internationally, clinical practice guideline developers have in the past used a variety of systems to rate the quality of the evidence that underpins recommendations within the guideline and the strength of the recommendation that is being made.[20] The different systems use varying combinations of letters and numbers to communicate the methodological quality of the underlying evidence and the strength of the recommendation. This variety of systems can be extraordinarily confusing for users of guidelines, since the same evidence and recommendation could be graded as 'II-2, B', 'C+, 1' or 'strong evidence, strongly recommended' depending on which system is used.[21]

Methods for grading evidence and rating the strength of recommendations are continuing to evolve. One method that has now been adopted by several organisations and journals (including the Cochrane Collaboration) is the GRADE (Grading of Recommendations Assessment, Development and Evaluation) approach.[22] The working group that developed this system used the following definitions:

BOX 13.1

Domains and items contained in the AGREE II instrument

DOMAIN 1. SCOPE AND PURPOSE

1. The overall objective(s) of the guideline is (are) specifically described.
2. The health question(s) covered by the guideline is (are) specifically described.
3. The population (patients, public, etc.) to whom the guideline is meant to apply is specifically described.

DOMAIN 2. STAKEHOLDER INVOLVEMENT

4. The guideline development group includes individuals from all the relevant professional groups.
5. The views and preferences of the target population (patients, public, etc.) have been sought.
6. The target users of the guideline are clearly defined.

DOMAIN 3. RIGOUR OF DEVELOPMENT

7. Systematic methods were used to search for evidence.
8. The criteria for selecting the evidence are clearly described.
9. The strengths and limitations of the body of evidence are clearly described.
10. The methods for formulating the recommendations are clearly described.
11. The health benefits, side effects and risks have been considered in formulating the recommendations.
12. There is an explicit link between the recommendations and the supporting evidence.
13. The guideline has been externally reviewed by experts prior to its publication.
14. A procedure for updating the guideline is provided.

DOMAIN 4. CLARITY OF PRESENTATION

15. The recommendations are specific and unambiguous.
16. The different options for management of the condition or health issue are clearly presented.
17. Key recommendations are easily identifiable.

DOMAIN 5. APPLICABILITY

18. The guideline describes facilitators and barriers to its application.
19. The guideline provides advice and/or tools on how the recommendations can be put into practice.
20. The potential resource implications of applying the recommendations have been considered.
21. The guideline presents monitoring and/or auditing criteria.

DOMAIN 6. EDITORIAL INDEPENDENCE

22. The views of the funding body have not influenced the content of the guideline.
23. Competing interests of guideline development group members have been recorded and addressed.

OVERALL GUIDELINE ASSESSMENT

1. Rate the overall quality of this guideline (Scale of 1 to 7 with 1 being lowest possible quality and 7 being highest possible quality).
2. I would recommend this guideline for use (Options: Yes, Yes with modifications, No).

Source: AGREE Next Steps Consortium. 2009. *The AGREE II Instrument* [electronic version]. Online. Available: www.agreetrust.org; 20 Nov 2012.

- the **quality of evidence** indicates the extent to which one can be confident that an estimate of effect is adequate to support a particular recommendation
- the **strength of a recommendation** indicates the extent to which one can be confident that adherence to the recommendation will do more good than harm.

The GRADE system takes several elements into account when judging quality of the evidence, including: *study design* (for example, is the study an observational study or a randomised controlled trial?); *study quality* (the detailed study methods and execution); consistency (the similarity of estimates of effects across studies); and *directness* (the extent to which the people, interventions, and outcome measures are similar to those of interest). Judgments about the strength of recommendations take into consideration the balance between desirable and undesirable consequences of alternative management strategies, as well as the quality of evidence, applicability and the certainty of the baseline risk.

The GRADE Working Group website (www.gradeworkinggroup.org) has a number of resources for people wanting to learn more about the GRADE system, with a comprehensive list of published papers, presentations and aids to using the GRADE system. The *quality of evidence* grading used by GRADE is as follows:[21]

- **high**—further research is very unlikely to change our confidence in the estimate of effect
- **moderate**—further research is likely to have an important impact on our confidence in the estimate of effect and may change the estimate
- **low**—further research is very likely to have an important impact on our confidence in the estimate of effect and is likely to change the estimate
- **very low**—any estimate of effect is very uncertain.

Within many countries, guideline organisations set standards for guideline development. For example, in Australia the NHMRC sets standards in clinical practice guideline development[23] and can approve selected clinical practice guidelines developed by other organisations. To meet the NHMRC standards, clinical practice guidelines must:

- provide guidance on a clearly defined clinical problem based on an identified need
- be developed by a multidisciplinary group that includes relevant experts, end users and consumers affected by the clinical practice guideline
- include a transparent process for declaration and management of potential conflicts of interest by each member of the guideline development group
- be based on the systematic identification and synthesis of the best available scientific evidence
- make clear and actionable recommendations in plain English for health professionals practising in an Australian healthcare setting
- be easy to navigate for end-users
- undergo a process of public consultation and independent external clinical expert review
- incorporate a plan for dissemination, including issues for consideration in implementation.

The NHMRC standards cover requirements in seven domains;[23] and within these domains, some items are mandatory if the guideline is to be approved by NHMRC while some are desirable but not mandatory. The NHMRC requires guideline developers to engage reviewers who will assess the guideline using the AGREE II instrument and requires use of either the GRADE approach or an NHMRC-approved evidence rating system to grade recommendations.[24]

The NHMRC approach requires grading of the evidence according to the following components:

- the **evidence base**, in terms of the *number* of studies, *level* of evidence and the *quality* of studies (that is, their risk of bias)

- the **consistency** of the study results between studies
- the **potential clinical impact** of the proposed recommendation (for example, effect size, precision of the effect size estimate, clinical significance, balance of risks and benefits)
- the **generalisability** of the body of evidence to the target population for the guideline
- the **applicability** of the body of evidence to the Australian healthcare context.

For each 'body of evidence' that is being evaluated, each of these components should be given a rating of A (excellent), B (good), C (satisfactory) or D (poor). Using this system, the developers of guidelines can then determine an overall grade, from A to D, for each of the recommendations that are contained in the guidelines, where:

A = Body of evidence can be trusted to guide practice.

B = Body of evidence can be trusted to guide practice in most situations.

C = Body of evidence provides some support for recommendation(s) but care should be taken in its application.

D = Body of evidence is weak and the recommendations must be applied with caution.

HOW TO USE A GUIDELINE IN PRACTICE

By now, it should be clear that there are many circumstances where you may wish to seek out a guideline to answer a clinical question. When searching for relevant guidelines, you should frame your clinical question of interest in a way that will help you to efficiently locate relevant information. The PICO method of formulating clinical questions, which was explained in Chapter 2, can also be used when searching for guidelines. Once you have located and appraised a guideline and decided that it is valid, as with other types of evidence, you then need to assess its applicability. That is, **is the guideline applicable to your patient/clinical scenario?** A key question that you need to ask is whether your patient is similar to the clinical population to which the guidelines apply. For example, your patient may have different risk factors to the clinical population who are the target group for the guidelines and, therefore, the guidelines cannot be applied to this patient. You should also **consider whether the setting for health care is similar to the setting to which the guidelines apply.** There are also **organisational factors** to bear in mind when considering implementing a guideline, such as whether the appropriate resources are available (for example, specialised equipment or staff with the necessary skills). Another issue to consider is whether the **values that are associated with a guideline** (either explicitly or implicitly) match the values of your patient or your community.[19] Your patient may have different values, preferences and beliefs to those that were assumed in the guideline.

A clinical guideline is not a mandate for practice. Regardless of the strength of the evidence on which the guideline recommendations are made, it is the responsibility of the individual health professional to interpret their application for each particular situation. Application involves taking account of patient preferences as well as local circumstances.[25] For example, while two patients may have exactly the same risks for a particular health condition, we should not assume that they will react in the same way to a suggestion about interventions which are recommended in the guideline. As the two patients are likely to have different values, beliefs and preferences, one patient may wish to proceed with the intervention that the guideline recommends, whereas the other patient may decide not to.

DO CLINICAL GUIDELINES CHANGE PRACTICE AND IMPROVE CARE?

The use of clinical guidelines is not without some controversy. A large amount of human and financial resources have been devoted to developing guidelines on a wide range of topics, but production and dissemination of a guideline alone has limited effect on uptake by health professionals.[26] It is clear that the effort and rigorous approach that goes into guideline development needs to be matched by similar investment of time and resource into guideline implementation. Implementing guideline recommendations often requires both a change in human behaviour and a change in the way systems work to deliver care, and this can be a difficult process. The process for implementing evidence into clinical practice, along with some of the barriers that may be encountered during the process and strategies for overcoming them, is discussed in Chapters 16 and 17.

Unfortunately there is a relative lack of high quality research evidence on the impacts of guideline implementation, but there is some evidence that, when implemented, use of guidelines can improve care processes and outcomes. Studies have documented improvements in specific areas of care such as cardiovascular disease and diabetes when guidelines are used.[27–30] A systematic review of studies evaluating the effects of Dutch evidence-based guidelines both on the process and structure of care and on patient outcomes showed that guidelines can be effective in improving the process and structure of care, although the effects on patient health outcomes were studied far less and data were less convincing.[31]

LEGAL ISSUES SURROUNDING THE USE OF CLINICAL GUIDELINES

We have seen that clinical guidelines are not a foolproof method of providing clinical care. Guidelines have, in the past, been criticised as being 'recipe book medicine' due to concerns that the rigid following of algorithms or care plans has the potential to de-skill health professionals. However, after reading this chapter, it should be clear that no matter how well clinical guidelines and their recommendations are linked to evidence, their interpretation and application should be guided by the health professional's clinical experience and judgment and the patient's preferences and values. Clinical guidelines are a standardised approach to care that apply to general conditions (such as a person who has had a stroke) and not necessarily to the particular clinical situation at hand (for example, a 43-year-old woman who has had a cerebellar infarction and also has diabetes, osteoarthritis and a history of smoking). Therefore, health professionals should interpret the guidelines within the context of an individual patient's circumstances.

The legal issues that surround the use of clinical guidelines can vary greatly between countries because of different laws that exist in each country. Under common law in Australia, minimum acceptable standards of clinical care derive from responsible customary practice, not from guidelines. In England and Wales, the National Health Service Executive has stated that clinical guidelines cannot be used to mandate, authorise or outlaw treatment options.[32] While clinical guidelines may be used as evidence in court (either supporting or not supporting the actions of the health professional involved), they are unlikely to alter the usual evidentiary processes in litigation as, currently, the testimony of experts is used to help the courts to decide what is reasonable and accepted practice.[33] In other words, court decisions about whether a health professional provided reasonable care and skill are typically based on expert opinion rather than the contents of a clinical guideline. So, while guidelines may be introduced into courts by expert witnesses as evidence of accepted and customary standards of care, they cannot, as yet, be introduced as a substitute for expert testimony.

Although guidelines currently do not set legal standards for clinical care, they provide the courts with a benchmark by which to judge clinical conduct.[34] Because evidence-based clinical guidelines can set normative standards for practice, departure from them may require some explanation.[34] In clinical situations where there is a serious departure from guidelines, this will need to be well documented in the patient's clinical records. The documentation should emphasise that the departure from the guidelines, and the possible consequences of this, have been thoroughly discussed and understood by the patient and the relevant clinical, or other (for example, patient choice), reasons for this departure provided.

SUMMARY POINTS OF THIS CHAPTER

- Clinical guidelines are systematically developed statements that are designed to help health professionals and their patients make decisions about patients' health care. Guidelines aim to reduce unnecessary variations in care, encourage best practice and facilitate more informed and meaningful involvement of patients in making decisions about their health care.

- Clinical guidelines can be a useful tool for evidence-based practice. They translate evidence into actionable recommendations that can be applied to clinical situations. They do not take the place of informed clinical judgment and patient choice in determining care, but can provide a useful adjunct to care.

- Clinical guidelines can be located using a variety of online resources, such as guideline-specific databases, bibliographic databases and the websites of disease-specific organisations.

- Clinical guidelines are typically developed by a range of stakeholders, including clinical experts, researchers and patients. Ideally, the development of guidelines should follow a rigorous process. However, the quality of guidelines varies according to the processes that occurred during their development.

- Because guidelines vary in quality, you should know how to appraise clinical guidelines and recognise the key features that discriminate high quality guidelines that can be used to guide practice from low quality clinical guidelines that should be dismissed. The AGREE II instrument is a useful tool for appraising guidelines and helping you to determine if you can trust the recommendations that are in a clinical guideline.

- Medico-legal considerations in relation to guidelines need to be taken into account. If a considerable departure from guideline recommendations is agreed on by the patient and the health professional, it is good practice to state the reason for this in the patient's clinical records.

References

1. Institute of Medicine. Field M, Lohr K, editors. Guidelines for clinical practice: from development to use. Washington DC: National Academy Press; 1992.
2. Institute of Medicine. Graham R, Mancher M, Wolman D, et al, editors. Clinical practice guidelines we can trust. Washington DC: National Academy Press; 2011.
3. Ward J, Grieco V. Why we need guidelines for guidelines: a study of the quality of clinical practice guidelines in Australia. Med J Aust 1996;165:574–6.
4. Buchan H, Currie K, Lourey E, et al. Australian clinical practice guidelines: a national study. Med J Aust 2010;192:490–4.
5. Feder G, Eccles M, Grol R, et al. Clinical guidelines: using clinical guidelines. BMJ 1999;318:728–30.
6. Menendez R, Torres A, Zalacain R, et al. Guidelines for the treatment of community-acquired pneumonia: predictors of adherence and outcome. Am J Respir Crit Care Med 2005;172:757–62.
7. Fonarow G, Abraham W, Albert N, et al. Association between performance measures and clinical outcomes for patients hospitalised with heart failure. JAMA 2007;297:61–70.
8. Du Pen S, Du Pen A, Polissar N, et al. Implementing guidelines for cancer pain management: results of a randomised controlled clinical trial. J Clin Oncol 1999;17:361–70.
9. Grimshaw J, Eccles M, Tetroe J. Implementing clinical guidelines: current evidence and future implications. J Contin Educ Health Prof 2004;24(Suppl 1):S31–7.
10. Craig J, Irwig L, Stockler M. Evidence-based medicine: useful tools for decision making. Med J Aust 2001;174:248–53.
11. Wilczynski N, Haynes R, Lavis J, et al. Optimal search strategies for detecting health services research studies in MEDLINE. CMAJ 2004;171:1179–85.
12. National Institute for Health and Clinical Excellence. Clinical guidelines development methods, 2009. Online. Available: www.nice.org.uk/aboutnice/howwework/developingniceclinicalguidelines/ clinicalguidelinedevelopmentmethods/clinical_guideline_development_methods.jsp; 20 Feb 2012.

13. Scottish Intercollegiate Guidelines Network. SIGN 50: a guideline developer's handbook, 2011. Online. Available: www.sign.ac.uk/guidelines/fulltext/50/index.html; 20 Feb 2012.

14. Graham I, Harrison M. Evaluation and adaptation of clinical practice guidelines. Evid Based Nurs 2005;8:68–72.

15. Shekelle P, Kravitz R, Beart J, et al. Are nonspecific practice guidelines potentially harmful? A randomised comparison of the effect of nonspecific versus specific guidelines on physician decision making. Health Serv Res 2000;34:1429–48.

16. Vlayen J, Aertgeerts B, Hannes K, et al. A systematic review of appraisal tools for clinical practice guidelines: multiple similarities and one common deficit. Int J Qual Health Care 2005;17:235–42.

17. The AGREE Collaboration. Development and validation of an international appraisal instrument for assessing the quality of clinical practice guidelines: the AGREE project. Qual Saf Health Care 2003;12:18–23.

18. Brouwers M, Kho M, Browman G, et al and the AGREE Next Steps Consortium. AGREE II: advancing guideline development, reporting and evaluation in health care. CMAJ 2010;182(18):E839–42. doi: 10.1503/cmaj.090449.

19. Straus S, Richardson W, Glasziou P, et al. Evidence-based medicine: how to practice and teach EBM. 4th ed. Edinburgh: Churchill Livingstone; 2011.

20 Atkins D, Eccles M, Flottorp S, et al, for GRADE Working Group. Systems for grading the quality of evidence and the strength of recommendations. I: critical appraisal of existing approaches. BMC Health Serv Res 2004;4:38.

21. GRADE Working Group. Grading the quality of evidence and the strength of recommendations, no date. Online. Available: www.gradeworkinggroup.org/intro.htm; 23 Nov 2011.

22. GRADE Working Group. Grading quality of evidence and strength of recommendations. BMJ 2004;328:1490–7.

23. National Health and Medical Research Council (NHMRC). Procedures and requirements for meeting the 2011 NHMRC standard for clinical practice guidelines, 2011. Online. Available: www.nhmrc.gov.au/guidelines/publications/cp133-and-cp133a; 20 Feb 2012.

24. National Health and Medical Research Council (NHMRC). NHMRC additional levels of evidence and grades for recommendations for developers of guidelines, 2009. Online. Available: www.nhmrc.gov.au/_files_nhmrc/file/guidelines/developers/nhmrc_levels_grades_evidence_120423.pdf; 11 Mar 2012.

25. Scalzitti D. Evidence-based guidelines: application to clinical practice. Phys Ther 2001;81:1622–8.

26. Grimshaw J, Thomas R, MacLennan G, et al. Effectiveness and efficiency of guideline dissemination and implementation strategies. Health Technol Assess 2004;8:iii–iv, 1–72.

27. LaBresh K, Fonarow G, Smith S Jr, et al, and the Get With The Guidelines Steering Committee. Improved treatment of hospitalised coronary artery disease patients with the Get With The Guidelines program. Crit Pathw Cardiol 2007;6:98–105.

28. Reeves M, Grau-Sepulveda M, Fonarow G, et al. Are quality improvements in the Get With The Guidelines—Stroke program related to better care or better data documentation? Circ Cardiovasc Qual Outcomes 2011;4:503–11.

29. Schwamm L, Fonarow G, Reeves M, et al. Get With The Guidelines—Stroke is associated with sustained improvement in care for patients hospitalised with acute stroke or transient ischemic attack. Circulation 2009;119:107–15.

30. Chin M, Cook S, Drum M, et al. Improving diabetes care in Midwest community health centers with the health disparities collaborative. Diabetes Care 2004;27:2–8.

31. Lugtenberg M, Burgers J, Westert G. Effects of evidence-based clinical practice guidelines on quality of care: a systematic review. Qual Saf Health Care 2009;18:385–92.

32. Hurwitz B. Clinical guidelines: legal and political considerations of clinical practice guidelines. BMJ 1999;318:661–4.

33. Dwyer P. Legal implications of clinical practice guidelines. Med J Aust 1998;169:292–3.

34. Hurwitz B. How does evidence based guidance influence determinations of medical negligence? BMJ 2004;329:1024–8.

Chapter 14

Talking with patients about evidence

Tammy Hoffmann and Leigh Tooth

LEARNING OBJECTIVES

After reading this chapter, you should be able to:

- Describe why it is important that health professionals communicate effectively with their patients
- Understand what is meant by the term patient-centred care
- Explain what is meant by shared decision making and discuss some of the challenges associated with it and the strategies that can be used to facilitate it
- List the key communication skills needed by health professionals when talking with patients about evidence
- Describe the various methods that can be used for communicating information to patients, the main considerations associated with each method, and the major factors that should be considered when deciding which communication tool(s) to use with a patient
- Explain how to effectively communicate statistical information to patients

At the heart of the definition of evidence-based practice that was provided in Chapter 1 lies the involvement of patients and the consideration of their values and preferences when making decisions regarding their health care. As part of the health care that they are receiving, patients often need to make decisions about aspects of their health care, such as whether to proceed with a particular intervention. Many patients and their families find it difficult to take an active part in healthcare decisions.[1] A health professional's ability to communicate effectively with patients and, often, also their family members is crucial to the successful involvement of patients in these decisions.[1] For these decisions to be fully informed and ones with which the patient is involved, patients need to know about the benefits, harms and risks and uncertainties associated with the various intervention options.[1] Even when a decision about intervention is not needed, there are often many other aspects of their health care that patients can benefit from being knowledgeable about. Many patients and their families have only a limited understanding about health and its determinants, and do not know where to find information that is clear, trustworthy and easy to understand.[1] Individualised education that is specific to the disease and the patient is able to improve a patient's self-efficacy to manage chronic conditions, assist with short-term behaviour change, improve quality of life and reduce morbidity and healthcare utilisation.[2] Effective communication can also help to build trust between patients and health professionals, make clinical practice more effective and reduce clinical mishaps and errors.[3]

Despite its importance, many health professionals are not specifically trained in how to effectively communicate with patients, and many patients do not know how to communicate with health professionals. Therefore, we have devoted a chapter of this book to this topic so that, when you are interacting with patients, you are aware of the importance of talking with your patients about evidence and are knowledgeable about the skills and resources that can assist you to do this successfully. In this chapter, we will discuss why effective communication is important, outline the steps to communicating effectively with patients and discuss some of the key communication skills that health professionals need, including sections on how to decide which communication method and tool(s) to use and how to communicate statistical information to patients. We will also outline the concept of patient-centred care and one of the skills that is often central to achieving this, namely shared decision making.

WHY IS EFFECTIVE COMMUNICATION SO IMPORTANT?

Many people do not think of communication as a particularly important or specialised skill for health professionals to have, and often health professionals do not give it the emphasis that it needs. Health professionals often think of communication as secondary to their 'real' job of caring for patients. However, the success of an intervention is frequently dependent on the health professional successfully providing the patient with appropriate information. In addition, health professionals often do not realise that, as with many of the other interventions that they provide to patients, there are theories and principles that should be used to guide communication with patients.

Effective communication is central to a 'patient-centred' approach by health professionals. The evolution and benefits of patient-centred care are discussed in the following section.

PATIENT-CENTRED CARE

Patient-centred care (also commonly referred to as *client-centred care* or *patient-centred practice*) is a broad umbrella term reflecting a particular approach to the health-professional–patient relationship that implies communication, partnerships, respect, choice and empowerment and a focus on the patient rather than their specific clinical condition.[4] Patient-centred practice by health professionals reflects their commitment to quality care by the way they respect patients' needs, goals, values, expectations and preferences and involve patients in the decision-making process.[5]

Central to patient-centred care is treating patients with dignity, responding quickly and effectively to patients' needs and concerns[6] and providing patients with enough information to enable them to make informed choices about their health care.[7] Patient-centred care has become the model that is advocated by health professionals and health professional associations. This model of care sits between the 'paternalistic' and 'informed patient or independent choice' models of care.[8,9] In the traditional 'paternalistic' model of care, the health professional is in control, discloses information as and when suitable and makes the decisions for the patient who is expected to be passive, unquestioning and compliant. At the other end of the spectrum is the 'informed patient or independent choice' model, in which health professionals present the facts and leave the decision making solely up to the patient.[8]

There is emerging evidence of the benefits of patient-centred care to health professionals and patients. Patient-centred practice can increase patient satisfaction and quality of life, reduce patient anxiety and improve symptom resolution, pain control, function and physiological measures and improve adherence to long-term medication use.[4,10] For health professionals, patient-centred practice can contribute to more appropriate and cost-effective use of health services, such as reducing the number of diagnostic tests and unnecessary referrals.[10,11] Features of patient-centred practice include shared decision making and tailoring communication and education to the needs, abilities and preferences of the patient, each of which will be discussed in the following sections of this chapter.

SHARED DECISION MAKING

Shared decision making refers to clinical decision making as a partnership between the patient and the health professional, with communication focused on achieving shared understanding of treatment goals and plans.[12] The ultimate goal of shared decision making is for health professionals to make decisions that are consistent with the wishes of patients,[13] and ones which respect patients' autonomy.[14] Shared decision making allows patients the opportunity to ask questions and to express their values, preferences and personal circumstances.[1] Patient involvement in the decision-making process often extends beyond just choosing treatment options and can also involve:[8]

- recognition and clarification of the health issue
- identification of possible solutions
- appraisal of possible solutions
- implementation of the chosen solution
- evaluation of the solution.

Many leading health organisations now advocate patient participation in clinical decision making. These include the National Health and Medical Research Council of Australia,[3] the USA Preventive Services Taskforce,[8] the American Medical Association[15] and the General Medical Council of the UK.[16] In 2011, the Salzburg Global Seminar published the Salzburg Statement on Shared Decision Making, which calls on patients and health professionals to work together to be co-producers of health.[1]

Shared decision making between patients and health professionals has been linked with improved patient outcomes, for example improved control of hypertension,[17] better compliance,[18,19] greater family satisfaction with communication,[20] improved emotional status[21] and reduced visits to emergency departments,[22] use of medications,[22] hospital admissions[23] and total medical costs.[23] However, shared decision making is not possible in all clinical encounters, nor is it welcomed or desired by all patients. The next section presents some of the challenges that can be associated with shared decision making.

Shared decision making: the challenges

Challenges related to the availability of evidence

Sometimes shared decision making can be relatively straightforward, for example in common health problems where there is only one course of action or where the evidence is clear and most informed health professionals and patients would agree that the benefits outweigh the harms.[24] In other situations, shared decision making can be more difficult. For example, with some chronic conditions the research evidence that is provided by randomised controlled trials and systematic reviews often fails to endorse one intervention, and instead highlights the benefits and harms of a number of interventions. While difficult, shared decision making can be particularly valuable in these situations, with health professionals helping patients to understand the risks, benefits and trade-offs of the various interventions.[18] Finally, for some medical conditions there may not be sufficient evidence about the benefits and harms of intervention options, in which case the health professional needs to assist the patient to assess this uncertainty against the patient's values and preferences.[24]

Patients' involvement in shared decision making

Shared decision making is not always possible, for example in medical emergencies or with patients who do not have the cognitive capacity to participate. Further, shared decision making is not always welcomed or desired by patients. In a nationally representative sample of 2750 adults in the USA, it was found that while 96% of the participants wanted to be asked for their opinions and offered choices, half preferred to rely on their doctors for information and half wanted to leave the final decisions up to their doctors.[25] Patients' preferences for involvement in decision making were found to differ by health status and socio-demographic characteristics. For example, patients who were in poorer health, male, older than 45 years of age and with fewer years of education were less likely to want to participate in shared decision making. More recently, in a 2010 patient survey by the Care Quality Commission in the United Kingdom, 48% of inpatients reported wanting more involvement in decisions about their care.[26] A systematic review of studies on patient preferences for shared decision making found that in 63% of studies, the majority of patients preferred to participate in shared decision making with their health professionals. Furthermore, the number of patients who prefer to make shared decisions appears to have increased over time. The majority of patients want to discuss their options and receive information, even though they may not wish to be responsible for making the final decision.[27]

Individual patients may also vary in the degree to which they want to participate in shared decision making, depending upon the specific clinical situation.[3] Indeed, shared decision making may be more easily conceptualised as a continuum, whereby decision making can be health professional or patient driven (at extreme ends of the continuum) or driven by the many combinations in between.[13] This illustrates the need for you, as a health professional, to determine the role that each of your patients wishes to take in the management of their health. A simple question that you can ask to help establish this is *'How do you feel about being involved in making decisions about your treatment?'*[28]

It is worth pointing out that shared decision making may also have unwanted effects. For example, once patients are fully informed about benefits, harms and risks, they may still decide not to undertake treatment for a health condition or to have a screening test because they are at low risk of developing future problems.[29] It has been suggested that this expression of 'fully informed choice may sometimes frustrate the health professional',[29] as it can lead to some patients choosing a path that results in harm or death. A clear example of this is when patients reject the need for blood transfusions due to religious beliefs.

Shared decision making also has legal implications, in particular concerning informed consent. Health professionals have been found legally liable for damages in instances where inadequate information has been provided to patients and harm has arisen following intervention.[30] The High Court of Australia has referred to the importance of shared decision making, defining it as 'a shared exercise in which healthcare practitioners are obliged to take active steps to ensure that patients are empowered to make their own decisions about important procedures to be undertaken on their bodies'.[30]

The complexities of patient and health professional involvement in shared decision making

Shared decision making is a complex process which involves not only the patient's values and preferences, but also their feelings and views about their relationship with the health professional and the degree of effort that both parties put into the decision-making process and the communication between them.[8] Box 14.1 provides some examples of the complexities in health-professional–patient relationships that can influence shared decision making.[8]

Strategies to assist shared decision making

As a health professional, there are various strategies that you can use to facilitate effective shared decision making and these are presented in Box 14.2.[13,18,20,21,31–33] Central to successful shared decision making is effective communication, which involves communicating the evidence to patients and actively listening to patients' concerns. Effective communication is informed by how patients prefer to receive information and their ability to understand it. These issues are described in more detail later in this chapter.

Assessment tools for health professionals to use in shared decision making

A number of scales have been developed to assess the involvement of patients and health professionals in shared decision making. The scales in these two areas will be discussed separately and one example of each will be described in detail. These scales can also assist you by providing examples of questions that you can ask and competencies you can aim for in your own clinical practice.

BOX 14.1

Examples of the complexities in the health-professional–patient relationship[7]

- Patients who believe that the health professional cares about them and is collaborating with them and making an effort on their behalf may be more likely to be encouraged to do their own bit in relation to their health care.
- Patients who doubt that their health professional likes them or doubt that their health professional is focused on their best interests may be less confident about the recommended intervention options.
- Health professionals who have positive views of their patients as partners who are capable and able to be trusted are more likely to facilitate the involvement of patients in the decision-making process.
- Health professionals who are mentally disengaged from patients or the decision-making process may be less likely to facilitate other aspects of patient involvement in the decision-making process.

BOX 14.2

Strategies to facilitate shared decision making

- Attend to the whole of patients' problems and take account of their expectations, feelings and ideas.
- Value patients' contributions, for example the life experiences and values that patients bring to the decision-making process.
- Provide clear, honest and unbiased information.
- Be an active listener.
- Assess the degree to which your patients understand the information that you have provided to them.
- Assess the degree to which your patients want to be involved in decision making.
- Provide a caring, respectful and empowering context in which patients can be enabled to participate in decision making.
- Be well informed about the most current evidence, particularly regarding issues such as diagnosis and intervention.
- Do not assume that your patients will make the same decisions as you just because the evidence has been provided to them in a manner that they can understand.

Scales to measure health professionals' involvement in shared decision making

In a 2001 systematic review, eight instruments that assess various aspects of clinical decision making were described, but the authors of the review concluded that none of the eight instruments sufficiently captured the concept of whether the health professional encouraged patient 'involvement' in the decision-making process.[33] The authors of the review subsequently developed and revised the 12-item OPTION (Observing Patient Involvement in Decision Making) scale to measure the extent that a health professional engages in shared decision making during patient consultations.[34,35] Examples of the 12 'competencies' that are assessed in OPTION are:

- Item 1: The health professional draws attention to an identified problem as one that requires a decision-making process.
- Item 3: The health professional assesses the patient's preferred approach to receiving information to assist decision making.
- Item 5: The health professional explains the pros and cons of options to the patient (taking 'no action' is an option).
- Item 10: The health professional elicits the patient's preferred level of involvement in decision making.

Each 'competency' is rated by observers on a scale that measures the order of magnitude to which the health professional demonstrates the skill. The scale is as follows:

0—'The behaviour is not observed'

1—'A minimal attempt is made to exhibit the behaviour'

2—'The health professional asks the patient about their preferred way of receiving information to assist decision'

3—'The behaviour is exhibited to a good standard'

4—'The behaviour is observed and executed to a high standard'.

Scales to measure patients' involvement in shared decision making

Questionnaires have been developed to assess patients' satisfaction with decision making,[36] degree of decisional conflict,[37] perceived involvement in care,[38] risk communication and confidence in decision making[28] and the extent of shared decision making.[39] One of these will now be further described.

The COMRADE (Combined Outcome Measure for Risk Communication and Treatment Decision Making Effectiveness) was developed by combining items from some existing shared decision-making scales and constructs identified by patients during focus groups.[28] It consists of 20 statements that represent two broad aspects of decision-making effectiveness—risk communication and confidence in the decision.

Each statement is scored on a five-point Likert scale from 1 (strongly agree) to 5 (strongly disagree). While the original scale statements use the term 'doctor', the COMRADE can be used by all health professionals. Examples of the 20 statements are as follows.

Statements about risk communication:

- The health professional gave me enough information about the treatment choices available.
- The health professional gave me the chance to express my opinions about the different treatments available.
- The health professional gave me the chance to decide which treatment I thought was best for me.

Statements about confidence in decision making:

- I am satisfied that I am adequately informed about the issues important to the decision.

- I am satisfied with the way the decision was made in the consultation.
- I am sure that the decision is the right one for me personally.

The COMRADE is intended to be used in conjunction with three other relevant instruments, the SF-12 measure of quality of life, the short-form anxiety instrument and the patient enablement instrument (see the reference that describes the COMRADE[28] for more details).

KEY STEPS TO COMMUNICATING EVIDENCE TO PATIENTS EFFECTIVELY

A five-step model for communicating evidence to patients in a way that facilitates shared decision making has been proposed[40] and is presented below. Although the model was developed as a guide for medical practitioners who are consulting with patients and helping them to make healthcare decisions, the key principles of the model can be used as a guide for any health professional who is communicating evidence to a patient.

1. **Understand the patient's (and family members') experiences and expectations.**

   You need to take the time and make the effort to understand the needs, fears, experiences, expectations and values of your patient.

2. **Build partnerships.**

   Rather than just providing information to your patient in an old-style paternalistic manner, you should try to gain your patient's trust and build a partnership with them. Activities that may assist with this include: encouraging partnership (for example, 'This is a decision that we need to make together'), acknowledging the difficulty of the situation/decision that is being discussed, expressing empathy and expressing mutual understanding (for example, 'I think I understand …').[40]

3. **Discuss the evidence, including a balanced discussion about uncertainties.**

   In addition to answering your patient's questions, you should also discuss issues that they may not have thought to ask or are reluctant to bring up. A discussion of the evidence needs to include a simple explanation of the uncertainties surrounding the evidence, but be aware that overemphasising the uncertainty can cause some patients to lose confidence.[40] Using an appropriate method to communicate statistical information can be beneficial at this stage and a discussion of the various methods for doing this are explained in a later section of this chapter.

4. **Present recommendations.**

   Obviously a healthcare decision does not need to be made every time that you communicate evidence to a patient, particularly if it is evidence related to a prognostic or qualitative information need that you or your patient had. However, when the clinical question is about the effect of an intervention, a decision may need to be made. This step should only occur after you have integrated the best quality clinical evidence that is available for the issue with your patient's values and preferences. You should explain how your recommendation has been generated from both the evidence and your patient's values.[40] In situations where the evidence is uncertain or contradictory and you do not have a specific recommendation, you should present each of the options neutrally.

5. **Check for understanding and agreement.**

   It is important to confirm that your patient has understood the information that you have presented to them. You may wish to ask your patient to briefly summarise their understanding of the information for you. You may need to repeat the information, explain it in a different way or provide more-detailed information. There are various communication tools that can be used to share information with patients and, in some cases, help them to make decisions. These tools are discussed in a later section of this chapter.

KEY COMMUNICATION SKILLS NEEDED BY HEALTH PROFESSIONALS

In addition to the general communication and relationship-building skills that you should have as a health professional, some of the key skills that you need when talking with your patients about evidence are listed in Box 14.3.

METHODS FOR COMMUNICATING INFORMATION

There are various formats that you can choose to use when providing patients with information with the aim of increasing their knowledge and understanding of the evidence related to their situation. Using more than one method to provide the information can be a valuable way of increasing patients' retention of the information.[41]

Verbal information

Verbal education is the method that is most commonly used by health professionals for providing information. There are some general points that you should follow when providing patients with information verbally to improve the effectiveness of the information exchange[42] and these are listed in Box 14.4.

One of the major limitations of providing information verbally is that people often forget what they have been told. It has been estimated that most people remember less than a quarter of what they have been told.[43] For this reason, using written materials to supplement or reinforce information that has been presented verbally is recommended.[44]

BOX 14.3

Key skills needed by health professionals when talking with their patients about evidence

- Ability to communicate complex information using non-technical language.
- Tailoring the amount and pace of information to the patient's needs and preferences.
- Drawing diagrams to aid comprehension.
- Understanding the principles of shared decision making and how and when to implement this with patients.
- Ability to determine how much involvement in decision making patients desire.
- Considering the patient's preferences and values and integrating this with the clinical evidence for the various treatment options.
- Understanding the factors that can impede information exchange and shared decision making.
- When a healthcare decision needs to be made, the ability to clearly explain the probability and risk for each option.
- Facilitative skills to encourage patient involvement.
- Evaluation of internet information that patients might bring with them.
- Creating an environment in which patients feel comfortable asking questions.
- Giving patients time to take in the information.
- Declaration of 'equipoise' when present—equipoise exists when there is uncertainty about which treatment option, including the option of no further treatment, will benefit a patient the most.
- Checking patient understanding.
- Negotiation skills.

Adapted with permission from Ford S, Schofield T, Hope T. What are the ingredients for a successful evidence-based patient choice consultation? A qualitative study; published by Social Science and Medicine, 2003.[32]

BOX 14.4

Strategies for clearly and effectively providing information verbally to patients

- Sit down with the patient, maintain eye contact, remove any distractions and give the patient your full attention.
- Use effective communication skills such as active listening, gesturing and responding to the patient's non-verbal cues to facilitate communication.
- Do not speak too quickly.
- Use clear and simple language. Avoid jargon where possible. Explain any medical terminology that is used.
- Where possible, use the same terms consistently throughout the discussion rather than using a range of different terms that mean the same thing.
- Present the most important information first.
- Do not provide too much information at once. Present a few points and then pause to check that the patient understands.
- Observe for indicators that the patient may not have understood, such as a look of confusion or a long pause before responding to a question.
- Have the patient indicate their level of understanding. Having them repeat the main points of what you have said in their own words can often be more valuable than just asking 'Do you understand?'

Combination of verbal and written information

The combination of verbal and written information has the potential to maximise a patient's knowledge.[36,45] For example, a Cochrane systematic review that evaluated the effect of providing written summaries or recordings (such as an audiotape) of consultations for people with cancer found that the majority of participants in the trials who received recordings or summaries used and valued them as a reminder of what was said during the consultation.[46] Most studies found that patients who were given the summaries demonstrated better recall of information and reported greater satisfaction with the information received during the consultations.[46] However, none of the studies in the review found that the summaries had a statistically significant effect on anxiety, depression or quality of life.[46]

Written information

Appropriate readability and design of written materials

There are many forms that written information can take, such as a pamphlet, booklet, printed information sheet or information from internet sites. Regardless of the form, for written information to be useful to patients they need to notice, read, understand, believe and remember it. Many written materials that health professionals use with patients are written and designed in a way that can make it difficult for patients to understand the content they contain. One of the most common problems is that many health education materials are written at a reading level that is too high for the majority of the patients who receive them.[47,48] A fifth- to sixth-grade reading level (approximately a 10- to 11-year-old reading age in countries such as Australia) is recommended for written health information. There are various readability formulas that can be used to quickly and easily assess the readability of written information, including the SMOG[49] and the Flesch Reading Ease formula[50] (available in Microsoft Word).

In addition to readability, there are many other features of written patient health education materials that need to be given appropriate consideration in order to maximise the usefulness of the materials for patients. This includes features such as:

- the content in the material (for example, is it evidence-based?)
- the language used (for example, what types of words are used and how are sentences structured?)
- the organisation of content (for example, are bulleted lists used where possible?)
- the layout and typography throughout the material (for example, is an appropriate font size used throughout?)
- the illustrations within the material (for example, is each illustration appropriately labelled and explained in the text?)
- the incorporation of learning and motivation features into the content (for example, are there features in the material that actively engage the reader?)

It is beyond the scope of this chapter to discuss these features in detail. However, summaries of this information are readily available,[51] and there are a number of checklists that can be used to assess the quality of the written information that is used with patients.[51-53]

Assessing the quality of written information about treatment choices

In addition to having appropriate readability and design, it is important that written health information is evidence-based. DISCERN is a questionnaire designed to assess the quality of written information on treatment choices for a health problem. It consists of 16 items, each scored on a 5-point scale. Box 14.5 lists the main points that are covered in the DISCERN questionnaire.[54] The full questionnaire is available on the DISCERN website (www.discern.org.uk).

BOX 14.5

Issues covered by DISCERN–a questionnaire for assessing the quality of written information on treatment choices for a health problem

- Is the publication reliable?
  - Are the aims clear?
  - Does it achieve its aims?
  - Is it relevant?
  - Is it clear what sources of information were used to compile the publication?
  - Is it clear when the information used or reported in the publication was produced?
  - Is it balanced and unbiased?
  - Does it provide details of additional sources of support and information?
  - Does it refer to areas of uncertainty?
- How good is the quality of the information on treatment choices?
  - Does it describe how each treatment works?
  - Does it describe the benefits of each treatment?
  - Does it describe the risks of each treatment?
  - Does it describe what would happen if no treatment was used?
  - Does it describe how the treatment choices affect overall quality of life?
  - Is it clear that there may be more than one possible treatment choice?
  - Does it provide support for shared decision making?
- Overall rating of the publication as a source of information about treatment choices.

Source: www.discern.org.uk/discern_instrument.php.

Computer-based information

In addition to accessing health information from the internet, there are other ways that computers can be used as a health information resource for patients. For example, providing patients with computer-generated interactive patient education materials (see, for example, the systematic review by Treweek and colleagues[55]) or with tailored printed information (see, for example, the system described by Hoffmann and colleagues[56]). There is preliminary evidence that computer-tailored education materials can be effective in changing various behaviours such as physical activity, short-term dietary behaviour and safe-sex behaviours,[57–60] although intervention features such as intensity can influence whether this type of intervention is effective. Interactive computer-based health information interventions can have a positive effect on health knowledge, social support and behavioural outcomes (such as changes in diet and exercise) for patients with chronic diseases.[61] Computer-based materials can also be used to assist patients to make health-related decisions. More information about this is provided in the later section of this chapter about decision aids.

Internet-based health information

As much health information is obtained from the internet,[62] you should be prepared to evaluate health information from the internet that patients may bring with them and also to evaluate health information websites prior to recommending them to patients. There are various criteria that can be used to evaluate health information websites, and these criteria relate to the content of the website including an evaluation of its descriptive content, accuracy and completeness;[63] the credibility of the website's authors, disclosure on the website and the design and aesthetics of the website.[41] For internet sites that contain information about treatment options for a health problem, the DISCERN questionnaire (as shown in Box 14.5) can also be used to evaluate these sites.

As recommending health information websites to patients is now a common occurrence during health-professional–patient consultations, the following resources may be of use to you:

- The Cochrane Consumer Network (www.consumers.cochrane.org)—is aimed at helping patients to make informed decisions and provides a plain language summary of Cochrane reviews.

- MedlinePlus (www.nlm.nih.gov/medlineplus)—a free service provided by the US National Library of Medicine that offers web links that meet pre-established quality criteria to health information on the internet. It is designed to help provide high quality health information to patients and their families. Health professionals can also use this site to obtain quick and easy access to images or videos to help when providing information to patients.

- Health on the Net (HON) Foundation (www.hon.ch)—a foundation aimed at guiding internet users to reliable, understandable, accessible and trustworthy sources of health information. Using the HONcode (which consists of eight principles), the foundation evaluates websites and those that meet the criteria become accredited websites and can display the HON logo. On this site you can also access HONmedia (www.hon.ch/HONmedia), which contains a wide selection of medical illustrations that can be used when educating patients.

- HealthFinder (www.healthfinder.gov)—a US government gateway site to reliable health information resources that have been reviewed by HealthFinder staff.

Interactive computer-based information

Compared with standard verbal or written methods of providing information, interactive computer-based information has been found to significantly increase patients' knowledge, understanding and satisfaction.[64,65] The use of computer programs to provide patients with interactive health information is generally well accepted by patients[65] and often preferred to reading a booklet or watching a videotape.[66]

Tailored print information

Tailored information is information which is customised according to an individual's characteristics or preferences. Although it is not essential to use a computer to provide patients with tailored information, doing so can make the process of tailoring information to individual patients' needs quick and easy. There is evidence that, compared with non-tailored information, tailored print information is better remembered, read and perceived as relevant and/or credible.[67] Tailored information is also more likely to influence changes in health behaviour[67,68] and result in greater patient satisfaction with the information that is provided and in better-met informational needs.[69] However, the effectiveness of tailored information is moderated by a number of variables such as the type of health behaviour, patient population and theoretical concepts which are being tailored.[67]

DVDs/videotapes and audiotapes

Use of media such as digital video discs (DVDs), videotapes and/or audiotapes can be a useful method for providing information to patients, particularly patients who have a low literacy level or English as a second language, or those who have an auditory (if audiotape) or visual (if DVD) learning style. There is some evidence that using formats such as videotapes or DVDs can improve patient outcomes such as knowledge and satisfaction,[70] and clinical outcomes such as reducing in-hospital falls.[71]

Decision aids

What are decision aids?

For people who are facing decisions about the best way to manage their health, whether it is a decision about treatment or about screening, decision aids are a communication tool that may be of some assistance for patients in certain situations. Decision aids are interventions designed to help patients make decisions by providing them with information about the options and about the personal importance of possible benefits and harms, and encouraging their active participation in the decision-making process together with their health professional.[72] Decision aids may be paper-based (such as a pamphlet) or involve a video (often with accompanying printed information). However, the majority of decision aids are internet-based.

What outcomes can decision aids have an effect on?

A Cochrane systematic review that evaluated the effectiveness of decision aids concluded that, compared with usual care, decision aids assist patients to have a greater knowledge of their options, more-realistic expectations of possible benefits and harms and make choices which better reflect their personal values and preferences, with no adverse effect on their health outcomes or satisfaction.[72] Decision aids were also found to increase patient communication with health professionals and participation in collaborative decision making.[72]

Finding decision aids

Currently, the majority of decision aids that exist are on topics that are most appropriate for medical practitioners to discuss with their patients (for example, deciding between various treatments for cancer or deciding whether to receive hormone replacement therapy). However, other health professionals such as nurses and allied health professionals may find some of the decision aids that are currently available also useful in their clinical practice. For example, there are decision aids available on topics such as deciding about nursing-home care for a family member who has dementia, options for managing back pain and options for managing carpal tunnel syndrome.

New decision aids are continually being developed, so when you have a patient who needs to make a healthcare decision it is worth searching on the internet to see if there is a relevant decision aid. A recommended resource is the Ottawa Health Research Institute (www.ohri.ca/decisionaid), which maintains an inventory of decision aids. The Wiser Choices Program from the Mayo Clinic Shared Decision Making National Resource Center (kercards.e-bm.info) has also developed a number of useful decision aids.[73]

Using decision aids

As with other patient-education resources, if you are considering using a decision aid with a patient there are a number of factors that you need to take into account. These are detailed in the section below. If you choose to use a decision aid with a patient, you need to ensure that it is of good quality. A set of criteria, known as the CREDIBLE criteria, has been developed for assessing the quality of decision aids; full details of the criteria are available in the Cochrane review on decision aids that was discussed earlier.[72] The main criteria are:

C—competently developed

R—recently updated

E—evidence-based

DI—devoid of conflicts of interest

BL—balanced presentation of options, benefits and harms

E—decision aid is efficacious at improving decision making.

Decision aids, particularly internet-based ones, are a relatively new tool that can be used for communicating evidence to patients and enabling them to participate in making decisions about their health care. However, there are many gaps in the research related to decision aids, such as how they affect health-professional–patient communication, factors that determine the successful use of decision aids in practice, and what types of decision aids work best with different types of patients.[72]

DECIDING WHICH COMMUNICATION TOOL(S) TO USE WITH YOUR PATIENTS

As discussed earlier in this chapter, there are various communication tools that you may choose to use when providing patients with information. Your choice will be influenced by a number of factors, including:

- patient's preference—this may also be influenced by your patient's preferred learning style (for example, visual or auditory), cultural background, level of motivation, cultural background and primary language
- patient's literacy level and education level—see below for more information
- patient's cognitive ability and any impairments they have that may affect their ability to communicate, understand or recall information or make decisions—see below for more information
- the educational resources/communication tools that are available to you
- time-related issues—see below for more information.

Literacy levels

If written (or printed or computer-based) health-education materials are used to provide information or supplement information that is provided verbally, the literacy levels of the patients who are receiving the information need to be considered. Written materials will not benefit patients if they are unable to understand them. However, health literacy encompasses more than general literacy skills. There are various definitions of health literacy. The US Institute of Medicine has defined health literacy as the degree to which individuals have the capacity to obtain, process and understand the basic information needed to make appropriate decisions about their health.[74] You should be aware of your patient's literacy skills so that you can alter the educational intervention accordingly.[75] There are a number of resources that provide strategies for how to do this—for example, see the publication by Fischoff and colleagues.[76] Be aware that people with poor literacy often use a range of strategies to hide literacy problems[75] and are often reluctant to ask questions so as not to appear ignorant.[77]

Although literacy levels can be influenced by educational level, low health-literacy levels can be found at all levels of educational attainment.[78] Therefore, it is recommended that you assess patients' reading skills using one of the published tests that have been designed to do this, rather than relying only on their self-reported level of education.[77,78] Commonly used tests include: the Rapid Estimate of Adult Literacy in Medicine (REALM),[79] the Test of Functional Health Literacy in Adults (TOFHLA)[80] and the Medical Achievement Reading Test (MART).[81] Recently, the use of a brief and simple screening tool to assess health literacy has been developed and validated among patients with heart failure.[82] This tool consists of the three items, each scored on a 5-point scale (with higher scores indicating lower literacy): (1) How often do you have someone help you read hospital materials?; (2) How often do you have problems learning about your medical condition, because of difficulty reading hospital materials?; and (3) How confident are you filling out forms by yourself? All of these tests evaluate a patient's ability to understand medical terminology and are quick and straightforward to administer and score.

Impairments which may affect communication

Your patient may have one or more impairments that can affect how they are able to process information. This can include cognitive, hearing, visual or speech and language impairments. You need to consider how the presence of one or more of these impairments may result in the need for you to alter how you communicate with your patient and which communication tool(s) you choose to use. There are various strategies that you can use to facilitate communication with patients who have one or more of these impairments; however, it is beyond the scope of this chapter to detail these. Further reading about strategies specific to different impairments is recommended; for example, refer to the patient education book by McKenna and Tooth.[83]

Time-related issues

Time-related issues include both the amount of time that is available for communicating with your patient and the timing of communicating with your patient. Patients' needs vary at different times. For example, patients' informational needs during an initial consultation are different to their needs after a diagnosis or during follow-up consultations or treatment sessions. There may be various points in time (for example, after a diagnosis or when feeling acutely unwell) when patients are unable to process much information. You should be sensitive to when this may be the case and adapt your communication with the patient accordingly. Providing only the most essential information may be sufficient initially. More-detailed information can be provided to your patient at a later, more appropriate time.

Various communication tools may also be indicated at different times. For example, verbal information is usually the main format that is used during initial consultations with patients, but in between subsequent consultations, patients may be given written information or referred to recommended internet sites. This may be useful as a reinforcement of information already provided, to answer some of the patient's questions and/or to generate more questions which can be discussed the next time that they see you.

COMMUNICATING STATISTICAL INFORMATION TO PATIENTS

Patients expect information about benefits and risks that is (as far as possible) accurate, unbiased, personally relevant to them and presented in a way that they can understand.[3]

Communicating statistical information, most notably information about probabilities and risks, in a manner that patients can understand is an area that health professionals need to be aware of. There are many examples of statistical information about health being presented in a non-transparent and/or incorrect manner by health professionals, public figures and journalists who write stories about health (for a good overview, see the article by Gigerenzer and colleagues;[84] Gigerenzer has also written an excellent book which is recommended at the end of this chapter). The impacts of incorrectly presented and/ or misunderstood health statistics are many, including:

- incorrectly heightened or lowered appreciation of risk and the associated emotional reactions and health decisions that can occur
- impediments to shared decision making and informed consent procedures, and
- incorrect diagnosis[84] or overdiagnosis.[85]

There are often differences between how health professionals and patients understand probability and risk. Many health professionals have been trained to understand these as mathematical probabilities of an event happening within a whole population. Health professionals subsequently tend to view these statistics as objective and impersonal. Conversely, patients' views and understanding of these concepts are commonly influenced by emotions, anxieties, concerns about the future, what they have seen and heard reported in the media and by the views of their social networks. Indeed, patients often personalise risk and are less interested in what happens to 'populations'.[3] Information about risks can also be hard for patients to understand when they do not have previous experience to compare the numbers against; for example, if the risk of an event is 20%, patients may not know whether this is relatively high or low.[3] Finally, for allied health professionals the responsibility for a good health-professional–patient information exchange process may be even greater in cases where patients have not had a prior referral from a medical practitioner and may have no understanding about the possible risks of treatments.[30]

There are different types of statistical information that health professionals need to communicate to patients. The next section describes frequently used statistics and how patients may misinterpret the meanings. Table 14.1 presents strategies that you can use to simplify how you present this information.

TABLE 14.1: THE PROBLEM OF PROBABILITIES AND RISK AND HOW USING NATURAL FREQUENCIES CAN HELP WHEN EXPLAINING THIS TYPE OF INFORMATION			
The clinical scenario	Expressed as a probability	How probabilities may be incorrectly understood	Expressed as natural frequencies (event rates)
Patient needs to have a particular treatment but there is a 20% risk of a side effect	Single probability commonly expressed as 'There is a 20% chance that you will have a particular side effect if you follow the treatment'	That they will have the side effect 20% of the time	Of every 100 patients who have this treatment, 20 patients will experience this side effect
The clinical scenario	Expressed as a relative risk	How relative risks may be incorrectly understood	Expressed in natural frequencies as an absolute risk
By undergoing a particular screening test, the patient's risk of dying from a disease may be reduced	For example, 'By having a screening test your risk of dying from the disease is reduced by 50%'	The large percentage may mislead the patient into thinking that the reduction in the risk of their own possible death is large	The patient's baseline risk of dying from the disease is 1 out of 1000. By undergoing the screening test, this is reduced by half, or to 0.5 in 1000

Types of data that health professionals use and how to present them to patients

Probability

Probability refers to the chance of an event occurring. Values for probability lie between 0 and 1 and are often presented as a percentage. For example, a probability of 0.5 may be expressed as 50%.

Probability can occur as a single probability or as a conditional probability. Consider the situation where a patient wants to know the likelihood of side effects that they might experience in relation to an intervention. An example of *single probability* is that there is a 20% chance that the patient will have a particular side effect if they receive a certain intervention. The problem with this concept is that how it should be interpreted may be confusing.[86] For example, a patient may interpret this as meaning that 20% of patients will have the side effect or that all patients will have the side effect 20% of the time. The latter interpretation reflects the 'personal' as opposed to 'population' view that patients tend to have.[87] *Conditional probability* refers to the probability of an event, given that another event has occurred. An example of conditional probability is if a person has a disease, the probability that a screening test will be positive for the disease is 90%.

Risk of disease/side effect

Risk of disease (or side effect) refers to the probability of developing the disease (or side effect) in a stated time period. As we saw in Chapter 4, risk is often presented either as absolute risk or relative risk. When referring to the risk of a disease or a side effect, these concepts can be interpreted as follows:

- *Absolute risk* refers to the incidence (or natural frequency) of the disease or event in the population.
- *Relative risk* is the ratio of two risks (or, as we saw in Chapter 4, the flip side of the concept of relative risk is relative benefit): the risk in the population exposed to some factor (for example, having received a particular intervention) divided by the risk of those not exposed. Relative risk gives an indication of the degree of risk.
  - If the relative risk is *equal to 1*, the risk in the exposed population is *the same* as the unexposed population.
  - If the relative risk is *greater than 1*, the risk in the exposed population is *greater than* it is for those in the unexposed population.
  - If the relative risk is *less than 1*, the risk in the exposed population is *less than* it is for those in the unexposed population.

Box 14.6 illustrates an example of *relative* risk.

BOX 14.6

Example of relative risk

Incidence of a side effect among people exposed to medication $A = \dfrac{34}{1000} = 0.034$

Incidence of a side effect among people not exposed to medication $A = \dfrac{22}{1000} = 0.022$

Relative risk $= \dfrac{\text{Incidence in exposed}}{\text{Incidence in unexposed}} = \dfrac{0.034}{0.022} = 1.5$

Therefore, in people who have taken the medication, the risk of having the side effect is 1.5 times greater (or a relative risk increase of 50%) than in those people who have not taken the medication.

Absolute risk: natural frequencies (incidence) versus probabilities (chance)

There is a general consensus that presenting natural frequencies (for example, 5 out of every 100 people) is preferable to probabilities or percentages (for example, 5%). A recent Cochrane systematic review of alternative statistical formats for presenting risk and risk-reduction information found that natural frequencies were better understood by health consumers and health professionals than probabilities/percentages in the context of making decisions about diagnostic or screening tests.[88] This review included eight trials and the authors concluded that there was a moderate effect size for this finding. However, a recent randomised trial of community-based adults found percents to be better understood than natural frequencies.[89] It also found that presenting both formats together led to better comprehension than natural frequencies alone. An important limitation to this trial was that it did not test comprehension in a setting of medical decision making and was an internet-based cross-sectional survey. Thus, while more research is obviously needed on determining the optimal way to present information, it would seem that having a flexible approach which utilises combined formats and assesses patients' comprehension of the content that is presented is warranted.

Relative risk reductions (or increases) versus absolute risk reductions (or increases)

This same Cochrane systematic review of alternative statistical formats[88] also assessed the impact of presenting absolute risk reduction versus relative risk reduction on understanding, perception and persuasiveness. The settings were clinical decision making scenarios regarding diagnostic and screening tests by health consumers and health professionals.[88] The review found moderate to strong evidence that while absolute risk reduction and relative risk reduction were equally understood, health consumers and health professionals were likely to perceive interventions to be more effective and be more persuaded to use or prescribe a treatment when presented with relative risk reductions. However, the review also found that relative risks were also more likely to lead to misinterpretation. The potential for relative risk to be misleading, to either patients or health professionals, was pointed out in Chapter 4.

As shown in the example in Box 14.6, while patients who take a medication may have a 50% higher risk of experiencing a side effect, in absolute terms, if a patient's initial risk was only 22 in 1000 (or 2.2%), then taking the medication would increase this risk to only 34 in 1000 people (or 3.4%). An important factor to note is to avoid using qualitative descriptors, such as 'low', 'high', 'rare' and 'frequent', to quantify risk without clear explanation, as patients' and health professionals' perceptions of what such descriptors actually mean can vary dramatically.[40]

The importance of baseline risk was explained in Chapter 4. When explaining absolute and relative risk reduction (or increase) to patients, the baseline or starting level of risk to the patient should also be presented to help the patient interpret the risks appropriately.[90] For example, a 1995 warning by the Committee on Safety in the USA stated that third-generation oral contraceptive drugs were associated with twice the risk compared with second-generation contraceptives. This was reported by the media and it led to a dramatic reduction in the use of oral contraceptives and a subsequent increase in pregnancies and terminations. However, what the media did not inform people of was that the baseline risk was extremely low, at 15 cases per year per 100,000 users, and that the increased risk was still extremely low, at 25 cases per year.[90,91]

Number needed to treat

The concept of number needed to treat was explained in Chapter 4 and we saw that it can be a clinically useful concept for health professionals. However, you should be aware that studies which evaluated patients' understanding and ability to use the concept of number needed to treat have mostly found that it is a difficult concept for patients to understand and may have limited use as a communication tool during shared decision making.[92]

Table 14.1 above provides two examples of the issues surrounding the presentation of probability and risk to patients, and shows how using natural frequencies or plain numbers (for example, '8 out of 100') can aid patients' understanding.

Factors for health professionals to consider when presenting statistical information to patients

Framing

Framing of information refers to whether the information is presented in a positive or a negative manner. If information is positively framed, it is presented in terms of who will benefit. For example, out of 1000 patients who have this treatment, 800 (or 80%) will benefit. If information is negatively framed, it is presented in terms of who will not benefit (or possibly be harmed). For example, out of 1000 patients who have this treatment, 200 (or 20%) will experience an adverse side effect.

How information is framed has been found to influence patients' perceptions of test or treatment options and confidence in medical decision making.[87] However, a recent Cochrane review concluded that the effect of framing on actual health behaviour is not consistent, based on the available trials.[93] Positive framing has been linked with patients being more willing to undertake risky treatments.[87] Information can also be framed in terms of a gain or loss with respect to screening; for example, gain or loss framing concerns the outcomes from having (*gain*) or not having (*loss*) a screening test. Loss framing, which outlines the possible adverse outcomes from not having the test, has been linked with a higher uptake by patients of screening tests than gain framing, which outlines the advantages of having the test.[87]

Current recommendations are that health professionals be unbiased and present patients with both the positive and the negative aspects of an intervention by using the same statistical denominator; for example, telling a patient that the risk of developing a disease is 34 in 1000 people who follow the treatment and that the risk of not developing the disease is 966 in 1000 people who follow the treatment. Gigerenzer and Edwards[87] describe an example of poor practice in an information brochure for patients about a particular screening test. In the brochure, health professionals presented information using relative risk statistics to make the benefits appear large presenting the risks of undertaking screening using absolute risk statistics (which were smaller).

Using graphs and pictures

Using graphs or pictures can assist patients to understand the information that you are presenting. For example, a pictograph of a population of 1000 people (represented by circles) which you can colour in to show how many will benefit (or be harmed) by a particular intervention is one way of showing data in an absolute manner. Figure 14.1 shows how a pictograph can be used, using a hypothetical example. Pictographs have been found to be more easily and accurately understood when the data are presented along the horizontal axis of the pictograph.[94] This presentation can assist patients to see the overall picture and help them put the information into perspective. For example, they can see the baseline level of risk and how much the level of risk changes following the intervention.

The pictograph in Figure 14.1 illustrates that:

- of 1000 people aged between 50 and 60 years, the chance of dying is 20 in 1000 if the medication is *not* taken (see second bottom row of the pictograph)
- of 1000 people aged between 50 and 60 years, the chance of dying is reduced to 5 in 1000 if the medication *is* taken (see bottom row of the pictograph).

Graphs representing benefit and harm can also be prepared. Figure 14.2 shows a hypothetical example of a graphical representation of risk for experiencing a side effect from taking a particular medication.

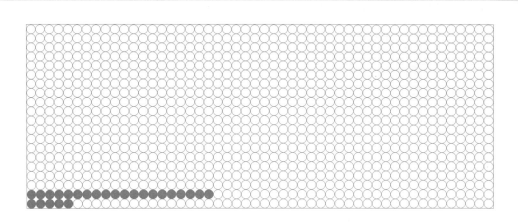

Figure 14.1
Pictograph of a population of 1000 people that can be used to illustrate the risk of a certain intervention.

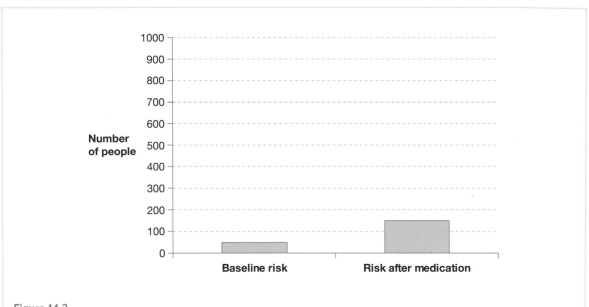

Figure 14.2
Graphical representation of the risk of side effects after taking a particular medication.

The vertical (y) axis shows the number of patients per 1000 who experience this side effect. The horizontal (x) axis shows two groups. Group one is the general population (to represent baseline risk), and group two represents the patients who take the medication. The graph clearly shows the increased risk of experiencing the side effect for patients who take this particular medication, in comparison with the general population. Using this approach, graphs of benefit and harm can be presented side by side. However, if graphs of benefit and harm are presented side by side, the same y-axis should be used in both graphs to ensure consistency.[87] There is some evidence that vertical bar graphs are better than horizontal bars, pie charts and systematic or random ovals in helping to explain differences in proportions to patients.[95,96]

As we saw in Chapter 8, survival curves can sometimes be used to display prognostic information. A study that investigated using survival curves to inform patients found that survival curves were understood by patients if they were given more than one opportunity to see and discuss them.[95] However, a more recent study found that mortality rates are better understood by patients rather than survival curves.[84]

Consider timeframes and social factors

You should be aware that how patients perceive probabilities and risks can differ according to their age. A lifetime risk may not mean much to a young person, whereas a risk over the next 5 years may mean more to an older person.[3] There are also many social factors that can influence how patients interpret risk information. Patients can be influenced by the social context of the information, for example the perceived relevance of it and the extent to which they trust the source. Health professionals need to understand that they are just one source of information about risk and may not be the source that patients trust the most.[97] In previous sections of this chapter we have described strategies that health professionals can use to help develop a relationship of trust with patients. These included: engaging in shared decision making; respecting the patient's needs, views and preferences; and using effective communication techniques.

The nature of the risk also influences how patients may react. For example, patients may be more sensitive to high-consequence risks (such as being struck by lightning) than by the consequences of disease/disability from smoking.[97] These types of high-consequence, but rare, risks often evoke a strong emotional reaction and a disproportionately large popular media coverage. To help patients put risk numbers into perspective, it can be useful to compare risk numbers with other, more familiar risks, for example dying of any cause in the next year. Figure 14.3 provides an example of a perspective chart

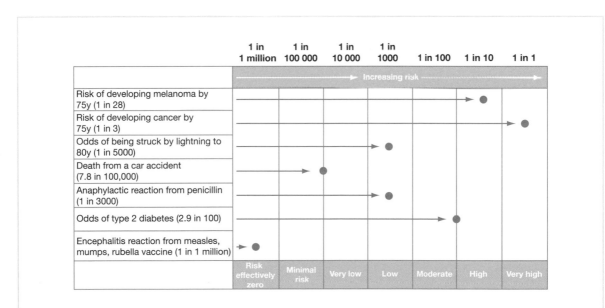

Figure 14.3
Presenting risk information in a way that gives perspective to the probability of an outcome.
Based on: Risk Communication Format, © John Paling, 2000 (see www.riskcomm.com*); reproduced with permission.*

(based on one developed by Paling[98]) that can be used by health professionals when educating patients about the probability of developing melanoma. The chart provides the estimated risk of developing melanoma as well as the estimated risk of other events such as death by car accident, developing type 2 diabetes and being struck by lightning.

Less is more

Finally, health professionals should attempt to reduce the amount of statistical information they present to patients. Research has shown that limiting the amount to a few key points may results in higher comprehension, and therefore better and higher quality decision making by patients.[99,100] Box 14.7 summarises the strategies that health professionals can use to ensure that statistical information about health is presented in the best possible way for patients to understand.

One final comment—we have focused in this chapter on the crucial role and, indeed, responsibility that health professionals have in assisting patients to understand and use health information and participate in the decision-making process. However, at a broader level, we should also, at every opportunity, be helping the public in general to gain the skills and knowledge needed to be critical consumers of health information, make informed decisions and also understand issues such as how research knowledge is generated and presented. As a starting point, some highly recommended resources that have been written on these topics (and, wonderfully, are free to download as PDFs) include: *Testing Treatments* (www.testingtreatments.org), *Smart Health Choices* (www.sensiblehealthadvice.org) and *Know your Chances: Understanding Health Statistics* (www.jameslindlibrary.org/documents/KnowYourChances_000.pdf). Additionally, the book *Better Doctors, Better Patients, Better Decisions: Envisioning health care 2020* by Gerd Gigerenzer and Muir Gray is extremely well worth reading (mitpress.mit.edu/books/better-doctors-better-patients-better-decisions).

BOX 14.7

How to present statistical information to patients

- Be open about uncertainties surrounding benefits and risks.
- Give information in terms of both positive and negative outcomes to avoid bias.
- Use the same denominator when presenting positive and negative outcomes.
- Present natural frequencies (that is, plain numbers) rather than percentages or relative risks.
- If you need to use relative statistics, supplement with absolute risks (natural frequencies) or benefits.
- Use multiple formats: for example, verbal and written descriptions and, where possible, simple visual aids such as graphs.
- Avoid using descriptors, for example 'high', 'low', 'rare' and 'frequent'.
- Use visual aids such as graphs, pictures or perspective charts to aid in understanding where possible.
- Less is more: avoid presenting too much information.

SUMMARY POINTS OF THIS CHAPTER

- It is important that health professionals communicate effectively with their patients for many reasons, such as obtaining fully informed consent, enabling patients to be involved in making decisions about their health care, building trust between the patient and health professional and maximising the effectiveness of particular interventions.

- Patient-centred care is an approach to the health-professional–patient relationship that can have benefits for both the patient and the health professional. This approach involves forming a partnership with the patient, engaging in shared decision making and responding effectively to the patient's needs and concerns.

- In shared decision making, the patient and the health professional form a partnership to make decisions about the patient's health care. Shared decision making is not always possible, and sometimes there can be a number of challenges involved with achieving it. There are various strategies that health professionals can use to facilitate shared decision making. There are also tools that can be used to measure the extent of both patient and health professional involvement in decision making.

- The steps involved in effectively communicating evidence to patients can include: understanding the patient's experiences and expectations, building a partnership with them, discussing the evidence, presenting the recommendations and confirming the patient's understanding and agreement.

- There is a range of formats that can be used when providing patients with information, including verbal information, written information, computer-based information, DVDs and audiotapes and decision aids. Before using any of these formats with a patient, there are issues that need to be considered, such as the quality, credibility and presentation of the information and the suitability of the format for that patient and their needs, abilities and clinical circumstances.

- It can be difficult to communicate statistical information, such as risks and probabilities, to patients in a way that they will understand. There is a range of strategies, such as using natural frequencies, visual aids and framing information correctly, that can be used to aid patients' understanding.

References

1. Salzburg Global Seminar. The Salzburg statement on shared decision making. BMJ 2011;342:d1745. doi: 10.1136/bmj.d1745.
2. Tooth L, Refshauge K. The effectiveness of client education: a review of the evidence and future challenges. In: McKenna K, Tooth L, editors. Client education: a partnership approach for health practitioners. Sydney: University of New South Wales Press; 2006. pp. 22–56.
3. National Health and Medical Research Council of Australia. Making decisions about tests and treatments: principles for better communication between healthcare consumers and healthcare professionals. Canberra: Australian Government Printer; 2006.
4. Groves J. International Alliance of Patients' Organisations perspectives on person-centred medicine. Int J Integr Care 2010;10(Suppl):27–9.
5. Bergeson S, Dean J. A systems approach to patient-centered care. JAMA 2006;296:2848–51.
6. Coulter A. After Bristol: putting patients at the centre. BMJ 2002;324:648–51.
7. McKenna T, Tooth L. Client education: a partnership approach for health practitioners. Sydney: University of New South Wales Press; 2006.
8. Entwistle V, Watt I. Patient involvement in treatment decision-making: the case for a broader conceptual framework. Patient Educ Couns 2006;63:268–78.

9. Quill T, Brody H. Physician recommendations and patient autonomy: finding a balance between physician power and patient choice. Ann Intern Med 1996;125:763–9.

10. Kahn K, Schneider E, Malin J, et al. Patient centred experiences in breast cancer: predicting long-term adherence to tamoxifen use. Med Care 2007;45:431–9.

11. Coulter A. What do patients and the public want from primary care? BMJ 2005;331:1199–201.

12. Trevena L, Barratt A. Integrated decision making: definitions for a new discipline. Patient Educ Couns 2003;50:265–8.

13. Kon A. The shared decision making continuum. JAMA 2010;304:903–4.

14. Elwyn G, Laitner S, Coulter A, et al. Implementing shared decision making in the NHS. BMJ 2010;341:971–3.

15. American Medical Association. Policy H-373.997 Shared Decision-Making, no date. Online. Available: www.ama-assn.org/resources/doc/cms/a10-cms-rpt-7.pdf; 5 May 2012.

16. General Medical Council of the United Kingdom. Good medical practice: relationships with patients, 2006. Online. Available: www.gmc-uk.org/static/documents/content/GMP_0910.pdf; 5 May 2012.

17. Naik A, Kallen M, Walder A, et al. Improving hypertension control in diabetes mellitus: the effects of collaborative and proactive health communication. Circulation 2008;117:1361–8.

18. Frosch D, Kaplan R. Shared decision making in clinical medicine: past research and future directions. Am J Prev Med 1999;17:285–94.

19. Wilson S, Strub P, Buist S, et al. Shared treatment decision making improves adherence and outcomes in poorly controlled asthma. Am J Respir Crit Care Med 2010;181:566–77.

20. White D, Braddock C, Bereknyei S, et al. Toward shared decision making at the end of life in intensive care units: opportunities for improvement. Arch Intern Med 2007;167:461–7.

21. Stewart A. Effective physician–patient communications and health outcomes: a review. CMAJ 1995;152:1423–33.

22. McWilliams D, Jacobson R, Van Houten H, et al. A program of anticipatory guidance for the prevention of emergency department visits for ear pain. Arch Paediatr Adolesc Med 2008;162:151–6.

23. Wennberg D, Marr A, Lang L, et al. A randomised trial of a telephone care-management strategy. New Engl J Med 2010;363:1245–55.

24. O'Connor A, Legare F, Stacey D. Risk communication in practice: the contribution of decision aids. BMJ 2003;327:736–40.

25. Levinson W, Kao A, Kuby A, et al. Not all patients want to participate in decision making: a national study of public preferences. J Gen Intern Med 2005;20:531–5.

26. Care Quality Commission. The state of health care and adult social care in England: an overview of key themes in care 2010/11. Online. Available: www.cqc.org.uk/sites/default/files/media/documents/state_of_care_2010_11.pdf; 20 Oct 2011.

27. Chewning B, Bylund C, Shah B, et al. Patient preferences for shared decisions: a systematic review. Patient Educ Couns 2012;86:9–18.

28. Edwards A, Elwyn G, Hood K, et al. The development of COMRADE: a patient-based outcome measure to evaluate the effectiveness of risk communication and treatment decision making in consultations. Patient Educ Couns 2003;50:311–22.

29. Bauman A, Fardy H, Harris P. Getting it right: why bother with patient centred care? Med J Aust 2003;179:253–6.

30. Delany C. Cervical manipulation: how might informed consent be obtained before treatment? J Law Med 2002;10:174–86.

31. Lockwood S. 'Evidence of me' in evidence based medicine? BMJ 2004;329:1033–5.

32. Ford S, Schofield T, Hope T. What are the ingredients for a successful evidence-based patient choice consultation? A qualitative study. Soc Sci Med 2003;56:589–602.

33. Elwyn G, Edwards A, Mowle S, et al. Measuring the involvement of patients in shared decision making. Patient Educ Couns 2001;43:5–22.

34. Elwyn G, Edwards A, Wensing M. Shared decision making: developing the OPTION scale for measuring patient involvement. Qual Saf Health Care 2003;12:93–9.

35. Elwyn G, Hutchings H, Edwards A, et al. The OPTION scale: measuring the extent that health professionals involve patients in decision-making tasks. Health Expect 2005;8:34–42.

36. Holmes-Rovner M, Kroll J, Schmitt N, et al. Patient satisfaction with health care decisions: the satisfaction with decision scale. Med Decis Making 1996;16:58–64.

37. O'Connor A. Validation of a decisional conflict scale. Med Decis Making 1995;15:25–30.

38. Lerman C, Brody D, Caputo G, et al. Patients' perceived involvement in care scale: relationship to attitudes about illness and medical care. J Gen Intern Med 1990;5:29–33.

39. Simon D, Schorr G, Wirtz M, et al. Development and first validation of the shared decision-making questionnaire (SDM-Q). Patient Educ Couns 2006;63:319–27.

40. Epstein R, Alper B, Quill T. Communicating evidence for participatory decision making. JAMA 2004;291:2359–66.

41. McKenna K, Tooth L. Deciding the content and format of educational interventions. In: McKenna K, Tooth L, editors. Client education: a partnership approach for health practitioners. Sydney: University of New South Wales Press; 2006. pp. 128–58.

42. Tse S, Lloyd C, McKenna K. When clients are from diverse linguistic and cultural backgrounds. In: McKenna K, Tooth L, editors. Client education: a partnership approach for health practitioners. Sydney: University of New South Wales Press; 2006. pp. 307–26.

43. Boundouki G, Humphris G, Field A. Knowledge of oral cancer, distress and screening intentions: longer term effects of a patient information leaflet. Patient Educ Couns 2004;53:71–7.

44. Hill J. A practical guide to patient education and information giving. Baillières Clin Rheumatol 1997;11:109–27.

45. Johnson A, Sandford J, Tyndall J. Written and verbal information versus verbal information only for patients being discharged from acute hospital settings to home. Cochrane Database Syst Rev 2008;CD003716. doi: 10.1002/14651858.CD003716.

46. Pitkethly M, MacGillivray S, Ryan R. Recordings or summaries of consultations for people with cancer. Cochrane Database Syst Rev 2008;CD001539. doi: 10.1002/14651858.CD001539.

47. Griffin J, McKenna K, Tooth L. Discrepancy between older clients' ability to read and comprehend and the reading level of written educational materials used by occupational therapists. Am J Occup Ther 2006;60:70–80.

48. Hoffmann T, McKenna K. Analysis of stroke patients' and carers' reading ability and the content and design of written materials: recommendations for improving written stroke information. Patient Educ Couns 2006;60:286–93.

49. McLaughlin H. SMOG grading: a new readability formula. J Reading 1969;12:639–46.

50. Flesch R. A new readability yardstick. J Appl Psychol 1948;32:221–33.

51. Hoffmann T, Worrall L. Designing effective written health education materials: considerations for health professionals. Disabil Rehabil 2004;26:1166–73.

52. Doak C, Doak L, Root J. Teaching patients with low literacy skills. 2nd ed. Philadelphia: J.B. Lippincott; 1996.

53. Paul C, Redman S, Sanson-Fisher R. The development of a checklist of content and design characteristics for printed health education materials. Health Promot J Aust 1997;7:153–9.

54. Charnock D, Sheppard S, Needham G, et al. DISCERN: an instrument for judging the quality of written consumer health information on treatment choices. J Epidemiol Commun Hlth 1999;53:105–11.

55. Treweek S, Glenton C, Oxman A, et al. Computer-generated patient education materials: do they affect professional practice? A systematic review. J Am Med Inform Assoc 2002;9:346–58.

56. Hoffmann T, Russell T, McKenna K. Producing computer-generated tailored written information for stroke patients and their carers: system development and preliminary evaluation. Int J Med Inform 2004;73:751–8.

57. Kroeze W, Werkman A, Brug J. A systematic review of randomised trials on the effectiveness of computer-tailored education on physical activity and dietary behaviours. Ann Behav Med 2006;31:205–23.

58. Neville L, O'Hara B, Milat A. Computer-tailored dietary behaviour change interventions: a systematic review. Health Educ Res 2009;24:699–720.

59. Short C, James E, Plotnikoff R, et al. Efficacy of tailored-print interventions to promote physical activity: a systematic review of randomised trials. Int J Behav Nutr Phys Act 2011;17.113.

60. Bailey J, Murray E, Rait G, et al. Interactive computer-based interventions for sexual health promotion. Cochrane Database Syst Rev 2010;CD006483. doi: 10.1002/14651858.CD006483.pub2.

61. Murray E, Burns J, Tai S, et al. Interactive health communication applications for people with chronic disease. Cochrane Database Syst Rev 2009;CD004274. doi: 10.1002/14651858.CD004274.pub4.

62. McMullan M. Patients using the Internet to obtain health information: how this affects the patient–health professional relationship. Patient Educ Couns 2006;63:24–8.

63. Zun L, Downey L, Brown S. Completeness and accuracy of emergency medical information on the web: update 2008. West J Emerg Med 2011;12:448–54.

64. Tait A, Voepel-Lewis T, Moscucci M, et al. Patient comprehension of an interactive, computer-based information program for cardiac catheterisation: A comparison with standard information. Arch Intern Med 2009;169:1907–14.

65. Beranova E, Sykes C. A systematic review of computer-based softwares for educating patients with coronary heart disease. Patient Educ Couns 2007;66:21–8.

66. Stromberg A, Ahlen H, Fridlund, B. Interactive education on CD-ROM: a new tool in the education of heart failure patients. Patient Educ Couns 2002;46:75–81.

67. Noar S, Benac C, Harris M. Does tailoring matter? Meta-analytic review of tailored print health behavior change interventions. Psych Bull 2007;133:673–93.

68. Krebs P, Prochaska J, Rossi J. A meta-analysis of computer-tailored interventions for health behavior change. Prev Med 2010;51:214–21.

69. Hoffmann T, McKenna K, Worrall L, et al. Randomised controlled trial of a computer-generated tailored written education package for patients following stroke. Age Ageing 2007;36:280–6.

70. Gysels M, Higginson I. Interactive technologies and videotapes for patient education in cancer care: systematic review and meta-analysis of randomised trials. Support Care Cancer 2007;15:7–20.

71. Haines T, Hill A, Hill D, et al. Patient education to prevent falls among older hospital inpatients: a randomised controlled trial. Arch Intern Med 2011;171:516–24.

72. Stacey D, Bennet C, Barry M, et al. Decision aids for people facing health treatment or screening decisions. Cochrane Database Syst Rev 2011;CD001431. doi: 10.1002/14651858.CD001431.pub3.

73. Mayo Clinic. Knowledge and Education Research Unit (KER), no date. Online. Available: mayoresearch.mayo.edu/mayo/research/ker_unit/index.cfm; 6 May 2012.

74. Institute of Medicine (IOM). Health literacy: a prescription to end confusion. Washington: IOM; 2004.

75. Weiss B, Coyne C, Michielutte R, et al. Communicating with patients who have limited literacy skills: report of the National Work Group on Literacy and Health. J Fam Pract 1998;46:168–75.

76. Fischoff B, Brewer N, Downs J. Communicating risks and benefits: an evidence-based user's guide. Silver Spring, MD: US Department of Health and Human Services, Food and Drug Administration; 2011. Online. Available: www.fda.gov/AboutFDA/ReportsManualsForms/Reports/ucm268078.htm; 15 Nov 2012.

77. Wilson F, McLemore R. Patient literacy levels: a consideration when designing patient education programs. Rehabil Nurs 1997;22:311–17.

78. Australian Bureau of Statistics (ABS). Health Literacy. Report No. 4233.0. Canberra: ABS; 2008.

79. Murphy P, Davis T, Long S, et al. REALM: a quick reading test for patients. J Reading 1993;37:124–30.

80. Parker R, Baker D, Williams M, et al. The Test of Functional Health Literacy in Adults: a new instrument for measuring patients' literacy skills. J Gen Intern Med 1995;10:537–41.

81. Hanson-Divers E. Developing a medical achievement reading test to evaluate patient literacy skills: a preliminary study. J Health Care Poor Underserved 1997;8:56–9.

82. Peterson P, Shetterly S, Clarke C, et al. Health literacy and outcomes among patients with heart failure. JAMA 2011;305:1695–701.

83. McKenna K, Tooth L, editors. Client education: a partnership approach for health practitioners. Sydney: University of New South Wales Press; 2006.

84. Gigerenzer G, Gaissmaier W, Kurz-Milcke E, et al. Helping doctors and patients make sense of health statistics. Psychol Sci Public Interest 2008;8:53–96. Online. Available: www.psychologicalscience.org/journals/pspi/pspi_8_2_article.pdf; 15 Nov 2012.

85. Welch HG, Schwartz L, Woloshin S. Over-diagnosed: making people sick in the pursuit of health. Boston: Beacon Press; 2012.

86. Gigerenzer G. Why do single event probabilities confuse patients? BMJ 2012;344:245.

87. Gigerenzer G, Edwards A. Simple tools for understanding risks: from innumeracy to insight. BMJ 2003;327:741–4.

88. Akl EA, Oxman AD, Herrin J, et al. Using alternative statistical formats for presenting risks and risk reductions. Cochrane Database Syst Rev 2011;(3):CD006776. doi: 10.1002/14651858.CD006776.pub2.

89. Woloshin S, Schwartz L. Communicating data about the benefits and harms of treatment: a randomised trial. Ann Intern Med 2011;155:87–96.

90. Berry D, Knapp P, Raynor T. Expressing medicine side effects: assessing the effectiveness of absolute risk, relative risk and number needed to harm and the provision of baseline risk information. Patient Educ Couns 2006;63:89–96.

91. Edwards R, Cohen J. The recent saga of cardiovascular disease and safety of oral contraceptives. Hum Reprod Update 1999;5:565–620.

92. Halvorsen P, Kristiansen I. Decisions on drug therapies by numbers needed to treat: a randomised trial. Arch Int Med 2005;165:1140–6.

93. Akl EA, Oxman AD, Herrin J, et al. Framing of health information messages. Cochrane Database Syst Rev 2011;(12):CD006776. doi: 10.1002/14651858.CD006777.pub2.

94. Price M, Cameron R, Butow P. Communicating risk information: the influence of graphical display format on quantitative information perception—accuracy, comprehension and preferences. Patient Educ Couns 2007;69:121–8.

95. Trevena L, Davey H, Barratt A, et al. A systematic review on communicating with patients about evidence. J Eval Clin Pract 2006;12:13–23.

96. Carling C, Kristoffersen D, Flottorp S, et al. The benefits of alternative graphical displays used to present the benefits of antibiotics for sore throat on decisions about whether to seek treatment: a randomised trial. PLoS Med 2009;6:e1000140.

97. Alaszewski A, Horlick-Jones T. How can doctors communicate information about risk more effectively? BMJ 2003;327:728–31.

98. Paling J. Strategies to help patients understand risks. BMJ 2003;327:745–8.

99. Peters E, Dieckmann N, Dixon A, et al. Less is more in presenting quality information to consumers. Med Care Res Rev 2007;64:169–90.

100. Zikmund-Fisher B, Fagerlin A, Ubel P. Improving understanding of adjuvant therapy options by using simpler risk graphics. Cancer 2008;113:3382–90.

Chapter 15

Clinical reasoning and evidence-based practice

Merrill Turpin and Joy Higgs

LEARNING OBJECTIVES

After reading this chapter, you should be able to:

- Describe some of the complexities and uncertainties of clinical practice
- Understand what is meant by the term clinical reasoning
- Be aware of the different perspectives about the concept of 'evidence'
- Understand the importance of clinical experience for evidence-based practice
- Understand what is meant by the term professional practice
- Explain how clinical reasoning can be used to integrate information and knowledge from the different sources that are required for evidence-based practice
- Understand what is meant by critical reflection and how it might support evidence-based practice

Evidence-based practice aims to improve outcomes for patients.[1] This goal appears uncontentious and would generally be accepted by a range of stakeholders in health. Patients, health professionals, funding bodies and policy makers all share in this aim. However, a range of issues make it problematic to uncritically adopt an evidence-based practice approach, and the complexity of the problem becomes clearer when we question *how* best to achieve optimal health care.

Patient outcomes are dependent on a range of factors, such as:

- the nature of the patient's health problem
- the types of services that are available to and accessible by the patient
- the practices of the health professionals working in those services
- the nature and quality of the interaction between the patient and the health professional
- the attitudes of the patient towards the services offered
- the patient's own conceptualisation of the health problem
- the ease with which any service recommendations that are made can be carried out by patients within the broader context of their lives.

This list illustrates the complexity of the issue of improving patient outcomes. If all of these issues interact together to affect the health outcomes for a particular patient, where should planned improvements focus? Will a change in one factor be sufficient to obtain the desired result, or do factors need to be considered in an integrated way? Health professionals face these kinds of questions on a daily basis, as well as the ever-present question, 'What can and should I do in this specific situation?'

Professional practice is complex and health professionals need to consider the range of factors that affect patient outcomes when planning and delivering services. They are required to make decisions about what services they can and should offer, given the particular needs of, and circumstances surrounding, the individual patient and the broader organisational and societal context. Making these kinds of decisions requires complex thinking processes, as the 'problem' or situation about which decisions have to be made is often poorly defined and the desired outcomes are often unclear.[2] This thinking process is often referred to as *clinical or professional reasoning, decision making,* or *professional judgment.*

Health professionals need to use their clinical reasoning to gather and interpret different types of information and knowledge from a range of sources to make judgments and decisions regarding complex situations under conditions of uncertainty. In addition to the logical decisions that health professionals make, they also have to make ethical and pragmatic ones. They have to ask themselves questions like: 'What is the most effective thing I could do?', 'What is most likely to work in this situation?', 'What is the patient most likely to accept and do?' and 'What should I do (ethically) in this situation?'.

This chapter aims to explore the relationship between clinical reasoning and evidence-based practice. As you have seen throughout this book, evidence-based practice is a movement in health that aims to improve patient outcomes by supporting health professionals to incorporate research evidence into their practice. Evidence-based practice also recognises that research evidence alone is not sufficient for addressing the complex nature of professional practice and that the ability to integrate different types of information and knowledge from different sources is also required. Therefore, to practise in an evidence-based way, health professionals need to integrate research with their clinical experience, an understanding of the preferences and circumstances of their patients and the demands and expectations of the practice context. Clinical reasoning is the process by which health professionals integrate this information and knowledge.

In this chapter, we explore the notion of evidence-based practice and the roles that different forms of knowledge and information play in providing evidence for practice; and we highlight how the concept of practice should be viewed as being embedded within particular contexts. We also explore the clinical reasoning processes that occur within practice and provide some brief suggestions for you to consider when critically reflecting on your own practice from the perspective of making it evidence-based.

THE EVIDENCE-BASED PRACTICE MOVEMENT'S CONCEPT OF EVIDENCE

The assumption underpinning the perceived need for an evidence-based practice is that basing practice on rigorously produced information (often referred to as *data*) will lead to enhanced patient outcomes. Given the complex range of factors that can affect patient outcomes, how can we be sure that basing our practice on such evidence will improve them, and what kinds of information or knowledge constitutes appropriate and sufficient evidence? These are important questions for health professionals to ask.

The first question about whether basing practice on evidence does lead to better patient outcomes has been examined widely in relation to specific interventions and specific outcomes.

The second key question is: what constitutes evidence? As we saw in Chapter 1, evidence-based practice across the health professions evolved from its medical counterpart, evidence-based medicine, and as a consequence, many of the assumptions of medicine have been adopted in evidence-based practice. In the definition of evidence-based practice by Sackett and colleagues[3] that was examined in Chapter 1, the term 'current best evidence' was introduced as the criterion for evidence. Predictably, clarifying the nature of 'best' evidence has become the central concern of the evidence-based practice and evidence-based medicine movements. As the empirico-analytic paradigm is the dominant philosophy that underpins medicine, this also became the assumed perspective of the evidence-based practice movement.

The **empirico-analytic paradigm** is also known as the scientific paradigm or the empiricist model of knowledge creation. According to Higgs, Jones and Titchen,[4] this paradigm 'relies on observation and experiment in the empirical world, resulting in generalisations about the content and events of the world which can be used to predict the future' (p. 155). From the perspective of the empirico-analytic paradigm, the best form of evidence is that produced through rigorous scientific enquiry. It has been assumed that such rigour can be achieved best through the methods of research, especially quantitative research.[5]

Therefore, information and knowledge generated from research is the concept of evidence that is used by the evidence-based practice movement and is the approach taken throughout this text. Many people take this assumption for granted, and this is highlighted by the fact that some professions use the clarifying term 'research-based practice' rather than 'evidence-based practice'.

The position that scientific knowledge is the sole key to evidence has been questioned by a number of writers[5–7] who have argued that research evidence alone is not sufficient for addressing the complexities of professional practice and that the ability to generate and integrate different types of evidence from different sources is also required. While the evidence based practice movement is centred on evidence derived from rigorously conducted research, early definitions of evidence-based medicine did clearly emphasise that, to practise in an evidence-based way, professionals need to integrate research findings with practical knowledge derived from their clinical experience and an understanding of the preferences and circumstances of their patients.

In some ways, the assumption that 'evidence equals research findings' has been problematic for the evidence-based practice movement and has probably contributed to a strong division between those who align themselves with the evidence-based practice movement and those who oppose it. Critics of evidence-based practice argue that there are problems with the production, relevance and availability of research evidence and that it has limited capacity to address the problems of practice and enhance decision making in the context of complex practice and life situations.[8] Examples of criticisms include: that the research that is undertaken is often dependent on funding and, therefore, factors other than need and importance can influence what is researched; that the research undertaken can reflect what is easier to measure more than what is important to understand or most important to professional practice; and that, often, research findings are not presented in forms that are easily accessible to health professionals.

Perhaps the situation is summed up best by Naylor[9] who, in relation to evidence-based medicine (and his comments are just as relevant to evidence-based practice), stated that 'A backlash is not surprising in view of the inflated expectations of outcomes-oriented and evidence-based medicine and the fears of some clinicians that these concepts threaten the art of patient care' (p. 840). Exploring the assumptions about what is meant by the notion of 'evidence' can be a good start to examining what evidence-based practice is, and we do this in the next section.

EVIDENCE OF WHAT?

What is evidence? The *Heinemann Australian Student's Dictionary* defines evidence as 'anything which provides a basis for belief'[10] and the *Macquarie Dictionary* defines it as 'grounds for belief'.[11] In this context, *belief* refers to acceptance of the credibility or substantiation of a position or argument, for instance providing support for a course of action. Using this definition, evidence would be information or knowledge that supports some sort of belief; and an evidence-based practice, therefore, would be a practice that is based on such information and knowledge. But whose beliefs are referred to? Is it an individual health professional's beliefs, the beliefs of a particular health profession or the beliefs that underpin a particular health service or model of service delivery? Is it the beliefs of those receiving care from a particular service or those funding or providing the service? Are the beliefs of all of these stakeholders in health the same and of equal value?

These questions highlight the argument that the types of information and knowledge that are seen as potentially appropriate to use as evidence for health practice can vary among different stakeholders. For example, if a service measures patient outcomes in terms of reducing (or eliminating) impairments, then it is information about the effectiveness of interventions in reducing impairments that will be used most often as evidence, regardless of the functional and practical implications of using those interventions. However, people using health services might employ other criteria to measure outcomes. For example, they might value services that make an appreciable difference to their health experience, are accessible (physically and financially) and use interventions that are easy to implement within their own life contexts. Healthcare funding bodies might be most concerned with value-for-money and might seek information that substantiates the cost-effectiveness of interventions or services. That is, they might only look favourably on interventions and service provision models that have both evidence to support the effectiveness of the intervention in improving patient outcomes *and* an acceptable financial cost.

From the perspective of the empirico-analytic paradigm

As explained in the previous section, the evidence-based practice movement has primarily taken its understanding of evidence from the empirico-analytic paradigm that underpins the assumptions of medicine. This paradigm aims to develop a knowledge base generated from a positivist perspective about 'reality' or 'how the world is' in which the world is taken to be observable (often with the assistance of technology), and information that is valued as knowledge is reliably generated and reproducible. In this perspective, to be dependable as evidence of reality (including how people's health responds to intervention), research data need to be free of bias when collected, the potential effects of the information collection process on the phenomena needs to be minimised and any changes observed must be able to be reliably attributed to particular factors or variables.

To make the empirico-analytic concept of best evidence explicit, a number of hierarchies have been developed, based on the methodology that is used to generate research data. In Chapter 2 the authors explored the hierarchies and levels of evidence for questions about intervention, diagnosis and prognosis in detail. Developing levels of evidence was a strategy used to establish the degree to which information and research findings could be trusted as 'evidence'. For example, the top two levels of evidence in the hierarchy for intervention effectiveness are randomised controlled trials and their systematic reviews. As we saw in Chapter 4, randomised controlled trials (individual and systematically reviewed) generate knowledge that is considered to have a high degree of validity. By eliminating potential bias and controlling for variables that might influence the outcome, the confidence that any observed change can be attributed to one particular factor is very high. Therefore, in the empirico-analytic paradigm, this study design represents the most trustworthy type of research-generated knowledge to use as 'evidence'.

Understanding the origins of the evidence-based practice movement in the empirico-analytic paradigm helps to explain its assumption that 'evidence equals research findings' and its emphasis on quantitative research methods. However, within the evidence-based practice movement, there are calls to acknowledge the value of other types of research methods such as qualitative research,[12] but acceptance of methods other than quantitative research is at times still contested (although acceptance is growing, as explained in Chapters 10 and 12). As the imperative to identify 'current best evidence' remains a core value of the evidence-based practice movement, determining ways to assess the quality of such research remains a central endeavour (to ensure that it is 'best' evidence). Concern for the development and identification of critical-appraisal tools and strategies of metasynthesis of qualitative research (like the systematic review of quantitative research) are examples.

While the empirico-analytic paradigm focuses on generating knowledge through the rigorous scientific methods with which research is often associated, other stakeholders might value other types of knowledge as evidence. The sections that follow explore some of the other types of information and knowledge that are valued as evidence on which to base practice. As we will discuss later in the chapter, the professional's task of integrating these different types of 'evidence' in order to make practice decisions can be difficult.

From the perspective of technical rationality

Technical rationality is a second approach that addresses the type of information that is considered as appropriate evidence for professional practice. This approach aims to improve patient outcomes by regulating practice in order to enhance its efficiency and cost-effectiveness. Schön[13] explained that, from the perspective of technical rationality, professional activity involves 'instrumental problem solving made rigorous by the application of scientific theory and technique' (p. 21). The major elements of this definition are problem solving and the rigorous use of scientific theory and technique. Whereas the empirico-analytic approach emphasises the trustworthiness of information in representing phenomena, this approach focuses on the problem solving of health professionals. Therefore, a major difference between these two approaches is that the former centres on the *quality* of the information whereas the latter targets the process of *using* the information.

From a technical rationalist perspective, human reasoning and judgment is understood in health care as problem solving, which requires the framing and definition of a problem and the search for a solution within a defined problem space. From this approach, efficiency and cost-effectiveness can be improved by providing tools that support the problem-solving process and minimise the likelihood of reasoning errors. As the technical rationalist approach values the rigorous use of the scientific method and technique, information that is generated using this method is incorporated into routines and procedures that aim to lessen and support the professional judgment required. The influence of technical rationality on health care is evident in the use of clinical pathways, protocols, decision trees and other tools that aim to systematise practice decisions. For example, the typical path to be taken by a health professional is clarified when a standard problem definition (often based on a medical diagnosis) can be used. Decision trees work in this way.

A major aim of using reasoning tools and research evidence is to reduce reasoning errors and the potentially biasing effects that can come from clinical opinions. An example of this type of bias is that health professionals can overemphasise the effectiveness of their own interventions because they might only see the short-term effects of the intervention. In addition, they might be overly influenced by situations and outcomes that they have access to, while potentially being unaware of or undervaluing other possibilities (such as interventions offered by other health professionals). In contrast, clinical protocols and research findings are generated from data that are gathered from a broader range of sources. For example, protocols are often developed using information such as research evidence, broader trends in patient outcomes or statistics about adverse incidents, epidemiological trends in population health and patients' opinions and experiences.

The technical rationalist approach shares a similar definition of evidence with the empirico-analytic approach. Both approaches value information that is generated using rigorous scientific methods and consider it to be appropriate evidence upon which to base clinical practice. While they share a concern for effectiveness, they often differ in relation to cost-effectiveness. In the empirico-analytic approach it might be argued that an effective intervention is essential, regardless of the cost. A technical rationalist approach would also include as evidence outcomes such as the reduction of health service costs and adverse incidents that occur during service delivery. However, a criticism of the technical rationalist approach is that it fails to give due attention to the complexity of professional practice and the individual nature of patient experience.[14] This criticism is derived from the argument that the problems of professional practice are both specific and varied, which makes it impossible to develop protocols and procedures to cover the variety of situations that health professionals face.

What information helps health professionals to address the dilemmas of their practice?

A third approach to the matter of what constitutes evidence is to consider the question, 'What information helps professionals to address the specific and varied dilemmas of their practice?' Health professionals use judgment to deal with the complexity of professional practice,[15] which relies on their clinical or professional expertise. The concept of professional expertise is central to the evidence-based practice process. This is illustrated in Sackett and colleagues' 1996[3] definition of evidence-based medicine that was presented in Chapter 1. The beginning of this definition of evidence-based medicine, pertaining to the judicious and conscientious use of research evidence, is well known. However, the section that follows has been quoted infrequently when definitions of evidence-based medicine (or practice) are presented. It reads:

> The practice of evidence based medicine means integrating individual clinical expertise with the best available external clinical evidence from systematic research. By individual clinical expertise we mean the proficiency and judgement that individual clinicians acquire through clinical experiences and clinical practice. Increased expertise is reflected in many ways, but especially in more effective and efficient diagnosis and in the more thoughtful identification and compassionate use of individual patients' predicaments, rights, and preferences in making clinical decisions about their care. (p. 71)

As was pointed out in Chapter 1, this definition makes it clear that an evidence-based practice requires professional expertise, which includes thoughtfulness and compassion as well as effectiveness and efficiency.

Socio-cultural theories of learning suggest that professional expertise is developed through interaction with communities of practice.[16,17] Health professionals learn the practices, activities and ways of thinking and knowing of their profession through participation in the community of practice. Expertise develops 'as an individual gains greater knowledge, understanding and mastery' (p. 24)[17] in their practice area.

The work of Dreyfus and Dreyfus[18] has been widely used to understand the concept of professional expertise developing with experience. The different ways that professionals think as they gain experience have been characterised into five stages, namely: novice, advanced beginner, competent, proficient and expert. Essentially these five stages reflect a movement from a practice that is based on context-free information and generalised rules to a sophisticated and 'embodied' understanding of the specific context in which the practice occurs. While the earlier stages focus on the application of generalised knowledge, in the proficient and expert stages health professionals are able to recognise (often subtle) similarities between the current situation and previous ones and use their knowledge of the previous outcomes to make judgments about what might be best in the current situation.

Professional expertise is difficult to quantify, as it is partly determined by the understandings that are shared by members of the community of practice. For example, Craik and Rappolt[1] selected health professionals who were 'deemed by their peers to be educationally influential practitioners' as a criterion for inclusion into their research study of 'elite' practitioners. In nursing, expertise has been associated with holistic practice, holistic knowledge, salience, knowing the patient, moral agency and skilled know-how.[19] Fleming[20] reported that occupational therapists described expert practitioners (on videotapes) as appearing 'elegant and effortless' (p. 27). Jensen and colleagues[21] developed a grounded theory of expert practice in physiotherapy and proposed that expertise in physiotherapy is a combination of multi-dimensional knowledge, clinical reasoning skills, skilled movement and virtue and that all four of these dimensions contribute to the therapist's philosophy of practice. It appears that members of a community of practice are able to recognise expertise, even though it involves unstated and embodied knowledge, skills and attributes that can be difficult to quantify.

As professionals often have to make decisions about what action to take with a particular patient in a particular organisational context, appropriate information could be conceptualised as including health professionals' memories of previous experiences and their specific outcomes. This is not to suggest that expert health professionals no longer use knowledge that is generated from research. Professional communities of practice have codes of ethics that usually include the need to maintain up-to-date knowledge of the field, and some professional bodies require members to undertake formal accreditation processes. Health professionals meet this ethical requirement through a range of activities such as attending conferences and workshops, reading professional journals, sharing this information with one another and discussing cases and experiences with one another. All of these activities can increase professional knowledge through exposure to findings from systematic research as well as expanding practice knowledge through experiential learning. Thus, the use of both knowledge that is generated from research and knowledge that is generated from practical experience is important for health professionals to be more able to undertake practice that is based on a rich evidence base.

Considering evidence from the patient's perspective

A fourth approach is brought into focus when we ask the question, 'What is going to make the biggest difference to my patient's life and health?' This question helps to turn our attention to the patient's perspective. The definition of evidence-based medicine by Sackett and colleagues,[3] quoted earlier in the chapter, includes the 'thoughtful identification and compassionate use of individual patients' predicaments, rights, and preferences in making clinical decisions about their care' (p. 71). Patients seek professional services because they need something that they cannot obtain in other ways. Professional services often come at substantial financial costs (and other costs such as time and effort) to patients. Attending to patients' predicaments, rights and preferences requires a developed ability to understand people, both as individuals and as members of groups within the overall population. Examples of understanding preferences and rights include giving patients choices in relation to interventions (that is, considering their preferences) and understanding and advocating for the rights of marginalised people to participate in social roles such as work. Understanding 'predicaments' requires the ability to imagine patients within the context of their living situations and social roles (not just the service contexts in which they are seen). For example, a health professional might have to consider the need for support from a patient's carer, the logistics of whether a patient is able to follow an intervention recommendation when the patient returns to daily life, and the opportunities for social participation that he/she has.

While patients expect health professionals to offer them services that will be effective, they also expect them to listen to their concerns and validate their experiences of health. Therefore, in addition to the effectiveness of the interventions, patients might seek 'evidence' of a health professional's interpersonal skills (e.g. a professional's ability to listen to their concerns), 'value for money' and the accessibility (physical and temporal) of the services that are being offered. Patients might seek this kind of information from sources such as the internet; friends, relatives and neighbours; and/or another trusted health professional. The importance of health professionals being able to communicate effectively with their patients was discussed in Chapter 14.

Evidence of what? A summary

In summary, asking the question 'Evidence of what?' can emphasise the fact that different stakeholders seek different types of information. People who work from an empirico-analytic paradigm are likely to seek information that is accepted as reliable representations of the world. Starting from this position, they are likely to value one kind of information (research findings) over other types of information, as illustrated by the established hierarchies of evidence. People who work from a technical rationalist perspective are most likely to seek information that provides a combination of evidence of efficiency and cost-effectiveness and will aim to use this information to develop tools and strategies to standardise practice according to what is considered best practice. Health professionals are most likely to value and seek information that provides evidence to support the decisions that they need to make about what they, as a member of a specific health profession in a particular organisational context, should offer a certain patient, given his or her life circumstances. Finally, patients are most likely to value and seek information that provides evidence of services and health professionals that offer effective, accessible, value-for-money interventions that they are likely to be able to incorporate into the context of their daily life.

All of these different perspectives are important when considering what an evidence-based practice might look like for health professionals, because they highlight the complexity of professional practice. Health professionals are influenced by and need to consider in their practice all of the different types of knowledge and the different types of information or 'evidence' that different stakeholders might consider relevant and valid. Using information that can be 'trusted' is a key concern of the evidence-based practice movement and will remain so as the movement explores a broader base upon which to make practice decisions.

In 2000, Sackett and colleagues[22] provided a more succinct definition of evidence-based medicine that emphasised the complexity of the task that faces health professionals in striving to create and sustain a practice that is evidence-based. The definition succinctly stated that the process of evidence-based medicine requires 'the integration of best research evidence with clinical expertise and patient values' (p. 1). To understand this process of integration, it is important to contextualise professional practice as requiring art, science and ethics. In the following section, we explore this process of integration.

INTEGRATING INFORMATION AND KNOWLEDGE: THE FORGOTTEN ART?

Current conceptualisations of evidence-based practice define it as a process that requires the integration of information from different sources. However, an understanding of how such integration occurs is still evolving. As discussed, much of the early attention of the evidence-based practice movement centred on the nature of evidence that is appropriate for health practice (mainly research evidence), and little systematic investigation was undertaken into how health professionals integrate knowledge and information from different sources such as research, clinical expertise, patient values and preferences, and the practice context. Conceptualising evidence-based practice as a process of integration requires a focus on the activities of health professionals. This section of the chapter will explore the nature of professional practice.

Health professionals provide services to their patients. They think and act within particular contexts, which have been established to provide a particular type of service, and remain accountable to their patients, employers and funding bodies. Health professionals also belong to particular professional groups or communities of practice. Therefore, professional practice needs to be understood within its social, organisational and professional contexts.

Professional practice has been described as a dynamic, creative and constructive phenomenon that flows constantly, like a river that shapes and is shaped by the landscape over which it flows.[23] It is more than just a rational or routine practice. It requires the interaction between professions and patients and among professionals from different disciplines, as well as ethical and professional behaviour. As Fish and Higgs[24] have stated, 'as responsible members of a profession, [the] role [of health professionals] is precisely to argue their moral position, utilise their abilities to wear an appropriate variety of hats on different occasions with proper transparency and integrity and exercise their clinical thinking and professional judgement in the service of differing individuals while making wise decisions about the relationship between the privacy of individuals and the common good' (p. 21).

These descriptions illustrate the complexity of professional practice. It is not just a problem-solving exercise (as technical rationalists might argue), although it requires problem solving. It is not just a process of applying theories and research-generated knowledge to practice (as an empirico-analytic approach emphasises), although these are vital in guiding practice. It includes the fulfilment of role expectations, professional judgment, ethical conduct and the delivery of patient-centred services. As Coles[15] has stated, 'professionals are asked to engage in complex and unpredictable tasks on society's behalf, and in doing so must exercise their discretion, making judgements' (p. 3). Professional practice requires systematic thinking, social and contextual understanding, deep listening, good communication and the ability to deal creatively and ethically with uncertainty. Examples of the uncertainty of medical practice that have been described[25] include uncertainties about diagnosis, the accuracy of diagnostic tests, the natural history of diseases/disabilities and the effects of interventions on groups and populations. Each health profession has its own complexity and areas of uncertainty.

Health professionals need to use their judgment to make decisions about the best course of action to take under conditions of uncertainty. Part of the complexity is dealing with different and often competing understandings from a variety of data and knowledge sources and considering the individual nature of patient circumstances, needs and preferences. Professional practice is an ethical endeavour tailored to the individual patient that requires the credible use of theory and research, good judgment and problem solving and the ability to implement protocols and procedures. Integrating information from research, clinical expertise, patient values and preferences, and information from the practice context requires judgment and artistry as well as science and logic.

Strategies for combining science and art in practice are embedded in the way that health professionals think about their work. For example, in reference to occupational therapists, it has been stated that 'when occupational therapists refer to the paired concepts of art and science, they express their moral dissatisfaction with being constrained by either. In isolation, art somehow seems too soft and unquantifiable and science too hard and unyielding' (p. 482).[26] While science is generally associated with rigour, reliability and predictability, artistry is associated with judgment and being able to deal with unpredictability. In Sackett's 1996 definition of evidence-based medicine,[3] artistry is evident in the reference to 'thoughtful identification and compassionate use' of information that pertains to a particular patient.

While various health professions emphasise art and science to different degrees, they all appear to accept that a balance of these approaches is required for professional practice.

Professional practice could be characterised as reasoned action, as it requires both knowing and doing. The concept of 'art and science' highlights that different types of knowledge are required for health professionals to undertake such reasoned action. Three types of knowledge that are required for practice can be described as:[27]

- **Propositional knowledge**, also known as theoretical knowledge, is an explicit and formal type of knowledge that is generated through research and scholarship and is associated with knowing 'what'. This type of knowledge is often thought of as 'scientific knowledge' and has been emphasised in the main conceptualisation of evidence-based practice to date.

- **Professional craft knowledge** refers to knowing 'how' to carry out the tasks of the profession. It is often associated with the idea of an 'art' of practice and includes the particular perspectives that characterise each profession.

- **Personal knowledge** refers to an individual health professional's knowledge about his or her self in relation to others. This type of knowledge is important for professional practice as the relationships that health professionals build with their patients are often central to that practice.

The last two types of knowledge above 'may be tacit and embedded either in practice itself or in who the person is' (p. 5)[23] and have been referred to collectively as 'non-propositional' knowledge.

Different types of knowledge can be gained from different sources. The definition of evidence-based practice that was explained in Chapter 1 and shown in Figure 1.1 included four sources: research, clinical expertise, the patient's values and circumstances, and the practice context. The practice context, which does not occur in any of Sackett's definitions[3,22] as a knowledge source, provides important information about the local context.[5] This source draws attention to the context-specific nature of professional practice, to which insufficient attention has been paid historically when conceptualising a practice that is based on evidence. Health professionals need to know what and how things work in a particular context (relating to both the setting and the patient). Taken together, these four sources of knowledge provide objective, experiential and contextual information from researchers, health professionals and patients.

The complexity of professional practice becomes evident if you consider that it requires the ability to obtain and use different types of information from a range of sources; to meet the demands of particular practice environments; to fulfil roles consistent with the perspectives of the professional communities of practice to which the health professional belongs; and to consider the predicaments, preferences and values of individual patients. Thus, the creation of a practice that is 'evidence-based', for the purpose of improving patient outcomes, is equally complex. 'Evidence' and 'practice' are both important for understanding evidence-based practice. The study of clinical reasoning highlights one aspect of practice. As this investigation was initiated by medicine, the term *clinical reasoning* was used. However, as many of the settings within which various health professionals work are not considered 'clinical', the term *professional reasoning* or *professional decision making* has also been used.

APPROACHES TO CLINICAL REASONING

Higgs[28] defined clinical reasoning (or practice decision making) as:

> a context-dependent way of thinking and decision making in professional practice to guide practice actions. It involves the construction of narratives to make sense of the multiple factors and interests pertaining to the current reasoning task. It occurs within a set of problem spaces informed by practitioners' unique frames of reference, workplace contexts and practice models, as well as by patients or patients' contexts.

It utilises core dimensions of practice knowledge, reasoning and meta-cognition and draws upon these capacities in others. Decision making within clinical reasoning occurs at micro-, macro- and meta-levels and may be individually or collaboratively conducted. It involves the meta-skills of critical conversation, knowledge generation, practice model authenticity, and reflexivity. (p. 1)

Earlier approaches to the study of clinical reasoning were influenced by investigations into artificial intelligence, and conceptualised clinical reasoning as a purely cognitive process. These emphasised the iterative process of obtaining cues or information about the clinical situation, forming hypotheses about possible explanations and courses of action, interpreting information in light of these hypotheses and testing them. This process is referred to as hypothetico-deductive reasoning. Beyond this, Higgs' definition[28] emphasises that clinical reasoning is a process that involves cognition, meta-cognition (that is, the process of reflective self-awareness) and interactive and narrative ways of thinking.

The work of Higgs and Jones[29] presents a current approach to clinical reasoning. They broadly categorised approaches to clinical reasoning as *cognitive* and *interactive*. Table 15.1 outlines the main types of thinking that health professionals use. The wide range of clinical reasoning approaches presented in this table is related to the following factors:

1. **The inherently complex nature of clinical reasoning as a phenomenon.** Clinical reasoning models are essentially an interpretation or an approximation of a very complex set of thinking processes at both cognitive and meta-cognitive levels. These processes use both domain-specific and generic knowledge. They operate in conjunction with other abilities such as communication and interpersonal interaction and are framed by the health professional's individual values, interests and practice model.

2. **The multiple, multi-dimensional ways of reasoning that evolve with growing expertise.** Health professionals, both within and across various health professions, do not reason in the same way. The assumption that there is one way of representing clinical reasoning expertise or a single correct way to solve a problem has been challenged.[30] The different ways that health professionals think as they gain expertise was explained earlier in this chapter.

3. **The embedding of clinical reasoning in decision–action cycles.** As discussed, professional practice inherently deals with actions. Decisions and actions in professional practice influence each other. Decision making is a dynamic, reciprocal process of making decisions and implementing an optimal course of action.[31] These decision–action cycles form the basis for professional judgment.

4. **The influence of contextual factors.** It is important to remember that, in practice, health professionals are required to make decisions about particular actions that are going to be taken with particular patients in particular practice settings. The influence of context on clinical decision making has been examined, and it was identified that the nature of the task (such as its difficulty, complexity and uncertainty), the characteristics of the decision maker (including frames of reference, individual capabilities and experience) and the external decision-making context (such as professional ethics, disciplinary norms and workplace policies) all influence the decision-making process.[32]

5. **The nature of collaborative decision making.** As presented in Chapter 14, there is a growing trend, and indeed societal pressure, for patients and health professionals to adopt a collaborative approach to clinical reasoning which increases the patient's role and power in decision making.[33] Shared decision making and being able to work together are important for creating and providing services that result in satisfactory outcomes for patients.

An interpretative model of clinical reasoning

The above factors attest to the complexity and fluid nature of professional practice, which requires more than just cognitive processes. A model that views clinical reasoning as a contextualised interactive phenomenon has been developed by Higgs and Jones.[29]

TABLE 15.1:
SUMMARY OF CLINICAL REASONING APPROACHES

Model	Description
Hypothetico-deductive reasoning[34-36]	The generation of hypotheses based on clinical data and knowledge and testing of these hypotheses through further inquiry. It is used by novices and in problematic situations by experts.[37]
Pattern recognition[38]	Expert reasoning in non-problematic situations resembles pattern recognition or direct automatic retrieval of information from a well-structured knowledge base.[39] Through the use of inductive reasoning, pattern recognition/interpretation is a process characterised by speed and efficiency.[40]
Forward reasoning; backward reasoning[40,41]	Forward reasoning describes inductive reasoning in which data analysis results in hypothesis generation or diagnosis, utilising a sound knowledge base. Forward reasoning is more likely to occur in familiar cases with experienced health professionals, and backward reasoning with inexperienced health professionals or in atypical or difficult cases.[41] Backward reasoning is the re-interpretation of data or the acquisition of new clarifying data invoked to test a hypothesis.
Knowledge reasoning integration[42,43]	Clinical reasoning requires domain-specific knowledge and an organised knowledge base. A stage theory which emphasises the parallel development of knowledge acquisition and clinical reasoning expertise has been proposed.[43] Clinical reasoning involves the integration of knowledge, reasoning and meta-cognition.[44]
Intuitive reasoning[45,46]	'Intuitive knowledge' is related to 'instance scripts' or past experience with specific cases which can be used unconsciously in inductive reasoning.
Multidisciplinary reasoning[47]	Occurs when members of a multidisciplinary team work together to make clinical decisions for the patient, for example at case conferences and in multidisciplinary clinics.
Conditional reasoning[48-50]	Used by health professionals to estimate a patient's response to intervention and the likely outcomes of management and to help patients consider possibilities and reconstruct their lives following injury or the onset of disease.
Narrative reasoning[48,51,52]	The use of stories regarding past or present patients to further understand and manage a clinical situation. Telling the story of patients' illness or injury to help them make sense of the illness experience.
Interactive reasoning[48,49]	Interactive reasoning occurs between health professional and patient to understand the patient's perspective.
Collaborative reasoning[20,48,53,54]	The shared decision making that ideally occurs between health professionals and their patients. The patient's opinions as well as information about the problem are actively sought and utilised.
Ethical reasoning[48,55-57]	Those less recognised but frequently made decisions regarding moral, political and economic dilemmas which health professionals regularly confront, such as deciding how long to continue an intervention for.
Teaching as reasoning[48,58]	When health professionals consciously use advice, instruction and guidance for the purpose of promoting change in the patient's understanding, feelings and behaviour.

Figure 15.1 portrays the characteristics of this model, which include:

1. **Three core dimensions**
    a. **Discipline-specific knowledge**—propositional knowledge (derived from theory and research) and non-propositional knowledge (derived from professional and personal experience)
    b. **Cognition**—the thinking skills used to process clinical data against the health professional's existing discipline-specific and personal knowledge base in consideration of the patient's needs and the clinical problem
    c. **Meta-cognition**—reflective self-awareness enables health professionals to identify limitations in the quality of information obtained, monitor errors and credibility in their reasoning and practice and recognise inadequacies in their knowledge and reasoning.
2. **Interactive/contextual dimensions**
    a. **Mutual decision making**—the role of the patient in the decision-making process
    b. **Contextual interaction**—the interactivity between the decision makers and the decision-making situation
    c. **Task impact**—the influence of the nature of the clinical problem or task on the reasoning process.
3. **Four meta-skills**
    a. The ability to derive knowledge from reasoning and practice
    b. The capacity to locate reasoning within the health professional's chosen practice models
    c. The reflexive ability to promote patients' and health professionals' wellbeing and development
    d. The use of critical, creative conversations[28] to make clinical decisions.

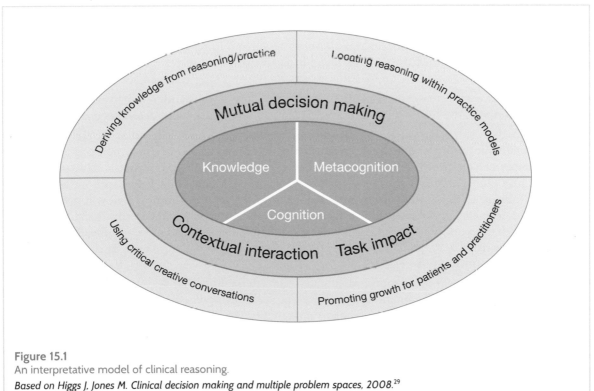

Figure 15.1
An interpretative model of clinical reasoning.
Based on Higgs J, Jones M. Clinical decision making and multiple problem spaces, 2008.[29]

As this model demonstrates, health professionals use a range of cognitive, meta-cognitive and interactive skills to obtain and combine knowledge and data from a range of sources when making clinical judgments. They need access to propositional knowledge that is appropriate to their professional discipline as well as knowledge about health and wellbeing more generally. This type of knowledge has been emphasised in conceptualisations of evidence-based practice to date. They also need access to non-propositional knowledge that is derived from professional and personal experience. They need the cognitive abilities to combine this information and the meta-cognitive skills to evaluate the trustworthiness and relevance of knowledge from these different sources and apply it to the practice decisions they have to make and to make changes to their practice accordingly. The capacity of health professionals to implement practice that aims to improve patient outcomes through the use of 'evidence' to substantiate that practice must be developed over time as experience grows and through critical appraisal of one's practice.

HOW DO I MAKE MY PRACTICE EVIDENCE-BASED?

In this chapter, we have presented professional practice as a complex and fluid process that is characterised by high levels of uncertainty that arise from the context-dependent nature of the tasks that are undertaken. Professional practice is difficult to describe specifically, as it involves fulfilling particular professional roles with particular patients within particular contexts. Each of these factors contributes a unique aspect to the phenomenon, leading to a complex range of variations to what might be considered 'standard practice'. Therefore, there is no easy answer to the question, 'How do I make my practice evidence-based?' However, a number of principles and tools can provide health professionals with strategies for working towards improved patient outcomes through a practice that is evidence-based. The following list provides some ideas that you may wish to use as your practice and professional development requires. The principle of critically reflecting on your practice underpins these ideas. Critical reflection refers to the process of analysing, reconsidering and questioning your experiences within a broad context of issues.

- Be systematic in the way you collect and use information and knowledge so that you can be sure that the information and knowledge you are using is trustworthy and relevant to the decisions you have to make.

- Use sound and logical reasoning as well as compassion and understanding when making decisions, and be clear about the information and knowledge you are basing those decisions on.

- Have a good working knowledge of the current propositional knowledge that is relevant to your professional community of practice or profession and the type of practice in which you are engaged (for example, if you are working as a rehabilitation therapist where you primarily treat people who have neurological disorders, you need to know the propositional knowledge appropriate to your work). Be aware of the limits of your propositional knowledge and plan how you will systematically expand this knowledge to better inform your practice. Plan how you will determine the relevance of this knowledge to your practice more generally and to individual patients more specifically. Remember that evidence from a range of research approaches forms a key component of the propositional knowledge relevant to your practice.

- Be aware of your current non-propositional knowledge. Remember that non-propositional knowledge includes your professional craft knowledge (for example, knowing *how* to do things) and your personal knowledge (for example, understanding of your strengths, weaknesses, preferences and interests). Ask yourself questions like: How have I systematically tested my practice experiences and derived knowledge from these experiences? Can I communicate this knowledge with credibility to my colleagues and patients and use it as sound evidence to support my practice? Is there personal knowledge derived from my life experiences (for example, working with people from different cultures) that I can use in my practice? What have I learned about communicating with people who speak different languages to me or who experience hardship, disability or illness/injury that I can use to enhance my practice? Planning to systematically enhance or expand this type of knowledge is an excellent way of drawing on your practice expertise and individualising the services that you provide to patients.

- Engage in empathic visioning and collaborative questioning with patients about their experiences, knowledge and values. Listen to your patients' stories and experiences and try to understand their experience of and perspective on the situation. Ask them what they think would make the biggest difference in their life. Practise problem solving and mutual decision making with your patients to expand your collaboration skills and improve your decision making.

- Be aware of the degree to which your actions are informed by the different sources of information and knowledge: research evidence; your own clinical expertise; the patients' values, preferences and circumstances; and an understanding of the practice context and how it shapes your practice (for example, what demands and expectations it places on you; in what ways is constrains what you can and cannot do).

- Critically reflect on and practise articulating your reasoning and your professional practice model.

Much professional expertise becomes 'embodied' knowledge or practice wisdom. You might not be aware of the details of this knowledge or be able to articulate this knowledge. To utilise this knowledge effectively as evidence for practice, it is important to raise awareness of those aspects of professional and personal thinking and action that have become taken for granted. This includes an ability to critically evaluate the types of knowledge that are available to health professionals, including the assumptions about knowledge that are unquestioned. By engaging in critical reflection, you can become more systematic in your collection and use of the knowledge upon which you base your practice. To conduct truly evidence-based practice, you need to be aware of the types of knowledge that you are using and how you are using them, and asking yourself whether this constitutes appropriate evidence for the particular questions and problems about which you seek to be informed. You also need to be aware of the cognitive and meta-cognitive processes that you are using to combine information from different sources within the context of your discipline and practice context.

SUMMARY POINTS OF THIS CHAPTER

- Health professionals need to use clinical reasoning to collect, interpret and combine different types of information and knowledge from a range of sources to make judgments and decisions in professional practice, particularly in complex and uncertain situations.

- Clinical reasoning is a process that involves cognition, meta-cognition (that is, the process of reflective self-awareness) plus interactive and narrative ways of thinking.

- Integrating knowledge from research, clinical expertise, patient values and preferences, and knowledge from practice requires judgment and artistry as well as science and reasoning.

- Critical reflection refers to the process of analysing, reconsidering and questioning your experiences within a broad context of issues. By engaging in critical reflection, you can become more systematic in your collection and use of the information upon which you base your practice and more aware of your decision making processes.

References

1. Craik J, Rappolt S. Theory of research utilisation enhancement: a model for occupational therapy. Can J Occup Ther 2003;70:266–75.
2. Robertson L. Clinical reasoning, part 1: the nature of problem solving; a literature review. Br J Occup Ther 1996;59:178–82.

3. Sackett D, Rosenberg W, Gray J, et al. Evidence based medicine: what it is and what it isn't: it's about integrating individual clinical expertise and the best external evidence. BMJ 1996;312:71–2.
4. Higgs J, Jones M, Titchen A. Knowledge, reasoning and evidence for practice. In: Higgs J, Jones M, Loftus S, et al. editors. Clinical reasoning in the health professions. 3rd ed. Edinburgh: Elsevier; 2008. pp. 151–61.
5. Rycroft-Malone J, Seers K, Titchen A, et al. What counts as evidence in evidence-based practice? J Adv Nurs 2004;47:81–90.
6. Higgs J, Andresen L, Fish D. Practice knowledge—its nature, sources and contexts. In: Higgs J, Richardson B, Abrandt Dahlgren M, editors. Developing practice knowledge for health professionals. Oxford: Butterworth–Heinemann; 2004. pp. 51–69.
7. Jones M, Grimmer K, Edwards I, et al. Challenges in applying best evidence to physiotherapy. Internet J Allied Health Sci Pract 2006;4(3). Online. Available: ijahsp.nova.edu/articles/vol4num3/jones.pdf; 13 Nov 2012.
8. Small N. Knowledge, not evidence, should determine primary care practice. Clin Governance 2003;8:191–9.
9. Naylor C. Grey zones of clinical practice: some limits to evidence-based medicine. Lancet 1995;345:840–1.
10. Heinemann Australian Student's Dictionary. Melbourne: Reed Educational and Professional Publishing; 1992.
11. The Macquarie Concise Dictionary. 3rd ed. Sydney: Macquarie Library; 1998.
12. Pearson A. Balancing the evidence: incorporating the synthesis of qualitative data into systematic reviews. JBI Reports 2004;2:45–64.
13. Schön D. The reflective practitioner: how professionals think in action. New York: Basic Books; 1983.
14. Fish D, Coles C. Developing professional judgement in health care: learning through the critical appreciation of practice. Oxford: Butterworth–Heinemann; 1998.
15. Coles C. Developing professional judgement. J Contin Educ Health Prof 2002;22:3–10.
16. Lave J, Wenger E. Situated learning: legitimate peripheral participation. Cambridge: Cambridge University Press; 1991.
17. Walker R. Social and cultural perspectives on professional knowledge and expertise. In: Higgs J, Titchen A, editors. Practice knowledge and expertise in the health professions. Oxford: Butterworth–Heinemann; 2001. pp. 22–8.
18. Dreyfus H, Dreyfus S. Mind over machine. New York: Free Press; 1986.
19. McCormack B, Titchen A. Patient-centred practice: an emerging focus for nursing expertise. In: Higgs J, Titchen A, editors. Practice knowledge and expertise in the health professions. Oxford: Butterworth–Heinemann; 2001. pp. 96–101.
20. Fleming M. The search for tacit knowledge. In: Mattingly C, Fleming M, editors. Clinical reasoning: forms of inquiry in a therapeutic practice. Philadelphia: F A Davis; 1994. pp. 22–34.
21. Jensen G, Gwyer J, Hack L, et al. Expertise in physical therapy practice. Boston: Butterworth–Heinemann; 1999.
22. Sackett D, Straus S, Richardson W, et al. Evidence-based medicine: how to practice and teach EBM. 2nd ed. Edinburgh: Elsevier Churchill Livingstone; 2000.
23. Higgs J, Titchen A, Neville V. Professional practice and knowledge. In: Higgs J, Titchen A, editors. Practice knowledge and expertise in the health professions. Oxford: Butterworth–Heinemann; 2001. pp. 3–9.
24. Fish D, Higgs J. The context for clinical decision making in the 21st century. In: Higgs J, Jones M, Loftus S, editors. Clinical reasoning in the health professions. 3rd ed. Edinburgh: Elsevier; 2008. pp. 19–30.
25. Hunink M, Glasziou P, Siegel J, et al. Decision making in health and medicine: integrating evidence and values. New York: Cambridge University Press; 2001.
26. Turpin M. The issue is … recovery of our phenomenological knowledge in occupational therapy. Am J Occup Ther 2007;61:481–5.
27. Higgs J, Titchen A. Propositional, professional and personal knowledge in clinical reasoning. In: Higgs J, Jones M, editors. Clinical reasoning in the health professions. Oxford: Butterworth–Heinemann; 1995. pp. 129–46.
28. Higgs J. The complexity of clinical reasoning: exploring the dimensions of clinical reasoning expertise as a situated, lived phenomenon. CPEA, Occasional Paper 6. Collaborations in Practice and Education Advancement. Australia: The University of Sydney; 2007.
29. Higgs J, Jones M. Clinical decision making and multiple problem spaces. In: Higgs J, Jones M, Loftus S, editors. Clinical reasoning in the health professions. 3rd ed. Edinburgh: Elsevier; 2008. pp. 3–17.
30. Norman G. Research in clinical reasoning: past history and current trends. Med Educ 2005;39:418–27.
31. Smith M, Higgs J, Ellis E. Factors influencing clinical decision making. In: Higgs J, Jones M, Loftus S, editors. Clinical reasoning in the health professions. 3rd ed. Edinburgh: Elsevier; 2008. pp. 89–100.
32. Smith M. Clinical decision making in acute care cardiopulmonary physiotherapy. Unpublished doctoral thesis. Sydney: The University of Sydney; 2006.
33. Trede F, Higgs J. Re-framing the clinician's role in collaborative clinical decision making: re-thinking practice knowledge and the notion of clinician–patient relationships. Learning Health Social Care 2003;2:66–73.
34. Barrows H, Feightner J, Neufield V, et al. An analysis of the clinical methods of medical students and physicians. Report to the Province of Ontario Department of Health McMaster University Hamilton, Ont.; 1978.
35. Elstein A, Shulman S, Sprafka S. Medical problem solving: an analysis of clinical reasoning. Cambridge, MA: Harvard University Press; 1978.

36. Feltovich P, Johnson P, Moller J, et al. LCS: The role and development of medical knowledge in diagnostic expertise. In: Clancey W, Shortliffe E, editors. Readings in medical artificial intelligence: the first decade. Reading, MA: Addison-Wesley; 1984. pp. 275–319.
37. Elstein A, Shulman L, Sprafka S. Medical problem solving: a ten year retrospective. Eval Health Prof 1990;13:5–36.
38. Barrows H, Feltovich P. The clinical reasoning process. Med Educ 1987;21:86–91.
39. Groen G, Patel V. Medical problem-solving: some questionable assumptions. Med Educ 1985;19:95–100.
40. Arocha J, Patel V, Patel Y. Hypothesis generation and the coordination of theory and evidence in novice diagnostic reasoning. Med Decis Making 1993;13:198–211.
41. Patel V, Groen G. Knowledge-based solution strategies in medical reasoning. Cogn Sci 1986;10:91–116.
42. Schmidt H, Norman G, Boshuizen H. A cognitive perspective on medical expertise: theory and implications. Acad Med 1990;65:611–21.
43. Boshuizen H, Schmidt H. On the role of biomedical knowledge in clinical reasoning by experts, intermediates and novices. Cogn Sci 1992;16:153–84.
44. Higgs J, Jones M. Clinical reasoning. In: Higgs J, Jones M, editors. Clinical reasoning in the health professions. Oxford: Butterworth–Heinemann; 1995. pp. 3–23.
45. Agan R. Intuitive knowing as a dimension of nursing. Adv Nurs Sci 1987;10:63–70.
46. Rew L. Intuition in critical care nursing practice. Dimens Crit Care Nurs 1990;9:30–7.
47. Loftus S. Language in clinical reasoning: learning and using the language of collective clinical decision making. PhD Thesis. Australia: The University of Sydney; 2006. Online, Available: http://ses.library.usyd.edu.au/handle/2123/1165; 13 Nov 2012.
48. Edwards I, Jones M, Carr J, et al. Clinical reasoning in three different fields of physiotherapy—a qualitative study. In: Proceedings of the Fifth International Congress of the Australian Physiotherapy Association, Melbourne; 1998. pp. 298–300.
49. Fleming M. The therapist with the three track mind. Am J Occup Ther 1991;45:1007–14.
50. Hagedorn R. Clinical decision making in familiar cases: a model of the process and implications for practice. Br J Occup Ther 1996;59:217–22.
51. Benner P, Tanner C, Chesla C. From beginner to expert: gaining a differentiated clinical world in critical care nursing. Adv Nurs Sci 1992;14:13–28.
52. Mattingly C, Fleming MH. Clinical reasoning: forms of inquiry in a therapeutic practice. Philadelphia: F A Davis; 1994.
53. Coulter A. Shared decision-making: the debate continues. Health Expect 2005;8:95–6.
54. Beeston S, Simons H. Physiotherapy practice: practitioners' perspectives. Physiother Theory Pract 1996;12:231–42.
55. Barnitt R, Partridge C. Ethical reasoning in physical therapy and occupational therapy. Physiother Res Int 1997;2:178–94.
56. Gordon M, Murphy C, Candee D, et al. Clinical judgement: an integrated model. Adv Nurs Sci 1994;16:55–70.
57. Neuhaus B. Ethical considerations in clinical reasoning: the impact of technology and cost containment. Am J Occup Ther 1988;42:288–94.
58. Sluijs EM. Patient education in physiotherapy: towards a planned approach. Physiotherapy 1991;77:503–8.

Chapter 16

Implementing evidence into practice

Annie McCluskey

LEARNING OBJECTIVES

After reading this chapter, you should be able to:

- Describe the process of transferring evidence into practice
- Explain what is meant by an evidence–practice gap and describe methods that can be used to demonstrate an evidence-based gap
- Explain various types of barriers to successfully implementing evidence and how barriers and enablers can be identified
- Describe strategies and interventions that can be used to facilitate the implementation of evidence
- Describe theories which can inform the development of implementation strategies and help explain behaviour change as it relates to the implementation of evidence

As we have seen throughout this book, searching for and appraising research articles are key components of evidence-based practice. However, while they are worthy activities, on their own they do not change patient outcomes. To improve outcomes, health professionals need to do more than read the evidence. Transferring the evidence into practice is also required. Professionals need to translate research that has proven value, for example evidence from evidence-based clinical guidelines, systematic reviews and high quality randomised controlled trials. Findings from research projects which have involved years of hard work, many participants and often substantial costs should not remain hidden in journals. Translating or implementing evidence into practice is the final step in the process of evidence-based practice, but it is often the most challenging step.

Implementation is a complex but active process which involves individuals, teams, systems and organisations. Translating evidence into practice requires careful forward planning.[1] While some planning usually does occur, the process is often intuitive.[2] There may be little consideration of potential problems and barriers. As a consequence, the results may be disappointing. To help increase the likelihood of success when implementing evidence, this chapter provides a checklist for individuals and teams to use when planning the implementation of evidence.

In this chapter, definitions of implementation 'jargon' are provided, followed by examples of evidence that different disciplines have applied in practice. A description is provided of the steps that health professionals follow when translating evidence into practice. Steps include collecting and analysing local data (gap analysis) and identifying possible barriers and enablers to change. Barriers might include negative attitudes, limited skills and knowledge, or limited access to medical records and equipment. A menu of implementation strategies is presented, along with a review of the evidence for the effectiveness of these strategies. Finally, theories which can help us predict and explain individual and group behaviour change are considered.

IMPLEMENTATION TERMINOLOGY

A number of confusing terms appear in the implementation literature. Different terms may mean the same thing in different countries. To help you navigate this new terminology, definitions relevant to the chapter are provided in Box 16.1.

IMPLEMENTATION CASE STUDIES

To help you understand the process of implementation, we now consider three case studies. The first case study involves reducing referrals for a test procedure (X-rays) by general practitioners for people who present with acute low back pain.[7] This case example involves the overuse of X-rays. The other two case studies involve increasing the uptake of two under-used interventions: cognitive–behavioural therapy for adolescents with depression,[8] and community travel and mobility training for people with stroke.[9,10]

Case study 1. Reducing the use of X-rays by general practitioners for people with acute low-back pain

Low back pain is one of the most common musculoskeletal conditions seen not only by general practitioners,[11] but also by allied health practitioners such as physiotherapists, chiropractors and osteopaths. Clinical guidelines released in Australia in mid-2005 recommend that people presenting with an episode of acute non-specific low back pain should *not* be sent for an X-ray because of the limited diagnostic value of this test for this condition.[12] In Australia, about 25% of people who visited their local general practitioner with acute low back pain between 2005 and 2008 were referred for an X-ray[13] after release of the guidelines. Even higher proportions are reported in the United States and Europe.[7] Put simply, X-rays are over-prescribed and costly. Instead of recommending an X-ray, rest and passive interventions, general practitioners should advise people with acute low back pain to remain active.[12]

Definitions of implementation terminology

Implementation of evidence–A planned and active process of using published research in practice. For example, delivering an effective therapy from a randomised controlled trial to patients in a local setting.

Implementation science–The science of applying ideas, innovations and practices within the constraints of real healthcare settings. Implementation scientists typically use theories (for example, behaviour theory) to help explain why some ideas fail and others succeed, and which professionals or teams are more likely to adopt an evidence-based intervention than others. Implementation also involves a systematic (and scientific) approach, with careful planning and preparation.[3]

Diffusion of innovations–The process of spreading new ideas, behaviours or routines across a population. The adoption of new ideas typically starts with a slow initial phase, followed by a period of acceleration as more people adopt the behaviours of the innovators, then a corresponding period of deceleration with adoption by the last few individuals.[4] Examples of health 'innovations' include the introduction of a new outcome measure, screening procedure or intervention.

Translational (or implementation) research–The scientific study of methods to promote the translation (or uptake) of research knowledge into practice. The aim is to ensure that new interventions or practices reach intended patient groups and are implemented routinely. This type of research typically involves studying the process of behaviour change, barriers to change, and the place of reminders and decision-support tools.[5]

Knowledge transfer (or translation)–A process of synthesising and exchanging knowledge between researchers and users (professionals, patients and policy makers). A primary aim of knowledge transfer is to accelerate the use of research by professionals, in order to improve health outcomes.[6] Multiple disciplines, such as health informatics, health education and organisational theory, are involved in the knowledge translation process, to help close evidence–practice gaps.

Evidence–practice gaps–Areas of practice where routines or behaviour differ from clinical guideline recommendations or known best practice. Areas of practice where quality improvement is required. For example, patients may be referred for an unnecessary and costly test procedure, while others may not be receiving an intervention that could improve their health.

Practice behaviour–A routine used by health professionals which can be observed. Practice behaviours include the ordering of diagnostic tests, use of assessments and outcome measures, clinical note writing, and the delivery of interventions to patients and carers.

In this instance, the evidence–practice gap is the overuse of a costly diagnostic test which can delay recovery. Recommendations about the management of acute low back pain, including the use of X-rays, have been made through the national clinical guidelines.[12] A program to change practice, in line with guideline recommendations, is the focus of one implementation study in Australia[7] and will be discussed further throughout this chapter.

Case study 2. Increasing the delivery of cognitive–behavioural therapy to adolescents with depression by community mental health professionals

Cognitive–behavioural therapy has been identified as an effective intervention for adolescents with depression, a condition that is on the increase in developed countries.[14] Outcomes from cognitive–behavioural therapy that is provided in the community are superior to usual care for this population.[15] Clinical guidelines recommend that young people who are affected by depression should receive a series of cognitive–behavioural therapy sessions. However, a survey of one group of health professionals in North America found that two-thirds had no formal training in cognitive–behavioural therapy, and no prior experience using an intervention manual for cognitive–behavioural therapy.[8] In other words, they were unlikely to deliver cognitive–behavioural therapy if they did not know much about it. Furthermore, almost half of the participants in that study reported that they never or rarely used evidence-based interventions for youths with depression, and a quarter of the group had no plans to use evidence-based intervention in the following 6 months. Subsequently, that group of mental health professionals was targeted with an implementation program to increase the uptake of the underused cognitive–behavioural therapy. The randomised controlled trial that describes this implementation program[8] and the evidence–practice gap (underuse of cognitive–behavioural therapy) will also be discussed throughout this chapter.

Case study 3. Increasing the delivery of travel and mobility training by community rehabilitation therapists to people who have had a stroke

People who have had a stroke typically have difficulty accessing their local community. Many experience social isolation. Approximately 50% of people who complete an on-road driving test after their stroke pass this test and resume driving,[16] but many do not return to driving[17] and up to 50% experience a fall at home in the first 6 months.[18] Australian clinical guidelines recommend that community-dwelling people with stroke should receive up to seven escorted journey sessions and transport information from a rehabilitation therapist, to help increase outdoor journeys.[19] Although that recommendation is based on a single randomised controlled trial,[20] the size of the intervention effect was large. The intervention doubled the proportion of people with stroke who reported getting out as often as they wanted and doubled the number of monthly outdoor journeys, compared with participants in the control group.[20]

In order to see whether people with stroke were receiving this intervention from community-based rehabilitation teams in a region of Sydney, local therapists and the author of this chapter conducted a retrospective file audit. The audit revealed that therapists were documenting very little about outdoor journeys and transport after stroke. Documented information about the number of weekly outings was present in only 14% of files (see Table 16.1). Furthermore, only 17% of people with stroke were receiving six or more sessions of intervention that targeted outdoor journeys, which was the 'dose' of intervention provided in the original trial by Logan and colleagues.[20,21] The audit data highlighted an

TABLE 16.1: SUMMARY OF BASELINE FILE AUDITS (n = 77) INVOLVING FIVE COMMUNITY REHABILITATION TEAMS DESCRIBING SCREENING AND PROVISION OF AN EVIDENCE-BASED INTERVENTION* FOR PEOPLE WITH STROKE		
	n	%
Screening for outdoor mobility and travel		
Driving status documented (pre-stroke or current)	37	48%
Preferred mode of travel documented	27	35%
Reasons for limited outdoor journeys documented	26	34%
Number of weekly outdoor journeys documented	11	14%
Outdoor journey intervention		
At least 1 session provided	44	57%
2 sessions or more provided	27	35%
6 sessions or more provided	13	17%
*Intervention to help increase outdoor journeys as described by Logan and colleagues[20,21]		

evidence–practice gap, specifically the underuse of an evidence-based intervention. This example will be used as the third case study throughout the chapter, to illustrate the process of implementation.

THE PROCESS OF IMPLEMENTATION

The following section summarises two models that may help you better understand the steps and factors involved in implementing evidence.

Model 1. The evidence-to-practice pipeline

The 'evidence pipeline' described by Glasziou and Haynes[22] and shown in Figure 16.1 provides a helpful illustration of steps in the implementation process. This metaphorical pipeline highlights how leakage can occur, drip by drip, along the way from awareness of evidence to the point of delivery to patients. First, there is an ever-expanding pool of published research to read, both original and synthesised research. This large volume of information causes busy professionals to miss important, valid evidence (*awareness*). Then, assuming that they have heard of the benefits of a successful intervention (or the overuse of a test procedure), professionals may need persuasion to change their practice (*acceptance*). They may be more inclined to provide familiar interventions with which they are confident, and which patients expect and value. Hidden social pressure from patients and other team members can make practice changes less likely to occur. Busy professionals also need to recognise appropriate patients who

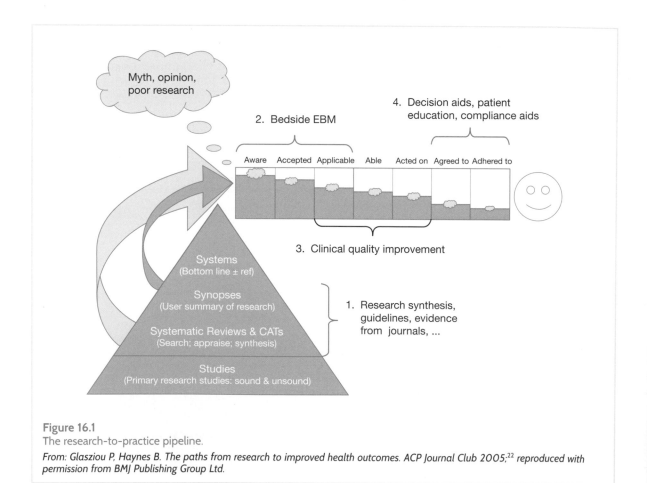

Figure 16.1
The research-to-practice pipeline.

From: Glasziou P, Haynes B. The paths from research to improved health outcomes. ACP Journal Club 2005;[22] reproduced with permission from BMJ Publishing Group Ltd.

should receive the intervention (or not receive a test procedure). Professionals then need to apply this knowledge in the course of a working day (*applicability*).

Some test procedures and interventions will require new skills and knowledge. For example, the delivery of cognitive–behavioural therapy to adolescents with depression involves special training, instruction manuals, extra study and supervision. A lack of skills and knowledge may be a barrier to practice change for professionals who need to deliver the intervention (*able*). A further challenge is that while we may be aware of an intervention, accept the need to provide it and are able to deliver it, we may not act on the evidence all of the time (*acted on*). We may forget—or, more likely, we may find it difficult to change well-established habits. For example, general practitioners who have been referring people with acute back pain for an X-ray for many years may find this practice difficult to stop.

The evidence-to-practice pipeline illustrates the steps involved in maximising the acceptance and uptake of research findings. The final two steps rely on patients agreeing to a different test procedure than they expect (*agree*) and changing their behaviour to comply with an intervention. For example, people with low back pain will need to stay active within the level of comfort permitted by their low back pain (*adherence*). Any intervention that involves a major change in behaviour, for example exercise or the use of cognitive–behavioural therapy principles, is likely to be difficult for many people to adopt and maintain. These last two steps highlight the important role that shared decision making and clear communication of evidence to patients (which were explained in Chapter 14) have in the process of implementing evidence into practice.

Model 2. Plan and prepare model

A different process of implementation has been proposed by Grol and Wensing.[3] Their bottom line is 'plan and prepare'. While intended for the implementation of clinical guidelines, the principles apply equally well to the implementation of test ordering, outcome measurement or interventions and for procedures that are either underused or overused. The 'plan and prepare' model involves five key steps:

1. **Write** a proposal for change with clear aims and target groups.
2. **Analyse** the target groups and setting for barriers, problems, enablers and other factors that may hinder or help the change process.
3. **Decide** on implementation strategies to help professionals learn about, adopt and sustain the practice change.
4. **Execute** the implementation plan, documenting a list of activities, tasks and a timeline.
5. **Evaluate**, revise if necessary and continuously monitor the implementation plan, using clinical indicators to measure ongoing success.

Using the travel and mobility study as an example, the two primary aims were:

- to increase the use of the underused intervention by rehabilitation therapists, as recommended by a national guideline recommendation
- to increase community participation, and the number of outdoor journeys, by people with stroke who received the evidence-based intervention.

The two target groups were:

- rehabilitation professionals (occupational therapists, physiotherapists and therapy assistants)
- community-dwelling people with stroke.

Examples of 'targets' or indicators of implementation success were also documented early in this project for both groups.[9] The first target was that rehabilitation therapists would deliver an outdoor mobility and travel training intervention[20,21] to 75% of people with stroke who were referred to the service (that is, a change in professional behaviour). The second target was that 75% of people with stroke who received the intervention would report getting out of the house as often as they wanted, and take more outdoor journeys per month compared with pre-intervention.

Other steps in the 'plan and prepare' model (identifying barriers and enablers, selecting implementation strategies) are discussed, using examples, in the following sections.

Demonstrating an evidence–practice gap (gap analysis)

A common first step is to identify and clarify the research–practice gap which needs to be bridged. Most health professionals who seek funding for an implementation project, and post-graduate students who write research proposals, will demonstrate their evidence–practice gap using simple data collection methods. Surveys and file audits are the most popular methods.

Surveys for gap analysis

A survey can be developed and used, with health professionals or patients, to explore attitudes, knowledge and current practices. If a large proportion of health professionals admit to knowing little about, or rarely using, an evidence-based intervention, this information represents the evidence–practice gap. In the cognitive–behavioural therapy example discussed earlier,[8] a local survey was used to explore attitudes to, knowledge of and use of cognitive–behavioural therapy by community mental health professionals.

The process of developing a survey to explore attitudes and behavioural intentions has been well documented in a manual by Jill Francis and colleagues.[23] The manual is intended for use by health service researchers who want to predict and understand behaviour, and measure constructs associated with the Theory of Planned Behaviour. Behavioural theories are discussed in a later section of this chapter. If you intend to develop your own local survey or questionnaire, whether the survey is for gap analysis or barrier analysis, it is recommended that you consult this excellent resource (freely available online; see reference 23). Sample questions include: 'Do you intend to do (intervention X) with all of your patients?' and 'Do you believe that you will be able to do X with your patients?'.

Audits for gap analysis

Audit is another method which can be used to demonstrate an evidence–practice gap. A small file audit can be conducted using local data (for example, 10 files may be selected, reflecting consecutive admissions over 3 months). The audit can be used to determine how many people with a health condition received a test or an evidence-based intervention. For example, we could determine the proportion of people with acute back pain for whom an X-ray had been ordered in a general practice over the previous 3 months. We could also count how frequently (or rarely) an intervention was used.

In the travel and mobility study, it was possible to determine the proportion of people with stroke who had received one or more sessions with an occupational therapist or physiotherapist to help increase outdoor journeys.[9] Baseline file audits of 77 consecutive referrals across five services in the previous year revealed that 44 out of 77 (57%) people with stroke had received at least one session targeting outdoor journeys, but 22 out of 77 (35%) had received two or more sessions, and only 13 out of 77 (17%) had received six or more sessions. In the original randomised controlled trial that evaluated this intervention,[20,21] a median of six sessions targeting outdoor journeys had been provided by therapists. This number of sessions was considered the optimal 'dose' (or target) of intervention.

It has been recommended that more than one method should be used to collect data on current practice, as part of a gap analysis (for example, an audit and a survey).[2] Collecting information from a small but representative sample of health professionals or patients, using both qualitative and quantitative methods, can be useful.[2]

In Australia, examples of evidence–practice gaps in healthcare have been summarised by the National Institute of Clinical Studies (NICS).[24] This organisation highlights gaps between what is known and what is practised. For example, projects have investigated evidence–practice gaps in the following areas: underuse of smoking cessation programs by pregnant mothers, suboptimal management of acute pain and cancer pain in hospitalised patients and underuse of preventative interventions for venous thrombo-embolism in hospitalised patients.[25]

After collating quantitative and qualitative information from a representative sample of health professionals, and/or patients in a facility, the next step is to identify potential barriers and enablers to implementation.

Identifying barriers and enablers to implementation (barrier analysis)

Barriers are factors or conditions that may prevent successful implementation of evidence. Conversely, enablers are factors that increase the likelihood of success. Barriers and enablers can be attributed to individuals (for example, attitudes or knowledge), groups and teams (for example, professional roles) or patients (for example, expectations about intervention). When barriers and enablers have been identified, a tailored program of strategies can be developed.

Attitudinal barriers are easy to recognise. Most health professionals will know someone in their team or organisation that resists change. Perhaps they have been exposed to too much change and innovation. Knowledge, skill and systems barriers are often less obvious (for example, do team members know how to deliver cognitive–behavioural therapy? Do they have access to manuals, video-recorders or vehicles for community visits?). Experienced health professionals may be reluctant to acknowledge a lack of skills, knowledge or confidence. Qualitative methods such as interviews can be useful for investigating what people know, how confident they feel and what they think about local policies, procedures and systems. Social influences can also be a barrier (or an enabler), but may be invisible. For example, patients may expect, and place pressure on, health professionals to order tests or deliver particular interventions.

Methods for identifying barriers are similar to those used for identifying evidence–practice gaps: surveys, individual and group interviews (or informal chats), and observation of practice.[26,27] Sometimes it may be useful to use two or more methods. The choice of method will be guided by time and resources, as well as local circumstances and the number of health professionals involved.

The travel and mobility study involved community occupational therapists, physiotherapists and therapy assistants from two different teams. Individual interviews were conducted with these health professionals. Interviews were tape-recorded with their consent (ethics approval was obtained), and the content was transcribed and analysed. The decision to conduct individual interviews was based on a desire to find out what professionals in different disciplines knew and thought about the planned intervention, and about professional roles and responsibilities. Rich and informative data were obtained;[10] however, this method produced a large quantity of information which was time-consuming to collect, transcribe and analyse. A survey or focus group would be more efficient for busy health professionals to use in practice. Examples of quotes from the interviews and four types of barriers from this study are presented in Figure 16.2.

Examples of questions to ask during interviews or in a survey, and potential barriers and enablers to consider, are listed in Box 16.2. The list has been adapted from a publication by Michie and colleagues.[28]

While patient expectations of intervention can be sought, this step often appears to be omitted during barrier analysis. A systematic review of treatment expectations confirmed that most people with acute low back pain who consult their general practitioner expect additional diagnostic tests to be ordered, and a referral to be made to specialists.[29] General practitioners in another study also reported a tendency

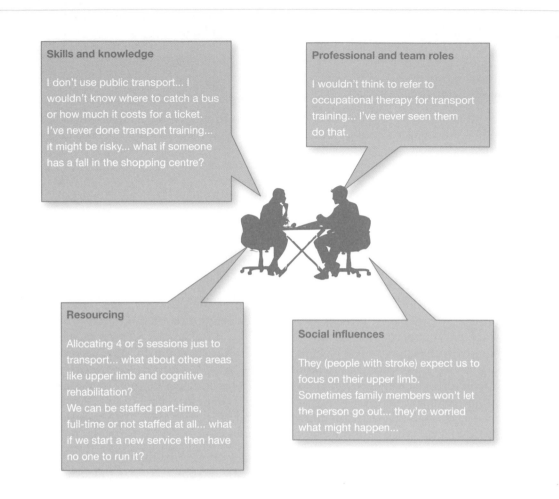

Figure 16.2
Barriers to the delivery of a community-based outdoor journey intervention for people with stroke, identified through qualitative interviews with allied health professionals (*n* = 13).

BOX 16.2

Example of questions to ask during an interview or in a survey when identifying potential barriers and enablers

- Do health professionals know about, accept and believe the evidence? (**knowledge, attitudes, values**)
- Does the original research describe what to do, and how to do it in sufficient detail? Is there a protocol for the intervention? Do health professionals know what to do? (**knowledge, skills, abilities**)
- Are health professionals confident that they can provide the intervention? (**attitudes, capabilities, confidence**)
- Do health professionals want to provide the intervention? (**motivation**)
- Do health professionals intend to provide the intervention? (**intention**)
- Is there an expectation from other team members or patients that the intervention will be provided? (**social influence**)
- Do health professionals have the necessary equipment, space, manuals and staff to provide the intervention routinely? (**resources and staffing**)

to 'give in' to patients' demands for an X-ray and referral to a physiotherapist.[30] McKenzie and colleagues[7] targeted this lack of confidence as part of their implementation strategy. To help practitioners refer fewer patients for an X-ray, workshops were conducted to model, rehearse and practise persuasive communication techniques during patient consultations. Such strategies targeted the skills, knowledge and confidence of health professionals who had to overcome pressure and social influence from patients.

Resources which can be used to identify barriers and enablers include those produced by the National Institute for Health and Clinical Excellence (NICE) in England[26] and the National Institute of Clinical Studies (NICS) in Australia.[27] An important next step is selecting evidence-based strategies to target identified barriers.

Implementation strategies and interventions

A range of strategies and interventions have been used to target barriers, help health professionals change their behaviour and get evidence into practice. The list is extensive. Frequently used strategies are listed below:

- educational materials[31,32]
- educational meetings[33]
- educational outreach visits,[34,35] including academic detailing (face-to-face education of health professionals, typically pharmacists and doctors, to change their clinical habits, such as prescribing habits, so that they are in line with best evidence)
- the use of external facilitators[36]
- the use of opinion leaders
- reminders,[37,38] including patient-mediated and computer-aided interventions
- audit and feedback[39,40]
- team building/practice development
- tailored (targeted) interventions or strategies that are planned and take account of prospectively identified barriers to change[41]
- multifaceted interventions, including several of the above strategies.[42]

Only some of these strategies have been evaluated for effectiveness and summarised in systematic reviews, or 'overviews' of reviews.[43,44] Some of the commonly used strategies, and findings from systematic reviews, are discussed next.

Educational materials

This strategy includes the distribution of published or printed materials such as clinical guideline summaries and guideline recommendations. Some authors also include audio-visual materials and electronic publications in their definition of educational materials. Content may be delivered personally or through mass mailouts. Materials may or may not target known knowledge and skill barriers. Such materials are relatively low-cost and feasible to provide, but are unlikely to be effective if they do not target local knowledge barriers.

In Chapter 13, the potential value of evidence-based clinical guidelines was explained. In an attempt to get health professionals to use clinical guidelines, they are often printed and mailed out to health professionals. Alone, mailed dissemination of guidelines is known to have little or no effect on behaviour. Consequently, this process of mailing out guidelines to professionals is often used with control groups in cluster randomised controlled trials. For example, in the study by McKenzie and colleagues,[7] doctors in the control group of practices received guideline recommendations about the management of acute low back pain. These guidelines were not expected to change doctors' X-ray ordering behaviour.

A Cochrane review on the effect of printed educational materials located and appraised 23 studies.[31] When randomised controlled trials were analysed alone ($n = 6$), the median effect was 4% absolute improvement (interquartile range −8% to 10%) for categorical outcomes such as X-ray requests and smoking cessation. The relative risk difference for continuous process outcomes such as medication change and X-ray requests per practice was greater (median change 14%, interquartile range −5% to 27%) based on four randomised controlled trials. However, there was no positive effect on patient outcomes. Indeed, a negative effect or deterioration in patient outcomes was reported when data were analysed. The median effect was −4% (interquartile range −1% to −5%) for categorical outcomes such as return to work, screening for a health condition, or smoking cessation. The authors concluded that when compared with no intervention, printed educational materials may positively influence practitioner behaviour but they do not improve patient outcomes.

The overall effect that may be expected from using educational materials to change practice is less than 10% improvement. As this chapter will show, few interventions to change practitioner behaviour result in changes greater than 10%.

Educational meetings

This strategy includes workshops, conferences, meetings and in-service sessions, intended to increase awareness, impart knowledge and develop skills. Meetings can be interactive or didactic. The former may target skills, attitudes and knowledge, whereas didactic sessions mainly target knowledge barriers. Ideally, these sessions target identified skills or knowledge barriers. If practitioners indicate lack of confidence with a new practice, such as cognitive–behavioural therapy in the study by Kramer and Burns,[8] educational meetings can help to address the need. In response to therapists' preferences, Kramer and Burns provided a one-day training session which prepared therapists to deliver motivational interviewing and cognitive behavioural therapy, educate adolescents about depression, promote medication adherence and assess ongoing suicide risk.

In the travel and mobility study, occupational therapists and physiotherapists indicated a lack of awareness about the published evidence, as well as a need for information about local transport systems (for example, local bus routes and ticketing systems) and risk management strategies when escorting a person with stroke across roads, to local shops and on public transport.[10] They also indicated a preference for a half-day workshop, which was provided.

The most recent review to examine the effect of educational meetings is a 2009 Cochrane review.[33] Its findings were consistent with the 2001 review which it replaced, but 49 new trials (total of 81 trials) were added. In most studies, the health professionals were doctors, particularly general practitioners. Targeted behaviours included delivery of preventative health education to patients, such as smoking cessation and exercise, test ordering, screening for disease and prescribing. Median follow-up time was 6 months. Appraisal of the 81 trials revealed much variation in the complexity of behaviours targeted, characteristics of interventions used and results. The median improvement in compliance with practice with any type of educational meeting compared with no intervention was 6% (interquartile range 2% to 16%). Educational meetings can result in small to moderate improvements in professional practice, with smaller improvements in patient outcomes. The 2001 review found interactive education meetings to be more effective than didactic meetings. The 2009 review found mixed interactive *and* didactic education to be most effective, not interactive education alone. No significant difference was found between multifaceted interventions (those with more than one component) and single interventions. Higher attendance at educational meetings was also associated with greater effects.

Educational outreach visits

An educational outreach visit is defined as a face-to-face visit by a trained person to the practice setting of health professionals, with the intent of improving practice.[32,35] This strategy is also known as educational or academic detailing and educational visiting.[35] The aim may be to decrease prescribing or test-ordering behaviours, and/or increase screening practices, and/or the routine delivery of an evidence-based intervention. This strategy is derived from social marketing and uses social persuasion methods to target individual knowledge and attitudes. Sessions aim to transmit a small number of messages (two or three) in 15 to 20 minutes, using an approach tailored to individual professionals or practices. Typically, the focus is on simple behaviours such as medication prescribing habits.

An example of the use of outreach visits to change practice was where a trained pharmacist visited general practitioners to discuss childhood asthma management, while also leaving educational materials about best practice. The effect of the educational outreach visits was tested using a cluster randomised controlled trial design, and involved multiple general practices in a township near Cape Town, South Africa.[34] Parents of children provided survey data on asthma severity and symptom frequency. Asthma symptom scores declined by 0.8 points more (on a 9-point scale, $p = 0.03$) in children whose doctor had received outreach visits compared with the control group of children. For every child with asthma seen in a practice which received outreach visits, the authors report that one extra child will experience substantially reduced symptoms.

A systematic review of studies published up until 1998 examined the effect of outreach visits on professional practice.[32] This review located and analysed 13 cluster randomised controlled trials, and five controlled before and after studies, with most evaluating outreach visits as part of a multifaceted intervention. When outreach visits were provided as part of a multifaceted intervention, they improved practice by a median of 6% (interquartile range −4% to 17%). The reviewers suggested that organisations should carefully consider the resources and cost involved in providing outreach visits for this modest (6%) change in behaviour. The Cochrane review on the effect of educational outreach visits was last updated in 2007.[35] This review appraised 69 studies published up until March 2007, involving more than 15,000 health professionals; 28 studies contributed to the median effect size. The reviewers reported a median (adjusted risk) difference in practice of 6% (interquartile range 3% to 9%). Many of the studies evaluated the effect of outreach visits on prescribing practice. The median effect was more varied when other types of professional practice were examined (median 6%, interquartile range 4% to 16%). The effect of outreach visits was slightly superior to audit and feedback when the two strategies were compared (in eight trials). When individual visits were compared with group visits (three trials), the results were mixed.

Reminders

Reminders aim to prompt a health professional to recall information, such as performing or avoiding some action, to improve individual patient care. A reminder can be provided verbally, on paper or via computer screen. Reminders can be encounter-specific, patient-mediated and/or involve computer-aided decision support.

'Encounter-specific' refers to reminders that are delivered to a health professional and associated with particular encounters such as breast screening or dental reviews, or a particular test result. In one example, educational messages about diabetes care were delivered to general practitioners with laboratory test results to help improve the quality of diabetes care.[37] Two examples of messages attached to HbA_{1c} (haemoglobin/blood test) reports were: 'If HbA_{1c} <6.5% = within target for type 2 diabetes'; and 'If HbA_{1c} 6.5–7.0% = for type 2 diabetes, consider increasing oral therapy'. Other messages targeted blood pressure control and foot inspection. Statistically significant reductions were reported in mean diastolic but not systolic blood pressure following the brief educational messages. The odds of achieving target blood pressure control and receiving a foot inspection during a consultation were increased. However, there was no effect on mean HbA_{1c} or cholesterol levels.

'Patient-mediated' reminders involve the person with the health condition taking information to the treating professional to help prompt a practice behaviour. One example is the use of a 'diabetes passport',[45] a patient-held record. The patient takes a passport with them to appointments, to help prompt monitoring by health professionals of blood pressure and foot health care, amongst other health indicators. After introducing the passports to patients and embedding the passport into general practices in the Netherlands, the effect on patient health outcomes was evaluated using a randomised controlled trial.[46] Diabetes passports were issued to 87% of eligible patients. After 15 months, 76% of patients reported that the passport was being used, and referred to, during clinic visits. Process measures of diabetes care improved significantly in intervention practices compared with control practices; for example, HbA_{1c}, creatinine, cholesterol, weight and glucose were examined more often, although blood pressure and foot inspections were not conducted more often. There were no significant differences in patient outcomes such as quality of life, self-advocacy or diabetes knowledge.

In the travel and mobility study, fluorescent pink stickers were provided as a reminder to therapists, containing the messages 'Screened for outdoor journeys' and 'Intervention provided targeting outdoor journeys'. These stickers were placed on the desks of occupational therapists and physiotherapists. The first sticker reminded therapists to ask a series of screening questions about driving status and community outings, complete a screening form and place the form in the patient's file, accompanied by the sticker and a file entry. The second sticker prompted therapists to deliver an outdoor journey intervention to people with stroke who were not getting out as often as they wanted, then document the content of sessions in the patient's file, accompanied by the sticker.

Evidence for the effectiveness of reminders is higher than for most other implementation strategies, but rehabilitation therapists have not been the focus of studies to date. The most recent Cochrane review only examined the effect of pop-up computer screen reminders when used with doctors.[38] That study found 28 studies that evaluated the effects of different on-screen computer reminders, for prescribing medications, warning the doctors about drug interactions, providing vaccinations and ordering tests. The review found small to moderate benefits; reminders improved doctors' practices by a median of 4%, with patients' health improving by a median of 3% in eight of the 28 studies. No specific reminders or features of reminders were consistently associated with these larger benefits.

Audit and feedback

Audit refers to any summary of clinical performance over a specified period of time. Feedback about audit findings may be written or oral, and the summary may or may not include details of compliance with audit criteria and recommendations for action. Audit information can be obtained from medical records, computerised databases or by observing patients and professionals. Implementation literature describes audit and feedback together, because there is limited value in conducting an audit if the target professionals do not receive feedback about the findings. Thus, some form of feedback about audit findings is needed.

One aim of audit and feedback is to create some urgency in the health professionals about the need for change. Without objective data from audits, health professionals are likely to perceive that their practice is within acceptable levels. However, it has been demonstrated that self-reports of behaviour are likely to overestimate performance by up to 27%.[47]

Audits are the mainstay of quality-improvement activities, yet surprisingly few health professionals have conducted an audit. If they have, the audit has typically focused on compliance with note writing and record keeping. Rarely do file audits focus on the content of the interventions. Even fewer audits seem to focus on evidence-based interventions. Audits conducted as part of an implementation process focus on evidence-based processes. For example: 'Of 50 files audited, what proportion of patients was asked screening questions, as recommended in a clinical guideline?' or 'What proportion of patients received written educational materials, as recommended in a clinical guideline?'

A Cochrane review of 118 trials investigated the effect of clinical audits, with or without feedback.[39] Feedback after an audit does improve practice, but the effects are small to moderate. The primary outcome of interest was practice change where audit and feedback were used as part of an intervention, for example in combination with an educational meeting. Comparison of dichotomous outcome data (for example, practice changed yes/no) resulted in a median-adjusted risk difference in compliance with desired practice of 5% (interquartile range 3% to 11%). That is, the probability of compliance with desired practice following audit and feedback was approximately 5% greater, compared with other interventions or no intervention. For continuous outcomes such as number of tests or prescriptions, the median-adjusted risk percentage change in practice for professionals who received audit and feedback compared with no intervention was 16% (interquartile range 5% to 37%).

Jamtvedt and colleagues[39] did not find a significant difference in the relative effectiveness of audit and feedback, with or without educational meetings or multifaceted interventions. When audit and feedback were used alone (which is rare in clinical practice), the median effect was greater (median-adjusted risk difference of 11.9% for continuous outcomes, interquartile range 5% to 22%) than no intervention. Larger effects were seen if baseline adherence to recommended practice was low and feedback intensity was greater. Audit and feedback should therefore be viewed as a helpful quality-improvement strategy, but caution is required during implementation projects because of the costs associated with data extraction and analysis of audit data. A promising cluster trial is currently underway,[40] exploring how feedback can be used to increase acceptability and usability in primary care. The trial aims to determine whether a theory-informed worksheet attached to feedback reports can help general practitioners improve the quality of care provided to patients with diabetes and/or ischaemic heart disease.

In summary, the effectiveness of several implementation strategies has been evaluated in systematic reviews. Most strategies lead to a small change in practice (typically no greater than 10%). Larger changes can be expected if compliance with practice at baseline is low. Health professionals and service managers who evaluate change due to implementation of evidence should not be surprised by changes of this magnitude. A process of continuous quality improvement is the best way to improve practice in line with the evidence, and discussion about this is included in Chapter 17. For updates on the effectiveness of these and other strategies to change behaviour, the website of the Cochrane Effective Practice and Organisation of Care review group (www.epoc.cochrane.org) is a useful resource.

THE USE OF THEORY TO SUPPORT EVIDENCE IMPLEMENTATION

Implementation of evidence is a complex process involving change in attitudes, systems and behaviour. Theories and frameworks are helpful for explaining complex processes. Thus it is helpful to theorise about why a person, organisation or profession succeeded or had difficulty with change, such as delivering an intervention or ceasing to use a test procedure. Theories can also be used for planning. We can anticipate potential problems, such as a change in professionals' (or patient) roles, and target these in advance.

The use of a theory or theoretical framework is now recommended to help identify and address factors that influence the adoption of a new practice behaviour.[48,49] Change theories can help us predict who might change, who might be resistant to change, how change might be experienced and the stages of change that most people will move through. Theories can also help inform the development of survey instruments[23,50] and interview questions about barriers to evidence uptake.[28] Researchers seeking funding, and postgraduate students investigating the implementation of innovations, are now expected to use theories to guide their research.

Grol and colleagues[49] have proposed a taxonomy of theories which aim to explain or predict: (1) individual behaviour change (for example, attitudes, routines, motivation); (2) the effect of social context on change (for example, social/peer pressure, opinion leaders, role models); and (3) organisational or team behaviour change (for example, culture, systems, resources). The authors note that most theories overlap, sometimes to a large extent. Grol and colleagues summarised each 'type' of theory. *Behaviour theories* aim to explain behaviour. *Cognitive theories* aim to explain thought processes, attitudes and values. *Social theories* aim to explain how social groups or systems operate. Problems can occur at any level. For more in-depth information about this, you may wish to read their summary.[49]

Theories which explain behaviour change

Some theories explain how change is experienced and factors which promote change. Examples include the transtheoretical stages of change theory by Prochaska and DiClemente[51] and the diffusions of innovation theory by Rogers.[52]

The **stages of change theory** has been used to guide many implementation studies, particularly those targeting public health behaviours such as cigarette smoking and alcohol consumption.[51] Individuals at each of the stages (for example pre-contemplation, contemplation, preparation and action) are typically targeted with different behaviour-change strategies. However, a systematic review which examined the body of research on interventions based on the stages of change theory found no difference in outcomes (amount of behaviour change) in studies using this theory, compared with studies that were not based on this theory.[53]

Another use of the stages of change theory has been for the development of an instrument to measure attitudes and readiness to change (Clinician Readiness to Measure Outcomes Scale, CReMOS).[50] The aim of the CReMOS is to measure clinicians' attitudes to outcome measurement and self-reported changes in attitude and practice, as a result of learning about standardised outcome measures. Sample statements from the 26-item CReMOS questionnaire, associated with the five stages of change, include:

- 'I know my interventions work. I do not need to measure them.' *(Precontemplation)*
- 'Measuring outcomes would be good if it did not mean spending time doing extra paperwork.' *(Contemplation)*
- 'I have had someone teach me how to search electronic databases to locate relevant outcome measures for my patients.' *(Preparation)*
- 'I have trialled some outcome measures with my patients.' *(Action)*
- 'I have been measuring outcomes with my patients for at least 6 months.' *(Maintenance)*

The highly influential **theory of diffusion of innovations** has been used to help spread many innovations in health services and has been comprehensively reviewed by Greenhalgh and colleagues.[4,54] Diffusion is a passive process of social influence, whereas dissemination and implementation are active, planned processes that aim to encourage the adoption of an innovation. The original theory proposed that the spread or diffusion of ideas about a new practice could be achieved by harnessing the influence of opinion leaders and change agents. The social networks of targeted individuals could be mapped and targeted during the diffusion process (who knows whom, and who copies whom). Some individuals lead the adoption (innovators), while others become champions and opinion leaders (the early adopters). A large proportion of individuals adopt the change in practice when change becomes inevitable (the early majority) and can be used to encourage and persuade others (the late majority). And finally, there are always non-adopters who will only change when forced to do so by policy or performance review (the laggards).

Studies and organisations which talk about using 'opinion leaders' and 'champions' are using ideas from the diffusions of innovation theory. One such study in occupational therapy[55] involved using a local opinion leader to teach therapists about evidence-based practice when the phenomenon was new and considered an 'innovation'. Funding was obtained to train 100 occupational therapists how to search for, and critically appraise, research evidence. The local opinion leader delivered a two-day workshop and encouraged therapists to become 'champions' of evidence-based practice in their organisation. To help spread the innovation, therapists provided in-service training at work for other staff and established journal clubs.[56]

Theories which predict behaviour change

Theories which can help us to anticipate or predict behaviour change include Ajzen's theory of planned behaviour[57] and a psychological theory of behaviour change developed by Michie and colleagues.[28] When planning to implement evidence, we are often interested in theories which help predict who will, and will not, adopt new practice behaviours. Questions and topics derived from these theories have been used in surveys and interviews, and to map results.

The **Theory of Planned Behaviour**[23,57] is one of the most frequently used theoretical frameworks. This theory proposes that intention and perceived control over behaviour are proximal predictors of behaviour; and while these constructs cannot be directly observed, they can be inferred from survey or questionnaire responses.[23] To predict whether a person intends to do something, we need to know whether that person is in favour of doing it ('attitude'), how much the person feels social pressure to do it ('subjective norm') and whether they feel in control of the action in question ('perceived behavioural control'). The Theory of Planned Behaviour proposes that these three constructs—attitudes, subjective norms and perceived behavioural control—predict the intention to perform a behaviour. Recent systematic reviews have confirmed that there is, indeed, a predictable relationship between the intentions of a health professional and their subsequent behaviour.[58,59] However, the review by Godin and colleagues[59] suggests that the Theory of Planned Behaviour helps predict *behaviour*, while other theories better capture *intentions*. Surveys and questionnaires based on the Theory of Planned Behaviour have been developed and used to investigate attitudes to and beliefs about the uptake of evidence.[23]

The **Psychological Theory of Behaviour Change**[28] is a more recent addition to the list of theories and also aims to help professionals and researchers anticipate and predict behaviour change. Michie and colleagues[28] proposed 12 domains and developed an interview profile which can be used to inform the implementation of evidence, in particular for identifying barriers and strategies to target known barriers. The domains are shown in Table 16.2.

As an example, in the travel mobility study involving occupational therapists and physiotherapists,[10] interview questions probed for therapists' attitudes, skills and knowledge, as well as role expectations about an outdoor journey intervention for people with stroke. The Psychological Theory of Behaviour Change provided a structure during interviews and, later, during analysis. Some brief examples of comments from therapists are presented in Figure 16.2. The majority of comments made during the 13 interviews could be mapped to two domains: beliefs about capabilities and social influences.

- **Beliefs about capabilities:**

    'It's quite a time-consuming intervention, in terms of the number of patients you can see, and the number of hours. I think it would be hard to get to the six [sessions of the outdoor journey intervention].'

    'The whole scooter thing is still something they [occupational therapists] are nervous about. How do we know the person's appropriate for a scooter? How do you assess a person …? and stuff around insurance and all that sort of thing … A lot of therapists don't get much exposure (to motorised scooters). I've never done a scooter prescription.'

    'Asking about driving, when someone is so unwell, can be an area that you don't want to go to. It can be the last thing on their mind, and the carers' mind. "Oh no! He won't get back to driving!" These sort of things could be a bit difficult to initiate in conversation.'

- **Social influence** (from patients and carers):

    'Sometimes they (people with stroke) are completely focused on their mobility, and tend to think of it (an outdoor journey intervention) as more of a physio thing. Maybe they won't bring it up with us (the

TABLE 16.2:
EXAMPLES OF QUESTIONS TO ASK ABOUT BARRIERS TO IMPLEMENTATION BASED ON TWO THEORIES OF BEHAVIOUR CHANGE

Focus/domain of question	Theory of planned behaviour[23]	Psychological theory of behaviour change[28]
Knowledge		Do you know about the evidence/guideline? Do you know you should be doing X?
Skills		Do you know how to deliver X? How easy or difficult do you find performing X? How confident are you about being able to perform X to the required standard in the required context?
Intentions, motivations and goals	Do you intend to do X with all of your patients? Of the next 10 patients you see with a diagnosis of X, for how many would you expect to do X?	How much do you want to do X? How much do you feel a need to do X? Are there other things you want to do or achieve that might interfere with X? Does the evidence/guideline conflict with other interventions you want to deliver? Are there incentives to do X?
Attitudes and emotions	Are there any issues that come to mind when you think about doing X? Overall do you think that doing X is harmful/pleasant; the right thing to do; the wrong thing to do/good practice?	Does doing X evoke an emotional response? To what extent do emotional factors facilitate or hinder X?
Professional/ social roles	Is it expected that you will do X?	Do you think guidelines or evidence should determine your behaviour? Is doing X compatible or in conflict with your professional role/standards/identity? Would this be true for all professional groups involved?
Beliefs about capabilities	Do you believe that you will be able to do X with the patient?	How easy or difficult it is it for you to do X? How confident are you that you can do X in spite of the difficulties? What would help you do X? How capable are you of maintaining X? How well equipped/comfortable do you feel about doing X?
Beliefs about consequences		What do you think will happen (to yourself, patients, colleagues and the organisation, positive and negative, short- and long-term consequences) if you do X? What are the costs of X? What do you think will happen if you do not do X? Do the benefits of doing X outweigh the costs? Does the evidence suggest that doing X is a good thing?
Memory, attention and decision processes		Is X something you usually do? Will you think or remember to do X? How much attention will you have to pay to doing X? Might you decide not to do X? Why?
Environmental context and resources		To what extent do physical or resource factors facilitate or hinder X? Are there competing tasks and time constraints? Are the necessary resources (staff, equipment etc) available to you and others who are expected to do X?

TABLE 16.2:
EXAMPLES OF QUESTIONS TO ASK ABOUT BARRIERS TO IMPLEMENTATION BASED ON TWO THEORIES OF BEHAVIOUR CHANGE—CONT'D

Focus/domain of question	Theory of planned behaviour[23]	Psychological theory of behaviour change[28]
Social influence or pressure	Are there any individuals or groups who would approve or disapprove of you doing X? Do you feel under any social pressure to do X with your patients? Do your patients expect or want X?	To what extent do social influences (for example peers, managers, other professional groups, patients, patients' relatives) facilitate or hinder X? Do you observe others performing X? (that is, do you have role models?)
Behavioural regulation		What preparatory steps (individual or organisational) are needed to do X? Are there procedures or ways of working that encourage you to do X?
Nature of the behaviours		What is the proposed behaviour? Who needs to do what differently, when, where, how, how often and with whom? What do you currently do? Is this a new behaviour, or an existing behaviour that needs to become a habit? Are there systems for maintaining longer-term change?

occupational therapists). Others are more focused on getting their arm to work again. Trying to identify goals different from that can be hard. Usually they've been told "We're referring you for upper limb therapy" and they become very focused on that. They don't want to look at getting out and about.'

'We could only achieve the goals he wanted to (work on) and would agree to.'

'His wife isn't confident that he can do it. She says "No, he won't be able to do it." Last week they had the opportunity to catch the train into the therapy session here, but the wife called the son to tell him to take the day off work to bring him in. So we've planned a visit to the coffee shop that he went to. It means catching a train, getting him to buy the tickets, and so on. It's cognitive as well as language. But his wife isn't confident he can do it ...'

Michie and colleagues[60] have recently added to the behaviour change literature with their 'behaviour change wheel'. The wheel comprises a hub and three essential conditions for change (capability, opportunity and motivation), nine intervention strategies to address deficits in these conditions and seven categories of policy to enable interventions to occur. The authors suggest that the wheel can be used by health services and policy makers to design more effective, targeted interventions.

Francis and colleagues used this theory and interview schedule with intensive-care consultants and neonatologists to determine which domains might prevent or enable behaviour change.[61] The domains relevant to this specialty group were: knowledge, beliefs about capabilities, beliefs about consequences, social influences and behavioural regulation. In another study, doctors' beliefs about consequences and their capabilities were likely determinants of lumbar spine X-ray referrals for patients presenting with low back pain.[62]

In summary, psychological theories can help service providers to predict who might be resistant to change, and why. Barriers and enablers to change can be identified more accurately, including intentions, attitudes, beliefs, skills and knowledge. These domains can then be targeted using evidence-based interventions as suggested in this chapter. There is supporting evidence that strategies which are tailored to these barriers (for example, education to address a knowledge or skills gap) can change practice.[41]

SUMMARY POINTS OF THIS CHAPTER

- Implementation is a planned and active process of using published research in practice. Another term for implementation is knowledge transfer. Both processes aim to help close evidence–practice gaps.

- The process of implementation involves a series of steps which include demonstrating an evidence–practice gap; identifying barriers and enablers to implementation; deciding on the best strategies and interventions to help health professionals learn about, adopt and sustain behaviour change; and then executing and evaluating the implementation plan.

- Surveys and medical record audits are popular methods for identifying an evidence–practice gap. These methods explore and measure attitudes, knowledge and practice behaviours. More than one method should be used to collect data on current practice for a gap analysis from a small but representative sample of health professionals and/or patients, preferably using both qualitative and quantitative methods.

- Common barriers to evidence implementation include: attitudes, beliefs, skills and knowledge of professionals; role expectations (professional and social); influences of other professionals, patients and family members; systems; and policies. Barriers are unique to local teams and organisations and time should be spent identifying local barriers. These can then be targeted with tailored implementation strategies.

- Strategies for implementing evidence in practice include, but are not limited to, educational materials, meetings and outreach visits, external facilitators, local opinion leaders, reminders, and audit and feedback.

- None of these implementation strategies is likely to change practice by more than 10% at any one time. Behaviours with low baseline compliance are likely to change the most.

- Surveys and questionnaires, as well as focus groups and interviews, should be informed by theoretical constructs from behaviour, cognitive or social theories. This means that questions should ask about intentions, beliefs, attitudes, values, expectations, social systems and networks.

References

1. Grol R. Implementation of changes in practice. In: Grol R, Wensing M, Eccles M, editors. Improving patient care: the implementation of change in clinical practice. Edinburgh: Elsevier Butterworth–Heinemann; 2005. pp. 6–15.
2. van Bokhoven M, Kok G, Weijden V. Designing a quality improvement intervention: a systematic approach. Qual Saf Health Care 2003;12:215–20.
3. Grol R, Wensing M. Effective implementation: a model. In: Grol R, Wensing M, Eccles M, editors. Improving patient care: the implementation of change in clinical practice. Edinburgh: Elsevier Butterworth–Heinemann; 2005. pp. 41–57.
4. Greenhalgh T, Robert G, Bate P, et al. Diffusions of innovations in health service organisations: a systematic review. Oxford, UK: BMJ Books; 2005.
5. Woolf S. The meaning of translational research and why it matters. JAMA 2008;299:211–13.
6. Davis D, Evans M, Jadad A, et al. The case for knowledge translation: shortening the journey from evidence to effect. BMJ 2003;327:33–5.
7. McKenzie J, French S, O'Connor D, et al. IMPLEmenting a clinical practice guideline for acute low back pain evidence-based manageMENT in general practice (IMPLEMENT): Cluster randomised controlled trial study protocol. Implement Sci 2008;3:11.
8. Kramer T, Burns B. Implementing cognitive behavioural therapy in the real world: a case study of two mental health centres. Implement Sci 2008;3:14.
9. McCluskey A, Middleton S. Feasibility of implementing an outdoor journey intervention to people with stroke: a feasibility study involving five community rehabilitation teams. Implement Sci 2010;5:59.

10. McCluskey A, Middleton S. Delivering an evidence-based outdoor journey intervention to people with stroke: barriers and enablers experienced by community rehabilitation teams. BMC Health Serv Res 2010;10:18.

11. Britt H, Miller G, Charles J, et al. General practice activity in Australia 2009–10. General Practice Series No 27. AIHW Cat No GEP 27. Canberra: Australian Institute of Health and Welfare; 2010.

12. National Health and Medical Research Council and Australian Acute Musculoskeletal Pain Guidelines Group. Evidence-based management of acute musculoskeletal pain: a guide for clinicians. Bowen Hills, Qld: Australian Academic Press; 2004.

13. Williams C, Maher C, Hancock M, et al. Low back pain and best practice care: a survey of general practice physicians. Arch Int Med 2010;170:271–7.

14. Klein J, Jacobs R, Reinecke M. Cognitive-behavioural therapy for adolescent depression: a meta-analytic investigation of changes in effect-size estimates. J Am Acad Child Adoles Psychiatry 2007;46:1403–13.

15. Weersing V, Weisz J. Community clinic treatment of depressed youth: benchmarking usual care against CBT clinical trials. J Consult Clin Psychol 2002;70:299–310.

16. Chua M, McCluskey A, Smead J. Retrospective analysis of factors that affect driving assessment outcomes after stroke. Aust J Occ Ther 2012;59:121–30.

17. Fisk G, Owsley C, Pulley L. Driving after stroke: driving exposure, advice and evaluations. Arch Phys Med Rehabil 1997;78:1338–45.

18. Mackintosh S, Goldie P, Hill K. Falls incidence and factors associated with falling in older, community-dwelling, chronic stroke survivors (>1 year after stroke) and matched controls. Aging Clin Exp Res 2005;17:74–81.

19. National Stroke Foundation. Clinical guidelines for stroke management. Melbourne: National Stroke Foundation; 2010.

20. Logan P, Gladman J, Avery A, et al. Randomised controlled trial of an occupational therapy intervention to increase outdoor mobility after stroke. BMJ 2004;329:1372–7.

21. Logan P, Walker M, Gladman, J. Description of an occupational therapy intervention aimed at improving outdoor mobility. Br J Occup Ther 2006;69:2–6.

22. Glasziou P, Haynes B. The paths from research to improved health outcomes. ACP J Club 2005;142:A8–9.

23. Francis J, Eccles M, Johnstone M, et al. Constructing questionnaires based on the theory of planned behaviour: a manual for health services researchers. Newcastle upon Tyne, UK: Centre for Health Services Research, University of Newcastle; 2004. Online. Available: pages.bangor.ac.uk/~pes004/exercise_psych/downloads/tpb_manual.pdf; 23 Nov 2012.

24. National Institute of Clinical Studies (NICS). Evidence–practice gaps report (volumes 1 and 2). Melbourne: NICS; 2005.

25. National Institute of Clinical Studies (NICS). Evidence–practice gaps report, volume 1: a review of developments 2004–7. Melbourne: NICS; 2008.

26. National Institute for Health and Clinical Excellence (NICE). How to change practice: understand, identify and overcome barriers to change. London: NICE; 2007. Online. Available: www.nice.org.uk/usingguidance/implementationtools/howtoguide/barrierstochange.jsp; 14 Nov 2012.

27. National Institute of Clinical Studies (NICS). Identifying barriers to evidence uptake. Melbourne: NICS; 2006. Online. Available: www.nhmrc.gov.au/nics/materials-and-resources/identifying-barriers-evidence-uptake; 14 Nov 2012.

28. Michie S, Johnston M, Abraham C, et al. Making psychological theory useful for implementing evidence based practice: a consensus approach. Qual Saf Health Care 2005;14:26–33.

29. Verbeek J, Sengers M, Riemens L, et al. Patient expectations of treatment for back pain: a systematic review of qualitative and quantitative studies. Spine 2004;29:2309–18.

30. Schers H, Wensing M, Huijsmans Z, et al. Implementation barriers for general practice guidelines on low back pain: a qualitative study. Spine 2001;26:E348–53.

31. Farmer A, Legare F, Turcot K, et al. Printed educational materials: effects on professional practice and health care outcomes. Cochrane Database Syst Rev 2008;(3):CD004398. doi: 10.1002/14651858.CD004398.pub2.

32. Grimshaw J, Eccles M, Thomas R, et al. Toward evidence-based quality improvement: evidence (and its limitations) of the effectiveness of guideline dissemination and implementation strategies 1966–1998. J Gen Intern Med 2006;21:S14–20.

33. Forsetlund L, Bjorndal A, Rashidian A, et al. Continuing education meetings and workshops: effects on professional practice and health care outcomes. Cochrane Database Syst Rev 2009;(2):CD003030. doi: 10.1002/14651858.CD003030.pub2.

34. Zwarenstein M, Bheekie A, Lombard C, et al. Educational outreach to general practitioners reduces children's asthma symptoms: a cluster randomised controlled trial. Implement Sci 2007;2:30.

35. O'Brien M, Rogers S, Jamtvedt G, et al. Educational outreach visits: effects on professional practice and health care outcomes. Cochrane Database Syst Rev 2007;(4):CD000409. doi: 10.1002/14651858.CD000409.pub2.

36. Stetler C, Legro M, Rycroft-Malone J, et al. Role of 'external facilitation' in implementation of research findings: a qualitative evaluation of facilitation experiences in the Veterans Health Administration. Implement Sci 2006;1:23.

37. Foy R, Eccles M, Hrisos S, et al. A cluster randomised trial of educational messages to improve the primary care of diabetes. Implement Sci 2011;6:129.

38. Shojania KG, Jennings A, Mayhew A, et al. The effects of on-screen, point of care computer reminders on processes and outcomes of care. Cochrane Database Syst Rev 2009;(3):CD001096. doi: 10.1002/14651858.CD001096.pub2.

39. Jamtvedt G, Young J, Kristoffersen D, et al. Audit and feedback: effects on professional practice and health care outcomes. Cochrane Database Syst Rev 2010;(2):CD000259. doi: 10.1002/14651858.CD000259.pub2.

40. Ivers NM, Tu K, Francis J, et al. Feedback GAP: study protocol for a cluster-randomised trial of goal setting and action plans to increase the effectiveness of audit and feedback interventions in primary care. Implement Sci 2010;41:5, 98.

41. Baker R, Camosso-Stefinovic J, Gillies C. et al. Tailored interventions to overcome identified barriers to change: effects on professional practice and health care outcomes. Cochrane Database Syst Rev 2010;(3):CD005470. doi: 10.1002/14651858.CD005470.pub2.

42. Wright J, Bibby J, Eastham J, et al. Multifaceted implementation of stroke prevention guidelines in primary care: cluster-randomised evaluation of clinical and cost effectiveness. Qual Saf Health Care 2007;16:51–9.

43. Bero L, Grilli R, Grimshaw J, et al. Closing the gap between research and practice: an overview of systematic reviews of interventions to promote the implementation of research findings. BMJ 1998;317:465–8.

44. Grimshaw J, Shirran L, Thomas R, et al. Changing provider behavior: an overview of systematic reviews of interventions. Med Care 2001;39:II2–45.

45. Dijkstra R, Braspenning J, Huijsmans Z, et al. Introduction of diabetes passports involving both patients and professionals to improve hospital outpatient diabetes care. Diabetes Res Clin Pract 2005;68:126–34.

46. Dijkstra R, Braspenning J, Grol R. Implementing diabetes passports to focus practice reorganisation on improving diabetes care. Int J Qual Health Care 2008;20:72–7.

47. Adams A. Evidence of self-report bias in assessing adherence to guidelines. Int J Qual Health Care 1999;11:187–92.

48. Ceccato N, Ferris L, Manuel D, et al. Adopting health behaviour change theory through the clinical practice guideline process. J Contin Educ Health Prof 2007;27:201–7.

49. Grol R, Wensing M, Hulscher M, et al. Theories of implementation of change in healthcare. In: Grol R, Wensing M, Eccles M, editors. Improving patient care: the implementation of change in clinical practice. Edinburgh: Elsevier Butterworth–Heinemann; 2005. pp. 15–40.

50. Bowman J, Lannin N, Cook C, et al. Development and psychometric testing of the Clinician Readiness for Measuring Outcomes Scale (CReMOS). J Eval Clin Pract 2009;15:76–84.

51. Prochaska J, DiClemente C. In search of how people change: applications to addictive behaviours. Am Psychol 1992;47:1102–14.

52. Rogers EM. Diffusion of innovations. 4th ed. New York: Free Press; 1995.

53. Reisma R, Pattenden J, Bridle C, et al. A systematic review of the effectiveness of interventions based on a stages of change approach to promote individual behaviour change. Health Technol Assess 2002;6:1–243.

54. Greenhalgh T, Robert G, Macfarlane F, et al. Diffusion of innovations in service organisations: systematic review and recommendations. Milbank Q 2004;82:581–629.

55. McCluskey A, Lovarini M. Providing education on evidence-based practice improved knowledge but did not change behaviour: a before and after study. BMC Med Educ 2005;5:40.

56. McCluskey A, Home S, Thompson L. Becoming an evidence-based practitioner. In: Law M, MacDermid J, editors. Evidence-based rehabilitation: a guide to practice. 2nd ed. Thorofare, NJ: Slack; 2008. pp. 35–60.

57. Ajzen I. The theory of planned behaviour. Organ Behav Hum Decis Process 1991;50:179–211.

58. Eccles M, Hrisos S, Francis J, et al. Do self-reported intentions predict clinicians' behaviour: a systematic review. Implement Sci 2006;1:28.

59. Godin G, Belanger-Gravel A, Eccles M, et al. Healthcare professionals' intentions and behaviours: a systematic review of studies based on social cognitive theories. Implement Sci 2008;3:36.

60. Michie S, van Stralen M, West R. The behaviour change wheel: a new method for characterising and designing behavior change interventions. Implement Sci 2011;6:42.

61. Francis J, Stockton C, Eccles M, et al. Evidence-based selection of theories for designing behaviour change interventions: using methods based on theoretical construct domains to understand clinicians' blood transfusion behaviour. Br J Health Psychol 2009;14:625–46.

62. Grimshaw J, Eccles M, Steen N, et al. Applying psychological theories to evidence-based clinical practice: identifying factors predictive of lumbar spine x-ray for low back pain in UK primary care practice. Implement Sci 2011;6:55.

Chapter 17

Embedding evidence-based practice into routine clinical care

Ian Scott, Chris Del Mar, Tammy Hoffmann and Sally Bennett

LEARNING OBJECTIVES

After reading this chapter, you should be able to:

- Understand that evidence-based practice occurs at micro, meso and macro levels of organisations
- Explain why organisations should promote evidence-based practice
- Describe the characteristics of organisations which integrate evidence-based practice
- Describe specific strategies that organisations might use to support evidence-based practice

Evidence-based practice can be conceptualised as operating at three organisational levels:

- *microsystems* of clinical departments, units, wards or clinical practices
- *mesosystems* such as hospitals and large group-practices
- *macrosystems* of health departments, general practice governing organisations, professional societies and clinical service networks.

Microsystems can be regarded as first-order units of practice in which health professionals, either as individuals or as tightly connected small groups, directly confront challenges in integrating evidence into the routine care of individual patients. This can occur at the bedside, clinic, community and through regular interactions with nearby colleagues. Until this chapter, this book has primarily focused on the skills required to undertake evidence-based practice at this level and described the use of the five-step process for evidence-based practice.

Barriers to evidence-based practice at the microsystem level have been explored in many studies, across many settings and many professional groups, and in various countries (see for example references 1–5). There is remarkable consistency in the major barriers that have been identified, and some of these are summarised in Table 17.1.

But health professionals, as either individuals or small groups, do not work in a vacuum. They operate within the **mesosystems** of large organisations. These, in turn, are influenced by external forces which come from the **macrosystems** level of government and professional governance bodies which define healthcare policies, standards and norms of practice. All three levels are interdependent and this is reflected in the evolution of our understanding of, and approach towards, translating evidence into practice over the last 20 years or so.[6]

The complexity and interrelatedness of these three levels was acknowledged in the previous chapter (Chapter 16), where we examined strategies which could be used to more consistently incorporate evidence into practice (either to accelerate the adoption of evidence-based practices or to discontinue interventions or assessment practices that are not supported by appropriate evidence). We overviewed strategies that can be used to narrow the gaps between current practice and practice that is based on the most rigorous evidence available, and also highlighted the influences and involvements of individuals, organisations and systems to achieve this aim.

Similarly, successfully using the steps of evidence-based practice in routine clinical work (as opposed to translating specific research evidence into practice, as discussed in Chapter 16) is not solely a function

TABLE 17.1: COMMONLY IDENTIFIED BARRIERS TO EMBEDDING EVIDENCE-BASED PRACTICE INTO ROUTINE CLINICAL PRACTICE	
Barrier	**Description**
Skills	A lack of skills in searching for, interpreting and applying research among health professionals means that they are insecure about changing practice from what they have read. There is also often too little support for doing so (including from senior colleagues with skills in evidence-based practice).
Time	In the chaos of everyday clinical practice, 'running behind', or dealing with urgent clinical situations, is common. The time pressure of administration and other responsibilities that health professionals have, coupled with the time taken for finding, let alone reading and appraising, the evidence, means that evidence-based practice is all too easily a casualty of being busy.
Attitudes	The traditional view of knowledge attainment (and thus, by extension, evidence-based practice) is that it is *separate* from clinical practice. That is, it is the responsibility of the individual health professional and, often, to be undertaken at the health professional's own expense and time. These attitudes may be held by both health professionals and the organisations where they work.

of behaviour or responsibility of individual health professionals. It also requires enablers and reinforcers which operate throughout different levels of the system of care in which health professionals work. There are enablers and reinforcers for each of the three major types of barriers to evidence-based practice listed in Table 17.1 (that is, skills, time and attitudes). The prime focus of this chapter is the organisational settings (or systems of care) that determine the extent to which evidence-based practice becomes more (much more for some) an *everyday* part of the clinical work that is done at the level of individuals and small groups.

WHY IS A SYSTEMS APPROACH IMPORTANT?

A systems approach examines what can be done at the organisational level to foster evidence-based practice as a core component of organisational activity. What can we do to make evidence-based practice part of the mission statement or *modus operandi*, or even the 'brand', of an organisation? How do we systematise the strategies for improving translation of evidence into practice (that were discussed at the health professional level in Chapter 16) at the level of the organisation?

The premise is that if organisations endorse evidence-based practice as 'the way we do things around here', then their policies, procedures, infrastructure and governance are more likely to support evidence-based practice. This then makes it easier for the individuals within the organisation to practise this way. Organisations need structures, processes and cultures that can accommodate the complexity of implementing evidence-based practice in daily operations.

WHY SHOULD ORGANISATIONS *WANT* TO PROMOTE EVIDENCE-BASED PRACTICE?

1. Maintaining reputation and 'market share'

Organisations—not just the individual health professionals who work within them—are now held more accountable for ensuring that the care they provide is safe, effective and of high quality. It is no longer the sole responsibility of individual health professionals to provide good care: the organisation itself can now suffer loss of reputation, staff and revenue if it is not seen as proactively nurturing evidence-based practice. Moreover, organisations do not operate in isolation, but instead in a constantly changing environment of new healthcare and information technologies, novel multidisciplinary models of care and changing societal expectations. All this necessitates clinical practice to be constantly informed (and re-informed) by good evidence if the organisation is to retain respect and authority within the community at large. Organisations also need to do this if they want to entice increasingly sophisticated and demanding recipients of care to pass through their doors.

2. Innovation is associated with better delivery of care

Organisations which foster evidence-based practice are more likely to be innovative, challenge orthodox practice and be ready to adopt new safety and quality initiatives that benefit patients. They are also more exciting and professionally satisfying to work in. A large-scale empirical study among the entire population of public hospital organisations ($n = 173$) that are part of the English National Health Service revealed a significant positive relationship between science- and practice-based innovation and clinical performance.[7] Other studies have revealed an association between evidence-based practice support systems and improved patient safety, reduced complications and shorter length of stay among Medicare beneficiaries in acute care hospitals in the United States.[8] An organisation's receptivity to, and readiness for, change are key determinants to how quickly and successfully new innovations in practice are adopted.[9] This is illustrated in Figure 17.1. Importantly, theories around organisational change readiness and implementation emphasise that change is both a social and a technical innovation. That is, whether change occurs or not depends just as much on group psychology and mindsets, internal and external

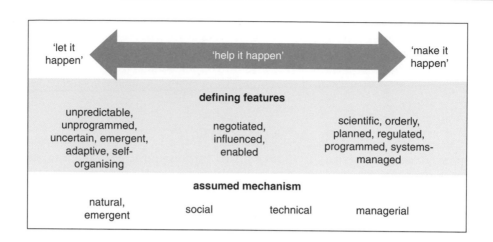

Figure 17.1
The spread of innovation in an organisation: its defining features and assumed mechanism.

Adapted from Greenhalgh T, et al. Diffusion of innovations in service organizations: systematic review and recommendations. Milbank Quarterly 2004; Fig 2.[9] Copyright 2004 Milbank Memorial Fund. Published by Blackwell Publishing; reproduced with permission.

socio-political influences, peer pressures and cultural attitudes as it does on implementing data systems or reconfiguring equipment and service resources.

3. Efficiency

In an era of limited resources but expanding demand for health care, organisations must learn to do more with less. This means they must discontinue—and disinvest from—clinical practices which consume resources but do not add value to patient care. Various ways of doing this have been proposed, including:

- eliminating waste—for example, stopping waste such as duplicated tests as well as unnecessary tests, procedures and treatments that confer no health benefit.[10] It has been estimated that this may account for as much as 30% of healthcare costs;[11,12]

- reducing diagnostic and treatment variation among health professionals and between communities; and

- reforming medical liability laws to decrease the practice of defensive medicine.

Many of these approaches (for example, reducing overuse, avoiding preventable complications and improving inefficient processes) are under way in many organisations, in both private and public sectors.[13] Greater alignment of clinical practice with evidence-based practice could result in significant savings in healthcare expenditure[14] or, at the very least, better value care for the monies spent.

CULTURE AND CHARACTERISTICS OF ORGANISATIONS WHICH INTEGRATE EVIDENCE-BASED PRACTICE

Introducing any innovation, including evidence-based practice, is challenging and occurs within a complex organisational context. The culture of an organisation influences attitudes towards the use of evidence-based practice and the change process itself.[15] An organisation's culture refers to the norms and expectations about how things are done in an organisation[16] or, more simply: 'how things are done around here'. An organisation's culture can affect staff attitudes, perceptions and behaviour.[15] Therefore, fostering a culture which is constructive and supportive of evidence-based practice is a key enabler of evidence-based practice. Some of the key characteristics of organisations that support the use of evidence-based practice are outlined below.

1. Active senior leadership commitment and support for evidence-based practice

Organisationally-driven evidence-based practice is more likely when senior leaders (such as clinical directors and managerial executives) promote change and foster a learning environment.[17,18] Leadership styles that positively influence the use of evidence-based practice have been described as transactional and/or transformative.[19] Transformative leadership supposes a strong attachment between the leader and their 'followers', such that the leader is then able to inspire and motivate others through role-modelling and mentoring.[20] Role models are very powerful change agents in the behaviour of health professionals. If senior health professionals perform evidence-based practice as part of routine care themselves, this is an important influence on other staff. For this reason alone, organisations should expect competence in evidence-based practice in their senior staff when offering appointments. Competency in this should be evaluated when undertaking professional performance reviews (perhaps based on documented evidence-based audits of clinical practice and 360° feedback from working colleagues). By spending their own time and effort on activities that directly support evidence-based continuous improvement and quality of care, senior leaders demonstrate the personal commitment and investment needed for sustained improvement.[17]

Transactional leadership makes use of rewards for meeting specific goals or performance criteria.[21] Examples of transactional leadership strategies that foster evidence-based practice include: performance appraisals for reviewing staff members' goals and learning needs *for evidence-based practice*; rostering time; providing remuneration; and organising physical resources (meeting rooms, audio-visual equipment, data systems, etc) which encourage staff to undertake a myriad of activities that foster evidence-based practice. Examples of these are journal clubs, practice reviews, bedside teaching, seminars and workshops, clinical audits and quality and safety improvement projects. Leaders may also create opportunities to communicate successes and failures and reward those who have championed evidence-based practice. Examples of rewards include: academic or peer commendations, sponsorship of presentations at professional meetings, awarding credits for maintenance of professional standard programs or continuing professional development schemes[20] and providing further training and leadership opportunities.[22]

2. Infrastructure of clinical informatics

For evidence-based practice to work, health professionals need ready access to three forms of data:

A. evidence in response to specific clinical questions posed during the course of doing routine clinical work;

B. guidelines and other forms of evidence guidance (for example clinical decision support systems) which can inform commonly performed clinical decisions; and

C. metrics of current practice for the purposes of conducting audits and identifying evidence–practice gaps—that is, the gaps between current practice (what we are doing) and best practice as defined by best available evidence (what we should be doing).

A. Access to evidence to answer specific questions

It is essential that organisations provide access to the relevant electronic literature databases for searching. This is normally provided through an organisation's library. In the community or smaller organisations, library services can be more of a problem. Obtaining full-text papers may have to rely on professional organisations (colleges, societies, associations or academies). Nevertheless, off-site access to free databases is becoming more easily achieved (see Chapter 3).

Health and medical librarians (now increasingly called 'clinical informationists') are important in helping to seek out the evidence that is requested by health professionals. Information requests (in the form of clinical questions) received from health professionals are reformatted into 'answerable questions', evidence is searched for, critically appraised (sometimes) and then returned to the health professional. Health professionals can then decide how to apply the evidence in the clinical setting from which the questions originated. In some cases, clinical informationists actually attend ward rounds and clinics, recording questions as they arise and then finding relevant evidence. Experiments featuring standardised literature searches and feedback of results to practising health professionals have changed practice for the better.[23] These services, in one form or another, exist in many organisations and target not only health professionals but also managers and policy-makers.[24]

Several services have been established, some more successful than others. One of the most enduring is the ATTRACT service (www.attract.wales.nhs.uk), which runs in Wales, UK.[25] It has become embedded into the routine of many health professionals in the country, and the database of questions asked, and their answers, have themselves become a valuable resource—the TRIP database (www.tripdatabase.com), which was explained in Chapter 3. Question-answering services have been trialled in other countries, such as Australia and Canada.[26,27] However, these services come at a cost and although they are probably cost-effective in terms of cost-savings resulting from better care,[28] budgetary constraints probably act as a barrier to their wholesale introduction. They can also fail from poor demand, possibly because the culture of asking questions (itself an evidence-based practice skill, as discussed in Chapter 2) is underdeveloped in many organisations.

B. Access to clinical decision support systems

Such systems, especially if computerised, have great potential to assist evidence-based practice. If they are well designed and field-tested with health professional input,[29] they can significantly improve quality of care and patient outcomes. The information devices which underpin clinical decision support systems are moving away from fixed desktop computers to more-portable and -personal digital devices such as notebooks, tablets and smart-phones. This technology now allows instant availability of evidence search engines, evidence-based clinical guidelines and pathways and clinical prediction rules. Research is starting to show benefits in terms of better and more-timely care.[30,31] This technology places the individual health professional firmly in the driver's seat for accessing and applying evidence to patient care.

However, organisations must commit to resourcing and maintaining the physical devices (such as repairing and renewing them) and the quality of the content found on them (such as ensuring that evidence resources are valid and up-to-date), and ensuring a proficient skill level of those who use them (such as by mandating ongoing health professional training and assessment). It has been shown that when given access to online information sources, health professionals from different disciplines are able to find correct answers to at least half of their clinical questions.[32]

C. Access to databases for auditing current practice

In most healthcare facilities, data are collected routinely for non-clinical purposes (often financial reasons!). In hospitals, different clinical units centralise collection of discrete data that reflect the single focus of the clinical activity (for example, postoperative wound infections). In contrast, in community clinical settings, data are usually routinely collected only for individual patients. This presents challenges to getting aggregate data on outcomes. Aggregating data can also be complicated (for example, by ethical issues) by the use of electronic patient-held records which are being introduced in some settings (www.ehealthinfo.gov.au). In addition, community health settings usually deal with a far greater range of clinical problems (because there is less specialisation in community-based care). This means there are many more *categories* of care, with fewer *components* in each category. Both of these elements combine to mean that if data are needed to identify evidence–practice gaps, or to decide about the adoption of a change in practice based on new evidence, then the data may have to be collected as an independent effort rather than using data that is routinely collected for other purposes. However, in the near future, electronic health records, which are already extensively employed in many primary care settings, may offer the ability to quickly extract de-identified clinical data that examines routine care with reference to evidence-based standards.

3. Provision of training

Organisations must provide the necessary education and training to enable all health professionals to have skills in evidence-based practice. A systematic review of interactive teaching of evidence-based practice around clinical cases (that is, clinically integrated with everyday work) found that this style of teaching changes knowledge and skills much more effectively than didactic lectures or tutorials.[33] Focused teaching in evidence-based practice (and access to electronic searching facilities) has been shown to improve the quality of care and the number of evidence-based interventions used by health professionals.[34] When considering which educational format to use for learning about evidence-based practice, small-group interaction, role-play and simulation of real-world learning environments, mentorship, and high educator to learner ratios have been found to be associated with more-effective learning.[35,36] In addition to the general evidence-based practice skills, health professionals also need to learn skills in decision making (that is, placing the evidence in perspective against the circumstances and needs of the patient)[37] and skills in communicating evidence to patients (which were described in Chapter 14).

Organisations need to maximise evidence-based practice learning opportunities. Some suggestions for ways of doing this are by:

- quarantining a little 'offline' time, away from clinical duties (perhaps weekly);
- expecting health professionals to attend courses/workshops to learn evidence-based practice skills; and
- supporting *evidence-based* journal clubs.

Evidence-based journal clubs (as opposed to the traditional, and more common, journal club which is typically *not* evidence-based) are especially important. They focus on 'pull' strategies (see Chapter 2), in which health professionals bring along questions that have arisen during routine clinical work, search for the answers in the form of evidence and critically appraise the evidence. Such exercises require support from the organisation if they are to work well. Some examples of the support needed are outlined in Table 17.2.

4. Using evidence-based practice to improve quality and safety

Evidence-based practice and the new science of quality and safety improvement (QSI) complement each other. New evidence will drive new QSI initiatives. Conversely, QSI aspirations will need best available evidence. How you decide what changes to make takes you to the growing literature around evidence-based QSI interventions itself. One approach to QSI is predicated on the use of evidence, as shown in Figure 17.2.[39]

The focus of evidence-based practice is on 'doing the right things', whereas quality improvement focuses more on 'doing things right'. Combined, these processes help us to 'do the right things right'.[40] The implication is that those who work in quality-improvement teams need to consider the validity, applicability and value of the change being introduced, and those who work from an evidence-based practice perspective need to look beyond the evidence to consider how change might be introduced in the local context.

In recent times, several developments have consolidated the linking of evidence-based practice with QSI:

TABLE 17.2:
ORGANISATIONAL SUPPORT REQUIRED FOR RUNNING EVIDENCE-BASED JOURNAL CLUBS

Type of support	Details
Roster journal clubs	Minimise appointment conflicts so that as many members of the ward/team/practice as possible can attend. Enable 'pairing up' of more- and less-experienced appraisers for support and training. Periodically allow time for club members to prioritise topics/questions to be answered over the coming meetings (and advertise this 'schedule' in advance if possible).
Pragmatic resources	A (booked!) room. Data-projector, whiteboard or large flip-chart (so everyone can see). Online access to databases (such as PubMed). Sandwiches or other bring-your-own meal (to save time).
Organisation of the actual meeting	Ensure all members of the club get the chance to be involved in different roles. Consider all of the roles that are involved, such as: • managing the group process (such as who will lead the club process, each topic/article, etc) • recording the discussion (writing on a whiteboard, for example) • storing and disseminating the 'findings' of the meeting • doing 'homework' for any tasks (like getting full-text articles) before the next meeting At the beginning of each meeting (or every alternate meeting), consider allowing time for discussion about 'what now'. That is, discuss what to do with the topic/question just covered and, if needed, devise a plan to implement desired changes in practice.[38] Also consider scheduling a 'follow-up' session for each topic/question some time later (such as 6 months after the topic was initially discussed) to see what changes were made, how they are working, any refinements/further action needed, etc.
Share knowledge and experience	Librarians—if available—can provide enormous help with searching. Student health professionals can be included to experience the role-modelling (and often can be great contributors, particularly if their evidence-based practice knowledge is fresh from a recent course/subject!).
Record notes	Provide a means for storing and disseminating the 'findings' of the club, so that others learn from the exercise and a sense of continuity is established, aided by a record of why clinical changes were considered desirable. Discuss ways to disseminate any practice-changing findings.

A. **Clinical registries:** registries which collect and analyse process and outcome data on large cohorts of patients from multiple hospitals and practices have grown in number in recent years[41] and provide an objective, audit-based window into real-world clinical practice and its possible shortcomings. Organisations which participate in such registries demonstrate evidence-based practice in action and are associated with higher-quality care. Registries can also generate new knowledge about effectiveness of care in unselected patients that may not be obvious in the results of randomised trials that seek to determine efficacy in highly selected populations.

B. **Quality improvement collaborations:** hospitals and other healthcare organisations can share data and experiences about care for specific patient populations and learn from each other about how to improve care and close evidence–practice gaps. Such collaborations can achieve substantial improvement in evidence-based care processes within relatively short time spans at relatively low cost.[42–44]

C. **Health service accreditation:** this is increasingly looking not just at structures (such as buildings, staffing levels, physical infrastructure) but also at outcomes (quality of care). Accreditation teams now expect healthcare organisations to integrate an evidence-based quality improvement framework into their operations with proactive remediation of identified instances of suboptimal care. To date, particular attention has been given to the care of common presentations which are associated with high morbidity or high resource utilisation.

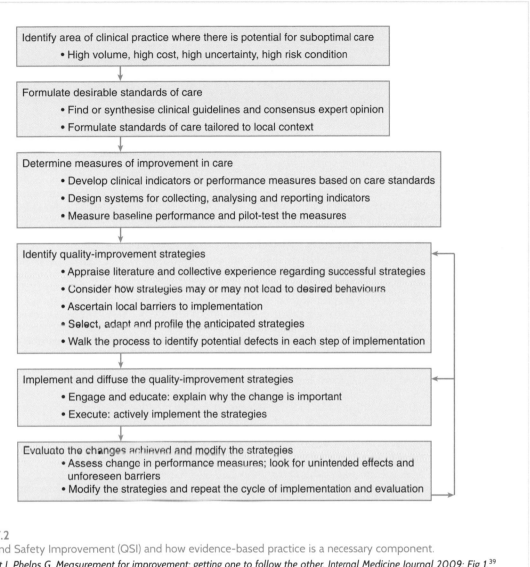

Figure 17.2
Quality and Safety Improvement (QSI) and how evidence-based practice is a necessary component.
From Scott I, Phelps G. Measurement for improvement: getting one to follow the other. Internal Medicine Journal 2009; Fig 1.[39]
© 2009 Royal Australasian College of Physicians; reproduced with permission.

There is also a Cochrane group ('The Cochrane Effective Practice and Organisation of Care Group; epoc. cochrane.org) which reports on what QSI interventions are effective.

5. Changing clinical processes

Finding and doing better ways to do things is dependent on the ability to change. The success and the speed of adoption of evidence-based practice are related. Successful adoption of evidence-based practice in an organisation requires an organisational ethos and governance structure which are committed to the ongoing redesign of clinical care processes in response to new evidence about patient need and the effectiveness of interventions. Importantly, clinical process redesign, if it is to be successful and sustained, has to be driven and owned internally by the members of the organisation, not imposed or led by

BOX 17.1

Examples of large-scale clinical process redesign

VETERANS AFFAIRS HEALTHCARE SYSTEM

The Veterans Affairs healthcare system in the USA underwent major transformation during the late 1990s and early 2000s.[48] This included implementation of a systematic approach to measuring, managing and accounting for quality improvement. The focus was on high-priority conditions (such as diabetes and coronary artery disease), and emphasised health maintenance and management of care. Performance contracts held managers accountable for meeting improvement goals. An integrated and comprehensive electronic medical record system was instituted at all Veterans Affairs medical centres. This enabled performance data to be made public, and key stakeholders such as veterans' service organisations and politicians were targeted. Payment policies for care delivery were aligned according to evidence of effectiveness. Health services, including ambulatory care, were integrated to achieve continuous and timely care. The widespread adoption of evidence-based practice was one of the central tenets of the new system of care.[49] Quality of care in the Veterans Affairs healthcare system substantially improved between 1997 and 2000, when the proportion of patients who received appropriate care was 90% or greater for 9 of 17 quality-of-care indicators, and exceeded 70% for 13. Compared against the Medicare fee-for-service program, the Veterans Affairs system performed significantly better on all 11 comparable quality indicators from 1997 to 1999, and in 2000 the Veterans Affairs system outperformed Medicare on 12 of 13 indicators.[50]

KAISER PERMANENTE HEALTH MAINTENANCE ORGANISATION (USA)

A performance-improvement system was introduced in 2006, after variations in performance in quality, safety, service and efficiency in the organisation were recognised. This led to a strategy for continuous improvement systems: six 'building blocks' were identified to enable Kaiser Permanente to become a learning organisation: (1) real-time sharing of performance data; (2) training in problem-solving methods and adoption of evidence-based practice; (3) workforce engagement and informal knowledge sharing; (4) investing in leadership structures, beliefs and behaviours; (5) internal and external benchmarking; and (6) technical knowledge sharing. This required multiple complex strategies which combined top-down and bottom-up approaches.[51] Performance improvements were assessed in the 22 medical centres (in four of the eight regions) after implementation between January 2008 and September 2009. They achieved a 61% improvement in selected capabilities and 84% of initial projects were successfully completed.[52] This was a cost saving—for each dollar invested in this, there was an estimated return of $2.36 surplus. Critical factors included: adequate dedicated time for performance improvement activities for staff, expert support, alignment of projects with regional and national strategic priorities, and a close working relationship between performance improvement staff and those who provide clinical care.

INTERMOUNTAIN HEALTHCARE (USA)

This is a conglomerate of hospitals and primary care organisations in Utah, USA. A process management theory (W Edwards Deming's theory; which says that the best way to reduce costs is to improve quality) was applied after 1988 to its healthcare delivery.[53] Data systems and management structures were created to increase accountability, drive improvement and produce savings. All participants (patients, providers and systems) were involved, especially health professionals. They were intimately involved in planning, implementing, analysing and educating others in evidence-based practice, assessing and refining guidelines and in reassessing and continually modifying the care map. This redesign has been very successful. For example, a new delivery protocol helped to reduce rates of elective induced labour, unplanned Caesarean sections and admissions to newborn intensive care units. Implementation of this one protocol alone saves an estimated $US50m every year.

GROUP HEALTH COOPERATIVE OF PUGET SOUND (USA)

The Chronic Care Model was developed initially across a large health maintenance organisation as a way of improving the ambulatory care of patients with chronic disease: better disease control, higher patient satisfaction and better adherence to guidelines.[54] Redesign processes cluster in six areas: (1) healthcare organisation; (2) community resources; (3) self-management support; (4) delivery-system design; (5) evidence-based decision support; and (6) clinical information systems. The model stresses continuous relationships with the care team (which is very relevant to chronic care); individualising care according to patients' needs and values; providing care that anticipates patients' needs; providing services which are based on evidence; and cooperation among health professionals. Assessment of the model's processes shows that 51 organisations were able to effect 48 practice changes relating to evidence-based processes of care, and that in 75% of cases these changes were sustained for at least 12 months.[55] This assessment suggests that this redesign process has led to improved patient care and better health outcomes, although this assessment is only preliminary and cost–effectiveness work has not yet been undertaken.

external agencies.[45] What should change is determined by evidence.[21] Clinical redesign is made up of several stages:

- providing a platform for building evidence-based practice reliably into routine work, rather than layering it on top of existing work as an added demand;[46]
- facilitating change by engaging health professionals in high-priority problem-solving around concrete and meaningful issues and providing them with the training and information necessary to effect change;[17,47] and
- maintaining momentum for further change and improvement. Success motivates staff to go further with improvement to achieve more success.

Successful clinical process redesign relies on having all the enabling organisational characteristics that have already been discussed operating simultaneously within the one organisation. To illustrate this, several exemplars of large-scale clinical process redesign are described in Box 17.1.

6. Organisational policies which embrace evidence-based practice

An organisation's policies can influence the extent to which evidence-based practice is embraced within the organisation. Policy statements indicate an organisation's position or principles regardless of whether this organisation is at the level of government, a profession, a healthcare agency or a non-profit health organisation. Many organisations now incorporate the principle of evidence-based practice as part of their policies. In turn this can influence governance structures, purchasing decisions and expectations for employees. Some organisations have position statements which are supportive of evidence-based practice that are designed to be visionary. However, other organisations go further and provide policies which inform governance structures that include expectations that employees will engage in evidence-based practice (for example, by meeting competency requirements or to support credentialling).[56] This is not to be confused with evidence-based policy which concerns the use of research evidence to inform policy development.

Most health professionals have an organisation (College, Association or Academy) to support them in their professional development. Some have developed resources and methods of facilitating skill development related to evidence-based practice, especially upskilling in question-asking, searching and critical appraisal. Maintenance of professional standards schemes also give increasing levels of credit points to audit and practice review activities that seek to align and remediate evidence–practice gaps. Many health professional organisations also have specific policy statements about evidence-based practice in the form of position statements. A few extracts from position statements from different disciplines are provided in Box 17.2 as examples.

BOX 17.2

Examples of position statements from different discipline-specific organisations

- **Physiotherapy** (The World Confederation for Physical Therapy):

  'The World Confederation for Physical Therapy (WCPT) believes that physical therapists have a responsibility to use evidence to inform practice and ensure that the management of patients, carers, and communities is based on the best available evidence'. http://www.wcpt.org/policy/ps-EBP

- **Nursing** (The Honor Society of Nursing, Sigma Theta Tau International):

  'As a leader in the development and dissemination of knowledge to improve nursing practice, the Honor Society of Nursing, Sigma Theta Tau International supports the development and implementation of evidence-based nursing (EBN). The society defines EBN as an integration of the best evidence available, nursing expertise, and the values and preferences of the individuals, families and communities who are served'. http://www.nursingsociety.org/aboutus/PositionPapers/Pages/EBN_positionpaper.aspx

BOX 17.3

Organisational strategies for supporting evidence-based practice

ACTIVE COMMITMENT AND SUPPORT FROM SENIOR MANAGERS

- Direct and open endorsement of evidence-based learning and continuous quality improvement within mission statements and operations of boards, directorships, and other sub-agencies of the organisation.
- Provide dedicated time, resources, and remuneration for health professionals to practice evidence-based care:
  - Clinical decision support, evidence databases, other information technology infrastructure.
  - Resources (staff and physical resources such as meeting rooms) for conduct of evidence-based practice journal clubs, seminars and workshops.
  - Scheduling of 10% of normal working hours to be spent on evidence-based practice-related activities (journal clubs, clinical audits, quality and safety reviews, etc).
- Recognise those who have championed evidence-based practice within the organisation and grant recognition awards.
- Sponsor presentations at professional meetings and/or attendance at professional development courses.

USE OF EVIDENCE TO INFORM CARE DELIVERY

- Establish interdisciplinary panels for developing and updating evidence-based clinical standards (or guidelines or pathways) applicable to key areas of practice within the organisation.
- Develop easily accessible and searchable electronic repositories of evidence-based clinical standards (or guidelines or pathways) for use by health professionals and policy-makers.
- Establish organisation-wide literature search services which staff can use to retrieve relevant and high-quality evidence to answer important clinical questions directly related to routine care.
- Sponsor clinician-led and organisation-wide restructuring of care processes and service delivery systems according to evidence of effectiveness in optimising care.
- Mandate that submissions for new clinical interventions or services include a rationale based on a systematic review of evidence of effectiveness compared with existing (or usual) care.
- Develop payment formulae that fully remunerate evidence-based practices while withholding payments for interventions for which robust evidence shows no benefit.
- Penalise providers financially for care which is consistently in violation of accepted evidence-based standards.
- Deploy performance appraisal and credentialling policies which restrict scope of practice of health professionals whose practice is consistently in violation of accepted evidence-based standards.
- Waiver professional indemnity from litigation in cases where care resulting in serious patient harm was in clear violation of accepted evidence-based standards.
- Provide legal protection from defamation proceedings for whistleblowers who expose colleagues whose practice is consistently in violation of accepted evidence-based standards.

ALIGNMENT OF EVIDENCE-BASED PRACTICE WITH QUALITY AND SAFETY IMPROVEMENT

- Foster system-wide recognition that evidence-based practice and quality and safety improvement are symbiotic–they complement and reinforce one another.
- Establish evidence-based quality and safety teams at the level of clinical microsystems (group practices, hospital units or departments) which involve practising health professionals in identifying and remediating shortfalls in care.
- Provide the necessary resources for establishing quality and safety measurement and feedback systems for defined sets of key clinical indicators for commonly encountered conditions and procedures.
- Support the creation of clinical registries which collect and analyse process and outcome data on cohorts of patients which relate to key areas of practice within the organisation.
- Maintain an up-to-date inventory of evidence-based quality and safety improvement interventions relevant to key areas of practice within the organisation.
- Participate in evidence-based quality and safety improvement collaborations with other like-minded organisations.
- Seek organisational accreditation that recognises the integration of an evidence-based quality and safety improvement framework with all mainstream organisational activities.

Organisational policies which support evidence-based practice (however specific this may be) are an essential means by which the organisation communicates a willingness to embrace a culture of evidence-based practice, and helps to establish the norms and expectations about how things are to be done.

CONCLUSION

In this chapter we have explained why promoting evidence-based practice is important to organisations and how they might go about it. Box 17.3 summarises the most pertinent strategies for supporting evidence-based practice.[57–59] Ensuring that patients receive evidence-based healthcare requires healthcare organisations to be proactive in adopting evidence-based practice across the spectrum of their activities. This requires:

- active top leadership commitment and support
- managerial support
- a well-developed and user-friendly infrastructure of clinical informatics
- dedicated training of health professionals in the direct application of evidence to clinical care
- alignment of evidence-based practice with quality and safety improvement frameworks
- systematised clinical process redesign in response to new evidence-based clinical practices
- evidence-based health policy-making at the level of senior executives.

Professional organisations also have a role in promoting evidence-based practice by developing resources and methods in question-asking, searching and critical appraisal relevant to their members. While the key factor in advancing evidence-based practice will always remain the individual health professional, the existence of an organisational environment which recognises the value of, and encourages, evidence-based practice will add immeasurable value in accelerating and expanding the benefits of evidence-based practice to all who seek care within our healthcare organisations.

SUMMARY POINTS OF THIS CHAPTER

- Evidence-based practice needs to be implemented into organisations at all levels: microsystems (such as the clinic/ward); mesosystems (such as hospitals or community practices); and macro-systems (such as health departments, professional societies and governing organisations). There is complexity at each level and interrelatedness of these levels.

- Evidence-based practice should be endorsed and actively supported at the organisational level. Organisations that foster a culture that is supportive of evidence-based practice often have some key characteristics, such as: (1) active senior leadership commitment and support for evidence-based practice; (2) appropriate clinical informatics infrastructure; (3) providing and supporting learning relevant to evidence-based practice (including support of *evidence-based* journal clubs); (4) alignment of evidence-based practice with quality and safety improvement (that is, 'doing the right things right'); (5) the ability to change and redesign clinical processes on the basis of evidence and patient need; and (6) organisational policies which embrace evidence-based practice.

- Put simply, organisations need to provide the right culture and appropriate leadership, and set the policies which enable health professionals to have the skills, time and attitude to provide evidence-based practice. The benefits of doing this are immense: success means building reputation, improving morale and delivering better care more safely and efficiently.

References

1. McColl A, Smith H, White P, et al. General practitioners' perceptions of the route to evidence based medicine: a questionnaire survey. BMJ 1998;316:361–5.
2. Burkiewicz J, Zgarrick D. Evidence-based practice by pharmacists: utilisation and barriers. Ann Pharmacother 2005;39:1214–19.
3. Bennett S, Tooth L, McKenna K, et al. Perceptions of evidence based practice: a survey of occupational therapists. Aust Occup Ther J 2003;50:13–22.
4. Al-Almaie S, Al-Baghli N. Barriers facing physicians practicing evidence-based medicine in Saudi Arabia. J Contin Educ Health Prof 2004;24:163–70.
5. Lai N, Teng C, Lee M. The place and barriers of evidence based practice: knowledge and perceptions of medical, nursing and allied health practitioners in Malaysia. BMC Res Notes 2010;3:279.
6. Scott I. The evolving science of translating research evidence into clinical practice. Evid Based Med 2007;12:4–7.
7. Salge T, Vera O. Hospital innovativeness and organizational performance: evidence from English public acute care. Health Care Manage Rev 2009;34:54–67.
8. Bonis P, Pickens G, Rind D, et al. Association of a clinical knowledge support system with improved patient safety, reduced complications and shorter length of stay among Medicare beneficiaries in acute care hospitals in the United States. Int J Med Inform 2008;77:745–53.
9. Greenhalgh T, Robert G, Macfarlane F, et al. Diffusion of innovations in service organizations: systematic review and recommendations. Milbank Q 2004;82:581–629.
10. American College of Physicians. How can our nation conserve and distribute health care resources effectively and efficiently? Policy paper. Philadelphia: American College of Physicians; 2011. Online. Available: www.acponline.org/advocacy/where_we_stand/policy/health_care_resources.pdf; 29 May 2012.
11. Al-Khatib S, Hellkamp A, Curtis J, et al. Non-evidence-based ICD implantations in the United States. JAMA 2011;305:43–9.
12. Wennberg J, Fisher E, Skinner J. Geography and the debate over Medicare reform. Suppl web exclusive. Health Aff (Millwood) 2002:W96–114.
13. Swensen S, Kaplan G, Meyer G, et al. Controlling healthcare costs by removing waste: what American doctors can do now. BMJ Qual Saf 2011;20:534–7.
14. Marshall M, Ovretveit J. Can we save money by improving quality? BMJ Qual Saf 2011;20:293–6.
15. Aarons G. Measuring provider attitudes toward evidence-based practice: consideration of organisational context and individual differences. Child Adolesc Psychiatr Clin N Am 2005;14:255–71.
16. Glisson C, James L. The cross-level effects of culture and climate in human service teams. J Organ Behav 2002;23:767–94.
17. Sirio C, Segel K, Keyser D, et al. Pittsburgh regional healthcare initiative: a systems approach for achieving perfect patient care. Health Aff (Millwood) 2003;22:157–65.
18. Lukas C, Holmes S, Cohen A, et al. Transformational change in health care systems: an organizational model. Health Care Manage Rev 2007;32:309–20.
19. Aarons G. Transformational and transactional leadership: association with attitudes toward evidence-based practice. Psychiatr Serv 2006;57:1162–9.
20. Bradley E, Webster T, Baker D, et al. Translating research into practice: speeding the adoption of innovative health care programs. Issue Brief (Commonw Fund) 2004;724:1–12.
21. Jung D. Transformational and transactional leadership and their effects on creativity in groups. Creat Res J 2001;13:185–95.
22. Caldwell E, Whitehead M, Fleming J, et al. Evidence-based practice in everyday clinical practice: strategies for change in a tertiary occupational therapy department. Aust Occup Ther J 2008;55:79–84.
23. Lucas B, Evans A, Reilly B, et al. The impact of evidence on physicians' inpatient treatment decisions. J Gen Intern Med 2004;19:402–9.
24. Davidoff F, Miglus J. Delivering clinical evidence where it's needed: building an information system worthy of the profession. JAMA 2011;305:1906–7.
25. Brassey J, Elwyn G, Price C, et al. Just in time information for clinicians: a questionnaire evaluation of the ATTRACT project. BMJ 2001;322:529–30.
26. Del Mar C, Silagy C, Glasziou P, et al. Feasibility of an evidence-based literature search service for general practitioners. Med J Aust 2001;175:134–7.
27. McGowan J, Hogg W, Campbell C, et al. Just-in-time information improved decision-making in primary care: a randomised controlled trial. PLoS ONE 2008;3:e3785.
28. McGowan J, Hogg W, Zhong J, et al. A cost–consequences analysis of a primary care librarian question and answering service. PLoS ONE 2012;7:e33837.
29. Kawamoto K, Houlihan C, Balas E, et al. Improving clinical practice using clinical decision support systems: a systematic review of trials to identify features critical to success. BMJ 2005;330:765.

30. McCord G, Smucker W, Selius B, et al. Answering questions at the point of care: do residents practice EBM or manage information sources? Acad Med 2007;82:298–303.

31. Lindquist A, Johansson P, Petersson G, et al. The use of the Personal Digital Assistant (PDA) among personnel and students in health care: a review. J Med Internet Res 2008;10:e31.

32. Westbrook J, Coiera E, Gosling A. Do online information retrieval systems help experienced health professionals answer clinical questions? J Am Med Inform Assoc 2005;12:315–21.

33. Coomarasamy A, Khan K. What is the evidence that postgraduate teaching in evidence-based medicine changes anything? A systematic review. BMJ 2004;329:1017.

34. Straus S, Ball C, Balcombe N, et al. Teaching evidence-based medicine skills can change practice in a community hospital. J Gen Intern Med 2005;20:340–3.

35. Murad M, Montori V, Kunz R, et al. How to teach evidence-based medicine to teachers: reflections from a workshop experience. J Eval Clin Pract 2009;15:1205–7.

36. Menon A, Korner-Bitensky N, Kastner M, et al. Strategies for rehabilitation professionals to move evidence-based knowledge into practice: a systematic review. J Rehabil Med 2009;41:1024–32.

37. Slawson D, Shaughnessy A. Teaching evidence-based medicine: should we be teaching information management instead? Acad Med 2005;80:685–9.

38. Glasziou P. ACP Journal Club. Applying evidence: what's the next action? Ann Intern Med 2009;150:JC1–2, JC1–3.

39. Scott I, Phelps G. Measurement for improvement: getting one to follow the other. Intern Med J 2009;39:347–51.

40. Glasziou P, Ogrinc G, Goodman S. Can evidence-based medicine and clinical quality improvement learn from each other? BMJ Qual Saf 2011;20(Suppl 1):i13–17.

41. Evans S, Scott I, Johnson N, et al. Development of clinical-quality registries in Australia: the way forward. Med J Aust 2011;194:360–3.

42. Scott I, Denaro C, Bennett C, et al. for the Brisbane Cardiac Consortium Leadership Group. Achieving better in-hospital and post-hospital care of patients recently admitted with acute cardiac disease. Med J Aust 2004;180:S83–8.

43. Scott I, Darwin I, Harvey K, et al. Multisite, quality-improvement collaboration to optimise cardiac care in Queensland public hospitals. Med J Aust 2004;180:392–7.

44. Schouten L, Hulscher M, van Everdingen J, et al. Evidence for the impact of quality improvement collaboratives: systematic review. BMJ 2008;336:1491–4.

45. Scott I, Guyatt G. Clinical practice guidelines: the need for greater transparency in formulating recommendations. Med J Aust 2011;195:29–33.

46. Bradley E, Holmboe E, Mattera J, et al. Data feedback efforts in quality improvement: lessons learned from US hospitals. Qual Saf Health Care 2004;13:26–31.

47. Beer M, Eisenstat R, Spector B. Why change programs don't produce change. Harv Bus Rev 1990;68:158–66.

48. Kizer K. The 'new VA': a national laboratory for health care quality management. Am J Med Qual 1999;14:3–20.

49. Demakis J, McQueen L, Kizer K, et al. Quality Enhancement Research Initiative (QUERI): a collaboration between research and clinical practice. Med Care 2000;38(Suppl 1):I-17–25.

50. Jha A, Perlin J, Kizer K, et al. Effect of the transformation of the Veterans Affairs health care system on the quality of care. N Engl J Med 2003;348:2218–27.

51. Schilling L, Dearing J, Staley P, et al. Kaiser Permanente's performance improvement system, part 4: creating a learning organization. Jt Comm J Qual Patient Saf 2011;37:532–43.

52. Schilling L, Deas D, Jedlinsky M, et al. Kaiser Permanente's performance improvement system, part 2: developing a value framework. Jt Comm J Qual Patient Saf 2010;36:552–60.

53. James B, Savitz L. How Intermountain trimmed health care costs through robust quality improvement efforts. Health Aff (Millwood) 2011;30:1185–91.

54. Wagner E, Austin B, Davis C, et al. Improving chronic illness care: translating evidence into action. Health Aff (Millwood) 2001;20:64–78.

55. Coleman K, Austin B, Brach C, et al. Evidence on the Chronic Care Model in the new millennium. Health Aff (Millwood) 2009;28:75–85.

56. Oman K, Duran C, Fink R. Evidence-based policy and procedures: an algorithm for success. J Nurs Admin 2008;38:47–51.

57. Wensing M, Wollersheim H, Grol R. Organisational interventions to implement improvements in patient care: a structured review of reviews. Implement Sci 2006;1:2.

58. Lukas C, Engle R, Holmes S, et al. Strengthening organisations to implement evidence-based clinical practices. Health Care Manage Rev 2010;35:235–45.

59. Powell B, McMillen J, Proctor E, et al. A compilation of strategies for implementing clinical innovations in health and mental health. Med Care Res Rev 2012;69:123–57.

Index

Page numbers followed by 'f' indicate figures, 't' indicate tables, and 'b' indicate boxes.

THE
PRACTICE OF
NURSING RESEARCH

Appraisal, Synthesis, and Generation of Evidence

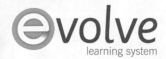 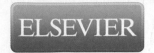
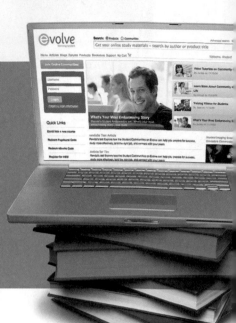

**SEVENTH
EDITION**

THE
PRACTICE OF
NURSING RESEARCH

Appraisal, Synthesis, and Generation of Evidence

Susan K. Grove, PhD, RN, ANP-BC, GNP-BC
Professor
College of Nursing
The University of Texas at Arlington
Arlington, Texas;
Adult Nurse Practitioner
Family Practice
Grand Prairie, Texas

Nancy Burns, PhD, RN, FCN, FAAN
Professor Emeritus
College of Nursing
The University of Texas at Arlington
Arlington, Texas;
Faith Community Nurse
St. Matthew Cumberland Presbyterian Church
Burleson, Texas

Jennifer Gray, PhD, RN
George W. and Hazel M. Jay Professor
College of Nursing
Associate Dean and Chair
Department of MSN Administration, Education, and PhD Programs
The University of Texas at Arlington
Arlington, Texas

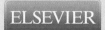

SAUNDERS

3251 Riverport Lane
St. Louis, Missouri 63043

THE PRACTICE OF NURSING RESEARCH: APPRAISAL, SYNTHESIS,   978-1-455-70736-2
AND GENERATION OF EVIDENCE, SEVENTH EDITION
Copyright © 2013, 2009, 2005, 2001, 1997, 1993, 1987 by Saunders, an imprint of Elsevier Inc.

Notices

Knowledge and best practice in this field are constantly changing. As new research and experience
broaden our understanding, changes in research methods, professional practices, or medical treatment may
become necessary.

Practitioners and researchers must always rely on their own experience and knowledge in evaluating
and using any information, methods, compounds, or experiments described herein. In using such
information or methods they should be mindful of their own safety and the safety of others, including
parties for whom they have a professional responsibility.

With respect to any drug or pharmaceutical products identified, readers are advised to check the most
current information provided (i) on procedures featured or (ii) by the manufacturer of each product to be
administered, to verify the recommended dose or formula, the method and duration of administration, and
contraindications. It is the responsibility of practitioners, relying on their own experience and knowledge
of their patients, to make diagnoses, to determine dosages and the best treatment for each individual
patient, and to take all appropriate safety precautions.

To the fullest extent of the law, neither the Publisher nor the authors, contributors, or editors, assume
any liability for any injury and/or damage to persons or property as a matter of products liability,
negligence or otherwise, or from any use or operation of any methods, products, instructions, or ideas
contained in the material herein.

Library of Congress Cataloging-in-Publication Data

Grove, Susan K.
  The practice of nursing research : appraisal, synthesis, and generation of evidence / Susan K. Grove,
Nancy Burns, Jennifer Gray.—7th ed.
      p. ; cm.
  Nancy Burns is first named author on previous edition.
  Includes bibliographical references and index.
  ISBN 978-1-4557-0736-2 (pbk.)
  I. Burns, Nancy, Ph.D.   II. Gray, Jennifer, 1955-   III. Title.
  [DNLM: 1. Nursing Research—methods.   2. Evidence-Based Nursing.   WY 20.5]
  610.73072—dc23
                                                                                2012019862

Executive Content Strategist: Lee Henderson
Associate Content Development Specialist: Julia Curcio
Publishing Services Manager: Jeff Patterson
Production Manager: Hemamalini Rajendrababu
Senior Project Manager: Antony Prince
Design Direction: Karen Pauls

Printed in China

Last digit is the print number: 9 8 7 6 5 4 3 2 1

To our readers and researchers, nationally and internationally, who will provide the science to develop an evidence-based practice for nursing.

*To our family members for their constant input, support, and love,
especially our husbands
Jay Suggs,
Jerry Burns,
and
Randy Gray*

Susan, Nancy, and Jennifer

Contributors

Daisha J. Cipher, PhD
Clinical Associate Professor
College of Nursing
University of Texas at Arlington
Arlington, Texas
Chapters 22, 23, 24 & 25

Kathryn M. Daniel, PhD, RN
Assistant Professor
College of Nursing
University of Texas Arlington
Arlington, Texas

Diane Doran, RN, PhD, FCAHS
Professor
Scientific Director, Nursing Health Services
    Research Unit (University of Toronto site)
Lawrence S. Bloomberg Faculty of Nursing
University of Toronto
Toronto, Ontario
Canada
Chapter 13

Kathryn Aldrich Lee, RN, PhD
Professor and Associate Dean for Research
James and Marjorie Endowed Chair in Nursing
Family Health Care Nursing
University of California
San Francisco
San Francisco, California
Chapters 20 & 27

Judy L. LeFlore PhD, RN, NNP-BC, CPNP-PC & AC, ANEF
Director
Pediatric, Acute Care Pediatric, Neonatal Nurse
    Practitioner Programs
Nursing
University of Texas at Arlington
Arlington, Texas
Nurse Practitioner
Advanced Practice Services
Children's Medical Center, Dallas
Dallas, Texas
Chapters 10 & 11

Christine Miaskowski, RN, PhD, FAAN
Professor & Associate Dean
Physiological Nursing
University of California
San Francisco, California
Chapter 29

Rosemary C. Polomano, PhD, RN, FAAN
Associate Professor of Pain Practice
Department of Biobehavioral Health Sciences
University of Pennsylvania School of Nursing
Philadelphia, Pennsylvania
Clinical Educator Faculty
Department of Nursing
Hospital of the University of Pennsylvania
Philadelphia, Pennsylvania
Associate Professor of Anesthesiology and Critical
    Care
Department of Anesthesiology and Critical Care
University of Pennsylvania School of Medicine
Philadelphia, Pennsylvania
Chapter 14

Reviewers

Lisa D. Brodersen ED, RN
Allen College
Waterloo, Iowa

Sara L. Clutter, PhD, RN
Associate Professor of Nursing
Waynesburg University
Waynesburg, Pennsylvania

Josephine DeVito, PhD, RN
Associate Professor
College of Nursing
Seton Hall University
South Orange, New Jersey

Jacalyn P. Dougherty, PhD, RN
Aurora, Colorado

Betsy Frank, RN, PhD
College of Nursing, Health, and Human Services
Indiana State University
Terre Haute, Indiana

Sharon Kitchie, RN, PhD, CNS-BC
Patient Education and Interpreter Services Specialist
Upstate University Hospital
Syracuse, New York

Madelaine Lawrence, PhD, RN
Queens University of Charlotte
Charlotte, NC

Ida Slusher, RN, DSN, CNE
Professor & Nursing Education Coordinator
Department of Baccalaureate & Graduate Nursing
Eastern Kentucky University
Richmond, Kentucky

Jeanne M. Sorrell, PhD, RN, FAAN
Cleveland Clinic
Cleveland, Ohio

Molly J. Walker, PhD, RN. CNS, CNE
Associate Professor, Angelo State University
San Angelo, Texas

Angela F. Wood RN, NNP-BC, PhD
Carson-Newman College
Jefferson City, Tennesse

Fatma A. Youssef, RN, MPH, DNSc
Professor of Nursing, Marymount University
Arlington, VA

Mary Beth Zeni, MSN, ScD, RN
Senior Nurse Researcher, Cleveland Clinic
Cleveland, Ohio

Preface

Research is a major force in the nursing profession that is used to change practice, education, and health policy. Our aim in developing the seventh edition of *The Practice of Nursing Research: Appraisal, Synthesis, and Generation of Evidence* is to increase excitement about research and to facilitate the development of evidence-based practice for nursing. It is critically important that all nurses, especially those in advanced-practice roles (nurse practitioners, clinical nurse specialists, nurse anesthetists, and nurse midwives) and those assuming roles as administrators and educators, have a strong understanding of the research methods conducted to generate evidence-based knowledge for nursing practice. Graduate and undergraduate nursing students and practicing nurses need to be actively involved in critically appraising and synthesizing research evidence for the delivery of quality, cost-effective care. This text provides detailed content and guidelines for implementing critical appraisal and synthesis processes. The text also contains extensive coverage of the research methods—quantitative, qualitative, outcomes, and intervention—commonly conducted in nursing. Doctoral students might use this text to facilitate their conduct of quality studies essential for generating nursing knowledge.

The depth and breadth of content presented in this edition reflect the increase in research activities and the growth in research knowledge since the previous edition. Nursing research is introduced at the baccalaureate level and becomes an integral part of graduate education (master's and doctoral) and clinical practice. We hope that this new edition might raise the number of nurses at all levels involved in research activities to improve the outcomes for nursing practice.

The seventh edition is written and organized to facilitate ease in reading, understanding, and implementing the research process. The major strengths of this text are as follows:

- State-of-the-art coverage of EBP—a topic of vital and growing importance in a healthcare arena focused on quality, cost-effective patient care.
- A clear, concise writing style that is consistent among the chapters to facilitate student learning.
- Comprehensive coverage of quantitative, qualitative, outcomes, and intervention research methods.
- A balanced coverage of qualitative and quantitative research methodologies.
- Electronic references and websites that direct the student to an extensive array of information that is important for conducting studies and using research findings in practice.
- Rich and frequent illustration of major points and concepts from the most current nursing research literature from a variety of clinical practices areas.
- A strong conceptual framework that links nursing research with EBP, theory, knowledge, and philosophy.

Our text provides a comprehensive introduction to nursing research for graduate and practicing nurses. For use at the master's and doctoral level, the text provides not only substantive content related to research but also practical applications based on the authors' experiences in conducting various types of nursing research, familiarity with the research literature, and experience in teaching nursing research at various educational levels.

The seventh edition of this text is now organized into 5 units and 29 chapters. Unit One introduces the reader to the world of nursing research. The content and presentation of this unit have been designed to introduce EBP, quantitative research, and qualitative research.

Unit Two provides an in-depth presentation of the research process for both quantitative and qualitative research. As with previous editions, this text provides extensive coverage of the many types of quantitative and qualitative research.

Unit Three addresses the implications of research for the discipline and profession of nursing. Content is provided to direct the student in conducting critical appraisals of both quantitative and qualitative research. A detailed discussion of types of research synthesis and strategies for promoting EBP is provided.

Unit Four gives students and practicing nurses the content they need for implementing studies. This unit includes chapters focused on data collection, statistical analysis, interpretation of research outcomes, and dissemination of research finding.

Unit Five addresses proposal development and seeking support for research. Readers are given direction for developing quantitative and qualitative research proposals and seeking funding for their research.

The changes in the seventh edition of this text reflect the advances in nursing research and also incorporate comments from outside reviewers, colleagues, and students. Our desire to promote the continuing development of the profession of nursing was the incentive for investing the time and energy required to develop this new edition.

New Content

The seventh edition provides current comprehensive coverage of nursing research and is focused on the learning needs and styles of today's nursing students and practicing nurses. Several exciting new areas of content based on the changes and expansion in the field of nursing research are included in this edition. Some of the major changes from the previous edition are as follows:

- Chapter 1, "Discovering the World of Nursing Research," is a strong introduction to evidence-based practice (EBP) that is linked to nursing research using a revised framework model for this edition of the text.
- Chapter 2, "Evolution of Research in Building Evidence-Based Nursing Practice," has a new title and is focused on building an EBP for nursing. This chapter introduces the most current processes for synthesizing research knowledge, which are systematic reviews, meta-analyses, meta-syntheses, and mixed method systematic reviews. The chapter includes a table that presents the purposes of these syntheses, the types of research they include (the "sampling frame"), and the analysis for achieving the different types of syntheses. A model of the continuum of the levels of research evidence, from strongest to weakest evidence, is provided.
- Chapter 4, "Introduction to Qualitative Research," describes the philosophical perspectives that guide the following five approaches to qualitative research: (1) phenomenology, (2) grounded theory, (3) ethnography, (4) exploratory-descriptive qualitative research, and (5) historical research. Excerpts from qualitative studies are provided to emphasize the contributions researchers using each approach have made to nursing science.
- Chapter 6, "Review of Relevant Literature," provides current, comprehensive strategies for searching the literature to identify relevant sources.
- Chapter 9, "Ethics in Research," features updated coverage of (1) the Health Insurance Portability

and Accountability Act (HIPAA), (2) U.S. Department of Health and Human Services (DHHS) regulations for protection of human subjects in research, and (3) U.S. Food and Drug Administration (FDA) regulations for protection of research subjects. This chapter also details the escalating problem of research misconduct in all healthcare disciplines and the actions that have been taken to manage this problem.

- Chapter 10, "Understanding Quantitative Research Designs," provides new content on mixed-methods designs that include both quantitative and qualitative research methods. Four common mixed-method research strategies conducted in nursing are discussed: sequential explanatory strategy, sequential exploratory strategy, sequential transformative strategy, and concurrent triangulation strategy. These strategies are presented using models, narrative descriptions, and examples.
- Chapter 11, "Selecting a Quantitative Research Design," describes many currently used designs that are not covered in other leading texts but that are important to the generation of nursing knowledge. It contains a detailed discussion of randomized controlled trials (RCTs) along with the Consolidated Standards for Reporting Trials (CONSORT, 2010) guidelines.
- Chapter 12, "Qualitative Research Methodology," is completely reorganized to address each step of the research process from writing the problem statement to interpreting the findings for qualitative studies. The data collection methods of observing, interviewing, and conducting focus groups are described in depth. In addition, examples of using photovoice, videos, and electronic communication are given. Methods specific to each philosophical approach are also discussed.
- Chapter 13, "Outcomes Research," a unique feature of our text, was significantly rewritten to promote understanding of the history, significance, and impact of outcomes research on nursing and health care, for both students and nurses in clinical practice. New content is included on nurse-sensitive patient outcomes, advanced-practice nursing outcomes, and databases used in conducting outcomes research. In addition, the methodologies for conducting outcomes research have been updated and expanded. This chapter was revised by a leading authority in the conduct of outcomes research, Dr. Diane Doran.
- Chapter 14, "Intervention-Based Research," was extensively rewritten to focus on the conduct of intervention-based research. It offers students and

practicing nurses detailed, current content and guidelines for critically appraising and conducting intervention studies. The chapter was revised by Dr. Rosemary Polomano, an authority in the conduct of intervention research.

- Chapter 15, "Sampling," contains extensive coverage of current sampling methods and the processes for determining sample size for quantitative and qualitative studies. This chapter includes formulas for calculating the acceptance and refusal rates for potential study participants and the retention and attrition rates for subjects participating in a study. Additional current content is provided to assist researchers in determining sample size for quantitative and qualitative research and for recruiting and retaining subjects for their studies.

- Chapter 16, "Measurement Concepts," features detailed information for examining the reliability and validity of measurement methods and the precision and accuracy of physiological measures used in nursing studies. Students are provided a background for understanding sensitivity, specificity, and likelihood ratios used to determine the quality of diagnostic tests.

- Chapter 17, "Measurement Methods Used in Developing Evidence for Practice," provides more detail on the use of physiological measurement methods in research. A growing number of nursing studies are focused on the measurement of the outcomes from interventions using physiological measurement methods, and this chapter equips the reader to understand and participate in these studies.

- Chapter 18, "Critical Appraisal of Nursing Studies," has a more refined process for critically appraising quantitative studies that consists of the following steps: (1) identifying the steps of the research process, (2) determining the study strengths and weaknesses, and (3) evaluating the credibility and meaning of a study for nursing knowledge and practice. The process of critically appraising qualitative studies was revised to evaluate studies using the standards of philosophical congruence, methodological coherence, intuitive comprehension, and intellectual contribution.

- Chapter 19, "Evidence Synthesis with Strategies for Promoting Evidence-Based Practice," has undergone extensive revision to achieve a completely new focus on how to conduct research syntheses and use the best research evidence in practice. The chapter now contains extensive details for conducting systematic reviews, meta-analyses, meta-syntheses, and mixed-method

systematic reviews. Guidelines are also provided to direct students in evaluating these research syntheses, which are appearing more frequently in the nursing and healthcare literature. Current information is given on the activities of Evidence-Based Practice Centers and the new initiative for funding translation research through the National Institutes of Health to increase the implementation of evidence-based interventions in practice.

- Chapter 20, "Collecting and Managing Data," now covers practical aspects of developing a data collection plan, including formatting instruments, creating a data flow chart, and training data collectors. In addition, common problems that occur during data collection are described, with possible solutions.

- Major revisions have been made in the chapters focused on statistical concepts and analysis techniques (Chapters 21 through 25). The content is presented in a clear, concise manner and supported with examples of analyses conducted on actual clinical data. Dr. Daisha Cipher, a noted statistician and healthcare researcher, assisted with the revision of these chapters.

- Chapter 27, "Disseminating Research Findings," features expanded and updated content on communicating study findings through oral and poster presentations and publications.

- Chapter 29, "Seeking Funding for Research," provides current strategies to assist students and practicing nurses in obtaining funding for their studies.

Student Ancillaries

An **Evolve Resources website,** which is available at http://evolve.elsevier.com/Grove/practice/, features a wealth of assets, including the following:

- Interactive Review Questions
- Data Sets and Data Set Activities
- Sample Research Proposals

An electronic **Study Guide** accompanies this edition of *The Practice of Nursing Research.* This study guide is keyed chapter-by-chapter to the text. It includes the following:

- *Relevant Terms* activities that help students understand and apply the language of nursing research
- *Key Ideas* exercises that reinforce essential concepts
- *Making Connections* activities that give students practice in the higher-level skills of comprehension and content synthesis
- *Crossword Puzzles* that serve not only as a clever learning activity but also as a welcome "fun" activity for busy adult learners

- *Exercises in Critical Appraisal* that provide experiences for students and practicing nurses to critically evaluate both quantitative and qualitative studies
- *Going Beyond* activities that provide suggestions for further study
- An Answer Key is provided at the end of each chapter that offers immediate feedback to reinforce learning
- A Published Studies appendix is provided for the critical appraisal exercises in the study guide, and other current studies are included on the Evolve website for faculty to use in providing learning experiences for their students.

Instructor Ancillaries

The **Instructor Resources** are available on Evolve, at http://evolve.elsevier.com/Grove/practice/. Instructors also have access to the online student resources. The Instructor Resources are an Instructor's Manual, an expanded Test Bank including 600 questions, Power-Point Presentations totaling more than 700 slides, and an Image Collection consisting of most images from the text.

Acknowledgments

Writing the seventh edition of this textbook has allowed us the opportunity to examine and revise the content of the previous edition based on input from a number of scholarly colleagues, the literature, and our graduate and undergraduate students. A textbook such as this requires synthesizing the ideas of many people and resources. For the first time, expert contributors have revised key chapters of this textbook. These experts have added invaluable content in critical areas of outcomes research, intervention research, design, data collection, and statistics. We thank these scholars for sharing their expertise.

We have also attempted to extract from the nursing and healthcare literature the essence of knowledge related to the conduct of nursing research. Thus we would like to thank those scholars who shared their knowledge with the rest of us in nursing and who have made this knowledge accessible for inclusion in this textbook. The ideas from the literature were synthesized and discussed with our colleagues and students to determine the revisions needed for the seventh edition.

We would also like to express our appreciation to Dean Elizabeth Poster and faculty members of the College of Nursing at The University of Texas at Arlington, for their support during the long and sometimes arduous experiences that are inevitable in developing a book of this magnitude. We would also like to thank Dr. Julie Barroso for her suggestions regarding the qualitative research content in this text. We particularly value the questions raised by our students regarding the content of this text, which allow us a unique view of our learners' perceptions.

We would also like to recognize the excellent reviews of the colleagues who helped us make important revisions in this text. These reviewers are located in large and small universities across the United States and provided a broad range of research expertise.

Finally, we thank the people at Elsevier, who have been extremely helpful to us in producing a scholarly, attractive, appealing text. We extend a special thank you to the people most instrumental in the development and production of this book: Lee Henderson, Executive Content Strategist; and Julia Curcio, Associate Content Development Specialist. We also want to thank others involved with the production and marketing of this book—Antony Prince, Project Manager; Karen Pauls, Designer; and Pat Crowe, Marketing Manager.

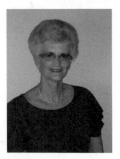

Susan K. Grove,
PhD, RN, ANP-BC, GNP-BC

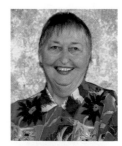

Nancy Burns,
PhD, RN, FAAN

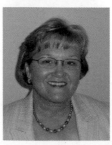

Jennifer Gray,
PhD, RN

Contents

1

Discovering the World of Nursing Research

evolve http://evolve.elsevier.com/Grove/practice/

Welcome to the world of nursing research. You might think it is strange to consider research a "world," but research is truly a new way of experiencing reality. Entering a new world requires learning a unique language, incorporating new rules, and using new experiences to learn how to interact effectively within that world. As you become a part of this new world, your perceptions and methods of reasoning will be modified and expanded. Understanding the world of nursing research is critical to providing evidence-based care to your patients. Since the 1990s, there has been a growing emphasis for nurses—especially advanced practice nurses (nurse practitioners, clinical nurse specialists, nurse anesthetists, and nurse midwives), administrators, educators, and nurse researchers—to promote an evidence-based practice in nursing (Brown, 2009; Craig & Smyth, 2012; Melnyk & Fineout-Overholt, 2011). Evidence-based practice in nursing requires a strong body of research knowledge that nurses must synthesize and use to promote quality care for their patients, families, and communities. We developed this text to facilitate your understanding of nursing research and its contribution to the implementation of evidenced-based nursing practice.

This chapter broadly explains the world of research. A definition of nursing research is provided followed by the framework for this textbook that connects nursing research to the world of nursing. The chapter concludes with a discussion of the significance of research in developing an evidence-based practice for nursing.

Definition of Nursing Research

The root meaning of the word research is "search again" or "examine carefully." More specifically,

research is the diligent, systematic inquiry or investigation to validate and refine existing knowledge and generate new knowledge. The concepts *systematic* and *diligent* are critical to the meaning of research because they imply planning, organization, and persistence. Many disciplines conduct research, so what distinguishes nursing research from research in other disciplines? In some ways, there are no differences, because the knowledge and skills required to conduct research are similar from one discipline to another. However, when one looks at other dimensions of research within a discipline, it is clear that research in nursing must be unique to address the questions relevant to the profession. Nurse researchers need to implement the most effective research to develop a unique body of knowledge for nursing.

The American Nurses Association (ANA, 2012) developed the following definition of nursing that identifies the unique body of knowledge needed by the profession: "Nursing is the protection, promotion, and optimization of health and abilities, prevention of illness and injury, alleviation of suffering through the diagnosis and treatment of human response, and advocacy in the care of individuals, families, communities, and populations." On the basis of this definition, nursing research is needed to generate knowledge about human responses and the best interventions to promote health, prevent illness, and manage illness (ANA, 2010b).

Many nurses hold the view that nursing research should focus on acquiring knowledge that can be directly implemented in clinical practice, which is sometimes referred to as applied research or practical research (Brown, 2009; Mackay, 2009). However, another view is that nursing research should include studies of nursing education, nursing administration, health services, and nurses' characteristics and roles as well as clinical situations. Riley, Beal, Levi, and McCausland (2002) support this second view and believe nursing scholarship should include education, practice, and service. Research is needed to identify teaching-learning strategies to promote nurses' management of practice. Thus, nurse researchers are involved in building a science for nursing education so the teaching-learning strategies used are evidence-based (National League for Nursing [NLN], 2009). Nurse administrators are involved in research to enhance nursing leadership and the delivery of quality, cost-effective patient care. Studies of health services and nursing roles are important to promote quality outcomes in the nursing profession and the healthcare system (Doran, 2011).

Thus, the knowledge generated through nursing research provides the scientific foundation essential for all areas of nursing. In this text, **nursing research** is defined as a scientific process that validates and refines existing knowledge and generates new knowledge that directly and indirectly influences the delivery of evidence-based nursing.

Framework Linking Nursing Research to the World of Nursing

To best explore nursing research, we have developed a framework to help establish connections between research and the various elements of nursing. The framework presented in the following pages links nursing research to the world of nursing and is used as an organizing model for this textbook. In the framework model (see Figure 1-1), nursing research is not an entity disconnected from the rest of nursing but rather is influenced by and influences all other nursing elements. The concepts in this model are pictured on a continuum from concrete to abstract. The discussion introduces this continuum and progresses from the concrete concept of the empirical world of nursing practice to the most abstract concept of nursing philosophy. The use of two-way arrows in the model indicates the dynamic interaction among the concepts.

Concrete-Abstract Continuum

As previously mentioned, Figure 1-1 presents the components of nursing on a concrete-abstract continuum. This continuum demonstrates that nursing thought flows both from concrete to abstract thinking and from abstract to concrete. **Concrete thinking** is oriented toward and limited by tangible things or by

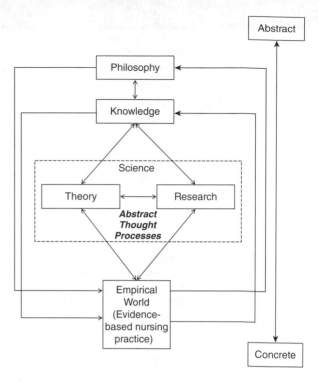

Figure 1-1 Framework linking nursing research to the world of nursing.

events that we observe and experience in reality. Thus, the focus of concrete thinking is immediate events that are limited by time and space. Most nurses believe they are concrete thinkers because they focus on the specific actions in nursing practice. **Abstract thinking** is oriented toward the development of an idea without application to, or association with, a particular instance. Abstract thinkers tend to look for meaning, patterns, relationships, and philosophical implications. This type of thinking is independent of time and space. Currently, graduate nursing education fosters abstract thinking, because it is an essential skill for developing theory and creating an idea for study. Nurses assuming advanced roles and registered nurses (RNs) need to use both abstract and concrete thinking. For example, a nurse practitioner must explore the best research evidence about a practice problem (abstract thinking) before using his or her clinical expertise to diagnose and manage an individual patient's health problem (concrete thinking). RNs also use abstract and concrete thinking to develop and refine protocols and policies based on current research to direct patient care.

Nursing research requires skills in both concrete and abstract thinking. Abstract thought is required to identify researchable problems, design studies, and interpret findings. Concrete thought is necessary in both planning and implementing the detailed steps of data collection and analysis. This back-and-forth flow between abstract and concrete thought may be one reason why nursing research seems complex and challenging.

Empirical World

The empirical world is what we experience through our senses and is the concrete portion of our existence. It is what we often call *reality*, and "doing" kinds of activities are part of this world. There is a sense of certainty about the empirical or real world; it seems understandable, predictable, controllable. Concrete thinking focuses on the empirical world; words associated with this thinking include "practical," "down-to-earth," "solid," and "factual." Concrete thinkers want facts. They want to be able to apply whatever they know to the current situation.

The practice of nursing takes place in the empirical world, as demonstrated in Figure 1-1. The scope of nursing practice varies for the RN and the advanced practice nurse (APN). RNs provide care to and coordinate care for patients, families, and communities in a variety of settings. They initiate interventions as well as carry out treatments authorized by other healthcare providers (ANA, 2010a). APNs, such as nurse practitioners, nurse anesthetists, nurse midwives, and clinical nurse specialists, have an expanded practice. Their knowledge, skills, and expertise promote role autonomy and overlap with medical practice. APNs usually concentrate their clinical practice in a specialty area, such as acute care, pediatrics, gerontology, adult or family primary care, psychiatric-mental health, women's health, maternal child, or anesthesia (ANA, 2010b). You can access the most current nursing scope and standards for practice from the ANA (2010a). Within the empirical world of nursing, the goal is to provide evidence-based practice to improve the health outcomes of individuals, families, and communities (see Figure 1-1). The aspects of evidence-based practice and the significance of research in developing evidence-based practice are covered later in this chapter.

Reality Testing Using Research

People tend to *validate* or test the reality of their existence through their senses. In everyday activities, they constantly check out the messages received from their senses. For example, they might ask, "Am I really seeing what I think I am seeing?" Sometimes their senses can play tricks on them. This is why

instruments have been developed to record sensory experiences more accurately. For example, does the patient just feel hot or actually have a fever? Thermometers were developed to test this sensory perception accurately. Through research, the most accurate and precise measurement devices have been developed to assess the temperature of patients on the basis of age and health status (Waltz, Strickland, & Lenz, 2010). Thus, research is a way to test reality and generate the best evidence to guide nursing practice.

Nurses use a variety of research methods to test their reality and generate nursing knowledge, including quantitative research, qualitative research, outcomes research, and intervention research. Quantitative research, the most frequently conducted method, is a formal, objective, systematic methodology to describe variables, test relationships, and examine cause-and-effect interactions (Kerlinger & Lee, 2000; Shadish, Cook, & Campbell, 2002). Since the 1980s, nurses have been conducting qualitative research to generate essential theories and knowledge for nursing. Qualitative research is a rigorous, interactive, holistic, subjective research approach used to describe life experiences and give them meaning (Marshall & Rossman, 2011; Munhall, 2012). Both quantitative and qualitative research methods are important to the development of nursing knowledge (Fawcett & Garity, 2009; Munhall, 2012; Shadish et al., 2002). Some researchers effectively combine these two methods in implementing mixed method research to address selected nursing research problems (Creswell, 2009).

Medicine, healthcare agencies, and now nursing are focusing on the outcomes of patient care. Outcomes research is an important scientific methodology that has evolved to examine the end results of patient care and the outcomes for healthcare providers, such as RNs, APNs, and physicians, and for healthcare agencies (Doran, 2011). Nurses are also engaged in intervention research, a methodology for investigating the effectiveness of nursing interventions in achieving the desired outcomes in natural settings (Forbes, 2009). These different types of research are all essential to the development of nursing science, theory, and knowledge (see Figure 1-1). Nurses have varying roles related to research that include conducting research, critically appraising research, and using research evidence in practice.

Roles of Nurses in Research

Generating a scientific knowledge base with implementation in practice requires the participation of all

TABLE 1-1 Nurses' Participation in Research at Various Levels of Education	
Educational Preparation	**Research Functions**
BSN	Read and critically appraise studies. Use best research evidence in practice with guidance. Assist with problem identification and data collection.
MSN	Critically appraise and synthesize studies to develop and revise protocols, algorithms, and policies for practice. Implement best research evidence in practice. Collaborate in research projects and provide clinical expertise for research.
DNP	Participate in evidence-based guideline development. Develop, implement, evaluate, and revise as needed protocols, policies, and evidence-based guidelines in practice. Conduct clinical studies, usually in collaboration with other nurse researchers.
PhD	Major role in conducting independent research and contributing to the empirical knowledge generated in a selected area of study. Obtain initial funding for research. Coordinate research teams of BSN, MSN, and DNP nurses.
Post-doctorate	Assume a full researcher role with a funded program of research. Lead and/or participate in nursing and interdisciplinary research teams. Identified as experts in their areas of research. Mentor PhD-prepared researchers.

nurses in a variety of research activities. Some nurses are developers of research and conduct studies to generate and refine the knowledge needed for nursing practice. Others are consumers of research and use research evidence to improve their nursing practice. The American Association of Colleges of Nursing (AACN, 2006) and ANA (2010a, 2010b) have published statements about the roles of nurses in research. No matter their education or position, all nurses have roles in research and some ideas about those roles are presented in Table 1-1. The research role a nurse assumes usually expands with his or her advanced education, expertise, and career path. Nurses with a Bachelor of Science in Nursing (BSN) degree have knowledge of the research process and skills in reading and critically appraising studies. They assist with the implementation of evidence-based guidelines, protocols, algorithms, and policies in practice. In addition, these nurses might provide valuable assistance in identifying research problems and collecting data for studies.

Nurses with a Master of Science in Nursing (MSN) have undergone the educational preparation to critically appraise and synthesize findings from studies to revise or develop protocols, algorithms, or policies for use in practice. They also have the ability to identify and critically appraise the quality of evidence-based guidelines developed by national organizations. APNs and nurse administrators have the ability to lead healthcare teams in making essential changes in nursing practice and in the healthcare system on the basis of current research evidence. Some MSN-prepared nurses conduct studies but usually do so in collaboration with other nurse scientists (AACN, 2006; ANA 2010a).

The doctorate in nursing can be practice focused (doctorate of nursing practice [DNP]) or research focused (doctorate of philosophy [PhD]). Nurses with DNPs are educated to have the highest level of clinical expertise, with the ability to translate scientific knowledge for use in practice. These doctorally prepared nurses have advanced research and leadership knowledge to develop, implement, evaluate, and revise evidence-based guidelines, protocols, algorithms, and policies for practice (Clinton & Sperhac, 2006). In addition, DNP-prepared nurses have the expertise to conduct and/or collaborate with clinical studies.

PhD-prepared nurses assume a major role in the conduct of research and the generation of nursing knowledge in a selected area of interest (Brar, Boschma, & McCuaig, 2010). These nurse scientists often coordinate research teams that include DNP-, MSN-, and BSN-prepared nurses to facilitate the conduct of high-quality studies in a variety of healthcare agencies. Postdoctorate nurses usually assume full-time researcher roles and have funded programs of research. They lead interdisciplinary teams of researchers and sometimes conduct studies in multiple settings. These scientists often are identified as experts in selected areas of research and provide mentoring of new PhD-prepared researchers (AACN, 2006) (see Table 1-1).

Abstract Thought Processes

Abstract thought processes influence every element of the nursing world. In a sense, they link all the elements together. Without skills in abstract thought, we are trapped in a flat existence; we can experience the empirical world, we cannot explain or understand it (Abbott, 1952). Through abstract thinking, however, we can test our theories (which explain the nursing world) and then include them in the body of scientific knowledge (Smith & Liehr, 2008). Abstract thinking also allows scientific findings to be developed into theories (Munhall, 2012). Abstract thought enables both science and theories to be blended into a cohesive body of knowledge, guided by a philosophical framework, and applied in clinical practice (see Figure 1-1). Thus, abstract thought processes are essential for synthesizing research evidence and knowing when and how to use this knowledge in practice.

Three major abstract thought processes— introspection, intuition, and reasoning—are important in nursing (Silva, 1977). These thought processes are used in critically appraising and applying best research evidence in practice, planning and implementing research, and developing and evaluating theory.

Introspection

Introspection is the process of turning your attention inward toward your own thoughts. It occurs at two levels. At the more superficial level, you are aware of the thoughts you are experiencing. You have a greater awareness of the flow and interplay of feelings and ideas that occur in constantly changing patterns. These thoughts or ideas can rapidly fade from view and disappear if you do not quickly write them down. When you allow introspection to occur in more depth, you examine your thoughts more critically and in detail. Patterns or links between thoughts and ideas emerge, and you may recognize fallacies or weaknesses in your thinking. You may question what brought you to this point and find yourself really enjoying the experience.

Imagine the following clinical situation. You have just left John Brown's home. John has a colostomy and has been receiving home health care for several weeks. Although John is caring for his colostomy, he is still reluctant to leave home for any length of time. You are irritated and frustrated with this situation. You begin to review your nursing actions and to recall other patients who reacted in similar ways. What were the patterns of their behavior?

You have an idea: Perhaps the patient's behavior is linked to the level of family support. You feel unsure about your ability to help the patient and family deal with this situation effectively. You recall other nurses describing similar reactions in their patients, and you wonder how many patients with colostomies have this problem. Your thoughts jump to reviewing the charts of other patients with colostomies and reading relevant ideas discussed in the literature. Some research has been conducted on this topic recently, and you could critically appraise these findings to determine the level of evidence for possible use of the ideas in practice. If the findings are inadequate, perhaps other nurses would be interested in studying this situation with you.

Intuition

Intuition is an insight into or understanding of a situation or event as a whole that usually cannot be logically explained (Smith, 2009). Because intuition is a type of knowing that seems to come unbidden, it may also be described as a "gut feeling" or a "hunch." Because intuition cannot be explained with ease scientifically, many people are uncomfortable with it. Some even say that it does not exist. Sometimes, therefore, the feeling or sense is suppressed, ignored, or dismissed as silly. However, intuition is not the lack of knowing; rather, it is a result of deep knowledge— tacit knowing or personal knowledge (Benner, 1984; Polanyi, 1962, 1966). The knowledge is incorporated so deeply within that it is difficult to bring it consciously to the surface and express it in a logical manner. One of the most commonly cited examples of nurses' intuition is their recognition of a patient's physically deteriorating condition. Odell, Victor, and Oliver (2009) conducted a review of the research literature and described nurses' use of intuition in clinical practice. They noted that nurses have an intuition or a knowing that something is not right with their patients by recognizing changes in behavior and physical signs. Through clinical experience and the use of intuition, nurses are able to recognize patterns of deviations from the normal clinical course and to know when to take action.

Intuition is generally considered unscientific and unacceptable for use in research. In some instances, that consideration is valid. For example, a hunch about significant differences between one set of scores and another set of scores is not particularly useful as an analysis technique. However, even though intuition is often unexplainable, it has some important scientific uses. Researchers do not always need to be able to explain something in order to use it. A burst of intuition may identify a problem for study, indicate important variables to measure, or link two ideas together in interpreting the findings. The trick is to recognize the feeling, value it, and hang on to the idea long enough to consider it. Some researchers keep a journal to capture elusive thoughts and hunches as they think about their phenomenon of interest. These intuitive hunches often become important later as they conduct their studies.

Imagine the following situation. You have been working in an oncology center for the past 3 years.

You and two other nurses working in the center have been meeting with the acute care nurse practitioner to plan a study to determine which factors are important for promoting positive patient outcomes in the center. The group has met several times with a nursing professor at the university, who is collaborating with the group to develop the study. At present, the group is concerned with identifying the outcomes that need to be measured and how to measure them.

You have had a busy morning. Mr. Green, a patient, stops by to chat on his way out of the clinic. You listen, but not attentively at first. You then become more acutely aware of what he is saying and begin to have a feeling about one variable that should be studied. Although he didn't specifically mention fear of breaking the news about having cancer to his children, you sense that he is anxious about conveying bad news to his loved ones. You cannot really explain the origin of this feeling, something in the flow of Mr. Green's words has stimulated a burst of intuition. You suspect other patients diagnosed with cancer face similar fear and hesitation about informing their family members of bad news, that they have cancer or that their cancer has spread. You believe the variable "fear of breaking bad news to loved ones" needs to be studied. You feel both excited and uncertain. What will the other nurses think? If the variable has not been studied, is it really significant? Somehow, you feel that it is important to consider.

Reasoning

Reasoning is the processing and organizing of ideas in order to reach conclusions. Through reasoning, people are able to make sense of their thoughts and experiences. This type of thinking is often evident in the verbal presentation of a logical argument in which each part is linked together to reach a logical conclusion. Patterns of reasoning are used to develop theories and to plan and implement research. Barnum (1998) identified four patterns of reasoning as being essential to nursing: (1) problematic, (2) operational, (3) dialectic, and (4) logistic. An individual uses all four types of reasoning, but frequently one type of reasoning is more dominant than the others. Reasoning is also classified by the discipline of logic into inductive and deductive modes (Chinn & Kramer, 2008).

Problematic Reasoning

Problematic reasoning involves (1) identifying a problem and the factors influencing it, (2) selecting solutions to the problem, and (3) resolving the problem. For example, nurses use problematic reasoning in the nursing process to identify diagnoses and to implement nursing interventions to resolve these problems. Problematic reasoning is also evident when one identifies a research problem and successfully develops a methodology to examine it.

Operational Reasoning

Operational reasoning involves the identification of and discrimination among many alternatives and viewpoints. It focuses on the process (debating alternatives) rather than on the resolution (Barnum, 1998). Nurses use operational reasoning to develop realistic, measurable health goals with patients and families. Nurse practitioners use operational reasoning to debate which pharmacological and nonpharmacological treatments to use in managing patient illnesses. In research, operationalizing a treatment for implementation and debating which measurement methods or data analysis techniques to use in a study require operational thought (Kerlinger & Lee, 2000; Waltz et al., 2010).

Dialectic Reasoning

Dialectic reasoning involves looking at situations in a holistic way. A dialectic thinker believes that the whole is greater than the sum of the parts and that the whole organizes the parts (Barnum, 1998). For example, a nurse using dialectic reasoning would view a patient as a person with strengths and weaknesses who is experiencing an illness, and not just as the "stroke in room 219." Dialectic reasoning also involves examining factors that are opposites and making sense of them by merging them into a single unit or idea that is greater than either alone. For example, analyzing studies with conflicting findings and summarizing these findings to determine the current knowledge base for a research problem require dialectic reasoning. Analysis of data collected in qualitative research requires dialectic reasoning to gain an understanding of the phenomenon being investigated (Munhall, 2012).

Logistic Reasoning

Logic is a science that involves valid ways of relating ideas to promote understanding. The aim of logic is to determine truth or to explain and predict phenomena. The science of logic deals with thought processes, such as concrete and abstract thinking, and methods of reasoning, such as logistic, inductive, and deductive.

Logistic reasoning is used to break the whole into parts that can be carefully examined, as can the relationships among the parts. In some ways, logistic reasoning is the opposite of dialectic reasoning. A logistic reasoner assumes that the whole is the sum of the parts and that the parts organize the whole. For example, a patient states that she is cold. You logically examine the following parts of the situation and their relationships: (1) room temperature, (2) patient's temperature, (3) patient's clothing, and (4) patient's activity. The room temperature is 65° F, the patient's temperature is 98.6° F, and the patient is wearing lightweight pajamas and drinking ice water. You conclude that the patient is cold because of external environmental factors (room temperature, lightweight pajamas, and drinking ice water). Logistic reasoning is used frequently in quantitative, outcomes, and intervention research to develop a study design, plan and implement data collection, and conduct statistical analyses.

Inductive and Deductive Reasoning

The science of logic also includes inductive and deductive reasoning. People use these modes of reasoning constantly, although the choice of types of reasoning may not always be conscious (Kaplan, 1964). Inductive reasoning moves from the specific to the general, whereby particular instances are observed and then combined into a larger whole or general statement (Chinn & Kramer, 2008). An example of inductive reasoning follows:

A headache is an altered level of health that is stressful.

A fractured bone is an altered level of health that is stressful.

A terminal illness is an altered level of health that is stressful.

Therefore, all altered levels of health are stressful.

In this example, inductive reasoning is used to move from the specific instances of altered levels of health that are stressful to the general belief that all altered levels of health are stressful. By testing many different altered levels of health through research to determine whether they are stressful, one can confirm the general statement that all types of altered health are stressful.

Deductive reasoning moves from the general to the specific or from a general premise to a particular situation or conclusion. A premise or hypothesis is a statement of the proposed relationship between two or more variables. An example of deductive reasoning follows:

PREMISES:

All human beings experience loss.

All adolescents are human beings.

CONCLUSION:

All adolescents experience loss.

In this example, deductive reasoning is used to move from the two general premises about human beings experiencing loss and adolescents being human beings to the specific conclusion, "All adolescents experience loss." However, the conclusions generated from deductive reasoning are valid only if they are based on valid premises. Consider the following example:

PREMISES:

All health professionals are caring.

All nurses are health professionals.

CONCLUSION:

All nurses are caring.

The premise that all health professionals are caring is not necessarily valid or an accurate reflection of reality. Research is a means to test and confirm or refute a premise so that valid premises can be used as a basis for reasoning in nursing practice.

Science

Science is a coherent body of knowledge composed of research findings and tested theories for a specific discipline (see Figure 1-1). Science is both a product (end point) and a process (mechanism to reach an end point) (Silva & Rothbart, 1984). An example from the discipline of physics is Newton's law of gravity, which was developed through extensive research. The knowledge of gravity (product) is a part of the science of physics that evolved through formulating and testing theoretical ideas (process). The ultimate goal of science is to explain the empirical world and thus to have greater control over it. To accomplish this goal, scientists must discover new knowledge, expand existing knowledge, and reaffirm previously held knowledge in a discipline (Greene, 1979). Health professionals integrate this evidence-based knowledge to control the delivery of care and thereby improve patient outcomes (evidence-based practice).

The science of a field determines the accepted process for obtaining knowledge within that field. Research is an important process for obtaining scientific knowledge in nursing. Some sciences rigidly limit the types of research that can be used to obtain knowledge. A valued method for developing a science is the traditional research process, or quantitative research. According to this process, the information gained from one study is not sufficient for its inclusion in the body of science. A study must be replicated several times and must yield similar results each time before that information can be considered to be sound empirical evidence (Fahs, Morgan, & Kalman, 2003).

Consider the research on the relationships between smoking, lung damage, and cancer. Numerous studies conducted on animals and humans over the past decades indicate causative relationships between smoking and lung damage and between smoking and lung cancer. Everyone who smokes experiences lung damage; and although not everyone who smokes gets lung cancer, smokers are at a much higher risk for cancer. Extensive, quality research has been conducted to generate empirical evidence about the health hazards of smoking, and this evidence guides the actions of nurses in practice. We provide smoking cessation education, emotional support, and drugs like nicotine patches and Chantix (Varenicline) to assist individuals to stop smoking. On the basis of this scientific evidence about the hazards of smoking, society has moved toward providing many smoke-free environments.

Findings from studies are systematically related to one another in a way that seems to best explain the empirical world. Abstract thought processes are used to make these linkages. The linkages are called *laws* or *principles*, depending on the certainty of the facts and relationships within the linkage. Laws express the most certain relationships and provide the best research evidence for use in practice. The certainty depends on the amount of research conducted to test a relationship and, to some extent, on the skills in abstract thought processes to link the research findings to form meaningful evidence. The truths or explanations of the empirical world reflected by these laws and principles are never absolutely certain and may be disproved by further research.

Nursing is in the beginning stages of developing a science for the profession, and additional original and replication studies are needed to develop the knowledge necessary for practice (Fahs et al., 2003; Melnyk & Fineout-Overholt, 2011). As discussed earlier, nursing science is being developed with the use of a variety of research methodologies, including quantitative, qualitative, outcomes, and intervention. The focus of this textbook is to increase your understanding of these different types of research used in the development and testing of nursing theory.

Theory

A **theory** is a creative and rigorous structuring of ideas used to describe, explain, predict, or control a particular phenomenon or segment of the empirical world (Chinn & Kramer, 2008; Smith & Liehr, 2008). A theory consists of a set of concepts that are defined and interrelated to present a systematic view of a phenomenon. A classic example is the theory of stress developed by Selye (1976) to explain the physical and emotional affects of illness on peoples' lives. This theory of stress continues to be important in understanding the affects of health changes on patients and families. Extensive research has been conducted to detail the types, number, and severity of stressors experienced in life and the effective interventions for managing these stressful situations.

A theory is developed from a combination of personal experiences, research findings, and abstract thought processes. The theorist may use findings from research as a starting point and then organize the findings to best explain the empirical world. This is the process Selye used to develop his theory of stress. Alternatively, the theorist may use abstract thought processes, personal knowledge, and intuition to develop a theory of a phenomenon. This theory then requires testing through research to determine whether it is an accurate reflection of reality. Thus, research has a major role in theory development, testing, and refinement. Some forms of qualitative research focus on developing new theories or extending existing theories. Quantitative, outcomes, and intervention methods of research are often implemented to test the accuracy of theory. The study findings either support or fail to support the theory, providing a basis for refining the theory (Chinn & Kramer, 2008; Fawcett & Garity, 2009).

Knowledge

Knowledge is a complex, multifaceted concept. For example, you may say that you *know* your friend John, *know* that the earth rotates around the sun, *know* how to give an injection, and *know* pharmacology. These are examples of knowing—being familiar with a person, comprehending facts, acquiring a psychomotor skill, and mastering a subject. There are differences in types of knowing, yet there are also similarities. Knowing presupposes order or imposes order on thoughts and ideas (Engelhardt, 1980). People have a desire to know what to expect. There is a need for certainty in the world, and individuals seek it by trying to decrease uncertainty through knowledge. Think of the questions you ask a person who has presented some bit of knowledge: "Is it true?" "Are you sure?" "How do you know?" Thus, the knowledge that we acquire is expected to be an accurate reflection of reality.

Ways of Acquiring Nursing Knowledge

We acquire knowledge in a variety of ways and expect it to be an accurate reflection of the real world (White, 1982). Nurses have historically acquired knowledge through (1) traditions, (2) authority, (3) borrowing,

(4) trial and error, (5) personal experience, (6) role-modeling and mentorship, (7) intuition, (8) reasoning, and (9) research. Intuition, reasoning, and research were discussed earlier in this chapter; the other ways of acquiring knowledge are briefly described in this section.

Traditions

Traditions consist of "truths" or beliefs that are based on customs and past trends. Nursing traditions from the past have been transferred to the present by written and verbal communication and role-modeling and continue to influence the present practice of nursing. For example, some of the policies and procedures in hospitals and other healthcare facilities contain traditional ideas. In addition, some nursing interventions are transmitted verbally from one nurse to another over the years or by the observation of experienced nurses. For example, the idea of providing a patient with a clean, safe, well-ventilated environment originated with Florence Nightingale (1859).

However, traditions can also narrow and limit the knowledge sought for nursing practice. For example, tradition has established the time and pattern for providing baths, evaluating vital signs, and allowing patient visitation on many hospital units. The nurses on these units quickly inform new staff members about the accepted or traditional behaviors for the unit. Traditions are difficult to change because people with power and authority have accepted and supported them for a long time. Many traditions have not been tested for accuracy or efficiency and require research for continued use in practice.

Authority

An authority is a person with expertise and power who is able to influence opinion and behavior. A person is thought of as an authority because she or he knows more in a given area than others do. Knowledge acquired from authority is illustrated when one person credits another person as the source of information. Nurses who publish articles and books or develop theories are frequently considered authorities. Students usually view their instructors as authorities, and clinical nursing experts are considered authorities within their clinical settings. However, persons viewed as authorities in one field are not necessarily authorities in other fields. An expert is an authority only when addressing his or her area of expertise. Like tradition, the knowledge acquired from authorities sometimes has not been validated through research and is not considered the best evidence for practice.

Borrowing

As some nursing leaders have noted, knowledge in nursing practice is partly made up of information that has been borrowed from disciplines such as medicine, psychology, physiology, and education (McMurrey, 1982; Walker & Avant, 2011). Borrowing in nursing involves the appropriation and use of knowledge from other fields or disciplines to guide nursing practice.

Nursing practice has borrowed knowledge in two ways. For years, some nurses have taken information from other disciplines and applied it directly to nursing practice. This information was not integrated within the unique focus of nursing. For example, some nurses have used the medical model to guide their nursing practice, thus focusing on the diagnosis and treatment of physiological diseases with limited attention to the patient's holistic nature. This type of borrowing continues today as nurses use technological advances to focus on the detection and treatment of disease, to the exclusion of health promotion and illness prevention.

Another way of borrowing, which is more useful in nursing, is the integration of information from other disciplines within the focus of nursing. Because disciplines share knowledge, it is sometimes difficult to know where the boundaries exist between nursing's knowledge base and the knowledge bases of other disciplines. Boundaries blur as the knowledge bases of disciplines evolve (McMurrey, 1982). For example, information about self-esteem as a characteristic of the human personality is associated with psychology, but this knowledge also directs the nurse in assessing the psychological needs of patients and families. However, borrowed knowledge has not been adequate to answer many questions generated in nursing practice.

Trial and Error

Trial and error is an approach with unknown outcomes that is used in a situation of uncertainty when other sources of knowledge are unavailable. The nursing profession evolved through a great deal of trial and error before knowledge of effective practices was codified in textbooks and journals. The trial-and-error way of acquiring knowledge can be time-consuming, because multiple interventions might be implemented before one is found to be effective. There is also a risk of implementing nursing actions that are detrimental to a patient's health. Because each patient responds uniquely to a situation, however, uncertainty in nursing practice continues. Because of the uniqueness of patient response and the resulting uncertainty, nurses must use trial and error in providing care. The trial-and-error approach to developing knowledge would be more efficient if nurses documented the patient and situational characteristics that provided the context for the patient's unique response.

Personal Experience

Personal experience is the knowledge that comes from being personally involved in an event, situation, or circumstance. In nursing, personal experience enables one to gain skills and expertise by providing care to patients and families in clinical settings. The nurse not only learns but is able to cluster ideas into a meaningful whole. For example, students may be told how to give an injection in a classroom setting, but they do not *know* how to give an injection until they observe other nurses giving injections to patients and actually give several injections themselves.

The amount of personal experience you have will affect the complexity of your knowledge base as a nurse. Benner (1984) described five levels of experience in the development of clinical knowledge and expertise that are important today. These levels of experience are (1) novice, (2) advanced beginner, (3) competent, (4) proficient, and (5) expert. *Novice nurses* have no personal experience in the work that they are to perform, but they have preconceived notions and expectations about clinical practice that are challenged, refined, confirmed, or contradicted by personal experience in a clinical setting. The *advanced beginner* has just enough experience to recognize and intervene in recurrent situations. For example, the advanced beginner nurse is able to recognize and intervene to meet patients' needs for pain management.

Competent nurses frequently have been on the job for 2 or 3 years, and their personal experiences enable them to generate and achieve long-range goals and plans (Benner, 1984). Through experience, the competent nurse is able to use personal knowledge to take conscious, deliberate actions that are efficient and organized. From a more complex knowledge base, the *proficient nurse* views the patient as a whole and as a member of a family and community. The proficient nurse recognizes that each patient and family have specific values and needs that lead them to respond differently to illness and health.

The *expert nurse* has had extensive experience and is able to identify accurately and intervene skillfully in a situation (Benner, 1984). Personal experience increases an expert nurse's ability to grasp a situation intuitively with accuracy and speed. Lyneham, Parkinson, and Denholm (2009) studied Benner's fifth stage of practice development and noted the links of intuition, science, knowledge, and theory to expert clinical

practice. The clinical expertise of the nurse is a critical component of evidence-based practice. It is the expert nurse who has the greatest skill and ability to implement the best research evidence in practice to meet the unique values and needs of patients and families.

Role-Modeling and Mentorship

Role-modeling is learning by imitating the behaviors of an exemplar. An exemplar or role model knows the appropriate and rewarded roles for a profession, and these roles reflect the attitudes and include the standards and norms of behavior for that profession (ANA, 2010a). In nursing, role-modeling enables the novice nurse to learn from interacting with expert nurses or following their examples. Examples of role models are admired teachers, expert practitioners, researchers, and illustrious individuals who inspire students, practicing nurses, educators, and researchers through their examples.

An intense form of role-modeling is mentorship. In a mentorship, the expert nurse, or mentor, serves as a teacher, sponsor, guide, exemplar, and counselor for the novice nurse (or mentee). Both the mentor and the mentee or protégé invest time and effort, which often result in a close, personal mentor-mentee relationship. This relationship promotes a mutual exchange of ideas and aspirations relative to the mentee's career plans. The mentee assumes the values, attitudes, and behaviors of the mentor while gaining intuitive knowledge and personal experience. Mentorship is essential for building research competence in nursing (Byrne & Keefe, 2002).

To summarize, in nursing, a body of knowledge must be acquired (learned), incorporated, and assimilated by each member of the profession and collectively by the profession as a whole. This body of knowledge guides the thinking and behavior of the profession and of individual practitioners. It also directs further development and influences how science and theory are interpreted within the discipline (see Figure 1-1). This knowledge base is necessary in order for health professionals, consumers, and society to recognize nursing as a science.

Philosophy

Philosophy provides a broad, global explanation of the world. It is the most abstract and most all-encompassing concept in the model (see Figure 1-1). Philosophy gives unity and meaning to the world of nursing and provides a framework within which thinking, knowing, and doing occur (Kikuchi & Simmons, 1994). Nursing's philosophical position influences its knowledge base. How nurses use science and theories to explain the empirical world depends on their philosophy. Ideas about truth and reality, as well as beliefs, values, and attitudes, are part of philosophy. Philosophy asks questions such as, "Is there an absolute truth, or is truth relative?" and "Is there one reality, or is reality different for each individual?"

Everyone's world is modified by her or his philosophy, as a pair of eyeglasses would modify vision. Perceptions are influenced first by philosophy and then by knowledge. For example, if what you see is not within your ideas of truth or reality, if it does not fit your belief system, you may not see it. Your mind may reject it altogether or may modify it to fit your philosophy (Scheffler, 1967). For example, you might believe that education is not effective in promoting smoking cessation, so you do not provide your patients this education. As you start to discover the world of nursing research, it is important for you to keep an open mind to the value of research and your future role in the development or use of research evidence in practice.

Philosophical positions commonly held within the nursing profession include the view that human beings are holistic, rational, and responsible. Nurses believe that people desire health, and health is considered to be better than illness. Quality of life is as important as quantity of life. Good nursing care facilitates improved patterns of health and quality of life (ANA, 2010a, 2010b). In nursing, truth is relative, and reality tends to vary with perception (Kikuchi, Simmons, & Romyn, 1996; Silva, 1977). For example, because nurses believe that reality varies with perception and that truth is relative, they would not try to impose their views of truth and reality on patients. Rather, they would accept patients' views of the world and help

them seek health from within those worldviews, an approach that is a critical component of evidence-based practice.

Significance of Research in Building an Evidence-Based Practice for Nursing

The ultimate goal of nursing is to provide evidence-based care that promotes quality outcomes for patients, families, healthcare providers, and the healthcare system (Craig & Smyth, 2012; Melnyk & Fineout-Overholt, 2011). **Evidence-based practice** (EBP) evolves from the integration of the best research evidence with clinical expertise and patient needs and values (Sackett, Straus, Richardson, Rosenberg, & Haynes, 2000). Figure 1-2 demonstrates the major contribution of the best research evidence to the delivery of EBP. **Best research evidence** is the empirical knowledge generated from the synthesis of quality study findings to address a practice problem. A discussion of the levels of best research evidence and the sources for this evidence is presented in Chapter 2. A team of expert researchers, healthcare professionals, policy makers, and consumers often synthesizes the best research evidence for developing standardized guidelines for clinical practice. For example, research related to the chronic health problem of hypertension (HTN) has been conducted, critically appraised, and synthesized by experts to develop a practice guideline for implementation by APNs, such as nurse practitioners, and physicians to ensure that patients with HTN receive quality, cost-effective care (Chobanian

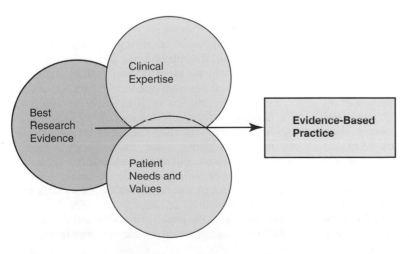

Figure 1-2 Model of evidence-based practice.

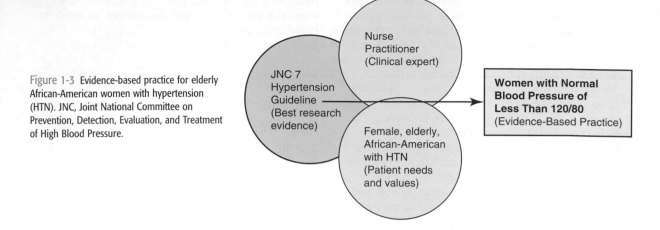

Figure 1-3 Evidence-based practice for elderly African-American women with hypertension (HTN). JNC, Joint National Committee on Prevention, Detection, Evaluation, and Treatment of High Blood Pressure.

et al., 2003). The most current guidelines for the diagnosis and management of HTN, "The Seventh Report of the Joint National Committee on Prevention, Detection, Evaluation, and Treatment of High Blood Pressure: The JNC 7 Report," were published in 2003 (Chobanian et al., 2003) and are available online at www.nhlbi.nih.gov/guidelines/hypertension. The JNC 8 Report is currently under development, with projected publication of the revised HTN guidelines in 2012 or 2013 (see http://www.nhlbi.nih.gov/guide lines/hypertension/jnc8). Many national standardized guidelines are available through the Agency for Healthcare Research and Quality (AHRQ) and professional organizations, which are discussed in more detail in Chapters 2 and 19.

Clinical expertise is the knowledge and skills of the healthcare professional providing care. A nurse's clinical expertise is determined by his or her years of practice, current knowledge of the research and clinical literature, and educational preparation. The stronger the nurse's clinical expertise, the better his or her clinical judgment is in the delivery of quality care (Craig & Smyth, 2012; Eizenberg, 2010). The patient's need(s) might focus on health promotion, illness prevention, acute or chronic illness management, or rehabilitation (see Figure 1-2). In addition, patients bring values or unique preferences, expectations, concerns, and cultural beliefs to the clinical encounter. With EBP, patients and their families are encouraged to take an active role in managing their health care. In summary, expert clinicians use the best research evidence available to deliver quality, cost-effective care to a patients and families with specific health needs and values to achieve EBP (Brown, 2009; Craig & Smyth, 2012; Sackett et al., 2000).

Figure 1-3 provides an example of the delivery of evidence-based care to women with HTN. In this example, the best research evidence on HTN is the JNC 7 National Standardized Guideline (Chobanian et al., 2003). An expert nurse practitioner translates this guideline to meet the needs (chronic illness management) and values of elderly African-American women with HTN. In this case, the outcome of EBP is women with a normal blood pressure, less than 120 mm Hg systolic/80 mm Hg diastolic (see Figure 1-3). A detailed discussion of how to locate, critically appraise, and use national standardized guidelines in practice is presented in Chapter 19.

In nursing, the research evidence must focus on the description, explanation, prediction, and control of phenomena important to practice. The following sections address the types of knowledge that need to be generated in these four areas as nursing moves toward EBP.

Description

Description involves identifying and understanding the nature of nursing phenomena and, sometimes, the relationships among them (Chinn & Kramer, 2008; Munhall, 2012). Through research, nurses are able to (1) explore and describe what exists in nursing practice, (2) discover new information, (3) promote understanding of situations, and (4) classify information for use in the discipline. Some examples of clinically important research evidence developed from research focused on description include the following:

- Identification of the responses of individuals to a variety of health conditions
- Description of the health promotion and illness prevention strategies used by various populations

- Determination of the incidence of a disease locally, nationally, and internationally
- Identification of the cluster of symptoms for a particular disease
- Description of the effects and side effects of selected pharmacological agents in a variety of populations

For example, Imes, Daugherty, Pyper, and Sullivan (2011, p. 208) conducted "a qualitative study to describe the experience of living with heart failure (HF) from the perspective of the partner." These researchers synthesized their findings as follows: "The severity of the patient's disease limited the partner's lifestyle, resulting in social isolation and difficulties in planning for the future for both the patient and the partner. The partners were unprepared to manage the disease burden at home without consistent information and assistance by healthcare providers. Moreover, end-of-life planning was neither encouraged by healthcare providers nor embraced by patients or partners" (Imes et al., 2011, p. 208).

The findings from this study provide insights into the experience of HF by a loved one and their experiences with healthcare providers. This type of research, focused on description, is essential groundwork for studies that will help to explain, predict, and control nursing phenomena.

Explanation

Explanation clarifies the relationships among phenomena and clarifies why certain events occur. Research focused on explanation provides the following types of evidence essential for practice:

- Determination of the assessment data (both subjective data from the health history and objective data from physical examination) needed to address a patient's health need
- Link of assessment data to determine a diagnosis (both nursing and medical)
- Link of causative risk factors or etiologies to illness, morbidity, and mortality
- Determine the relationships among health risks, health status, and healthcare costs

For example, Manojlovich, Sidani, Covell, and Antonakos (2011) conducted an outcomes study to examine the links between a "nurse dose" (nurse characteristics and staffing) and adverse patient outcomes. The nurse characteristics examined were education, experience, and skill mix. The staffing variables included full-time employees, RN:patient ratio, and RN hours per patient day. The adverse outcomes examined were methicillin-resistant *Staphylococcus aureus* (MRSA) infections and reported patient falls

for a sample of inpatient adults in acute care units. The researchers found that the nurse characteristics and staffing variables were significantly correlated with MRSA infections and reported patient falls. Thus, the nursing characteristics and staffing were potential predictors of MRSA infections and patient falls. This study illustrates how explanatory research can identify relationships among nursing phenomena that are the basis for future research focused on prediction and control.

Prediction

Through prediction, one can estimate the probability of a specific outcome in a given situation (Chinn & Kramer, 2008). However, predicting an outcome does not necessarily enable one to modify or control the outcome. It is through prediction that the risk of illness is identified and linked to possible screening methods that will identify the illness. Knowledge generated from research focused on prediction is critical for EBP and includes the following:

- Prediction of the risk for a disease in different populations
- Prediction of the accuracy and precision of a screening instrument, such as mammogram, to detect a disease
- Prediction of the prognosis once an illness is identified in a variety of populations
- Prediction of the impact of nursing actions on selected outcomes
- Prediction of behaviors that promote health and prevent illness
- Prediction of the health care required based on a patient's need and values

For example, Scheetz and Kolassa (2007, p. 399) examined "crash scene variables to predict the need for trauma center care in older persons." The researchers analyzed 26 crash scene variables and developed triage decision rules for managing persons with severe and moderate injuries. Further research is needed to determine whether the triage decision rules improve the health outcomes of the elderly following trauma. Predictive studies isolate independent variables that require additional research to ensure that their manipulation or control results in successful outcomes for patients, healthcare professionals, and healthcare agencies.

Control

If one can predict the outcome of a situation, the next step is to control or manipulate the situation to produce the desired outcome. Dickoff, James, and Wiedenbach (1968) described control as the ability to write a prescription to produce the desired results. Using the best research evidence, nurses could prescribe specific interventions to meet the needs of patients. Nurses need this type of research evidence to provide EBP (see Figure 1-2). Research in the following areas is important for generating EBP in nursing:

- Testing interventions to improve the health status of individuals, families, and communities
- Testing interventions to improve healthcare delivery
- Determining the quality and cost-effectiveness of interventions
- Implementing an evidence-based intervention to determine whether it is effective in managing a patient's health need (health promotion, illness prevention, acute and chronic illness management, and rehabilitation) and producing quality outcomes

Yoo, Kim, Hur, and Kim (2011) conducted a study that examined the effect of a prescribed animation distraction intervention on the pain response of preschool children during venipuncture. The intervention or independent variable was a 3-minute animation video that could be downloaded from the Internet and shown to the child using a laptop computer. The pain response was measured by the following dependent variables: "self-reported pain response, behavioral pain response, blood cortisol, and blood glucose" (Yoo et al., 2011, p. 94). The researchers found a significant difference between the experimental and control groups for all four dependent variables of pain response. Thus, the animation distraction intervention was determined to be an effective method of managing children's pain during venipuncture. The researchers concluded that this intervention required minimal effort and time and might be a convenient and cost-effective intervention to be used in clinical settings to reduce children's pain.

Many more studies need to be conducted to generate the research evidence in the areas of prediction and control (Brown, 2009; Craig & Smyth, 2012; Melnyk & Fineout-Overholt, 2011). This need for additional nursing research provides you with many opportunities to be involved in the world of nursing research. This chapter introduced you to the world of nursing research and the significance of research in developing an EBP for nursing. The following chapters will expand your understanding of different research methodologies so you can critically appraise studies, synthesize research findings, and use the best research evidence available in clinical practice. This text also gives you a background for conducting research in collaboration with expert nurse researchers. We think you will find that nursing research is an exciting adventure that holds much promise for the future practice of nursing.

KEY POINTS

- This chapter introduces you to the world of nursing research.
- Nursing research is defined as a scientific process that validates and refines existing knowledge and generates new knowledge that directly and indirectly influences the delivery of evidence-based nursing practice (EBP).
- This chapter presents a framework that links nursing research to the world of nursing and organizes the content presented in this textbook (see Figure 1-1). The concepts in this framework range from concrete to abstract and include concrete and abstract thinking, the empirical world (evidence-based nursing practice), research, abstract thought processes, science, theory, knowledge, and philosophy.
- The empirical world is what we experience through our senses and is the concrete portion of our existence where nursing practice occurs.
- Research is a way to test reality, and nurses use a variety of research methods to test their reality and generate nursing knowledge, such as quantitative, qualitative, outcomes, and intervention.
- All nurses have a role in research—some are developers of research and conduct studies to generate and refine the knowledge needed for nursing practice, and others are consumers of research and use research evidence to improve their nursing practice.
- Three major abstract thought processes—introspection, intuition, and reasoning—are important in nursing.
- A theory is a creative and rigorous structuring of ideas used to describe, explain, predict, or control a particular phenomenon or segment of the empirical world.
- Reliance on tradition, authority, trial and error, and personal experience is no longer an adequate basis for sound nursing practice.
- The goal of nurses and other healthcare professionals is to deliver evidence-based health care to patients and their families.
- EBP evolves from the integration of best research evidence with clinical expertise and patient needs and values (see Figure 1-2).
- The best research evidence is the empirical knowledge generated from the synthesis of quality studies to address a practice problem.

- The clinical expertise of a nurse is determined by his or her years of clinical experience, current knowledge of the research and clinical literature, and educational preparation.
- The patient brings values—such as unique preferences, expectations, concerns, and cultural beliefs, and health needs—to the clinical encounter, which are important to consider in providing evidence-based care.
- The knowledge generated through research is essential for describing, explaining, predicting, and controlling nursing phenomena.
- Nursing practice based on synthesized research findings can have a powerful, positive impact on patient outcomes and the healthcare system.

REFERENCES

Abbott, E. A. (1952). *Flatland*. New York, NY: Dover.

American Association of Colleges of Nursing (AACN, 2006). *AACN Position statement on nursing research*. Washington, DC: AACN. Retrieved from *http://www.aacn.nche.edu/Publications/positions/NsgRes.htm*.

American Nurses Association (ANA, 2012). *What is nursing?* Retrieved from *http://www.nursingworld.org/EspeciallyForYou/StudentNurses/WhatisNursing.aspx*.

American Nurses Association. (2010a). *Nursing: Scope and standards of practice* (2nd ed.). Silver Spring, MD: Author.

American Nurses Association. (2010b). *Nursing's social policy statement: The essence of the profession*. Silver Spring, MD: Author.

Barnum, B. S. (1998). *Nursing theory: Analysis, application, evaluation* (5th ed.). Philadelphia, PA: Lippincott Williams & Wilkins.

Benner, P. (1984). *From novice to expert: Excellence and power in clinical nursing practice*. Menlo Park, CA: Addison-Wesley.

Brar, K., Boschma, G., & McCuaig, F. (2010). The development of nurse practitioner preparation beyond the master's level: What is the debate about? *International Journal of Nursing Education Scholarship*, 7(1), Article 9.

Brown, S. J. (2009). *Evidence-based nursing: The research-practice connection*. Sudbury, MA: Jones and Bartlett.

Byrne, M. W., & Keefe, M. R. (2002). Building research competence in nursing through mentoring. *Journal of Nursing Scholarship*, 34(4), 391–396.

Chinn, P. L., & Kramer, M. K. (2008). *Theory and nursing: Integrated knowledge development* (6th ed.). St. Louis, MO: Mosby.

Chobanian, A.V., Bakris, G. L., Black, H. R., Cushman, W. C., Green, L. A., Izzo, J. L., et al. (2003). The seventh report of the Joint National Committee on prevention, detection, evaluation, and treatment of high blood pressure: The JNC 7 report. *Journal of the American Medical Association*, 289(19), 2560–2572.

Clinton, P., & Sperhac, A. M. (2006). National agenda for advanced practice nursing: The practice doctorate. *Journal of Professional Nursing*, 22(1), 7–14.

Craig, J. V., & Smyth, R. L. (2012). *The evidence-based practice manual for nurses* (3rd ed.). Edinburgh, Scotland: Churchill Livingstone.

Creswell, J. W. (2009). *Research design: Qualitative, quantitative, and mixed methods approaches* (3rd ed.). Los Angeles, CA: Sage.

Dickoff, J., James, P., & Wiedenbach, E. (1968). Theory in a practice discipline: Practice oriented theory (Part I). *Nursing Research*, 17(5), 415–435.

Doran, D. M. (2011). *Nursing-sensitive outcomes: State of the science*. Sudbury, MA: Jones & Bartlett.

Eizenberg, M. M. (2010). Implementation of evidence-based nursing practice: Nurses' personal and professional factors? *Journal of Advanced Nursing*, 67(1), 33–42.

Engelhardt, H. T., Jr. (1980). Knowing and valuing: Looking for common roots. In H. T. Engelhardt & D. Callahan (Eds.), *Knowing and valuing: The search for common roots* (Vol. 4, pp. 1–17). New York: Hastings Center.

Fahs, P. S., Morgan, L. L., & Kalman, M. (2003). A call for replication. *Journal of Nursing Scholarship*, 35(1), 67–71.

Fawcett, J., & Garity, J. (2009). *Evaluating research for evidence-based nursing practice*. Philadelphia, PA: F. A. Davis.

Forbes, A. (2009). Clinical intervention research in nursing. *International Journal of Nursing Studies*, 46(4), 557–568.

Greene, J. A. (1979). Science, nursing and nursing science: A conceptual analysis. *Advances in Nursing Science*, 2(1), 57–64.

Imes, C. C., Dougherty, C. M., Pyper, G., & Sullivan, M. D. (2011). Care of patients with heart failure: Descriptive study of partners' experiences of living with severe heart failure. *Heart & Lung*, 40(3), 208–216.

Kaplan, A. (1964). *The conduct of inquiry*. New York, NY: Harper & Row.

Kerlinger, F. N., & Lee, H. B. (2000). *Foundations of behavioral research* (4th ed.). Fort Worth, TX: Harcourt College Publishers.

Kikuchi, J. F., & Simmons, H. (1994). *Developing a philosophy of nursing*. Thousand Oaks, CA: Sage.

Kikuchi, J. F., Simmons, H., & Romyn, D. (1996). *Truth in nursing inquiry*. Thousand Oaks, CA: Sage.

Lyneham, J., Parkinson, C., & Denholm, C. (2009). Expert nursing practice: A mathematical explanation of Benner's 5th stage of practice development. *Journal of Advanced Nursing*, 65(11), 2477–2484.

Mackay, M. (2009). Why nursing has not embraced the clinician-scientist role. *Nursing Philosophy*, 10(4), 287–296.

Manojlovich, M., Sidani, S., Covell, C. L., & Antonakos, C. L. (2011). Nurse dose: Linking staffing variables to adverse patient outcomes. *Nursing Research*, 60(4), 214–220.

Marshall, C., & Rossman, G. B. (2011). *Designing qualitative research* (5th ed.). Los Angeles, CA: Sage.

McMurrey, P. H. (1982). Toward a unique knowledge base in nursing. *Image-Journal of Nursing Scholarship*, 14(1), 12–15.

Melnyk, B. M., & Fineout-Overholt, E. (2011). *Evidence-based practice in nursing & healthcare: A guide to best practice* (2nd ed.). Philadelphia, PA: Lippincott Williams & Wilkins.

Munhall, P. L. (2012). *Nursing research: A qualitative perspective* (5th ed.). Sudbury, MA: Jones & Bartlett Learning.

National League for Nursing (NLN, 2009). *Building a science of nursing education: Foundation for evidence-based teaching and learning*. New York, NY: Author.

Nightingale, F. (1859). *Notes on nursing: What it is, and what it is not*. Philadelphia, PA: Lippincott.

Odell, M., Victor, C., & Oliver, D. (2009). Nurses' role in detecting deterioration in ward patients: Systematic literature review. *Journal of Advanced Nursing*, 65(10), 1992–2006.

Polanyi, M. (1962). *Personal knowledge*. Chicago, IL: University of Chicago Press.

Polanyi, M. (1966). *The tacit dimension*. New York, NY: Doubleday.

Riley, J. M., Beal, J., Levi, P., & McCausland, M. P. (2002). Revisioning nursing scholarship. *Journal of Nursing Scholarship*, 34(4), 383–389.

Sackett, D. L., Straus, S. E., Richardson, W. S., Rosenberg, W., & Haynes, R. B. (2000). *Evidence-based medicine: How to practice & teach EBM* (2nd ed.). London, England: Churchill Livingstone.

Scheetz, L. J., & Kolassa, J. E. (2007). Using crash scene variables to predict the need for trauma center care in older persons. *Research in Nursing & Health*, 30(4), 399–412.

Scheffler, I. (1967). *Science and subjectivity*. Indianapolis, IN: Bobbs-Merrill.

Selye, H. (1976). *The stress of life*. New York, NY: McGraw-Hill.

Shadish, W. R., Cook, T. D., & Campbell, D. T. (2002). *Experimental and quasi-experimental designs for generalized causal inference*. Chicago, IL: Rand McNally.

Silva, M.C. (1977). Philosophy, science, theory: Interrelationships and implications for nursing research. *Image-Journal of Nursing Scholarship*, 9(3), 59–63.

Silva, M. C., & Rothbart, D. (1984). An analysis of changing trends in philosophies of science on nursing theory development and testing. *Advances in Nursing Science*, 6(2), 1–13.

Smith, A. (2009). Exploring the legitimacy of intuition as a form of nursing knowledge. *Nursing Standard*, 23 (40), 35–40.

Smith, M. J., & Liehr, P. R. (2008). *Middle range theory for nursing* (2nd ed.). New York, NY: Springer Publishing Company.

Walker, L. O., & Avant, K. C. (2011). *Strategies for theory construction in nursing* (5th ed.). Norwalk, CT: Appleton & Lange.

Waltz, C. F., Strickland, O. L., & Lenz, E. R. (2010). *Measurement in nursing and health research* (4th ed.). New York, NY: Springer Publishing Company.

White, A. R. (1982). *The nature of knowledge*. Totowa, NJ: Rowman & Littlefield.

Yoo, H., Kim, S., Hur, H., & Kim, H. (2011). The effects of an animation distraction intervention on pain response of preschool children during venipuncture. *Applied Nursing Research*, 24(2), 94–100.

2

Evolution of Research in Building Evidence-Based Nursing Practice

Initially, nursing research evolved slowly, from Florence Nightingale's investigations of patient mortality in the nineteenth century to the studies of nursing education in the 1930s and 1940s. Nurses and nursing roles were the focus of research in the 1950s and 1960s. However, in the late 1970s and 1980s, many researchers designed studies aimed at improving nursing practice. This emphasis continued in the 1990s with research focused on testing the effectiveness of nursing interventions and examining patient outcomes. The goal in this millennium is the development of an evidence-based practice for nursing, with the current best research evidence being used to deliver quality health care.

Evidence-based practice (EBP) is the conscientious integration of best research evidence with clinical expertise and patient values and needs in the delivery of quality, cost-effective health care. Chapter 1 presents a model depicting the elements of EBP and provides an example (see Figures 1-2 and 1-3). You probably have many questions about EBP because it is an evolving concept in nursing and health care. What does "best research evidence" mean? How is research evidence developed? Are there levels of quality in the types of research evidence? This chapter will increase your understanding of how nursing research has evolved over the past 150 years and of the current movement of the profession toward EBP. The chapter describes the historical events relevant to nursing research in building an EBP, identifies the methodologies used in nursing to develop research evidence, and concludes with a discussion of the best research evidence needed to build an EBP.

Historical Development of Research in Nursing

Some people think that research is relatively new to nursing, but Florence Nightingale initiated nursing research more than 150 years ago (Nightingale, 1859). Following Nightingale's work (1840-1910), nursing research received minimal attention until the mid-1900s. In the 1960s, nurses gradually recognized the value of research, but few had the educational background to conduct studies until the 1970s. However, in the 1980s and 1990s, research became a major force in developing a scientific knowledge base for nursing practice. Today, nurses obtain federal, corporate, and foundational funding for their research, conduct complex studies in multiple settings, and generate sound research evidence for practice. Table 2-1 identifies key historical events that have influenced the development of nursing research and the movement toward EBP. These events are discussed in the following section.

Florence Nightingale

Nightingale has been described as a reformer, reactionary, and researcher who influenced nursing specifically and health care in general. Nightingale's book, *Notes on Nursing* (1859), described her initial research activities, which focused on the importance of a healthy environment in promoting the patient's physical and mental well-being. She identified the need to gather data on the environment, such as ventilation, cleanliness, temperature, purity of water, and diet, to determine their influence on the patient's health (Herbert, 1981).

Nightingale is also noted for her data collection and statistical analyses during the Crimean War. She gathered data on soldier morbidity and mortality rates and the factors influencing them and presented her results in tables and pie charts, a sophisticated type of data presentation for the period (Cohen, 1984; Palmer, 1977). Nightingale was the first woman elected to the Royal Statistical Society (Oakley, 2010), and her research was highlighted in the periodical *Scientific American* in 1984 (Cohen, 1984).

TABLE 2-1	Historical Events Influencing Research in Nursing
Year	**Event**
1850	Florence Nightingale is recognized as the first nurse researcher.
1900	*American Journal of Nursing* is published.
1923	Teachers College at Columbia University offers the first educational doctoral program for nurses.
1929	First Master's in Nursing Degree is offered at Yale University.
1932	Association of Collegiate Schools of Nursing is organized to promote conduct of research.
1950	American Nurses Association (ANA) publishes study of nursing functions and activities.
1952	First research journal in nursing, *Nursing Research,* is published.
1953	Institute of Research and Service in Nursing Education is established.
1955	American Nurses Foundation is established to fund nursing research.
1957	Southern Regional Educational Board (SREB), Western Interstate Commission on Higher Education (WICHE), Midwestern Nursing Research Society (MNRS), and New England Board of Higher Education (NEBHE) are developed to support and disseminate nursing research.
1963	*International Journal of Nursing Studies* is published.
1965	ANA sponsors the first nursing research conferences.
1967	Sigma Theta Tau International Honor Society of Nursing publishes *Image,* emphasizing nursing scholarship; now entitled *Journal of Nursing Scholarship.*
1970	ANA Commission on Nursing Research is established.
1972	Cochrane published *Effectiveness and Efficiency,* introducing concepts relevant to evidence-based practice (EBP). ANA Council of Nurse Researchers is established.
1973	First Nursing Diagnosis Conference is held, which evolved into North American Nursing Diagnosis Association (NANDA).
1976	Stetler/Marram Model for Application of Research Findings to Practice is published.
1978	*Research in Nursing & Health* and *Advances in Nursing Science* are published.
1979	*Western Journal of Nursing Research* is published.
1980s-1990s	Sackett and colleagues developed methodologies to determine "best evidence" for practice.
1982-1983	Conduct and Utilization of Research in Nursing (CURN) Project is published.
1983	*Annual Review of Nursing Research* is published.
1985	National Center for Nursing Research (NCNR) is established to support and fund nursing research.
1987	*Scholarly Inquiry for Nursing Practice* is published.
1988	*Applied Nursing Research* and *Nursing Science Quarterly* are published.
1989	Agency for Health Care Policy and Research (AHCPR) is established and publishes EBP guidelines.
1990	*Nursing Diagnosis,* official journal of NANDA, is published; now entitled *International Journal of Nursing Terminologies and Classifications.* ANA established the American Nurses Credentialing Center (ANCC), which implemented the Magnet Hospital Designation Program for Excellence in Nursing Services.
1992	*Healthy People 2000* is published by the U.S. Department of Health and Human Services (DHHS). *Clinical Nursing Research* is published.
1993	NCNR is renamed the National Institute of Nursing Research (NINR) to expand funding for nursing research. *Journal of Nursing Measurement* is published. Cochrane Collaboration is initiated providing systematic reviews and EBP guidelines (http://www.cochrane.org/).
1994	*Qualitative Health Research* is published.
1999	AHCPR is renamed Agency for Healthcare Research and Quality (AHRQ).
2000	*Healthy People 2010* is published by DHHS. *Biological Research for Nursing* is published.
2001	Stetler publishes her model Steps of Research Utilization to Facilitate Evidence-Based Practice.
2002	Joint Commission revises accreditation policies for hospitals supporting evidence-based health care. NANDA becomes international—NANDA-I.
2004	*Worldviews on Evidence-Based Nursing* is published.
2011	NINR identifies mission and funding priorities (http://www.ninr.nih.gov/). *Healthy People 2020* is published; available at DHHS website http://www.healthypeople.gov/2020/topicsobjectives2020/default.aspx.
2012	AHRQ identifies mission and funding priorities (http://www.ahrq.gov/). American Nurses Association (ANA) Research Agenda is published.

Nightingale's research enabled her to instigate attitudinal, organizational, and social changes. She changed the attitudes of the military and society toward the care of the sick. The military began to view the sick as having the right to adequate food, suitable quarters, and appropriate medical treatment, a change that greatly reduced the mortality rate (Cook, 1913). Nightingale improved the organization of army administration, hospital management, and hospital construction. Because of Nightingale's research evidence and influence, society began to accept responsibility for testing public water, improving sanitation, preventing starvation, and decreasing morbidity and mortality rates (Palmer, 1977).

Early 1900s

From 1900 to 1950, research activities in nursing were limited, but a few studies advanced nursing education. These studies included the Nutting Report, 1912; Goldmark Report, 1923; and Burgess Report, 1926 (Abdellah, 1972; Johnson, 1977). On the basis of recommendations of the Goldmark Report, more schools of nursing were established in university settings. The baccalaureate degree in nursing provided a basis for graduate nursing education, with the first master of nursing degree offered by Yale University in 1929. Teachers College at Columbia University offered the first doctoral program for nurses in 1923 and granted a degree in education (Ed.D.) to prepare teachers for the profession. The Association of Collegiate Schools of Nursing, organized in 1932, promoted the conduct of research to improve education and practice. This organization also sponsored the publication of the first research journal in nursing, *Nursing Research*, in 1952 (Fitzpatrick, 1978).

A research trend that started in the 1940s and continued in the 1950s focused on the organization and delivery of nursing services. Studies were conducted on the numbers and kinds of nursing personnel, staffing patterns, patient classification systems, patient and nurse satisfaction, and unit arrangement. Types of care such as comprehensive care, home care, and progressive patient care were evaluated. These evaluations of care laid the foundation for the development of self-study manuals, which are similar to the quality assurance manuals of today (Gortner & Nahm, 1977).

Nursing Research in the 1950s and 1960s

In 1950, the American Nurses Association (ANA) initiated a 5-year study on nursing functions and activities. The findings were reported in *Twenty Thousand Nurses Tell Their Story*, and this study enabled the

ANA to develop statements on functions, standards, and qualifications for professional nurses. Also during this time, clinical research began expanding as specialty groups, such as community health, psychiatric, medical-surgical, pediatric, and obstetrical nurses, developed standards of care. The research conducted by ANA and the specialty groups provided the basis for the nursing practice standards that currently guide professional nursing practice (Gortner & Nahm, 1977).

Educational studies were conducted in the 1950s and 1960s to determine the most effective educational preparation for the registered nurse. A nurse educator, Mildred Montag, developed and evaluated the 2-year nursing preparation (associate degree) in junior colleges. Student characteristics, such as admission and retention patterns and the elements that promoted success in nursing education and practice, were studied for both associate and baccalaureate degree–prepared nurses (Downs & Fleming, 1979).

In 1953, an Institute for Research and Service in Nursing Education was established at Teachers College, Columbia University, which provided research-learning experiences for doctoral students (Werley, 1977). The American Nurse's Foundation, chartered in 1955, was responsible for receiving and administering research funds, conducting research programs, consulting with nursing students, and engaging in research. In 1956, a Committee on Research and Studies was established to guide ANA research (See, 1977).

A Department of Nursing Research was established in the Walter Reed Army Institute of Research in 1957. This was the first nursing unit in a research institution that emphasized clinical nursing research (Werley, 1977). Also in 1957, the Southern Regional Educational Board (SREB), the Western Interstate Commission on Higher Education (WICHE), Midwest Nursing Research Society (MNRS), and the New England Board of Higher Education (NEBHE) were developed. These organizations are actively involved in promoting research and disseminating the findings today. ANA sponsored the first of a series of research conferences in 1965, and the conference sponsors required that the studies presented be relevant to nursing and conducted by a nurse researcher (See, 1977). During the 1960s, a growing number of clinical studies focused on quality care and the development of criteria to measure patient outcomes. Intensive care units were being developed, promoting the investigation of nursing interventions, staffing patterns, and cost-effectiveness of care (Gortner & Nahm, 1977).

Nursing Research in the 1970s

In the 1970s, the nursing process became the focus of many studies, with the investigations of assessment techniques, nursing diagnoses classification, goal-setting methods, and specific nursing interventions. The first Nursing Diagnosis Conference, held in 1973, evolved into the North American Nursing Diagnosis Association (NANDA). In 2002, NANDA became international and is now known as NANDA-I. NANDA-I supports research activities focused on identifying appropriate diagnoses for nursing and generating an effective diagnostic process. NANDA's journal, *Nursing Diagnosis,* was published in 1990 and was later renamed *International Journal of Nursing Terminology and Classifications*. Details on NANDA-I can be found on their website at http://www.nanda.org/.

The educational studies of the 1970s evaluated teaching methods and student learning experiences. The National League for Nursing (NLN), founded in 1893, has had a major role in the conduct of research to shape nursing education. Currently, NLN provides programs, grants, and resources to advance nursing education research in "pursuit of quality nursing education for all types of nursing education programs" (NLN, 2011; http://www.nln.org/aboutnln/index.htm/). A number of studies were conducted to differentiate the practices of nurses with baccalaureate and associate degrees. These studies, which primarily measured abilities to perform technical skills, were ineffective in clearly differentiating between the two levels of education.

Primary nursing care, which involves the delivery of patient care predominantly by registered nurses (RNs), was the trend for the 1970s. Studies were conducted to examine the implementation and outcomes of primary nursing care delivery models. The number of nurse practitioners (NPs) and clinical nurse specialists (CNSs) with master's degrees increased rapidly during the 1970s. Limited research has been conducted on the CNS role; however, the NP and nurse midwifery roles have been researched extensively to determine their positive impact on productivity, quality, and cost of health care. In addition, those clinicians with master's degrees acquired the background to conduct research and to use research evidence in practice.

In the 1970s, nursing scholars began developing models, conceptual frameworks, and theories to guide nursing practice. The works of these nursing theorists also directed future nursing research. In 1978, a new journal, *Advances in Nursing Science*, began publishing the works of nursing theorists and the research

related to their theories. The number of doctoral programs in nursing and the number of nurses prepared at the doctoral level greatly expanded in the 1970s (Jacox, 1980). Some of the nurses with doctoral degrees increased the conduct and complexity of nursing research; however, many doctorally prepared nurses did not become actively involved in research. In 1970, the ANA Commission on Nursing Research was established; in turn, this commission established the Council of Nurse Researchers in 1972 to advance research activities, provide an exchange of ideas, and recognize excellence in research. The commission also prepared position papers on subjects' rights in research and on federal guidelines concerning research and human subjects, and it sponsored research programs nationally and internationally (See, 1977).

Federal funds for nursing research increased significantly, with a total of slightly more than $39 million awarded for research in nursing from 1955 to 1976. Even though federal funding for nursing studies rose, the funding was not comparable to the $493 million in federal research funds received by those doing medical research in 1974 alone (de Tornyay, 1977).

Sigma Theta Tau, the International Honor Society for Nursing, sponsored national and international research conferences, and the chapters of this organization sponsored many local conferences to promote the dissemination of research findings. *Image* was a journal initially published in 1967 by Sigma Theta Tau now titled *Journal of Nursing Scholarship,* the journal publishes many nursing studies and articles about research methodology. A major goal of Sigma Theta Tau is to advance scholarship in nursing by promoting the conduct, communication, and use of research evidence in nursing. The addition of two new research journals in the 1970s, *Research in Nursing & Health* in 1978 and *Western Journal of Nursing Research* in 1979, also increased the communication of nursing research findings. However, the findings of many studies conducted and published in the 1970s were not being used in practice, so Stetler and Marram (1976) developed a model to promote the communication and use of research findings in practice.

Professor Archie Cochrane originated the concepts of evidence-based practice with a book he published in 1972 titled *Effectiveness and Efficiency: Random Reflections on Health Services*. Cochrane advocated the provision of health care based on research to improve the quality of care and patient outcomes. To facilitate the use of research evidence in practice, the Cochrane Center was established in 1992, and the Cochrane Collaboration in 1993. The Cochrane Collaboration and Library house numerous resources to promote EBP, such as systematic reviews of research and evidence-based guidelines for practice (discussed later in this chapter) (see the Cochrane Collaboration at www.cochrane.org/).

Nursing Research in the 1980s and 1990s

The conduct of clinical nursing research was the focus in the 1980s and 1990s. A variety of clinical journals (*Achieves of Psychiatric Nursing; Cancer Nursing; Cardiovascular Nursing; Dimensions of Critical Care Nursing; Heart & Lung; Journal of Neurosurgical Nursing; Journal of Obstetric, Gynecologic, and Neonatal Nursing; Journal of Pediatric Nursing; Oncology Nursing Forum;* and *Rehabilitation Nursing*) published a growing number of studies. One new research journal was started in 1987, *Scholarly Inquiry for Nursing Practice,* and two in 1988, *Applied Nursing Research* and *Nursing Science Quarterly.*

Even though the body of empirical knowledge generated through clinical research grew rapidly in the 1970s and 1980s, little of this knowledge was used in practice. Two major projects were launched to promote the use of research-based nursing interventions in practice: the Western Interstate Commission for Higher Education (WICHE) Regional Nursing Research Development Project and the Conduct and Utilization of Research in Nursing (CURN) Project. In these projects, nurse researchers, with the assistance of federal funding, designed and implemented strategies for using research findings in practice. The WICHE Project participants selected research-based interventions for use in practice and then functioned as change agents to implement the selected intervention in a clinical agency. Because of the limited amount of research that had been conducted, the project staff and participants had difficulty identifying adequate clinical studies with findings ready for use in practice (Krueger, Nelson, & Wolanin, 1978).

The CURN Project was a 5-year venture (1975-1980) directed by Horsley, Crane, Crabtree, and Wood (1983) to increase the utilization of research findings by (1) disseminating findings, (2) facilitating organizational modifications necessary for implementation, and (3) encouraging collaborative research that was directly transferable to clinical practice. Research utilization was seen as a process to be implemented by an organization rather than by an individual nurse. The Project team identified the activities of research utilization to involve identification and synthesis of multiple studies in a common conceptual area (research base) as well as transformation of the knowledge derived from a research base into a solution or clinical protocol. The clinical protocol was then transformed

into specific nursing actions (innovations) that were administered to patients. The implementation of the innovation was to be followed by clinical evaluation of the new practice to ascertain whether it produced the predicted result (Horsley et al., 1983). The clinical protocols developed during the project were published to encourage nurses in other healthcare agencies to use these research-based intervention protocols in their practice (CURN Project, 1981-1982).

To ensure that the studies were incorporated into nursing practice, the findings needed to be synthesized for different topics. In 1983, the first volume of the *Annual Review of Nursing Research* was published (Werley & Fitzpatrick, 1983). This annual publication contains experts' reviews of research in selected areas of nursing practice, nursing care delivery, nursing education, and the profession of nursing. The *Annual Review of Nursing Research* continues to be published each year to (1) expand the synthesis and dissemination of research findings, (2) promote the use of research findings in practice, and (3) identify directions for future research.

Many nurses obtained master's and doctoral degrees during the 1980s and 1990s, and postdoctoral education was encouraged for nurse researchers. The ANA (1989) stated that nurses at all levels of education have a role in research, which extends from reading research to conducting complex, funded programs of research (see Chapter 1). Another priority of the 1980s and 1990s was to obtain greater funding for nursing research. Most of the federal funds in the 1980s were designated for studies involving the diagnosis and cure of diseases. Therefore, nursing received a small percentage of the federal research and development (R&D) funds (approximately 2% to 3%) compared with medicine (approximately 90%), even though nursing personnel greatly outnumbered medical personnel (Larson, 1984). However, in 1985, the ANA achieved a major political victory for nursing research with the creation of the National Center for Nursing Research (NCNR) within the National Institutes of Health (NIH). This center was created after years of work and two presidential vetoes (Bauknecht, 1986). The purpose of the National Center was to support the conduct of basic and clinical nursing research and the dissemination of findings. With its creation, nursing research had visibility at the federal level for the first time. In 1993, during the tenure of its first director, Dr. Ada Sue Hinshaw, the NCNR became the National Institute of Nursing Research (NINR). This change in title enhanced the recognition of nursing as a research discipline and expanded the funding for nursing research.

Outcomes research emerged as an important methodology for documenting the effectiveness of healthcare services in the 1980s and 1990s. This type of research evolved from the quality assessment and quality assurance functions that originated with the professional standards review organizations (PSROs) in 1972. During the 1980s, William Roper, the director of the Health Care Finance Administration (HCFA), promoted outcomes research for determining the quality and cost-effectiveness of patient care (Johnson, 1993).

In 1989, the Agency for Health Care Policy and Research (AHCPR) was established to facilitate the conduct of outcomes research (Rettig, 1991). This Agency also had an active role in communicating research findings to healthcare practitioners and was responsible for publishing the first evidence-based national clinical practice guidelines in 1989. Several of these guidelines, including the latest research findings with directives for practice, were published in the 1990s. The Healthcare Research and Quality Act of 1999 reauthorized the AHCPR, changing its name to the Agency for Healthcare Research and Quality (AHRQ, 2012). This significant change positioned the AHRQ as a scientific partner with the public and private sectors to improve the quality and safety of patient care by promoting the use of the best research evidence available in practice.

Building on the process of research utilization, physicians, nurses, and other healthcare professions focused on the development of EBP during the 1990s. A research group led by Dr. David Sackett at McMaster University in Canada developed explicit research methodologies to determine the "best evidence" for practice. The term *evidence based* was first used by David Eddy in 1990, with the focus on providing EBP for medicine (Craig & Smyth, 2012; Sackett, Straus, Richardson, Rosenberg, & Haynes, 2000).

In 1990, the ANA leaders established the American Nursing Credentialing Center (ANCC) and approved a recognition program for hospitals called the Magnet Hospital Designation Program for Excellence in Nursing Services (ANCC, 2012). This program has evolved over the last 20 years but has remained true to its commitment to promote research conducted by nurses in clinical settings and to support implementation of care based on the best current research evidence.

Nursing Research in the 21st Century

The vision for nursing research in the 21st century includes conducting quality studies through the use of a variety of methodologies, synthesizing the study findings into the best research evidence, using this research evidence to guide practice, and examining the outcomes of EBP (Brown, 2009; Craig & Smyth, 2012; Doran, 2011; Melnyk & Fineout-Overholt, 2011). The focus on EBP has become stronger over the last decade. In 2002, the Joint Commission on Accreditation of Healthcare Organizations (JCAHO) revised the accreditation policies for hospitals to support the implementation of evidence-based health care. To facilitate the movement of nursing toward EBP in clinical agencies, Stetler (2001) developed her Research Utilization to Facilitate EBP Model (see Chapter 19 for a description of this model). The focus on EBP in nursing was supported with the initiation of the *Worldviews on Evidence-Based Nursing* journal in 2004.

The focus of healthcare research and funding has expanded from the treatment of illness to include health promotion and illness prevention. *Healthy People 2000* and *Healthy People 2010,* documents published by the U.S. Department of Health and Human Services (U.S. DHHS 1992, 2000), have increased the visibility of health promotion goals and research. *Health People 2020* (U.S. DHHS, 2012) information is now available at the department's website, http://www.healthypeople.gov/2020/. Some of the new topics covered by *Healthy People 2020* include: adolescent health; blood disorders and blood safety; dementias; early and middle childhood; genomics; global health; healthcare-associated infections; lesbian, gay, bisexual, and transgender health; older adults; preparedness; sleep health; and social determinants of health. In the next decade, nurse researchers will have a major role in the development of interventions to promote health and prevent illness in individuals, families, and communities.

The AHRQ has been designated the lead agency supporting research designed to improve the quality of health care, reduce its cost, improve patient safety, decrease medical errors, and broaden access to essential services. The AHRQ sponsors and conducts research that provides evidence-based information on healthcare outcomes, quality, cost, use, and access. This research information promotes effective healthcare decision making by patients, clinicians, health system executives, and policy makers. The three future goals of the AHRQ are focused on the following:

Safety and quality: Reduce the risk of harm by promoting delivery of the best possible health care.

Effectiveness: Improve healthcare outcomes by encouraging the use of evidence to make informed healthcare decisions.

Efficiency: Transform research into practice to facilitate wider access to effective healthcare services and reduce unnecessary costs. (AHRQ, 2012)

AHRQ identifies funding priorities and research findings on their website at http://www.ahrq.gov/. Currently, the AHRQ and NINR work collaboratively to promote funding for nursing studies. These agencies often jointly call for proposals for studies of high priority to both agencies.

NINR is one of the most influential organizations committed to providing funding, support, and education to advance research in nursing. The current mission, goals, research priorities, and strategies of NINR are as follows:

The mission of the NINR is to promote and improve the health of individuals, families, communities, and populations. NINR supports and conducts clinical and basic research and research training on health and illness across the lifespan. The research focus encompasses health promotion and disease prevention, quality of life, health disparities, and end-of-life. NINR seeks to extend nursing science by integrating the biological and behavioral sciences, employing new technologies to research questions, improving research methods, and developing the scientists of the future. (NINR, 2011; http:// www.ninr.nih.gov/AboutNINR/NINRMissionand StrategicPlan/)

The NINR has supported the development of nurse scientists in genetics and genomics and sponsored the Summer Genetics Institute to expand nurses' contributions to genetic research. The funding priorities, funding process, and current research findings are available on the NINR website at http://www.ninr.nih.gov/.

The mission of ANA is to ensure the advancement of nurses in their profession to improve health for all. Central to this mission is the promotion of quality outcomes that require the use of research to provide EBP. ANA's (2012) research agenda can be viewed online. To accomplish this agenda, we need to ensure an effective research enterprise in nursing by (1) creating a research culture; (2) providing quality educational (baccalaureate, master's, doctoral, and post-doctoral) programs to prepare a workforce of nurse scientists; (3) developing a sound research infrastructure; and (4) obtaining sufficient funding for essential research (ANA, 2012; AACN, 1999, 2012). With this professional support, nurses can conduct studies using a variety of research methodologies to generate the essential knowledge needed to promote EBP and quality health outcomes for all.

Methodologies for Developing Research Evidence in Nursing

Scientific method incorporates all procedures that scientists have used, currently use, or may use in the future to pursue knowledge (Kaplan, 1964). This broad definition dispels the belief that there is one way to conduct research and embraces the use of both quantitative and qualitative research methodologies in developing research evidence for practice.

Since the 1930s, many researchers have narrowly defined scientific method to include only quantitative research. This research method is based on the philosophy of logical empiricism or positivism (Norbeck, 1987; Scheffler, 1967). Therefore, scientific knowledge is generated through an application of logical principles and reasoning whereby the researcher adopts a distant and noninteractive posture with the research subject to prevent bias (Silva & Rothbart, 1984). Thus, quantitative research is best defined as a formal, objective, systematic process implemented to obtain numerical data for understanding aspects of the world. This research method is used to describe variables, examine relationships among variables, and determine cause-and-effect interactions between variables (Kerlinger & Lee, 2000; Shadish, Cook, & Campbell, 2002). Currently, the predominantly used method of scientific investigation in nursing is quantitative research.

Qualitative research is a systematic, interactive, subjective, holistic approach used to describe life experiences and give them meaning (Marshall & Rossman, 2011; Munhall, 2012). Qualitative research is not a new idea in the social and behavioral sciences (Baumrind, 1980; Glaser & Strauss, 1967). This type of research is conducted to explore, describe, and promote understanding of human experiences, events, and cultures over time.

Comparison of Quantitative Research and Qualitative Research

The quantitative and qualitative types of research complement each other because they generate different kinds of knowledge that are useful in nursing practice. The problem and purpose to be studied determine the type of research to be conducted, and the researcher's knowledge of both types of research promotes

TABLE 2-2 Characteristics of Quantitative and Qualitative Research Methods

Characteristic	Quantitative Research	Qualitative Research
Philosophical origin	Logical positivism, post positivism	Naturalistic, interpretive, humanistic
Focus	Concise, objective, reductionistic	Broad, subjective, holistic
Reasoning	Logistic, deductive	Dialectic, inductive
Basis of knowing	Cause-and-effect relationships	Meaning, discovery, understanding
Theoretical focus	Tests theory	Develops theory and frameworks
Researcher involvement	Control	Shared interpretation
Methods of measurement	Structured interviews, questionnaires, observations, scales, physiological measures	Unstructured interviews, observations, focus groups
Data	Numbers	Words
Analysis	Statistical analysis	Text-based analysis
Findings	Acceptance or rejection of theoretical propositions Generalization	Uniqueness, dynamic, understanding of phenomena, new theory, models, and/or frameworks

accurate selection of the methodology for the problem identified (Creswell, 2009). Quantitative and qualitative research methodologies have some similarities, because both require researcher expertise, involve rigor in implementation, and result in the generation of scientific knowledge for nursing practice. Some of the differences between the two methodologies are presented in Table 2-2. Some researchers include both quantitative and qualitative research methodologies in their studies, an approach referred to as mixed methods research (see Chapter 10).

Philosophical Origins of Quantitative and Qualitative Research Methods

The quantitative approach to scientific inquiry emerged from a branch of philosophy called logical positivism, which operates on strict rules of logic, truth, laws, axioms, and predictions. Quantitative researchers hold the position that truth is absolute and that there is a single reality that one could define by careful measurement. To find truth as a quantitative researcher, you need to be completely objective, meaning that your values, feelings, and personal perceptions cannot enter into the measurement of reality. Quantitative researchers believe that all human behavior is objective, purposeful, and measurable. The researcher needs only to find or develop the "right" instrument or tool to measure the behavior.

Today, however, many nurse researchers base their quantitative studies on more of a postpositivist philosophy (Clark, 1998). This philosophy evolved from positivism but focuses on the discovery of reality that is characterized by patterns and trends that can be used to describe, explain, and predict phenomena. With

postpositivism, "truth can be discovered only imperfectly and in a probabilistic sense, in contrast to the positivist ideal of establishing cause-and-effect explanations of immutable facts" (Ford-Gilboe, Campbell, & Berman, 1995, p. 16). The postpositivist approach also rejects the idea that the researcher is completely objective about what is to be discovered but continues to emphasize the need to control environmental influences (Newman, 1992; Shadish et al., 2002).

Qualitative research is an interpretive methodological approach that values more of a subjective science than quantitative research. Qualitative research evolved from the behavioral and social sciences as a method of understanding the unique, dynamic, holistic nature of human beings. The philosophical base of qualitative research is interpretive, humanistic, and naturalistic and is concerned with helping those involved to understand the meaning of their social interactions. Qualitative researchers believe that truth is both complex and dynamic and can be found only by studying persons as they interact with and within their sociohistorical settings (Marshall & Rossman, 2011; Munhall, 2012).

Focuses of Quantitative and Qualitative Research Methods

The focus or perspective for quantitative research is usually concise and reductionistic. Reductionism involves breaking the whole into parts so that the parts can be examined. Quantitative researchers remain detached from the study and try not to influence it with their values (objectivity). Researcher involvement in the study is thought to bias or sway the study toward the perceptions and values of the researcher, and biasing a study is considered poor scientific technique (Creswell, 2009; Kerlinger & Lee, 2000; Shadish et al., 2002).

The focus of qualitative research is usually broad, and the intent is to give meaning to the whole (holistic). The qualitative researcher has an active part in the study and acknowledges that personal values and perceptions may influence the findings. Thus, this research approach is subjective, because the approach assumes that subjectivity is essential for understanding human experiences (Marshall & Rossman, 2011; Munhall, 2012).

Uniqueness of Conducting Quantitative Research and Qualitative Research

Quantitative research describes and examines relationships and determines causality among variables. Thus, this method is useful for testing a theory by testing the validity of the relationships that compose the theory (Creswell, 2009). Quantitative research incorporates logistic, deductive reasoning as the researcher examines particulars to make generalizations about the universe.

Qualitative research generates knowledge about meaning through discovery. Inductive reasoning and dialectic reasoning are predominant in these studies. For example, the qualitative researcher studies the whole person's response to pain by examining premises about human pain and determining the meaning that pain has for a particular person. Because qualitative research is concerned with meaning and understanding, researchers using qualitative approaches may identify relationships among the variables, and these relational statements may be used to develop and extend theories.

Quantitative research requires control (see Table 2-2). The investigator uses control to identify and limit the problem to be researched and attempts to limit the effects of extraneous or other variables that are not the focus of the study. For example, as a quantitative researcher, you might study the effects of nutritional education on serum lipid levels (total serum cholesterol, low-density lipoprotein [LDL] cholesterol, high-density lipoprotein [HDL] cholesterol, and triglycerides). You would control the educational program by manipulating the type of education provided, the teaching methods, the length of the program, the setting for the program, and the instructor. The nutritional program might be consistently implemented with the use of DVDs shown to subjects in a structured setting. You could also control other extraneous variables, such as participant's age, history of cardiovascular disease, and exercise level, because these extraneous variables might affect the serum lipid levels. The intent of this control is to more precisely examine the effects of nutritional education on serum lipid levels.

Quantitative research also requires the use of (1) structured interviews, questionnaires, or observations, (2) scales, and (3) physiological measures that generate numerical data. Statistical analyses are conducted to reduce and organize data, describe variables, examine relationships, and determine differences among groups. Control, precise measurement methods, and statistical analyses are used to ensure that the research findings accurately reflect reality so that the study findings can be generalized. Generalization involves the application of trends or general tendencies (which are identified by studying a sample) to the population from which the research sample was drawn. Researchers must be cautious in making generalizations, because a sound generalization requires the support of many studies with a variety of samples (Shadish et al., 2002).

Qualitative researchers use observations, interviews, and focus groups to gather data. The interactions are guided but not controlled in the way that quantitative data collection is controlled. For example, the researcher may ask subjects to share their experiences of powerlessness in the healthcare system. Qualitative researchers would begin interpreting the subjective data during data collection, recognizing that their interpretation is influenced by their own perceptions and beliefs (Munhall, 2012).

Qualitative data take the form of words and are analyzed according to the qualitative approach that is being used. The intent of the analysis is to organize the data into a meaningful, individualized interpretation, framework, or theory that describes the phenomenon studied. The findings from a qualitative study are unique to that study, and it is not the researcher's intent to generalize the findings to a larger population. Qualitative researchers are encouraged to question generalizations and to interpret meaning based on individual study participants' perceptions and realities (Munhall, 2012).

Classification of Research Methodologies Presented in this Text

Research methods used frequently in nursing can be classified in different ways, so a classification system was developed for this textbook and is presented in Box 2-1. This textbook includes quantitative, qualitative, outcomes, and intervention methods of research. The quantitative research methods are classified into four categories: (1) descriptive, (2) correlational, (3) quasi-experimental, and (4) experimental. Types of quantitative research are used to test theories and generate and refine knowledge for nursing practice. Quantitative research methods are introduced in this section and described in more detail in Chapter 3.

The qualitative research methods included in this textbook are (1) phenomenological research, (2) grounded theory research, (3) ethnographic research, (4) exploratory-descriptive qualitative research, and (5) historical research. These approaches, all methodologies for discovering knowledge, are introduced in this section and described in depth in Chapters 4 and 12. Unit Two of this textbook focuses on understanding the research process and includes discussions of both quantitative and qualitative research.

Quantitative Research Methods

Descriptive Research
Descriptive research provides an accurate portrayal or account of characteristics of a particular individual, situation, or group (Kerlinger & Lee, 2000). Descriptive studies offer researchers a way to (1) discover new meaning, (2) describe what exists, (3) determine the frequency with which something occurs, and (4) categorize information. Descriptive studies are usually conducted when little is known about a phenomenon and provide the basis for the conduct of correlational,

quasi-experimental, and experimental studies (Creswell, 2009).

Correlational Research
Correlational research involves the systematic investigation of relationships between or among two or more variables that have been identified in theories, observed in practice, or both. If the relationships exist, the researcher determines the type (positive or negative) and the degree or strength of the relationships. The primary intent of correlational studies is to explain the nature of relationships, not to determine cause and effect. However, correlational studies are the means for generating hypotheses to guide quasi-experimental and experimental studies that focus on examining cause-and-effect interactions.

Quasi-Experimental Research
The purposes of quasi-experimental studies are (1) to identify causal relationships, (2) to examine the significance of causal relationships, (3) to clarify why certain events happened, or (4) a combination of these objectives (Shadish et al., 2002). These studies test the effectiveness of nursing interventions that can then be implemented to improve patient and family outcomes in nursing practice.

Quasi-experimental studies are less powerful than experimental studies because they involve a lower level of control in at least one of three areas: (1) manipulation of the treatment or independent variable, (2) manipulation of the setting, and (3) selection of subjects. When studying human behavior, especially in clinical areas, researchers are commonly unable to manipulate or control certain variables. Also, subjects are usually not randomly selected but are selected on the basis of convenience. Thus, as a nurse researcher you will probably conduct more quasi-experimental than experimental studies.

Experimental Research
Experimental research is an objective, systematic, controlled investigation conducted for the purpose of predicting and controlling phenomena. This type of research examines causality (Shadish et al., 2002). Experimental research is considered the most powerful quantitative method because of the rigorous control of variables. Experimental studies have three main characteristics: (1) a controlled manipulation of at least one treatment variable (independent variable), (2) administration of the treatment to some of the subjects in the study (experimental group) and not to others (control group), and (3) random selection of subjects or random assignment of subjects to groups,

or both. Experimental studies usually are conducted in highly controlled settings, such as laboratories or research units in clinical agencies. A randomized controlled trial (RCT) is a type of experimental research that produces the strongest research evidence for practice.

Qualitative Research Methods

Phenomenological Research

Phenomenological research is a humanistic study of phenomena. The aim of phenomenology is to explore an experience as it is lived by the study participants and interpreted by the researcher. During the study, the researcher's experiences, reflections, and interpretations influence the data collected from the study participants (Munhall, 2012). Thus, the participants' lived experiences are expressed through the researcher's interpretations that are obtained from immersion in the study data and the underlying philosophy of the phenomenological study. Phenomenological research is an effective methodology for discovering the meaning of a complex experience as it is lived by a person, such as the lived experience of chronic illness.

Grounded Theory Research

Grounded theory research is an inductive research method initially described by Glaser and Strauss (1967). This research approach is useful for discovering what problems exist in a social setting and the processes people use to handle them. Grounded theory is particularly useful when little is known about the area to be studied or when what is known does not provide a satisfactory explanation. Grounded theory methodology emphasizes interaction, observation, and development of relationships among concepts. Throughout the study, the researcher explores, proposes, formulates, and validates relationships among the concepts until a theory evolves. The theory developed is "grounded," in or has its roots in, the data from which it was derived (Wuest, 2012).

Ethnographic Research

Ethnographic research was developed by anthropologists to investigate cultures through in-depth study of the members of the cultures. This type of research attempts to tell the story of people's daily lives while describing the culture in which they live. The ethnographic research process is the systematic collection, description, and analysis of data to develop a description of cultural behavior. The researcher (ethnographer) actually lives in or becomes a part of the cultural setting to gather the data. Through the use of

ethnographic research, different cultures are described, compared, and contrasted to add to our understanding of the impact of culture on human behavior and health (Wolf, 2012).

Exploratory-Descriptive Qualitative Research

Exploratory-descriptive qualitative research is conducted to address an issue or problem in need of a solution and/or understanding. Qualitative nurse researchers explore an issue or problem area using varied qualitative techniques with the intent of describing the topic of interest and promoting understanding. Although the studies result in descriptions and could be labeled as descriptive qualitative studies, most of the researchers are in the exploratory stage of studying the area of interest. This type of qualitative research usually lacks a clearly identified qualitative methodology, such as phenomenology, grounded theory, or ethnography. In this text, studies that the researchers identified as being qualitative without indicating a specific approach like phenomenology or grounded theory will be labeled as being exploratory-descriptive qualitative studies.

Historical Research

Historical research is a narrative description or analysis of events that occurred in the remote or recent past. Data are obtained from records, artifacts, or verbal reports. Through historical research, nursing has a way of understanding the discipline and interpreting its contributions to health care and society. Initial historical research focused on nursing leaders, such as Nightingale, and her contributions to nursing research and practice. In addition, the mistakes of the past can be examined to help nurses understand and respond to present situations affecting nurses and nursing practice. Thus, historical research has the potential to provide a foundation for and to direct the future movements of the profession (Lundy, 2012).

Outcomes Research

The spiraling cost of health care has generated many questions about the quality and effectiveness of healthcare services and the patient outcomes. Consumers want to know what services they are buying and whether these services will improve their health. Healthcare policy makers want to know whether the care is cost-effective and high quality. These concerns have promoted the development of **outcomes research**, which examines the results of care and measures the changes in health status of patients (AHRQ, 2012; Doran, 2011). Key ideas related to outcomes research are addressed throughout the text, and Chapter 13 contains a detailed discussion of this methodology.

Intervention Research

Intervention research investigates the effectiveness of a nursing intervention in achieving the desired outcome or outcomes in a natural setting. "Interventions are defined as treatments, therapies, procedures, or actions implemented by health professionals to and with clients, in a particular situation, to move the clients' condition toward desired health outcomes that are beneficial to the clients" (Sidani & Braden, 1998, p. 8). An intervention can be a specific treatment implemented to manage a well-defined patient problem or a program. A program intervention, such as a cardiac rehabilitation program, consists of multiple nursing actions that are implemented as a package to improve the health conditions of the participants (Brown, 2002; Forbes, 2009). The goal of intervention research is to generate sound scientific knowledge for actions or interventions that nurses can use to provide evidence-based nursing care. The details of intervention research are presented in Chapter 14. In summary, nurse researchers conduct a variety of research methodologies (quantitative, qualitative, outcomes, and intervention research) to develop the best research evidence for practice.

Introduction to Best Research Evidence for Practice

EBP involves the use of best research evidence to support clinical decisions in practice. As a nurse, you make numerous clinical decisions each day that affect the health outcomes of your patients and their families. By using the best research evidence available, you can make quality clinical decisions that will improve the health outcomes for patients, families, and communities. This section introduces you to the concept of best research evidence for practice by providing (1) a definition of the term *best research evidence*, (2) a model of the levels of research evidence available, and (3) a link of the best research evidence to evidence-based guidelines for practice.

Definition of Best Research Evidence

Best research evidence is a summary of the highest-quality, current empirical knowledge in a specific area of health care that is developed from a synthesis of quality studies (quantitative, qualitative, outcomes, and intervention) in that area. The synthesis of study

findings is a complex, highly structured process that is conducted most effectively by at least two researchers or even a team of expert researchers and healthcare providers. There are various types of research syntheses, and the type of synthesis conducted varies according to the quality and types of research evidence available.

The quality of the research evidence available in an area depends on the number and strength of the studies. Replicating or repeating of studies with similar methodology adds to the quality of the research evidence. The strengths and weaknesses of the studies are determined by critically appraising the validity or credibility of the study outcomes (see Chapter 18). The types of research commonly conducted in nursing were identified earlier in this chapter as quantitative, qualitative, outcomes, and intervention (see Box 2-1). The research synthesis process used to summarize knowledge varies for quantitative and qualitative research methods. In building the best research evidence for practice, the quantitative experimental study, such as an RCT, has been identified as producing the strongest research evidence for practice (Craig & Smyth, 2012; Institute of Medicine, 2001; Melnyk & Fineout-Overholt, 2011; Sackett et al., 2000).

Research evidence in nursing and health care is synthesized by using the following processes: (1) systematic review, (2) meta-analysis, (3) meta-synthesis, and (4) mixed methods systematic review. Depending on the quantity and strength of the research findings available, nurses and healthcare professionals use one or more of these four synthesis processes to determine the current best research evidence in an area. Table 2-3 identifies the processes used in research synthesis, the purpose of each synthesis process, the types of research included in the synthesis (sampling frame), and the analysis techniques used to achieve the synthesis of research evidence (Craig & Smyth, 2012; Sandelowski & Barroso, 2007; Whittemore, 2005).

A systematic review is a structured, comprehensive synthesis of the research literature to determine the best research evidence available to address a healthcare question. A systematic review involves identifying, locating, appraising, and synthesizing quality research evidence for expert clinicians to use to promote an EBP (Craig & Smyth, 2012; Higgins & Green, 2008). Teams of expert researchers, clinicians, and sometimes students conduct these reviews to determine the current best knowledge for use in practice. Systematic reviews are also used in the development of national and international standardized guidelines for managing health problems such as depression, hypertension, and type 2 diabetes. The

TABLE 2-3 Processes Used to Synthesize Research Evidence			
Synthesis Process	Purpose of Synthesis	Types of Research Included in the Synthesis (Sampling Frame)	Analysis for Achieving Synthesis
Systematic review	Use of specific, systematic methods to identify, select, critically appraise, and synthesize research evidence to address a particular problem in practice (Craig & Smyth, 2012; Higgins & Green, 2008).	Usually includes quantitative studies with similar methodology, such as randomized controlled trials (RCTs), and can also include meta-analyses focused on an area of the practice problem.	Narrative and statistical
Meta-analysis	Synthesis or pooling of the results from several previous studies using statistical analysis to determine the effect of an intervention or the strength of relationships (Higgins & Green, 2008).	Includes quantitative studies with similar methodology, such as quasi-experimental and experimental studies focused on the effect of an intervention or correlational studies focused on relationships.	Statistical
Meta-synthesis	Systematic compiling and integration of qualitative studies to expand understanding and develop a unique interpretation of the studies' findings in a selected area (Barnett-Page & Thomas, 2009; Finfgeld-Connett, 2010; Sandelowski & Barroso, 2007).	Uses original qualitative studies and summaries of qualitative studies to produce the synthesis.	Narrative
Mixed methods systematic review	Synthesis of the findings from independent studies conducted with a variety of methods (both quantitative and qualitative) to determine the current knowledge in an area (Higgins & Green, 2008).	Synthesis of a variety of quantitative, qualitative, and mixed methods studies.	Narrative

processes for critically appraising and conducting systematic reviews are detailed in Chapter 19.

A meta-analysis is conducted to statistically pool the results from previous studies into a single quantitative analysis that provides one of the highest levels of evidence about an intervention's effectiveness (Andrel, Keith, & Leiby, 2009; Craig & Smyth, 2012; Higgins & Green, 2008). The studies synthesized are usually quasi-experimental or experimental types of studies. In addition, a meta-analysis can be performed on correlational studies to determine the type (positive or negative) or strength of relationships among selected variables (see Table 2-3). Because meta-analyses involve statistical analysis to combine study findings, it is possible to be objective rather than subjective in synthesizing research evidence. Some of the strongest evidence for using an intervention in practice is generated from a meta-analysis of multiple, controlled quasi-experimental and experimental studies. Thus, many systematic reviews conducted to generate evidence-based guidelines include meta-analyses. The process for conducting a meta-analysis is presented in Chapter 19.

Qualitative research synthesis is the process and product of systematically reviewing and formally integrating the findings from qualitative studies (Sandelowski & Barroso, 2007). The process for conducting a synthesis of qualitative research is still in the developmental phase, and a variety of synthesis methods have appeared in the literature (Barnett-Page & Thomas, 2009; Finfgeld-Connett, 2010; Higgins & Green, 2008). In this text, the concept meta-synthesis is used to describe the process for synthesizing qualitative research. Meta-synthesis is defined as the systematic compiling and integration of qualitative study results to expand understanding and develop a unique interpretation of study findings in a selected area. The focus is on interpretation rather than the combining of study results as with quantitative research synthesis (see Table 2-3). The process for conducting a meta-synthesis is presented in Chapter 19.

Over the past 10 to 15 years, nurse researchers have conducted mixed methods studies (previously referred to as triangulation studies) that include both quantitative and qualitative research methods (Creswell, 2009). In addition, determining the current research evidence in an area might require synthesizing both quantitative and qualitative studies. Higgins and Green (2008) refer to this synthesis of quantitative, qualitative, and mixed methods studies as a mixed methods systematic review (see Table 2-3). Mixed methods systematic reviews might include a variety of study designs, such as qualitative research and quasi-experimental, correlational, and/or descriptive studies (Higgins & Green, 2008). Some researchers have conducted syntheses of quantitative and/or qualitative studies and called them "integrative reviews of research." In this text, the synthesis of a variety of quantitative and qualitative study findings is referred to as *mixed methods systematic reviews*. The value of these reviews depends on the standards used to the conduct them. The process for conducting a mixed method systematic review is discussed in Chapter 19.

Levels of Research Evidence

The strength or validity of the best research evidence in an area depends on the quality and quantity of the

studies conducted in the area. Quantitative studies, especially experimental studies like RCTSs, are thought to provide the strongest research evidence. In addition, the replication of studies with similar methodology increases the strength of the research evidence generated. The levels of the research evidence can be visualized as a continuum with the highest quality of research evidence at one end and weakest research evidence at the other (see Figure 2-1) (Craig & Smyth, 2012; Higgins & Green, 2008; Melnyk & Fineout-Overholt, 2011). The systematic research reviews and meta-analyses of high-quality experimental studies provide the strongest or best research evidence for use by expert clinicians in practice. Meta-analyses and integrative reviews of quasi-experimental and experimental studies also provide

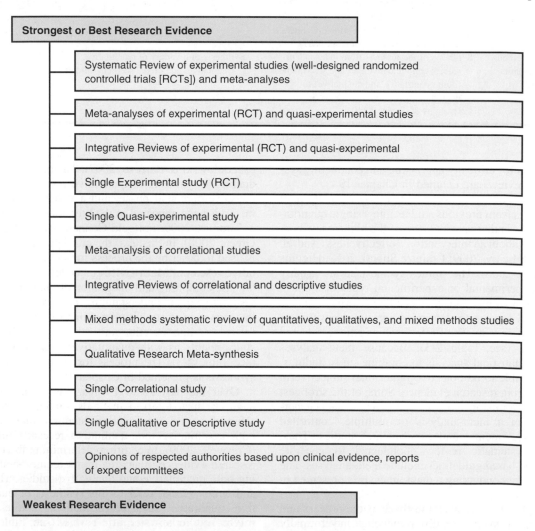

Strongest or Best Research Evidence

Systematic Review of experimental studies (well-designed randomized controlled trials [RCTs]) and meta-analyses

Meta-analyses of experimental (RCT) and quasi-experimental studies

Integrative Reviews of experimental (RCT) and quasi-experimental

Single Experimental study (RCT)

Single Quasi-experimental study

Meta-analysis of correlational studies

Integrative Reviews of correlational and descriptive studies

Mixed methods systematic review of quantitatives, qualitatives, and mixed methods studies

Qualitative Research Meta-synthesis

Single Correlational study

Single Qualitative or Descriptive study

Opinions of respected authorities based upon clinical evidence, reports of expert committees

Weakest Research Evidence

Figure 2-1 Levels of research evidence.

strong research evidence for managing practice problems. Correlational, descriptive, and qualitative studies direct further research and provide some useful findings for practice (see Figure 2-1). The weakest evidence comes from expert opinions, which can include expert clinicians' opinions or the opinions expressed in committee reports. When making a decision in your clinical practice, be sure to base your decision on the best research evidence available.

The levels of research evidence identified in Figure 2-1 help nurses determine the quality and validity of the evidence that is available for them to use in practice. Advance practice nurses must seek out the best research knowledge available in an area to ensure that they manage patients' acute and chronic illnesses with quality care (Craig & Smyth, 2012; Higgins & Green, 2008; Melnyk & Fineout-Overholt, 2011). This best research evidence generated from systematic reviews, meta-analyses, and mixed methods systematic reviews is used most often to develop standardized or evidence-based guidelines for practice.

Introduction to Evidence-Based Practice Guidelines

Evidence-based practice guidelines are rigorous, explicit clinical guidelines that are based on the best research evidence available in that area. These guidelines are usually developed by a team or panel of expert researchers; expert clinicians (physicians, nurses, pharmacists, and other health professionals); and sometimes consumers, policy makers, and economists. The expert panel seeks consensus on the content of the guideline to provide clinicians with the best information for making clinical decisions in practice. There has been a dramatic growth in the production of EBP guidelines to assist healthcare providers in building an EBP and in improving healthcare outcomes for patients, families, providers, and healthcare agencies.

Every year, new guidelines are developed, and some of the existing guidelines are revised on the basis of new research evidence. These guidelines have become the gold standard (or standard of excellence) for patient care, and nurses and other healthcare providers are encouraged to incorporate these standardized guidelines into their practice. Expert national and international government agencies, professional organizations, and centers of excellence have made many of these evidence-based guidelines available online. When selecting a guideline for practice, be sure that a credible agency or organization developed the guideline and that the reference list reflects the synthesis of extensive research evidence.

An extremely important source for evidence-based guidelines in the United States is the National Guideline Clearinghouse (NGC), which was initiated in 1998 by the AHRQ. The Clearinghouse started with 200 guidelines and has expanded to contain more than 1500 EBP guidelines (see http://www.guideline.gov/). Another excellent source of systematic reviews and EBP guidelines is the Cochrane Collaboration and Library in the United Kingdom, which can be accessed at http://www.cochrane.org/. The Joanna Briggs Institute has also been a leader in developing evidence-based guidelines for nursing practice (http://www.joannabriggs.edu.au/). In addition, professional nursing organizations, such as the Oncology Nursing Society (http://www.ons.org/) and the National Association of Neonatal Nurses (http://www.nann.org/), have developed EBP guidelines for their specialties. These websites will introduce you to some of guidelines that exist nationally and internationally. Chapter 19 will help you to critically appraise the quality of an EBP guideline and implement that guideline in your practice.

--- **KEY POINTS** ---

- Florence Nightingale initiated nursing research more than 150 years ago; this start was followed by decades of limited research. During the 1950s and 1960s, research became a higher priority, with the development of graduate programs in nursing that increased the number of nurses with doctorates and master's degrees. In the 1970s and 1980s, the major focus was on the conduct of clinical research to improve nursing practice.
- Outcomes research emerged as an important methodology for documenting the effectiveness of healthcare service in the 1980s and 1990s. In 1989, the Agency for Health Care Policy and Research (later renamed the Agency for Healthcare Research and Quality [AHRQ]) was established to facilitate the conduct of outcomes research.
- The vision for nursing in the 21st century is the development of a scientific knowledge base that enables nurses to implement an EBP.
- Nursing research incorporates quantitative, qualitative, outcomes, and intervention research methodologies.
- Quantitative research is classified into four types for this textbook: descriptive, correlational, quasi-experimental, and experimental.
- Qualitative research is classified into five types for this textbook: phenomenological research,

grounded theory research, ethnographic research, exploratory-descriptive qualitative research, and historical research.

- Outcomes research focuses on determining the end results of care or a measure of the change in health status of the patient and family.

- Intervention research involves the investigation of the effectiveness of a nursing intervention in achieving the desired outcomes in a natural setting.

- Best research evidence is a summary of the highest-quality, current empirical knowledge in a specific area of health care that is developed from a synthesis of high-quality studies (quantitative, qualitative, outcomes, and intervention) in that area.

- Research evidence in nursing and health care is synthesized using the following processes: (1) systematic review, (2) meta-analysis, (3) meta-synthesis, and (4) mixed methods systematic review.

- The levels of the research evidence can be thought of as a continuum with the highest quality of research evidence at one end and the weakest at the other. The best research evidence is synthesized by a team or panel of experts to develop evidence-based guidelines for clinicians in practice.

- EBP guidelines are rigorous, explicit clinical guidelines that are based on the best research evidence available in that area.

- EBP guidelines have become the gold standard (or standard of excellence) for patient care, and nurses and other healthcare providers are encouraged to incorporate them into their practice.

REFERENCES

Abdellah, F. G. (1972). Evolution of nursing as a profession. *International Nursing Review, 19*(3), 219–235.

Agency for Healthcare Research and Quality (AHRQ, 2012). *AHRQ at a glance.* Retrieved http://www.ahrq.gov/about/ataglance.htm/.

American Association of Colleges of Nursing (AACN, 1999). Position statement on nursing research. *Journal of Professional Nursing, 15*(4), 253–257.

American Association of Colleges of Nursing (AACN, 2012). *Missions and values.* Retrieved from *http://www.aacn.nche.edu/about-aacn/mission-values/.*

American Nurses Association (ANA, 1950). *Twenty thousand nurses tell their story.* Kansas City, MO: Author.

American Nurses Association (ANA, 1989). *Education for participation in nursing research.* Kansas City, MO: Author.

American Nurses Association (ANA, 2012). *American Nurses Association Research Agenda.* Retrieved from *http://www.nursingworld.org/MainMenuCategories/ThePracticeofProfessionalNursing/PatientSafetyQuality/Research-Measurement/Research-Agenda-.asp/.*

American Nurses Credentialing Center (ANCC, 2012). *Magnet Program Overview.* Retrieved from http://www.nursecredentialing.org/Magnet/ProgramOverview.aspx.

Andrel, J. A., Keith, S. W., & Leiby, B. E. (2009). Meta-analysis: A brief introduction. *Clinical & Translational Science, 2*(5), 374–378.

Barnett-Page, E., & Thomas, J. (2009). Methods for the synthesis of qualitative research: A critical review. *BMC Medical Research Methodology, 9,* 59. DOI: 10.1186/147–2288-9-59.

Bauknecht, V. L. (1986). Congress overrides veto, nursing gets center for research. *American Nurse, 18*(1), 24.

Baumrind, D. (1980). New directions in socialization research. *American Psychologist, 35*(7), 639–652.

Brown, S. J. (2002). Focus on research methods. Nursing intervention studies: A descriptive analysis of issues important to clinicians. *Research in Nursing & Health, 25*(4), 317–327.

Brown, S. J. (2009). *Evidence-based nursing: The research-practice connection.* Sudbury, MA: Jones and Bartlett Publishers.

Clark, A. M. (1998). The qualitative-quantitative debate: Moving from positivism and confrontation to post-positivism and reconciliation. *Journal of Advanced Nursing, 271*(6), 1242–1249.

Cohen, B. (1984). Florence Nightingale. *Scientific American, 250*(3), 128–137.

Conduct and Utilization of Research in Nursing (CURN) Project. (1981-1982). *Using research to improve nursing practice.* New York, NY: Grune & Stratton.

Cook, Sir E. (1913). *The life of Florence Nightingale (Vol. 1).* London, England: Macmillan.

Craig, J. V., & Smyth, R. L. (2012). *The evidence-based practice manual for nurses* (3rd ed.). Edinburgh, Scotland: Churchill Livingstone.

Creswell, J. W. (2009). *Research design: Qualitative, quantitative, and mixed methods approaches* (3rd ed.). Los Angeles, CA: Sage.

de Tornyay, R. (1977). Nursing research—the road ahead. *Nursing Research, 26*(6), 404–407.

Doran, D. M. (2011). *Nursing-sensitive outcomes: State of the science.* Sudbury, MA: Jones & Bartlett.

Downs, F. S., & Fleming, W. J. (1979). *Issues in nursing research.* New York, NY: Appleton-Century-Crofts.

Finfgeld-Connett, D. (2010). Generalizability and transferability of meta-synthesis research findings. *Journal of Advanced Nursing, 66*(2), 246–254.

Fitzpatrick, M. L. (1978). *Historical studies in nursing.* New York, NY: Teachers College Press.

Forbes, A. (2009). Clinical intervention research in nursing. *International Journal of Nursing Studies, 46*(4), 557–568.

Ford-Gilboe, M., Campbell, J., & Berman, H. (1995). Stories and numbers: Coexistence without compromise. *Advances in Nursing Science, 18*(1), 14–26.

Glaser, B. G., & Strauss, A. L. (1967). *The discovery of grounded theory: Strategies for qualitative research.* Chicago, IL: Aldine.

Gortner, S. R., & Nahm, H. (1977). An overview of nursing research in the United States. *Nursing Research, 26*(1), 10–33.

Herbert, R. G. (1981). *Florence Nightingale: Saint, reformer or rebel?* Malabar, FL: Robert E. Krieger.

Higgins, J. P. T., & Green, S. (2008). *Cochrane handbook for systematic reviews of interventions.* West Sussex, England: Wiley-Blackwell and The Cochrane Collaboration.

Horsley, J. A., Crane, J., Crabtree, M. K., & Wood, D. J. (1983). *Using research to improve nursing practice: A guide; CURN Project*. New York, NY: Grune & Stratton.

Institute of Medicine. (2001). *Crossing the quality chasm: A new health system for the 21ˢᵗ century*. Washington, DC: National Academy Press.

Jacox, A. (1980). Strategies to promote nursing research. *Nursing Research, 29*(4), 213–218.

Johnson, J. E. (1993). Outcomes research and health care reform: Opportunities for nurses. *Nursing Connections, 6*(4), 1–3.

Johnson, W. L. (1977). Research programs of the National League for Nursing. *Nursing Research, 26*(3), 172–176.

Kaplan, A. (1964). *The conduct of inquiry: Methodology for behavioral science*. New York, NY: Chandler.

Kerlinger, F. N., & Lee, H. B. (2000). *Foundations of behavioral research* (4th ed.). Fort Worth, TX: Harcourt.

Krueger, J. C., Nelson, A. H., & Wolanin, M. A. (1978). *Nursing research: Development, collaboration, and utilization*. Germantown, MD: Aspen.

Larson, E. (1984). Health policy and NIH: Implications for nursing research. *Nursing Research, 33*(6), 352–356.

Lundy, K. S. (2012). Historical research. In P. L. Munhall (Ed.), *Nursing research: A qualitative perspective* (5th ed., pp. 381–397). Sudbury, MA: Jones & Bartlett Learning.

Marshall, C., & Rossman, G. B. (2011). *Designing qualitative research* (5th ed.). Los Angeles, CA: Sage.

Melnyk, B. M., & Fineout-Overholt, E. (2011). *Evidence-based practice in nursing & healthcare: A guide to best practice* (2nd ed.). Philadelphia, PA: Lippincott Williams & Wilkins.

Munhall, P. L. (2012). *Nursing research: A qualitative perspective* (5th ed.). Sudbury, MA: Jones & Bartlett Learning.

National Institute of Nursing Research (NINR, 2011). *NINR mission and strategic plan*. Retrieved from *http://www.ninr.nih.gov/AboutNINR/NINRMissionandStrategicPlan/*

National League for Nursing (NLN; 2011). *About the NLN*. Retrieved from *http://www.nln.org/aboutnln/index.htm*.

Newman, M. A. (1992). Prevailing paradigms in nursing. *Nursing Outlook, 40*(1), 10–13, 32.

Nightingale, F. (1859). *Notes on nursing: What it is, and what it is not*. Philadelphia, PA: Lippincott.

Norbeck, J. S. (1987). In defense of empiricism. *Image—Journal of Nursing Scholarship, 19*(1), 28–30.

Oakley, K. (2010). Nursing by the numbers. *Occupational Health, 62*(4), 28–29.

Palmer, I. S. (1977). Florence Nightingale: Reformer, reactionary, researcher. *Nursing Research, 26*(2), 84–89.

Rettig, R. (1991). History, development, and importance to nursing of outcomes research. *Journal of Nursing Quality Assurance, 5*(2), 13–17.

Sackett, D. L., Straus, S. E., Richardson, W. S., Rosenberg, W., & Haynes, R. B. (2000). *Evidence-based medicine: How to practice & teach EBM* (2nd ed.). London, England: Churchill Livingstone.

Sandelowski, M., & Barroso, J. (2007). *Handbook for synthesizing qualitative research*. New York, NY: Springer.

Scheffler, I. (1967). *Science and subjectivity*. Indianapolis, IN: Bobbs-Merrill.

Shadish, S. R., Cook, T. D., & Campbell, D. T. (2002). *Experimental and quasi-experimental designs for generalized causal inference*. Boston, MA: Houghton Mifflin Company.

See, E. M. (1977). The ANA and research in nursing. *Nursing Research, 26*(3), 165–171.

Sidani, S., & Braden, C. P. (1998). *Evaluating nursing interventions: A theory-driven approach*. Thousand Oaks, CA: Sage.

Silva, M. C., & Rothbart, D. (1984). An analysis of changing trends in philosophies of science on nursing theory development and testing. *Advances in Nursing Science, 6*(2), 1–13.

Stetler, C. B. (2001). Updating the Stetler Model of research utilization to facilitate evidence-based practice. *Nursing Outlook, 49*(6), 272–279.

Stetler, C. B., & Marram, G. (1976). Evaluating research findings for applicability in practice. *Nursing Outlook, 24*(9), 559–563.

U.S. Department of Health and Human Services (DHHS, 1992). *Healthy People 2000*. Washington, D.C.: Author.

U.S. Department of Health and Human Services (DHHS, 2000). *Healthy People 2010*. Washington, D.C.: Author.

U.S. Department of Health and Human Services (DHHS, 2012). *Health People 2020 topics and objectives*. Retrieved from http://www.healthypeople.gov/2020/topicsobjectives2020/default.aspx.

Werley, H. H. (1977). Nursing research in perspective. *International Nursing Review, 24*(3), 75–83.

Werley, H. H., & Fitzpatrick, J. J. (Eds.) (1983). *Annual review of nursing research* (Vol. 1). New York, NY: Springer.

Wolf, Z. (2012). Ethnography: The method. In P. L. Munhall (Ed.), *Nursing research: A qualitative perspective* (5th ed., pp. 285–338). Sudbury, MA: Jones & Bartlett Learning.

Wuest, J. (2012). Grounded theory: The method. In P. L. Munhall (Ed.), *Nursing research: A qualitative perspective* (5th ed., pp. 225–256). Sudbury, MA: Jones & Bartlett Learning.

Whittemore, R. (2005). Combining evidence in nursing research: Methods and implications. *Nursing Research, 54*(1), 56–62.

3

CHAPTER

Introduction to Quantitative Research

What do you think of when you hear the word *research*? Frequently, the word *experiment* comes to mind. One might equate experiments with randomizing subjects into groups, collecting data, and conducting statistical analyses. Many people believe that an experiment is conducted to answer a clinical question, such as "Is one pain medicine more effective than another?" These ideas are associated with the classic experimental design originated by Sir Ronald Fisher (1935). Fisher is noted for adding structure and control to the steps of the quantitative research process to decrease the potential for error and improve the accuracy of study findings.

Four types of quantitative research are included in this text: descriptive, correlational, quasi-experimental, and experimental. Fisher's experimentation provided the groundwork for what is now known as experimental research. Throughout the years, other quantitative approaches have been developed. Campbell and Stanley (1963) are noted for developing quasi-experimental designs for conducting quantitative research. Karl Pearson (Kerlinger & Lee, 2000) developed statistical approaches for examining relationships among variables, which increased the conduct of correlational research. The fields of sociology, education, and psychology are noted for their development and expansion of strategies for conducting descriptive research. The steps of the research process used in these different types of quantitative study are the same, but the philosophy and strategies for implementing these steps vary with the approach.

Many quantitative research approaches and designs are essential to develop the body of knowledge needed for evidence-based practice. Thus, quantitative research is a major focus throughout this textbook. This chapter provides an overview of quantitative research by (1) discussing concepts relevant to quantitative research, (2) identifying the steps of the quantitative research process, and (3) providing examples of different types of quantitative studies.

Concepts Relevant to Quantitative Research

Some concepts relevant to quantitative research are basic research, applied research, rigor, and control. These concepts are defined here, and the major points are reinforced with examples from quantitative studies.

Basic Research

Basic, or pure, research is a scientific investigation that involves the pursuit of "knowledge for knowledge's sake," or for the pleasure of learning and finding truth (Nagel, 1961). The purpose of basic research is to generate and refine theory and build constructs; thus, the findings are frequently not directly useful in practice. However, because the findings are more theoretical in nature, they can be generalized to various settings (Wysocki, 1983).

Basic research also examines pathological and physiological responses as well as underlying mechanisms of actions of an intervention or outcome (Fawcett & Garity, 2009). Often basic research is conducted in a laboratory with animals or human tissues. For example, cachexia in cancer patients clinically manifests as anorexia, weight loss, and wasting of skeletal muscles that decrease patients' functioning and quality of life. Cachexia is a very complex process that has been studied for many years, but the knowledge of the specific causes and progression of this condition is still evolving. Thus, additional basic research is needed to examine the pathology of cancer cachexia with skeletal muscle wasting. For example, Byerley et al. (2010) conducted a basic study to examine the causes of body fat loss early in the development of cancer cachexia in male rats. Their study findings are summarized in the following excerpt:

"We provide evidence that a factor other than the previously identified lipid mobilizing factor, zinc alpha-2 glycoprotein, promotes lipolysis in the … sarcoma-bearing cachexia model.… We compared tumor-bearing ad lib fed (TB) animals to nontumor-bearing ad lib fed (NTB) animals.… Prior to cachexia, the TB animals lost more than $10 \pm 0.7\%$ of their body fat before losing protein mass and decreasing their food intake. Fat loss occurred because adipocyte size, not number, was reduced.… Yet circulating levels of norepinephrine, epinephrine, and TNF-α [tissue necrosing factor-alpha], and zinc alpha-2 glycoprotein were not increased prior to the loss of fat mass. We provide evidence for a serum factor(s), other than zinc alpha-2 glycoprotein, that stimulates release of glycerol from 3T3-L1 adipocytes and promotes the loss of stored adipose lipid prior to the loss of lean body mass in this model." (Byerley et al., 2010, p. 484)

Byerley and colleagues' (2010) study demonstrates the importance of genetic research in understanding disease pathology. It provides the basis for further research to isolate and characterize the lipolytic protein causing loss of body fat in animals with cancer. This basic research in animals provides the basis for human research in this area. A major force in genetic research is the National Human Genome Research Institute (NHGRI) (2012), which plans and conducts a broad program of laboratory research to improve our understanding of the human genetic makeup, genetics of diseases, and potential gene therapy. This basic research provides a basis for conducting applied "clinical research to translate genomic and genetic research into a greater understanding of human genetic disease, and to develop better methods for the detection, prevention, and treatment of heritable and genetic disorders" (NHGRI, 2012).

Applied Research

Applied, or practical, research is a scientific investigation conducted to generate knowledge that will directly influence or improve clinical practice. The purpose of applied research is to solve problems, to make decisions, or to predict or control outcomes in real-life practice situations. Because applied research focuses on specific problems, the findings are less generalizable than those from basic research. Applied research is also used to test theory and validate its usefulness in clinical practice. Often, the new knowledge discovered through basic research is examined for usefulness in practice by applied research, making these approaches complementary (Bond & Heitkemper, 1987; NHGRI, 2012).

Artinian et al. (2007) conducted an applied study to determine the effectiveness of a nurse-managed telemonitoring (TM) program on the blood pressure (BP) of urban African Americans. The TM program (1) provided BP equipment for patients to monitor their BPs at home, (2) improved access to care by sending patients' BP readings via telephone to healthcare agencies, and (3) increased monitoring of the patients' BPs by a care provider with immediate feedback to the patients. The treatment group received the nurse-managed TM intervention or treatment, and the comparison group received usual care (UC). The TM intervention group had a significant reduction in systolic BP in comparison with the UC group, and diastolic BP was greatly reduced but was not statistically significant from that of the UC group at 12 months. Thus, the TM intervention did have a positive impact on the BPs of African Americans, and additional research is needed to determine whether the intervention has a long-term effect on BPs and improves hypertension control in this population. The findings from this applied study do have implications for practice, because this nurse-managed TM intervention significantly affected BP in a population with a high incidence of hypertension. On the basis of Artinian and colleagues' (2007; 2004; Artinian, Washington, & Templin, 2001) research and the research of others documenting the importance of home BP monitoring, a scientific statement from the American Heart Association, American Society of Hypertension, and Preventive Cardiovascular Nurses Association recommended the use of and reimbursement for home BP monitoring (Pickering et al., 2008). Artinian was a member of the group making this recommendation about home BP monitoring. For more information about the home BP monitoring recommendation, you can view an article on the American Heart Association (2011) website, at http://my.americanheart.org/professional/General/Call-to-Action-on-Use-and-Reimbursement-for-Home-Blood-Pressure-Monitoring_UCM_423866_Article.jsp.

Many nurse researchers have conducted applied studies to produce findings that directly affect clinical practice. Usually, applied studies focus on developing and testing the effectiveness of nursing interventions in the treatment of patient and family health problems.

In addition, most previous federal funding for nursing has been granted for applied research. However, the National Institute of Nursing Research (NINR, 2012) recognizes the importance of basic research to nursing and has made it a funding priority. Basic research is needed to expand our understanding of several pathophysiological variables, such as impaired oxygenation and perfusion, fluid and electrolyte imbalance, altered neurological function, impaired immune system, nutritional disorders, and sleep disturbance. NHGRI (2012) priorities include the identification of the genes responsible for numerous human genetic diseases and the generation of animal models essential for the study of human inherited disorders. Because the future of any profession rests on its research base, both basic and applied studies are needed to develop knowledge for evidence-based practice (EBP) in nursing (Brown, 2009; Melnyk & Fineout-Overholt, 2011).

Rigor in Quantitative Research

Rigor is the striving for excellence in research and involves discipline, scrupulous adherence to detail, and strict accuracy. A rigorous quantitative researcher constantly strives for more precise measurement methods, structured treatments, representative samples, and tightly controlled study designs (Borglin & Richards, 2010; Shadish, Cook, & Campbell, 2002). Characteristics valued in these researchers include critical examination of reasoning and attention to precision.

Logistic reasoning and deductive reasoning are essential to the development of quantitative research. The research process consists of specific steps that are developed with meticulous detail and logically linked together. These steps are critically examined and reexamined for errors and weaknesses in areas such as design, intervention development and implementation, measurement, sampling, statistical analysis, and generalization. Reducing these errors and weaknesses is essential to ensure that the research findings are an accurate reflection of reality and can be generalized. Generalizing research findings involves applying the findings from a particular study sample to a large population of similar individuals (Borglin & Richards, 2010). For example, the findings from the study by Artinian et al. (2007) could be generalized from the African American study participants with hypertension to the larger population of African Americans with hypertension.

Another aspect of rigor is precision, which encompasses accuracy, detail, and order. Precision is evident in the concise statement of the research purpose, the detailed development of the study design, and the formulation of explicit treatment protocols. The most explicit use of precision, however, is evident in the measurement of the study variables (Borglin & Richards, 2010). Measurement involves objectively experiencing the real world through the senses: sight, hearing, touch, taste, and smell. The researcher continually searches for new and more precise ways to measure elements and events of the world (Waltz, Strickland, & Lenz, 2010).

Control in Quantitative Research

Control occurs when the researcher imposes "rules" to decrease the possibility of error and thus increase the probability that the study's findings are an accurate reflection of reality. The rules used to achieve control are referred to as design. Through control, the researcher can reduce the influence or confounding effect of extraneous variables on the study variables. For example, in a study focused on the effect of relaxation therapy on the perception of incisional pain, the extraneous variables, such as type of surgical incision and the timing, amount, and type of pain medication administered after surgery, would have to be controlled to prevent them from influencing the patient's perception of pain.

Controlling extraneous variables enables the researcher to identify relationships among the study variables accurately and examine the effects of one variable on another. Researchers can control extraneous variables with sampling criteria by selecting a certain type of subject, such as only those individuals who are having abdominal surgery or those with a certain medical diagnosis. Using a random sampling method also improves the control of extraneous variables and reduces the potential for bias in the study sample. The setting can also be structured to control extraneous variables such as temperature, noise, and interactions with other people. The data collection process can be sequenced to control extraneous variables such as fatigue and discomfort (Borglin & Richards, 2010).

Quantitative research requires varying degrees of control, ranging from minimal control to highly controlled, depending on the type of study (Table 3-1). Descriptive studies are usually conducted with minimal control of the study design, because subjects are examined as they exist in their natural setting, such as home, work, or school. However, the researcher still hopes to achieve the most precise measurement of the research variables as possible. Experimental studies are highly controlled and often conducted on animals in laboratory settings to determine the underlying mechanisms for and effectiveness of a treatment.

TABLE 3-1	Control in Quantitative Research
Type of Research	**Level of Control in Development of the Research Design**
Descriptive research	Minimal or partial control
Correlational research	Minimal or partial control
Quasi-experimental research	Moderate to high control
Experimental research	High control

Some common areas in which control might be enhanced in quantitative research are (1) selection of subjects (sampling), (2) reduction of subject or participant attrition, (3) selection of the research setting, (4) development and implementation of the intervention, (5) measurement of study variables, and (6) subjects' knowledge of the study (Borglin & Richards, 2010; Forbes, 2009; Shadish et al., 2002). Nurses are being encouraged to develop more powerful, controlled, rigorous quantitative studies (NINR, 2012).

Sampling and Attrition

Sampling is a process of selecting subjects, events, behaviors, or elements for participation in a study. In performing quantitative research, you will use a variety of random and nonrandom sampling methods to obtain study samples. Random sampling methods usually provide a sample that is representative of a population, because each member of the population has a probability greater than zero of being selected for a study. Thus, random or probability sampling methods require greater researcher control and rigor than nonrandom or nonprobability sampling methods. Sample sizes in quantitative studies are usually determined with a power analysis to ensure adequate numbers of study participants throughout the study. Researchers are rigorous in reducing attrition, or loss of study subjects needed to describe variables, examine relationships, and determine the effect of interventions (Aberson, 2010; Thompson, 2002). Chapter 15 provides a detailed discussion of the sampling process and determining sample size for quantitative studies.

Research Settings

There are three common settings for conducting research: natural, partially controlled, and highly controlled. Natural settings are uncontrolled, real-life settings where studies are conducted (Fawcett & Garity, 2009; Kerlinger & Lee, 2000). Descriptive and correlational types of quantitative research are often conducted in natural settings. A partially controlled setting is an environment that the researcher

manipulates or modifies in some way. A growing number of quasi-experimental studies are being conducted to test the effectiveness of nursing interventions, and these studies are often conducted in partially controlled settings. For example, hospitals, clinics, or rehabilitation centers might be manipulated in selected ways to control for extraneous variables, such as type of care, medications, and family interactions. Highly controlled settings are artificially constructed environments that are developed for the sole purpose of conducting research. Laboratories, experimental centers, and research units are highly controlled settings often used for the conduct of experimental research. Chapter 15 discusses the process for selecting a setting for the conduct of quantitative research.

Development and Implementation of Study Interventions or Treatments

Quasi-experimental and experimental studies examine the effect of an independent variable or intervention on a dependent variable or outcome. More intervention studies are being conducted in nursing to establish an EBP. Controlling the development and implementation of a study intervention increases the validity of the study design and the credibility of the findings. A study intervention needs to be (1) clearly and precisely developed, (2) consistently implemented, and (3) examined for effectiveness through quality measurement of the dependent variables (Forbes, 2009; Morrison et al., 2009; Santacroce, Maccarelli, & Grey, 2004). The detailed development of a quality intervention and the consistent implementation of this intervention are known as intervention fidelity. Chapter 14 provides detailed directions for the development and implementation of a study intervention. Artinian et al. (2007) provided the following detailed description of the implementation of the nurse-managed TM (telemonitoring) intervention to improve the BPs of African Americans:

"Participants in the TM group received UC [usual care] plus nurse-managed TM. Specially trained registered nurses delivered the intervention. During a prescheduled appointment, the intervention nurse delivered the BP monitor and TM link device (device that links BP monitor to the telephone) to the participant's home. At the time of the home visit, an intervention nurse taught participants how to self-monitor BP in accordance with The Seventh Report of the Joint National Committee on Prevention, Detection, Evaluation, and Treatment of High Blood

Pressure (JNC-VII) guidelines (Chobanian et al., 2003), set up the home TM system, demonstrated the system, had participants practice using the BP monitor, and answered questions. Given the memory in the BP monitor and that all BPs recorded by the monitor were telephonically sent to care providers and the principal investigator, participants received verbal and written reminders that the BP monitor was exclusively for their use.... LifeLink Monitoring, Inc. (Bearsville, NY) provided TM services for this study.... Telemonitoring participants were also asked to telephonically send their BP readings to the intervention nurse and their care providers.... Once the intervention nurses received the BP reports, they telephoned each participant to provide feedback in relation to the target goals and to provide telecounseling about lifestyle modification and medication adherence in accordance with JNC-VII guidelines (Chobanian et al., 2003)." (Artinian et al., 2007, p. 315)

Measurement of Study Variables

When you are conducting a quantitative study, you will attempt to use the most precise instruments available to measure the study variables. Using a variety of quality measurement methods promotes an accurate and comprehensive understanding of the study variables. In addition, researchers want to rigorously control the process for measuring study variables to improve the design validity and quality of the study findings (Waltz et al., 2010). Measurement concepts, process, and strategies are the foci of Chapters 16 and 17.

Nursing studies often include the measurement of biophysical variables, which require precise, accurate physiological measures (Ryan-Wenger, 2010). For example, Artinian et al. (2007) described their precise measurement of the dependent physiological variable, BP, with an accurate, nationally standardized device as follows:

"The outcome measure of the BP was measured with electronic BP monitor (Omron HEM-737 Intellisense, Omron Healthcare, Inc., Vernon Hills, IL) that has been validated in accordance with the criteria of the British Hypertension Society and the Association of the Advancement of Medical Instrumentations (Dabl Educational Trust, 2005)." (Artinian et al., 2007, p. 316)

Subjects' Knowledge of a Study

Subjects' knowledge of a study could influence their behavior and possibly alter the research outcomes. This possibility threatens the validity or accuracy of the study design. An example of this type of threat to design validity is the **Hawthorne effect**, which was identified during the classic experiments at the Hawthorne plant of the Western Electric Company during the late 1920s and early 1930s. The employees at this plant exhibited a particular psychological response when they became research participants: They changed their behavior simply because they were subjects in a study, not because of the research treatment. In these studies, the researcher manipulated the working conditions (altered the lighting, decreased work hours, changed payment, and increased rest periods) to examine the effects on worker productivity (Homans, 1965). The subjects in both the treatment group (whose work conditions were changed) and the control group (whose work conditions were not changed) increased their productivity. The subjects seemed to change their behaviors (increase their productivity) solely in response to being part of a study. In the study by Artinian et al. (2007, p. 321), both the treatment and the comparison groups experienced decreases in their BPs, and the researchers indicated "the Hawthorne effect may have been a factor, with participants paying more attention to their BP and hypertension self-care behaviors because they were aware of their participation in the study."

There are several ways to strengthen a study, decreasing the threats to design validity and selecting the strongest design for the proposed study. Chapter 10 addresses design validity, and Chapter 11 focuses on the process for selecting an appropriate study design. Your understanding of rigor and control provide the basis for the implementation of the steps of the quantitative research process, which are precisely executed in descriptive, correlational, quasi-experimental, and experimental research.

Steps of the Quantitative Research Process

The quantitative research process consists of conceptualizing a research project, planning and implementing that project, and communicating the findings. Figure 3-1 identifies the steps of the quantitative research process and shows the logical flow of this process as each step progressively builds on the

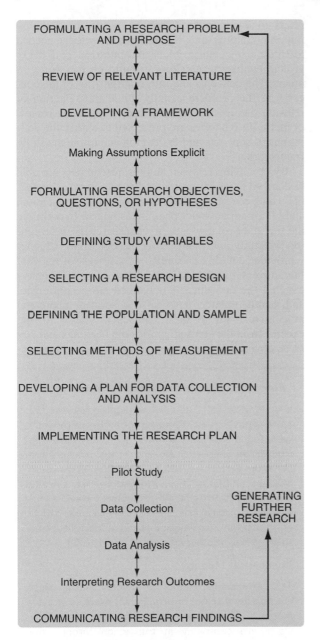

FORMULATING A RESEARCH PROBLEM
AND PURPOSE

REVIEW OF RELEVANT LITERATURE

DEVELOPING A FRAMEWORK

Making Assumptions Explicit

FORMULATING RESEARCH OBJECTIVES,
QUESTIONS, OR HYPOTHESES

DEFINING STUDY VARIABLES

SELECTING A RESEARCH DESIGN

DEFINING THE POPULATION AND SAMPLE

SELECTING METHODS OF MEASUREMENT

DEVELOPING A PLAN FOR DATA COLLECTION
AND ANALYSIS

IMPLEMENTING THE RESEARCH PLAN

Pilot Study

Data Collection

Data Analysis

Interpreting Research Outcomes

COMMUNICATING RESEARCH FINDINGS

GENERATING
FURTHER
RESEARCH

Figure 3-1 **Steps of the quantitative research process.**

previous steps. This research process is also flexible and fluid, with a flow back and forth among the steps as researchers strive to clarify the steps and strengthen the proposed study. This back-and-forth flow among the steps is indicated in the figure by the two-way arrows connecting the steps of the process. Figure 3-1

also contains a feedback arrow, indicating that the research process is cyclical, for each study provides a basis for generating further research in the development of knowledge for EBP.

In this chapter, you are briefly introduced to the steps of the quantitative research process that are presented in detail in Unit Two, The Research Process, and Unit Four, Collecting and Analyzing Data to Determine Research Outcomes for Dissemination. The descriptive correlational study conducted by Gill and Loh (2010), on the relationships of perceived stress, optimism, and health-promoting behaviors in new primiparous mothers, is presented as an example for introducing the steps of the quantitative research process. Quotations from this study appear throughout this section, in shaded boxes, to clarify the steps of the quantitative research process. The bracketed words are inserted in the quotations to clarify the key concepts and steps of the quantitative research process.

Formulating a Research Problem and Purpose

A **research problem** is an area of concern or phenomenon of interest in which there is a gap in the knowledge base needed for nursing practice. The problem identifies an area of concern or phenomenon of interest for a particular population and often indicates the concepts to be studied. The major sources for nursing research problems include (1) nursing practice, (2) literature review, (3) research priorities for funding agencies and professional organizations, (4) researcher and peer interactions, and (5) theory testing. The research problem usually indicates significance to nursing, background knowledge in the area, and problem statement of what is not known (Fawcett & Garity, 2009). As a researcher, you will use deductive reasoning to generate a research problem from a research topic or a broad problem area of personal interest that is relevant to nursing.

The **research purpose** is generated from the problem and identifies the specific focus or aim of the study. The focus of the study might be to identify, describe, explain, or predict a solution to a situation. The purpose often indicates the type of study to be conducted (descriptive, correlational, quasi-experimental, or experimental) and usually includes the variables, population, and setting for the study. Chapter 5 provides a background for formulating a research problem and purpose. Gill and Loh (2010) identified the following problem and purpose for their study of new primiparous mothers as follows:

Problem

"The transition to motherhood is considered to be one of the most stressful and disruptive life transitions (Chen, Kuo, Chou, & Chen, 2007; Warren, 2005).... Additional competing priorities may include learning the maternal role, experiencing physical changes, and learning how to care for their own needs.... These different roles and priorities may be perceived by the new mother as highly stressful, particularly as many of these stressors occur simultaneously (Warren, 2005).... Specifically, perceived stress can occur when the demands of a particular situation are assessed by the individual as greater than their coping attributes [*problem significance*]....

"Past research has found that perceived stress may lead a new mother to neglect personal health-promoting behaviors in her effort to balance the competing priorities of being a first-time mother (Chen et al., 2007; Walker, 1989).... Optimism and perceived stress have an inverse relationship (Brissette, Scheier, & Carver, 2002).... Optimistic people cope better with stressful situations and thereby report fewer physical health symptoms [*problem background*]....

"Perceived stress has been associated with fewer health-promoting behaviors in new primiparous mothers, but less is known about the mechanisms responsible for such effects" [*problem statement*]. (Gill & Loh, 2010, pp. 348–349)

Purpose

"This investigation was conducted to examine the potential role of optimism as a partial mediator of the relationship between perceived stress and health-promoting behaviors in new primiparous mothers." (Gill & Loh, 2010, p. 350)

The research problem is significant and is based on pervious research. The problem statement indicates what is not known and provides a basis for the study purpose. The research purpose clearly indicates that the focus of this study is to describe and examine relationships among the variables optimism, perceived stress, and health-promoting behavior in new first-time mothers.

Review of Relevant Literature

A **review of relevant literature** is conducted to generate an understanding of what is known about a particular situation, phenomenon, or problem and to identify the knowledge gaps that exist. **Relevant literature** refers to those sources that are pertinent or highly important in providing the in-depth knowledge needed to study a selected problem and purpose. This background enables researchers to build on the works of others. The concepts and interrelationships of the concepts in the problem usually guide the selection of relevant theories and studies presented in the review of literature. Theories are presented to clarify the definitions of concepts and to develop and refine the study framework.

By reviewing relevant studies, researchers are able to clarify (1) which problems have been investigated, (2) which require further investigation or replication, and (3) which have not been investigated. In addition, the literature review can direct researchers in designing the study and interpreting the outcomes. Chapter 6 provides details for conducting a review of relevant literature. Gill and Loh's (2010) literature review covered the concepts of perceived stress, optimism, and health practice. They also described theoretical models relevant to these concepts. The following excerpt from the study identifies the headings and key ideas covered by the review of relevant literature:

"Perceived Stress and Health Practices

In a longitudinal study from midpregnancy to 12 months postpartum, American primiparous mothers were found to decline gradually in healthy behaviors after birth, with exercise and stress management behaviors performed least by these women (Patteson & Killien, 2001).... There are also significant health benefits in practicing health-promoting behaviors. For example, exercise has been shown to have a dual effect of promoting weight loss and reducing reported stress in new mothers (Groth & David, 2008)....

Theoretical Models

The transactional model for understanding stress emphasizes that the environmental event (e.g., new motherhood) and the cognitive faculties of the individual are constantly in transaction through the process of appraisal (Lazarus & Folkman, 1984).... According to the transactional model of stress and coping, individuals adopt different coping mechanisms to deal with the perceived stress they encounter....

There are widespread observations that people with optimism generally tend to use less avoidant and more goal-directed coping mechanisms.... In this study, optimism (i.e., dispositional optimism) refers to a personality variable where individuals believe that good outcomes rather than bad will occur in one's life

(Scheier & Carver, 1992). Optimists tend to have an internal locus of control and believe that events result primarily from their own behaviors and actions....

Perceived Stress and Optimism

Another study assessing constructive thinking during pregnancy found that optimism helped in the adjustment to stressful situations during this time and reduced the level of stress experienced (Park, Moore, Turner, & Adler, 1997). An optimistic disposition can therefore be seen to reduce perceived stress and encourage more positive appraisals of situations....

Optimism and Health Practices

Optimism was found also to diminish the impact of depression in pregnant women and up to 3 weeks postpartum (Carver & Gaines, 1987)....

Optimism as a Mediator

Substantial research exists where optimism has served as a mediator of a stress relationship.... In a study with pregnant women, optimism was found to confer positive benefits through constructive thinking in decreasing perceived stress, anxiety, and substance abuse.... Despite these findings, previous studies have not investigated how optimism might mediate the relationships between perceived stress and health-promoting behaviors in new mothers. This is important because health-promoting behaviors have the potential to help new mothers cope with the daily stress of parenthood and define maternal identity (Walker, 1989)." (Gill & Loh, 2010, pp. 348–350)

Gill and Loh (2010) clearly cover relevant studies related to the concepts of stress, health practices, and optimism in pregnant women and new mothers. They also cover relevant theories that describe the relationships among key concepts. The literature review summarizes what is known in the areas of stress, health practices, and optimism in new mothers and clearly indicates what is not known. The study purpose focuses on what is not known, which is how optimism mediates the relationship between perceived stress and health-promoting behaviors.

Developing a Framework

A **framework** is the abstract, logical structure of meaning that will guide the development of a study and enable the researcher to link the findings to the body of nursing knowledge. In quantitative research, the framework is often a testable midrange theory that

has been developed in nursing or in another discipline, such as psychology, physiology, or sociology (Smith & Liehr, 2008). The framework may also be developed inductively from clinical observations.

The terms related to frameworks are *concept, relational statement, theory,* and *framework model or map.* A **concept** is a term to which abstract meaning is attached. A **relational statement** or proposition declares that a relationship of some kind exists between or among two or more concepts. A **theory** consists of an integrated set of defined concepts and propositions that present a view of a phenomenon and can be used to describe, explain, predict, or control the phenomenon. The propositions or relationship statements of the theory, not the theory itself, are tested through research.

A study framework can be expressed as a **model** or a diagram of the relationships that provide the basis for a study and/or can be presented in narrative format. The steps for developing a framework are described in Chapter 7. The framework for Gill and Loh's (2010) study is presented in Figure 3-2 and is described in the following quote. The framework model identifies the relationships that are examined in this study, and the description of the framework identifies the proposition that was tested by this study.

"It was speculated that maternal perceived stress would inversely affect a new primiparous mother's health-promoting behaviors. However, this relationship would be mediated partially by a new mother's sense of optimism. In other words, on the basis of work by Scheier and Carver (1992) the protective role of optimism would enable a new mother to self-regulate her perception of stress positively and help her to engage in health-promoting behaviors to maintain her sense of well-being and control [see Figure 3-2].

It is important to note that partial mediation (as opposed to full mediation) was proposed because optimism was hypothesized to be only one of a number of possible variables that contribute to the associate between maternal perceived stress and health-promoting behaviors" [*proposition*]. (Gill & Loh, 2010, p. 350)

Making Assumptions Explicit

Assumptions are statements that are taken for granted or are considered true, even though they have not been scientifically tested. Assumptions are often embedded (unrecognized) in thinking and behavior, and uncovering them requires introspection. Sources of assumptions include universally accepted truths (e.g., all

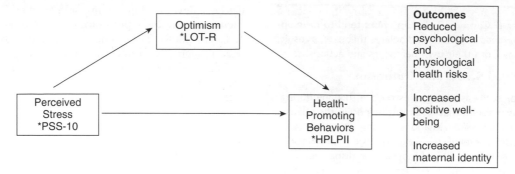

Figure 3-2 Theoretical model outlining the relationships between predictor variables and proposed outcomes.
*Instruments used to measure study variables: HPLPII, Health-Promoting Lifestyle Profile II; LOT-R, Life Orientation Test–Revised; PSS-10, Perceived Stress Scale. (From Gill, R. M., & Loh, J. M. (2010). The role of optimism in health-promoting behaviors in new primiparous mothers. *Nursing Research, 59*(5), 350.)

humans are rational beings), theories, previous research, and nursing practice (Myers, 1982).

In studies, assumptions are embedded in the philosophical base of the framework, study design, and interpretation of findings. Theories and instruments are developed on the basis of assumptions that the researcher may or may not recognize. These assumptions influence the development and implementation of the research process. Because researchers' assumptions influence the logic of the study, their recognition leads to more rigorous study development.

Researchers often do not identify assumptions that provide a basis for their study in their research report; but if assumptions are included, they are usually part of the framework discussion. Gill and Loh (2010) did not clearly identify the assumptions for their study, but the following assumptions seem to provide a basis for it: (1) stress needs to be managed to promote health, (2) people's psychological perspectives influence their actions, and (3) health is a priority for most people.

Formulating Research Objectives, Questions, or Hypotheses

Research objectives, questions, and hypotheses bridge the gap between the more abstractly stated research problem and purpose and the study design and plan for data collection and analysis. Objectives, questions, and hypotheses are narrower in focus than the research purpose and often (1) specify only one or two research variables, (2) identify the relationship between the variables, and (3) indicate the population to be studied.

Some quantitative studies do not include objectives, questions, or hypotheses; the development of such a study is directed by the research purpose. Many descriptive studies include only a research purpose, and other descriptive studies include a purpose and

objectives or questions. Some correlational studies include a purpose and specific questions or hypotheses. Quasi-experimental and experimental studies often use hypotheses to direct the development and implementation of the studies and the interpretation of findings. Chapter 8 examines the development of research objectives, questions, and hypotheses. Gill and Loh (2010) predicted relationships among the study variables that were examined with a predictive correlational design (Kerlinger & Lee, 2000; see Figure 11-9). With this type of design, researchers often formulate hypotheses to predict the outcomes for their study as was done by Gill and Loh:

"Four hypotheses were proposed for the current study.

1. Perceived stress will be related negatively to health-promoting behaviors in new primiparous mothers.
2. Perceived stress will be related negatively to optimism in new primiparous mothers.
3. Optimism will be related positively to health-promoting behaviors in new primiparous mothers.
4. Optimism will mediate the relationship between perceived stress and health-promoting behaviors partially in new primiparous mothers." (Gill & Loh, 2010, p. 350)

Defining Study Variables

The research purpose and the objectives, questions, or hypotheses identify the variables that are examined in a study. **Study variables** are concepts of various levels of abstraction that are measured, manipulated, or controlled in a study. The more concrete concepts, such as temperature, weight, and blood pressure, are referred to as "variables." The more abstract concepts, such as creativity, empathy, and social support, are sometimes referred to as "research concepts."

The variables or concepts in a study are operationalized when they are conceptually and operationally defined. A **conceptual definition** provides a variable or concept with theoretical meaning (Fawcett & Garity, 2009) and either is derived from a theorist's definition of the concept or is developed through concept analysis. An **operational definition** indicates how a variable will be measured or manipulated in a study. The knowledge you gain from studying the variable will increase your understanding of the concept that the variable represents (see Chapter 8).

Gill and Loh (2010) provided conceptual and operational definitions of the study variables identified in their purpose and hypotheses: perceived stress, health-promoting behaviors, and optimism. The conceptual definitions for these variables are provided in the review of literature and are reflective of the framework that includes Lazarus and Folkman's (1984) transactional model and the role of optimism by Scheier and Carver (1992). The operational definitions indicate how the variables were measured and are linked to the study variables in the framework model (see Figure 3-2) and detailed in the measures section of the study methodology.

Perceived Stress

Conceptual Definition

"Perceived stress may be defined as the degree to which individuals appraise events in their life as overwhelming and insurmountable. Specifically, perceived stress can occur when the demands of a particular situation are assessed by the individual as greater than their coping attributes." (Gill & Loh, 2010, p. 348)

Operational Definition

Perceived stress was measured by the Perceived Stress Scale (PSS-10) (Cohen & Williamson, 1988).

Health-Promoting Behavior

Conceptual Definition

"Health-promoting behaviors are defined as a pattern of actions and cognitions that aim to augment the level of wellness, self-actualization, and fulfillment of an individual." (Gill & Loh, 2010, p. 348)

Operational Definition

The Health-Promoting Life-Style Profile II (HPLPII) (Walker & Hill-Polerecky, 1996) was used to measure the new primiparous mothers' health-promoting behaviors.

Optimism

Conceptual Definition

"In this study, optimism (i.e., dispositional optimism) refers to a personality variable where individuals believe that good outcomes rather than bad will occur in one's life (Scheier & Carver, 1992)." (Gill & Loh, 2010, p. 349)

Operational Definition

"The revised Life Orientation Test (Scheier et al., 1994) was used to measure optimism exhibited by the mothers in this study." (Gill & Loh, 2010, p. 351)

Selecting a Research Design

A **research design** is a blueprint for maximizing control over factors that could interfere with a study's desired outcome. The type of design directs the selection of a population, sampling process, methods of measurement, and a plan for data collection and analysis. The choice of research design depends on the researcher's expertise, the problem being examined, the purpose for the study, and the desire to generalize the findings.

Designs have been developed to meet unique research needs as they emerge; thus, a variety of descriptive, correlational, quasi-experimental, and experimental designs have been generated over time. In descriptive and correlational studies, no treatment is administered, so the study design centers on describing variables, examining relationships, and improving the precision of measurement (Waltz et al., 2010). Quasi-experimental and experimental study designs usually involve treatment and control groups and focus on achieving high levels of control as well as precision in measurement (Cook & Campbell, 1979; Kerlinger & Lee, 2000; Shadish et al, 2002). Chapter 10 covers the purpose of a design and the threats to design validity. Chapter 11 presents models and descriptions of several types of descriptive, correlational, quasi-experimental, and experimental designs.

Gill and Loh (2010) conducted a descriptive correlational study that involved a cross-sectional, predictive correlational design. Cross-sectional design is used to examine groups of subjects in various stages of development, trends, patterns, and changes simultaneously with the intent to describe changes in the phenomenon across stages. The researchers provide very little detail of the cross-sectional aspect of this study design but do mention examining primiparous mothers with babies varying in age from 2 to 12 months. The predictive correlational design is clearly addressed in the study. Relationships among study variables perceived stress, optimism, and health-promoting behaviors are examined. The predictor or independent variables, perceived stress and optimism, are used to predict the criterion or dependent variable, health-promotion behavior.

Defining the Population and Sample

The **population** is all the elements (individuals, objects, or substances) that meet certain criteria for inclusion in a given universe (Kaplan, 1964; Thompson, 2002). For example, suppose you wanted to conduct a study to describe patients' responses to nurse practitioners as their primary care providers. You could define the population in different ways: It could include all patients being seen for the first time in (1) a single clinic, (2) all clinics in a specific network in one city, or (3) all clinics in that network nationwide. Your definition of the population would depend on the sample criteria and the similarity of subjects in these various settings. The researcher needs to determine which population is accessible and can be best represented by the study sample.

A **sample** is a subset of the population that is selected for a particular study, and sampling defines the process for selecting a group of people, events, behaviors, or other elements with which to conduct a study. As mentioned earlier in this chapter, nursing studies use both probability (random) and nonprobability (nonrandom) sampling methods, and sample size is usually determined by conduction of a power analysis. The following quote identifies the sample size, population, sample criteria, and sample characteristics for the study conducted by Gill and Loh (2010). The study would have been strengthened by identification of the sampling method, which appears to be a nonprobability sample of convenience, whereby subjects are selected because they happen to be in a given place at a given time.

> **"Participants**
>
> Participants were 174 new primiparous mothers [*sample size; population*] recruited from online baby forums [*setting*]. Tabachnick and Fidell's (2007) rule of thumb was applied to calculate the power required for this study. With two predictors, 106 participants were required, and the study was therefore adequately powered [*power analysis*]. Only primiparous mothers with babies up to and including 12 months of age were eligible to complete the study [*sample criteria*]. Demographic information for the participants is displayed in a table" [see Table 3-2] [*sample characteristics*]. (Gill & Loh, 2010, p. 350)

Selecting Methods of Measurement

Measurement is the process of assigning "numbers to objects (or events or situations) in accord with some rule" (Kaplan, 1964, p. 177). A component of measurement is **instrumentation**, which is defined as the application of specific rules to the development of a measurement device or instrument. An instrument is

TABLE 3-2   **Means, Standard Deviations, Potential Range, Obtained Range, and Cronbach's Alpha of the Scores for Main Study Variables**

Measure	n	M	SD	Potential Range	Obtained Range	Cronbach's Alpha
1. Perceived stress	174	13.62	6.83	0-40	0-29	.75
2. Optimism	174	17.74	4.51	0-24	0-24	.89
3. Health-promoting behavior	174	2.74	0.58	1-4	1.54-3.92	.97
4. Income*	174	4.44	0.89	1-5	1-5	—
5. Age	174	31.5	4.44	18-40+	18-42	—
6. Months since birth	174	6.17	3.28	0-12	−.20-12	—

*1 = <$20,000; 2 = $20,001-35,000; 3 = $35,001-50,000; 4 = $50,001-75,000; 5 = >$75,000. Income reported in Australian dollars.
n = Sample size for calculations.
M = Mean.
SD = standard deviation.
Cronbach's alpha (α) = reliability of the measurement methods for this study.
From Gill, R. M., & Loh, J. M. (2010). The role of optimism in health-promoting behaviors in new primiparous mothers. *Nursing Research, 59*(5), 348–355. The table is on page 352.

selected to measure a specific variable in a study. Data generated with an instrument are at the nominal, ordinal, interval, or ratio level of measurement. The level of measurement, with nominal being the lowest form of measurement and ratio being the highest, determines the type of statistical analyses that you can perform on the data (Grove, 2007).

Selection of an instrument requires extensive examination of its reliability and validity. **Reliability** assesses how consistently the measurement technique measures a concept. The **validity** of an instrument is the extent to which it actually reflects the abstract concept being examined (Waltz et al., 2010). Chapter 16 introduces the concepts of measurement and explains the different types of reliability and validity for instruments and precision and accuracy for physiological measures (Ryan-Wenger, 2010). Chapter 17 provides a background for selecting measurement methods for a study. Gill and Loh (2010) provided the following description of the three Likert scales that were used to measure their study variables:

"Measures

Perceived Stress The Perceived Stress Scale (PSS-10; Cohen & Williamson, 1988) was used to measure stress in the mothers. This scale contains 10 items that measure perceived stress experienced within the last month. Participants were asked to indicate on a 5-point Likert-type scale (0 = *never* to 4 = *very often*) their response to each item. A sample questions was, 'In the last month, how often have you found that you could not cope with all the things that you had to do?' High scores on the scale indicated higher levels of perceived stress. Internal reliability of the PSS-10 for this study was found to be .78, and adequate construct validity was reported (Cohen & Williams, 1988). Cronbach's alpha (α) for perceived stress in the current study was .75.

Health-Promoting Behaviors The Health-Promoting Lifestyle Profile II [HPLPII] (Walker & Hill-Polerecky, 1996) was used to measure new primiparous mothers' health-promoting behaviors. Participants were asked to indicate on a 4-point scale (1 = *never* to 4 = *routinely*) the frequency with which they engaged in the behavior indicated. Sample items include 'I discuss my health concerns with health professionals' and 'I follow a planned exercise program.' In the original study, internal consistency was found to be .94 for the global scale, and construct validity was .68 (Walker & Hill-Polerecky, 1996). Cronbach's alpha in the current study was .97.

Optimism The revised Life Orientation Test [LOT-R] (Scheier et al., 1994) was used to measure optimism exhibited by the mothers in this study. Participants were asked to rate their agreement with the statements on a 5-point Likert scale (0 = *strongly disagree* to 4 = *strongly agree*). A sample item was, 'In uncertain times, I usually expect the best.' In a study with 2,055 undergraduate students, the revised Life Orientation Test reported internal consistency was .78 for the six items used and adequate construct validity (Scheier et al., 1994). Internal consistency in the current study was .89 for the six items." (Gill & Loh, 2010, p. 351)

The three Likert scales used in this study seemed to have strong reliability from previous research (Cronbach's alpha = 0.78 to 0.94) and were reliable in this study (Cronbach's alpha = 0.75 to 0.97). However, the researchers provide very limited specific information about the validity of the scales, especially the PSS-10 and LOT-R.

Developing a Plan for Data Collection and Analysis

Data collection is the precise, systematic gathering of information relevant to the research purpose or the specific objectives, questions, or hypotheses of a study. The data collected in quantitative studies are usually numerical. Planning data collection will enable you to anticipate problems that are likely to occur and to explore possible solutions. Usually, detailed procedures for implementing a treatment and collecting data are developed, with a schedule that identifies the initiation and termination of the process (see Chapter 20).

Planning data analysis is the final step before the study is implemented. The analysis plan is based on (1) the research objectives, questions, or hypotheses, (2) the data to be collected, (3) research design, (4) researchers' expertise, and (5) availability of computer resources. Several statistical analysis techniques are available to describe the sample, examine relationships, or determine significant differences within studies. Most researchers consult a statistician for assistance in developing an analysis plan.

Implementing the Research Plan

Implementing the research plan involves intervention implementation, data collection, data analysis, interpretation of research findings, and, sometimes, a pilot study.

Pilot Study

A *pilot study* is commonly defined as a smaller version of a proposed study that is conducted to refine the methodology. It is developed much like the proposed study, using similar subjects, the same setting, the same treatment, and the same data collection and analysis techniques. However, you could use a pilot study to develop various steps in the research process. For example, you could conduct a pilot study to develop and refine an intervention, a measurement method, a data collection tool, or the data collection process. Thus, a pilot study could be used to develop a research plan rather than to test an already developed plan.

Some of the reasons for conducting pilot studies are as follows (Arain, Campbell, Cooper, & Lancaster, 2010; Feeley et al., 2009; Hertzog, 2008; Prescott & Soeken, 1989):

- To determine whether the proposed study is feasible (e.g., are the subjects available, does the researcher have the time and money to do the study?).
- To develop or refine a research treatment or intervention (see Chapter 14).
- To develop a protocol for the implementation of an intervention.
- To identify problems with a study design.
- To determine whether the sample is representative of the population or whether the sampling technique is effective.
- To examine the reliability and validity of the research instruments.
- To develop or refine data collection instruments.
- To refine the data collection and analysis plan.
- To give the researcher experience with the subjects, setting, methodology, and methods of measurement.
- To try out data analysis techniques.

Hayward et al. (2007) believed that conducting a pilot study improved the strength of their study design and directed their development of a quality proposal for a large multisite clinical trial that received external grant support. Thus, conducting pilot studies has the potential to improve the development, funding, and implementation of future studies.

Data Collection

In quantitative research, **data collection** involves obtaining numerical data to address the research objectives, questions, or hypotheses. To collect data, you must obtain consent or permission from the setting or agency where the study is to be conducted and from potential subjects. Frequently, study participants are asked to sign a consent form, which describes the study, promises the subjects confidentiality, and indicates that they can stop participation at any time (see Chapter 9).

During data collection, the study variables are measured through a variety of techniques, such as observation, interview, questionnaires, scales, and physiological measurement methods. In a growing number of studies, nurses measure physiological variables with high-technology equipment. The data are collected and recorded systematically for each subject and are organized to facilitate computer entry or are directly recorded in the computer (Ryan-Wenger, 2010). The procedure for data collection is usually identified in the Methods section of a study report. Gill and Loh (2010) provided the following description of their data collection process. This section would have been strengthened by a more detailed discussion of the online survey format and the process for collection and management of data.

> **"Procedure**
>
> New primiparous mothers were asked to complete an online anonymous survey that could be accessed from a link available from an online baby forum Web page. This survey took approximately 20 minutes to complete. Implied consent was given by the participant on the completion and submission of the online questionnaire; this was stated explicitly in the introductory sheet on the first page of the online survey. Ethics approval was granted for this study and all requirements pertaining to this approval were met."
> (Gill & Loh, 2010, pp. 350–351)

Data Analysis

Data analysis reduces, organizes, and gives meaning to the data. The analysis of data from quantitative research involves the use of (1) descriptive analysis techniques (see Chapter 22) to describe demographic variables and study variables; (2) statistical techniques to test proposed relationships among variables (see Chapter 23); (3) analysis techniques to make predictions (see Chapter 24); and (4) analysis techniques to examine group differences, such as the difference between the experimental or intervention group and the control group (see Chapter 25). Computers are used to perform most statistical analyses, so Chapter 21 provides a discussion of the computer software programs used for conducting data analysis.

The choice of analysis techniques implemented is determined primarily by the research objectives, questions, or hypotheses; the research design; and the level of measurement achieved by the research instruments. Gill and Loh (2010) used frequencies and percentages to analyze the demographic variables of marital status, nationality, employment, education, and income. The age and months since the baby's birth were described with the use of means and standard deviations (see Table 3-2). Perceived stress, optimism, and health-promoting behavior variables were (1) described with means, standard deviations, and ranges, (2) examined for relationships with Pearson product-moment correlation, and (3) examined for prediction with regression analysis.

The Results Section in the Gill and Loh (2010) article was clearly organized by the study hypotheses. All four of the hypotheses were supported, indicating support for the study framework. These analyses are somewhat complicated at this point in the text, but we encourage you to examine each of the tables for key ideas. Table 3-3 presents a correlation matrix of the results obtained from Pearson correlation analysis of the study variables (perceived stress, optimism, and health-promoting behaviors) and the demographic variables (income, age, and months since birth) (see Chapter 23). These results were examined for significance using the t-test (t value), and the significant

"Analysis Approach

The means [M], standard deviations [SD], ranges, and Cronbach's α of the study ... variables are presented in Table 3-2. Correlations between the main study variables are depicted in Table 3-3. All correlations were in the predicted direction. [Perceived stress was significantly negatively correlated with optimism, −.60* and health-promoting behaviors, −.67*. Optimism and health-promoting behaviors were significantly positively correlated, .70*. The * indicates the results were significant at $p < .01$]. On average, participants had missing data on 22.8% of the variables. The missing data in the sample were assessed to be missing at random.... Fifteen cases were deleted for having excessive ... missing data on greater than 50% of the variables." (Gill & Loh, 2010, p. 351)

"Results

... Results indicated that perceived stress was significantly negatively related to health-promoting behaviors, $\beta = -.60$, $t(167) = -10.27$, and uniquely accounted for 33% of the variance [change] in health-promoting behaviors, $F(6,167) = 25.74$, $p < .001$ [see regression

analysis in Table 3-4]. Hypothesis 1 was therefore supported because perceived stress was related inversely to health-promoting behaviors.

Hypothesis 2 was supported because perceived stress was related inversely to optimism, $\beta = -.55$, $t(167) = -8.56$, and uniquely accounted for 27% of the variance in optimism, $F(6,167) = 17.50$, $p < .001$.

In the third analysis, optimism positively influenced health-promoting behaviors, after controlling for the effects of perceived stress on health-promoting behaviors, $\beta = .46$, $t(166) = 7.36$, and uniquely accounted for 13% of the variance in optimism, $F(7,166) = 36.38$, $p < .001$.... Hypothesis 3 therefore was supported because optimism was related positively to health-promoting behaviors after controlling for perceived stress.

In the fourth analysis, perceived stress was related to health-promoting behaviors after controlling for the effects of optimism, $\beta = -.35$, $t(166) = -5.77$, and explained an additional 8% of the variance in health-promoting behaviors, optimism, $F(7,166) = 36.83$, $p < .001$ [see Table 3-4]... Hence Hypothesis 4 was supported." (Gill & Loh, 2010, p. 352)

TABLE **3-3** Correlations among the Main Study Variables ($N = 174$)					
Variable	1	2	3	4	5
1. Perceived stress					
2. Optimism	−.60*	—			
3. Health-promoting behavior	−.67	.70*	—		
4. Income	−.30*	.26*	.38*	—	
5. Age	−.21*	−.34*	.27*	.45*	—
6. Months since birth	−.08	−.03	.02	—	—

Asterisk (*) indicates a significant correlation.

From Gill, R. M., & Loh, J. M. (2010). The role of optimism in health-promoting behaviors in new primiparous mothers. *Nursing Research, 59*(5), 348–355. Table is on page 352.

TABLE 3-4 Standard Multiple Regression Testing the Direct Effects of Perceived Stress and Optimism on Health-Promoting Behaviors: Test of Mediation (N = 174)

Analysis and Predictor Variable	β	SE	R^2	F	Criterion Variable
Analysis 1*: Perceived stress	−.60	0.42	.48	25.74[§]	HPB
Analysis 2[†]: Perceived stress	−.55	3.44	.39	17.50*	Optimism
Analysis 3: Optimism	.46				
Analysis 4[‡]: Perceived stress	−.35	0.37	.61	36.83*	HPB

HPB, health-promoting behavior.
*Effect of predictor variable on criterion at df = 6,167.
[†]Effect of predictor variable on mediator at df = 6,167.
[‡]Effects of predictor variable and mediator on criterion variable at df = 7,166.
[§]$P < .01$ level.
N = Sample size for regression analysis calculation.
df = Degrees of freedoms for regression analysis.
β = Beta coefficients for regression analysis.
SE = Standard error.
R^2 = Square of Regression statistic R to determining percent of variance explained by predictor variables.
F = Statistic for Analysis of Variance to determine significance of predictor variables.
From Gill, R. M., & Loh, J. M. (2010). The role of optimism in health-promoting behaviors in new primiparous mothers. *Nursing Research, 59*(5), 353.

correlations have an asterisk (*). Table 3-4 presents the regression analysis results, predicting the effects of perceived stress and optimism on health-promoting behaviors in new first-time mothers. The significance of the regression analysis results was demonstrated with F-values (see Chapter 24). The amount of missing data for the study variables was a concern, and it is unclear how this lack might have influenced the study results.

Interpreting Research Outcomes

The results obtained from data analysis require interpretation to be meaningful. **Interpretation of research outcomes** involves (1) examining the results from data analysis, (2) exploring the significance of the findings, (3) identifying study limitations, (4) forming conclusions, (5) generalizing the findings, (6) considering the implications for nursing, and (7) suggesting further studies. The study results from data analyses are translated and interpreted to become **findings**, and these findings are synthesized to form **conclusions**. Study conclusions are influenced by the limitations of the study. **Limitations** are restrictions or problems in a study that may decrease the generalizability of the findings. Study limitations often include a combination of theoretical and methodological weaknesses. Theoretical weaknesses in a study might include a poorly developed study framework and unclear conceptual definitions of variables. The limited conceptual

definitions of the variables might decrease the operationalization or measurement of the study variables. Methodological limitations result from factors such as nonrepresentative samples, weak designs, a single setting, limited control over treatment (intervention), instruments with limited reliability and validity, limited control over data collection, and improper use of statistical analyses. These study limitations can limit the credibility of the findings and conclusions and restrict the population to which the findings can be generalized. The study conclusions provide a basis for identifying nursing implications and suggesting further studies (see Chapter 26). In the excerpts that follow, Gill and Loh (2010) discuss their study findings, limitations, conclusions, suggestions for further research, and implications for practice for their study. Because of the study limitations, the researchers limit the generalization of the findings and provide direction for further research. The discussion section would have been strengthened by a clarification of the implications of the study findings for practice.

"Discussion

... Finally, results indicated that optimism partially mediated the relationship between perceived stress and health-promoting behaviors, suggesting a protective role of dispositional optimism in the sample of new primiparous mothers. This finding is consistent with previous research, in which optimism has served as a mediator of a stress relationship ... and promoted positive psychological and behavioral health outcomes in mothers.... Caution must be observed when interpreting the results of this study. Given the cross-sectional data, a causal relationship cannot be confirmed between perceived stress and optimism in new mothers [*findings*]. In addition, the sample group predominantly consists of high-income, well-educated, and computer-literate women who may not be representative of most new primiparous mothers. Expanding on this sample group may be an area for future research. Additional limitations include using retrospective reporting and self-reporting scales, which can lead to response bias. A further limitation is the use of the PSS-10, which measures perceptions of stress that have occurred during the last month. Stress relating to the mothers' daily lives may be perceived differently, depending on how long ago they gave birth and subsequently how old their child is [*limitations*].... Therefore, although assessing the perceived stress of the new mother is interesting, it may be more useful for future research to use a measure specifically designed to capture stress response at different milestones of the baby's development....

The results indicated that optimism only partially mediated the relationship between perceived stress and health-promoting behaviors in new primiparous mothers.... Social support received from family or new mother groups also may influence positive well-being in new mothers. Further research is therefore recommended to explore some of these issues.

In summary, optimism serves as a partial mediator for new primiparous mothers to self-regulate their perceptions of stress positively and thereby to facilitate their involvement in health-promoting behaviors. Health-promoting actions have many positive benefits for new mothers [*conclusion*], including building identity as a mother, enhancing positive well-being, and minimizing the risk of future illness outcomes through exercise" [*implications for practice*]. (Gill & Loh, 2010, p. 354)

Communicating Research Findings

Research is not considered complete until the findings have been communicated. **Communicating research findings** involves developing and disseminating a research report to appropriate audiences; the research report is disseminated through presentations and publication (see Chapter 27). The Gill and Loh (2010) study was published in one of the most prestigious nursing journals, *Nursing Research*.

Types of Quantitative Research

This textbook deals with four types of quantitative research: (1) descriptive, (2) correlational, (3) quasi-experimental, and (4) experimental. The level of existing knowledge for the research problem influences the type of research planned. When little knowledge is available, descriptive studies are often conducted. As the knowledge level increases, correlational, quasi-experimental, and experimental studies are implemented. This section builds on the content in Chapter 2 and identifies the purpose of each quantitative research approach. The chapter concludes with the steps of the research process from a published quasi-experimental study.

Descriptive Research

The purpose of **descriptive research** is to explore and describe phenomena in real-life situations. This approach is used to generate new knowledge about concepts or topics about which limited or no research has been conducted. Through descriptive research, concepts are described and relationships are identified that provide a basis for further quantitative research and theory testing. The study by Gill and Loh (2010) presented earlier in this chapter has a descriptive component, which included description of the study variables optimism, perceived stress, and health-promoting behaviors of new first-time mothers. The descriptive results of this study can be clearly identified in Table 3-2.

Correlational Research

Correlational research examines linear relationships between or among two or more variables and determines the type (positive or negative) and degree (strength) of the relationship. The strength of a relationship varies from −1 (perfect negative correlation) to +1 (perfect positive correlation), with 0 indicating no relationship. The positive relationship indicates that the variables vary together—that is, the two variables either increase or decrease together. The negative or inverse relationship indicates that the variables vary in opposite directions; thus, as one variable increases, the other decreases (see the results presented earlier from Gill & Loh, 2010 study). The descriptive correlational study conducted by Gill and Loh (2010), presented earlier in this chapter, provides an example of the steps of the quantitative research process for correlational research with a predictive correlational design. The results of the relationships among the study variables are clearly presented in Table 3-3. Regression analysis results in Table 3-4 indicated that perceived stress and optimism significantly predicted health-promoting behaviors of primiparous mothers in this study.

Quasi-Experimental Research

The purpose of quasi-experimental research is to examine cause-and-effect relationships among selected independent and dependent variables. Quasi-experimental studies in nursing are conducted to determine the effects of nursing interventions or treatments (independent variables) on patient outcomes (dependent variables) (Cook & Campbell, 1979; Shadish et al., 2002). Artinian et al. (2007) conducted a quasi-experimental study to determine the effects of nurse-managed telemonitoring (TM) on the BPs of African Americans. The steps for this study are described here and illustrated with excerpts from the example study.

Steps of the Research Process in a Quasi-Experimental Study

Research Problem

"Nearly one in three, or approximately 65 million adults in the United States have hypertension, defined as (a) having systolic blood pressure (SBP) of 140 mm Hg or higher or diastolic blood pressure (DBP) of at least 90 mm Hg or higher, (b) taking antihypertensive medication, or (c) being told at least twice by a physician or other health professional about having high blood pressure (BP) (American Heart Association [AHA], 2004; AHA Statistics Committee & Stroke Statistics Subcommittee [AHASC], 2006; Fields et al., 2004).... Estimated direct and indirect costs associated with hypertension total $63.5 billion (AHA, 2004).... The crisis of high BP (HBP) is particularly apparent among African Americans; their prevalence of HBP is among the highest in the world.... Unless healthcare professionals can improve care for individuals with hypertension, approximately two thirds of the population will continue to have uncontrolled BP and face other major health risks (Chobanian et al., 2003) [*problem significance*].... Self-monitoring of BP has been shown to lead to improved BP control.... The efficacy of BP TM has been tested using a randomized controlled design, but the sample was small (Artinian et al., 2001) [*problem background*].... The influence of TM on BP control warrants further study" [*problem statement*]. (Artinian et al., 2007, pp. 312–314)

Research Purpose

"The purpose of this randomized controlled trial with urban African Americans was to compare usual care (UC) only with BP telemonitoring (TM) plus UC to determine which leads to greater reduction in BP from baseline over 12 months of follow-up, with assessments at 3, 6, and 12 months postbaseline." (Artinian et al., 2007, p. 313)

Review of Literature

The literature review for this study included relevant, current studies that the researchers summarized to identify what is known and not known about the impact of TM on BP. The sources were current and ranged in publication dates from 1998 to 2005, with the majority of the studies published in the last 5 years. The study was accepted for publication on May 31, 2007, and published in the September/October 2007 issue of *Nursing Research*. Artinian et al. (2007, p. 314) summarized the current knowledge about the effect of TM on BP by stating, "Although promising, the effects of TM on BP have been tested in small, sometimes nonrandomized, samples, with one study suggesting that patients may not always adhere to measuring their BP at home. The influence of TM on BP control warrants further study."

Framework

Artinian et al. (2007) developed a model that identified the theoretical basis for their study. The model presented in Figure 3-3 indicates that "nurse-managed TM is an innovative strategy that may offer hope to hypertensive African Americans who have difficulty accessing care for frequent BP checks.... In other words, TM may lead to a reduction in opportunity costs or barriers for obtaining follow-up care by minimizing the contextual risk factors that interfere with frequent healthcare visits.... Combined with information about how to control hypertension, TM may both help individuals gain conscious control over their HBP and contribute to feelings of confidence for carrying out hypertension self-care actions.... Home TM appeared to contribute to individuals' increased personal control and

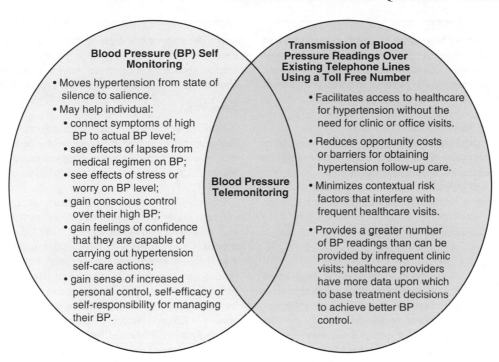

Figure 3-3 Theoretical basis for the effects of telemonitoring on blood pressure (BP). (From Artinian, N. T., Flack, J. M., Nordstrom, C. K., Hockman, E. M., Washington, O. G. M., Jen, K. C., et al. [2007]. Effects of nurse-managed telemonitoring on blood pressure at 12-month follow-up among urban African Americans. *Nursing Research, 56*[5], 313.)

self-responsibility for managing their BP, which ultimately led to improved BP control (Artinian et al., 2004; Artinian et al., 2001)." (Artinian et al., 2007, pp. 313–314)

The framework for this study was based on tentative theory that was developed from the findings of previous research by Artinian et al. (2004; 2001) and other investigators. This framework map (see Figure 3-3) and description provide a basis for interpreting the study findings and giving them meaning. The framework mainly provides a basis for the TM intervention and would be strengthened by including concepts to represent the outcomes or more of a discussion of the SBP and DBP.

Hypothesis Testing

"H1: Individuals who participate in UC plus nurse-managed TM will have a greater reduction in BP from baseline at 3-, 6-, and 12-month follow-up than would individuals who receive UC only." (Artinian et al., 2007, p. 317)

Variables

The independent variable was the TM Program and the dependent variables were SBP and DBP. Only the TM Program, SBP, and DBP conceptual and operational definitions are presented as examples. The conceptual definitions are derived from the study framework and/or are included as part of the literature review. In this study, the operational definitions for the dependent variables are found in the methods section under "Outcome Measurement," and the independent variable is operationalized under an "Intervention" heading.

Independent Variable: TM Program

Conceptual Definition: TM program is an innovative strategy that may offer hope to hypertensive African Americans to reduce their opportunity costs and barriers for obtaining follow-up care for BP management (Artinian et al., 2007).

Operational Definition: TM "refers to individuals self-monitoring their BP at home, then transmitting the BP readings over existing telephone lines using a toll-free number" (Artinian et al., 2007, p. 313). The BP readings were reviewed by the care providers, with immediate feedback provided to the patients about their treatment plan.

Dependent Variables: SBP and DBP

Conceptual Definition: SBP and DBP are an indication of the patient's blood pressure control and ultimately the management of his or her hypertension.

Operational Definition: The outcome of SBP and DBP were measured with the electronic BP monitor (Omron HEM-737 Intellisense, Omron Health Care, Inc.) (Artinian et al., 2007).

Design

"A randomized, two-group, experimental, longitudinal design was used. The treatment group received nurse-managed TM and the control group received enhanced UC. Data were collected at baseline and 3-, 6-, and 12-month follow-ups. Follow-up periods were chosen to allow some comparisons of findings from this study with those from other TM studies that have been reported in the literature.…

Because imbalances in the number of participants assigned to each group could occur with simple randomization, block stratified randomization for antihypertensive medication use was performed to ensure an equal number of participants taking antihypertensive medications in each group. It was important to avoid an imbalance in the number of participants taking antihypertensive medications in one of the groups because an imbalance could confound the effects of the TM intervention.

Sequentially numbered computer-generated randomization assignments were determined prior to the start of data collection, but participants were not notified of the group assignment until after baseline data were collected. To keep data collectors blinded to group assignment, the study's project manager informed the participants of their group assignment by mail or telephone within a week of their baseline interview. Data collectors were trained not to ask participants about group assignment and to ask participants not to reveal their assignment to them." (Artinian et al., 2007, pp. 314–315)

This study has a strong design with groups stratified according to hypertension medication use. The stratification ensured that the TM group was similar to the UC group regarding the number of participants taking hypertension medications. Thus, differences found between the groups would be due to the treatment and

not to differences in the group participants. The participants were randomly assigned to the treatment or comparison groups by a computer with the data collectors blinded to, or kept unaware of, the group assignment.

Sample

"African Americans with hypertension [*population*] were recruited through free BP screenings offered at community centers, thrift stores, drug stores, and grocery stores located on the east side of Detroit [*natural settings*]….

Inclusion criteria were ≥18 years of age; SBP ≥ 140 mm Hg or DBP ≥ 90 mm Hg, unless self-identified as a diabetic or with a history of chronic kidney disease, then SBP ≥ 130 mm Hg or DBP ≥ 80 mm Hg; access to a land-based telephone in own residence (owned or rented) [*natural setting*]; oriented to person, time, and place; English speaking; and intent to remain in Detroit for the next year. Exclusion criteria were arm circumference > 17.5 in.; history of dementia, mental illness, terminal cancer, advanced liver disease, or hemodialysis; and self-reported illicit drug use or alcohol abuse as measured by the CAGE (Cut, Annoyed, Guilty, Eye-opener) questions." (Artinian et al., 2007, p. 315)

The population and the recruitment process are clearly described. The sample criteria for including and excluding subjects from the study were detailed and provided a means of identifying patients with hypertension. The sample size was 387 (194 in the TM group and 193 in the UC group), and there was a 13% attrition, or loss of subjects, over the 12-month study, which are both study strengths. The original sample was a nonrandom sample of convenience, and the subjects were recruited through free BP screenings offered at a variety of locations. The nonrandom sampling introduces a potential for sampling bias, because not all potential subjects had an equal chance to participate in the study. . The subjects participating in free BP screenings might differ in some way from those who do not seek screening. These study elements are more characteristic of a quasi-experimental study, but the study does have an experimental type of design (Kerlinger & Lee, 2000; Shadish et al., 2002).

Procedures

Artinian et al. (2007) detailed the nurse-managed TM intervention that was presented earlier in this chapter and provided in entirety on pages 315-316 in the research article. The outcome measure of BP was measured with the electronic Omron BP monitor "after a 5-minute rest period; at least two BPs were measured, and the average of all was used for analyses. Participants wore unrestrictive clothing and sat next to the interviewer's table, their feet on the floor; their back supported; and their arm abducted, slightly flexed, and supported at heart level by the smooth, firm surface of a table" (Artinian et al., 2007, pp. 316–317).

"Most of the data were collected during 2-hour structured face-to-face interviews and brief physical exams, which were conducted by trained interviewers in a private room at one of the project-affiliated neighborhood community centers. Mailed postcards provided interview appointment reminders 1 week before the scheduled interview; telephone call reminders were made the evening before the interview.... Participants were compensated $25.00 after the completion of each interview" (Artinian et al., 2007, p. 316). The study was approved by the Wayne State University Human Investigation Committee, and all participants signed consent forms indicating their willingness to participate in this study.

Results

"The hypothesis was supported partially by the data. Overall, the TM intervention group had a greater reduction in SBP (13.0 mm Hg) than the UC group did (7.5 mm Hg; $t = -2.09$, $p = 0.04$) from baseline to the 12-month follow-up. Although the TM intervention group had a greater reduction in the DBP (6.3 mm Hg) compared with the UC group (4.1 mm Hg), the differences were not statistically significant ($t = -1.56$, $p = 0.12$)" (Artinian et al., 2007, pp. 317–318). The study results were clearly presented in tables and figures.

Discussion

"The nurse-managed TM group experienced both clinically and statistically significant reductions in SBP (13.0 mm Hg) and clinically significant reductions in DBP (6.3 mm Hg) over a 12-month monitoring period [*study conclusions*].... The BP reductions achieved here are important results, which, if maintained over time, could improve care and outcomes significantly for urban African Americans with hypertension.... This may mean that an individual could avoid starting a drug regimen or may achieve BP control using a one-drug regimen rather than a two-drug regimen and thus be at risk for fewer medication side effects [*implications of the findings for nursing practice*].... Future research needs to determine if this intervention effect maintained over time leads to reducing the number of complications associated with uncontrolled BP and if it leads to reducing the number of drugs necessary to achieve BP control." (Artinian et al., 2007, pp. 320–321)

Experimental Research

The purpose of experimental research is to examine cause-and-effect relationships between independent and dependent variables under highly controlled conditions (Shadish et al., 2002). Researchers exert high control over the planning and implementation of experimental studies, including experimental designs, random samples, highly structured interventions, and quality measurement methods. Often these studies are conducted in highly controlled settings, such as laboratories or research units, with humans or animals. The study by Byerley et al. (2010) introduced earlier in this chapter is an experimental study to examine the causes of cancer-related cachexia using male rats that was conducted in a laboratory setting. To improve your understanding of the steps of the research process, read this study and identify the steps of quantitative research process outlined in this chapter.

--------- **KEY POINTS** ---------

- Nurses use a broad range of quantitative approaches—including descriptive, correlational, quasi-experimental, and experimental—to develop nursing knowledge.
- Some of the concepts relevant to quantitative research are (1) basic research, (2) applied research, (3) rigor, and (4) control.
- Basic, or pure, research is a scientific investigation that involves the pursuit of "knowledge for knowledge's sake" or for the pleasure of learning and finding truth.
- Applied, or practical, research is a scientific investigation conducted to generate knowledge that will directly influence or improve clinical practice.
- Rigor involves discipline, scrupulous adherence to detail, and strict accuracy.
- Control involves the imposing of "rules" by the researcher to decrease the possibility of error and thus increase the probability that the study's findings are an accurate reflection of reality.
- The quantitative research process involves conceptualizing a research project, planning and implementing that project, and communicating the findings.
- The steps of the quantitative research process are as follows:

1. *Formulating a research problem and purpose* identifies an area of concern and the specific focus or aim of the study.

2. *Reviewing relevant literature* allows the researcher to build a picture of what is known about a particular situation or phenomenon and identify the knowledge gaps that exist.

3. *Developing a framework* guides the development of the study and enables the researcher to link the findings to the body of knowledge in nursing.

4. *Formulating research objectives, questions, or hypotheses* allows the researcher to bridge the gap between the more abstractly stated research problem and purpose and the study design and plan for data collection and analysis.

5. *Operationalizing study variables* involves developing a conceptual definition and operational definition for each variable.

6. *Selecting a research design* directs the selection of a population, sampling procedure, implementation of the intervention, methods of measurement, and a plan for data collection and analysis.

7. *Defining the population and sample* determines who will participate in the study.

8. *Implementation of the study intervention* involves the detailed development of the steps or elements of the intervention and the consistent implementation of the intervention during the study.

9. *Selecting methods of measurement* involves determining the best method(s) to measure each study variable.

10. *Developing a plan for data collection and analysis* directs the precise, systematic gathering of information relevant to the research purpose or the specific objectives, questions, or hypotheses of a study and involves the selection of appropriate statistical techniques to analyze the study data.

11. *Implementing the research plan* involves intervention implementation, data collection, data analysis, and interpretation of research outcomes.

12. *Interpreting the research outcomes* involves examining the results from data analysis, exploring the significance of the findings, identifying study limitations, forming conclusions, generalizing findings as appropriate, considering implications for nursing practice, and suggesting further studies.

13. *Communicating findings* includes the development and dissemination of a research report to appropriate audiences through presentations and publication.

- This chapter introduces four types of quantitative research: descriptive, correlational, quasi-experimental, and experimental. Examples from published studies are used to illustrate the steps of the quantitative research process for these different types of quantitative research.

REFERENCES

Aberson, C. L. (2010). *Applied power analysis for the behavioral sciences*. New York, NY: Routledge Taylor & Francis Group.

American Heart Association (AHA). (2004). *Heart disease and stroke statistics–2005 update*. Dallas, TX: Author.

American Heart Association (AHA). (2011). Call to action on use and reimbursement for home blood pressure monitoring. Retrieved from http://my.americanheart.org/professional/General/Call-to-Action-on-Use-and-Reimbursement-for-Home-Blood-Pressure-Monitoring_UCM_423866_Article.jsp/.

American Health Association Statistics Committee and Stoke Statistics Subcommittee. (2006). Heart disease and stroke statistics—2006 update. *Circulation, 113*(6), e85–e152.

Arain, M., Campbell, M. J., Cooper, C. L., & Lancaster, G. A. (2010). What is a pilot or feasibility study? A review of current practice and editorial policy. *BMC Medical Research Methodology, 10*(1), 67.

Artinian, N. T., Flack, J. M., Nordstrom, C. K., Hockman, E. M., Washington, O. G. M., Jen, K. C., et al. (2007). Effects of nurse-managed telemonitoring on blood pressure at 12-month follow-up among urban African Americans. *Nursing Research, 56*(5), 312–322.

Artinian, N. T., Washington, O. G., Klymko, K. W., Marbury, C. M., Miller, W. M., & Powell, J. L. (2004). What you need to know about home blood pressure telemonitoring, but may not know to ask. *Home Healthcare Nurse, 22*(10), 680–686.

Artinian, N. T., Washington, O. G., & Templin, T. N. (2001). Effects of home telemonitoring and community-based monitoring on blood pressure control in urban African Americans: A pilot study. *Heart & Lung, 30*(3), 191–199.

Bond, E. F. & Heitkemper, M. M. (1987). Importance of basic physiologic research in nursing science. *Heart & Lung, 16*(4), 347–349.

Borglin, G. & Richards, D. A. (2010). Bias in experimental nursing research: Strategies to improve the quality and explanatory power of nursing science. *International Journal of Nursing Studies, 47*(1), 123–128.

Brissette, I., Scheier, M. F., & Carver, C. S. (2002). The role of optimism in social network development, coping, and psychological adjustment during a life transition. *Journal of Personality and Social Psychology, 82*(1), 102–111.

Brown, S. J. (2009). *Evidence-based nursing: The research-practice connection*. Sudbury, MA: Jones and Bartlett.

Byerley, L. O., Lee, S. H., Redmann, S., Culberson, C., Clemens, M., & Lively, M. O. (2010). Evidence for a novel serum factor distinct from zinc alpha-2 glycoprotein that promotes body fat loss early in the development of cachexia. *Nutrition and Cancer*, 62(4), 484–494.

Campbell, D. T. & Stanley, J. C. (1963). *Experimental and quasi-experimental designs for research*. Chicago, IL: Rand McNally.

Carver, C. S. & Gaines, J. G. (1987). Optimism, pessimism, and postnatal depression. *Cognitive Therapy and Research*, 11(4), 449–462.

Chen, C. M., Kuo, S. F., Chou, Y. H., & Chen, H. C. (2007). Post-partum Taiwanese women: Their postpartum depression, social support and health-promoting lifestyle profiles. *Journal of Clinical Nursing*, 16(8), 1550–1560.

Chobanian, A., Bakris, G., Black, H., Cushman, W., Green, L., Izzo, J., Jr., et al. (2003). Seventh report of the Joint National Committee on Prevention, Detection, Evaluation, and Treatment of High Blood Pressure. *Hypertension*, 42(6), 1206–1252.

Cohen, S. & Williamson, G. (1988). Perceived stress in a probability sample of the United States. In S. Spacapam & S. Oskamp (Eds.), *The social psychology of health* (pp. 31–67). Newbury Pare, CA: Sage.

Cook, T. D. & Campbell, D. T. (1979). *Quasi-experimentation: Design and analysis issues for field settings*. Chicago, IL: Rand McNally.

Dabl Educational Trust. (2005). Device table: Upper arm devices for self-measurement of blood pressure. Retrieved from http://www.dableducational.com/sphygmomanometers.html/.

Fawcett, J. & Garity, J. (2009). *Evaluating research for evidence-based nursing practice*. Philadelphia, PA: F. A. Davis.

Feeley, N., Cossette, S., Côté, J., Héon, M., Stremler, R., Martorella, G., et al. (2009). The importance of piloting an RCT intervention. *Canadian Journal of Nursing Research*, 41(2), 85–99.

Fields, L., Burt, V., Cutler, J., Hughers, J., Roccella, E., & Sorlie, P. (2004). The burden of adult hypertension in the United States 1999 2000: A rising tide. *Hypertension*, 44(4), 398–404.

Fisher, Sir, R. A. (1935). *The designs of experiments*. New York, NY: Hafner.

Forbes, A. (2009). Clinical intervention research in nursing. *International Journal of Nursing Studies*, 46(4), 557–568.

Gill, R. M. & Loh, J. M. (2010). The role of optimism in health-promoting behaviors in new primiparous mothers. *Nursing Research*, 59(5), 348–355.

Groth, S. W. & David, T. (2008). New mothers' views of weight and exercise. *American Journal of Maternal Child Nursing*, 33(6), 364–370.

Grove, S. K. (2007). *Statistics for health care research: A practical workbook*. St. Louis, MO: Saunders Elsevier.

Hayward, K., Campbell-Yeo, M., Price, S., Morrison, D., Whyte, R., Cake, H., et al. (2007). Cobedding twins: How pilot study findings guided improvements in planning a larger multicenter trial. *Nursing Research*, 56(2), 137–143.

Hertzog, M. A. (2008). Considerations in determining sample size for pilot studies. *Research in Nursing & Health*, 31(2), 180–191.

Homans, G. (1965). Group factors in worker productivity. In H. Proshansky & B. Seidenberg (Eds.), *Basic studies in social psychology* (pp. 592–604). New York, NY: Holt, Rinehart & Winston.

Kaplan, A. (1964). *The conduct of inquiry: Methodology for behavioral science*. New York. NY: Chandler.

Kerlinger, F. N. & Lee, H. B. (2000). *Foundations of behavioral research* (4th ed.). New York, NY: Harcourt Brace.

Lazarus, R. S. & Folkman, S. (1984). *Stress, appraisal and coping*. New York, NY: Springer.

Melnyk, B. M. & Fineout-Overholt, E. (2011). *Evidence-based practice in nursing & healthcare: A guide to best practice* (2nd ed.). Philadelphia, PA: Lippincott, Williams, & Wilkins.

Morrison, D. M., Hoppe, M. J., Gillmore, M. R., Kluver, C., Higa, D., & Wells, E. A. (2009). Replicating an intervention: The tension between fidelity and adaptation. *AIDS Education and Prevention*, 21(2), 128–140.

Myers, S. T. (1982). The search for assumptions. *Western Journal of Nursing Research*, 4(1), 91–98.

Nagel, E. (1961). *The structure of science: Problems in the logic of scientific explanation*. New York, NY: Harcourt, Brace & World.

National Human Genome Research Institute (NHGRI). (2012). *An overview of the division of intramural research*. Retrieved from http://www.genome.gov/10001634/.

National Institute of Nursing Research (NINR). (2012). *Research and funding*. Retrieved from http://www.ninr.nih.gov/Research AndFunding/

Park, C. L., Moore, P. J., Turner, R. A., & Alder, N. E. (1997). The roles of constructive thinking and optimism in psychological and behavioral adjustment during pregnancy. *Journal of Personality and Social Psychology*, 73(3), 584–592.

Patteson, D. & Killien, M. G. (2001). The working mother's study: Health promoting behaviors of employed mothers. *Communicating Nursing Research*, 34(9), 179.

Pickering, T. G., Miller, N. H., Ogedegbe, G., Krakoff, L. R., Artinian, N. T., & Goff, D. (2008). Call to action on use and reimbursement for home blood pressure monitoring: A joint scientific statement from the American Heart Association, American Society of Hypertension, and Preventive Cardiovascular Nurses Association. *Journal of Cardiovascular Nursing*, 23(4), 299–323.

Prescott, P. A. & Soeken, K. L. (1989). Methodology corner: The potential uses of pilot work. *Nursing Research*, 38(1), 60–62.

Ryan-Wenger, N. A. (2010). Evaluation of measurement precision, accuracy, and error in biophysical data for clinical research and practice. In C. F. Waltz, O. L. Strickland, & E. R. Lenz (Eds.), *Measurement in nursing and health research* (4th ed.) (pp. 371–383). New York, NY: Springer Publishing Company.

Santacroce, S. J., Maccarelli, L. M., & Grey, M. (2004). Methods: Intervention fidelity. *Nursing Research*, 53(1), 63–66.

Scheier, M. F. & Carver, C. S. (1992). Effects of optimism on psychological and physical well-being: Theoretical overview and empirical update. *Cognitive Therapy and Research*, 16(2), 201–228.

Scheier, M. F., Carver, C. S., & Bridges, M. W. (1994). Distinguishing optimism from neuroticism (trait anxiety, self-mastery, and self-esteem): A re-evaluation of the life orientation test. *Journal of Personality and Social Psychology*, 67(6), 1063–1078.

Shadish, W. R., Cook, T. D., & Campbell, D. T. (2002). *Experimental and quasi-experimental designs for generalized causal inference*. Chicago, IL: Rand McNally.

Smith, M. J. & Liehr, P. R. (2008). *Middle range theory for nursing* (2nd ed.). New York, NY: Springer Publishing Company.

Tabachnick, B. G. & Fidell, L. S. (2007). *Using multivariate statistics* (5th ed.). Boston, MA: Allyn & Bacon.

Thompson, S. K. (2002). *Sampling* (2nd ed.). New York, NY: John Wiley & Sons.

Walker, L. O. (1989). Stress process among mothers of infants: Preliminary model testing. *Nursing Research*, *38*(1), 10–16.

Walker, S. & Hill-Polerecky, D. M. (1996). *Psychometric evaluation of the Health-Promoting Lifestyle Profile II*. (Unpublished manuscript.) University of Nebraska, Omaha, NE.

Waltz, C. F., Strickland, O. L., & Lenz, E. R. (2010). *Measurement in nursing and health research* (4th ed.). New York, NY: Springer.

Warren, P. L. (2005). First-time mothers: Social support and confidence in infant care. *Journal of Advanced Nursing*, *50*(5), 479–488.

Wysocki, A. B. (1983). Basic versus applied research: Intrinsic and extrinsic considerations. *Western Journal of Nursing Research*, *5*(3), 217–224.

Introduction to Qualitative Research

Qualitative research is a scholarly approach to describe life experiences from the perspective of the persons involved. It is a way to give significance to the subjective human experience as well as gain insights to guide nursing practice (ZuZelo, 2012). These insights are gained not through measuring concepts or establishing causality but through improving our comprehension of a phenomenon of interest. Within a naturalistic holistic framework, qualitative research allows us to explore the depth, richness, and complexity inherent in the lives of human beings. The insights from this process can foster an understanding of patient needs and problems, guide emerging theories, and build nursing knowledge (Munhall, 2012). Although qualitative research is somewhat flexible, qualitative researchers use rigorous and systematic processes that require conceptualization, imaginative reasoning, and elegant expression.

To critically appraise studies in publications, use the findings in practice, and develop the skills needed to conduct qualitative research, you must comprehend qualitative research methodologies. Nurse researchers conducting qualitative studies are contributing important information to our body of knowledge unobtainable by quantitative means. The terminology used in qualitative research and the methods of reasoning are different from those of quantitative research and are reflections of the philosophical orientations of the different types of qualitative research. Each qualitative approach flows from a specific philosophical orientation that directs the methodology and interpretation of data. This chapter presents a general overview of the following qualitative approaches: phenomenological research, grounded theory research, ethnographic research, exploratory-descriptive qualitative research, and historical research. Many other approaches to qualitative research have been developed, but these are the approaches and methods most frequently used by nurse researchers. Although each qualitative approach is unique, there are many commonalities. These commonalities constitute the perspective of the qualitative researcher.

Perspective of the Qualitative Researcher

All scientists approach problems from a philosophical stance or perspective. The **philosophical perspective** of the researcher guides the questions asked and the methods selected for conducting a specific study. Both quantitative and qualitative researchers have philosophical perspectives. Quantitative studies are based primarily on the philosophy of logical positivism that values logic, empirical data, and tightly controlled methods (see Chapter 3) (Kerlinger & Lee, 2000; Shadish, Cook, & Campbell, 2002). Qualitative studies are based on a wide range of philosophies, such as phenomenology, symbolic interactionism, constructivism, and hermeneutics, each of which espouses slightly different approaches to gaining new knowledge (Liamputtong & Ezzy, 2005).

Philosophy Describes a View of Science

Qualitative researchers ascribe to a view of science that values the uniqueness of the individual and the holistic approach to understanding human experiences. The philosophical perspective of the researcher is consistent with research questions that seek the participant's perspective of a phenomenon or experience. Figure 4-1 demonstrates this idea, as the arrow on the left of the figure ("Philosophy") shapes and fits with the next arrow ("View of Science"). Because of their philosophical perspectives, quantitative researchers hold views of science that value tightly controlled studies and generalizable numerical findings. In contrast, the philosophical perspectives of qualitative

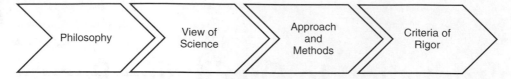

Figure 4-1 Valid science is based on congruence from philosophy to rigor.

researchers influence their views of science. As a result, qualitative researchers value rigorous, but flexible designs to identify study findings. Through the study findings, we are able to increase our understanding of an experience using a discovery process that allows a complex picture to emerge (Forman, Creswell, Damschroder, Kowalski, & Krein, 2008).

The primary thinking process used in quantitative studies is deduction; in contrast, qualitative researchers tend to be inductive thinkers (Forman et al., 2008). **Deductive thinking** begins with a theory or abstract principle that guides the selection of methods to gather data to support or refute the theory or principle. Forman et al. (2008) call this a "top-down" approach. **Inductive thinking** involves perceptually putting insights and pieces of information together and identifying abstract themes or working from the bottom up. From this inductive process, meanings emerge. Because the perception of each qualitative researcher is unique, the meanings identified within the data may vary from researcher to researcher. However, others should be able to retrace the analysis and thinking processes that resulted in the researcher's conclusions. In order to do this, readers must be aware of the underlying philosophical perspective of the study being reviewed.

Philosophy Guides Methods

Each type of qualitative research is consistent with a particular philosophical perspective (see Figure 4-1). The philosophy shapes the view of science that in turn shapes the approaches and methods selected for the study, just as the arrows in Figure 4-1 fit together like the pieces of a puzzle. The philosophical perspective includes an **epistemology,** a view of knowing and knowledge (Munhall, 2012). As a result, the philosophy directs the research questions and the collection and interpretation of the data. Creswell (2009) emphasizes this point by stating that the assumptions of the specific philosophical approach cannot be separated from the methods. For example, researchers who hold to a phenomenological philosophy of science will ask research questions about the "lived experiences" of persons. They will analyze the data in such a way as to develop a rich, deep description of an experience

from the perspective of the participants. Although the researcher does not always clearly state the philosophical stance on which the study is based, a knowledgeable reader can recognize the philosophy through the description of the problem, formulation of the research questions, and selection of the methods to address the research questions. A well-designed qualitative study is congruent at each stage with the underlying philosophical perspective as identified by the researcher.

Qualitative researchers use open-ended methods to gather descriptions of health-related experiences from participants (Fawcett & Garity, 2009). These open-ended methods include interviews, focus groups, observation, and document review (Speziale & Carpenter, 2007). When oral methods are used, the researcher will usually capture the interaction by an audio or video recording so that a transcript of the communication can be prepared for analysis. These methods are discussed in detail in Chapter 12.

Philosophy Guides Criteria of Rigor

Scientific rigor is valued because it is associated with the worth of the research outcomes. The **rigor** of qualitative studies is appraised differently from the rigor of quantitative studies because of the differences in the underlying philosophical perspectives. Quantitative studies are considered rigorous when the procedures for the study are prescribed prior to data collection, the sample is large enough to represent the population, and researchers tightly control the collection and analysis of the data. A quantitative researcher expects that another researcher could replicate or repeat the study with a similar sample and receive similar results. This is desirable because quantitative researchers define rigor to include objectivity and generalizability. Rigorous qualitative researchers, however, are characterized by openness and demonstrate methodological congruence, scrupulous adherence to a philosophical perspective, thoroughness in collecting data, consideration of all the data in the analysis process, and self-understanding. The researcher's self-understanding is important because qualitative research is an interactive process shaped by the researcher's personal history, biography, gender, social class, race, and ethnicity as well as by those of the study participants (Creswell, 2009; Marshall & Rossman, 2011). Self-understanding allows the researcher to have insight into his or her potential biases related to the phenomenon of interest and prevent these biases from interfering with the voices of the participants being heard. These characteristics of qualitative researchers are essential to produce a valid study. Critical appraisal of the rigor of qualitative studies is discussed in more detail in Chapter 18.

To reinforce the key points of Figure 4-1 that philosophy shapes one's view of science, the methods, and criteria of rigor, a study of families with asthmatic children are presented as an example.

Meah, Callery, Milnes, and Rogers (2009) explored how parents and preadolescent children shared the responsibility for asthma management. The researchers had noted a gap in knowledge about the transfer of responsibility from parents to children. The purpose of the study was to "examine meaning of responsibility in children's lives and how parents and children negotiate these responsibilities over time" (Meah et al., 2009, p. 1953). An exploratory-descriptive qualitative study was conducted because quantitative studies had produced diverse results that did not provide adequate understanding of the transfer of responsibility. The study included a framework of responsibility, and the researchers designed the study to be consistent with feminist philosophy and sociological perspectives:

> "Interpretation of the data drew upon both feminist epistemology and sociological understandings of children, health, and the body which relocate subjective experience at the heart of scientific inquiry." (Meah et al., 2009, p. 1954)

Consistent with sociological perspectives, the familial unit was the focus, instead of only the child or only the parents. The researchers' methods included conducting "open-ended, conversational-style interviews" with 18 children and their parents (Meah et al., 2009, p. 1954). The researchers also interviewed the parents separately. The recordings of the interviews were transcribed and "descriptive codes were developed from the transcripts" (p. 1954). The researchers briefly described how they displayed excerpts from the transcripts on charts that "enabled comparison of the children's and adults' perceptions while simultaneously facilitating comparison within children's accounts and those of their parents"

(p. 1954). The study results revealed the of allowing children to manage their asthma grow older:

> "For many of the children in our study, their ability to take responsibility for their condition was often dependent on what they were both allowed and encouraged to do by their parents/carers. Clearly then, we must understand this as a negotiated process and to appreciate its full complexity, we must also look at how parents approached the sharing of responsibility regarding their children's asthma." (Meah et al., 2009, p. 1955)

The researchers concluded that their findings were consistent with the theoretical framework of responsibility that they introduced at the beginning of the study report. The implementation of the study and its findings were also consistent with the philosophical perspectives that the researchers explicitly identified. The approach and methods allowed for children and parents to share their thoughts and feelings in a nonthreatening setting. The data analysis involved strategies that allowed the perspectives of the participants to be described. The researchers could have strengthened the report by providing details about how rigor was ensured. Additional information about the rigor of the methods would increase the validity of the findings.

This example confirms that philosophy shapes one's view of science, which in turn shapes the methods used in a study and the criteria by which the rigor of the study will be evaluated (see Figure 4-1). Because qualitative studies emerge from several philosophies, an understanding of different approaches to qualitative research is needed as a foundation for appraising the rigor of research and making appropriate application of the findings.

Approaches to Qualitative Research

Five approaches to qualitative research commonly conducted and published in the nursing literature are: phenomenological research, grounded theory research, ethnographic research, exploratory-descriptive qualitative research, and historical research (see Table 4-1). Although the five approaches have the commonalities already discussed, these approaches are different, in great part because researchers in different disciplines

TABLE 4-1 Philosophical Orientations Supporting Qualitative Approaches to Nursing Research	
Philosophical and Theoretical Orientations	**Qualitative Approach**
Phenomenology	Phenomenological research
Symbolic interaction theory	Grounded theory research
Naturalism and ethical principles	Ethnographic research
Interpretive and naturalistic perspectives; pragmatism	Exploratory-descriptive qualitative research
Historicism, pragmatism	Historical research

developed them. For example, the social and psychological scientists developed the approaches known as phenomenological research and grounded theory research (Giorgi, 2010; Reed, 2010). Anthropologists developed ethnography with its focus on culture (Morse & Richards, 2002). Exploratory-descriptive qualitative research has emerged from the disciplines of nursing and medicine and has a pragmatic focus on using the knowledge gained to benefit patients and families and improve health outcomes. Historians developed methods to analyze source documents, artifacts, and interviews of witnesses to summarize the knowledge gained by studying the past (Lewenson & Herrmann, 2008). Nurse researchers adapted these methods to understand changes within nursing and health care. The common purpose among the methods, however, is to examine the meaning of human experiences from the perspective of the "knower," the person (or persons) to whom the experiences belong (Bassett, 2004).

Although the data are gathered with openness to the individual experiences of study participants, this fact does not mean that the interpretation is value-free. Each approach is based on a philosophical orientation that influences the study design from the wording of the research question through the interpretation of the data (see Figure 4-1). Thus, you as a consumer of qualitative research must be aware of the guiding principles of the philosophical perspective of a study and use these principles to critically appraise a qualitative study. The discussion of each approach will cover its philosophical perspective or orientation, methodology, and contribution to nursing knowledge.

Phenomenological Research

Phenomenology is both a philosophy and a research method. The purpose of phenomenological research is to describe experiences (or phenomena) as they are lived-in phenomenological terms, to capture the "lived experience" of study participants (Fawcett & Garity, 2009; Munhall, 2012). The philosophical positions taken by phenomenological researchers are very different from those common in the culture and research traditions of the nursing field, which value large samples and generalizable findings.

Philosophical Orientation

Phenomenologists view the person as integral with the environment. The world is shaped by the self and shapes the self. At this point, however, phenomenologists diverge in their beliefs according to adherence to a particular phenomenological philosopher. The key philosophers used by nurse researchers adhering to phenomenology are Husserl and Heidegger.

Philosopher Edmund Husserl (1859-1938) is considered the father of modern phenomenology (Phillips-Pula, Strunk, & Pickler, 2011). Husserl wrote *Logical Investigations* (1901/1970), in which he developed his ideas about phenomena in an effort to resolve the conflict in thought between human sciences (primarily psychology) and the basic sciences (such as physics). Phenomena make up the world of experience. These experiences cannot be explained by examining causal relations but need to be studied as the very things they are. A phenomenon occurs only when there is a person who experiences it. Thus, the experience must be described, not studied using statistics or the researcher's preconceived ideas. To describe the experience, the researcher must be open to the participant's worldview, set aside personal perspectives, and allow meanings to emerge. Husserlian phenomenologists believe that although self and world are mutually shaping, it is possible to separate oneself from one's beliefs or set aside one's beliefs to see the world firsthand in a naive way (Dowling, 2007). Setting aside one's beliefs during qualitative research is called "bracketing."

Researchers who follow the philosophy proposed by Heidegger do not agree, taking the position that bracketing is not possible. Martin Heidegger (1889-1976) was a student of Husserl but expanded the goal of phenomenology from description of lived experience to the interpretation of lived experiences (Earle, 2010). Heidegger's seminal work was *Being and Time* (1927/1962). Heideggerian phenomenologists believe that the person is a self within a body, or is embodied (Munhall, 2012). Munhall describes embodiment as "the unity of body and mind" that eliminates the "the idea of a subjective and objective world" (p. 127). She goes on to say, "the world is knowable only through the subjectivity of being in the world" (p. 127). For example, the interaction between the sensory input that your body sends to your brain and your brain's thinking processes determines your perceptions of the world in which you exist. A depressed person may not notice the color of sunset or the joy in a child's laughter. Another person may not be able to see the sunset because of blindness but may find special meaning in the nuances of the child's laughter. In each situation, the person's being in the world is shaped by the unity of body and mind.

Heideggerian phenomenologists posit that the person is situated in specific context and time that shapes his or her experiences, paradoxically freeing and constraining the person's ability to establish meanings through language, culture, history, purposes, and values (Munhall, 2012). For example, a 50-year-old man diagnosed with aggressive cancer in the United States would experience the diagnosis differently from a 20-year-old woman in rural Ethiopia receiving the same diagnosis. The body, the world, and the concerns, unique to each person, are the context within which that person can be understood. Heideggerians believe that the person experiences being within the framework of time, also called being-in-time. The contexts of the man and the woman with cancer would have different meanings, depending on whether they lived during the 1960s or the 2010s. The availability of treatment, financial resources, and gender roles are only a few of the factors that would shape the cancer experience for these individuals. Each of them has only situated freedom, not total freedom. The man has the freedom to choose physicians from among those who will accept his insurance. The woman may have the freedom only to choose whether she will use a traditional healer or not seek treatment at all. Until a disruption such as an expected diagnosis of cancer occurs, the person may not have considered the limits on meaning imposed by the context and the time.

Other philosophers have built on Husserl and Heidegger's perspectives and refined phenomenological methods. Merleau-Ponty (1908-1961) was among the French philosophers who further developed the Heideggerian concepts of being-in-time and embodiment (Munhall, 2012). He wrote *The Phenomenology of Perception* (1945/2002). Colaizzi (1973), Giorgi (1985), and van Manen (1990) proposed research guidelines for phenomenological research focused on procedural interpretations of the phenomenological method (Speziale & Carpenter, 2007). The novice nurse researcher interested in phenomenology should expand his or her knowledge in this area through immersion in the original writings of these philosophers (Munhall, 2012).

All phenomenologists agree that there is not a single reality; each individual has his or her own reality. Reality is considered subjective, and as a result, unique to the individual. The researcher's experiences in collecting data and analyzing the data during a study are also unique. The researcher must invest considerable time exploring the various philosophical stances within phenomenology to select one compatible with his or her perspective and the research question being asked. More detail on the conduct of phenomenological research is provided in Chapter 12.

Phenomenology's Contribution to Nursing Science

Phenomenology is the philosophical base for three nursing theories and studies that have explored these theories. These theories include the theory of humanistic nursing (Paterson & Zderad, 1976), the theory of human becoming (Parse, 1981, 1992), and the theory of caring (Watson, 1999). Paterson and Zderad emphasized in their theory of humanistic nursing that phenomenology shapes the nurse and the patient as they share experiences in the context of health care. The theory is applicable to research because the researcher meets the participant with openness and respect for uniqueness.

On the basis of the values of Paterson and Zderad's (1976) theory, Lesniak (2010) conducted a study with adolescent females who deliberately injure themselves by cutting. She interviewed six young women who described their experiences, including what they would like emergency nurses to know about self-cutting. From their interviews, the researchers identified "an element of loneliness," "an overall meaning of angst and desperation," and "a recovery process after the cutting is over" (Lesniak, 2010, p. 146). Emergency nurses adhering to Paterson and Zderad's caring values who are alert to signs of self-cutting will assess the adolescent and identify strategies to "protect the adolescent from future self-injury" (p. 146). Lesniak noted that the sample was limited to white, middle-class adolescents and could not be generalized to adolescents of other races/ethnicities or income levels.

In 1981, Parse described her theory of man-living-health as evolving from the foundation of existential phenomenology. As she conducted studies congruent with the theory, she refined her ideas into the human becoming theory (Parse, 1992). According to her theory, human beings co-create reality with the environment and structure meaning through images, words, and actions. Parse proposes research methods consistent with phenomenology, the philosophical foundation for her theory (Parse, 2001, 2011). Using Parse's research methods, Chen (2010) conducted a study of the lived experience of moving forward among persons who had experienced a spinal cord injury. Chen collected data from 15 persons through "dialogical engagement, in which the true presence of the researcher was with the participant" (p. 1134). From the stories of the participants and the recordings of the research interactions, Chen extracted three core concepts that she reframed within Parse's theory: "confronting difficulties," "going on and finding self-value and confidence," and "co-creating successes amid opportunities and restrictions" (pp. 1137-1138). The use of Parse's theory during the interpretation of the data was consistent with her research approach but somewhat of a departure from remaining open to the meanings that emerge from qualitative data.

Watson's (1999) theory of caring is also congruent with phenomenology. She describes values of nurses that produce caring actions and an intersubjective experience shared by the nurse and patient. She proposes 10 carative factors that provide a structure for caring as the core of nursing. Transpersonal caring relationships and the carative factors "potentiate therapeutic healing processes and relationships: they affect the one caring and the one-being-cared-for" (Watson, 1997). Byers and France (2008) conducted a phenomenological study using Watson's theory with nurses who care for patients with dementia hospitalized on medical-surgical units. From their interviews with nine nurses, they extracted a "synthesis of unity," a sentence that captured the experience, which they stated as "They stay with you: they come home with you every day" (p. 47). High nurse-patient ratios and the needs of dementia patients challenged the nurses and resulted in stress. Because of their commitment to caring, the nurses were frustrated by giving what they perceived to be care that did not meet their personal standards. Byers and France conclude by noting that "the essence of caring is revealed as it is manifested in the RN caring for the patients with dementia yet it is also the RN who needs to be cared for" (p. 48). An appraisal can be made of this study similar to that of the Chen (2010) study. The use of a theory within a phenomenological approach has the potential to interfere with the emergence of the participants' perspectives.

Shorter and Stayt (2010) conducted a phenomenological study of the experiences of grief and coping mechanisms of nurses in an adult intensive care unit. The philosophical perspective, the methodology, and the contributions to nursing knowledge of this study are presented as an example of a phenomenological study. Shorter and Stayt designed their study to be consistent with the Heideggerian phenomenological perspective (Johnson, 2000) and to "explore critical care nurses' experiences of grief and their coping

mechanisms when a patient dies" (p.160). The researchers' methodology included interviewing eight nurses and analyzing the narratives of the interviews according to Colaizzi's guidelines, a specific approach to phenomenological data analysis (Dowling, 2007). The researchers found clusters of data around two phases in the experience—"the death experience" and "the death thereafter." In describing the death experience, one nurse commented "I hate it when the patient dies suddenly—everything seems just so disorganized. … It makes me feel awful when that happens.... I like to feel that I have done everything that I can" (p. 162). Another nurse talking about the death thereafter said, "You do have to keep a distance in a way, because death happens so often on our unit. You'd be an emotional wreck if you let it bother you or affect you all the time" (Shorter & Stayt, 2010, p. 164).

The death experience was described with the phrases "expectedness, control and good care," "striking a chord," and "meaningful engagement" (Shorter & Stayt, 2010, pp. 162-163). The phrases "formal support," "informal support," "normalization of death," and "emotional dissociation" (pp. 163-164) described the death thereafter. Shorter and Stayt concluded that the grief and coping strategies of nurses are complex and may vary by type of care setting.

Shorter and Stayt (2010) clearly identified the philosophical perspective and methods of their study, although they did not cite primary sources for either Heidegger or Colaizzi. Consistent with the Heideggerian perspective, they collected and analyzed data simultaneously. They used Colaizzi's framework to cluster common meanings and identify themes from the transcripts of the interviews they had conducted. Shorter and Stayt explicitly noted adherence to the Heidegerrian tenets when they discussed the rigor of the study to include "co-construction of knowledge between researcher and participant" (p. 161). The researchers proposed that additional studies are needed to explore whether the coping strategies of nurses affect the quality of care they provide.

Grounded Theory Research

Grounded theory research is an inductive research technique developed by Glaser and Strauss (1967) through their study of the experience of dying. The method's name means that the findings are grounded in the concrete world as experienced by the participants and are interpreted at a more abstract theoretical level. The desired outcome of grounded theory studies is a middle range or substantive theory (Fawcett & Garity, 2009; Marshall & Rossman, 2011; Munhall, 2012).

Philosophical Orientation

Grounded theory is congruent with symbolic interaction theory, which holds many views in common with phenomenology. George Herbert Mead (1863-1931), a social psychologist, developed the principles of interaction theory that were posthumously published (Mead, 1934). His principles were shaped and refined by other social psychologists and became known as *symbolic interaction theory* (Crossley, 2010). Symbolic interaction theory explores how perceptions of interactions with others shape one's view of self and subsequent interactions. One's view of self influences subsequent interactions and creates meaning. People create reality by attaching meanings to situations. Meaning is expressed in terms of symbols, such as words, religious objects, and clothing. These symbolic meanings are the basis for actions and interactions.

Symbolic meanings are different for each individual. We cannot completely know the symbolic meanings of another individual. In social life, groups share meanings. They communicate these shared meanings to others through socialization processes. Group life is based on consensus and shared meanings. Interaction among people may lead to redefinition of experiences, new meanings, and possibly a redefinition of self. Because of its theoretical importance, the interactions among the person and other individuals in social contexts are the focus of observation in grounded theory research.

Grounded Theory's Contribution to Nursing Science

Grounded theory researchers have contributed to our understanding of the patient experience across a wide range of settings. Giske and Artinian (2008) helped us understand how gastroenterology patients undergoing diagnostic testing were balancing between hope and despair. Balancing was the primary theoretical code in the resulting theory of preparative waiting. On similar themes of waiting and balance, Trimm and Sanford (2010) described the family experience of waiting during surgery as maintaining balance during the wait. In cardiac care settings, researchers have described the inner strength of women following placement of a coronary artery stent (Mendes, Roux, & Ridosh, 2010) and the "dialogue around maintaining and renegotiating normality" following a coronary artery bypass graft procedure (Banner, 2010, p. 3123). Noiseux and Ricard (2008) conducted a grounded theory study to develop a theory describing the experience of recovery from schizophrenia from the perspectives of patients, their families, and healthcare professionals.

Maliski, Connor, Williams, and Litwin (2010) conducted a grounded theory study to understand the experiences of low-income, uninsured African American men diagnosed with prostate cancer. These researchers noted that African American men were disproportionately affected by prostate cancer and often were faced with a "death sentence" due to an unwelcomed and unexpected diagnosis of cancer. The methodology of the study was secondary analysis of transcripts from a larger study (Maliski, Rivera, Connor, Lopez, & Litwin, 2008). The sample for the original study included 60 Latina and 35 African American men who had undergone treatment for prostate cancer. When the transcripts were analyzed for the original study, the researchers noted that spiritual concepts emerged in the interviews with some of the African American men. Thus, Maliski et al. (2010, p. 471) analyzed the transcripts from in-depth interviews with 18 African American men from the original study, "focusing on the role of faith in coping with their prostate cancer diagnosis, treatment, and adverse effects." The researchers did not specify the philosophical perspective upon which the study was developed; however, they did indicate that they used grounded theory analytic strategies to analyze the data.

Listen to the voice of one participant as he used his faith to conquer his fear. "As long as my heart and spirit are good, I can keep going. Good things can happen in the future, and I was put on Earth for a reason so I'm not afraid of death" (Maliski et al., 2010, p. 474).

As you can see, grounded theory research examines experiences and processes with a breadth and depth not usually possible with quantitative research. The reader can intuitively verify these findings through her or his own experiences. Through the rigorous conduct of grounded theory research, these investigators were able to conclude that faith was a spiritual coping strategy for those men of limited resources (Maliski et al., 2010). The contribution to nursing science is that a clear, cohesive description of the phenomenon allows greater understanding. Although a theory was not developed, the improved understanding can guide nursing interventions that meet the needs of patients in ways that they value.

Ethnographic Research

Ethnographic research provides a framework for studying cultures. The word ethnography is derived by combining the Greek roots *ethno* (folk or people) and *graphy* (picture or portrait). Ethnographies are the written reports of a culture from the perspective of insiders. These reports were initially the products of anthropologists who studied primitive, foreign, or remote cultures. Now, however, a number of other disciplines, including social psychology, sociology, political science, education, and nursing, promote cultural research (Wolf, 2012).

Ethnography does not require travel to another country or region; however, it requires spending considerable time in the setting observing and gathering data. A specific group or subculture is identified for study, such as women giving birth at home in Haiti or male nurses working in acute care settings. Ethnography can be used to describe and analyze aspects of the ways of life of a particular culture, even your own. McGibbon, Peter, and Gallop (2010) conducted an ethnographic study with pediatric intensive care nurses focusing on the social organization and the institutional context that contributed to the stress of the nurses. They identified "six main forms of nurses' stress, including emotional distress; constancy of presence; burden of responsibility; negotiating hierarchical power; engaging in bodily caring; and being mothers, daughters, aunts, and sisters" (p. 1357).

An appreciation of other cultures often begins with an examination of your own culture and identification of ethnocentric values that may influence your care of people of other cultures. The formal study of one's own culture or social context, **autoethnography**, involves critical reflection on your own life experiences as shaped by your culture (Wolf, 2012). For example, Brooks (2011) conducted an autoethnography of the mental illness of obsessive-compulsive disorder from her unique viewpoints as "an academic observer and an individual sufferer" (p. 251). Brooks, not a nurse, shared her autoethnography in part so nurses and other healthcare professionals could understand the ability of some obsessive-compulsive disorder sufferers to appear as though nothing is wrong. In her words, by "performing 'appropriately' and putting on my socially acceptable 'face,'" she "suppressed the personal and tragic reality of my illness" (p. 259). Her description of her experience reflected the performances required by her roles within the cultures of academia and mental health treatment.

Philosophical Orientation

Anthropologists seek to understand people: their ways of living, believing, acquiring information, transforming knowledge, and socializing the next generation. Studying a culture begins with the philosophical values of respecting, appreciating, and seeking to preserve the values and ways of life of the culture (Wolf, 2012). The philosophical bases of ethnography are naturalism and respect for others. The purpose of anthropological research is to describe a culture and

TABLE 4-2 Four Types of Ethnography

Type	Other Labels	Purpose
Classic	Traditional	Describe a foreign culture through immersion in the culture for an extended period
Systematic	Institutional	Describe the social organizational structure influencing a specific group of people
Interpretative		Interpret the values and attitudes shaping the behaviors of members of a specific group, in order to promote understanding of the context of culture
Critical	Disrupted	Examine the life of a group in the context of an alternative theory or philosophy, such as feminism or constructivism

explore "the meanings of social actions within cultures" (Wolf, 2012, p. 285).

Four schools of thought within ethnography have emerged from different philosophical perspectives: classic, systematic, interpretive, and critical ethnography (Speziale & Carpenter, 2007). Classic ethnography seeks to provide a comprehensive holistic description of a culture (Wolf, 2012). For example, researchers who conduct classic ethnographic studies live for extended periods outside of their own country in the environment of their study and write a factual description of the culture (see Table 4-2). In contrast, systematic ethnography explores and describes the structures of the culture with an increased focus on groups, patterns of social interaction, organizations, and institutions. The study by McGibbon et al. (2010, p. 1356), described earlier, is an example of a systematic ethnography as evidenced by exploring "nurses' everyday work with institutional structures that shape practice."

Interpretive ethnography has as its goal understanding the values and thinking that result in behaviors and symbols of the people being studied. Alexander (2003) identified his study of the black barbershop as an interpretive ethnography. Through observation, repeated interaction, and recall of childhood experiences, Alexander clarified the values of socializing young black men and creating community within a physical space. Critical ethnography has a political purpose of relieving oppression and empowering a group of people to take action on their own behalf. Wolf (2012) calls this type of ethnography "disrupted" or "disruptive," and identifies its philosophical foundation to be critical social theory (Boutain, 1999; Fontana, 2004). Gardezi and colleagues (2009) conducted a critical ethnography of interprofessional communication in the operating suite and analyzed data from 700 surgical procedures performed from 2005 through 2007. An unanticipated finding was the importance of silence, especially those silences that emerged during the analysis of episodes of ineffective communication. Consistent with critical ethnography, the researchers noted that policies and procedures are needed that encourage team members to speak up to protect the patients, but they also acknowledged the complex interaction of silence and speech in the operating room.

Ethnography's Contribution to Nursing Science

Madeline Leininger (1970) brought ethnography into nursing science by writing the first book linking nursing with anthropology. Leininger was first a nurse and then earned her doctoral degree in anthropology. In the 1950s, she began developing a framework for culture care that became the Sunrise Model (Clarke, McFarland, Andrews, & Leininger, 2009). The Sunrise Model identifies factors that affect health and illness, such as religion, income, kinship, education, values, and beliefs. Chapter 7 contains more information about the Theory of Culture Care developed by Leininger, so this section focuses on the qualitative method that she developed to be consistent with ethnonursing.

Ethnonursing research values the unique perspective of groups of people within their cultural context that is influenced at the macro-level by geographical location, political system, and social structures (see Table 4-1). Multiple levels of factors affect the culture and, consequently, the care expressions of the people. A Vietnamese family who is the only family in a small rural community in Georgia may have different care practices from those who live in New York City in a predominantly Vietnamese community. Leininger developed "enablers," sets of questions to guide the researcher's study of the culture (Leininger, 1997; 2002). The enablers provide a flexible framework for the researcher to use to collect and analyze the qualitative data. For example, one of the enablers is "Leininger's Observation-Participation-Reflection Enabler" (Leininger, 1997, p. 45), which reminds the researcher to use these three processes during a study. The method is naturalistic, meaning that the research is conducted in a natural setting without any attempt to control or alter the context. The researcher can be open to explore the insider perspective on health and well-being. The primary ethnonursing data collection method is participant-observation (Douglas et al., 2010). Participant-observation is defined as being present and interacting with participants in routine activities. At the same time, the researcher is paying attention to what is happening from the perspective of an outsider.

Schumacher (2010) conducted an ethnonursing study in a rural village in the Dominican Republic. She used Leininger's Observation-Participation-Reflection (OPR) Enabler (1997) to guide 28 days of data collection related to the different aspects of the Sunrise Model, such as technological, cultural, and religious factors. In addition to observing patterns of behavior related to health, she interviewed 29 people to learn more about the meaning of the observations. These people are called informants. The raw data were organized into 12 categories consistent with the model. From the categories, recurring patterns emerged that eventually led to three themes presented in the following quotations from the study:

> One informant said, "Family is everything. It is the most important and central thing in this culture.... Life is lived for the family.... Family is the basis of our society ..." (Schumacher, 2010, p. 98). This quotation was used as an exemplar of the first theme that family presence is necessary for cultural care of the community members. The second theme was caring as giving respect to the person and paying attention. "Respect and attention are central to the meaning of care for rural Dominicans" (p. 98). Schumacher noted that the people "both value and use generic (folk) care practices as well as professional care practices" (p. 99). This third theme was supported by interview data about using home remedies and faith healers and seeking treatment by a healthcare professional.

Congruent with Leininger's theory and ethnonursing method, Schumacher (2010, p. 99) discussed the findings using the theory's action modes of "culture care preservation/maintenance, culture care accommodation/negotiation, and culture care repatterning/restructuring." The methods were implemented with rigor and produced quality findings. Although this study was conducted in the Dominican Republic, the insights into these health values could promote culturally appropriate care for immigrants from that country in the United States.

Exploratory-Descriptive Qualitative Research

Qualitative nurse researchers have conducted studies with the purpose of exploring and describing a topic of interest but, at times, have not identified a specific qualitative methodology. Other researchers have identified their studies as grounded theory but have not identified theoretical elements and relationships in their findings. Some have identified their studies as phenomenology but have not provided a thick description of a lived experience in their findings. Qualitative descriptive research is a legitimate method of research that may be the appropriate "label" for studies that have no clearly specified method or in which the method was specified but that ended with "a comprehensive summary of an event in the everyday terms of these events" (Sandelowski, 2000, p. 336). Labeling a study as a specific type (grounded theory, phenomenology, or ethnographic) implies fixed categories of research with distinct boundaries, but the boundaries between methods are more appropriately viewed as permeable (Sandelowski, 2010). Although the studies result in descriptions and could be labeled as descriptive qualitative studies, most of the researchers are in the exploratory stage of studying the subject of interest. To decrease any confusion between quantitative descriptive studies and the discussion of this qualitative approach, we decided to call this approach exploratory-descriptive qualitative research. In this book, studies that the researchers identified as being qualitative without indicating a specific approach like phenomenology or grounded theory will be labeled as being exploratory-descriptive qualitative research.

Exploratory-descriptive qualitative studies are conducted to address an issue or problem in need of a solution. For example, Rohr, Adams, and Young (2010) recognized that nurses used inconsistent approaches to prevent and relieve oral discomfort of terminally ill patients. These researchers used interviews in their exploratory-descriptive qualitative study to gain the perspective of the patient receiving palliative care so that standards for oral care could be established for this unique population. They concluded that oral care must begin with structured assessment of patients' mouths every day and include recognition of the impact that oral discomfort has on the emotions and social life of patients receiving palliative care.

Philosophical Orientation

The philosophical orientation that supports exploratory-descriptive qualitative studies undergirds most methods of qualitative inquiry. In contrast to the received view of reality that is the foundation for quantitative methods, qualitative researchers ascribe to a perceived view of reality. The perceiver—the

person living the experience—is the source of information. Closely aligned with the perceived view is a general approach to science that Liamputtong and Ezzy (2005) call the "interpretive orientation." The interpretive orientation acknowledges that meaning is created and maintained in context. Other qualitative experts call the general qualitative approach "naturalistic inquiry." Naturalistic inquiry encompasses studies designed to study people and situations in their natural states (Sandelowski, 2000). Another broad philosophical orientation often inferred by exploratory-descriptive qualitative researchers is pragmatism. Pragmatism supports studies designed to gather data for transformation into information needed to solve a problem or offer a new strategy. "It [pragmatism] indicates that there is a goal, that what works is defined in practice and thus must be put into practice" (McCready, 2010, p. 192). Pragmatism was the philosophical orientation of the study conducted by Rohr et al. (2010).

Exploratory-Descriptive Qualitative Research's Contribution to Nursing Science

An exploratory-descriptive qualitative researcher often indicates that a study is needed with a specific population to understand the needs of, desired outcomes of, or views on appropriate interventions held by the members of the group. The goal is to create a program or an intervention to benefit the population. Exploratory-descriptive qualitative researchers identify a specific lack of knowledge that can be addressed only through seeking the viewpoints of the people most affected. After citing numerous quantitative studies on the topic, Swanlund (2010) wrote about the need for this approach in her study of medication adherence of the older cardiovascular patient:

> "Additionally, the research questions for these studies were derived from the healthcare provider's perspective. These studies have left many questions unanswered regarding the reasons for nonadherence from the perspective of the older adult. Information is needed that will help community-dwelling older adults be successful with their medication management." (Swanlund, 2010, p. 23)

Researchers who value the perspectives of participants may begin a program of research with qualitative methods to: (1) begin development of interventions, (2) evaluate the appropriateness of an intervention following implementation, or (3) develop participants' definitions of concepts that researchers would like to measure. For example, qualitative data were collected during a federally funded study of stress management interventions with healthy adults and persons living with HIV infection (Tuck & Thinganjana, 2007). The researchers sought to understand the participants' perspectives on spirituality as a first step in developing an operational definition for measurement of spirituality. Qualitative data have also been collected through interviews or focus groups to evaluate the cultural appropriateness of and participants' satisfaction with an intervention at the conclusion of a study. For example, Vincent (2009) conducted a focus group with Mexican-Americans with diabetes who had been the recipients of a tailored intervention for health behavior change. She found that the intervention group participants were satisfied with the intervention.

Health promotion within chronic obstructive pulmonary disease (COPD) was the focus of a qualitative study conducted by Caress, Luker, and Chalmers (2010). The philosophical orientation, methodology, and results of the study are discussed as an example of the exploratory-descriptive qualitative approach. Caress et al. described their study as an "exploratory, descriptive design … using semistructured interviews with patients and family caregivers" (p. 565). They did not specify the philosophical orientation; however, they noted that all interviews took place in the participants' homes, an approach consistent with a naturalistic orientation. In addition, the aim of the study, provided in the following quotations and summary, was consistent with a pragmatic philosophical perspective:

"The aim of this study was to generate in-depth insights into patients' and family members' understanding of the causation, progression, and prevention of COPD and the role of health promotion with this population" (Caress et al., 2010, p. 565). The interviews were digitally recorded and transcribed. Data analysis included measures to "ensure the congruence of the analysis amongst the investigators" such as "independent review and coding, discussion of the emerging themes, identification of the key themes, re-examination of the full data set to ensure the 'fit' of the codes to the data, and finally discussion of any discrepancies with a goal of achieving consensus" (Caress et al., 2010, p. 566). Additional measures that they used to enhance the rigor of the study and to protect the ethical rights of the participants were described in detail in this study.

From the transcribed interviews of 14 patients and 12 family members, Caress et al. (2010) identified three themes. The first theme, "Health promotion: What's that?" emerged from the limited spontaneous information about health promoting behaviors provided by the participants. The behaviors that were mentioned were more preventive in nature, rather than health promoting. The second theme, "Community resources for health promotion" (Caress et al., p. 569), was derived from participant statements that indicated limited knowledge of community resources, with the exception of pulmonary rehabilitation. The theme "It wasn't just the smoking: Patients' and family members' views on the causation of COPD" (p. 569) encompassed several participants' statements about the role tobacco played in the development of the disease. The researchers concluded the study's report by proposing a new approach to promoting health among the patients with COPD and their families:

"Our data suggest that a more wide-ranging approach, encompassing aspects of health promotion, might be welcomed by many patients and their family carers.… The findings from this study highlight gaps in patients' and carers' understanding of the potential role of health promotion in COPD and areas of intervention for health professionals." (Caress et al., 2010, pp. 571-772)

This study is a typical example of exploratory-descriptive qualitative research, in that the researchers reported the data without transforming the data into more abstract concepts or constructs. The study would have been strengthened by a clear discussion of the philosophical perspective of the study, which seems to be a mixture of naturalistic and pragmatic perspectives. The research report clearly identified the exploratory-descriptive qualitative methodology used to conduct this study. The researchers took extensive steps to ensure rigor in the data collection and analysis phase and the development of study findings. An unexpected finding was that patients reported anxiety and fear more frequently than depression. Prior to this study, researchers had focused their attention almost exclusively on depression. On the basis of these findings, the researchers would return to the literature to examine studies on anxiety and fear. They may have identified a gap in knowledge that warrants additional research. In addition to addressing anxiety and fear of patients with COPD, health professionals can use these findings as the justification for the development of a health promotion program for such patients and their family members.

Historical Research

Historical research examines events of the past. Historians describe events in the context of time, social structures, concurrent events, and key individuals. These descriptions can increase understanding and raise awareness of the forces shaping current events. Historical nursing research can do the same for the profession and its role in society (Lewenson & Herrmann, 2008). Nurse researchers using historical methods have examined the events and people that shaped health in different settings and countries as well as nursing as a profession. For example, Wood (2009) examined the role of the surgical nurse in Australia, Britain, and New Zealand in the era before antibiotics. Her data sources were nursing articles and textbooks published between 1895 and 1935. She noted that the surgical nurse's role was described in relation to the surgeon rather than the patient. The surgical nurse's role was described as supporter, scrubber, sentry, saboteur, and sloven. The last two descriptors were applied in cases of patient sepsis following a surgery. The relationship between the surgeon and the nurses went beyond simple subservience to include admiration for each other's skills and a conscientious approach to protecting the patient.

Wagner and Whaite (2010, p. 230) examined selected writings of Florence Nightingale using content analysis and identified five themes related to caring: "attend to, attention to, nurture, competent, and genuine." Other historical researchers examined recent events; for example, D'Antonio (2004) studied the push for higher education of nurses as affected by women's opportunities as members of racial/ethnic groups. These studies demonstrate the importance of historical research in describing the past to provide direction for the future in nursing education and practice (Lewenson & Herrmann, 2008).

Philosophical Orientation

History is a very old science that dates back to the beginnings of humankind, when people and groups of people asked, "Where have we come from?" Others asked, "Who are we?" and "Where are we going?" These questions have been asked throughout time. Although the questions do not change, the answers have changed because of the influence of social, cultural, and personal forces. History provides the context of experience (Lewenson & Herrman, 2008).

A primary assumption of historical philosophy is that we can learn from the past and that this knowledge can increase our understanding of the present and future. The philosophy of history is a search for wisdom. The historian examines what has been, what is, and what ought to be. Influenced by the values of the profession and the philosophy of pragmatism, historical nurse researchers often apply the lessons of the past to current events. Wagner and Whaite (2010, p. 233) end the report of their study of the writings of Florence Nightingale with these sentences: "These research findings and others encourage nurses to examine and reflect on how caring relationships impact their practice ... helping students to understand how caring relationships in nursing can occur in all practice settings."

Historical Research's Contribution to Nursing Science

Historical research, although viewed as a legitimate source of knowledge, has received less attention by funding agencies and nurse researchers in the past 10 years because of a shift toward studies that produce evidence to improve patient outcomes. The American Association for the History of Nursing is an organization with a focus on historical methodologies. The association's journal, *Nursing History Review,* serves as vehicle for continued knowledge development in this area. In this journal, Irwin (2011, p. 79) published "a study of U.S. nurses who worked across continents."

The philosophical orientation and methodology of the study received minimal attention, but the researcher noted the role documents played in the study. "The archives, sources, and figures that are central to the field provide a ready means to trace the spread of U.S. global influence in the early twentieth century" (Irwin, 2011, p. 80). Irwin could have strengthened the report by providing more detail on methods used to ensure rigor. Like most historical researchers, Irwin focused the report on the product and provided little information on the processes she used.

Irwin (2011) described four nurses who provided overseas service through the American Red Cross during World War I and in the immediate post-war era. The nurses cared for military personnel but were very involved also in relief efforts for citizens, refugees, and families. They participated in efforts to improve hygiene, care for those with tuberculosis, and open training schools for nurses. Irwin's contribution to nursing knowledge was to increase nurses' awareness of their potential influence. Building on this history of nurse reformers, nurses today can conceive of roles that extend beyond political borders.

KEY POINTS

- Qualitative research is a scholarly approach used to describe life experiences from the perspective of the persons involved.
- The philosophical foundation of qualitative research describes a view of science and guides both the selection of methods and the criteria of rigor.
- Quantitative research is guided by the philosophy of logical positivism. In contrast, qualitative research is guided by a wider range of philosophies.
- Qualitative researchers use open-ended methods to gather data, such as interviews, focus groups, observation, and examination of documents.
- The goal of phenomenological research is to describe experiences as they are lived. Phenomenology is the philosophy guiding these studies, a philosophy that began with the writings of Husserl.
- The goal of grounded theory research is to produce findings grounded in the concrete world as experienced by the participants that can be interpreted at a more abstract level of a theory. Symbolic interactionism is the underlying philosophical and theoretical perspective.
- Ethnographic research is the investigation of cultures through an in-depth study of the members of the culture. Nurse anthropologist Leininger developed the ethnonursing research method.
- Exploratory-descriptive qualitative research elicits the perceptions of participants to provide insights for understanding patients and groups, influencing practice, and developing appropriate programs for specific groups of people. The philosophy of pragmatism and the naturalistic and interpretive orientations guide exploratory-descriptive qualitative studies.
- Historical research is designed to analyze the interaction of people, events, and social context that occurred in the remote or recent past. The methodologies of historical research include interviewing people with knowledge of past events and examining documents describing the events.

REFERENCES

Alexander, B. K. (2003). Fading, twisting, and weaving: An interpretive ethnography of the Black barbershop as cultural space. *Qualitative Inquiry, 9*(1), 105–128.

Banner, D. (2010). Becoming a coronary artery bypass graft surgery patient: A grounded theory study of women's experiences. *Journal of Clinical Nursing, 19*(21/22), 3123–3133.

Bassett, D. (2004). Qualitative research. In C. Bassett (Ed.), *Qualitative research in health care* (pp. 1–5). London, England: Whurr Publishers Ltd.

Boutain, D. M. (1999). Critical nursing scholarship: Exploring critical social theory with African American studies. *Advances in Nursing Science, 21*(4), 37–47.

Brooks, C. F. (2011). Social performance and secret ritual: Battling against obsessive-compulsive disorder. *Qualitative Health Research, 21*(2), 249–261.

Byers, D. C., & France, N. E. M. (2008). The lived experience of registered nurses providing care to patients with dementia in the acute care setting: A phenomenological study. *International Journal of Caring, 12*(4), 44–49.

Caress, A., Luker, K., & Chalmers, K. (2010). Promoting health of persons with chronic obstructive pulmonary disease: Patients' and carers' views. *Journal of Clinical Nursing, 19*(19), 564–573.

Chen, H. (2010). The lived experience of moving forward for clients with spinal cord injury: A Parse research method study. *Journal of Advanced Nursing, 66*(5), 1132–1141.

Clark, P. N., McFarland, M. R., Andrews, M. M., & Leininger, J. (2009). Caring: Some reflections on the impact of the culture care theory by McFarland & Andrews and a conversation with Leininger. *Nursing Science Quarterly, 22*(3), 233–239.

Colaizzi, P. F. (1973). *Reflection and research in psychology: A phenomenological study of learning.* Dubuque, IA: Kendall Hunt.

Creswell, J. W. (2009). *Research design: Qualitative, quantitative, and mixed methods approaches* (3rd ed.). Los Angeles, CA: Sage.

Crossley, N. (2010). Networks and complexity: Directions for interactionist research? *Symbolic Interaction, 33*(3), 341–363.

D'Antonio, P. (2004). Women, nursing, and baccalaureate education in 20th century America. *Journal of Nursing Scholarship, 36*(4), 379–384.

Douglas, M. K., Kemppainen, J. K., McFarland, M. R., Papadopoulos, I., Ray, M. A., Roper, J. M., Scollan-Koliopoulos, M., Shapira, J., & Tsai, H-M. (2010). Chapter 10: Research methodologies for investigating cultural phenomena and evaluating interventions. *Journal of Transcultural Nursing, 21*(Suppl. 1), 3737–4055.

Dowling, M. (2007). From Husserl to van Manen: A review of different phenomenological approaches. *International Journal of Nursing Studies, 44*(1), 131–142.

Earle, V. (2010). Phenomenology as research method or substantive metaphysics? An overview of phenomenology's uses in nursing. *Nursing Philosophy, 11*(4), 286–296.

Fawcett, J., & Garity, J. (2009). *Evaluating research for evidence-based nursing practice.* Philadelphia, PA: F. A. Davis.

Fontana, J. S. (2004). A methodology for critical science in nursing. *Advances in Nursing Science, 27*(2), 93–101.

Forman, J., Creswell, J. W., Damschroder, L., Kowalski, C. P., Krein, S. L. (2008). Qualitative research methods: Key features and insights gained from use in infection prevention research. *American Journal of Infection Control, 36*(10), 764–771.

Gardezi, F., Lingard, L., Espin, L. S., Whyte, S., Orser, B., & Baker, R. (2009). Silence, power, and communication in the operating room. *Journal of Advanced Nursing, 65*(7), 1390–1399.

Giorgi, A. (1985). *Phenomenology and psychological research.* Pittsburg, PA: Duquesne University Press.

Giorgi, A. (2010). Phenomenological psychology: A brief history and its challenges. *Journal of Phenomenological Psychology, 41*(2), 145–179.

Giske, T., & Artinian, B. (2008). Patterns of "balancing between hope and despair" in the diagnostic phase: A grounded theory study of patients on a gastroenterology ward. *Journal of Advanced Nursing, 62*(1), 22–31.

Glaser, B. G., & Strauss, A. (1967). *The discovery of grounded theory: Strategies for qualitative research.* Chicago, IL: Aldine.

Heidegger, M. (1927/1962). *Being in time* (J. Macquarrie & E. Robinson, Trans.). New York, NY: Harper.

Husserl, E. (1901/1970). *Logical investigations: Vol. 1* (N. Findlay, Trans.). New York, NY: Routledge.

Irwin, J. F. (2011). Nurses without borders: The history of nursing as U.S. international history. *Nursing Historical Review, 19*(1), 78–102.

Johnson, M. (2000). Heidegger and meaning: Implications for phenomenological research. *Nursing Philosophy, 1*(2), 134–146.

Kerlinger, F. N., & Lee, H. P. (2000). *Foundations of behavioral research* (4th ed.). Fort Worth, TX: Harcourt College.

Leininger, M. M. (1970). *Nursing and anthropology: Two worlds to blend.* New York, NY: Wiley.

Leininger, M. M. (1997). Overview of the Theory of Culture Care with the ethnonursing research method. *Journal of Transcultural Nursing, 8*(2), 32–54.

Leininger, M. M. (2002). Culture care theory: A major contribution to advance transcultural nursing knowledge and practices. *Journal of Transcultural Nursing, 13*(3), 189–192.

Lesniak, R. G. (2010). The lived experience of adolescent females who self-injure by cutting. *Advanced Emergency Nursing Journal, 32*(2), 137–147.

Lewenson, S. B., & Herrmann, E. K. (2008). Why do historical research? In S. B. Lewenson & E. K. Hermann (Eds.), *Capturing nursing history* (pp. 1–10). New York, NY: Springer.

Liamputtong, P., & Ezzy, D. (2005). *Qualitative research methods* (2nd ed.). Melbourne, VIC, Australia: Oxford University Press.

Maliski, S. L., Connor, S. E., Williams, L., & Litwin, M. S. (2010). Faith among low-income, African American/Black men treated for prostate cancer. *Cancer Nursing, 33*(6), 470–478.

Maliski, S., Rivera, S., Connor, S., Lopez, G., & Litwin, M. (2008). Renegotiating masculine identity after prostate cancer treatment. *Qualitative Health Research, 18*(12), 1609–1620.

Marshall, C., & Rossman, G. B. (2011). *Designing qualitative research* (5th ed.). Los Angeles, CA: Sage.

McCready, J. S. (2010). Jamesian pragmatism: A framework for working towards unified diversity in nursing knowledge development. *Nursing Philosophy, 11*(3), 191–203.

McGibbon, E., Peter, E. & Gallop, R. (2010). An institutional ethnography of nurses' stress. *Qualitative Health Research, 20*(10), 1353–1378.

Mead, G. H. (1934). *Mind, self, and society.* Chicago, IL: University of Chicago Press.

Meah, A., Callery, P., Milnes, L., & Rogers, S. (2009). Thinking "taller": Sharing responsibility in the everyday lives of children with asthma. *Journal of Clinical Nursing, 19*(13/14), 1952–1959.

Mendes, B., Roux, G., & Ridosh, M. (2010). Phenomenon of inner strength in women post-myocardial infarction. *Critical Care Nursing Quarterly, 33*(3), 248–258.

Merleau-Ponty, M. (1945/2002). *Phenomenology of perception* (C. Smith, Trans.). London, England: Routledge Classics.

Morse, J., & Richards, L. (2002). *Readme first for a user's guide to qualitative methods.* Thousand Oaks, CA: Sage.

Munhall, P. L. (2012). *Nursing research: A qualitative perspective* (5th ed.). Sudbury, MA: Jones & Bartlett.

Noiseux, S., & Ricard, N. (2008). Recovery as perceived by persons with schizophrenia, family members, and health professionals: A grounded theory. *International Journal of Nursing Studies, 45*(8), 1148–1162

Parse, R. R. (1981). *Man-living-health: A theory of nursing.* New York, NY: Wiley.

Parse, R. R. (1992). Human becoming: Parse's theory of nursing. *Nursing Science Quarterly, 5*(1), 35–42.

Parse, R. R. (2001). *Qualitative inquiry: The path of sciencing.* New York, NY: National League for Nursing.

Parse, R. R. (2011). The human becoming modes of inquiry: Refinements. *Nursing Science Quarterly, 24*(1), 11–15.

Paterson, J. G., & Zderad, L. T. (1976). *Humanistic nursing.* New York, NY: Wiley.

Phillips-Pula, L., Strunk, J., & Pickler, R. H. (2011). Understanding phenomenological approaches to data analysis. *Journal of Pediatric Health Care, 25*(1), 67–71.

Reed, I. A. (2010). Epistemology contextualized: Social-scientific knowledge in a post-positivistic era. *Sociological Theory, 28*(1), 20–39.

Rohr, Y., Adams, J., & Young, L. (2010). Oral discomfort in palliative care: Results of an exploratory study of the experiences of terminally ill patients. *International Journal of Palliative Nursing, 16*(9), 439–444.

Sandelowski, M. (2000). What happened to qualitative description? *Research in Nursing & Health, 23*(4), 334–340.

Sandelowski, M. (2010). What's in a name? Qualitative description revisited. *Research in Nursing & Health, 33*(1), 77–84.

Schumacher, G. (2010). Culture care meanings, beliefs, and practices in rural Dominican Republic. *Journal of Transcultural Nursing, 21*(2), 93–103.

Shadish, W. R., Cook, T. D., & Campbell, D. T. (2001). *Experimental and quasi-experimental designs for generalization causal inference.* Chicago, IL: Rand McNally.

Shorter, M., & Stayt, L. C. (2010) Critical care nurses' experiences of grief in an adult intensive care unit. *Journal of Advanced Nursing, 66*(1), 159–167.

Speziale, H. J. S., & Carpenter, D. R. (2007). *Qualitative research in nursing: Advancing the humanistic perspective* (4th ed.). Philadelphia, PA: Lippincott Williams & Wilkins.

Swanlund, S. L. (2010). Successful cardiovascular medication management processes as perceived by community-dwelling adults over age 74. *Applied Nursing Research, 23*(1), 22–29.

Trimm, D. R., & Sanford, J. T. (2010). The process of family waiting during surgery. *Journal of Family Nursing, 16*(4), 435–461.

Tuck, I., & Thinganjana, W. (2007). An exploration of the meaning of spirituality voiced by persons living with HIV disease and health adults. *Issues in Mental Health Nursing, 28*(2), 151–166.

van Manen, M. (1990). *Researching lived experience: Human science for an action sensitive pedagogy.* Ontario, Canada: Althouse Press.

Vincent, D. (2009). Culturally tailored education to promote lifestyle change in Mexican Americans with type 2 diabetes. *Journal of the American Academy of Nurse Practitioners, 21*(9), 520–527.

Wagner, D. J., & Whaite, B. (2010). An exploration of the nurse of caring relationships in the writings of Florence Nightingale. *Journal of Holistic Nursing, 28*(4), 225–234.

Watson, J. (1997). Theory of human caring: Retrospective and prospective. *Nursing Science Quarterly, 10*(1), 49–52.

Watson, J. (1999). *Nursing: Human science and human care: A theory of nursing.* Boston, MA: Jones & Bartlett.

Wolf, Z. E. (2012). Ethnography: The method. In P. L. Munhall (Ed.). *Nursing research: A qualitative perspective* (5th ed.) (pp. 285–338). Sudbury, MA: Jones & Bartlett.

Wood, P. J. (2009). Supporting or sabotaging the surgeon's efforts: Portrayals of the surgical nurse's role in preventing wound sepsis, 1895-1935. *Journal of Clinical Nursing, 18*(19), 2739–2746.

Zuzelo, P. R. (2012). Evidence-based nursing and qualitative research: A partnership imperative for real-world practice. In P. L. Munhall (Ed.). *Nursing research: A qualitative perspective* (5th ed.) (pp. 533–552). Sudbury, MA: Jones & Bartlett.

Research Problem and Purpose

evolve http://evolve.elsevier.com/Grove/practice/

We are constantly asking questions to better understand ourselves and the world around us. This human ability to wonder and ask creative questions about behaviors, experiences, and situations in the world provides a basis for identifying research topics and problems. Identifying a problem is the initial step, and one of the most significant, in conducting quantitative, qualitative, outcomes, and intervention research. The research purpose evolves from the problem and directs the subsequent steps of the research process.

Research topics are concepts, phenomena of interest, or broad problem areas that researchers can focus on to enhance evidence-based nursing. Research topics contain numerous potential research problems, and each problem provides the basis for developing many purposes. Thus, the identification of a relevant research topic and a challenging, significant problem can facilitate the development of numerous study purposes to direct a lifetime program of research. However, the abundance of research topics and potential problems frequently is not apparent to nurses struggling to identify their first study problem.

This chapter differentiates a research problem from a purpose, identifies sources for research problems, and provides a background for formulating a problem and purpose for study. The criteria for determining the feasibility of a proposed study problem and purpose are described. The chapter concludes with examples of research topics, problems, and purposes from current quantitative, qualitative, outcomes, and intervention studies.

What Is a Research Problem and Purpose?

A research problem is an area of concern where there is a gap in the knowledge base needed for nursing

practice. Research is conducted to generate knowledge that addresses the practice concern, with the ultimate goal of providing evidence-based health care. A research problem can be identified by asking questions such as the following: What is wrong or is of concern in this clinical situation? What knowledge is needed to improve this situation? Will a particular intervention work in this clinical situation? What is known about this intervention's effectiveness? Would another intervention be more effective in producing the desired outcomes?

By questioning and reviewing the literature, researchers begin to recognize a specific area of concern and the knowledge gap that surrounds it. The knowledge gap, or what is not known about this clinical problem, determines the complexity and number of studies needed to generate essential knowledge for nursing practice (Craig & Smyth, 2012; Creswell, 2009). In addition to the area of concern, the research problem identifies a population and sometimes a setting for the study.

A research problem includes significance, background, and a problem statement. The significance of a problem indicates the importance of the problem to patients and families, nursing, healthcare system, and society. The background for a research problem briefly identifies what we know about the problem area. The problem statement identifies the specific gap in the knowledge needed for practice. A research problem from the study by Grady, Entin, Entin, and Brunye (2011) is presented as an example. This study was conducted to examine the effectiveness of educational messages or information on the knowledge, attitudes, and behaviors of people with diabetes.

"Diabetes prevalence has reached epidemic proportions in this country. The health and economic consequences for Americans with this disease are overwhelming and expected to grow as our population continues to age. Approximately 23.6 million people in the United States have diabetes and, despite the disease being underreported as a cause of death, diabetes was listed as the seventh leading cause of death in the United States in 2006 (Centers for Disease Control and Prevention, 2008a). The direct medical costs of diabetes care and complications of $116 billion, together with indirect costs of $58 billion related to disability and reduced productivity, resulted in an estimated economic cost of diabetes totaling $174 billion in 2007 (American Diabetes Association, 2009).... Complications contribute to a risk of death among individuals with diabetes that is about 2 times higher than that of individuals without diabetes (Centers for Disease Control and Prevention, 2008a).

Amputations and foot ulcerations are the most common consequences of diabetic neuropathy and the major causes of morbidity and disability in people with diabetes. Approximately 2% to 3% of individuals with diabetes develop one or more foot ulcers each year, and an estimated 15% will develop a foot ulcer during their lifetime (Singh, Armstrong, & Lipsky, 2005) [*problem significance*]....

As the cornerstone of diabetes treatment and an integral part of a self-management regime, education of patients with diabetes takes place in both inpatient and outpatient venues.... Patient education takes time in the continuum of care that an already overworked staff is challenged to provide.... The research cited in the reviews of Boren et al. (2006) and Jackson et al. (2006) provides evidence that delivery of healthcare information can be accomplished effectively without involving diabetes educators or nurses and offers support for the use of information-technology-based education as an alternative way to provide information and guidance to persons with diabetes [*problem background*]. However, regardless of whether the information is presented in person or via technology, a relevant and still-open question is how to present the information so as to foster positive attitudinal and behavioral change and maximize the long-term effectiveness of health management education [*problem statement*]." (Grady et al., 2011, pp. 22-23)

In this example, the research problem identifies an area of concern (incidence, costs, and complications of diabetes) for a particular population (persons with diabetes) in selected settings (inpatient and outpatient venues). Grady and colleagues (2011) clearly identified the significance of the problem, which is extensive and relevant to patients, families, nursing, healthcare system, and society. The problem background focuses on key research conducted to examine the effectiveness of health education on the management of diabetes. The last sentence in this example is the problem statement, which identifies the gap in the knowledge needed for practice. In this study, there is limited research on how to present diabetic education to maximize its effectiveness on attitudinal and behavioral change in people with this chronic illness.

The research problem in this example includes concepts or research topics such as diabetes prevalence, economic consequences, complications of diabetes, consequences of diabetic neuropathy, health management education, self-management, and attitudinal and behavioral changes. Health management education is an abstract concept, and a variety of nursing actions or interventions could be implemented to determine their effectiveness in promoting long-term attitudinal and behavioral changes in persons with diabetes. Thus, each problem may generate many research purposes. The knowledge gap regarding how to present information to foster positive attitudinal and behavioral changes in persons with diabetes provides clear direction for formulating the research purpose.

The **research purpose** is a clear, concise statement of the specific focus or aim of the study that is generated on the basis of the research problem. The purpose usually indicates the type of study (quantitative, qualitative, outcomes, or intervention) to be conducted and often includes the variables, population, and setting for the study. The goals of quantitative research include identifying and describing variables, examining relationships among variables, and determining the effectiveness of interventions in managing clinical problems (Creswell, 2009; Shadish, Cook, & Campbell, 2002). The goals of qualitative research include exploring a phenomenon, such as depression as it is experienced by pregnant women; developing theories to describe and manage clinical situations; examining the health practices of certain cultures; describing health-related issues, events, and situations; and determining the historical evolution of the profession (Marshall & Rossman, 2011; Munhall, 2012). The focus of outcomes research is to identify, describe, and improve the outcomes or end results of patient care (Doran, 2011). Intervention research focuses on investigating the effectiveness of nursing interventions in achieving the desired outcomes in natural settings (Forbes, 2009). Regardless of the type of research, every study needs a clearly expressed purpose statement to guide it. Grady et al. (2011) clearly identified their study purpose following their research problem statement of the gap in the knowledge base. Thus, the purpose of their study was to "examine the impact of information framing in an educational program about proper foot care and its importance for preventing diabetic complications on long-term changes in foot care knowledge, attitudes, and behavior" (Grady et al., 2011, p. 23).

This research purpose indicates that these investigators conducted a quantitative quasi-experimental study to determine the effectiveness of an independent variable or intervention (information framing educational program about diabetic foot care and prevention of complications) on the dependent or outcome variables (foot care knowledge, attitudes, and behaviors). The researchers also identified two hypotheses to direct their study, which included the four variables identified (see Chapter 8 for a discussion of hypotheses). The study findings indicated that the gain framed messages focused on the benefits of taking action were significantly more effective in promoting positive behavioral changes in people with diabetes than the loss-framed messages focused on the costs of not taking action. A gain-framed message might be stated as follows: "Achieving normal blood sugar increases your feelings of health and well being and promotes control of your illness." A loss-framed message might be worded as follows: "Poorly controlled blood sugars can lead to complications of neuropathy, foot lesions, and amputation." Grady et al. (2011) also found that changes in knowledge affected changes in attitudes and that attitudes were direct predictors of long-term behavior management of diabetes. The findings from this study and other research provide evidence of the effectiveness of information messages in sustaining health promoting behavior by people with diabetes.

Sources of Research Problems

Research problems are developed from many sources, but you need to be curious, astute, and imaginative to identify problems from the sources. The sources for research problems included in this text are (1) clinical practice, (2) researcher and peer interactions, (3) literature review, (4) theories, and (5) research priorities identified by funding agencies and specialty groups. Researchers often use more than one source to identify and refine their research problem.

Clinical Practice

The practice of nursing must be based on knowledge or evidence generated through research. Thus, clinical practice is an extremely important source for research problems. Problems can evolve from clinical observations. For example, while watching the behavior of a patient and family in crisis, you may wonder how you as a nurse might intervene to improve the family's coping skills. A review of patient records, treatment plans, and procedure manuals might reveal concerns or raise questions about practice that could be the basis for research problems. For example, you may wonder: What nursing intervention will open the lines of communication with a patient who has had a stroke? What is the impact of home visits on the level of function, readjustment to the home environment, and rehospitalization pattern of a child with a severe chronic illness? What is the most effective treatment for acute and chronic pain? What is the best pharmacological agent or agents for treating hypertension in elderly, diabetic patients—angiotensin-converting enzyme (ACE) inhibitor, angiotensin II receptor blocker (ARB), diuretic, beta blocker, calcium channel blocker, or alpha antagonist, or a combination of these drugs? What are the most effective pharmacological and nonpharmacological treatments for a patient with a serious and persistent mental illness? What are the needs of stroke survivors from their perspective? What are the cultural factors that promote better birth outcomes in Hispanic women? These clinical questions could direct you in identifying a significant research problem and purpose.

Extensive patient data, such as diagnoses, treatments, and outcomes, are now computerized. Analyzing this information might generate research problems that are significant to a clinic, community, or national healthcare system. For example, you may ask: Why has adolescent obesity increased so rapidly in the past 10 years, and what treatments will be effective in managing this problem? What pharmacological and nonpharmacological treatments have been most effective in treating common acute illnesses such as otitis media, sinusitis, and bronchitis in your practice or nationwide? What are the outcomes (patient health status and costs) for treating such chronic illnesses as type 2 diabetes, hypertension, and dyslipidemia in your practice? Review of agency patient data often reveals patterns and trends in a clinical setting and helps nurses and students to identify patient care problems.

Because health care is constantly changing in response to consumer needs and trends in society, the focus of current research varies according to these needs and trends. For example, research evidence is needed to improve practice outcomes for infants and new mothers, the elderly and residents in nursing homes, and persons from vulnerable and culturally diverse populations. Healthcare agencies would benefit from studies of varied healthcare delivery models. Society would benefit from interventions recognized to promote health and prevent illness. In summary, clinically focused research is essential if nurses are to develop the knowledge needed for evidence-based practice (EBP) (Brown, 2009; Melnyk & Fineout-Overholt, 2011).

Researcher and Peer Interactions

Interactions with researchers and peers offer valuable opportunities for generating research problems. Experienced researchers serve as mentors and help novice researchers to identify research topics and formulate problems. Nursing educators assist students in selecting research problems for theses and dissertations. When possible, students conduct studies in the same area of research as the faculty. Faculty members can share their expertise regarding their research program, and the combined work of the faculty and students can build a knowledge base for a specific area of practice. This type of relationship could also be developed between an expert researcher and a nurse clinician. Because nursing research is critical for designation as a Magnet facility by the American Nurses Credentialing Center© (ANCC, 2012), hospitals and healthcare systems employ nurse researchers for the purpose of guiding studies conducted by staff nurses. Building an EBP for nursing requires collaboration between nurse researchers and clinicians as well as with researchers from other health-related disciplines. Interdisciplinary research teams have the expertise to increase the quality and quantity of studies conducted. Being a part of a research team is an excellent way to expand your understanding of the research process.

Beveridge (1950) identified several reasons for discussing research ideas with others. Ideas are clarified and new ideas are generated when two or more people pool their thoughts. Interactions with others enable researchers to uncover errors in reasoning or information. These interactions are also a source of support in discouraging or difficult times. In addition, another person can provide a refreshing or unique viewpoint, which helps avoid conditioned thinking, or following an established habit of thought. A workplace that encourages interaction can stimulate nurses to identify research problems. Nursing conferences and professional meetings also provide excellent opportunities for nurses to discuss their ideas and brainstorm to identify potential research problems.

The Internet has greatly extended the ability of researchers and clinicians around the world to share ideas and propose potential problems for research. Most colleges or schools of nursing have websites that identify faculty research interests and provide mechanisms for contacting individuals who are conducting research in your area of interest. Thus, interactions with others are essential to broaden your perspective and knowledge base and to support you in identifying significant research problems and purposes.

Literature Review

Reviewing research journals, such as *Advances in Nursing Science, Applied Nursing Research, Clinical Nursing Research, Evidence-Based Nursing, International Journal of Psychiatric Nursing Research, Journal of Nursing Scholarship, Journal of Advanced Nursing, Journal of Research in Nursing, Nursing Research, Nursing Science Quarterly, Research in Nursing & Health, Scholarly Inquiry for Nursing Practice: An International Journal, Southern Online Journal of Nursing Research,* and *Western Journal of Nursing Research*, as well as theses and dissertations will acquaint novice researchers with studies conducted in an area of interest. The nursing specialty journals, such as *American Journal of Maternal Child Nursing, Archives of Psychiatric Nursing, Dimensions of Critical Care, Heart & Lung, Infant Behavior and Development, Journal of Pediatric Nursing,* and *Oncology Nursing Forum,* also place a high priority on publishing research findings. Reviewing research articles enables you to identify an area of interest and determine what is known and not known in this area. The gaps in the knowledge base provide direction for future research. (See Chapter 6 for the process of reviewing the literature.)

At the completion of a research project, an investigator often makes recommendations for further study. These recommendations provide opportunities for others to build on a researcher's work and strengthen the knowledge in a selected area. For example, the Grady et al. (2011, p. 27) study, introduced earlier in this chapter, provided recommendations for further research to examine "the longer term eventualities of gain- and loss-framed messages on preventative behaviors." They also recommended examining how long the gain-framed message might last and when it would be "necessary to provide another message presentation to bolster effective self-care behavior" (p. 27). These researchers also encouraged others to validate their findings through replication studies that varied the content and delivery format of educational messages provided persons with diabetes.

Replication of Studies

Reviewing the literature is a way to identify a study to replicate. **Replication** involves reproducing or repeating a study to determine whether similar findings will be obtained (Fahs, Morgan, & Kalman, 2003). Replication is essential for knowledge development because it (1) establishes the credibility of the findings, (2) extends the generalizability of the findings over a range of instances and contexts, (3) reduces the number of type I and type II errors, (4) corrects the limitations in studies' methodologies, (5) supports theory development, and (6) lessens the acceptance of erroneous results. Some researchers replicate studies because they agree with the findings and wonder whether the findings will hold up in different settings with different subjects over time. Others want to challenge the findings or interpretations of prior investigators. Some researchers develop research programs focused on expanding the knowledge needed for practice in an area. This program of research often includes replication studies that strengthen the evidence for practice.

Four different types of replications are important in generating sound scientific knowledge for nursing: (1) exact, (2) approximate, (3) concurrent, and (4) systematic extension (Haller & Reynolds, 1986). An **exact** (or identical) **replication** involves duplicating the initial researcher's study to confirm the original findings. All conditions of the original study must be maintained; thus, "there must be the same observer, the same subjects, the same procedure, the same measures, the same locale, and the same time" (Haller & Reynolds, 1986, p. 250). Exact replications might be thought of as ideal to confirm original study findings, but these are frequently not attainable. In addition, one would not want to replicate the errors in an original study, such as small sample size, weak design, or poor-quality measurement methods.

When conducting an **approximate** (or operational) **replication**, the subsequent researcher repeats the original study under similar conditions, following the methods as closely as possible. The intent is to determine whether the findings from the original study hold up despite minor changes in the research conditions. If the findings generated through replication are consistent with the findings of the original study, then the knowledge is considered more credible and has a greater probability of accurately reflecting the real world. If the replication fails to support the original

findings, the designs and methods of both studies should be examined for limitations and weaknesses, and further research must be conducted. Conflicting findings might also generate additional theoretical insights and provide new directions for research.

For a **concurrent** (or internal) **replication**, the researcher collects data for the original study and the replication study simultaneously thereby checking the reliability of the original study findings. The confirmation, through replication of the original study findings, is part of the original study's design. For example, your research team might collect data simultaneously at two different hospitals to compare and contrast the findings. Consistency in the findings increases the credibility of the study and the likelihood that others will be able to generalize the findings. Some expert researchers obtain funding to conduct multiple concurrent replications, in which a number of individuals conduct repetitions of a single study, but with different samples in different settings. Clinical trials that examine the effectiveness of the pharmacological management of chronic illnesses, such as diabetes, hypertension, and dyslipidemia, are examples of concurrent replication studies. As each study is completed, the findings are compiled in a report that specifies the series of replications that were conducted to generate these findings. Some outcome studies involve concurrent replication to determine whether the outcomes vary for different healthcare providers and healthcare settings across the United States (Brink & Wood, 1979; Brown, 2009; Doran, 2011).

A **systematic** (or constructive) **replication** is done under distinctly new conditions. The researchers conducting the replication do not follow the design or methods of the original researchers; rather, the second investigative team identifies a similar problem but formulates new methods to verify the first researchers' findings (Haller & Reynolds, 1986). The aim of this type of replication is to extend the findings of the original study and test the limits of the generalizability of such findings. Intervention research might use this type of replication to examine the effectiveness of various interventions devised to address a practice problem.

Nurse researchers need to actively replicate studies to develop strong research evidence for practice. However, the number of nursing studies replicated continues to be limited. The replications of studies might be limited because (1) some view replication as less scholarly or less important than original research, (2) the discipline of nursing lacks adequate resources and funding for conducting replication studies, and (3) editors of journals publish fewer replication studies than original studies (Fahs et al., 2003). However, the lack of replication studies severely limits the generation of sound research findings needed for EBP in nursing. Thus, replicating a study should be respected as a legitimate scholarly activity for both expert and novice researchers. Funding from both private and federal sources is needed to support the conduct of replication studies, with a commitment from journal editors to publish these studies.

Replication provides an excellent learning opportunity for the novice researcher to conduct a significant study, validate findings from previous research, and generate new research evidence about different populations and settings. Students studying for a master's of science in nursing degree could be encouraged to replicate studies for their theses, possibly to replicate faculty studies. Expert researchers, with programs of research, implement replication studies to generate sound evidence for use in practice. When publishing a replication study, researchers need to designate the type of replication conducted and the contribution the study made to the existing body of knowledge.

Theory

Theories are an important source for generating research problems because they set forth ideas about events and situations in the real world that require testing (Chinn & Kramer, 2008). In examining a theory, you may note that it includes a number of propositions and that each proposition is a statement of the relationship of two or more concepts. A research problem and purpose could be formulated to explore or describe a concept or to test a proposition from a theory. Middle range theories are the ones most commonly used as frameworks for quantitative studies and are tested as part of the research process (Smith & Liehr, 2008). In qualitative research, the purpose of the study might be to generate a theory or framework to describe a unique event or situation (Marshall & Rossman, 2011; Munhall, 2012).

Some researchers combine ideas from different theories to develop maps or models for testing through research. The map serves as the framework for the study and includes key concepts and relationships from the theories that the researchers want to study. Frenn, Malin, and Bansal (2003, p. 38) conducted a quasi-experimental study to examine the effectiveness of a "4-session Health Promotion/Transtheoretical Model-guided intervention in reducing percentage of fat in the diet and increasing physical activity among low- to middle-income culturally diverse middle school students." The intervention was based on the "components of two behaviorally based research models that have been well tested among

adults—Health Promotion Model (Pender, 1996) and Transtheoretical Model (Prochaska, Norcross, Fowler, Follick, & Abrams, 1992)—but have not been tested regarding low-fat diet with middle school-aged children" (Frenn et al., 2003, p. 36). They developed a model of the study framework (see Figure 5-1) and described the concepts and propositions from the model that guided the development of different aspects of their study.

"A combined Health Promotion/Transtheoretical Model guided the intervention designed for this study [see Figure 5-1]. The first individual characteristic examined in this study was temptation (low self-efficacy), defined as the inability to overcome barriers in sustaining a low-fat diet … and an intervention helping adolescents develop behavioral control may enhance self-efficacy and improve health habits.

The second characteristic common to both the Health Promotion and Transtheoretical Models was benefits/barriers. In a study of fifth- through seventh-grade children, Baranowski and Simons-Morton (1990) found the most common barriers to reducing saturated fat in the diet were (a) giving up preferred foods, (b) meals outside the home that contained fat, (c) not knowing what foods were low in fat, and (d) not wanting to take the time to read labels.

The last individual characteristic used in this study was access to low-fat foods. This concept from the Health Promotion Model is important in a middle school-aged population, as they are, to some extent, dependent on others for the types of food available." (Frenn et al., 2003, pp. 37-38)

Frenn et al. (2003) used the Pender (1996) Health Promotion Model and the Transtheoretical Model (Prochaska et al., 1992), which are middle range theories, to develop the following research questions to guide their study:

"(a) Do demographic variables, access to low-fat foods, perceived self-efficacy, benefits/barriers, and stages of change predict percentage of fat reported in the diet by middle school-aged children? (b) Does the application of a Health Promotion/Transtheoretical Model intervention in 4 classroom sessions significantly improve adoption of a diet lower in fat and duration of physical activity as compared with a control group of students not engaged with the program?" (Frenn et al., 2003, p. 39)

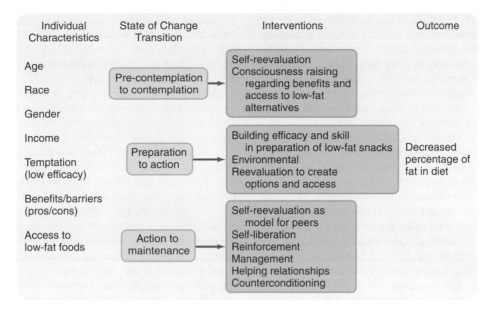

Figure 5-1 The health promotion stage of change model: A synthesis of health promotion and transtheoretical models guiding low-fat diet intervention for students in an urban middle school.

The findings from a study either support or do not support the relationships identified in the model. The study by Frenn et al. (2003) added support to the Health Promotion/Transtheoretical Model with their findings that the classroom intervention decreased dietary fat and increased physical activity for middle school–age adolescents. Further research is needed to determine whether classroom interventions over time reduce body mass index, body weight, and the percentage of body fat of overweight and obese adolescents. As a graduate student, you could use this model as a framework and test some of the relationships in your clinical setting.

Research Priorities

Since 1975, expert researchers, specialty groups, professional organizations, and funding agencies have identified nursing research priorities. The research priorities for clinical practice were initially identified in a study by Lindeman (1975). Those original research priorities included nursing interventions related to stress, care of the aged, pain management, and patient education. Developing evidence-based nursing interventions in these areas continues to be a priority.

Many professional nursing organizations use websites to communicate their current research priorities. For example, the American Association of Critical-Care Nurses (AACN) determined initial research priorities for this specialty in the early 1980s

(Lewandowski & Kositsky, 1983) and revised these priorities on the basis of patients' needs and the changes in health care. The current AACN (2011) research priorities are identified on this organization's website as (1) effective and appropriate use of technology to achieve optimal patient assessment, management, or outcomes, (2) creation of a healing, humane environment, (3) processes and systems that foster the optimal contribution of critical care nurses, (4) effective approaches to symptom management, and (5) prevention and management of complications. AACN (2011) has also identified future research needs under the following topics: medication management, hemodynamic monitoring, creating healing environments, palliative care and end-of-life issues, mechanical ventilation, monitoring of neuroscience patients, and noninvasive monitoring. If your specialty is critical care, this list of research needs might help you identify a priority problem and purpose for study.

The American Organization of Nurse Executives (AONE, 2012) provides a discussion of their education and research priorities online at http://www .aone.org/education/index.shtml/. For 2011-2012, AONE identified more than 25 research priorities in four strategic areas: (1) design of future patient care delivery systems, (2) healthful practice environments, (3) leadership, and (4) the positioning of nurse leaders as valued healthcare executives and managers. To promote the design of future patient care delivery systems, AONE encourages research focused on new technology, patient safety, and the work environment that allows strategies for improvement crucial to the success of the delivery system. In the area of healthful practice environments, AONE encourages research focused on practice environments that attract and retain nurses and that promote professional growth and continuous learning, including mentoring of staff nurses and nursing leaders. In the area of leadership, AONE encourages research focused on evidence-based leadership capacity, measurement of patient care quality outcomes, and technology to complement patient care. To promote the positioning of nurse leaders as valued healthcare executives and managers, AONE encourages research focused on patient safety and quality, disaster preparedness, and workforce shortages. AONE recognizes the importance of supporting education and research initiatives to create a healthy work environment, a quality healthcare system, and strong nurse executives. You can search online for the research priorities of other nursing organizations to help you identify priority problems for study.

A significant funding agency for nursing research is the National Institute of Nursing Research (NINR). A major initiative of the NINR is the development of a national nursing research agenda that involves identifying nursing research priorities, outlining a plan for implementing priority studies, and obtaining resources to support these priority projects. The NINR has an annual budget of more than $90 million, with approximately 74% of the budget used for extramural research project grants, 7% for predoctoral and postdoctoral training, 6% for research management and support, 5% for the centers program in specialized areas, 5% for other research including career development, 2% for the intramural program, and 1% for contracts and other expenses (see NINR at http://www.ninr.nih.gov/).

The NINR (2011) developed four strategies for building the science of nursing: "(1) integrating biological and behavior science for better health; (2) adopting, adapting, and generating new technologies for better health care; (3) improving methods for future scientific discoveries; and (4) developing scientists for today and tomorrow." The areas of research emphasis include: (1) promoting health and preventing disease, (2) improving quality of life, (3) eliminating health disparities, and (4) setting directions for end-of-life research (NINR, 2011). Specific research priorities were identified for each of these four areas of research emphasis and were included in the NINR Strategic Plan. These research priorities provide

important information for nurses seeking funding from the NINR. Details about the NINR mission, strategic plan, and areas of funding are available on its website at http://www.ninr.nih.gov/AboutNINR/NINRMissionandStrategicPlan/.

Another federal agency that is funding healthcare research is the Agency for Healthcare Research and Quality (AHRQ). The purpose of the AHRQ is to enhance the quality, appropriateness, and effectiveness of healthcare services, and access to such services, by establishing a broad base of scientific research and promoting improvements in clinical practice and in the organization, financing, and delivery of healthcare services. Some of the current AHRQ funding priorities are research focused on prevention; health information technology; patient safety; long-term care; pharmaceutical outcomes; system capacity and emergency preparedness; and the cost, organization, and socioeconomics of health care. For a complete list of funding opportunities and grant announcements, see the AHRQ website at http://www.ahrq.gov/.

The World Health Organization (WHO) is encouraging the identification of priorities for a common nursing research agenda among countries. A quality healthcare delivery system and improved patient and family health have become global goals. By 2020, the world's population is expected to increase by 94%, with the elderly population growing by almost 240%. Seven of every 10 deaths are expected to be caused by noncommunicable diseases, such as chronic conditions (heart disease, cancer, and depression) and injuries (unintentional and intentional). The priority areas for research identified by WHO are to (1) improve the health of the world's most marginalized populations, (2) study new diseases that threaten public health around the world, (3) conduct comparative analyses of supply and demand of the health workforce of different countries, (4) analyze the feasibility, effectiveness, and quality of education and practice of nurses, (5) conduct research on healthcare delivery modes, and (6) examine the outcomes for healthcare agencies, providers, and patients around the world (WHO, 2012). A discussion of WHO's mission, objectives, and research policies can be found online at http://www.who.int/rpc/en.

The *Healthy People 2020* website identifies and prioritizes health topics and objectives for all age groups over the next decade (U.S. Department of Health and Human Services, 2012). These health topics and objectives direct future research in the areas of health promotion, illness prevention, illness management, and rehabilitation and can be accessed

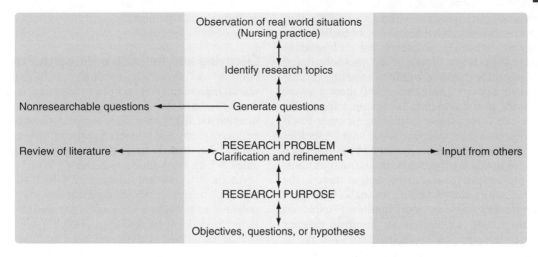

Figure 5-2 Formulating a research problem and purpose.

online at http://www.healthypeople.gov/2020/topics objectives2020/default.aspx/.

In summary, funding organizations, professional organizations, and governmental healthcare organizations, both national and international, are sources for identifying priority research problems and offer opportunities for obtaining funding for future research.

Formulating a Research Problem and Purpose

Potential nursing research problems often emerge from real-world situations, such as those in nursing practice. A *situation* is a significant combination of circumstances that occur at a given time. Inexperienced researchers tend to want to study the entire situation, but it is far too complex for a single study. Multiple problems exist in a single situation, and each can be developed into a study. A researcher's perception of what problems exist in a situation depends on that individual's clinical expertise, theoretical base, intuition, interests, and goals. Some researchers spend years developing different problem statements and new studies from the same clinical situation.

The exact thought processes used to extract problems from a situation have not been clearly identified because of the abstractness and complexity of the reasoning involved. However, in formulating their study problems, researchers often implement the following steps: (1) examine a real-world situation, (2) identify research topics, (3) generate questions, (4) review relevant literature, and (5) ultimately clarify and refine a research problem. From the problem, the researcher develops a specific focus or research purpose for study. The flow of these steps is presented in Figure 5-2 and described in the following sections.

Examining a Real-World Situation and Identifying Research Topics

A nursing situation often includes a variety of research topics or concepts that identify broad problem areas requiring investigation. Nurses frequently investigate patient- and family-related topics, such as stress, pain, coping patterns, the teaching and learning process, self-care deficits, health promotion, rehabilitation, prevention of illness, disease management, and social support. Other relevant research topics focus on the healthcare system and providers, such as cost-effective care; advanced practice nurse roles (nurse practitioner, clinical nurse specialist, midwife, and nurse anesthetist); managed care; and redesign of the healthcare system. Outcomes research focuses on topics of health status, quality of life, cost-effectiveness, and quality of care. A specific outcome study might focus on a particular condition, such as terminal cancer, and examine outcomes, such as nutrition, hygiene, skin integrity, and pain control with a variety of treatments (Doran, 2011).

Generating Questions and Reviewing the Literature

Situations encountered in nursing stimulate a constant flow of questions. The questions fit into three categories: (1) questions answered by existing knowledge, (2) questions answered with problem solving, and (3) research-generating questions. The first two types of questions are nonresearchable and do not facilitate the formulation of research problems that will generate knowledge for practice. Some of the questions raised have a satisfactory answer within the nursing profession's existing body of knowledge, and these answers are available in the literature and online, from EBP guidelines, or from experts in nursing or other disciplines. For example, suppose you have questions about performing some basic nursing skills, such as a protocol for taking a temperature or giving injections; you can find answers to questions such as these in the research literature and procedure manuals (see Figure 5-2). However, suppose your questions focus on investigating new techniques to improve existing skills, patient responses to techniques, or ways to educate patients and families to perform techniques. Your efforts to answer these types of questions could add to knowledge needed for EBP.

Some of the questions raised can be answered using problem-solving or evaluation projects. The problem-solving process addresses a particular problem situation, and the goal of the research process is the generation of knowledge to be generalized to other similar situations. Many evaluation projects are conducted with minimal application of the rigor and control required with research. These projects do not fit the criteria of research, and the findings are relevant for a particular situation. For example, quality assurance is an evaluation of the patient care implemented by a specific healthcare agency; the results of this evaluation project are usually relevant mainly to the agency conducting the review.

The type of question that can initiate the research process is one that requires further knowledge to answer it. Some of the questions that come to mind about situations include the following: Is there a need to explore or describe concepts, to know how they are related, or to be able to predict or control some event within the situation? What is known and what is not known about the concepts? What are the most urgent factors or outcomes to know? Is there a need to generate or test theory in an area important to practice? Is the patient's perspective in this situation needed to develop an intervention? Which intervention is most effective in achieving quality patient outcomes? Research experts have found that asking the right question is frequently more valuable than finding the solution to a problem. The solution identified in a single study might not withstand the test of time or might be useful in only a few situations. However, one well-formulated question can generate numerous research problems, direct a lifetime of research activities, and significantly contribute to a discipline's body of knowledge.

Clarifying and Refining a Research Problem

Fantasy and creativity are part of formulating a research problem, so you need to imagine prospective studies related to the situation. You also need to imagine the difficulties likely to occur with each study, but avoid being too critical of potential research problems at this time. Which studies seem the most workable? Which ones appeal intuitively? Which problem is the most significant to nursing? Which study is of personal interest? Which problem has the greatest potential to provide a foundation for further research in the field (Fawcett & Garity, 2009)?

The problems investigated need to have professional significance and potential or actual significance for society. A research problem is significant when it has the potential to generate or refine knowledge to build an EBP for nursing (Craig & Smyth, 2012; Melnyk & Fineout-Overholt, 2011). Nurse researchers believe that significant research problems need to focus on real-world concerns, to be methodologically sound, to build knowledge for nursing, to develop and/or test theory, and to focus on current or timely concerns (Alligood, 2010; Chinn & Kramer, 2008; Craig & Smyth, 2012; Smith & Liehr, 2008). The problems that are considered significant vary with time and the needs of society. The priorities identified earlier indicate some of the current, significant nursing research topics and problems.

Personal interest in a problem influences the quality of the problem formulated and the study conducted. A problem of personal interest is one that an individual has pondered for a long time or one that is especially important in the individual's nursing practice or personal life. For example, if you know someone who has had a mastectomy, you may be particularly interested in studying the emotional impact of a mastectomy or strategies for caring for mastectomy patients. This personal interest in the topic can become the driving force needed to conduct a quality study.

Answering these questions regarding significance and personal interest can often assist you in narrowing the number of problems. Without narrowing potential problems to only one idea, try some of the ideas out on colleagues (see Figure 5-2). Let them play the devil's advocate and explore the strengths and weaknesses of each idea. Then begin some preliminary reading in the area of interest. Examine literature related to the situation, the variables within the situation, measurement of the variables, previous studies related to the situation, and supportive theories. The literature review often enables you to refine the problem and clearly identify the gap in the knowledge base. Once you have identified the problem, you must frame it or ground it in past research, practice, and theory. The discussion of the problem must culminate in a problem statement that identifies the gap in the knowledge base that your proposed study will address. Thus, the refined problem has documented significance to nursing practice, is based on past research and theory, and identifies a gap in nursing knowledge that directs the development of the research purpose.

Research Purpose

The purpose is generated from the problem, identifies the focus, aim, or goal of the study, and directs the development of the study. In the research process, the purpose is usually stated after the problem, because the problem identifies the gap in knowledge in a selected area and the purpose clarifies the knowledge to be generated by the study. The research purpose must be stated *objectively*, that is, in a way that does not reflect particular biases or values of the researcher. Investigators who do not recognize their values might include their biases in the research. This situation can lead them to generate the answers they want or believe to be true and might add inaccurate information to a discipline's body of knowledge (Kaplan, 1964). Therefore, on the basis of your research purpose, you can develop specific research objectives, questions, or hypotheses to direct your study (see Chapter 8).

Example of Problem and Purpose Development

You might have observed the women receiving treatment at a mental health clinic and noted that many were withdrawn, depressed, and unable to discuss certain events in their lives. Their progress in therapy was usually slow, and they seemed to have similar physical and psychological symptoms. Often, after developing a rapport with a therapist, they would reveal that they were victims of sexual abuse as a child. This situation could lead you to identify research topics and generate searching questions. Research topics of interest include childhood sexual abuse, history and nature of abuse, parental characteristics, adult survivors of child sexual abuse, physical and psychological symptoms in adulthood, assessment and diagnosis of child sexual abuse history, therapeutic interventions to manage abuse history and symptoms, and psychological adjustment. Possible questions

include the following: What are the physical and psychological symptoms demonstrated by someone who has experienced childhood sexual abuse? How would one assess the occurrence, frequency, and impact of rape or incest on a woman? What influences do age, duration, and nature of abuse have on a woman's current behavior and psychological adjustment? How frequently is childhood sexual abuse a problem in the mentally disturbed adult female? How does a healthcare provider assess, diagnose, and manage the emotional problems of adult survivors of child sexual abuse? These are the types of questions that Zinzow, Seth, Jackson, Niehaus, and Fitzgerald (2010) might have raised as they developed the following problem and purpose for their study titled "Abuse and Parental Characteristics, Attributions of Blame, and Psychological Adjustments in Adult Survivors of Child Sexual Abuse":

Research Problem

"A history of childhood sexual abuse (CSA) has been consistently related to adult psychological symptomatology in women, including anxiety, depression, posttraumatic stress, interpersonal difficulties, sexual dysfunction, and somatization.... However, wide variability among the presence and severity of negative outcomes has been observed. Factors that have been found to account for some of this variation in adult adjustment include abuse characteristics (e.g., severity, number of incidents) (...Steel, Sanna, Hammond, Whipple, & Cross, 2004) and family characteristics such as parenting style and parental psychopathology.... Furthermore, an emerging body of research has demonstrated a link between cognitive mechanisms, such as attributions for abuse, and psychological outcomes in abuse survivors (see review by Valle & Silovsky, 2002).... However, little is known about the influence of abuse and parental characteristics on attributional content. Moreover, the relative contribution of self-blame, family blame, and perpetrator blame to the sequelae of CSA is poorly understood." (Zinzow et al., 2010, p. 80)

Research Purpose

"The purpose of this study was to examine the influence of abuse and parental characteristics on attributional content and determine the relative contribution of different attributions of blame in predicting psychological symptoms among adult survivors of childhood sexual abuse." (Zinzow et al., 2010, p. 79)

The research problem identified by Zinzow et al. (2010) included significance because CSA was linked to several psychological problems in adult women who suffered abuse. The key findings from previous research focused on the nature and duration of abuse, parental characteristics, and attributions of blame. However, the findings were varied regarding the psychological adjustment and outcomes of women who were adult survivors of CSA. The contributions of self-blame, family blame, and perpetrator blame to adult survivors' adjustment and symptoms are poorly understood. These gaps in the knowledge base provided a basis for the study purpose. The study purpose clearly identifies the focus or aim of the study. Zinzow et al. (2010) studied 83 female undergraduates with a history of CSA. They found that abuse characteristics such as severity and number of incidents were significantly related to attributions. Family- and perpetrator-blame accounted for significant variability in psychological symptoms and adjustments of the women in the sample, which were greater than the contributions of abuse characteristics, family environment, and self-blame. The findings from this study included implications for treatment of women who were adult survivors of CSA and directions for further research.

Feasibility of a Study

As the research problem and purpose increase in clarity and conciseness, the researcher has greater direction in determining the feasibility of a study. The feasibility of a study is determined by examining the time and money commitment; the researcher's expertise; availability of subjects, facility, and equipment; cooperation of others; and the study's ethical considerations (Creswell, 2009; Fawcett & Garity, 2009; Munhall, 2012; Rogers, 1987).

Time Commitment

Conducting research frequently takes longer than anticipated, making it difficult for any researcher, especially a novice, to estimate the time that will be involved. In estimating the time commitment, the researcher examines the purpose of the study; the more complex the purpose, the greater the time commitment. You can approximate the time needed to complete a study by assessing the following factors: (1) type and number of subjects needed, (2) number and complexity of the variables to be studied, (3) methods for measuring the variables (Are instruments available to measure the variables or must they be

developed?), (4) methods for collecting data, and (5) the data analysis process. Another factor that can increase the time needed for a study is obtaining institutional review board (IRB) approval, especially if more than one clinical agency is used for data collection in a study. Also, researchers often overlook the time commitment necessary to write the research report for presentation and publication. You must approximate the time needed to complete each step of the research process and determine whether the study is feasible.

Most researchers propose a designated time or set a specific deadline for their project. For example, an agency might set a 2-year deadline for studying the turnover rate of staff. The researcher must determine whether the identified purpose can be accomplished by the designated deadline; if not, the purpose could be narrowed or the deadline extended. Researchers are often cautious about extending deadlines because a project could continue for many years. The individual interested in conducting qualitative research frequently must make an extensive time commitment of 2 years or longer to allow for quality collection and analysis of data (Marshall & Rossman, 2011). Time is as important as money, and the cost of a study can be greatly affected by the time required to conduct it.

Money Commitment

The problem and purpose selected are influenced by the amount of money available to the researchers. Sources for nursing research funding include: (1) government funding from such offices as the NINR and AHRQ; (2) professional organizations such as AACN, AONE, and the Oncology Nursing Society; and (3) local clinical agencies, corporations, and universities (see Chapter 29). Potential sources for funding should be considered at the time the problem and purpose are identified. For example, Grady et al. (2011), who studied the effects of educational messages on health-related knowledge, attitudes, and behavior of persons with diabetes, was partially funded by an Office of Naval Research Award. Federal and private sources of funding greatly strengthen the feasibility of conducting a research project.

The cost of a research project can range from a few dollars for a student's small study to hundreds of thousands of dollars for complex projects, such as multisite clinical trials and major qualitative studies. In estimating the cost of a research project, the following questions need to be considered, in addition to other areas of expense based on the study being conducted:

Literature: What will the review of the literature—including computer searches, copying articles, and purchasing books—cost?

Subjects: How many subjects or study participants will need to be recruited for the study, and will the subjects have to be paid for their participation in the project? Grady et al. (2011) paid their approximately 155 study participants $25 at each of the three data collection periods. This resulted in an $11,625 expense that would require funding to accomplish.

Equipment: What will the equipment for the study cost? Can the equipment be borrowed, rented, bought, or obtained through donation? Is the equipment available, or will it need to be built? What type of maintenance will be required for the equipment during the study? What will the measurement instruments cost?

Personnel: Will assistants or consultants, or both, be hired to collect, computerize, and analyze the data and assist with the data interpretation? Will clerical help be needed to type and distribute the report and prepare a manuscript for publication?

Computer time: Will computer time be required to analyze the data? If so, what will be the cost?

Transportation: What will be the transportation costs for conducting the study and presenting the findings?

Supplies: Will any supplies—such as envelopes, postage, pens, paper, and photocopies—be needed? Will a cell phone be needed to contact the researcher about potential subjects? Will a survey or reminder postcard by mailed to participants? Will long-distance phone calls or overnight mailing be needed?

Researcher Expertise

A research problem and purpose must be selected on the basis of the ability of the investigator(s). Initially, you might work with another researcher (mentor) to learn the process and then investigate a familiar problem that fits your knowledge base or experience. Selecting a difficult, complex problem and purpose can only frustrate and confuse the novice researcher. However, all researchers need to identify problems and purposes that are challenging and collaborate with other researchers as necessary to build their research background.

When a team of researchers conducts a study, the team members often have a variety of research and clinical experiences that add to the quality of the study conducted. In the study conducted by Grady et al.

(2011), these investigators had research and clinical expertise in nursing, public health, psychology, and biostatistics. The researchers are all doctorally prepared, and Grady is a seasoned faculty member for the University of Pittsburgh. Eileen and Elliot Entin are both senior research psychologists with Aptima, Inc.; and Brunye is a cognitive psychologist for the U.S. Army. The credentials and employment sites for the investigators are identified under the title of the study article. These researchers all appear to have strong backgrounds for conducting research in the discipline of nursing, psychology, and health care. You can obtain more information about the authors by searching their names online. The researchers also acknowledged the support of the following in conducting their study: registered nurses, Conemaugh Diabetes Institute, Flipside Media, Inc., and Telehealth Department, Mount Aloysius College.

Availability of Subjects or Participants

In selecting a research purpose, you must consider the type and number of study participants needed. Finding a sample might be difficult if the study involves investigating a unique or rare population, such as quadriplegic individuals who live alone and are currently attending college. The more specific the population selected for study, the more difficult it is to find subjects. In addition, the Health Insurance Portability and Accountability Act (HIPAA) prevents clinical agencies from sharing lists of potential subjects with a researcher without specific stipulations (see Chapter 9). Potential subjects who are stigmatized, such as persons with HIV/AIDS, may be more difficult to access.

The money and time available to the researcher will affect the subjects selected. With limited time and money, the researcher might want to investigate subjects who are accessible and do not require payment for participation. Even if you identify a population with a large number of potential subjects, those individuals may be unwilling to participate in the study because of the topic selected. For example, nurses could be asked to share their experiences with alcohol and drug use, but many might fear that sharing this information would jeopardize their jobs and licenses. Researchers need to be prepared to pursue the attainment of study participants at whatever depth is necessary. Having a representative sample of reasonable size is critical for generating quality research findings (Aberson, 2010). Grady et al. (2011) selected a setting where they could obtain the sample size that they needed for their study, as identified in the following quotation:

"The study was conducted at the diabetes outpatient facility of an acute care hospital in west central Pennsylvania. After receiving institutional review board approval from the participating facility, participants were obtained through advertisements in local newspapers recruiting people older than 18 years, who have had diabetes for 5 years or more, and who have no known foot problems.... The final sample was composed of 64 men and 91 women." (Grady et al., 2011, p. 24)

Availability of Facilities and Equipment

Researchers need to determine whether their studies will require special facilities to implement. Will a special room be needed for an educational program, interview, or observations? If the study is conducted at a hospital, clinic, or college of nursing, will the agency provide the facilities that are needed? Setting up a highly specialized laboratory for the conduct of a study would be expensive and would probably require external funding. Most nursing studies are done in natural settings such as a hospital room or unit, a clinic, or a patient's home. Grady et al. (2011) conducted all their research activities in the diabetes outpatient facility (partially controlled setting).

Nursing studies frequently require a limited amount of equipment, such as a tape or video recorder for interviews or a physiological instrument, such as a scale or thermometer. Often you can borrow equipment from the facility where the study is conducted, or you can rent it. Some companies are willing to donate equipment if the study focuses on determining the effectiveness of the equipment and the findings are shared with the company. If specialized facilities or equipment are required for a study, you must be aware of the options available before actively pursuing the study. Grady et al. (2011) delivered their educational messages (either gain-framed or loss-framed) to each subject individually in the diabetes outpatient facility:

"Videos were watched from digital video disk (DVD) on a 19-inch television monitor. The inventories were presented one at a time on a personal computer, via ScoreMD Web-based assessment software. Participants controlled the pacing of the questions in the inventories; responses were automatically coded and stored in a database.... Participants were paid $25 at each of the three data collection periods." (Grady et al., 2011, p. 25)

The researchers did not indicate how they obtained the equipment for their study, making it difficult to determine the expenses related to the study. They did identify the software that was used for data collection and analysis but not the expenses related to using this software. You could contact the principal investigator, Grady, and obtain more details related to equipment costs and computer expenses for data collection and analysis. The contact information for Grady and E. B. Entin is provided on the first page of the study article.

Cooperation of Others

A study might appear feasible, but without the cooperation of others, it is not. Some studies are conducted in laboratory settings and require the minimal cooperation of others. However, most nursing studies involve human subjects and are conducted in hospitals, clinics, schools, offices, or homes. Having the cooperation of people in the research setting, the subjects, and the research assistants involved in data collection is essential. People are frequently willing to cooperate with a study if they view the problem and purpose as significant or if they are personally interested. Grady et al. (2011) acknowledged the support of nurses and other professional organizations and corporations that assisted with the study. The researchers seemed to have strong agency support and the support of relevant businesses. Having the cooperation of others can improve the subject participation and promote the successful completion of the study (see Chapter 20 for details on the data collection process).

Ethical Considerations

The purpose selected for investigation must be ethical, which means that the participants' rights and the rights of others in the setting are protected. If your purpose appears to infringe on the rights of the participants, you should reexamine that purpose; the investigation may have to be revised or abandoned. There are usually some risks in every study, but the value of the knowledge generated should outweigh the risks. Grady et al. (2011, p. 24) received institutional review board approval from the diabetes outpatient facility in Pennsylvania where the study was conducted, and "all eligible adults wishing to participate in the study provided informed consent." By taking these steps, the researchers attempted to implement an ethical study that protected the rights of the adults with diabetes who participated (see Chapter 9 for details on ethical conduct in research).

Example Research Topics, Problems, and Purposes for Different Types of Research

Quantitative Research

Quantitative and qualitative research approaches enable nurses to investigate a variety of research problems and purposes. Examples of research topics, problems, and purposes for some of the different types of quantitative studies are presented in Table 5-1. The research purpose usually reflects the type of study that is to be conducted. The purposes of descriptive research are to identify patterns of variables, to describe and define variables, to identify initial links among variables, and to compare and contrast groups on selected variables (Kerlinger & Lee, 2000). For example, Trotter, Gallagher, and Donoghue (2011) conducted their study to describe the patterns of anxiety and concerns of patients undergoing percutaneous coronary interventions (PCIs). The research topics, problems, and purposes for this study are presented in Table 5-1. Trotter et al. (2011) found that symptoms of anxiety were common before and after PCIs. They recommended that patients who had chest pain or were undergoing a first PCI should be targeted for an intervention to reduce anxiety during the recovery period and after discharge.

The purpose of correlational research is to examine the type (positive or negative) and strength of the relationships among study variables. In their correlational study, Houck, Kendall, Miller, Morrell, and Wiebe (2011) examined the relationship between behavior problems and self-concept in adolescents and children with attention deficit hyperactivity disorder (ADHD) (see Table 5-1). Houck et al. (2011, p. 239) found that it is important "to assess self-concept in children and adolescents with ADHD, especially those who are older and have comorbid conditions." These individuals with ADHD who have low self-concept require diagnosis and treatment as part of their care.

Quasi-experimental studies are conducted to determine the effect of an intervention or independent variable on designated dependent or outcome variables (Shadish et al., 2002). For example, Nyamathi et al. (2009) conducted a quasi-experimental study to examine the effects of a nurse-managed program (intervention) on the vaccine completion rates for hepatitis A and B vaccine series (outcomes) in a population of homeless adults. The research topics, problem, and purpose are identified in Table 5-1.

Nyamathi and colleagues found that a program that used nurse case management and tracking was essential in supporting the adherence and completion of 6-month hepatitis A and B vaccine series. This was especially important for white homeless persons, who were the least likely to complete their vaccine series without an intervention tailored to address their unique needs.

Experimental studies are conducted in highly controlled settings and under highly controlled conditions to determine the effect of one or more independent variables on one or more dependent variables (Shadish et al., 2002). Sharma, Ryals, Gajewski, and Wright (2010) conducted an experimental study to determine the effects of an aerobic exercise program on the pain-like behavior and neurotrophin-3 (NT-3) in mice with chronic widespread pain (see Table 5-1). These researchers found that moderate-intensity aerobic exercise had the effect of deep tissue mechanical hyperalgesia on chronic pain in mice. This finding provides a possible molecular basis for aerobic exercise training in reducing muscular pain.

Qualitative Research

The problems formulated for qualitative research identify an area of concern that requires investigation. The purpose of a qualitative study indicates the focus of the study and whether it is a subjective concept, an event, a phenomenon, experience, situation, or a facet of a culture or society (Marshall & Rossman, 2011; Munhall, 2012). Examples of research topics, problems, and purposes from some different types of qualitative studies are presented in Table 5-2 and in Chapter 12. Phenomenological research seeks an understanding of human experience from the researcher's perspective, such as children's experiences of living with asthma conducted by Trollvik, Nordbach, Silen, and Ringsberg (2011). The research topics, problem, and purpose for this study are presented in Table 5-2. The findings from the study by Trollvik et al. (2011, p. 295) "described two themes with five subthemes: fear of exacerbation (body sensations, frightening experiences, and loss of control) and fear of being ostracized (experiences of being excluded and dilemma of keeping the asthma secret or being open about it)."

In grounded theory research, the problem identifies the area of concern and the purpose indicates the focus of the theory to be developed from the research (Munhall, 2012). For example, El-Mallakh (2007) investigated the poverty and self-care among individuals with schizophrenia and diabetes mellitus. On the basis of findings from this grounded theory study,

Text continued on p. 92

TABLE 5-1 Quantitative Research: Topics, Problems, and Purposes

Type of Research	Research Topic	Research Problem and Purpose
Descriptive research	Anxiety, concerns, percutaneous coronary intervention, coronary heart disease	*Title of study:* "Care of patients with coronary heart disease: Anxiety in patients undergoing percutaneous coronary interventions" (Trotter, Gallagher, & Donoghue, 2011, p. 185). *Problem:* "Coronary artery disease (CAD) is a leading cause of mortality, morbidity, and loss of quality of life globally. One of the most common treatments for CAD is percutaneous transluminal coronary angioplasty/stent placement, collectively labeled percutaneous coronary intervention (PCI).... Although PCIs are common and relatively low risk, many patients undergoing these treatments experience clinically relevant anxiety, with an estimated prevalence rate of 24% to 72%.... Although anxiety levels decrease after a PCI, clinically relevant anxiety may still be common, with one study noting that 21% of patients remained anxious 6 to 8 weeks after the procedure (Astin, Jones, & Thompson, 2005).... Few studies have investigated anxiety levels and patients' expressed concerns in the very early recovery period within 24 hours after the procedure or the early recovery period in the week after discharge" (Trotter et al., 2011, p. 186). *Purpose:* The purpose of this study was "to determine the patterns of anxiety and concerns experienced by patients undergoing PCI..." (Trotter et al., 2011, 185).
Correlational research	Self-concept, attention deficit hyperactivity disorder, behavior problems	*Title of study:* "Self-concept in children and adolescents with attention deficit hyperactivity disorder" (Houck, Kendall, Miller, Morrell, & Wiebe, 2011, p. 239). *Problem:* "Attention deficit hyperactivity disorder (ADHD) is the most common mental health disorder of childhood, affecting approximately 3%–8.7% of children and adolescents in the United States (National Institutes of Mental Health, 2008). ADHD is a chronic and stigmatizing neurological disorder with deficits in the neurotransmitter systems that affect executive functioning.... People with ADHD have impairments in adaptive functioning, which is often manifested in difficult behaviors, such as aggression, poor rule-regulated behavior, inability to delay gratification, behavioral disinhibition, learning difficulties, poor impulse control and low motivation.... Findings from previous studies on the relationships between ADHD and self-concept are mixed, with some studies indicating that self-concept scores are higher in children with ADHD than in those without ADHD (Treuting & Hinshaw, 2001).... Understanding more specifically how self-concept and behavioral problems are related, given the behavioral disruption that accompanies ADHD, is important to support a child's social and emotional development" (Houck et al., 2011, pp. 239–240). *Purpose:* "The purpose of this study was to examine the relationship between behavioral problems and self-concept in children and adolescents with ADHD" (Houck et al., 2011, p. 241).

| Quasi-experimental research | Nurse-case-managed intervention, hepatitis A and B vaccine completion rate, socio-demographic factors, risk behaviors, homeless | *Title of study:* "Effects of a nurse-managed program on hepatitis A and B vaccine completion among homeless adults" (Nyamathi et al., 2009, p. 13).

 Problem: "Hepatitis B virus (HBV) infection poses a serious threat to public health in the United States. Recent estimates place the true prevalence of chronic HBV in the United States at approximately 1.6 cases per 100,000 persons (Centers for Disease Control and Preventions [CDC], 2008b). It is estimated that there were 51,000 new cases of HBV infection in 2005, a financial burden reaching \$1 billion annually (Cohen et al., 2007).... Homeless populations are at particularly high risk of HBV infection due to high rates of unprotected sexual behavior and sharing of needles and other IDU [injection drug user] paraphernalia. Previous studies have reported that HBV infection rates among homeless populations range from 17% to 31% (i.e., from 17,000 to 31,000 per 100,000...) compared with 2.1 per 100,000 in the general United States population.... Vaccination is the most effective way to prevent HBV infection (CDC, 2006).... Improving vaccination adherence rates among homeless persons is an important step toward reducing the high prevalence of HBV infection in this population.... Thus, little is known about adherence to HBV vaccination among community samples of urban homeless persons or about the effect of stronger interventions to incorporate additional strategies, such as nurse case management and targeted HBV education along with client tracking" (Nyamathi et al., 2009, pp. 13-14.)

 Purpose: The purpose of this study was to determine the "effectiveness of a nurse-case-managed intervention compared with that of two standard programs on completion of the combined hepatitis A virus (HAV) and HBV vaccine series among homeless adults and to assess socio-demographic factors and risk behaviors related to the vaccine completion" (Nyamathi et al., 2009, p. 13). |
| Experimental research | Chronic widespread pain, aerobic exercise, analgesia, neurotrophin-3 synthesis, pain management, animal model | *Title of study:* "Aerobic exercise alters analgesia and neurotrophin-3 [NT-3] synthesis in an animal model of chronic widespread pain" (Sharma, Ryals, Gajewski, & Wright, 2010, p. 714).

 Problem: "Chronic widespread pain is complex and poorly understood and affects about 12% of the adult population in developed countries (Rohrbeck, Jordan, & Croft, 2007).... Management of chronic pain syndromes poses challenges for healthcare practitioners, and pharmacological interventions offer limited efficacy.... Exercise training has been long suggested to reduce pain and improve functional outcomes (Whiteside, Hansen, & Chaudhuri, 2004).... Surprisingly, the current literature is mainly limited to human studies where the molecular basis for exercise training cannot be easily determined. Relatively few animal studies have addressed the effects and mechanisms of exercise on sensory modulation of chronic pain" (Sharma et al., 2010, p. 715).

 Purpose: "The purpose of the present study was to examine the effects of moderate-intensity aerobic exercise on pain-like behavior and NT-3 in an animal model of widespread pain" (Sharma et al., 2010, p. 714). |

TABLE 5-2 Qualitative Research: Topics, Problems, and Purposes

Type of Research	Research Topic	Research Problem and Purpose
Phenomenological research	Lived experience of children, asthma, health promotion, child health, chronic illness, fears of exacerbations, fears of being ostracized	*Title of study:* "Children's experiences of living with asthma: Fear of exacerbations and being ostracized" (Trollvik, Nordbach, Silen, & Ringsberg, 2011, p. 295). *Problem:* "Asthma is the most common childhood disease and long-term medical condition affecting children (Masoli, Fabian, Holt, Beasley, & Global Initiative for Asthma [GINA] Program, 2004). The prevalence of asthma is increasing, and atopic diseases are considered to be a worldwide health problem and an agent of morbidity in children.... Studies show that children with asthma have more emotional/behavioral problems than healthy children.... It has also been found that asthma control in children is poor and that healthcare professionals (HCPs) and children focus on different aspects of having asthma (Price et al., 2002).... Few studies have considered very young children's, 7-10 years old, perspectives; this study might contribute to new insights into their lifeworld experiences" (Trollvik et al., 2011, pp. 295-296). *Purpose:* "The aim of this study was to explore and describe children's everyday experiences of living with asthma to tailor an Asthma Education Program based on their perspectives.... In this study, a phenomenological and hermaneutical approach was used to gain an understanding of the children's lifeworld" (Trollvik et al., 2011, p. 296).
Grounded theory research	Self-care, poverty, schizophrenia, diabetes mellitus	*Title of study:* "Doing my best: Poverty and self-care among individuals with schizophrenia and diabetes mellitus" (El-Mallakh, 2007, p. 49). *Problem:* "Mental health clinicians and researchers increasingly recognize that individuals with schizophrenia have a high risk of developing diabetes mellitus (DM) (Bushe & Holt, 2004).... Whereas rates of diabetes in the general populations range from 2% to 6%, prevalence rates of diabetes among individuals with schizophrenia range from 15% to 18%, and up to 30% have impaired glucose tolerance (Bushe & Holt, 2004; Schizophrenia and Diabetes Expert Consensus Group, 2004).... The recent mental health literature has focused on the screening, diagnosis, and treatment of diabetes in this population, including discussions of the risks and benefits of atypical antipsychotic use.... However, few researchers have investigated the influence of social and demographic characteristics on diabetic self-care among individuals with schizophrenia and diabetes" (El-Mallakh, 2007, pp. 49-50). *Purpose:* "A grounded theory study was conducted to examine several aspects of diabetic self-care in individuals with schizophrenia and DM" (El-Mallakh, 2007, p. 50).
Ethnography research	Critical illness, mechanical ventilation, weaning, family presence	*Title of study:* "Family presence and surveillance during weaning from prolonged mechanical ventilation" (Happ et al., 2007, p. 47). *Problem:* "During critical illness, mechanical ventilation imposes physical and communication barriers between family members and their critically ill loved ones.... Most studies of family members in the intensive care unit (ICU) have focused on families' needs for information, access to the patient, and participation in decisions to withdraw or withhold life-sustaining treatment.... Although numerous studies have been conducted of patient experiences with short- and long-term mechanical ventilation (LTMV), research has not focused on family interactions with patients during weaning from mechanical ventilation. Moreover, the importance of family members' bedside presence and clinicians' interpretation of family behaviors at the bedside have not been critically examined" (Happ et al., 2007, pp. 47-48). *Purpose:* "With the use of data from an ethnographic study of the care and communication processes during weaning from LTMV, we sought to describe how family members interact with the patients and respond to the ventilator and associated ICU bedside equipment during LTMV weaning" (Happ et al., 2007, p. 48).

Exploratory-descriptive qualitative research	Intimate partner violence, abuse of spouse, supporting mothering, parent-child relationships, family health, providers' perspective, social support	*Title of study:* "Supporting mothering: Service providers' perspectives of mothers and young children affected by intimate partner violence" (Letourneau et al., 2011, p. 192). *Problem:* "Estimates of the percent of women with exposure to intimate partner violence (IPV) over their lifetimes by husbands, partners, or boyfriends range between 8% and 66%.... The high concentration of preschool-age children in households where women experience IPV... is a major concern.... Indeed, preschool-age children exposed to IPV may share many of the adjustment difficulties experienced by victims of direct physical and psychological abuse (Litrownik, Newton, Hunter, English, & Everson, 2003). The degree to which children from birth to 36 months of age are affected by IPV, however, is not well understood. Even less is known of effective services and supports that target mothers and their young children exposed to IPV" (Letourneau et al., 2011, p. 193). *Purpose:* "We conducted a qualitative descriptive study of service providers' understandings of the impact of IPV on mothers, young children (birth to 36 months), and mother-infant/child relationships, and of the support needs of these mothers and young children" (Letourneau et al., 2011, p. 192).
Historical research	History, Cold War, mass disaster preparation, nursing research, 1950s, Harriet H. Werley, Army Nurse Corps	*Title of study:* "Planning for mass disaster in the 1950s: Harriet H. Werley and nursing research" (Leifer & Glass, 2008, p. 237). *Problem:* "Americans were continually aware of the potential for nuclear disaster during the Cold War era.... Because the fear of nuclear war was ever present, military and civil defense programs were developed to help Americans prepare for disaster.... Military and civilian healthcare personnel were mobilized to prepare for any mass casualties caused by a nuclear attack. "In the 21st century, world events remind nurses of the need to be prepared to respond to disaster. Since the events of September 11, 2001; the Southeast Asian tsunami in 2004; and the Gulf Coast hurricanes in 2005, there has been an increased emphasis on preparedness and response planning for man-made or natural disasters.... During the turbulent Cold War era, Harriet H. Werley, an Army Nurse Corps (ANC) major, was a pioneer in mass disaster education and nursing research. She served as the first nursing consultant in the newly formed Department of Atomic Casualties Studies (DACS) from 1955-1958.... When working with military officials in Washington, DC, including the ANC, the Office of the Surgeon General, the Army Institute of Research, and the Walter Reed Army Hospital, Werley shared her vision of an evolving role for nurses that included increased opportunities for leadership, research, and expanded practice.... Primary and secondary sources regarding Werley's work in the DACS and the field of disaster nursing were examined to obtain data for this historical study" (Leifer & Glass, 2008, pp. 237-238). *Purpose:* The purpose of this historical study "was to analyze nurses' involvement in research and mass disaster preparations during the Cold War era and to describe the role of Harriet H. Werley and the Army Nurse Corps" (Leifer & Glass, 2008, p. 237).

El-Mallakh (2007, p. 49) developed a "model, Evolving Self-Care, that describes the process by which respondents developed health beliefs about self-care of dual illnesses. One subcategory of the model, 'Doing My Best,' was further analyzed to examine the social context of respondents' diabetic self-care."

In ethnographic research, the problem and purpose identify the culture and the specific attributes of the culture to be examined, described, analyzed, and interpreted. Happ et al. (2007) conducted an ethnographic study of family presence and surveillance during weaning of their family member from a ventilator (see Table 5-2). These researchers concluded that "this study provided a potentially useful conceptual framework of family behaviors with long-term critically ill patients that could enhance the dialogue about family-centered care and guide future research on family presence in the intensive care unit" (Happ et al., 2007, p. 47).

Exploratory-descriptive qualitative research is being conducted by several qualitative researchers to describe unique issues, health problems, or situations that lack clear description or definition. This type of research often provides the basis for future qualitative and quantitative research (Creswell, 2009). Letourneau et al. (2011) conducted an exploratory-descriptive qualitative study of service provider's understandings of the impact of intimate partner violence (IPV) on the mothers and their young children and to determine their needs for support (see Table 5-2). These researchers found that mothers experiencing such violence and their children require more support than is currently available. In addition, the service providers had difficulty in identifying interventions to promote and protect these mothers and their children.

The problem and purpose in historical research focus on a specific individual, a characteristic of society, an event, or a situation in the past and identify the period in the past that will be examined. For example, Leifer and Glass (2008) conducted a historical study of nurses' involvement in mass disaster preparations and research during the Cold War era in the 1950s (see Table 5-2). These researchers focused on the career of Harriet Werley and how her planning for mass disaster during the 1950s increased her emphasis on research and interdisciplinary collaboration. Werley's vision provides insights for today's nurses, who are once again faced with the challenges and demands of disaster management preparation.

Outcomes Research

Outcomes research is conducted to examine the end results of care (Doran, 2011). Table 5-3 summarizes the topics, problem, and purpose from an outcomes study by Bae, Mark, and Fried (2010). These researchers examined the impact of nursing unit turnover rates on patient outcomes in hospitals. They found that

TABLE 5-3 Outcomes Research: Topics, Problem, and Purpose		
Type of Research	**Research Topic**	**Research Problem and Purpose**
Outcomes research	Nurse turnover, workgroup processes, patient outcomes, quality of care, patient safety, patient satisfaction	*Title of study:* "Impact of nursing unit turnover on patient outcomes in hospitals" (Bae, Mark, & Fried, 2010, p. 40) *Problem:* "The adverse impact of nursing turnover on quality of patient care is a long-standing assumption, yet there is little understanding of the turnover-quality relationship or its underlying mechanisms. When turnover occurs, the remaining staff must adjust to newcomers, and turnover may affect the interaction and integration among staff members who remain.... Most empirical research on nursing turnover has focused on a direct relationship between turnover and patient outcomes; the underlying mechanisms of the turnover-outcomes relationship have not been explored (Alexander, Bloom, & Nuchols, 1994).... In order to understand the mechanisms by which nursing turnover is related to patient outcomes, it is necessary to explore the impact of nursing turnover on nursing units, which is the proximal context for individuals and a bounded interactive context created by nurses' attributes, interactions, and responses (Kozlowski, Steve, & Bell, 2003)" (Bae et al., 2010, pp. 40-41). *Purpose:* "The aim of this study was to examine how nursing unit turnover affects key workgroup processes and how these processes mediate the impact of nursing turnover on patient outcomes" (Bae et al., 2010, p. 40).

TABLE 5-4   Intervention Research: Topics, Problem, and Purpose

Type of Research	Research Topic	Research Problem and Purpose
Intervention research	Stress management, social support, nursing interventions, HIV/AIDS, psychoneuroimmunology (PNI), quality of life, coping, psychosocial functioning, immune status, somatic health, viral load	*Title of study:* "Effects of stress management on PNI-based outcomes in persons with HIV disease" (McCain et al., 2003, p. 102). *Problem:* "Although it remains potentially fatal, infection with the human immunodeficiency virus (HIV) has become eminently more treatable as a chronic illness with the advent of highly active antiretroviral therapies.... Insights as to the relationship of psychological and physiological health in HIV and other disease are emanating from research in psychoneuroimmunology (PNI).... A growing body of research with persons who have HIV disease, as well as those who have other chronic and potentially fatal illnesses such as cancer, indicates that not only can a variety of biobehavioral strategies for stress management mitigate psychological distress and improve coping skills, they also can enhance immune function through neuroendocrine–immune system modulation.... More recent work has continued to support the use of CBSM [cognitive-behavioral stress management] as an effective strategy in the management of distress associated with HIV disease.... Little comparative research has been done to determine the relative effect of these two types of interventions on either psychological or physiological status" (McCain et al., 2003, pp. 102-105). *Purpose:* "This study was undertaken to compare the effects of CBSM groups, social support groups (SSG), and a wait-listed control group on the outcomes of psychosocial functioning (perceived stress, coping patterns, social support, uncertainty, psychological distress), quality of life, neuroendocrine mediation (salivary cortisol, DHEA levels), and somatic health (disease progression, HIV-specific health status, viral load, and immune status)" (McCain et al., 2003, p. 105).

nursing unit turnover had a significant adverse affect on the workgroup processes on the unit where turnover took place. The negative effects on workgroup processes adversely impact continuity and quality of patient care and patient outcomes.

Intervention Research

Intervention research determines the interventions that are most effective in managing clinical problems. Some interventions might focus on risk reduction, prevention, treatment, or resolution of health-related problems or symptoms; management of a problem or symptom; or prevention of complications associated with a practice problem. In intervention research, the interventions might have more than one purpose and multiple outcomes. For example, McCain et al. (2003) examined the effectiveness of two complex interventions, cognitive-behavioral stress management (CBSM) and social support, on the multiple outcomes of patients with HIV infection. Table 5-4 lists the topics, problem, and purpose from the study by McCain et al. (2003). The outcomes measured in this study were many physiological and psychological variables, which are commonly used to determine the health status of patients with HIV. The CBSM intervention was found to be the most effective in producing positive physical and psychological outcomes for patients with HIV infection.

KEY POINTS

- A research problem is an area of concern where there is a gap in the knowledge base needed for nursing practice and includes significance, background, and problem statement.
- The major sources for nursing research problems include nursing practice; researcher and peer interactions; literature review; theories; and research priorities identified by individuals, specialty groups, professional organizations, and funding agencies.
- Replication is essential for the development of evidence-based knowledge for practice and consists of four types: exact, approximate, concurrent, and systematic.

- The research purpose is a concise, clear statement of the specific focus or aim of the study and usually indicates the type of study (quantitative, qualitative, outcomes, or intervention research) to be conducted.
- The researcher examines the real-world situation, identifies research topics, generates questions, and ultimately clarifies and refines a research problem.
- From the problem, a specific aim or research purpose is developed that provides a clear focus for the study.
- On the basis of the research purpose, specific research objectives, questions, or hypotheses are developed to direct the study.
- The feasibility of the research problem and purpose are determined by examination of the time and money commitments; researchers' expertise; availability of subjects, facility, and equipment; cooperation of others; and the study's ethical considerations.
- Quantitative, qualitative, outcomes, and intervention studies enable nurses to investigate a variety of research problems and purposes.

REFERENCES

Aberson, C. L. (2010). *Applied power analysis for the behavioral sciences*. New York, NY: Routledge Taylor & Francis Group.

Alexander, J. A., Bloom, J. R., & Nuchols, B. A. (1994). Nursing turnover and hospital efficiency: An organization-level analysis. *Industrial Relations*, *33*(4), 505.

Alligood, M. R. (2010). *Nursing theory: Utilization & application*. Maryland Heights, MO: Mosby Elsevier.

American Diabetes Association. (2009). Diabetes statistics. Retrieved from http://www.diabetes.org/diabetes-statistics.jsp/.

American Association of Critical-Care Nurses (AACN). (2011). AACN's identified research needs. Retrieved from http://www.aacn.org/WD/practice/docs/research/identified-research-needs.pdf.

American Nurses Credentialing Center (ANCC). (2012). Magnet© Program: Overview. Retrieved from http://www.nursecredentialing.org/Magnet/ProgramOverview.aspx/.

American Organization of Nurse Executives (AONE). (2012). AONE 2012 education and research priorities. Retrieved from http://www.aone.org/education/index.shtml/.

Astin, F., Jones, K., & Thompson, D. R. (2005). Prevalence and patterns of anxiety and depression in patients undergoing elective percutaneous transluminal coronary angioplasty. *Heart & Lung*, *34*(6), 393–401.

Bae, S., Mark, B., & Fried, B. (2010). Impact of nursing unit turnover on patient outcomes in hospitals. *Journal of Nursing Scholarship*, *42*(1), 40–49.

Baranowski, T., & Simons-Morton, B. (1990). A center-based program for exercise change among Black-Americans. *Health Education Quarterly*, *17*(3), 179–186.

Beveridge, W. I. B. (1950). *The art of scientific investigation*. New York, NY: Vintage.

Boren, S. A., Gunlock, T. L., Santosh, K., & Kramer, T. C. (2006). Computer-aided diabetes education: A synthesis of randomized controlled trials. *American Medical Informatics Association Annual Symposium Proceedings* (pp. 51–55).

Brink, P. J., & Wood, M. J. (1979). Multiple concurrent replications. *Western Journal of Nursing Research*, *1*(1), 117–118.

Brown, S. J. (2009). *Evidence-based nursing: The research-practice connection*. Sudbury, MA: Jones and Bartlett Publishers.

Bushe, C., & Holt, R. (2004). Prevalence of diabetes and impaired glucose tolerance in patients with schizophrenia. *British Journal of Psychiatry*, *184*(Suppl 47), S67–S71.

Centers for Disease Control and Prevention. (2006). A comprehensive immunization strategy to eliminate transmission of hepatitis B virus infection in the United States. *Morbidity and Mortality Weekly Report*, *55*(RR-16), 1–25.

Centers for Disease Control and Prevention. (2008a). *National diabetes fact sheet: General information and national estimates on diabetes in the United States, 2007*. Atlanta, GA: U.S. Department of Health and Human Services, Author.

Centers for Disease Control and Prevention. (2008b). Surveillance for acute viral hepatitis—United States, 2006. *Morbidity and Mortality Weekly Report*, *57*(SS02), 1–24.

Chinn, P. L., & Kramer, M. K. (2008). *Integrated theory and knowledge development* (7th ed.). St. Louis, MO: Mosby.

Cohen, C. A., London, W. T., Evans, A. A., Block, J., Conti, M. C., & Block, T. (2007). Underestimation of chronic hepatitis B in APIs: A call for advocacy and action [Abstract 149577]. Paper presented at the 135th American Public Health Association Annual Meeting & Exposition, Washington, DC.

Craig, J. V., & Smyth, R. L. (2012). *The evidence-based practice manual for nurses* (3rd ed.). Edinburgh, Scotland: Churchill Livingstone.

Creswell, J. W. (2009). *Research design: Qualitative, quantitative, and mixed methods approaches* (3rd ed.). Los Angeles, CA: Sage.

Doran, D. (2011). *Nursing-sensitive outcomes: The state of the science* (2nd ed.). Sudbury, MA: Jones & Bartlett Learning.

El-Mallakh, P. (2007). Doing my best: Poverty and self-care among individuals with schizophrenia and diabetes mellitus. *Archives of Psychiatric Nursing*, *21*(1), 49–60.

Fahs, P. S., Morgan, L. L., & Kalman, M. (2003). A call for replication. *Journal of Nursing Scholarship*, *35*(1), 67–71.

Fawcett, J., & Garity, J. (2009). *Evaluating research for evidence-based nursing practice*. Philadelphia, PA: F. A. Davis.

Forbes, A. (2009). Clinical intervention research in nursing. *International Journal of Nursing Studies*, *46*(4), 557–568.

Frenn, M., Malin, S., & Bansal, N.K. (2003). Stage-based interventions for low-fat diet with middle school students. *Journal of Pediatric Nursing*, *18*(1), 36–45.

Grady, J. L., Entin, E. B., Entin, E. E., & Brunye, T. T. (2011). Using message framing to achieve long-term behavioral changes in persons with diabetes. *Applied Nursing Research*, *24*(1), 22–28.

Haller, K. B., & Reynolds, M. A. (1986). Using research in practice: A case for replication in nursing: Part II. *Western Journal of Nursing Research*, *8*(2), 249–252.

Happ, M. B., Swigart, V. A., Tate, J. A., Arnold, R. M., Sereika, S. M., & Hoffman, L. A. (2007). Family presence and surveillance during weaning from prolonged mechanical ventilation. *Heart & Lung, 36*(1), 47–57.

Houck, G., Kendall, J., Miller, A., Morrell, P., & Wiebe, G. (2011). Self-concept in children and adolescents with attention deficit hyperactivity disorder. *Journal of Pediatric Nursing, 26*(3), 239–247.

Jackson, C. L., Bolen, S., Brancati, F. L., Batts-Turner, M. L., & Gary, T. L. (2006). A systematic review of interactive computer-assisted technology in diabetes care. *Journal of General Internal Medicine, 21*(2), 105–110.

Kaplan, B. A. (1964). *The conduct of inquiry: Methodology for behavioral science.* New York, NY: Harper & Row.

Kerlinger, F. N., & Lee, H. B. (2000). *Foundations of behavioral research* (4th ed.). Fort Worth, TX: Harcourt College Publishers.

Kozlowski, S. W. J., Steve, W. J., & Bell, B. S. (2003). Work groups and teams in organization. In W. C. Borman, D. R. Ilgen, & R. J. Klimoski (Eds.), *Comprehensive handbook of psychology: Industrial and organizational psychology.* New York, NY: Wiley.

Leifer, S. L., & Glass, L. K. (2008). Planning for mass disaster in the 1950s: Harriet H. Werley and nursing research. *Nursing Research, 57*(4), 237–244.

Letourneau, N., Young, C., Secco, L., Stewart, M., Hughes, J., & Critchley, K. (2011). Supporting mothering: Service providers' perspectives of mothers and young children affected by intimate partner violence. *Research in Nursing & Health, 34*(3), 192–203.

Lewandowski, A., & Kositsky, A. M. (1983). Research priorities for critical care nursing: A study by the American Association of Critical Care Nurses. *Heart & Lung, 12*(1), 35–44.

Lindeman, C.A. (1975). Delphi survey of priorities in clinical nursing research. *Nursing Research, 24*(6), 434–441.

Litrownik, A. J., Newton, R., Hunter, W. M., English, D., & Everson, M. D. (2003). Exposure to family violence in young at-risk children: A longitudinal look at the effects of victimization and witnessed physical and psychological aggression. *Journal of Family Violence, 18*(1), 59–73.

Marshall, C., & Rossman, G. B. (2011). *Designing qualitative research* (5th ed.). Los Angeles, CA: Sage.

Masoli, M., Fabian, D., Holt, S., Beasley, R., & Global Initiative for Asthma (GINA) Program. (2004). The global burden of asthma: Executive summary of the GINA Dissemination Committee Report. *Allergy, 59*(5), 469–478.

McCain, N. L., Munjas, B. A., Munro, C. L., Elswick, R. K., Robins, J. L. W., Ferreira-Gonzales, A., et al. (2003). Effects of stress management on the PNI-based outcomes in persons with HIV disease. *Research in Nursing & Health, 26*(2), 102–117.

Melnyk, B. M., & Fineout-Overholt, E. (2011). *Evidence-based practice in nursing & healthcare: A guide to best practice* (2nd ed.). Philadelphia, PA: Lippincott Williams & Wilkins.

Munhall, P. L. (2012). *Nursing research: A qualitative perspective* (5th. ed.). Sudbury, MA: Jones & Bartlett.

National Institute of Nursing Research (NINR). (2011). Strategic plan National Institute of Nursing Research: Areas of research emphasis. Retrieved from http://www.ninr.nih.gov/AboutNINR/NINRMissionandStrategicPlan/.

National Institutes of Mental Health (2008). Attention deficit hyperactivity disorder. Retrieved from http://www.nimh.nih.gov/health/publications/adhd-listing.shtml.

Nyamathi, A., Liu, Y., Marfisee, M., Shoptaw, S., Gregerson, P., Saab, S., et al. (2009). Effects of a nurse-managed program on hepatitis A and B vaccine completion among homeless adults. *Nursing Research, 58*(1), 13–22.

Pender, N. J. (1996). *Health promotion in nursing practice* (3rd ed.). Stamford, CT: Appleton & Lange.

Price, D., Ryan, D., Pearce, L., Bawden, R., Freeman, D., Thomas, M., et al. (2002). The burden of pediatric asthma is higher than health professionals think: Results from the Asthma In Real Life (AIR) study. *Primary Care Respiratory Journal, 11*(1), 30–33.

Prochaska, J. O., Norcross, J. C., Fowler, J. L., Follick, M. J., & Abrams, D. B. (1992). Attendance and outcome in a work site weight control program: Processes and stages of change as process and predictor variables. *Addictive Behaviors, 17*(1), 35–45.

Rogers, B. (1987). Research corner: Is the research project feasible? *AAOHN Journal, 35*(7), 327–328.

Rohrbeck, J., Jordan, K., & Croft, P. (2007). The frequency and characteristics of chronic widespread pain in general practice: A case-control study. *British Journal of General Practice, 57*(535), 109–115.

Schizophrenia and Diabetes Expert Consensus Group. (2004). Consensus summary. *British Journal of Psychiatry, 47*(2), S112–S114.

Shadish, W. R., Cook, T. D., & Campbell, D. T. (2002). *Experimental and quasi-experimental designs for generalized causal inference.* Chicago, IL: Rand McNally.

Sharma, N. K., Ryals, J. M., Gajewski, B. J., & Wright, D. E. (2010). Aerobic exercise alters analgesia and neurotrophin-3 synthesis in an animal model of chronic widespread pain. *Physical Therapy, 90*(5), 714–725.

Singh, N., Armstrong, D., & Lipsky, B. (2005). Preventing foot ulcers in patients with diabetes. *Journal of American Medical Association, 293*(2), 217–228.

Smith, M. J., & Liehr, P. R. (2008). *Middle range theory for nursing* (2nd ed.). New York, NY: Springer Publishing Company.

Steel, J., Sanna, L., Hammond, B., Wipple, J., & Cross, H. (2004). Psychological sequelae of childhood sexual abuse: Abuse-related characteristics, coping strategies, and attributional style. *Child Abuse & Neglect, 18*(7), 785–801.

Treuting, J., & Hinshaw, S. (2001). Depression and self-esteem in boys with ADHD: Associations with comorbid aggression and explanatory attributional mechanisms. *Journal of Abnormal Psychology, 29*(1), 23–39.

Trollvik, A., Nordbach, R., Silen, C., & Ringsberg, K. C. (2011). Children's experiences of living with asthma: Fear of exacerbations and being ostracized. *Journal of Pediatric Nursing, 26*(4), 295–303.

Trotter, R., Gallagher, R., & Donoghue, J. (2011). Care of patients with coronary heart disease: Anxiety in patients undergoing percutaneous coronary interventions. *Heart & Lung, 40*(3), 185–192.

U.S. Department of Health and Human Services (U.S. DHHS). (2012). Healthy people 2020: Topics and objectives. Retrieved from http://www.healthypeople.gov/2020/topicsobjectives2020/default.aspx/.

Valle, L. A., & Silovsky, J. F. (2002). Attributions and adjustment following child sexual and physical abuse. *Child Maltreatment*, *7*(1), 9–25.

Whiteside, A., Hansen, S., & Chaudhuri, A. (2004). Exercise lowers pain threshold in chronic fatigue syndrome. *Pain*, *109*(3), 497–499.

World Health Organization (WHO). (2012). World Health Organization research policy. Retrieved from http://who.int/rpc/en/.

Zinzow, H., Seth, P., Jackson, J., Niehaus, A., & Fitzgerald, M. (2010). Abuse and parental characteristics, attributions of blame, and psychological adjustment in adult survivors of child sexual abuse. *Journal of Child Sexual Abuse*, *19*(1), 79–98.

6

Review of Relevant Literature

You have been asked to present a lecture about home health care for undergraduate nursing students. Maybe you are concerned about the families of the patients in your critical care unit and want to devise a program to address their unique needs. Maybe you are a graduate nursing student and your teacher said your paper needed to include a review of the literature. Maybe you are in a Magnet hospital and the nurses on your unit are developing a proposal for a study. In each situation, you need to understand how to review the literature and to present the information you find in a logical, synthesized manner. By building on previous knowledge, nurse researchers can add to the evidence upon which we base our practice.

The rate of new knowledge being generated each year continues to grow. Early studies in the 1960s indicated that knowledge doubled every 13 to 15 years (Larsen & von Ins, 2010). The vast amount of information available within seconds implies that knowledge is doubling much more rapidly in the digital age. Bachrach (2001) noted that each new discipline launches new journals to develop its disciplinary knowledge. Computerized bibliographical databases have made the process of searching for relevant empirical or theoretical literature easier in some ways, but you are faced with the dilemma of selecting the most relevant sources from a much larger number of articles. The task of reading, critically appraising, analyzing, and synthesizing has expanded and can consume any time gained by more efficient searching. This chapter provides basic skills and knowledge to identify evidence for changing nursing practice, developing a research proposal, preparing a lecture, or writing a manuscript.

What Is "The Literature"?

"The literature" consists of all written sources relevant to the topic you have selected. The literature consists of newspapers, monographs, encyclopedias, conference papers, scientific journals, textbooks, other books, theses, dissertations, and clinical journals. Websites and reports developed by government agencies and professional organizations are also included. For example, to support the significance of diabetes mellitus as a topic for a research study, you could find statistics about the prevalence and cost of the disease from the Centers for Disease Control and Prevention (CDC) and the World Health Organization (WHO). Not every source that you find, however, will be valid and legitimate for scholarly use. The website of a company that sells insulin may not be an appropriate source for diabetes statistics. Online encyclopedias to which anyone can contribute, such as Wikipedia, are not considered scholarly sources. These websites might point you toward professional sources but should not be cited in a professional or academic paper. You should use primary, peer-reviewed, professional literature. New knowledge develops when researchers and scholars produce manuscripts for journals and books that are reviewed by peers to determine whether the manuscripts should be published.

What Is a Literature Review?

The literature review is an organized written presentation of what you find when you review the literature. The literature review is "central to scholarly work and disciplined inquiry" (Holbrook, Bourke, Fairbairn, & Lovat, 2007, p. 337); it summarizes what has been published on a topic by scholars and presents relevant research findings. Developing the ability to write coherently about what you have found in the literature requires time and guidance. The review should be organized into sections that present themes, identify trends, or examine variables. The purpose is not to list all the material published but, rather, to synthesize and evaluate it on the basis of the phenomenon of interest.

The focus of the review depends on the reason you are reviewing the literature. This overview describes common purposes for conducting literature reviews; however, the goal of this chapter is to provide specific guidance and practical suggestions related to reviewing research relevant to a proposed study. The three major stages of literature reviews are discussed: (1) searching the literature, (2) processing the literature, and (3) writing the literature review.

Purposes of Reviewing the Literature

Writing a Course Paper

For most course papers, your instructor will expect you to review published sources on the topic of your paper. Reviews of the literature for a course assignment will vary depending on the level of educational program, the purpose of the assignment, and the expectations of the instructor. The literature review for a graduate course is expected to have greater depth, scope, and breadth than a review for an undergraduate course (Hart, 2009). A paper in a nurse practitioner course might require that you review pharmacology and pathology reference books in addition to journal articles. In a nursing education course, you may review neurological development, cognitive science, and general education publications to write a paper on a teaching strategy. For a doctor of nursing practice course on clinical information systems, your review might need to extend into computer science and hospital management literature. For a theory course in a doctor of philosophy in nursing program, your review may need to include all the publications of a specific theorist or all the studies based on the theory. For each of these papers, your professor may specify the publication years and the type of literature to be included. Also, you must note the acceptable length of the written review of the literature to be submitted. Reviews of the literature for course assignments tend to focus on what is known, the strength of the evidence, the implications of the knowledge, and what is not known for the purpose of developing new studies.

Examining the Strength of the Evidence

Evidence-based practice guidelines are developed through the synthesis of the literature on the clinical problem. The purpose of the literature review designed to examine the strength of the evidence is to identify all studies that provide evidence of a particular intervention, to critically appraise the quality of each study, and to synthesize all of the studies providing evidence of the effectiveness of a particular intervention. It is also important to locate and include previous evidence-based papers that have examined the evidence of a particular intervention, because the conclusions of the authors of such papers are highly relevant. Literature syntheses related to promoting evidence-based nursing practice are described in Chapter 19.

Developing a Qualitative Research Proposal

In qualitative research, the purpose and timing of the literature review depend on the type of study to be conducted (see Chapter 12). Some phenomenologists believe that the literature should not be reviewed until after the data have been collected and analyzed, so that the literature does not interfere with the researcher's ability to suspend what is known and to approach the topic with openness (Munhall, 2012). In the development of a grounded theory study, a minimal review of relevant studies provides the beginning point of the inquiry, but this review is only a means of making the researcher aware of what studies have been conducted. This information, however, is not used to direct the collection of data or interpretation of the findings in a grounded theory study. During the data analysis stage, a core variable is identified and the researcher theoretically samples the literature for extant theories that may assist in explaining and extending the emerging theory (Munhall, 2012). In historical research, the initial review of the literature helps the researcher define the study questions and make decisions about relevant sources. The data collection is actually an intense review of published and unpublished documents that the researcher has found.

The purposes of reviewing the literature for ethnographic studies and for exploratory descriptive qualitative research are more similar to that for quantitative research. The researcher develops a general understanding of the concepts to be examined in relation to the selected culture or topic. The literature review also provides a background for conducting the study and interpreting the findings. Chapter 12 describes in more detail the role of the literature review in qualitative research.

Developing a Quantitative Study

The review of literature in quantitative research directs the development and implementation of a study. The focus of the major literature review at the beginning of the research process is to identify a gap in what is known. The study is designed to add knowledge in the

TABLE 6-1 The Role of the Literature Review in Developing a Quantitative Research Proposal

Phase of the Research Process	How Literature Is Used and Its Role
Research topic	Broad searches using keywords to understand the extent of what is known and what is not known; what concepts are related to the topic
Statement of the research purpose	From your synthesis of the literature, the specific gap in knowledge that this study will address
Background and significance	Searches of books and articles to provide an overview of the topic Identification of the size, cost, and consequences of the research problem
Research framework	Find and read relevant theories Facilitate development of the framework Develop conceptual definitions of concepts
Purpose of the study	On the basis of your knowledge of the literature, state the purpose of the study
Research objectives, questions, or hypotheses	On the basis of the knowledge gained from and examples found in the literature, write the objectives or questions of the study If sufficient literature allows a prediction, state the hypotheses of the study
Review of the literature	Find sources as evidence for logical argument for why this study and methodology are needed Summarize current empirical knowledge that is related to the topic
Methodology	Compare research designs of reviewed studies to select the most appropriate design for the proposed study Identify possible instruments or measures of variables Provide operational definitions of concepts Describe performance of measures in previous studies Develop sampling strategies based on what you have learned from the studies in the literature
Findings	Refer to statistical textbooks to explain the results of the data analysis
Discussion	Compare your findings with those of studies you have previously reviewed Return to the literature to find new references to interpret unexpected findings Identify limitations of the study Refer to theory sources to relate the findings to the research framework
Conclusions	On basis of your knowledge of the literature and your study's findings, draw conclusions Discuss implications for nursing clinical practice, administration, and education Propose future studies

area of the identified gap. For example, an intervention to prevent hospital-acquired infections related to intravenous infusions has been shown to reduce the incidence of these infections among postoperative patients who have no history of diabetes mellitus. After a thorough review of the literature, the researcher identifies a specific gap in knowledge. What is not known is whether this intervention will be equally effective for postoperative patients who have diabetes. After the data have been analyzed and the findings described, the researcher will return to the literature in the generalization phase of the research report to integrate knowledge from the literature with new knowledge obtained from the study. The purposes of the literature review are similar for the different types of quantitative studies (descriptive, correlational, quasi-experimental, and experimental).

Table 6-1 describes the role of the literature throughout the development and implementation of the study. The types of sources needed and how you will search the literature will vary throughout the study. The introduction section uses relevant sources to summarize the background and significance of the research problem. The review of the literature section includes both theoretical and empirical sources that document the current knowledge of the problem. The researcher develops the framework section from the theoretical literature and sometimes from empirical literature. If little theoretical literature is found, the researcher may need to develop a tentative theory to guide the study from the findings of previous research studies (see Chapter 7 for more information). The methods section describes the design, sample, measurement methods, treatment, and data collection process of the planned study and is based on previous research. Thus, previous studies may be cited in the methods section. In the results section, sources are included to document the different types of statistical analyses conducted and the computer software to conduct these analyses. The discussion section of the research report begins with what the results mean in light of the results of previous studies. Conclusions are drawn that are a synthesis of the cited findings from previous research and those from the present study.

Practical Considerations

What Types of Literature Can I Expect to Find?

Two broad types of literature are cited in the review of literature for research: theoretical and empirical. Theoretical literature consists of concept analyses, models, theories, and conceptual frameworks that support a selected research problem and purpose. Empirical literature comprises knowledge derived from research. The empirical literature reviewed depends on the study problem and the type of research conducted. Research problems that have been frequently studied or are currently being investigated have more extensive empirical literature than new or unique problems. If searching the empirical literature, you need to identify seminal and landmark studies. Seminal studies are the first studies that prompted the initiation of the field of research. Nurse researchers studying hearing loss in infants would need to review the seminal work of Fred H. Bess, an early researcher on this topic who advocated for effective screening tools (Gravel, 2009). Critical care nurses comparing correction formulas for QT intervals on electrocardiograms would want to refer to Bazet's correction formula. The development of the formula can be traced to his seminal paper, published in 1920, on time-relations in electrocardiograms (Roguin, 2011). Landmark studies are the studies that led to an important development or a turning point in the field of research. For example, researchers conducting studies related to glycemic control must be knowledgeable of the implications of the Diabetes Control and Complications Trial, a longitudinal study whose findings changed diabetic care beginning in the mid-1990s (Everett, Bowes, & Kerr, 2010).

Literature is disseminated in several different formats. Serials are published over time or may be in multiple volumes but do not necessarily have predictable publication dates. Periodicals are subsets of serials with predictable publication dates, such as journals, which are published over time and are numbered sequentially for the years published. This sequential numbering is seen in the year, volume, issue, and page numbering of a journal. Monographs, such as books, hard-copy conference proceedings, and pamphlets, are usually written once and may be updated with a new edition as needed. Conference proceedings can help you identify major researchers in your research area who have presented findings that may not yet be published. Periodicals and monographs are available in a variety of media, such as print, online, CD-ROM, and downloadable formats. Textbooks are monographs written to be used in formal education programs.

Entire volumes of books available in a digital or electronic format are called eBooks (Tensen, 2010). You may be familiar with digital books in the mass publication literature that are available to download to read on a special reading device, such as a Kindle or Nook. eBooks are also available for scholarly volumes and articles that can be downloaded to a reading device, cell phone, laptop, or other computer. Books that in the past would have been difficult to obtain through interlibrary loan are now available 24 hours a day, 7 days a week as eBooks.

To develop the significance and background section of a proposal, you may also need to search for government reports for the United States (U.S.) and other countries, if appropriate for your study. A researcher developing a proposal on task shifting in HIV care settings in low-resource countries would search the Ministry of Health websites for those countries to find official guidelines for this type of practice. Researchers developing a proposal in Wisconsin on the smoking cessation in adolescents would consult the Healthy People 2020 website for the national goals related to this topic (http://www.healthypeople.gov/2020/default.aspx/). They may also explore health-related agencies in Wisconsin to determine information specific to their state.

Position papers are disseminated by professional organizations and government agencies to promote a particular viewpoint on a debatable issue. Position papers, along with descriptions of clinical situations, may be included in the discussion of the background and significance of the research problem. A researcher developing a proposal on race-related differences in HIV treatment outcomes would want to review the Association of Nurses in AIDS Care position paper, "Health Disparities," which the organization's board approved in 2009.

Master's theses and doctoral dissertations are valuable literature as well but may not be published. A thesis is a research project completed as part of the requirements for a master's degree. A dissertation is an extensive, usually original research project that is completed as the final requirement for a doctoral degree. Theses and dissertations can be found by searching special databases that are available for these publications, such as ProQuest Dissertations and Theses (http://www.proquest.com/en-US/default .shtml/).

The published literature contains primary and secondary sources. A primary source is written by the person who originated, or is responsible for generating, the ideas published. A research publication published by the person or people who conducted the research is a primary source. A theoretical book or paper written by the theorist who developed the theory or conceptual content is a primary source. A secondary source summarizes or quotes content from primary sources. Thus, authors of secondary sources paraphrase the works of researchers and theorists. The problem with a secondary source is that its author has interpreted the works of someone else, and this interpretation is influenced by that author's perception and bias. Authors have sometimes spread errors and misinterpretations by using secondary sources rather than primary sources. You should use mostly primary sources to write literature reviews. Secondary sources are used only if primary sources cannot be located or if a secondary source contains creative ideas or a unique organization of information not found in a primary source. Citation is the act of quoting or paraphrasing a source, using it as an example, or presenting it as support for a position taken.

How Long Will the Review of the Literature Take?

The time required to review the literature is influenced by the problem studied, sources available, and goals of the reviewer. The literature review for a topic that is focused and somewhat narrow may require less time than one for a topic that is broad. The difficulty you experience identifying and locating sources and the number of sources to be located also influence the time involved, as does the intensity of effort. Only through experience does one become knowledgeable about the time needed for a literature review.

The novice reviewer requires more time to find the relevant literature than an experienced searcher, and the novice frequently underestimates the time needed for the review. An experienced librarian who works closely with nursing graduate students on a variety of course assignments recommends that the reviewer estimate the time required on the basis of the number of sources required and the reviewer's familiarity with the library's databases. The reviewer knows he or she needs at least 30 sources and that finding these sources may require 10 hours of searching. The reviewer estimates that it will take another 20 hours to read and synthesize the sources. The reviewer estimates that the review will require 30 hours. The reviewer should then multiply that number by four, making the estimated time required for the review 120 hours. This longer estimate is often more realistic. As searching skills are refined, the need to use this expanded estimate reduces. Often, the literature review is limited by the time that the reviewer can commit to the assignment. The conclusion related to the time issue is to start as early as possible and stay focused on the purpose of the review.

How Many Sources Do I Need to Review?

Students repeatedly ask, "How many articles should I have? How far back in years should I look to find relevant information?" The answer to both those questions is an emphatic "It depends." Course faculty for masters courses commonly require that you obtain full-text articles of all studies relevant to the variables in the proposed study that were published in the previous 10 years. The instructors often indicate, however, that the length of time may vary depending on the topic and the presence of classic studies. Doctoral students are expected to conduct a more extensive review for course papers. If you are writing a research proposal for a thesis or dissertation, the literature required will be extensive. You need to locate the key papers in the field of interest. After doing some initial searches, discuss what you find with your instructor, thesis chair, or dissertation chair, who will be able to help you determine a reasonable publication period for you to use in your review.

Am I Expected to Read Every Word of the Available Sources?

The answer is "No." If researchers attempted to read every word of every source that is somewhat related to a selected problem, they would be well read but would probably never complete their searches or move on to developing study proposals. Some individuals, even after a thorough literature review, continue to believe that they do not know enough about their area of interest, so they persist in their review; however, this activity ultimately becomes an excuse for not progressing with their work. The opposite of this situation is the individual who wants to move rapidly through the review of literature to reach the conclusion or get to the part of the work that is more enjoyable or important.

With the availability of full-text online articles, the researcher can easily get "lost in the literature" and forget the focus of the review. Becoming a skilled reviewer of the literature involves finding a balance and learning to identify the most pertinent and relevant sources. On the other hand, you cannot critically appraise and synthesize what you have not read. Avoid being distracted by nonrelevant information provided by the author. Learn to read with a purpose and involve multiple senses in your reading. Try reading aloud a section that you have difficulty understanding. Are you having difficulty following an author's presentation? Try writing an outline. Draw a diagram of key points. Audio record your thoughts on the content of an article. Listen to soothing music if you are tense or anxious. Listen to music with an upbeat tempo if you are tired and having trouble staying awake. Try reading in a quiet place outside or standing up with the copy of the article or your laptop on a counter or high table. Involving multiple senses while reading may help you stay awake and focused.

Stages of a Literature Review

The stages of a literature review reflect a systems model. Systems have input, throughput, and output. The *input* consists of the sources that you find through searching the literature. The *throughput* is the processes you use to read, critically appraise, analyze, and synthesize the literature you find. The written literature review is the *output* of these processes (see Figure 6-1). The quality of the input and throughput will determine the quality of the output. As a result, each stage of the literature review is critical to producing a high-quality literature review. Although these stages are presented here as sequential, you may go back to a previous stage. For example, during the analysis and

synthesis of your sources, you identify that the studies you are citing were conducted only in Europe. You might go back and search the literature again using the United States or another search term to ascertain that no studies have been done in that country. As you are writing your literature review, you may identify a problem with the logic of your presentation. To resolve it, you may return to the processing stage to clarify the presentation.

Searching the Literature

Before writing a literature review, you must first perform literature searches to identify sources relevant to your topic of interest. The literature review will help you narrow your topic and develop a feasible study (Hart, 2009). Whether you are a student, practicing nurse, or nurse researcher, your goal is to develop a search strategy designed to retrieve as much of the relevant literature as possible given the time and financial constraints of your project.

Libraries have become gateways to information or information resource centers, rather than storehouses of knowledge (Hart, 2009). High-quality libraries provide access to a large number of electronic databases that supply a broad scope of the literature available internationally, enabling library users not only to identify relevant sources quickly but also to read full-text versions of most of these sources immediately. When your library does not have the hard copy of a book or electronic access to a specific journal, the librarian can usually provide the book or an electronic copy of the article through interlibrary loan. All libraries, public, private, college, and university, have interlibrary loan capabilities. You may especially need to use interlibrary loan when sources relevant to your topic were published prior to the advent of electronic databases.

Consider consulting with an information professional, such as a subject specialist librarian, to develop a literature search approach (Booth, Colomb, & Williams, 2008; Tensen, 2010). Often these consultations can be performed via email or a web-based meeting, so that communication occurs at the convenience of both the researcher and the information professional. Many university libraries provide this consultation service whether or not the library user is affiliated with the university.

Develop a Search Plan

Before you begin searching the literature, you must consider exactly what information you are seeking. Expending time and effort in the early stage of a review to develop a search strategy is likely to save

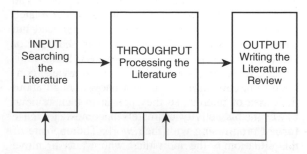

Figure 6-1 Systems model of the review of the literature.

TABLE 6-2	Plan and Record for Searching the Literature			
Database Searched	**Date of Search**	**Search Strategy and Limiters**	**Number and Type of Articles Found**	**Estimate of Relevant Articles**
Cumulative Index to Nursing and Allied Health Literature (CINAHL)				
MEDLINE				
Academic Search Premier				
Cochrane Library				

time and effort later (Hart, 2009). A written plan helps you to avoid duplication of effort, to return to a previously searched area with a different set of search terms or a different range of publication years. Your initial search should be based on the widest possible interpretation of your topic. This strategy enables you to envision the extent of the relevant literature. As you see the results of the initial searches and begin reading the material, you will refine your topic, and then you can narrow the focus of your searches.

As you search, add your selected search terms to your written search plan. As you search, add other terms that you discover from the references you locate. For each search, record (1) the name of the database, (2) the date, (3) search terms and searching strategy, (4) the number and types of articles found, and (5) an estimate of the proportion of the citations you retrieved that were relevant articles. Table 6-2 is an example of search history that you can use to record what and how you have searched the literature. Save the results of each search on your computer or external device. Some databases allow you to create an account and save your search history online (i.e., the record of what and how you searched).

Select Databases to Search

A database is computer data that have been collected and arranged to be searchable and automatically retrievable (Tensen, 2010). A **bibliographical database** is an "an electronic version of a bibliographic index" (p. 57) or compilation of citations. The database may consist of citations relevant to a specific discipline or may be a broad collection of citations from a variety of disciplines. Databases of periodical citations include the authors, title, journal, keywords, and usually an abstract of the article. Library databases contain titles and authors of hard copy books and documents, government reports, and reference books. Library databases also include a searchable list of the journals to which the library has a paper or electronic subscription. For example, your library

may have received paper copies of a monthly journal in the mail until 2006. The hard copies of the issues were bound to create annual volumes of the journal. Since 2006, the library has subscribed to the electronic journal or a journal database that provides access to specific issues.

Bibliographical databases provided by the same vendor, such as those databases affiliated with EBSCO Publishing, allow you to search multiple databases simultaneously to save time. Usually the search engine will automatically delete duplicates of the same study. You can also change the order in which the results of the search are shown. For example, with the EBSCO Publishing databases, you can sort the citations by relevance, date descending (most current first), or date ascending (oldest to more recent).

Older sources of reference indexes are useful for sources published prior to the electronic databases. Card catalogs, abstract reviews, and indexes were the only ways to search for nursing references until 1955, when the *Cumulative Index to Nursing and Allied Health Literature* (CINAHL) began being published. Because the printed editions had red covers, you still may hear more experienced scholars fondly refer to "the Red Books." The print version of CINAHL is still available in libraries, and you may find it useful when searching for citations published before 1982 or when bibliographic databases are not available (Tensen, 2010). In medicine, the *Index Medicus* (IM) was first published in 1879 and is the oldest health-related index. The *Index Medicus* includes some citations of nursing publications, with the number of nursing journals cited growing. CINAHL contains, however, a more extensive listing of nursing publications and uses more nursing terminology as subject headings. With the greater focus on interdisciplinary research, nurse researchers must also be consumers of the literature in the National Library of Medicine (MEDLINE), other government agencies, and professional organizations. Table 6-3 provides descriptions of commonly used bibliographical databases.

TABLE 6-3   **Bibliographical Databases**

Name of Database	Description of the Database by the Publisher*
Cumulative Index of Nursing and Allied Health Literature (CINAHL)	"Comprehensive source of full text for nursing & allied health journals, providing full text for more than 770 journals"
MEDLINE	"Information on medicine, nursing, dentistry, veterinary medicine, the health care system, pre-clinical sciences, and much more" Created and provided by the National Library of Medicine Uses Medical Subject Headings (MeSH terms) for indexing and searching of "citations from over 4,800 current biomedical journals"
PubMed	Free access to Medline that provides links to full-text articles when available
PsychARTICLES	15,000 "full-text, peer-reviewed scholarly and scientific articles in psychology" Limited to journals published by the American Psychological Association (APA) and affiliated organizations
PsychINFO	"Scholarly journal articles, book chapters, books, and dissertations, is the largest resource devoted to peer-reviewed literature in behavioral science and mental health" Supported by APA Covers over 3 million records
Academic Search Complete	"Comprehensive scholarly, multi-disciplinary full-text database, with more than 8,500 full-text periodicals, including more than 7,300 peer-reviewed journals"
Health Source Nursing/ Academic Edition	"Provides nearly 550 scholarly full text journals focusing on many medical disciplines" Also includes 1,300 patient education sheets for generic drugs
Psychological and Behavioral Sciences Collection	"Comprehensive database covering information concerning topics in emotional and behavioral characteristics, psychiatry & psychology, mental processes, anthropology, and observational & experimental methods" 400 journals indexed

*Direct quotations from EBSCO Publishing descriptions of the databases, available at http://www.ebscohost.com/academic/.

Search Strategies

Keywords

Keywords are the everyday words and phrases used for the major concepts or variables that must be included in your computer search (Tensen, 2010). To determine keywords, identify the concepts relevant to your study. Ascertain the populations that are of particular interest in your area of study or the specific interventions, measurement methods, or outcomes that are relevant. These databases have a thesaurus that the researcher, as well as anyone who reads an article, can use as keyword search terms. By logging on to the database, you can access the thesaurus to select relevant terms. The formal subject terms included in the thesaurus may encompass a number of the terms that you have identified and allow you to expand your search to obtain more references or to focus your search to be more specific to your interest. This expansion or focus occurs because someone who has already read the articles has grouped and linked all citations with similar concepts together.

A simple way to begin identifying a database's standardized subject terms is to search using one of your keywords and display full records of a few relevant citations. The *records* are the descriptions of the articles, not the articles themselves. The subject terms linked to that article are listed on the full record. Examine the terminology used to describe these articles, and use the terms in additional refined searches. Frequently, word-processing programs, dictionaries, and encyclopedias are helpful in identifying synonymous terms and subheadings. A combination of both keywords and formal subjects most often retrieves better search results.

The format and spelling of search terms can yield different results. Truncating words can allow you to locate more citations related to that term. For example, authors might have used intervene, intervenes, intervened, intervening, intervention, or intervenor. To capture all of these terms, you can use a truncated term in your search, such as *interven, interven*,* or *interven$*. The form or symbol used to truncate a search term depends on the rule of the search engine being used. Avoid shortening a search word to fewer than four letters. Otherwise, you will get far too many unwanted citations. Also, pay attention to variant spellings. You may need to search, for example, by *orthopedic* or *orthopaedic* (British spelling). Consider irregular plurals, such as *woman* and *women*.

Authors

If an author is cited frequently, you can perform a search using the author's name. In this case, you should identify the name as an author term, not a keyword term. Recognize that some databases list authors only under first and middle initials, whereas others use full first names. Identifying and using citations to seminal studies in various citation indexes or full-text databases can lead you to other, more current works that have also cited the seminal studies as references. Web of Knowledge, a database developed from the *Science Citation Index* and the *Social Science Citation Index,* focuses on the relationships among these citations. These indexes may require that your library subscribe to their services, however, Web of Knowledge does have a Facebook page (http://www.facebook.com/pages/Web-of-Knowledge/119687984715358/). Several other databases, depending on the vendor, may also have a function to search the references of articles.

Complex Searches

A complex search of the literature combines two or more concepts or synonyms in one search. There are several ways to arrange terms in a database search phrase or phrases. The three most common ways are by using (1) Boolean operators, (2) locational operators (field labels), and (3) positional operators. **Operators** permit you to group ideas, select places to search in a database record, and show relationships within a database record, sentence, or paragraph. Examine the Help screen of a database carefully to determine whether the operators you want to use are available and how they are used.

The **Boolean operators** are the three words AND, OR, and NOT. Often they must be capitalized. The Boolean operators AND and NOT are used with your identified concepts. Use AND when you want to search for the presence of two or more terms in the same citation. Use NOT when you want to search for one idea but not another in the same citation. NOT is rarely used because it is too easy to lose good citations. The Boolean operator OR is most useful with synonymous terms or concepts. Use OR when you want to search for the presence of any of a group of terms in the same search. Figure 6-2 shows the results

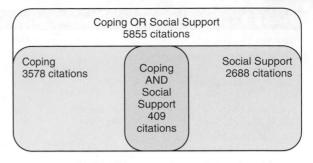

Figure 6-2 Example of search using social support and coping with different Boolean operators.

of searches using coping and social support as keywords alone and with Boolean operators.

Locational operators (field labels) identify terms in specific areas or fields of a record. These fields may be parts of the simple citation, such as the article title, author, and journal name, or they may be from additional fields provided by the database, such as subject headings, abstracts, cited references, publication type notes, instruments used, and even the entire article. In some databases, these specific fields can be selected by means of a drop-down menu in the database input area. In other databases, specific coding can be used to do the same thing. Do not assume that the entire article is being searched when you are using the default search; the default is usually looking for your terms in the title, abstract, and/or subject fields. You may choose to search for a concept only within the abstract of articles, on the basis of the logic that this strategy is less restrictive than searching for the concept only in article titles but more restrictive than searching for the concept in all the text of the article.

Positional operators are used to look for requested terms within certain distances of one another. Availability and phrasing of positional operators are highly dependent on the database search software. Common positional operators are NEAR, WITH, and ADJ; they also are often required to be capitalized and may have numbers associated with them. A positional operator is most useful in records with a large amount of information, such as those with full-text articles attached, and is often used with locational operators, either in an implied way or explicitly. For example, ADJ is an abbreviation for adjacent; it specifies that one term must be adjacent to another in the order entered. "ADJ2" commands that there must be no more than two intervening words between the search terms in the order entered. NEAR does not define the specific order of the terms; the command "term1 NEAR1 term2"

TABLE 6-4 Selected Internet-Only Nursing Journals	
Journal	**URL**
Online Journal of Issues in Nursing	http://nursingworld.org/MainMenuCategories/ANAMarketplace/ANAPeriodicals/OJIN.aspx/
Internet Journal of Advanced Nursing Practice	http://www.ispub.com/journal/the_internet_journal_of_advanced_nursing_practice.html/
Australian Electronic Journal of Nursing Education	http://www.scu.edu.au/schools/nhcp/aejne/
CONNECT: The World of Critical Care Nursing	http://en.connectpublishing.org/
Open Nursing Journal	http://www.benthamscience.com/open/tonursj/
International Journal of Nursing	http://www.ijnonline.com/index.php/ijn/index/

requires that the first term occur first and within two words of the second term. WITH often indicates that the terms must be within the same sentence, paragraph, or region (such as subject headings) of the record.

Limiting Your Search

You can use several strategies to limit your search if, after performing Boolean searches, you continue to get too many hits. The limits you can impose vary with the database. In CINAHL, for example, you may limit your search to English-language articles. You can also limit the years of your search. For example, you might choose to limit the search to articles published in the past 10 years. Searches can be limited to find only papers that are research, are reviews, are published in consumer health journals, include abstracts, or are available in full text. You may also narrow your search by adding your population or intervention to the search strategy.

Searching the Internet

A number of nursing journals are published only in electronic form. Table 6-4 contains selected online nursing journals with their URLs. Because of the high costs of publishing and distributing a printed journal, a publishing company risks losing money unless there is a large market for the journal. Most of the electronic journals are targeted to relatively small specialty audiences. These journals may have more current information on your topic than you will find in traditional journals, because articles submitted by authors to online journals are reviewed and published within 3 to 4 months. Articles submitted to printed journals are usually under review for an extended time and, if accepted, may not be seen in print for over a year. Faculty members at some universities have established online journals in a particular specialty area. In some cases, you may have to subscribe to the online journal to gain access to the articles. Some electronic journals are listed in available bibliographical

databases, and you can access full-text articles from an electronic journal through the database. However, many electronic journals are not yet in the bibliographical databases or may not be in the database you are using. Ingenta Connect (www.ingenta.com) is a commercial website that allows you to search more than 13,000 publications from many disciplines. Publications available through Ingenta include those that are free to download and those that require the reader to buy the article.

Metasearch engines, such as Google, allow you to search the Internet. Google Scholar is a specialized tool that allows you to focus your search on research and theoretical publications. With the exception of articles in online-only journals, scholarly sources are published first in traditional formats. Thus, what you find online will be older references. Especially early in your search, these older articles may point you to seminal and landmark studies or help you identify subject terms for new searches. Government reports and publications by professional organizations may also be found by searching the Internet. Prior to using a reference from the Internet, you must evaluate the reliability of the information and the potential for bias on the part of the author. There is no screening process for information placed on the World Wide Web. Thus, you find a considerable amount of misinformation as well as some "gems" you might not find elsewhere. It is important to check the source of any information you obtain from the Web so that you can judge its validity.

Locate Relevant Literature

Within each database, conduct your search of **relevant literature** using the strategies described in this chapter. Most databases provide abstracts of the articles in which the term is cited, allowing you to get some sense of their content so you may judge whether the information is useful in relation to your selected topic. If you find the information to be an important reference, save it to a file on your computer or in an online folder maintained by your employer or university, and/ or move it to a reference management program (next section). At this point in the process, do not try to examine all of the citations listed.

It is rarely, if ever, possible to identify every relevant source in the literature. The most extensive retrievals of literature are funded literature review projects focused on defining evidence-based practice or developing clinical practice guidelines (see Chapter 19). In these projects, a literature review coordinator manages the literature review process. The project employs several full-time, experienced, professional librarians as literature searchers. When these extensive literature reviews are completed, the results are published so that you may have access to them and to the citations from the review, either on the Internet or in journal articles.

Systematically Record References

The bibliographical information on a source should be recorded in a systematic manner, according to the format that you will use in the reference list. The purpose for carefully citing sources is that readers can retrieve the reference for themselves, confirm your interpretation of the findings, and gather additional information on the topic. Many journals and academic institutions use the format developed by the American Psychological Association (APA) (2010). Computerized lists of sources usually contain complete citations for references and should be saved electronically so you can access complete reference citations. The 6th edition of the APA's *Publication Manual* (2010) provides revised guidelines for citing electronic sources and direct quotations from electronic sources. Citing direct quotations from electronic sources has posed unique challenges. The APA standard for direct quotations from a print source is to cite the page of the source on which the quotation appears. The reference lists in this text are presented in APA format, with the exceptions that we have not included digital object identifiers (DOIs) and have slightly modified the citation of multiple authors.

DOIs have become the standard for the International Standards Organization (http://www.doi.org/) but have not yet received universal support. The use of DOIs seems to be gaining in credibility because the DOI "provides a means of persistent identification for managing information on digital networks" (APA, 2010, p. 188). CrossRef is an example of a registration agency for DOIs that enables citations to be linked across databases and disciplines (http://www.crossref.org/).

Each citation on the reference list is formatted as a paragraph with a *hanging indent,* meaning that the first line is on the left margin and subsequent lines are indented. If you do not know how to format a paragraph this way, search the Help tool in your word-processing program to find the correct command to use. When you retrieve an electronic source in portable document format (pdf), you cite the source the same as if you had made a copy of the print version of the article. When you retrieve an electronic source in html format, you will not have page numbers for the citation. The updated APA standard is to provide the URL for the home page of the journal from which the reader could navigate and find the source (APA, 2010). Providing the URL that you used to retrieve the article is not helpful because it is unique to the path you used to find the article and reflects your search engines and bibliographical databases. The following are examples for citing different types of articles:

Citation for the print copy or electronic pdf copy of an article:

Everett, J., Bowes, A., & Kerr, D. (2010). Barriers to achieving glycaemic control in CSII. *Journal of Diabetes Nursing,* 14(5), 176-181. doi:10.1177/ 1043659609357635.

Online full-text version of an article for which pdf was not available:

Scott, A. J., & Wilson, R. F. (2011). Social determinants of health among African Americans in a rural community in the Deep South: An ecological study. Rural and Remote Health, 11, 1634 (Online). Retrieved from http://www.rrh.org.au/

Use Reference Management Software

Reference management software can make tracking the references you have obtained through your searches considerably easier. You can use such software to conduct searches and to store the information on all search fields for each reference obtained in a search, including the abstract. Within the software, you can store articles in folders with other similar articles. For example, you may have a folder for theory sources, another for methodological sources, and a third for relevant research topics. When you export search results from the bibliographic database to your reference management software, all of the needed citation information and the abstract are readily available to you electronically when you write the literature review. As you read the articles, you can also insert comments into the reference file about each one.

Reference management software has been developed to interface directly with the most commonly used word processing software to organize the reference information using whatever citation style you stipulate. You may be familiar with APA format but want to submit a manuscript to a journal that uses another bibliographical style. Within these reference management programs, you can generate the reference list or bibliography in the format specific to the journal. You can insert citations into your paper with just a keystroke or two. The four most commonly used software packages, along with websites that contain information about them, are as follows:

EndNote (http://www.endnote.com/) has an inclusive format that is compatible with Windows and Mac computers.

RefWorks (www.refworks.com/) operates from the Web and can be accessed free by some universities' affiliates depending on the license.

Reference Manager (http://www.refman.com/) operates on your personal computer or you can use it to make your databases accessible to others in a Web environment.

Bookends (http://www.sonnysoftware.com/) is reference manager for Mac users that allows users to search bibliographical databases and download citations and full-text articles. Searches can also be downloaded from iPhone, iTouch, and iPad.

Saved Searches and Alerts

If you are working on a research project in which the literature review may take months or are engaged in a field of study that will interest you for years, you might want to repeat the same search regularly. Many databases permit you to create an account where you can save your search strategy so you can redo the same search with just a few clicks and without having to enter the entire strategy again. You might want to have just the new updates of a search strategy sent to you automatically by email without having to redo the entire search, even though this redo now entails just a few clicks. These Saved Search and Alert features may be available in your favorite databases. However, review your saved and alert strategies with some regularity to ensure you are obtaining what you really desire. Many journals also permit a table of contents to be sent to you automatically when new issues come out. Examine the database or journal home page help screens to determine how to create and use these features.

Processing the Literature

Reading and critically appraising sources promote understanding of the current knowledge of a research problem. It involves skimming, comprehending, analyzing, and synthesizing content from sources. Skills in reading and critically appraising sources are essential to the development of a high-quality literature review.

Reading

Skimming a source is quickly reviewing a source to gain a broad overview of its content. You would probably read the title, the author's name, and an abstract or introduction for the source. Then you would read the major headings and sometimes one or two sentences under each heading. Finally, you would review the conclusion or summary. Skimming enables you to make a preliminary judgment about the value of a source and to determine whether it is a primary or secondary source. Secondary sources are reviewed and used to locate cited primary sources, but they are seldom cited in a research proposal or report.

Comprehending a source requires that you read all of it carefully. Focus on understanding major concepts and the logical flow of ideas within the source. Highlight the content you consider important or make notes in the margins. Notes might be recorded on photocopies or electronic files of articles, indicating where the information will be used in developing a research proposal. The kind of information you highlight or note in the margins of a source depends on the type of study or source. The information highlighted on theoretical sources might include relevant concepts, definitions of those concepts, and relationships among them. The notes recorded in the margins of empirical literature might include relevant information about the researcher, such as whether the author is a major researcher of a selected problem and comparisons with other studies this individual has conducted. For a research article, the research problem, purpose, framework, major variables, study design, sample size, data collection, analysis techniques, and findings are usually highlighted. You may wish to record quotations (including page numbers) that might be used in a review of literature section. The decision to use or paraphrase these quotes can be made later.

You might also record creative ideas about content that develop while you are reading a source. At this point, you will identify relevant categories for sorting and organizing sources. These categories will ultimately guide you in writing the review of literature section, and some may even be major headings in this review.

Appraising and Analyzing Sources

Through analysis, you can determine the value of a source for a particular study. Analysis must take place in two stages. The first stage involves the critical appraisal of individual studies. The process of

TABLE 6-5 Literature Summary Table							
Author and Year	Purpose	Framework	Sample	Measurement	Treatment	Results	Findings

appraising individual studies, including the steps, is detailed in Chapter 18. During the critical appraisal, relevant content is clearly identified in the articles and sources are sorted into a sophisticated system of categories.

Conducting an **analysis of sources** to be used in a research proposal requires some knowledge of the subject to be critiqued, some knowledge of the research process, and the ability to exercise judgment in evaluation (Pinch, 1995, 2011). However, the critical appraisal of individual studies is only the first step in developing an adequate review of the literature. Any written literature review that simply appraises individual studies paragraph by paragraph is inadequate. A literature review that is a series of paragraphs, in which each paragraph is a description of a single study with no link to other studies being reviewed, does not provide evidence of adequate analysis of the literature.

Analysis requires manipulation of what you are finding, literally making it your own (Garrard, 2011). Pinch (1995) was the first nurse to publish a strategy to synthesize research findings using a literature summary table. We modified this table by adding two columns that are useful in sorting information from studies into categories for analysis (see Table 6-5). In 2001, Pinch published a modified table to use in translating research findings into clinical innovations. Hart (2009) provides examples of table formats that may be helpful at different points during the review. The reference management software may allow you to generate these tables from information you record about each study.

Another way to manipulate the information you have retrieved and transform it into knowledge is mapping (Hart, 2009). Nurse educators teach conceptual mapping to their students to encourage students to make connections among facts and principles that they are learning (Vacek, 2009). The same strategy applied to a literature review is to classify the sources and arrange them into some type of format that requires you to become familiar with key concepts (Hart, 2009). The map may connect studies with similar methodologies or key ideas.

The second stage of analysis involves making comparisons among studies. This analysis allows you to critically appraise the existing body of knowledge in relation to the research problem. You will be able to determine (1) theoretical formulations that have been used to explain how the variables in the problem influence one another, (2) what methodologies have been used to study the problem, (3) the methodological flaws in previous studies, (4) what is known about the problem, and (5) what the most critical gaps in the knowledge base are. The information gathered by using the table format shown in Table 6-5 or displayed in a conceptual map can be useful in making these comparisons. Various studies addressing a research problem have approached the examination of the problem from different perspectives. They may have organized the study from different theoretical perspectives, asked different questions related to the problem, selected different variables, or used different designs. Pay special attention to conflicting findings as they may provide clues for gaps in knowledge that represent researchable problems.

Sorting Your Sources

Relevant sources (theoretical and empirical) are organized for inclusion in the different chapters of the research proposal. The sources to be included in the review of literature chapter are organized to reflect the current knowledge about the research problem. Those sources that provide background and significance for the study are included in the introduction chapter. Certain theoretical sources establish the framework for the study. Other relevant sources become the basis for defining research variables and identifying assumptions and limitations. Content from methodologically strong studies is used to direct

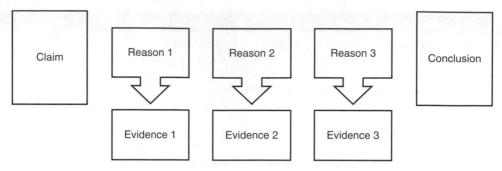

Figure 6-3 Building the logical argument. (Adapted from W. C. Booth, G. G. Colomb, & J. M. Williams [2008]. *The craft of research* [3rd ed.]. Chicago, IL: University of Chicago Press.)

the development of the research design, guide the selection of measurement methods, influence data collection and analysis, and provide a basis for interpretation of finding. (Refer back to Table 6-1 to review contributions of the literature to each part of the research process.)

Synthesizing Sources

Synthesis of sources involves clarifying the meaning obtained from the sources as a whole in the review of the literature section of your proposal. "Integration is making connections between ideas, theories, and experience" (Hart, 2009, p. 8).Through synthesis and integration, one can cluster and connect ideas from several sources to develop a personal overall view of the topic. Garrard (2011) describes this personal level of knowledge as ownership, as "being so familiar with what has been written by previous researchers that you know clearly how this area of research has progressed over time and across ideas" (p. 7). Synthesis is the key to the next step of the review process, which is developing the logical argument that supports the research problem you intend to address. Booth et al. (2008) details the process of constructing the argument as beginning with stating a claim and the supporting reasons. The reviewer must also include adequate information so that the reader agrees that the reasons are relevant to the claim. For each reason, the reviewer provides evidence to support the reasons. Thinking at this level and depth prepares you for outlining the written review. Figure 6-3 provides a visual representation of an argument that can be developed through a written review. The writer/reviewer supports each claim with evidence so that the reader can accept the conclusion the reviewer has made. For example, the reviewer has synthesized several sources related to medication adherence and is presenting the argument for developing patient-focused medication adherence

intervention. The following outline could be developed for this argument.

Claim 1: Interventions to promote medication adherence must incorporate the hypertensive patient's perspective.

> *Reason 1:* Provider-focused interventions have not resulted in long-term improvement in medication adherence.

> *Evidence 1:* Description of studies of provider-focused interventions and their outcomes

> *Reason 2:* Patients who do not adhere to an externally imposed medication regimen (the target population) may be less likely to use an intervention that is externally imposed.

> *Evidence 2:* Description of studies in which patients failed to return for appointments during a trial of an electronic device to promote adherence

> *Reason 3:* Medication adherence requires behavior change that must be incorporated into the patient's life.

> *Evidence 3:* Theoretical principles of behavior change that recommend individualization of interventions to meet unique patient needs

> *Conclusion 1:* Using a participatory approach to develop individual strategies for promoting medication adherence is an important first step to improving patient outcomes.

Writing the Review of Literature

Writing Suggestions

Clarity and cohesion are characteristics of scholarly writing. If you have followed the steps for reviewing the literature in this chapter, you want to demonstrate your synthesis and ownership of the literature by clearly presenting your argument. Rather than using direct quotes from an author, you should paraphrase his or her ideas. Paraphrasing involves expressing the ideas clearly and in your own words. The meanings of these sources are then connected to the proposed study. Last, the reviewer combines, or clusters, the meanings obtained from all sources to determine the current knowledge of the research problem (Pinch, 1995, 2001). Reviews that lack clarity and cohesion reflect deficits in synthesis more than deficits in written abilities.

Start each paragraph with a theme sentence that describes the main idea of the paragraph or makes a claim. Present the relevant studies as evidence of the main idea or claim and end the paragraph with a concluding sentence that transitions to the next claim. Each paragraph can be compared to a train with an engine (theme sentence), linked cargo cars (sentences with evidence), and a caboose (summary sentence linking to next paragraph).

Organization of Written Reviews

The readability and flow of a literature review are determined by its structure (Cronin, Ryan, & Coughlan, 2008). A review of the literature can be organized as series of claims with supporting reasons and claims (Booth et al., 2009) or it can be organized according to the research framework. Theories supporting the research framework may be presented in the first section. This then allows the writer/reviewer to use the framework as an outline for the section on empirical literature. In the section on empirical literature, subheading can identify each concept. Then in these subsections, studies most relevant to that concept can be discussed. The availability of studies will directly affect the length of the literature review. In newer areas of research, you may not have as many sources per concept.

The purpose of the written literature review is to establish a context for your study. The literature review for a study may have four major sections: (1) the introduction, (2) a discussion of theoretical literature, (3) a discussion of empirical literature, and (4) a summary. The introduction and summary are standard sections, but you will want to organize the discussion of sources in a way that makes sense for the topic. You may organize the discussion by themes, your logical argument, or your research framework.

Introduction

The introduction to the literature review indicates the focus or purpose of the study, identifies the purpose of the literature review, and presents the organizational structure of the review. You should make clear in this section what you will and will not cover. If you are taking a particular position or developing a logical argument for a particular perspective on the basis of the literature, make this position clear in the introduction.

Discussion of Theoretical Literature

The theoretical literature section contains concept analyses, models, theories, and conceptual frameworks that support the research purpose. Concepts, definitions of concepts, relationships among concepts, and assumptions are presented and analyzed to build a theoretical knowledge base for the study. This section of the literature review is sometimes used to present the framework for the study and may include a conceptual map that synthesizes the theoretical literature (see Chapter 7 for more detail on developing frameworks).

Discussion of Empirical Literature

The presentation of empirical literature should be organized by concepts or organizing topics. In the past, the researcher was expected to present the purpose, sample size, design, and specific findings for each study reviewed with a scholarly but brief critique of the study's strengths and weaknesses, This approach is expected less commonly now. Use the synthesis and key ideas related to each concept that you developed in the previous stage of the review to organize this section. In addition to the synthesis, you want to incorporate the strengths and weaknesses of the overall body of knowledge rather than a detailed presentation and critical appraisal of each study. The findings from the studies should logically build on each other so that the reader can see how the body of knowledge in the research area evolved.

Evidence from multiple studies is combined to reveal the current state of knowledge in relation to a particular concept or study focus (topic area). Conflicting findings and areas of uncertainty are explored. Similarities and differences in the studies should be identified. Gaps and areas needing more research are discussed. A summary of findings in the topic area is presented, along with inferences, generalizations, and conclusions you have drawn from your review of the literature. A conclusion is a statement about the state of knowledge in relation to the topic area. This should include a discussion of the strength of evidence available for each conclusion.

The reviewer who becomes committed to a particular viewpoint on the research topic must maintain the ethical standard of intellectual honesty. The content from reviewed sources should be presented honestly, not distorted to support the selected problem. Researchers frequently read a study and wish that the author had studied a slightly different problem or that the study had been designed or conducted differently. However, the reviewers must recognize their own opinions and must be objective in presenting information.

The defects of a study need to be addressed, but it is not necessary to be highly critical of another researcher's work. The criticisms must focus on the content that is in some way relevant to the proposed study and to be stated as possible or plausible explanations, so that the criticisms are more neutral and scholarly than negative and blaming.

Summary

The summary consists of a concise presentation of the current knowledge base for the research problem. Other literature reviews conducted in relation to your field of research should be discussed. The gaps in the knowledge base are identified, with a discussion of how the proposed study will contribute to the development of knowledge in the defined field of research. The summary concludes with a statement of how your study will contribute to the body of knowledge in this field of research.

Refining the Written Review

You complete the first draft of your review of the literature and breathe a sigh of relief before moving onto the next portion of the research proposal. Before moving on, you need to read, review, and refine your review. Set the review aside for 24 hours and then read it aloud. You may identify awkward sentences in this way that you might overlook when reading the review silently. Ask a fellow student or trusted colleague to read the review and provide constructive feedback. Use the criteria and guiding questions in Table 6-6 to evaluate your literature review.

Checking References

Sources that will be cited in a paper or recorded in a reference list should be cross-checked two or three times to prevent errors. Questions that will identify common errors are displayed in Box 6-1. To prevent these errors, check all the citations within the text of your literature review and each citation in your reference list. Typing or keyboarding errors may result in inaccurate information. You may omit some information, planning to complete the reference later, and then forget to do so. Downloading citations from a database directly into a reference management system and using the system's manuscript formatting functions

TABLE 6-6	Characteristics of High-Quality Literature Reviews
Criteria	**Guiding Questions**
Coverage	Did the writer provide evidence of having reviewed sufficient literature on the topic?
	Does the review indicate that the writer is sufficiently well informed about the topic and has identified relevant studies?
Understanding	Does the written review indicate that the writer has understood and synthesized what is being studied?
	Have similarities and differences of what was found been described?
Coherence	Does the writer make a logical argument related to the significance of the topic and the gap to be addressed by the proposed study?
Accuracy	Does the writer's attention to detail give the reader confidence in the conclusions of the review?

Box 6-1	Checking to Avoid Common Reference Citation Errors

Does every direct quotation have a citation that includes the author's name, year, and page number?

Are authors' names spelled the same way in the text and in the reference list?

Are the years on citations in the text the same as the years for the reference on the reference list?

Are the citations on the reference list complete so that the reference can be retrieved?

Does every source cited in the text have a corresponding citation on the reference list?

Is every reference on the reference list cited in the text?

reduces some errors but does not eliminate all of them. Use your knowledge and skills to enhance your technology use; relying on technology alone will not create a quality manuscript.

Example of a Literature Review

An excerpt from the literature review of the research report of a quasi-experimental study is provided here

"When comfort is enhanced, patients are better able to be successful in their health-seeking behaviors (HSBs). Scholtfeldt (1975) included internal behaviors and external behaviors in her definition of HSBs, and both of these behaviors are incorporated into Comfort Theory. Therefore, it was hypothesized that increased comfort would lead to a reduction in anxiety, stress, and depression.

Guided Imagery (GI)

"In the context of this study, GI is defined as the use of the imagination to bring about positive mind/body responses (Rossman, 2000). It is a cognitive process that evokes and uses many senses: sight, sound, smell, taste, and touch and also the senses of movement. All of these senses together produce regenerative changes in the mind and body (Achterberg, 1985). GI is a program of instructions meant to help people acquire a state of psychological and physiological ease through muscular relaxation and positive mental images, relieving the discomforts provoked by symptoms associated with mood disorders (Apóstolo, 2007). Increasing adaptive responses in depressive individuals requires replacing the negative processes of thinking with a more positive cognitive style (Achterberg, 1985; Rossman, 2000). GI is a complementary nursing intervention that can be implemented in addition to other therapeutic approaches to mood disorders. Studies show that focusing the imagination in a positive way can result in a state of ease, encouragement, and mood regulation, all of which allow the patient to reestablish a state of physical and mental health (Rossman, 2000).

Guided Imagery and Depression

"Currently, it is thought that good body functioning is accompanied by positive thoughts, whereas pathological body functioning is accompanied by negative and repetitive thoughts (Damásio, 2004). In the brain, a thought, idea, or mental image work as "emotionally competent stimuli." These stimuli, whether prescribed by biologic evolution or learned have the capacity to produce certain patterns of homeostasis. The state of sadness is accompanied by a reduced number of positive mental images and by more excessive attention to those images. When persons have the experience of positive thoughts, their mind represents more than well-being; it also represents well-thinking. On the contrary, feeling sadness is associated not only with sickliness but also with an inefficient way of thinking, concentrated around a limited number of ideas of loss (Damásio, 2004).

"In GI, positive mental images and positive affective experiences can counteract the depression rumination spiral (Folkman & Moskowitz, 2000). This process works as an adaptive alternative to decompensation, raising the mood, and relieving depressive symptoms. Therefore, GI contributes to antirumination strategies that, as Nolen-Hoeksema (1991, 2000) states, are debilitating. Positive mental images have a relaxing effect and, consequently, a psychophysiologic and cognitive effect (Singer, 2006). When depressed individuals have access to positive mental images and to a state of body relaxation, they are able to reorient their thoughts away from unpleasant stimuli. Thus, positive thoughts contribute to an improvement in feelings about oneself and the world.

"Results from the empirical literature indicated that GI was effective in improving mood states in individuals with a variety of illnesses. Sloman (2002) conducted a community-based nursing study in 56 people with advanced cancer. Progressive muscle relaxation and GI training revealed significant decreases in depression. Campbell-Gillies (2004) used a program including positive mental images and music with 45 women with breast cancer. Her findings revealed that GI decreased depression and anxiety over a six-cycle period of chemotherapy. McKinney, Antoni, Kumar, Times, and McCabe (1997) used GI combined with music with 28 healthy adults and reported significant decreases in depression, fatigue, and total mood disorders between pretest and posttest sessions. Identical outcomes were revealed in the study of Watanabe et al. (2006), with a sample of 148 healthy adults, using relaxation and positive mental images. After two sessions, positive mood increased, and negative mood decreased. Finally, in an experimental design, Kolcaba and Fox (1999) assessed the effects of GI for increasing comfort over time in patients with breast cancer going through radiation therapy. However, no experimental studies have been conducted for patients in a psychiatric context to increase their comfort." (Apostolo & Kolcaba, 2009, pp. 404-405) as an example of a review of the literature. Apóstolo and Kolcaba (2009) conducted a study to determine the effect of guided imagery on comfort, depression, anxiety, and stress among 60 hospitalized mental health patients. The researchers began the review with a presentation of Kolcaba's comfort theory, and then linked that theory to guided imagery and depression.

The guided imagery treatment group showed statistically significant improvement in their depression, anxiety, stress, and sense of comfort. Their results were compared with those in a matched control group. Apóstolo and Kolcaba (2009) indicated that GI was an effective intervention, supporting their findings with links back to their review of the literature. The strengths of the study were the use of matched controls that supported internal validity and the implementation of the study in three clinical facilities that supported the external validity of the study.

KEY POINTS

- Reviewing the existing literature related to your study is a critical step in the research process.
- A literature review is a written logical presentation of knowledge gained from reading and analyzing selected articles, books, conference proceedings, and other sources.
- Information from the literature guides the development and implementation of quantitative studies and is incorporated throughout the research proposal.
- With use of a systems approach, the three major stages of a literature review are searching the literature (input), processing the literature (throughput), and writing the literature review (output).
- The literature consists of all written sources relevant to the topic you have selected.
- Two types of literature are predominantly used in the review of literature for research: theoretical and empirical.
- Theoretical literature consists of concept analyses, models, theories, and conceptual frameworks that support a selected research problem and purpose.
- Empirical literature comprises relevant studies in journals and books as well as unpublished studies, such as master's theses and doctoral dissertations.
- Searching the literature begins with a written plan for the review that is maintained as a search history during the first stage of the literature review.
- Searching the literature requires use of bibliographical databases and reference management systems.

- Processing the literature requires the researcher to read the sources to be able to critically appraise, analyze, and synthesize the information that has been retrieved.
- A thorough, organized literature review facilitates the development of a research proposal.
- The well-written literature review presents a logical argument for why the research question should be studied and in the specific way that is being proposed.

REFERENCES

Achterberg, J. (1985). *Imagery in healing: Shamanism and modern medicine*. Boston: Shambhala.

American Psychological Association (2010). *Publication manual of the American Psychological Association* (6th ed.). Washington, DC: Author.

Apóstolo, J. L. A. (2007). *O imaginário conduzido no conforto de doentes em contexto psiquiátrico. Doctoral Dissertation*. Porto, PT: Porto University.

Apóstolo, J. L. A., & Kolcaba, K. (2009). The effects of guided imagery on comfort, depression, anxiety, and stress of psychiatric inpatients with depressive disorders. *Archives of Psychiatric Nursing*, 23(6), 403–411.

Association of Nurses in AIDS Care (2009). Position statement: Health disparities. Retrieved from http://www.proquest.com/en-US/default.shtml/.

Bachrach, S. (2001). Scientific journals of the future. In R. S. Berry & A. S. Moffat (Eds.), *The transition from paper: Where are we going and how will we get there?* Cambridge, MA: American Academy of Arts & Sciences. Online report. Retrieved from http://www.amacad.org/publications/trans.aspx/.

Booth, W. C., Colomb, G. G., & Williams, J. M. (2008). *The craft of research* (3rd ed.). Chicago, IL: University of Chicago Press.

Campbell-Gillies, L. (2004). Guided imagery as treatment for anxiety and depression in breast cancer patients: A pilot study [Online]. A dissertation submitted in partial fulfillment of the requirements for the degree of M.A. Psychology. Rand Afrikaans University. Retrieved from http://etd.rau.ac.za/theses/available/etd-10062004-095533/restricted/GIreviseddissert2003130304.pdf/.

Cronin, P., Ryan, F., & Coughlan, M. (2008). Undertaking a literature review: A step-by-step approach. *British Journal of Nursing*, 17(1), 38–43.

Damásio, A. R. (2004). *Ao encontro de Espinosa. As Emoções e a neurologia do sentir* (6th ed.). Mem Martins: Publicações Europa-América.

Everett, J., Bowes, A., & Kerr, D. (2010). Barriers to achieving glycaemic control in CSII. *Journal of Diabetes Nursing*, 14(5), 176–181.

Folkman, S., & Moskowitz, J. T. (2000). Positive affect and the other side of coping. *American Psychologist*, 55(6), 647–654.

Garrard, J. (2011). *Health sciences literature review made easy: The matrix method* (3rd ed.). Sudbury, MA: Jones & Bartlett.

Gravel, J. (2009). Bess and hearing screening: Portending the challenges in children. *Seminars in Hearing*, 30(2), 71–79.

Hart, C. (2009). *Doing a literature review: Releasing the social science imagination.* Los Angeles, CA: Sage.

Holbrook, A., Bourke, S., Fairbairn, H., & Lovat, T. (2007). Examiner comment on the literature review in Ph.D. theses. *Studies in Higher Education, 32*(3), 337–356.

Kolcaba, K. Y., & Fox, C. (1999). The effects of guided imagery on comfort of women with early stage breast cancer undergoing radiation therapy. *Oncology Nursing Forum, 26*(1), 67–72.

Larsen, P. O., & von Ins, M. (2010). The rate of growth in scientific publication and the decline in coverage provided by Scientific Citation Index. *Scientometrics, 84*(3), 575–603.

McKinney, C. H., Antoni, M. H., Kumar, M., Times, F. C., & McCabe, P. M. (1997). Effects of guided imagery and music (GIM) therapy on mood and cortisol in healthy adults. *Health Psychology, 16*(4), 390–400.

Munhall, P. L. (2012). *Nursing research: A qualitative perspective* (5th ed.). Sudbury, MA: Jones & Bartlett.

Nolen-Hoeksema, S. (1991). Responses to depression and their effects on the duration of depressive episodes. *Journal of Abnormal Psychology, 100*(4), 569–582.

Nolen-Hoeksema, S. (2000). The role of rumination in depressive disorders and mixed anxiety/depressive symptoms. *Journal of Abnormal Psychology, 109*(3), 504–511.

Pinch, W. J. (1995). Synthesis: Implementing a complex process. *Nurse Educator, 20*(1), 34–40.

Pinch, W. J. (2001). Improving patient care through use of research. *Orthopaedic Nursing, 20*(4), 75–81.

Roguin, A. (2011). Henry Cuthbert Bazett (1885-1950)—The man behind the QT interval correction formula. *Pace, 34*(3), 384–388.

Rossman, M. (2000). *Guided imagery for self-healing. An essential resource for anyone seeking wellness* (2nd ed.). Tiburon, CA: H.J. Kramer.

Scholtfeldt, R. (1975). The need for a conceptual framework. In P. Verhonic (Ed.), *Nursing research* (pp. 3–25). Boston: Little & Brown.

Scott, A. J., & Wilson, R. F. (2011). Social determinants of health among African Americans in a rural community in the Deep South: An ecological study. *Rural and Remote Health, 11*, 1634 (Online). Retrieved from http://www.rrh.org.au/.

Singer, J. L. (2006). *Imagery in psychotherapy.* Washington: American Psychological Association.

Sloman, R. (2002). Relaxation and imagery for anxiety and depression control in community patients with advanced cancer. *Cancer Nursing, 25*(6), 432–435.

Tensen, B. L. (2010). *Research strategies for the digital age* (3rd ed.). Boston, MA: Wadsworth.

Vacek, J. E. (2009) Using a conceptual approach with a concept map of psychosis as an exemplar of promote critical thinking. *Journal of Nursing Education, 48*(1), 49–53.

Watanabe, E., Fukuda, S., Hara, H., Maeda, Y., Ohira, H., & Shirakawa, T. (2006). Differences in relaxation by means of guided imagery in a healthy community sample. *Alternative Therapies in Health and Medicine, 13*(2), 60–66.

7

CHAPTER

Frameworks

A framework is an abstract, logical structure of meaning that guides the development of the study and enables you to link the findings to the body of knowledge in nursing. Frameworks are used in quantitative research and sometimes in qualitative research. In quantitative studies, the framework may be a testable theoretical structure or may be developed inductively from published research or clinical observations. In most qualitative studies, the researcher will not identify a theoretical framework. With a grounded theory study, the researcher is attempting to develop a theory as an outcome of the study.

Every quantitative study has a theoretical framework, although some researchers do not identify or describe the theoretical framework in the report of the study. For example, researchers may use anatomy and physiology knowledge to guide a study without identifying a framework. Ideally, the framework of a quantitative study is carefully structured, clearly presented, and well integrated with the methodology. When you critically appraise studies, you need to identify and evaluate the extent to which the framework guided the study methodology. Your ability to understand the study findings will depend on your ability to understand the logic within the framework and will determine how you will use the findings. In addition, when you develop a quantitative study, you will need to describe the study's theoretical framework. To help you build the knowledge and skills needed to critically appraise studies and describe or develop a framework for your own studies, this chapter begins by defining relevant terms. The chapter also describes processes used to examine and appraise the components of theories and presents approaches to identifying or developing a framework to guide a study.

Definition of Terms

The first step in understanding theories and frameworks is to become familiar with the terms related to

theoretical ideas and their application. This section is an introduction to key theoretical terms: concept, relational statement, conceptual model, theory, middle-range theory, and study framework. In response to the ongoing debate and varying opinions about the differences between a conceptual model and a theory or a conceptual model and a philosophy (Meleis, 2012), working definitions of these concepts are presented to facilitate the application of theoretical principles to research.

Concept

A concept is a term that abstractly describes and names an object, a phenomenon, or an idea, thus providing it with a separate identity or meaning. As a label for a phenomenon or composite of behavior and thoughts, a concept is a concise way to represent the experience or state (Meleis, 2012). An example of a concept is the term anxiety. The concept brings to mind a feeling of uneasiness in the stomach, a rapid pulse rate, and troubling thoughts about future negative outcomes. Consider the concept of hope. What feelings, expectations, and actions are expressed by this label?

Concepts can vary in their level of abstraction. At high levels of abstraction, concepts may have general meanings and are sometimes referred to as constructs. For example, a construct associated with the concept of anxiety might be "emotional responses." Constructs, because they are abstract, can subsume multiple concepts. For example, in addition to anxiety, emotional responses could include, grief, frustration, peace, hope, and confidence.

Relational Statements

A relational statement declares that a relationship of some kind exists between or among two or more concepts (Walker & Avant, 2011). Relational statements provide the skeleton of a framework. Clear relational statements are essential for constructing an integrated framework for guiding study design. The relationships expressed in your framework will direct the development of your study's objectives, questions, or hypotheses. The types of relationships described by the statements will determine the study design and the statistical analyses needed to address the study objectives, questions, or hypotheses. Mature theories, such as physiological theories, have measurable concepts and clear relational statements that can be tested through research.

Conceptual Models

A conceptual model, also known as a grand theory, is a set of highly abstract, related constructs. A conceptual model broadly explains phenomena of interest, expresses assumptions, and reflects a philosophical stance. Nurse scholars have expended time and effort to debate the distinctions between the definitions of theory, conceptual model, conceptual framework, and theoretical framework (Chinn & Kramer, 2011; Meleis, 2012). For example, Watson's theory of caring has been identified as a theory (Meleis, 2012), a philosophy (Alligood, 2010), and a conceptual model (Fitzpatrick & Whall, 2005). In this textbook, we are using the terms conceptual model, conceptual framework and grand nursing theory interchangeably because our purpose is not to classify theoretical thinking. The purpose of this chapter is to provide the information needed to use concepts, relational statements, and theories or theoretical structures to develop studies and interpret their findings.

Theory

A theory consists of an integrated set of defined concepts, existence statements, and relational statements that can be used to describe, explain, predict, or control the phenomenon being discussed. Existence statements within a theory declare that a given concept exists or that a given relationship occurs. For example, an existence statement might claim that a condition referred to as stress exists and that there is a relationship between stress and health. As discussed earlier, relational statements clarify the relationship that exists between or among concepts. It is the statements of a theory that are tested through research, not the theory itself. Thus, identifying statements within the theory is critical to the research endeavor and forms the basis of the study's framework.

Scientific theories are those for which repeated studies have validated the relationships among the concepts. These theories are sometimes called laws for this reason. Although few nursing and psychosocial theories have been validated to this extent, physiological theories have this level of evidence and can provide a strong basis for nursing studies.

Middle-Range Theories

Middle-range theories present a partial view of nursing reality. Proposed by Merton (1968), a sociologist, middle-range theories are less abstract and address more specific phenomena than grand theories do (Peterson, 2009). They directly apply to practice and focus on explanation and implementation. Middle-range theories may emerge from grand theories or may be developed inductively from research findings. Grounded theory studies are a scientific source of middle-range theory. Some middle-range theories have been developed by combining nursing theories with theories from other disciplines. Some middle-range theories have been developed from clinical practice guidelines. Whatever their source, middle-range theories are sometimes called substantive theories, because they are more concrete than grand theories.

Research Frameworks

One strategy for expressing the theoretical structure guiding a study is to present a map or diagram of the concepts and relational statements. Although some writers call these diagrams conceptual maps (Artinian, 1982; Fawcett, 1999; Newman, 1979, 1986), we are calling them research frameworks to indicate the purpose for which they were developed. A research framework summarizes and integrates what we know about a phenomenon more succinctly and clearly than a literary explanation and allows us to grasp the bigger picture of a phenomenon. A research framework should be supported by references from the literature. These frameworks vary in complexity and accuracy, depending on the available body of knowledge related to the phenomena they are describing. Mapping can also identify gaps in the logic of the theory being used as a framework and reveals inconsistencies, incompleteness, and errors. Now that this basic knowledge of the roles of concepts, relationships, and theories in research has been supplied, the next sections provide a discussion of the analysis and application of each of these components.

Understanding Concepts

Concepts are often described as the building blocks of theory. Abstract concepts are descriptive but may not be as applicable to clinical practice or research because of their abstractness. To make a concept more concrete, you can identify how the concept can be measured or observed. These measurable terms are referred to as **variables**. A variable is more specific than a concept and implies that the term is clearly defined and measurable. The word "variable" implies that the numerical values associated with the term **vary** from one instance to another. A variable related to anxiety might be "palmar sweating," which the researcher can measure by assigning a numerical value to the amount of sweat on the subject's palm. The links among constructs, concepts, and variables are displayed in Figure 7-1. On the left of the figure is the construct-to-variable continuum. The other two sets of shapes are examples of a construct, concept, and variable. Notice that a concept may have multiple ways of being measured. For example, anxiety could be measured by palmar sweating, the State-Trait Anxiety Scale, or a checklist of behaviors such as pacing, wringing one's hands, and expressing worries.

Defining concepts allows us to be consistent in the way we use a term in practice, apply it to a theory, and measure it in a study. A conceptual definition differs from the **denotative** (or dictionary) **definition** of a word. A **conceptual definition** (connotative meaning) is more comprehensive than a denotative definition because it includes associated meanings the word may have. For example, a connotative definition may associate the term "fireplace" with images of hospitality and warm comfort, whereas the dictionary definition would be a rock or brick structure in a house designed for burning wood. A conceptual definition can be established through concept synthesis, concept derivation, or concept analysis (Walker & Avant, 2011).

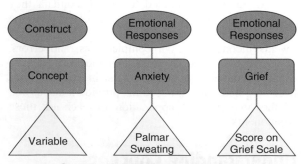

Construct-Concept-Variable Continuum

Figure 7-1 Links among constructs, concepts, and variables.

Concept Synthesis

In nursing, many phenomena have not yet been identified as discrete entities. Recognizing, naming, and describing these phenomena are often critical steps to understanding the process and outcomes of nursing practice. In your clinical practice, you may notice patterns of behavior or find patterns in empirical data. You may name a concept that emerges during data analysis in a qualitative study. The process of describing and naming a previously unrecognized concept is **concept synthesis**. Nursing studies often involve previously unrecognized and unnamed phenomena that must be named and carefully defined. Lee and Coakley (2011) conducted a concept synthesis of geropalliative care. Conceptual and philosophical works had examined gerontology and palliative care separately but the combined term lacked conceptual clarity. This lack of clarity was viewed as hindering progress in this interdisciplinary area of study. Lee and Coakley (2011) concluded that geropalliative care is "both a philosophical stance and structured interdisciplinary model of care delivery that guides care to patients and families during the last 5 years of life, irrespective of disease" (p. 247). They describe the critical attributes of geropalliative care as "high risk for ineffective pain management," "geriatric syndromes," "chronic, comorbid conditions," "risk for ineffective communication," and "beneficial in the absence of disease" (p. 247). The context of the concept includes end-of-life trajectories that are unpredictable, "shrinking social networks, insurance limitations," and "multiple settings" (p. 247). Concept synthesis can be an important element in the development of nursing theory (Walker & Avant, 2011).

Concept Derivation

Concept derivation may occur when the researcher or theorist finds no concept in nursing to explain a phenomenon (Walker & Avant, 2011). Concepts identified or defined in theories of other disciplines may provide insight. In **concept derivation**, one concept is transposed from one of field of knowledge to another. If a conceptual definition is found in another discipline, it must be examined to evaluate its fit with the new field in which it will be used. The conceptual definition may need to be modified so that it is meaningful within nursing and consistent with nursing thought (Walker & Avant, 2011). For example, the concept of weathering, from physical material science, means the alteration of a material exposed over time to sun, wind, and precipitation. Health researchers, including nurses, define *weathering* as the alteration of fundamental components of the human organism when exposed over time to stress, unsupportive environments, and limited resources (Holzman et al., 2009). Concept derivation is a creative process that can be fostered by thinking deeply and having a willingness to learn about processes and theories in other disciplines.

Concept Analysis

Concept analysis is a strategy that identifies a set of characteristics essential to the connotative meaning of a concept. The procedure will require you to explore the various ways the term is used and to identify a set of characteristics that clarify the range of objects or ideas to which that concept may be applied (Walker & Avant, 2011). These essential characteristics, called defining attributes or criteria, provide a means to distinguish the concept from similar concepts. Several approaches to concept analysis have been described in the nursing and healthcare literature. Because the approaches have varying philosophical foundations and products, nurse theorists and researchers must select the concept analysis approach that best suits their purposes in a specific situation. For example, a researcher attempting to measure the phenomenon of barriers may choose Walker and Avant's (2011) approach because of its product of a theoretical definition. Deepened understanding of the theoretical definitions allows the researcher to critically appraise the construct validity of instruments or methods being considered to measure the concept in a study. An emerging nurse theorist may choose Rodger's evolutionary approach to understand the contextual influences on and changes in the meaning of the concept over time. Several writers have compared the different types of concept analysis (Cronin, Ryan, & Coughlan, 2010; Duncan, Cloutier, & Bailey, 2007; Hupcey & Penrod, 2005; Risjord, 2009; Weaver & Mitcham, 2008). Several concept analysis strategies used in nursing and health care are listed in Table 7-1. In addition, a number of concept analyses have been published in the nursing literature, such as those listed in Table 7-2. The following section provides an example of how one group of researchers developed a conceptual definition for the concept frailty through an analysis of published definitions.

Importance of a Conceptual Definition: An Example

With the growth in the proportion of the population that are over age 65 years, there is increased urgency in preventing frailty among older people who live in the community (Gobbens, Luijkx, Wijnen-Sponselee,

TABLE 7-1 Methods of Concept Analysis

Type of Concept Analysis (Author[s], Date)	Unique Characteristics
Principle-based (Hupcey & Penrod, 2005)	Analysis guided by linguistic, epistemological, pragmatic, and logical principles
Ordinary use (Wilson, 1963)	Foci of analysis are exemplars (cases) that are used to identify criteria, antecedents, and consequences
Evolutionary method (Rodgers, 2000)	Contextual analysis of how the concept has developed over time in different settings
Hybrid (Schwartz-Barcott & Kim, 2000)	Contextual analysis and data collection in the field leading to conclusions about how concept has developed over time in different settings
Linguistic, pragmatic approach (Walker & Avant, 2011)	Analysis of explicit and implicit concept definitions in the literature to identify criteria, antecedents, and consequences for pragmatic purposes in practice and research
Simultaneous (Haase, Britt, Coward, Leidy, & Penn, 1992)	Examines closely related concepts to distinguish their unique meanings as well as areas of overlap

TABLE 7-2 Concept Analyses Using Different Methods

Concept Analyzed	Method of Concept Analysis
Advanced nursing practice (Ruel & Motyka, 2009)	Principle-Based (Hupcey & Penrod, 2005)
Dance in mental health nursing (Ravelin, Kylma, & Korhonen, 2006)	Hybrid (Schwartz-Barcott & Kim, 2000)
Clinical reasoning (Simmons, 2010)	Evolutionary method (Rodgers, 2000)
Acculturation in Filipino immigrants (Serafica, 2011)	Linguistic, Pragmatic (Walker & Avant, 2011)
Ethical demand in nursing (Mårtenson, Fägerskiöld, Runeson, & Berterö, 2009)	Simultaneous (Haase, Britt, Coward, Leidy, & Penn, 1992)

& Schols, 2010). An extensive literature review was done to identify conceptual and operational definitions of frailty. From their review of 18 conceptual definitions, Gobbens et al. concluded that "frailty is a dynamic state affecting an individual who experiences losses in one or more domains of human functioning (physical, psychological, social) that are caused by the influence of a range of variables and which increases the risk of adverse outcomes" (p. 85).

The definition allows researchers to distinguish frailty from disability and comorbidity. The refinement of the conceptual definition has limited value without a practical way to measure it (Gobbens et al., 2010). Having found no operational definition that was a logical fit with the conceptual definition proposed, the researchers identified their next step to be developing an operational definition of frailty consistent with the conceptual definition.

Examining Relational Statements

Understanding relational statements is essential for ensuring consistency between the research framework, study design, and statistical analyses. Relational statements in a research framework can be described by their characteristics.

Characteristics of Relational Statements

Relational statements describe the direction, shape, strength, symmetry, sequencing, probability of occurrence, necessity, and sufficiency of a relationship (Walker & Avant, 2011). One statement may have several of these characteristics; each characteristic is not exclusive of the others. Statements may be expressed as words in a sentence (literary form), as shapes and arrows (diagram form), or as equations (mathematical form). In nursing, the literary and diagrammatic forms of statements are used most frequently. Figure 7-2 displays the three forms of simple statements of relationships among spiritual perspective, social support, and coping. Notice in the diagram in Figure 7-2 that dotted arrows are used to indicate a relationship about which little is known. The mathematical form indicates the same relationships. Figure 7-3 provides literary, diagrammatic, and mathematical forms of a more complex statement among the previous concepts with the addition of perceived stress. Notice the change in the arrow between perceived stress and coping. The arrow is darker and heavier until spiritual perspective and social support modify the relationship. The mathematical form proposes that

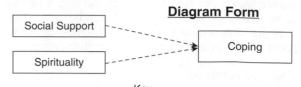

Literary Form

Social support and spirituality influence coping.

Diagram Form

Mathematical Form

$$SS(x) + SP(y) + K = C$$

Key
SS–Measurement of Social Support
SP–Measurement of Spirituality
C–Measurement of Coping
x–Strength of relationship between social support and coping
y–Strength of relationship between spirituality and coping

Figure 7-2 Literary, diagrammatic, and mathematical forms of a simple statement.

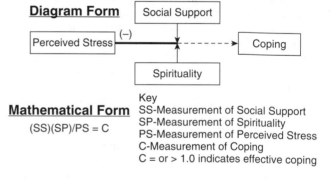

Literary Form

When social support and spirituality exceed perceived stress, effective coping occurs.

Diagram Form

Mathematical Form

$$(SS)(SP)/PS = C$$

Key
SS–Measurement of Social Support
SP–Measurement of Spirituality
PS–Measurement of Perceived Stress
C–Measurement of Coping
$C = $ or > 1.0 indicates effective coping

Figure 7-3 Literary, diagrammatic, and mathematical forms of a complex statement.

when the product of spiritual perspective and social support is greater than perceived stress, coping will be greater. When the product is less than perceived stress, coping is diminished.

Direction

The direction of a relationship may be positive, negative, or unknown (Fawcett, 1999). A positive linear relationship implies that as one concept changes (the value or amount of the concept increases or decreases), the second concept will also change in the same direction. For example, the literary statement, "As stress increases (A), the risk of illness (B) increases," expresses a positive relationship. This positive relational statement could also be expressed as "As stress decreases (A), the risk of illness (B) decreases."

A **negative linear relationship** implies that as one concept changes, the other concept changes in the opposite direction. For example, the statement "As relaxation (A) increases, blood pressure (B) decreases" expresses a negative linear relationship. The negative relationship could also be expressed as "As relaxation decreases (A), blood pressure (B) increases."

The nature of the relationship between two concepts may be unknown because it has not been studied or because study findings have been conflicting. For example, consider two studies that included the concepts of coping and social support. Tkatch et al. (2011) found that the number of people in the social networks of African American patients in cardiac rehabilitation (N = 115) and their health-related social support had weak, but statistically significant relationships with their coping efficacy. In contrast, Jackson et al. (2009) found nonsignificant relationships among social support and coping in a longitudinal study of 88 parents who had a child with a brain tumor. From the findings, we can conclude that although there is evidence that a relationship exists between these two concepts, the studies examining that relationship have conflicting findings. Conflicting findings may result from differences in the researchers' definitions and measurements of the two concepts in various studies. Another reason for conflicting findings may be that an unidentified confounding variable exists that changes the relationship between coping and social support. Whatever the reason, conflicting findings about a relationship between concepts could be indicated by a question mark. Figure 7-4 has diagrams representing the directional characteristics of relationships. More

details on diagramming relational statements are presented in Chapter 8.

Shape

Most relationships are assumed to be linear, and statistical tests are conducted to identify linear relationships. In a **linear relationship**, the relationship between the two concepts remains consistent regardless of the values of each of the concepts. For example, if the value of A increases by 1 point each time the value of B increases by 1 point, then the values continue to increase at the same rate whether the value is 2 or 200. The relationship can be illustrated by a straight line, as shown in Figure 7-5.

Relationships can also be curvilinear or form some other shape. In a **curvilinear relationship**, the relationship between two concepts varies according to the relative values of the concepts. The relationship between anxiety and learning is a good example of a curvilinear relationship. Very high or very low levels of anxiety are associated with low levels of learning, whereas moderate levels of anxiety are associated with high levels of learning (Bierman, Comijs, Rijmen, Jonker, & Beekman, 2008). This type of relationship is illustrated by a curved line, as shown in Figure 7-6.

Strength

The **strength of a relationship** is the amount of variation explained by the relationship. Some of the variation in a concept, but not all, is associated with variation in another concept (Fawcett, 1999). In discussing the strength of a relationship, researchers sometimes use the term **effect size**. The effect size explains how much "effect" variation in one concept has on variation in a second concept.

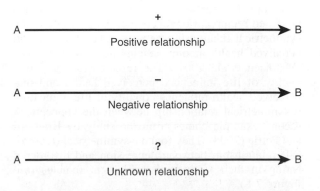

Figure 7-4 Directions of relational statements.

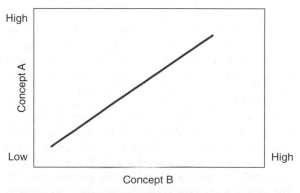

Figure 7-5 Linear relationship.

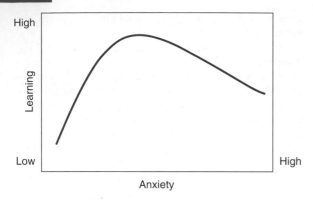

Figure 7-6 Curvilinear relationship.

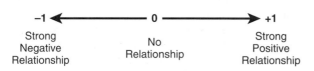

Figure 7-7 Relational statement strength.

Researchers usually determine the strength of the relationship between concepts by correlational analysis. The mathematical result of the analysis is a correlation coefficient such as the following:

$$r = 0.35$$

The statistic r is the coefficient obtained by performing the statistical procedure known as Pearson's product-moment correlation (see Chapter 23). A value of 0 indicates no strength, whereas a value of +1 or −1 indicates the greatest strength (see Figure 7-7).

When the correlation is large, a greater portion of the variation can be explained by the relationship; in others, only a moderate or a small portion of the variation can be explained by the relationship. For example, Tkatch et al. (2011) found a relationship of $r = 0.22$ ($p < 0.05$) between health-related social support and coping efficacy. The strength of the relationship meant that a small portion of the variance in coping was explained by variations in health-related social support (see Chapter 23 for additional information).

The + or − does not have an impact on the strength of the relationship. For example, $r = -0.35$ is as strong as $r = +0.35$. A weak relationship is usually considered one with an r value of 0.1 to 0.3; a moderate relationship is one with an r value of 0.31 to 0.5; and a strong relationship is one with an r value greater than 0.5. The greater the strength of a relationship, the easier it

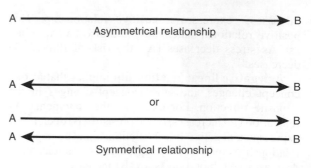

Figure 7-8 Relational statement symmetry.

is to detect relationships between the variables being studied. This idea will be explored further in the chapters on sampling, measurement, and data analysis (Chapters 15, 16, and 23, respectively).

Symmetry

Relationships may be symmetrical or asymmetrical. In an **asymmetrical relationship**, if A occurs (or changes), then B will occur (or change); but there may be no indication that if B occurs (or changes), A will occur (or change). An asymmetrical relationship is not reversible (Fawcett, 1999). You can think of this relationship as a one-way street, with influence going only in one direction. Bradford and Petrie (2008) found an asymmetrical relationship between internalized ideal of a thin body and body dissatisfaction in their study of disordered eating among 236 first-year, female college students. The internalized thin body ideal affected body dissatisfaction, but the reverse was not true (see Figure 7-8).

A **symmetrical relationship** is complex and contains two statements, such as if A changes, B will change and if B changes, A will change (Fawcett, 1999). You may think of the relationship between these concepts as a two-way street with influence going in both directions. These relationships may also be called reciprocal or reversible. An example is the symmetrical relationship between quality of life and perceived health among patients after heart surgery (Mathisen et al., 2007). The researchers found that quality of life influenced perceived health and that perceived health influenced quality of life, indicating a symmetrical relationship between the concepts. A second example comes from the study by Bradford and Petrie (2008). They found a symmetrical (reciprocal) relationship between depression and disordered eating in their study with adolescent females (see Figure 7-8).

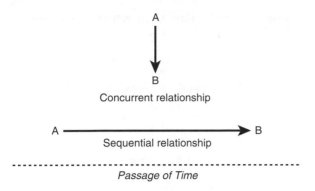

Figure 7-9 Relational statement sequencing.

Sequencing

The amount of time that elapses between one concept and another is stated as the sequential nature of a relationship. If the two concepts occur simultaneously, the relationship is **concurrent** (Fawcett, 1999). When there is a change in one concept, there is change in the other at the same time. If one concept changes and the second concept changes later, the relationship is **sequential**. Another example from Bradford and Petrie's study (2008) was a hypothesized concurrent relationship between internalizing the thin body ideal and dissatisfaction with one's body. Their findings provided mixed support for the relationship. They also hypothesized that depression would predict later pathological eating. This sequential relationship was supported by their findings. These relationships are diagrammed in Figure 7-9.

Probability of Occurrence

A relationship can be deterministic or probabilistic depending on the degree of certainty that it will occur. **Deterministic** (or **causal**) **relationships** are statements of what always occurs in a particular situation. For example, among Thai patients with heart failure, nurse researchers found that symptom status, social support, general health perception, and functional status had causal relationships with health-related quality of life (Phuangphaka, Veena, Chanokporn, & Sloan, 2008). Scientific laws are another example of deterministic relationships (Fawcett, 1999). A causal relationship is expressed as follows:

If A, then always B

A **probability statement** expresses the probability that something will happen in a given situation (Fawcett, 1999). This relationship is expressed as follows:

If A, then probably B

Probability statements are tested statistically to determine the extent of probability that B will occur in the event of A. For example, one could state that there is greater than a 50% probability that a patient who has an indwelling catheter for 1 week will experience a urinary bladder infection. This probability could be expressed mathematically as follows:

$$p > 0.50$$

The p is a symbol for probability. The $>$ is a symbol for "greater than." This mathematical statement asserts that there is more than a 50% probability that the relationship will occur.

Necessity

In a **necessary relationship**, one concept must occur for the second concept to occur (Fawcett, 1999). For example, one could propose that if sufficient fluids are administered (A), and only if sufficient fluids are administered, the unconscious patient will remain hydrated (B). This relationship is expressed as follows:

If A, and only if A, then B

In a **substitutable relationship**, a similar concept can be substituted for the first concept and the second concept will still occur. For example, a substitutable relationship might propose that if tube feedings are administered (A1), or if hyperalimentation is administered (A2), the unconscious patient can remain hydrated (B). This relationship is expressed as follows:

If A1, or if A2, then B

Sufficiency

A **sufficient relationship** states that when the first concept occurs, the second concept will occur, regardless of the presence or absence of other factors (Fawcett, 1999). A statement could propose that if a patient is immobilized in bed longer than a week, he or she will lose bone calcium, regardless of anything else. This relationship is expressed as follows:

If A, then B, regardless of anything else

A **contingent relationship** will occur only if a third concept is present. For example, a statement might claim that if a person experiences a stressor (A), the person will manage the stress (B), but only if she or he uses effective coping strategies (C). The third concept, in this case effective coping strategies, is referred to as an **intervening** (or **mediating**) **variable**.

TABLE 7-3 Characteristics of Relationships

Type of Relationship	Descriptive Statement
Positive linear	As A increases, B increases.
	As A decreases, B decreases.
Negative linear	As A increases, B decreases.
	As A decreases, B increases.
Unknown linear	As A changes, B may change.
Curvilinear	At a specific level, as A changes, B changes to a similar degree.
	At another specific level, as A changes, B changes to a greater or lesser extent.
Asymmetrical	As A changes, B changes.
	As B changes, A does not change.
Symmetrical	As A changes, B changes.
	As B changes, A changes.
Concurrent	When A changes, B changes at the same time.
Sequential	After A changes, B changes.
Causal	If A occurs, B always occurs.
Probabilistic	If A occurs, then probably B.
Necessary	If A occurs, and only if A occurs, B occurs.
Sufficient	If A occurs, and only if A, B occurs.
Substitutable	If A_1 or A_2 occurs, B occurs.
Contingent	If A occurs, then B occurs, but only if C occurs.

Intervening variables can affect the occurrence, strength, or direction of a relationship. A contingent relationship can be expressed as follows:

If A, then B, but only if C

Being able to describe relationships among the concepts is an important first step in identifying, evaluating, and developing research frameworks. Table 7-3 provides a summary of the characteristics of relational statements. Remember that a single statement may have multiple descriptive characteristics.

Statement Hierarchy

Statements about the same two conceptual ideas can be made at various levels of abstractness. The statements found in conceptual models and grand theories (**general propositions**) are at a high level of abstraction. Statements found in middle-range theories (**specific propositions**) are at a moderate level of abstraction. **Hypotheses**, which are a form of statement, are at a low level of abstraction and are specific. As statements become less abstract, they become narrower in scope (Fawcett, 1999), as shown in Figure 7-10.

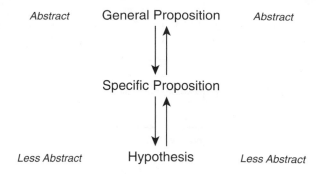

Figure 7-10 Abstract to concrete–general proposition to hypothesis.

Statements at varying levels of abstraction that express relationships between or among the same conceptual ideas can be arranged in hierarchical form, from general to specific. This arrangement allows you to see (or evaluate) the logical links among the various levels of abstraction. Statement sets link the relationships expressed in the framework with the hypotheses, research questions, or objectives that guide the methodology of the study. The following excerpts provide an example of the more abstract theoretical proposition that provided the basis for the hypothesis that was tested in a study by Xu, Floyd, Westmaas, and Aron (2010). These researchers asked 66 former and 74 current smokers to select self-expanding activities, such as a new romantic relationship or a new job, that occurred in the time immediately preceding attempts to stop smoking.

Proposition

"Because both self-expansion and nicotine appear to trigger feelings of reward that originate from the same parts of the brain, it is conceivable that the reward from self-expanding experiences could (at least partly) supplant or act as a substitute for the reward elicited by nicotine or other addictive drugs." (Xu et al., 2010, p. 296)

Hypothesis

"We hypothesized that smokers would report greater success abstaining from smoking if they had engaged in self-expanding activities prior to their quit attempt." (Xu et al., 2010, p. 296)

Xu and colleagues reported that, "former smokers reported a mean of 4.60 self-expanding events (*SD* = 4.1) in the 2-month period prior to their successful quit attempt" (p. 298).

Grand Theories

Most disciplines have several conceptual models, each with a distinctive vocabulary. Table 7-4 lists some of the conceptual models or grand theories in nursing. These philosophical theories of nursing vary in their level of abstraction and the breadth of phenomena they explain. Each provides an overall picture, or gestalt, of the phenomena they explain. It is not their purpose to provide detail or to be specific.

Nurses have developed a number of conceptual models or grand nursing theories. For example, Roy's (1988) model describes adaptation as the primary phenomenon of interest to nursing. This model identifies the constructs she considers essential to adaptation and how these constructs interact to produce adaptation (Roy & Andrews, 2008). Orem (2001) considered self-care to be the phenomenon central to nursing. Her model explains how nurses facilitate the self-care of clients. Rogers (1970, 1990) regarded human beings as the central phenomenon of interest to nursing. In her model, human beings are viewed as

energy fields interacting with the environmental energy fields.

In addition to concepts specific to the theory, nurse theorists include the metaparadigm or domain concepts of nursing: person, health, environment, and nursing (Chinn & Kramer, 2011). For example, Roy, Orem, and Rogers all include the construct health in their models but define it in different ways (see Table 7-5). The definitions inherent in grand nursing theories guide nursing practice by providing the characteristics of the person and environment that nurses should assess. For example, Orem's theory of self-care describes factors to be assessed as universal self-care requisites, developmental self-care requisites, and health deviation requisites. A nurse whose assessment is guided by Roy's theory would gather assessments related to the adaptive modes of physiological, self-concept, role function, and interdependence. Theories also guide nursing practice by defining the specific goal of practice (characteristics of health) and describing the nursing interventions (descriptions of nursing) to achieve the outcomes. Most are not directly testable through research and thus cannot be used alone as the framework for a study (Fawcett, 1999; Walker & Avant, 2011). Application of grand nursing theories to research is discussed later in this chapter.

Application of Middle-Range Theories

Middle-range theories are useful in both research and practice. Middle-range theories are less abstract than grand theories and closer to the day-to-day substance of clinical practice, a characteristic that explains why they can be called substantive theories. As a result, middle-range theories guide the practitioner to understanding the client's behavior, enabling interventions that are more effective. Because of their usefulness in practice, some writers refer to middle-range theories as **practice theories**. Middle-range theories are used more commonly than grand theories as frameworks for research. Researchers need to carefully consider which middle-range theory to use as a study framework and which aspects of this theory will be tested by their study. Tables 7-6 and 7-7 identify some of the middle-range theories more frequently used as frameworks in the past 10 years of nursing research.

Middle-range theories have been developed from clinical insights, elements of existing theories not previously related, outcomes of qualitative studies, or conceptual models. Kolcaba (2009) noted that, although comfort had been the goal of nursing interventions for

TABLE 7-4	Selected Grand Nursing Theories (in Alphabetical Order by Author Name)
Author (Year)	**Descriptive Label of the Theory**
Henderson, Virginia (1964)	Nursing as Promoting Patient Independence with 14 Activities of Daily Living
Johnson, Dorothy (1974)	Behavioral Systems
King, Imogene (1981)	Interacting Systems Theory of Nursing (includes middle-range theory of Goal Attainment)
Leininger, Madeline (1997)	Transcultural Nursing Care, Sunrise Model of Care
Orem, Dorothea (2001)	Self-Care Deficit Theory of Nursing
Neuman, Betty (Neuman & Fawcett, 2002)	Systems Model of Nursing
Newman, Margaret (1986)	Health as Expanding Consciousness
Nightingale, Florence (1859)	Environmental Health
Parse, Rosemarie (1992)	Human Becoming Theory
Peplau, Hildegard (1988, 1991)	Interpersonal Relations Theory
Rogers, Martha E (1970)	Unitary Human Beings
Roy, Calista (1988)	Adaptation Model
Watson, Jean (1979)	Philosophy and Science of Caring

TABLE 7-5 Comparison of the Domain Concepts—Person, Health, Environment, and Nursing—within Three Grand Theories

Domain Concept	Rogers: Unitary Human Beings	Roy: Adaptation Model	Orem: Self-Care Deficit Theory of Nursing
Person	Irreducible, indivisible energy fields; open systems that are integral with the environment	Biopsychosocial beings who adapt to their environment	Human beings with eight universal needs, two developmental needs, and the potential for six health deviation self-care needs; ability to provide self-care is affected by the conditioning factors of age, gender, health, and the availability of resources
Health	Symphonic interaction of the human and environment	Return to or maintenance of adaptation, through activation of the regulator and cognator systems and of the physiological, self-concept, role function, and interdependence adaptive modes	Extent to which person can meet own universal, development, and health-deviation self-care requisites
Environment	Irreducible, indivisible energy fields; open systems that are integral with the persons	Source of focal and contextual stimuli that may require responses by the person to maintain adaption	Source of resources and other factors that can affect person's ability to meet self-care needs
Nursing	Promote symphonic interaction in the human-environmental energy field	Promote the person's adaptation by modifying focal and contextual stimuli and facilitating use of the adaptive modes (physiological, self-concept, role function, interdependence)	Design and implement systems of care to decrease or remove the gap between self-care capacity and self-care needs; may provide wholly compensatory care, partially compensatory care, or supportive-educative care

Compiled from Banfield (2011); Denyes, Orem, & Bekel SozWiss (2001); and Rogers (1990).

many years, the concept had never been defined precisely. Her theory of comfort began with a concept analysis of comfort during her graduate nursing education (Kolcaba & Kolcaba, 1991). As she continued her doctoral studies, over the space of a year or more, she developed a taxonomy of comfort that provides the basis for describing types of comfort (Kolcaba, 1991) and an operational definition (Kolcaba, 1992). Through continued scholarly inquiry, Kolcaba's middle-range theory of comfort was developed (Kolcaba, 1994), as were several instruments to measure different types of comfort (http://www.thecomfortline.com/).

A more recent middle-range theory, the Synergy Model for Patient Care, was developed by members and leaders of the American Association of Critical Care Nurses to identify the unique contributions of nurses to patient and family outcomes (Hardin, 2009). The basic premise of the model is that "patient characteristics drive nurse competencies" (Curley, 2007, p. 2). The patient characteristics include stability, complexity, vulnerability, predictability, resiliency, resource availability, participation in care, and

participation in decision making. The nurse assesses the extent to which each of the characteristics are present in a specific patient and family. Based on the assessment, the nurse will use specific practice competencies. The practice competencies in the model are clinical judgment, clinical inquiry, caring practices, response to diversity, advocacy/moral agency, facilitation of learning, collaboration, and systems thinking. When synergy exists among the eight patient characteristics and eight nursing practice competencies, optimal patient outcomes are more likely to be found. Extensive work has been done applying the Synergy Model in practice, nursing education, and professional development (Curley, 2007).

A specific type of middle-range theory is intervention theory. Intervention theories seek to explain the dynamics of a patient problem and exactly how a specific nursing intervention is expected to change patient outcomes. Currently, these new theories are tentative, but some will likely become substantive in the future. Intervention theories are discussed in detail in Chapter 14.

TABLE 7-6 Selected Middle-Range Nursing Theories Developed 2001 through 2011	
Name of Theory	**Theorist Source**
Coping of relatives of patients in intensive care units	Johansson, I., Hildingh, C., Fridlund, B., & Ahlstrom, G. (2006). Theoretical model of coping among relatives of patients in intensive care units: A simultaneous concept analysis. *Journal of Advanced Nursing, 56*(5), 463-471.
Flight nursing expertise	Reimer, A. P., & Moore, S. M. (2011). Flight nursing expertise: Toward a theory of flight nursing. *Journal of Advanced Nursing, 66*(5), 1183-1192.
Humor in clinical nurse specialist–patient interactions	McCreaddie, M., & Wiggins, S. (2009). Reconciling the good patient persona with problematic and non-problematic humour: A grounded theory. *International Journal of Nursing Studies, 46*(8), 1079-1091.
Music, mood, and movement to improve health outcomes	Murrock, C. J., & Higgins, P. A. (2009). The theory of music, mood, and movement to improve health outcomes. *Journal of Advanced Nursing, 65*(10), 2249-2257.
Nursing intellectual capital	Covell, C. L. (2008). The middle-range theory of nursing intellectual capital. *Journal of Advanced Nursing, 63*(1), 94-103.
Nursing presence	McMahon, M., & Christopher, K. (2010). Toward a middle range theory of nursing presence. *Nursing Forum, 46*(2), 71-82.
Professional resilience and career persistence	Hodges, H. F., Troyan, P. J., & Keely, A. C. (2010). Career persistence in baccalaureate-prepared acute care nurses. *Journal of Nursing Scholarship, 42*(1), 83-91.
Quality oncology nursing practice	Radwin, L., Cabral, H., & Wilkes, G. (2009). Relationships between patient-centered cancer nursing interventions and desired health outcomes in the context of the health care system. *Research in Nursing & Health, 32*(1), 4-17.
Self-care management for vulnerable populations	Dorsey, C. J., & Murdaugh, C. L. (2003). Theory of self management for vulnerable populations. *Journal of Theory Construction and Testing, 7*(2), 43-49.
Story theory	Smith, M. J., & Liehr, P. (2005). Story theory: Advancing nursing scholarship. *Holistic Nursing Practice, 19*(6), 272-276.
Facilitated sense-making with families of patients in intensive care	Davidson, J. E. (2010). Facilitated sensemaking: A strategy and new middle-range theory to support families of intensive care unit patients. *Critical Care Nurse, 30*(6), 28-39.
Adaptation to chronic pain	Dunn, K. (2004). Toward a middle range theory of adaptation to chronic pain. *Nursing Science Quarterly, 17*(1), 78-84.
Caregiver stress	Tsai, P. (2003). A middle-range theory of caregiver stress. *Nursing Science Quarterly, 16*(2), 137-145.
Spiritual empathy	Chism, L., & Magnan, M. (2009). The relationship of nursing students' spiritual care perspectives to their expressions of spiritual empathy. *Nursing Science Quarterly, 48*(11), 597-605.

Appraising Theories and Research Frameworks

Nurses examine and evaluate theories to determine their maturity, applicability for practice, and usefulness for research. The evaluation of theories is complicated by the availability of at least seven sets of possible evaluative criteria (Fawcett, 2005). In keeping with the purpose of this book, we focus our discussion on critically appraising research frameworks in published studies.

Critical Appraisal of a Research Framework

During the process of critically appraising a study, *the first task related to the research framework is to describe it.* This task is easier when the researchers explicitly identified the framework. For example, Benkert, Hollie, Nordstrom, Wickson, and Bins-Emerick (2009) identified the Interactional Model of Client Health Behavior (IMCHB; Cox, 2003) as the theoretical framework for their study. This team of nurse researchers conducted a descriptive correlational study of patient satisfaction with the care provided by nurse practitioners (NPs) in primary care. The study participants ($N = 100$) were African American routinely seen by NPs in three urban clinics. Benkert et al. (2009) did not provide a diagram of the framework but carefully defined each of the framework's concepts and described the pencil-and-paper instruments used to measure them.

Other researchers, such as Dailey (2009), do not identify the frameworks in their studies. In Dailey's (2009) study of social stressors and strengths of low-income African American mothers and infant birth weight, the framework can be inferred from the literature review and the study variables. Consider the following excerpts from the literature review of the research report to identify the relational statements:

TABLE 7-7 Selected Middle-Range Nursing Theories Cited 2001 through 2011 but Developed Earlier

Name of Theory (Theorist[s], Year)	Recent Citation
Caring (Swanson, 1991)	Andershed, B., & Ollson, K. (2008). Review of literature related to Kristen Swanson's middle-range theory of caring. *Scandinavian Journal of Caring Sciences, 23*(3), 598-610.
Prescriptive pain management theory (Good & Moore, 1996)	Good, M., Anderson, G., Ahn, S., & Cong, X. (2005). Relaxation and music reduced pain following intestinal surgery. *Research in Nursing & Health, 28*(3), 240-251.
Theory of chronic sorrow (Eakes, Burke, & Hainsworth, 1998)	Gordon, J. (2009). An evidence-based approach for supporting parents experiencing chronic sorrow. *Pediatric Nursing, 35*(2), 115-119.
Theory of comfort (Kolcaba, 1994)	Kolcaba, K., & DiMarco, M. (2005). Comfort theory and its application to pediatric nursing. *Pediatric Nursing, 31*(3), 187-194.
Uncertainty in illness theory (Mishel, 1988)	Lin, L., Yeh, C., & Mishel, M. (2010). Evaluation of a conceptual model based on Mishel's theories of uncertainty in illness in a sample of Taiwanese parents of children with cancer: A cross-sectional questionnaire survey. *International Journal of Nursing Studies, 47*(12), 1510-1524.
Self-transcendence theory (Reed, 1991)	Reed, P. G., & Rousseau, E. (2007). Spiritual inquiry and well-being in life-limiting illness. *Journal of Religion, Spirituality, and Aging, 19*(4), 81-98.
Theory of unpleasant symptoms (Lenz, Pugh, Milligan, Gift, & Suppe, 1997)	Brant, J., Beck, S., & Miaskowski, C. (2010). Building dynamic models and theory to advance the science of symptom management research. *Journal of Advanced Nursing, 66*(1), 228-240.
Need-driven, dementia-compromised behavior (Algase et al., 1996).	Kovach, C. R., Noonan, P. E., Schlidt, A. M., & Wells, T. (2005). A model of consequences of need-driven, dementia-comprised behavior. *Journal of Nursing Scholarship, 37*(2), 134-140.
Experiencing transitions (Meleis, Sawyer, Im, Messiasis, & Schumacher, 2000)	Reedy, S., & Blum, K. (2010). Applying middle-range nursing theory to bariatric surgery patients: Experiencing transitions. *Bariatric Nursing and Surgical Patient Care, 5*(1), 35-43.

- The link between stressful life circumstances and birth outcomes...." (p. 340).
- "Several studies have identified associations between maternal experiences of racial discrimination and low-birth-weight deliveries...." (pp. 340-341).
- "Maternal stress associated with trauma exposure has been linked to ... health outcomes" (p. 341).
- "[J]ust as important to learn how women at risk adapt to the negative influences.... [E]ffects of maternal stress on health outcomes should be balanced by efforts to study personal resources that may be influential to maternal health" (p. 341).
- "Supportive networks contribute to the well being of African American women during pregnancy" (p. 341).
- "Levels of spirituality affect perinatal health" (p. 341).
- "Numerous researchers have studied socioeconomic status (SES), common medical conditions during pregnancy, and health practices in relation to birth weight outcomes" (p. 341).

Describing the research framework may be easier if you draw a diagram of the concepts and relationships among them. In the Dailey (2009) study, the study purpose contained four constructs. The purpose was to explore "the extent to which social stressors, personal resources, and known perinatal risk factors predict infant birth weight in a sample of urban low-income African American women" (Dailey, 2009, p. 341). These constructs were the basis for a conceptual map of the research framework. Figure 7-11 presents our diagrams of the constructs, concepts, and relationships among the concepts. In the figure, the first diagram shows that the constructs of social stressors, personal resources, and perinatal risk factors influence birth outcomes. The constructs were derived from the concepts discussed in the article. The second diagram identifies the concepts that Dailey (2009) used that were related to each construct. For example, the construct of social stressors was examined by measuring discrimination, trauma, and socioeconomic states. Although not identified as such, the conceptual and operational definitions of the concepts were easily identified in the article. Table 7-8 displays the definitions of three concepts as examples.

TABLE 7-8 Conceptual and Operational Definitions of Selected Concepts from Dailey's (2009) Study

Concept	Conceptual Definition	Operational Definition
Trauma	*Trauma* is experiencing, either as a witness or participant, an event that involves actual or threatened serious injury to or death of self or others (Dailey, 2009).	Trauma History Questionnaire guided the assessment of life trauma with a resulting score of 0-23, with higher scores indicative of more types of trauma.
Spirituality	*Spirituality* is defined as making meaning that empowers the self, supports coping, and promotes equanimity (Dailey, 2009).	Spirituality was measured using the Spiritual Perspective Scale (Reed, 1987). The operational definition is the summed score on the SPS, ranging from 10 to 60.
Discrimination	*Discrimination* is being excluded, exploited, or treated with prejudice and having one's rights and freedoms restricted.	Discrimination was measured using the Everyday Discrimination Scale. The operational definition is the summed score on the scale, ranging from 9-54.

Research Framework with Constructs

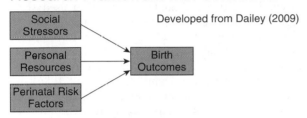

Developed from Dailey (2009)

Research Framework with Concepts

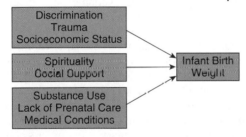

Figure 7-11 Derived research framework for Dailey's (2009) study of stressors and strengths that predict infant birth weight.

From your description of the framework, you are ready to *examine the logical structure of the framework*. Meleis's (2012) criteria for critically appraising theories include assessing the clarity and consistency of the logical structure. When the following questions about clarity and consistency can be answered "yes," the framework has a strong logical structure:

1. Are the definitions of constructs consistent with the theorist's definitions? This question is asked only if the researchers link their framework to a parent theory. (The *parent theory* is the theory from which the researchers have selected the constructs for their study.)

2. Do the concepts reflect the constructs identified in the framework? Some frameworks may not identify constructs and may have only concepts.
3. Do the variables reflect the concepts identified in the framework?
4. Are the conceptual definitions validated by references to the literature?
5. Are the propositions (relational statements) logical and defensible?

The next step in critically appraising a study framework is to *evaluate the extent to which the framework guided the methodology by asking the following question:*

1. Do the operational definitions reflect the conceptual definitions?
2. Do the hypotheses, questions, or objectives reflect the constructs and/or concepts in the propositions of the framework?
3. Is the design appropriate to test the propositions of the framework?

When a framework guides the methodology of a study, the answer to these questions will be "yes." Some researchers may describe a theory or theories to provide context for the study but may not use the framework to guide the methodology. Bond et al. (2011) conducted a study of how nurse researchers use theory by reviewing research reports in seven leading journals over 5 years. In 837 of the 2184 research reports (38%), the researchers included a theoretical framework, either a nursing theory or a theory from another discipline. Of these 837 reports, 93% contained evidence that the theory had been integrated into the study methodology. Bond et al. have documented that, when identified, the study framework most likely will be used to guide the methodology. The more prevalent problem is that nursing researchers often do not identify the theories guiding their studies.

The final step in critically appraising a study framework is to *decide the extent to which the researcher connected the findings to the framework* by asking the following questions:

1. Did the researcher interpret the findings in terms of the framework?
2. Are the findings for each hypothesis, question, or objective consistent with the relationships proposed by the framework?

Even in studies clearly guided by a research framework, the findings may not be discussed in terms of what they mean in relation to the framework. Findings that are consistent with the framework are evidence of the framework's validity, and this point should be noted in the discussion. When the findings are not consistent with the research framework, researchers should discuss the possible reasons for this disconnect. One reason may be a lack of construct validity (see Chapter 16). The instruments used may not have measured the constructs/concepts of the study framework adequately and accurately. Other possible reasons are that the framework was based on assumptions that were not true for the population being studied and that the framework does not represent the reality of the phenomena being studied in this specific sample.

Developing a Research Framework for Study

Developing a framework is one of the most important steps in the research process but, perhaps, also one of the most difficult. A research report in a journal often contains only a brief presentation of the study framework because of page limitations. As a result, you may gain little insight into the careful, thoughtful, prolonged work required to develop a research framework. Part of developing as a researcher is your commitment and motivation to learn the skills needed to perform this thoughtful work.

You have identified a research problem and are thinking about the proposed study's methodology. The guideline you are using for developing the proposal indicates that you need a research framework for a study. Where do you start? This section presents three basic approaches to beginning the process of constructing a study framework: (1) identifying an existing theory from nursing or another discipline, (2) synthesizing a framework from research findings, and (3) proposing a framework from clinical practice. The final steps of constructing a research framework are the same no matter the approach used to start the

construction and are discussed after the presentation of the approaches.

Identifying and Adapting an Existing Theory

Take another look at the research reports you have read related to your topic. Which theories have others used when studying this area? In your exploration, include studies on your topic of interest that have been done with populations other than your own. For example, researchers have used several health behavior and psychological theories to guide studies related to medication adherence. Kalichman et al. (2011) tested an adherence intervention based on the conflict theory of decision making with persons with HIV/AIDS. For her randomized controlled trial (RCT) of a nursing intervention to promote medication adherence in cardiac patients, Gould (2011, p.119) used self-regulation theory based on the "Common Sense Model of illness perception for self regulation of care" developed by Leventhal, Diefenbach, and Leventhal (1992). Schaffer and Tian (2004) used the protection motivation theory (Prentice-Dunn & Rogers, 1986) to examine adherence to preventive medication use of persons with asthma. Existing theories can provide insights into how the topic has been studied and the range of perspectives available on a given research topic.

Review theory textbooks and middle-range theory publications to examine the applicability of other nursing theories that might provide insight to your research problem (Tomey & Alligood, 2006). For example, Orem's (2001) theory of self-care could be used as a framework for a study of the effect of acuity-based staffing assignments on hospital length of stay for patients after a coronary artery bypass graft surgery. The acuity-based staff assignments could be supported by Orem's nursing systems—wholly compensatory care, partially compensatory care, and supportive-educative care. Examples of theories for specific topics are provided in Table 7-9. Prior to making a final decision about a theory, you should read primary sources written by the theorists to ensure that your topic is a conceptual and pragmatic fit with the concepts, definitions of concepts, assumptions, and propositions of the theory.

Synthesis from Research Findings

Developing a theory or a framework from research findings is the most accepted strategy of theory development (Meleis, 2012). The research-to-theory strategy, an inductive approach, begins by identifying relevant studies. For example, to develop a framework for a study of coping with HIV infection, Gray and

TABLE 7-9 Potential Theories for Different Research Topics	
Research Topic	**Theory (Theorist[s], Year)**
Light and noise as influences on patient recovery in acute care settings	Environmental theory (Nightingale, 1859, 1946, 1979)
Peer support group for adolescents to decrease their use of illegal substances	Roy's adaptation model (Roy & Andrews, 2008)
Sleep quality and dementia progression in long-term care facilities	Cognitive brain reserve (Stern, 2009)
Medication adherence of men on antihypertensive medications	Information motivation behavioral skills model (Fisher, Williams, Fisher, & Mallory, 1999)
Screening for diabetes mellitus among women with a history of gestational diabetes	Cardiometabolic Model (Ruhl, 2009)
Task shifting in low-resource settings	Theory of self-regulating teams (Millwood, Banks, & Riga, 2010)
Fear of HIV infection and sexual behavior of young gay men	Theory of planned behavior (Ajzen, 1991)
New graduate nurses' clinical competency and use of high-fidelity simulation in baccalaureate nursing education	NLN-Jeffries simulation framework (Jeffries et al., 2007)
Children's postoperative pain and parental anxiety	Philosophical approach: Externalist perceptual view of pain (Pesut & McDonald, 2007)
Nurse retention and environmental factors in rural hospitals	Theory of structural empowerment (Kanter, 1977)

Cason (2002) conducted an integrated review of 30 studies. Studies were included if the subjects were persons living with HIV infection, and the variables included coping and/or psychosocial factors related to coping. The researchers extracted study characteristics and documented them in a literature summary table (see Chapter 6). They carefully reviewed the findings of each study for relationships among concepts. The researchers became immersed in the published findings by diagramming the relationships on a large piece of paper and creating tables of each relational statement with the studies supporting the statement. Through this process, they identified concepts and relational statements for inclusion in the proposed study's framework.

Proposing a Framework from Practice Experiences

As members of a practice discipline, nurses may develop research frameworks from their clinical experiences. Nurses in practice may make generalizations about patients' responses as they repeatedly provide care to different types of patients. Nurses who reflect on practice may, over time, realize underlying principles of human behavior that guide their choices of interventions. Meleis (2012) notes that a nurse may have nagging questions about why certain situations persist or how to improve patient or organizational outcomes that lead to tentative theories. For example, a novice researcher who worked in a newborn intensive care unit was convinced from her clinical experiences that a mother's frequent visits to the hospital were related to her infant's weight gain. The nurse's

Research Framework from Clinical Practice

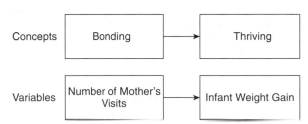

Figure 7-12   Research framework from clinical experience.

ideas could be diagrammed as the lower set of relationships shown in Figure 7-12.

The relationship she identified consisted of two concrete ideas: number of mother visits and weight gain. From the perspective of research, these ideas are variables. Instead of starting with a framework and linking the concepts of the framework to possible study variables, she was starting with variables and needed to identify the concepts that the variables represented. She reviewed the literature and looked for explanations for why visits by the mother were important and what happened when a mother visited the baby. As she reflected on what she read, she realized that maybe the visits promoted bonding or attachment. The researcher continued to reflect on her experiences and remembered that when babies failed to gain weight or lost weight, they were sometimes labeled as "failing to thrive." Wording that more positively, she decided the concept related to weight gain was thriving. On the basis of her clinical experiences and her thinking processes, the researcher began to learn more about theories of bonding and used what she learned to develop a framework for a study related to bonding and thriving of newborns in the neonatal intensive care (see Figure 7-12).

Research frameworks rarely develop from only one source of knowledge. Nurse researchers often combine existing theories, research findings, and insights from their clinical experiences into a framework for a study. For example, to study adherence to blood pressure medications among older Chinese immigrants, Li, Wallhagen, and Froelicher (2010) derived their model from Becker's Health Belief Model (1974), findings from preliminary studies, hypertension literature, and clinical experience. Whatever your approach to beginning the process, once you have possible concepts and relationships, you are ready to move through the remainder of the process to develop a framework that is explicitly expressed in the final research report. A study framework developed in this way is considered tentative theory until research findings provide evidence to support the relationships as diagrammed. *Tentative theories* are those that are developed from other theories, research findings, and clinical practice and that, as of yet, do not have new evidence to support their relational statements.

Defining Relevant Concepts

Concepts are selected for a framework on the basis of their relevance to the phenomenon you are studying. The concepts included in the research framework should reflect the problem statement and the literature review of the proposal. Each concept included in a framework must be defined conceptually. Conceptual definitions may be found in existing theoretical works and quoted in the proposal with sources cited. Conceptual definitions may also be found in published concept analyses, previous studies using the concept, or the literature associated with an instrument developed to measure the concept. Although the instrument itself is an operational definition of the concept, the writer will often provide a conceptual definition on which the instrument development was based. (See Chapter 8 for more extensive discussion of conceptual and operational definitions for study variables.) When acceptable conceptual definitions are not available, you should perform concept synthesis or concept analysis to develop them.

Developing Relational Statements

The next step in framework development is to link all of the concepts through relational statements. If you began with an existing theory, theoretical propositions

may have already been identified. If you synthesized research findings, you have evidence that supports relationships between or among some or all of the concepts. This evidence supports the validity of each relational statement. This support must include a discussion of previous quantitative or qualitative studies (or both) that have examined the proposed relationship and published observations from the clinical practice perspective.

Extracting relational statements from the literary text of an existing theory, published research, or clinical literature can be a daunting task. The following procedure describes how to do so: Select the portion of the theory, research report, or clinical literature that discusses the relationships among the concepts relevant to your study. Write single sentences that connect one concept to another. Change the sentence to a diagram of the relationship, similar to those presented earlier in this chapter (see Figures 7-3 and 7-4). Continue this process until all the relationships in the text have been expressed as diagrams. Burns and Grove (2011) illustrate this process in greater detail in Chapter 7 of their book.

If statements relating the concepts of interest are not available in the literature, statement synthesis is necessary. Develop statements that propose specific relationships among the concepts you are studying. You may gain the knowledge for your statement synthesis through clinical observation and integrative literature review (Walker & Avant, 2004).

Developing Hierarchical Statement Sets

A **hierarchical statement set** is composed of a specific proposition (relational statement) and a hypothesis or research question. The specific proposition may be preceded by a more general proposition when an existing theory was the source of the framework. The proposition is listed first, with the hypothesis or research question immediately following. In some cases, more than one hypothesis or research question may be developed for a single proposition. This statement set indicates the link between the framework and the methodology.

Constructing a Conceptual Map

A conceptual map is a visual representation of a research framework. With the concepts defined and the relational statements diagrammed, you are ready to visually represent the framework for your study. The framework may be limited to only the concepts that you are studying or may be inclusive of other related concepts that are not going to be studied or measured. When the framework includes concepts that are not included in the specific study being proposed, you must clearly identify the portion of the framework being used.

From a practical standpoint, first arrange the relational statements you have diagrammed from left to right with outcomes located at the far right. Concepts that are elements of a more abstract construct can be placed in a frame or box. Sets of closely interrelated concepts can be linked by enclosing them in a frame or circle. Second, using arrows, link the concepts in a way that is consistent with the statement diagrams you previously developed. Every concept should be linked to at least one other concept. Third, examine the framework diagram for completeness by asking yourself the following questions:

1. Are all of the concepts in the study also included on the map?
2. Are all the concepts on the map defined?
3. Does the map clearly portray the phenomenon?
4. Does the map accurately reflect all the statements?
5. Is there a statement for each of the links portrayed by the map?
6. Is the sequence of links in the map accurate?

Developing a well-constructed conceptual map requires repeated tries, but persistence pays off. You may need to reexamine the statements identified. Are there some missing links? Are some of the links inaccurately expressed?

As the map takes shape and begins to seem right, show it to trusted colleagues. Can they follow your logic? Do they agree with your links? Can they identify missing elements? Can you explain the map to them? Seek out individuals who have experienced the phenomenon you are mapping. Does the process depicted seem valid to them? Find someone more experienced than you in conceptual mapping to examine your map closely and critically.

Shanks (2010) conducted a pilot study of the quality of life of 15 patients with coronary artery disease who were receiving external counterpulsation (ECP). In the literature review section of the article, Shanks states, "According to Rector, Anand, and Cohn (2006), the effect of heart failure pathology on quality of life (QOL) is mediated by symptoms such as angina and decreased exercise tolerance" (p. 1). The model in the study by Rector et al. is shown in Figure 7-13. Shanks (2010) used some of these concepts and presented them in a more linear fashion in her simple conceptual framework (see Figure 7-14). She clearly identified the concepts of cardiac pathology,

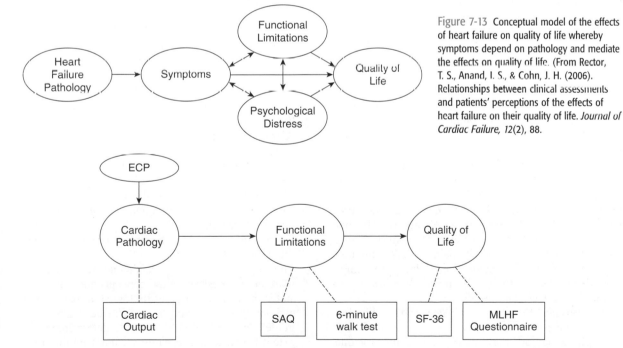

Figure 7-13 Conceptual model of the effects of heart failure on quality of life whereby symptoms depend on pathology and mediate the effects on quality of life. (From Rector, T. S., Anand, I. S., & Cohn, J. H. (2006). Relationships between clinical assessments and patients' perceptions of the effects of heart failure on their quality of life. *Journal of Cardiac Failure, 12*(2), 88.

Figure 7-14 The construct-concept-variable continuum. *ECP,* External counterpulsation; *MLHF,* Minnesota Living with Heart Failure; *SAQ,* Seattle Angina Questionnaire; SF-36 = Short Form 36 Health Survey. (From Shanks, L. C. [2010]. A pilot study to examine relationships among external counterpulsation, cardiac output, functional capacity, and quality of life [Online exclusive]. *Applied Nursing Research,* 2010 Dec 28. DOI: 10.1016/j.apnr.2010.09.002.)

functional limitations, and quality of life. Her diagram also includes the measurements for each concept, thus providing clear logical links to the study's methods. She described her conceptual framework as follows:

"[Figure 7-14] presents a conceptual model based on the model developed by Rector et al. (2006). This model focuses on the degree to which cardiac pathology influences functional limitations and QOL. One or two measures were obtained for each of the three concepts in this model." (Shanks, 2010, p. 2)

Her research questions reflected the conceptual model:

"1. What are the relationships among cardiac pathology, functional limitations, and QOL at Week 1 (entry into ECP) and Week 7 (end of ECP)?

2. Is there an improvement in cardiac output at the end of the 7-week ECP program?

3. Is there an improvement in functional limitations at the end of the 7-week ECP program?

4. Is there an improvement in perceived QOL at the end of the 7-week ECP program?" (Shanks, 2010, p. 2).

The participants in the study ranged in age from 50 to 75 years. Most were white, married men. More than 50% were retired and had annual incomes less than $50,000. Shanks (2010) found no significant correlations in response to research question 1. She also did not find evidence to support improvements in functional status or QOL, with one exception. There was a statistically significant improvement in the 6-minute walk test (research question 3). On the QOL measure, the improvement in the 6-minute walk was further supported by similar findings related to "physical role, physical function, and bodily pain" (p. 4). Although the small sample precluded generalizing the findings to other groups, the findings indicate a need for replication with larger samples.

The product of the creative and critical thinking that you have expended in the development of your research framework may provide a structure for one study or become the basis for a program of research. Continue to consider the framework as you collect and analyze data and interpret the findings. While you wait to hear whether your proposal has been funded or while your data are being collected, use the time to expand the written description of the framework and the evidence supporting its relationships into a manuscript for publication (see Chapter 27). When disseminated, your research framework has the potential to make a valuable contribution to nursing knowledge.

KEY POINTS

- A concept is a term that abstractly describes and names an object or a phenomenon, thus providing it with a separate identity or meaning.
- A relational statement declares that a relationship of some kind exists between two or more concepts.
- A conceptual model or grand theory broadly explains phenomena of interest, expresses assumptions, and reflects a philosophical stance.
- A theory is a set of concepts and relational statements explaining the relationships among them.
- Scientific theories have significant evidence and their relationships may be considered laws.
- Substantive theories are less abstract, can easily be applied in practice, and may be called middle-range theories.
- Middle-range theories may be developed from qualitative data, clinical experiences, clinical practice guidelines, or more abstract theories.
- Tentative theories are developed from research findings and clinical experiences and have not yet been validated.
- A framework is the abstract, logical structure of meaning that guides the development of the study and enables the researcher to link the findings to the body of knowledge used in nursing.
- Relational statements are the core of the framework; it is these statements that are examined through research.
- Every study has either an implicit or explicit theoretical framework.
- The steps of critically appraising a research framework are (1) describing the concepts and relational statements, (2) examining its logical structure, (3) evaluating the extent to which the framework guided the methodology, and (4) determining the extent to which the researcher connected the findings to the framework.
- The logical adequacy of a research framework is the extent to which the relational statements are clear and used consistently.

- The framework should be well integrated with the methodology, carefully structured, and clearly presented, whether the study is physiological or psychosocial.
- Study findings should be interpreted in light of the research framework.
- Research frameworks may start with existing theories, research findings, and/or clinical experiences.
- The remaining steps of the process are (1) selecting and defining concepts, (2) developing statements relating the concepts, (3) expressing the statements in hierarchical fashion, and (4) developing a conceptual map.
- Concepts and relational statements are visually represented by a diagram of the research framework, also called a conceptual map.
- Developing a framework for a study is one of the most important steps in the research process.

REFERENCES

Ajzen, I. (1991). The theory of planned behavior. *Organizational Behavior and Human Decisions Processes*, 50(2), 179–211.

Algase, D., Beck, C., Kolanowski, A., Whall, A., Berent, S., Richards, K., et al. (1996). Need-driven, dementia-compromised behavior: An alternative view of disruptive behavior. *American Journal of Alzheimer's Disease*, 11(6), 10, 12–19.

Alligood, M. R. (2010). *Nursing theory: Utilization & application* (4th ed.). Maryland Heights, MO: Mosby Elsevier.

Andershed, B., & Ollson, K. (2008). Review of literature related to Kristen Swanson's middle-range theory of caring. *Scandinavian Journal of Caring Sciences*, 23(3), 598–610.

Artinian, B. M. (1982) Conceptual mapping: Development of the strategy. *Western Journal of Nursing Research*, 4(4), 379–393.

Banfield, B. (2011). Nursing agency: The link between practical nursing science and nursing practice. *Nursing Science Quarterly*, 2(1), 42–47.

Becker, M. (1974). The Health Belief Model and sick role behavior. *Health Education Monographs*, 2(4), 409–462.

Benkert, R., Hollie, B., Nordstrom, C., Wickson, B., & Bins-Emerick, L. (2009). Trust, mistrust, racial identity and patient satisfaction in urban African American primary care patients of nurse practitioners. *Journal of Nursing Scholarship*, 4(2), 211–219.

Bierman, E., Comijs, H., Rijmen, F., Jonker, C., & Beekman, A. (2008). Anxiety symptoms and cognitive performance in later life: Results from the longitudinal aging study Amsterdam. *Aging & Mental Health*, 12(4), 517–523.

Bond, A., Eshah, N., Bani-Khaled, M., Hamad, A., Habashneh, S., Kataua, H., et al. (2011). Who uses nursing theory? A univariate descriptive analysis of five years' research articles. *Scandinavian Journal of Caring Sciences*, 25(2), 404–409.

Bradford, J., & Petrie, T. (2008). Sociocultural factors and the development of disordered eating: A longitudinal analysis of competing hypotheses. *Journal of Counseling Psychology*, 55(2), 246–262.

Burns, N., & Grove, S. K. (2011). *Understanding nursing research* (5th ed.). Maryland Heights, MO: Elsevier Saunders.

Chinn, P. L., & Kramer, M. K., (2011). *Integrated theory and knowledge development in nursing* (8th ed.). St. Louis, MO: Elsevier Mosby.

Cox, C. L. (2003). A model of health behavior to guide studies of childhood cancer studies (Online exclusive). *Oncology Nursing Forum*, 30(5), E92–E95. Retrieved from http://ons.metapress.com/content/c82737q205725174/fulltext.pdf/.

Cronin, P., Ryan, F., & Coughlan, M. (2010). Concept analysis in healthcare research. *International Journal of Therapy and Rehabilitation*, 17(2), 62–68.

Curley, M. (2007). *Synergy: The unique relationship between nurses and patients: The AACN Synergy Model for Patient Care.* Indianapolis, IN: Sigma Theta Tau International.

Dailey, D. (2009). Social stressors and strengths as predictors of infant birth weight in low-income African American women. *Nursing Research*, 58(5), 340–347.

Denyes, M. J., Orem, D., & Bekel SozWiss, G. (2001). Self care: A foundational science. *Nursing Science Quarterly*, 14(1), 48–54.

Duncan, C., Clouteir, J. D., & Bailey, P. H. (2007). Concept analysis: The importance of differentiating the ontological focus. *Journal of Advanced Nursing*, 58(3), 293–300.

Eakes, G. G., Burkes, M. L., & Hainsworth, M. A. (1998). Middle-range theory of chronic sorrow. *Image: Journal of Nursing Scholarship*, 30(2), 179–184.

Fawcett, J. (1999). *The relationship of theory and research* (3rd ed.). Philadelphia, PA: F. A. Davis Company.

Fawcett, J. (2005). Criteria for evaluation of theory. *Nursing Science Quarterly*, 18(2), 131–135.

Fisher, W. A., Williams, S. S., Fisher, J. D., & Malloy, T. E. (1999). Understanding AIDS risk behavior among sexually active urban adolescents: An empirical test of the Information-Motivation-Behavioral Skills Mode. *AIDS and Behavior*, 3(1), 13–23.

Fitzpatrick, J. J., & Whall, A. J. (2005). *Conceptual models of nursing: Analysis and application* (4th ed.). Upper Saddle River, NJ: Pearson Prentice Hall.

Gobbens, R. J., Luijkx, K. G., Wijnen-Sponselee, M. T., & Schols, J. M. (2010). Toward a conceptual definition of frail community dwelling older people. *Nursing Outlook*, 58(2), 76–86.

Good, M., & Moore, S. (1996). Clinical practice guidelines as a new source of middle-range theory: Focus on pain. *Nursing Outlook*, 44(2), 74–79.

Gould, K. (2011). A randomized controlled trial of a discharge nursing intervention to promote self regulation of care for early discharge interventional cardiology patients. *Dimensions of Critical Care Nursing*, 30(2), 117–125.

Gray, J., & Cason, C. L. (2002). Mastery over stress among women with HIV infection. *Journal of the Association of Nurses in AIDS Care*, 13(4), 43–57.

Haase, J., Britt, T., Coward, D., Leidy, N., & Penn, P. (1992). Simultaneous concept analysis of spiritual perspective, hope, acceptance, and self-transcendence. *Image: Journal of Nursing Scholarship*, 24(2), 141–147.

Hardin, S. (2009). The AACN Synergy Model. In S. J. Peterson & T. S. Bredow (Eds.), *Middle range theories: Application to nursing research* (2nd ed.) (pp. 99–114). Philadelphia, PA: Wolters Kluwer/Lippincott Williams & Wilkins.

Henderson, V. (1964). The nature of nursing. *American Journal of Nursing, 64*(8), 62–68.

Holzman, C., Eyster, J., Klevn, M., Messer, L. C., Kaufman, J. S., Laraia, B. A., et al. (2009). Maternal weathering and risk of preterm delivery. *American Journal of Public Health, 99*(10), 1864–1871.

Hupcey, J., & Penrod, J. (2005). Concept analysis: Examining the state of the science. *Research for Theory and Nursing Practice, 19*(2), 197–208.

Jackson, A., Enderby, K., O'Toole, M., Thomas, S., Ashley, D., Rosenfeld, J., et al. (2009). The role of social support in families coping with childhood brain tumor. *Journal of Psychosocial Oncology, 27*(1), 1–24.

Jeffries, P., Carter, N., Chambers, K., Childress, R. M., Childs, J., Decker, S., et al. (2007). *Simulation in nursing education: From conceptualization to evaluation.* New York City, NY: NLN Publications.

Johansson, I., Hildingh, C., Fridlund, B., & Ahlstrom, G. (2006). Theoretical model of coping among relatives of patients in intensive care units: A simultaneous concept analysis. *Journal of Advanced Nursing, 56*(5), 463–471.

Johnson, D. E. (1974). Development of theory: A requisite for nursing as a primary health profession. *Nursing Research, 23*(5), 372–377.

Kalichman, S., Cherry, C., Kalichman, M., Amaral, C., White, D., Pope, H., et al. (2011). Integrated behavioral intervention to improve HIV/AIDS treatment adherence and reduce HIV transmission. *American Journal of Public Health, 101*(3), 531–538.

Kanter, R. M. (1977). *Men and women of the corporation.* New York NY: Basic Books.

King, I. M. (1981). *A theory for nursing: Systems, concepts, and processes.* New York, NY: Wiley.

Kolcaba, K. (1991). A taxonomic structure for the concept comfort. *Image: The Journal of Nursing Scholarship, 23*(4), 237–240.

Kolcaba, K. (1992). Holistic comfort: Operationalizing the construct as a nurse-sensitive outcome. *Advances in Nursing Science, 15*(1), 1–10.

Kolcaba, K. (1994). A theory of holistic comfort for nursing. *Journal of Advanced Nursing, 19*(6), 1176–1184.

Kolcaba, K. (2009). Comfort. In S. J. Peterson & T. S. Bredow (Eds.), *Middle-range theories: Application to nursing research* (2nd ed.) (pp. 254–272). Philadelphia, PA: Wolters Kluwer/ Lippincott Williams & Wilkins.

Kolcaba, K., & Kolcaba, R. (1991). An analysis of the concept of comfort. *Journal of Advanced Nursing, 16*(11), 1301–1310.

Lee, S. M., & Coakley, E. E. (2011). Geropalliatative care: A concept synthesis. *Journal of Hospice and Palliative Care, 13*(4), 242–248.

Leininger, M. M. (1997). Overview of the Theory of Culture Care with the ethnonursing research method. *Journal of Transcultural Nursing, 8*(2), 32–54.

Lenz, E., Pugh, L. C., Milligan, R. A., Gift, A. G., & Suppe, E. (1997). The middle-range theory of unpleasant symptoms: An update. *Advances in Nursing Science, 19*(3), 14–27.

Leventhal, H., Diefenbach, M., & Leventhal, E. (1992). Illness cognition using common sense to understand treatment adherence and affect cognition interactions. *Cognitive Therapy Research, 16*(2), 143–163.

Li, W.-W., Wallhagen, M., & Froelicher, E. (2010). Factors predicting blood pressure control in older Chinese immigrants to the United States of America. *Journal of Advanced Nursing, 66*(10), 2202–2212.

Mårtenson, E. K., Fägerskiöld, A. M., Runeson, I. V., & Berterö, C. M. (2009). The ethical demand in nursing: The Scandinavian perspective. *Nursing Science Quarterly, 22*(3), 281–288.

Mathisen, L., Andersen, M., Veenstra, M., Wahl, A., Hanestad, B., & Fosse, E. (2007). Quality of life can both influence and be an outcome of general health perceptions after heart surgery. *Health & Quality of Life Outcomes, 5*(27). Retrieved from http://www.hqlo.com/content/5/1/27.

Meleis, A. I. (2012). *Theoretical nursing: Development and progress* (5th ed.). Philadelphia, PA: Wolters Kluwer/Lippincott Williams & Wilkins.

Meleis, A. I., Sawyer, A., Im, F., Messiasis, D., & Schumacher, K. (2000). Experiencing transitions: An emerging middle-range theory. *Advances in Nursing Science, 23*(1), 12–28.

Merton, R. K. (1968). *Social theory and social structure.* New York, NY: Free Press.

Millwood, L., Banks, A., & Riga, K. (2010). Effective self regulating teams: A generative psychological approach. *Team Performance and Management, 16*(1/2), 50–73.

Mishel, M. (1988). The theory of uncertainty in illness. *Image: Journal of Nursing Scholarship, 20*(4), 225–232.

Neuman, B., & Fawcett, J. (2002). *The Neuman Systems Model* (4th ed.). Upper Saddle River, NJ: Prentice-Hall.

Newman, M. (1979). *Theory development in nursing.* Philadelphia, PA: F.A. Davis.

Newman, M. (1986). *Health as expanding consciousness.* St. Louis, MO: Mosby.

Nightingale, F. (1859, 1946). *Notes on nursing: What it is and what it is not.* Philadelphia, PA: Lippincott.

Orem, D. E. (2001). *Nursing: Concepts for practice* (6th ed.) St. Louis, MO: Mosby Year-Book Inc.

Parse, R. (1992). Human becoming: Parse's theory of nursing. *Nursing Science Quarterly, 5*(1), 35–42.

Peplau, H. (1988, 1991). *Interpersonal relations in nursing: A conceptual frame of reference for psychodynamic nursing.* New York, NY: Springer Publisher.

Pesut, B., & McDonald, H. (2007). Connecting philosophy and practice: Implications of two philosophic approaches to pain for nurses' expert clinical decision making. *Nursing Philosophy, 8*(4), 256–263.

Peterson, S. (2009). Introduction to the nature of nursing knowledge. In S. J. Peterson & T. S. Bredow (Eds.), *Middle-range theories: Application to nursing research* (2nd ed.) (pp. 3–45). Philadelphia, PA: Wolters Kluwer/Lippincott Williams & Wilkins.

Phuangphaka, K., Veena, J., Chanokporn, J., & Sloan, R. (2008). Causal model of health-related quality of life in Thai patients with heart failure. *Journal of Nursing Scholarship, 40*(3), 254–260.

Prentice-Dunn, S., & Rogers, R. (1986). Protection motivation theory and preventive health: Beyond the health belief model. *Health Education Research, 1*(3), 153–161.

Ravelin, T., Kylma, J., & Korhonen, T. (2006). Dance in mental health nursing: A hybrid concept analysis. *Issues in Mental Health Nursing*, *27*(3), 307–317.

Rector, T. S., Anand, I. S., & Cohn, J. H. (2006). Relationships between clinical assessments and patients' perceptions of the effects of heart failure on their quality of life. *Journal of Cardiac Failure*, *12*(2), 87–92.

Reed, P. G. (1987). Spirituality and well-being in terminally ill hospitalized adults. *Research in Nursing & Health*, *10*(5), 335–344.

Reed, P. G. (1991). Toward a nursing theory of self-transcendence: Deductive reformulation using developmental theories. *Advances in Nursing Science 13*(4), 64–77.

Risjord, M. (2009). Rethinking concept analysis. *Journal of Advanced Nursing*, *65* (3), 684–691.

Rodgers, B. L. (2000). Concept analysis: An evolutionary view. In B. L. Rodgers (Ed.), *Concept development in nursing: Foundations, techniques, and applications* (2nd ed.) (pp. 77–102). Philadelphia, PA: W. B. Saunders.

Rogers, M. E. (1970). *An introduction to the theoretical basis of nursing*. Philadelphia, PA: Davis.

Rogers, M. E. (1990). Nursing: Science of unitary, irreducible human beings: Updated 1990. In E. A. M. Barrett (Ed.), *Visions of Rogers' science-based nursing* (pp. 5–11). New York, NY: National League for Nursing.

Roy, C. (1988). An explication of the philosophical assumptions of the Roy Adaptation Model. *Nursing Science Quarterly*, *1*(1), 26–34.

Roy, C., & Andrews, H. A. (2008). *Roy's Adaptation Model for Nursing* (3rd ed.). Location: Publisher?

Ruel, J., & Motyka, C. (2009). Advanced practice nursing: A principle-based concept analysis. *Journal of the American Academy of Nurse Practitioners*, *21*(17), 384–392.

Ruhl, C. (2009). Cardiometabolic health: Connecting the dots. *Nursing for Women's Health*, *13*(1), 78–82.

Schaffer, S. D., & Tian, L. (2004). Promoting adherence: Effects of theory-based asthma education. *Clinical Nursing Research*, *13*(1), 69–89.

Schwartz-Barcott, D., & Kim, H. S. (2000). An expansion and elaboration of the hybrid model of concept development. In B. L. Rogers & K. Knafl (Eds.), *Concept Development in Nursing: Foundations, Techniques, and Applications* (pp. 129–159). Philadelphia: W. B. Saunders Company.

Serafica, R. (2011). Concept analysis of acculturation in Filipino immigrants within health context. *Nursing Forum*, *46*(3), 128–136.

Shanks, L. C. (2010). A pilot study to examine relationships among external counterpulsation, cardiac output, functional capacity, and quality of life (Online exclusive). *Applied Nursing Research*, *23*, 1–6. Available online Dec 28. DOI: 10.1016/j.apnr.2010.09.002.

Simmons, B. (2010). Clinical reasoning: Concept analysis. *Journal of Advanced Nursing*, *66* (5), 1151–1158.

Stern, Y. (2009). Cognitive reserve. *Neuropsychologia*, *47*(10), 2015–2028.

Swanson, K. (1991). Empirical development of a middle-range theory of caring. *Nursing Research*, *40*(3), 161–166.

Tkatch, R., Artinian, N., Abrams, J., Mahn, J., Franks, M., Keteyian, S., et al. (2011). Social networks and health outcomes among African American cardiac rehabilitation patients. *Heart & Lung*, *40*(3), 193–200.

Tomey, A. M., & Alligood, M. R. (2006). *Nursing theorists and their work* (6th ed.). St. Louis, MO: Mosby Elsevier.

Walker, L. O., & Avant, K. C. (2011). *Strategies for theory construction in nursing* (5th ed.). Boston, MA: Prentice Hall.

Watson, J. (1979). *Nursing: The philosophy and science of caring*. Boston, MA: Little Brown and Company.

Weaver, K., & Mitcham, C. (2008). Nursing concept analysis in North America: State of the art. *Nursing Philosophy*, *9*(1), 180–194.

Wilson, J. (1963). *Thinking with concepts*. Cambridge, England: Cambridge University Press.

Xu, X., Floyd, A., Westmaas, J., & Aron, A. (2010). Self expanding and smoking abstinence. *Addictive Behaviors*, *35*(4), 295–301.

8
CHAPTER

Objectives, Questions, Hypotheses, and Study Variables

Researchers formulate objectives, questions, and hypotheses to bridge the gap between the more abstractly stated research purpose and the detailed plan for data collection and analysis. Objectives, questions, and hypotheses delineate the study variables, the relationships among the variables, and, often, the population to be studied.

Study variables are concepts at various levels of abstraction that are measured, manipulated, or controlled in a study. Concrete concepts, such as temperature, weight, and blood pressure, are referred to as *variables* in a study; abstract concepts, such as creativity, empathy, and social support, are sometimes referred to as *research concepts*. Research variables and concepts are conceptually defined, on the basis of the study framework, and are operationally defined to direct their measurement, manipulation, or control in a study.

In this chapter, you will explore when objectives, questions, or hypotheses might be developed to direct the conduct of a study. You will also learn how to formulate research objectives, questions, and hypotheses, especially how to test different types of hypotheses through research. This chapter concludes with a discussion of different types of variables and direction for conceptually and operationally defining variables for a study.

Formulating Research Objectives or Aims

Research objectives or aims are clear, concise, declarative statements expressed in the present tense that usually are presented following the study purpose to specify the study focus. For clarity, an objective usually focuses on one or two variables (or concepts) and indicates whether the variables are to be identified or described. Objectives can also identify relationships or associations among variables, determine differences between groups or compare groups on selected variables, and predict a dependent variable on the basis of selected independent variables.

A combination of the following formats might be used in developing objectives to guide a study. The focus of each objective is identified in the parentheses at the end of each statement. The objectives are placed in order from the least complex to the most complex in generating research evidence. Thus, the objectives or aims of studies might be to:

1. Identify the elements or characteristics of variable X in a selected population (*identification*).
2. Describe variable X in a selected population (*description*).
3. Determine the difference between groups 1 and 2 or to compare groups 1 and 2 on variable X in a selected population (*difference*).
4. Examine the relationship between variables X and Y in a selected population (*relational*).
5. Determine whether certain independent variables are predictive of a dependent variable in a selected population (*prediction*).

Formulating Objectives or Aims in Quantitative Studies

The objectives or aims in quantitative studies are developed on the basis of the research problem and purpose to clarify the study goals, variables, and population. The following excerpts, from a descriptive study of the symptom management strategies used by elderly patients after coronary artery bypass surgery (CABS), demonstrate the logical flow from research problem (including the problem significance, background, and statement) and purpose to research aims (Schulz, Zimmerman, Pozehl, Barnason, & Nieveen, 2011).

Research Problem

"A major component of nursing care after coronary artery bypass surgery (CABS) is focused on educating patients to recognize and manage postoperative symptoms [*problem significance*]. The symptoms commonly experienced have been well documented in the literature and include sleep disturbances (Tranmer & Parry, 2004; Zimmerman, Barnason, Nieveen, & Schmaderer, 2004), fatigue (Tranmer & Parry, 2004; Zimmerman et al., 2004), swelling (Tranmer & Parry, 2004; Zimmerman et al., 2004), shortness of breath (SOB), appetite problems, and chest and leg incision pain (Zimmerman et al., 2004) [*problem background*]. Although much has been done to document postoperative symptoms, very little has been done to describe the strategies that patients use to manage these symptoms [*problem statement*]." (Schulz et al., 2011, pp. 65-66)

Research Purpose

"The purpose of this study was to describe the symptom management strategies used by older adults after CABS." (Schulz et al., p. 66)

Research Aims

"The specific aims of this study were to examine data 3 and 6 weeks after CABS to (a) identify categories of symptom management strategies from patient's self report data; (b) describe symptom management strategies used for frequently reported symptoms including SOB, fatigue, incision pain, sleep disturbance, swelling, and appetite problems; and (c) determine if patients used appropriate strategies to manage symptoms by comparing reported symptom management strategies to current evidence." (Schulz et al., 2011, p. 66)

In this example, the problem provides a basis for the purpose, and the aims evolve from the purpose to clearly focus the conduct of the study. The first aim was focused on *identification* of the categories of symptom management strategies (*variable*) used by older adults (*population*) 3 and 6 weeks after CABS (*hospital and home settings*). The study participants were recruited from four Midwestern hospitals, but the majority of data collection took place in the participants' homes. The second aim was focused on *description* of the older adults' symptom management strategies (*variable*) used. The third objective was focused on *comparison of or differences in* patients' reported symptom management strategies and current

evidence-based guidelines developed by the American Heart Association. Schulz et al. (2011, p. 65) found, "Three weeks after surgery, the most frequently used strategies were rest to manage shortness of breath (53%) and fatigue (53%), medications for incision pain (24%), and repositioning for swelling (35%) and sleep disturbance (18%). Overall, fewer patients experiencing sleep disturbances (39%), incision pain (39%), swelling (46%), and appetite problems (17%) reported using a strategy to manage their symptoms." Thus, the researchers stressed the importance of nurses' education of patients about symptom identification and effective management strategies to improve recovery following CABS.

Formulating Objectives or Aims in Qualitative Studies

Many qualitative studies are guided by the study purpose and do not include research objectives or questions. However, some qualitative researchers do develop objectives to guide selected studies. The objectives in qualitative studies usually have a broader focus and include more abstract and complex variables or concepts than those in quantitative studies (Munhall, 2012). An ethnographic study by Happ, Swigart, Tate, Hoffman, and Arnold (2007) included objectives to direct their investigation of patients' involvement in health-related decisions during prolonged critical illness, as shown by the following excerpts.

Research Problem

"Clinicians increasingly recognize the need to involve patients in decision making before, and, if possible, during prolonged critical illness, but have little guidance as to how and when to do this most effectively [*problem significance*].... Prior reports of studies containing the number of patients able to communicate treatment preferences or to participate in decisions during an acute or critical illness vary from none to as high as 48% [*problem background*].... Moreover, few reports of studies of treatment decision making indicate the criteria used to make decisional capacity assessments.... Consequently, empirical knowledge of practice in this important area of patient care is limited [*problem statement*]." (Happ et al., 2007, pp. 361-362)

Research Purpose

The purpose of this study was to "describe patterns of communication of patients involved in health-related decision making during prolonged mechanical ventilation (PMV)" (Happ et al., 2007, p. 362).

Research Objectives

The objectives of this study were to "describe: (a) characteristics of patients who were involved in health-related decisions; (b) types of health-related decisions made with patient involvement; (c) how patient involvement occurred; and (d) the extent of patient involvement with health-related decisions during PMV" (Happ et al., 2007, p. 361).

In this ethnographic study, the problem statement indicated that inadequate research had been conducted on patient involvement in health-related decisions during critical illness, which provided a basis for the study purpose. All four objectives focused on detailed *descriptions* of the study *variables*: (1) characteristics of patients undergoing PMV, (2) health-related decision making of these patients, (3) how patient involvement in decision making occurred, and (4) extent of patient decision making. The findings from this study indicated that families, advanced practice nurses, and physicians were engaging critically ill patients in decision making whenever possible. However, most of the time the patients could not make independent decisions but were able to share decision making with their families and clinicians. These findings emphasize how important it is for families and clinicians to include critically ill patients in health-related decisions at whatever level possible (Happ et al., 2007).

Formulating Research Questions

A **research question** is a concise, interrogative statement that is worded in the present tense and includes one or more variables (or concepts). The research questions focus on the following: (1) the *identification* and/or *description* of the variable(s), (2) a determination of *differences* between two or more groups regarding selected variables, (3) an examination of relationships among variables (*relational*), and (4) the use of independent variables to *predict* a dependent variable.

You might use the following formats in developing research questions for a study (the focus for each question is shown in parentheses). The levels of evidence to be generated by the following research questions progress from simple (identification) to complex (prediction).

1. What are the elements or characteristics of variable *X* in a selected population (*identification*)?

2. How is variable *X* described by a selected population (*description*)?
3. Is there a difference between groups 1 and 2 regarding variable *X* (*difference*)?
4. What is the relationship between variables *X* and *Y* in a selected population (*relational*)?
5. Are independent variables *W*, *X*, and *Y* predictive of dependent variable *Z* (*prediction*)?

Formulating Questions in Quantitative Studies

Delaney, Apostolidis, Lachapelle, and Fortinsky (2011, p. 285) conducted a comparative descriptive study to examine "home care nurses' knowledge of evidence-based education topics for management of heart failure." The following excerpts from this study demonstrate the flow from research problem and purpose to research questions.

Research Problem

"Heart failure (HF), a chronic and disabling syndrome affecting adults of all ages and particularly older adults, is a major public health problem. An estimated 5.7 million Americans are currently affected by HF, and this figure is expected to double over the next 25 years, primarily because of the aging of the population and decreased mortality from other cardiovascular conditions (Hodges, 2009).... HF is characterized by poor posthospital discharge outcomes [*problem significance*].... Home care agencies are currently being challenged by Centers for Medicare and Medicaid Services (CMS) to improve outcomes in HF management.... Home care nurses play key roles in the delivery of education to patients and their families [*problem background*]. However, home care nurses face unique challenges compared with nurses at other sites of care in providing comprehensive education on managing HF. These challenges include a lack of access to detailed patient information (Bowles, Pham, O'Connor, & Horowitz, 2010), a focus on generalist rather than specialist practice, and few opportunities for continuing education in specialized knowledge such as managing HF [*problem statement*]." (Delaney et al., 2011, p. 286)

Research Purpose

The purpose of this study was to examine "home care nurses' knowledge of evidence-based HF education related to the disease process, its management, and patients' self-management" (Delaney et al., 2011, p. 286).

Research Questions

Research questions included the following:
"(1) What is the level of knowledge of home care nurses regarding evidence-based education topics for patients with HF?...
(2) Were differences evident in nurses' knowledge based on education and work experience?...
(3) What are home care nurses' self-reported knowledge needs related to the care of patients with HF?" (Delaney et al., 2011, p. 287)

Question 1 focused on *description* of the home care nurses' (*population*) knowledge about HF (*variable*). Question 2 focused on determining *differences* in the nurses' knowledge on the basis of educational level and years of work experience (*demographic variables*). Question 3 focused on *description* of the nurses' self-reported knowledge needs (*variable*) in managing patients with HF. Delaney et al. (2011) found that home care nurses were limited in their evidence-based knowledge for managing HF. There were no significance differences in the nurses' knowledge and their educational level and years of experience. The researchers concluded that the home care nurses needed educational programs focused on HF patient management to improve the quality of patient education they could provide.

Formulating Questions in Qualitative Studies

The questions in qualitative studies are often limited in number, have a broad focus, and include concepts that are more complex and abstract than those in quantitative studies. Marshall and Rossman (2011) noted that the questions in qualitative research either might be theoretical ones, which can be studied with different populations or in a variety of sites, or could be focused on a particular population or setting. Hudson et al. (2010) conducted an exploratory-descriptive qualitative study to examine the health-seeking challenges perceived by homeless young adults. The problem, purpose, and research questions used to direct this study are presented in the following excerpts.

Research Problem

"Adolescent homelessness is a distressing social problem. Approximately 1.5 to 2 million homeless adolescent persons live on the streets in the United States (Bucher, 2008); homelessness among young persons is more common than homelessness among older adults.... Homeless young adults are highly vulnerable to negative health consequences because of the realities of street life [*problem significance*].... Homeless young persons are at risk for sexual and physical abuse.... Other negative health consequences experienced by homeless young adults include sexually transmitted infections, poorly controlled chronic mental illness, and lack of immunization for conditions, such as hepatitis A and hepatitis B (Hudson, Nyamathi, & Sweat, 2008).... Homeless persons are more likely to be admitted to the hospital and have increased durations of hospitalization than those of nonhomeless persons due to negative health consequences associated with street living.... Nearly half of all homeless young persons have no regular source of health care (Sneller et al., 2008) [*problem background*].... The perceptions of how homeless persons view the health care system have not been well studied.... There is a growing assertion that improvements should be made with respect to the provision of quality care for the homeless young adults living in the United States.... One way to achieve high-quality programs designed to improve health care for homeless adults is to solicit these adults' input in program development [*problem statement*]." (Hudson et al., 2010, pp. 212-213)

Research Purpose

"The purpose of this article was to gain a further understanding of the perceptions of homeless youth regarding their healthcare-seeking behaviors" (Hudson et al., 2010, p. 213).

Research Questions

This study included the following research questions:
"1. What are homeless young adults' perspectives on facilitators and barriers to receiving health care?
2. How can existing homeless youth and young-adult-centered healthcare programs be improved?" (Hudson et al., 2010, 213)

The first study question focused on developing a *description* of the homeless young adults' (*population*) perspectives on facilitators and barriers to receiving health care (*research* concepts). The second question focused on *identifying* and *describing* how young-adult-centered healthcare programs can be improved (*research* concept). The study's "identified themes were failing access to care based on perceived structural barriers (limited clinic sites, limited hours of operation, priority health conditions, and long wait times) and social barriers (perception of discrimination by uncaring professionals, law enforcement, and society in general…)" (Hudson et al., 2010, p. 212). The researchers also gained insights into the programmatic and agency resources that are needed to promote health-seeking behaviors by homeless young adults.

Formulating Hypotheses

A hypothesis is the formal statement of the expected relationship or relationships between two or more variables in a selected population. The hypothesis translates the problem and purpose into a clear explanation or prediction of the expected results or outcomes of the study (Shadish, Cook, & Campbell, 2002). This section describes the purpose, sources, and types of hypotheses that are commonly developed by researchers. In addition, the process for developing and testing hypotheses in nursing studies is described.

Purpose of Hypotheses

The purpose of a hypothesis is similar to that of research objectives and questions. A hypothesis (1) specifies the variables you will manipulate or measure, (2) identifies the population you will examine, (3) indicates the type of research, and (4) directs the conduct of your study. Hypotheses direct the conduct of a study by influencing the study design, sampling technique, data collection and analysis methods, and interpretation of findings. Hypotheses differ from objectives and questions by predicting the outcomes of a study. Study hypotheses are used to organize the results section of a study, and the results indicate support or nonsupport of each hypothesis. Hypothesis testing allows us to generate knowledge by testing theoretical statements or relationships that were identified in previous research, proposed by theorists, or observed in practice (Chinn & Kramer, 2008; Fawcett & Garity, 2009).

Sources of Hypotheses

Research hypotheses can be generated by observing phenomena or problems in nursing practice, analyzing theory, and reviewing the research literature. Many hypotheses originate from real-life experiences. Clinicians and researchers observe events in practice and identify relationships among these events (theorizing), which are the bases for formulating hypotheses. For example, you may notice that the hospitalized patient who complains the most about pain receives the most pain medicine and other pain management strategies. The relationship identified is a prediction about events in clinical practice that has potential for empirical

testing, because certain patients might not be receiving adequate pain management.

You could conduct a literature review to identify a theory that supports this relationship. For example, Fagerhaugh and Strauss (1977) developed a theory of pain management and identified the following relationship or proposition: As expressions of pain increase, pain management increases. The researchers developed this proposition through the use of grounded theory research. Additional testing is necessary to determine its usefulness in describing how patients express pain and how that pain is managed in a variety of practice situations. On the basis of theory and clinical observation, the following hypothesis might be formulated: The more frequently a hospitalized patient verbalizes perceptions of pain, the greater the administration of analgesic medications by healthcare providers.

Some hypotheses are initially generated from relationships expressed in a theory, when the intent of the researcher is to test a theory. Usually, middle-range theories are tested in research, and a proposition or relationship from the theory provides the basis for the generation of one or more study hypotheses (Fawcett & Garity, 2009; Smith & Liehr, 2008). For example, Rungruangsiripan, Sitthimongkol, Maneesriwongul, Talley, and Vorapongsathorn (2011) tested the relationships in the Common-Sense Model of Illness Representation (Diefenbach & Leventhal, 1996) to examine the factors affecting medication adherence in individuals with schizophrenia. Figure 8-1 contains the framework model for this study based on the Common-Sense Model of Illness Representation, which has three stages: sources of information, illness representation, and coping. "Sources of information included social support variable, therapeutic alliance variable, and experience of medication side effects variable. Coping consisted of intention to change adherence behavior and adherence behavior" (Rungruangsiripan et al., 2011, p. 272). This model shows the direct and indirect relationships among the concepts that provide a basis for the study hypotheses. A direct relationship is when one concept links to another concept without an intervening concept. For example, the concept of social support is linked directly to illness representation. In an indirect relationship, one concept is linked to another concept through an intervening third concept. For example, the concept experience with medication side effects is indirectly linked to the concept intention to change adherence behavior through the concept of illness representation (see Figure 8-1). The Rungruangsiripan et al. (2011) study set the following hypotheses:

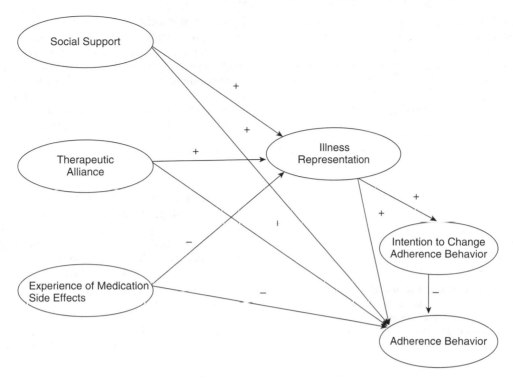

Figure 8-1 Hypothesized medication adherence model. (From Rungruangsiripan, M., Sitthimongkol, Y., Maneesriwongul, W., Talley, S., & Vorapongsathorn, T. [2011]. Mediating role of illness representation among social support, therapeutic alliance, experience of medication side effects, and medication adherence in persons with schizophrenia. *Archives of Psychiatric Nursing, 25*[4], 273.)

"(a) Social support and therapeutic alliance would have a positive direct effect on illness representation and adherence behavior in individuals with schizophrenia;

(b) Experience of medication side effects would have a negative direct effect on illness representation and adherence behavior in individuals with schizophrenia;

(c) Intention to change adherence behavior would have a negative direct effect on adherence behavior;

(d) Social support, therapeutic alliance, and experience of medication side effects would have an indirect effect on intention to change adherence behavior and adherence behavior through illness representation; and

(e) Illness representation would have a positive direct effect on intention to change adherence behavior and adherence behavior as well as an indirect effect on adherence behavior via intention to change adherence behavior."
(Rungruangsiripan et al., 2011, p. 272)

These hypotheses were formulated to test the propositions or relationships from the Common-Sense Model of Illness Representation (see Figure 8-1). The researchers found that "therapeutic alliance and the experience of medication side-effects enhanced illness representation, which in turn led to an intention to change adherence behavior. Social support did not alter illness representation or adherence behavior" (Rungruangsiripan et al., 2011, p. 269). *Illness representation* is the patients' perception of their schizophrenia and their ability to cope with the illness. Patients with a clear perception of their schizophrenia have strong intentions to change their adherence behaviors. Thus, mental health nurses need to promote the patients' understanding of their schizophrenia illness to enhance their adherence to their medications.

Reviewing the research literature and synthesizing findings from different studies can also be used to generate hypotheses. For example, Ross, Sawatphanit, Mizuno, and Takeo (2011) synthesized the findings from studies to identify the factors that predict depressive symptoms in postpartum women who are HIV-positive. They developed a conceptual framework for

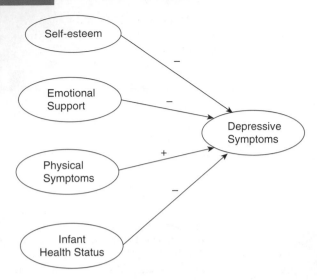

Figure 8-2 Conceptual framework of the study. (From Ross, R., Sawatphanit, W., Mizuno, M., & Takeo, K. [2011]. Depressive symptoms among HIV-positive postpartum women in Thailand. *Archives of Psychiatric Nursing, 25*[1], 37.)

their study that is presented in Figure 8-2. The researchers "hypothesized that depressive symptoms are negatively related to self-esteem, emotional support, and infant health status but positively associated with physical symptoms" (Ross et al., 2011, p. 37).

Ross et al. (2011) found that self-esteem and infant health status were significant predictors of postpartum women's depressive symptoms but physical symptoms and emotional support were not. The study results indicated that 74.1% of the HIV-positive postpartum women had symptoms of depression, and the researchers encouraged nurses to examine the self-esteem and infant health status of such women to increase identification of episodes of depression. The researchers also recommended further research to identify additional factors that might be predictive of depression in HIV-positive postpartum women. Thus, two relationships, those of self-esteem and infant health status to depressive symptoms, were supported in the framework model (see Figure 8-2). However, the other relationships, those of emotional support and physical symptoms to depressive symptoms, were not supported in this study. Additional research is needed to increase understanding of the factors that might be predictive of depression in postpartum women who are HIV-positive.

Types of Hypotheses

Hypotheses identify different types of relationships and include different numbers of variables. Studies might have one, three, or more hypotheses, depending on the complexity and scope of the study. The type of hypothesis developed is based on the problem and purpose of a study. The following four categories are used to describe types of hypotheses: (1) associative versus causal, (2) simple versus complex, (3) directional versus nondirectional, and (4) null versus research.

Associative versus Causal Hypotheses

The relationships in hypotheses are identified as associative or causal. An **associative relationship** identifies variables that occur or exist together in practice, and as one variable changes so does the other. For example, research indicates there is an associative relationship between anxiety and depression, and as a person's depression changes so does the anxiety level. Thus, **associative hypotheses** are developed to examine relationships among variables in a study. The formats used for expressing associative hypotheses follow:

1. Variable X is related to or associated with variable Y in a selected population. (Predicts a relationship between two variables but does not indicate the type of relationship.)
2. An increase in variable X is related to an increase in variable Y, or variable X is positively related to variable Y in a selected population. (Predicts a positive relationship.)
3. A decrease in variable X is related to a decrease in variable Y in a selected population. (Predicts a positive relationship.)
4. An increase in variable X is related to a decrease in variable Y, or variable X is negatively related to variable Y in a selected population. (Predicts a negative or inverse relationship.)
5. Variables X and Y are predictive of variable Z in a study. (The independent variables X and Y are used to predict the dependent variable Z in a predictive correlational study.)

Associative hypotheses identify relationships among variables in a study but do not indicate that one variable causes an effect on another variable. Researchers state associative hypotheses when the focus of their study is to examine relationships and not to determine cause and effect. For example, Reishtein (2005) conducted a predictive correlational study to examine the relationships between symptoms and functional performance in patients with chronic obstructed pulmonary disease

(COPD). Reishtein developed the following associative hypotheses to guide the study:

> "1. Positive relationships exist among dyspnea, fatigue, and sleep difficulty in people with COPD;
> 2. Dyspnea, fatigue, and sleep difficulty are related to functional performance; and
> 3. Dyspnea, fatigue, and sleep difficulty, taken together, will explain more of the variance in functional performance in people with COPD than any of these symptoms alone." (Reishtein, 2005, p. 40)

Hypothesis 1 predicts positive relationships or associations among the variables of dyspnea, fatigue, and sleep difficulty for patients with COPD. A positive relationship means that the variables change together; thus, they will all increase together in value or all decrease together. These relationships are depicted in the following diagram:

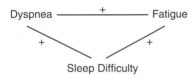

Hypothesis 2 predicts relationships between three variables—dyspnea, fatigue, and sleep difficulty—and the variable functional performance, but it does not identify the type of relationship. These relationships are shown in the following diagram:

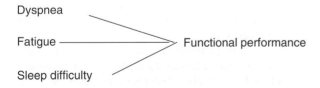

Hypothesis 3 uses the independent variables dyspnea, fatigue, and sleep difficulty to predict the dependent or outcome variable functional performance in COPD patients. The predictive relationship is shown in the following diagram:

$$\text{Dyspnea} + \text{Fatigue} + \text{Sleep Difficulty} \rightarrow$$
$$\text{Functional Performance}$$

The results from Reishtein's (2005) study partially supported hypothesis 1, in that dyspnea had positive, significant relationships with fatigue ($r = 0.43$, $p < 0.001$) and sleep difficulty ($r = 0.39$, $p < 0.001$), but fatigue and sleep difficulty were positively but not significantly related ($r = 0.19$). Hypothesis 2 was also partially supported in that dyspnea ($r = -0.54$, $p < 0.001$) and fatigue ($r = -0.24$, $p < 0.01$) were significantly, negatively related to functional performance, but sleep difficulty ($r = -0.17$) was not. Thus, in hypothesis 3, dyspnea was the most predictive of functional performance, with fatigue and sleep difficulty providing limited prediction. Thus, managing dyspnea may be the best way to improve the symptoms and functional performance in patients with COPD. Additional research may distinguish other symptoms that might predict functional performance in COPD patients and thereby help them and healthcare providers in managing this chronic disease.

Causal relationships identify a cause-and-effect interaction between two or more variables, which are referred to as independent and dependent variables. The **independent variable** (intervention, treatment, or experimental variable) is manipulated or varied by the researcher to have an effect on the dependent variable. The **dependent variable** (outcome or response variable) is measured to examine the effect created by the independent variable. A format for stating a causal hypothesis is as follows: Subjects experiencing the independent variable X demonstrate greater change in dependent variable Y than do the subjects in the control or comparison group. For example, cancer patients receiving a relaxation music intervention have less perceived pain than those receiving usual care.

Scott, Hofmeister, Rogness, and Rogers's (2010) review of the literature indicated that nurses working 12-hour shifts had difficulties staying awake on duty, reduced time for sleep, and significantly higher risk for errors. Thus, these researchers conducted a quasi-experimental study to determine the effect of a fatigue countermeasures program for nurses (FCMPN) on nurses' alertness and number of near and actual patient errors. A causal hypothesis was tested in the conduct of this study. The researchers hypothesized that implementing the FCMPN had the potential for improving sleep quality and sleep duration and decreasing daytime sleepiness, drowsiness episodes, risk for auto accidents, and actual and near reported work errors (Scott et al., 2010).

The independent variable or study intervention was the FCMPN that was implemented to determine its impact on the dependent or outcome variables sleep quality, sleep duration, daytime sleepiness, drowsiness episodes, auto accident risk, and work errors. The study population was hospital staff nurses, and the settings were medical-surgical units in three major acute care Michigan hospitals. Scott et al. (2010) found that the FCMPN significantly improved the hospital nurses' sleep duration, sleep quality, alertness (fewer episodes of drowsiness), and accident and error risk. However, there was not significant improvement in daytime sleepiness. Thus, the hypothesis was supported for five of the six dependent variables and not

supported for the outcome daytime sleepiness. The interpretation of the results might have been facilitated by the statement of additional hypotheses with fewer dependent variables in each hypothesis. A diagram of this hypothesis follows, with causal arrows (→) indicating the cause-and-effect relationship between the independent variable (IV) and dependent variables (DVs). Causal arrows indicate the effect of IV on the DV (see Chapter 7 for discussion of types of relationships). After each dependent variable is indicated whether this part of the hypothesis was supported or not supported.

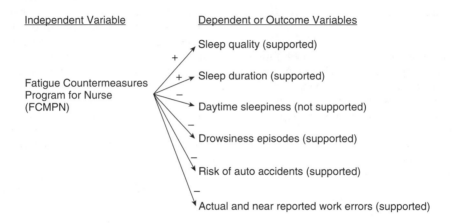

Simple versus Complex Hypotheses

A **simple hypothesis** predicts the relationship (associative or causal) between two variables. One format for stating a simple associative hypothesis is as follows: Variable *X* is related to variable *Y*. A simple causal hypothesis identifies the relationship between one independent variable and one dependent variable, for example, independent variable *X* causes a change in dependent variable *Y*. Vasan et al. (2003) studied the relationship of elevated plasma homocysteine levels with the risk for congestive heart failure (CHF) in adults without prior myocardial infarction (MI). A simple, associative hypothesis was developed to direct this study: "We hypothesized that elevated plasma homocysteine levels are associated with an increased risk for CHF" (Vasan et al., 2003, p. 1251). The following diagram demonstrates the positive relationship that was identified between the two study variables of plasma homocysteine level and risk for CHF:

The results of this 8-year study indicated that an elevated plasma homocysteine concentration was positively and strongly related to risk of CHF in both men and women who did not have a prior history of MI. The hypothesis was supported in this study, indicating that nurse practitioners and clinical nurse specialists need to examine plasma homocysteine levels in individuals with a family history of CHF and treat those levels as needed.

A **complex hypothesis** predicts the relationship (associative or causal) among three or more variables. A complex associative hypothesis predicts the relationships among three or more variables, such as the relationships among the variables *X, Y*, and *Z*. Complex causal hypotheses also include three or more variables but predict the effects of one independent variable on two (or more) dependent variables or predict the effects of two or more independent variables on one or more dependent variables. For example, Scott et al.

↑ Plasma homocysteine level ──────── + ──────── ↑ Risk for CHF

(2010) tested a complex causal hypothesis in their examination of the effects of the nurse fatigue intervention program (FCMPN) on the sleep duration, sleep quality, daytime sleepiness, drowsiness episodes, risk of auto accident, and actual and near reported work errors. The figure presented earlier demonstrating this causal hypothesis includes one independent variable, FCMPN, and six dependent or outcome variables. This intervention offers potential benefits for managing nurses' fatigue but requires additional investigation to determine its effectiveness in managing daytime sleepiness. Often, in practice situations, multiple variables cause an event, or an intervention results in multiple outcomes. Therefore, complex rather than simple associative or causal hypotheses are often more representative of nursing practice.

Nondirectional versus Directional Hypotheses

A nondirectional hypothesis states that a relationship exists but does not predict the nature of the relationship. If the direction of the relationship being studied is not clear in clinical practice or the theoretical or empirical literature, the researcher has no clear indication of the nature of the relationship and states a nondirectional hypothesis (Fawcett & Garity, 2009). For example, Reishtein's (2005, p. 4) second hypothesis (introduced earlier in this chapter) is nondirectional: "Dyspnea, fatigue, and sleep difficulty are related to functional performance." This hypothesis indicates that dyspnea, fatigue, and sleep difficulty are related to functional performance, but it does not indicate the direction or nature (positive or negative) of the relationship. This hypothesis is nondirectional, complex (four variables), and associative (indicating that a relationship exists).

A directional hypothesis states the nature or direction of the relationship between two or more variables. These hypotheses are developed from theoretical statements, findings of previous studies, and clinical experience. As the knowledge on which a study is based increases, the researcher is able to predict the direction of a relationship between the variables being studied. Terms such as *less, more, increase, decrease, positive, negative, greater*, and *smaller* indicate the directions of relationships in hypotheses. Directional hypotheses can be associative or causal and simple or complex. In a study introduced earlier, Ross et al. (2011) "hypothesized that depressive symptoms are negatively related to self-esteem, emotional support, and infant health status but positively associated with physical symptoms" based on their framework model [see Figure 8-2] (Ross et al., 2011, p. 37). This hypothesis is associative (examines relationships or

associations among variables), complex (includes five variables), and directional (identifies positive and negative associations among variables).

A causal hypothesis predicts the effect of an independent variable on a dependent variable, specifying the direction of the relationship. Thus, all causal hypotheses are directional. Efe and Özer (2007) examined the pain-relieving effect of breast-feeding during immunization injections in healthy neonates and used a causal hypothesis to direct their study. "The hypothesis tested was that breast-feeding would decrease the length of crying time, prevent an increase in heart rate, and prevent a decrease in oxygen saturation during vaccination as compared with the control condition (i.e., no breast-feeding)" (Efe & Özer, 2007, p. 11). This causal hypothesis predicted the effect of an intervention or independent variable, breast-feeding, during immunization injections on the dependent or outcome variables length of crying time, heart rate, and oxygen saturation. Thus, this is a complex (four variables), directional (decrease crying time and prevent increased heart rate and decreased oxygen saturation), causal hypothesis. The breast-feeding significantly decreased crying time but did not significantly affect the neonates' heart rate or oxygen saturation values. Because breast-feeding did decrease neonate crying time during immunizations, nurses might encourage mothers to implement this safe, easy, effective intervention in practice.

Null versus Research Hypotheses

The null hypothesis (H_0), also referred to as a statistical hypothesis, is used for statistical testing and interpretation of these results. Even if the null hypothesis is not stated, it is implied, because it is the converse of the research hypothesis (Kerlinger & Lee, 2000; Shadish et al., 2002). A null hypothesis can be simple or complex and associative or causal. An associative null hypothesis states that there is no relationship between the variables studied. A causal null hypothesis might be stated in one of the following formats:
1. The independent variable has no effect on the dependent variable.
2. The experimental group, who received the independent variable, is no different from the control or comparison group for the dependent variable.

Youngkin and Lester (2010, p. 5) conducted a study to "(a) determine if nonpregnant, childbearing-age women could accurately self-screen to predict BV [bacterial vaginosis] using a researcher-developed home self-test system comprised of three integrated components—education, application of self-test method, and scoring of self-test findings using a unique scoring system—and (b) determine if the women would seek early professional diagnosis and treatment." These researchers developed two hypotheses to direct their study:

> "The researchers expected to find a significant positive correlation between the self-screening scores from the women and the follow-up evaluation scores from the nurse researchers using the self-test system. It was further expected that there would be no significant differences between the women's scores on the criteria using the scoring method and the related researchers' scores." (Youngkin & Lester, 2010, p. 5)

The first hypothesis is associative (identifies a relationship between women's scores and researchers' scores on the self-test system), simple (includes two variables), and directional (examines positive correlation or relationship). The second hypothesis is a null hypothesis that states there is no difference between the women's and the researchers' scores on the basis of the scoring method. Null hypothesis is nondirectional since it states that no relationship exists between variables or that no difference exists between groups. Research hypotheses are supported or not supported and null hypotheses are accepted or rejected on the basis of statistical results. Youngkin and Lester (2010) stated a simple null hypothesis about no difference between the women's and researchers' scores on the basis of previous research and their clinical expertise. The researchers found that the women accurately tested themselves for BV using the self-test system and appropriately sought definitive professional diagnosis and treatment. Thus, the research hypothesis was supported and the null hypothesis was accepted on the basis of study results.

A **research hypothesis** is the alternative hypothesis (H_1 or H_a) to the null. The research hypothesis states that there is a relationship between two or more variables, and it can be simple or complex, nondirectional or directional, and associative or causal. The prediction in a research hypothesis might be based on theoretical statements, previous research findings, and/or clinical experience. All the previous examples of hypotheses presented in this chapter are research hypotheses except for the one null hypothesis formulated by Youngkin and Lester (2010).

Researchers have different beliefs about when to state a research hypothesis versus a null hypothesis. Some researchers state the null hypothesis because it is more easily interpreted on the basis of the results of statistical analyses. A researcher will also use the null hypothesis when she or he believes there is no relationship between two or more variables and when there is inadequate theoretical or empirical information to state a research hypothesis. Otherwise it is best to state a research hypothesis that clearly predicts the outcome of a study. As previously discussed, Youngkin and Lester (2010) stated both a research hypothesis and a null hypothesis based on previous research and clinical expertise. They expected both hypotheses to be supported by their study results, and they were.

Developing Hypotheses

Developing hypotheses requires inductive and deductive thinking. Most people have a predominant way of thinking and will use that thinking pattern in developing hypotheses. *Inductive* thinkers have a tendency to focus on the relationships they observe in clinical practice, and they synthesize these observations to formulate a general statement about the relationships. For example, inductive thinkers might note that elderly patients who are not instructed in the importance of early postoperative ambulation are slow to get out of bed. *Deductive* thinkers examine more abstract statements from theories or previous research and then formulate a hypothesis for study (Smith & Liehr, 2008). Deductive thinkers might translate a statement or proposition, such as "People who receive education about self-care are more capable in caring for themselves," from Orem's (2001) theory into a hypothesis.

The inductive thinker must link the relational statement or hypothesis that was developed from clinical observations with a theoretical framework. Making this connection with the framework requires deductive thinking and improves the usefulness of the study findings. The deductive thinker must use inductive thinking to determine whether the proposition from a theory accurately predicts the relationship of events in clinical practice. Without this real-world experience, the selection of subjects and the identification of ways to measure the variables would be unclear. An example hypothesis is, "Elderly patients receiving an activity educational program before surgery ambulate earlier and have a shorter hospital stay after surgery than elderly patients receiving standard care."

In formulating a hypothesis, you as a researcher will have several decisions to make. These decisions are directed by the problem studied and by your own expertise and preference. You must decide whether the problem is best investigated with the use of simple or complex hypotheses. Complex hypotheses frequently require complex methodology, and the outcomes may be difficult to interpret. Some beginning researchers prefer the clarity of simple hypotheses.

The research problem and purpose determine whether you will study an associative or a causal relationship. Testing a hypothesis that states a causal relationship requires expertise in implementing a treatment and controlling extraneous variables. Another decision you must make involves the formulation of a research or a null hypothesis. You must make this decision according to what you believe is the most accurate prediction of the relationship between the study variables.

A hypothesis that is clearly and concisely stated gives the greatest direction for conducting a study. For clarity, hypotheses are expressed as declarative statements written in the present tense. Thus, hypotheses are best developed without the phrase "There *will/will not be* a relationship…," because the future tense refers to the sample being studied. Hypotheses are statements of relationships about populations, not about study samples. According to mathematical theory regarding generalization, one cannot generalize to the future (Kerlinger & Lee, 2000).

Hypotheses are clearer without the phrase "There is no *significant* difference…," because the level of significance is only a statistical technique applied to sample data. In addition, hypotheses should not identify methodological points, such as techniques of sampling, measurement, and data analysis (Kerlinger & Lee, 2000). Therefore, a statement such as "*measured by*," "in a *random sample* of," or "*using ANOVA* (analysis of variance)" are not appropriate. Such a phrase limits the hypothesis to measurement methods, sampling methods, or data analysis techniques in a single study. A well-formulated hypothesis clearly identifies the relationship between the variables and the study population. There is no set number for how many hypotheses are needed to direct a study, but the number formulated usually reflects the researcher's expertise and the complexity of the problem and purpose being studied. However, most studies contain one to three hypotheses, and the relationships identified in these hypotheses set the limits for a study (Fawcett & Garity, 2009; Shadish et al., 2002).

Testing Hypotheses

A hypothesis's value is ultimately derived from whether or not it can be tested in the real world. A testable hypothesis contains variables that can be measured or manipulated in practice. For example, Efe and Özer (2007) manipulated the breast-feeding intervention in their study using set protocol so that the treatment was consistently manipulated for each study situation. They measured crying time in seconds and measured the heart rate and oxygen saturation with a pulse oximeter (Nellcor N180).

Hypotheses are evaluated with statistical analyses. If the hypothesis states an associative relationship, correlational analyses are usually conducted on the data. Spearman's rank order correlation coefficient is often used to analyze ordinal level data, and Pearson's product-moment correlation coefficient is used for interval and ratio level data (see Chapter 23). These correlational analyses determine the existence, type, and degree of the relationship between the variables studied.

A hypothesis that states a causal relationship is analyzed through the use of statistics that examine differences, such as the Mann-Whitney U test, the t test, and analysis of variance (ANOVA) (see Chapter 25). It is the null hypothesis (stated or implied) that is tested through statistical analysis. The intent is to determine whether the independent variable had a significant effect on the dependent variable. The level of significance, alpha (α) = 0.05, 0.01, 0.001, is set after the generation of causal hypotheses and before the conduct of the study. To learn more about selecting statistical tests and a level of significance for testing hypotheses, see Chapter 21.

The results obtained from testing a hypothesis are described with the use of certain terminology. Research findings do not prove hypotheses true or false; instead, hypotheses are statements of relationships or differences in populations. Even after a series of studies, the word *proven* is not used in scientific language because of the tentative nature of science. Research hypotheses are described as being *supported* or *not supported* in a study. When a null hypothesis is tested, it is either *rejected* or *accepted*. Accepting the null hypothesis indicates that no relationship or effect was found among the variables. Rejecting the null hypothesis indicates the possibility that a relationship or difference exists. A study might partially support a complex hypothesis. Efe and Özer's (2007, p. 11) hypothesis stated that "breast-feeding decreases the length of crying time, prevents an increase in heart rate, and prevents a decrease in oxygen saturation during vaccination as compared with the control condition (i.e., no breast-feeding)." Their study supported the decreased crying time part of the hypothesis, but it did not support the part of the hypothesis that focused on the prevention of increased heart rate and decreased oxygen saturation. However, the study did provide valuable evidence about the effectiveness of breast-feeding in reducing the pain of immunization injections in infants. In addition, this study provides direction for future research.

Selecting Objectives, Questions, or Hypotheses for Quantitative or Qualitative Research

Selecting objectives, questions, or hypotheses for a study is often based on (1) the number and quality of relevant studies conducted on a selected problem (existing knowledge base), (2) the framework of the study, (3) the expertise and preference of the researcher, and (4) the type of study to be conducted (quantitative or qualitative). Commonly, if minimal or no research has been conducted on a problem, investigators state objectives or questions because they do not have the knowledge necessary to formulate hypotheses. The framework for a study indicates whether the intent is to develop or to test theory. Objectives and questions are usually stated to guide theory development, and the focus of a hypothesis is to test theory.

Researcher expertise and preference can also influence the selection of objectives, questions, or hypotheses to direct a study. The number of nursing studies containing hypotheses continues to grow, and there appears to be a trend away from descriptive quantitative studies toward studies focused on examining relationships between variables and testing hypotheses. The greater use of hypotheses to direct quantitative, outcomes, and intervention research indicates growth of knowledge in selected problem areas and the increasing sophistication of nurse researchers (Doran, 2011; Forbes, 2009). However, it is important that researchers state hypotheses to direct their studies explicitly versus implicitly or through implication. An explicit statement of hypotheses is important to provide clear direction for the conduct of a study, the interpretation of the findings, and the use of the findings in practice (Brown, 2009; Craig & Smyth, 2012; Fawcett & Garity, 2009).

The objectives, questions, or hypotheses designated for study frequently indicate a pattern that the researcher uses in conducting investigations. Problems can be investigated in a variety of ways. Some researchers start at the core of a problem and work their way outward. Other investigators study a problem from the outside edge and work to the core (Kaplan, 1964). Each study must logically build on the other, as the researcher establishes a pattern for studying a problem area that will affect the quality and quantity of the knowledge generated in that area.

Researchers select objectives, questions, or hypotheses according to the type of study they plan to conduct. Objectives and questions are typically stated when the intent of the study is to identify or describe

TABLE 8-1	Selecting Objectives, Questions, or Hypotheses for Different Types of Research
Type of Research	**Objectives, Questions, or Hypotheses Commonly Developed**
Qualitative research	Objectives, questions, or none
Quantitative research:	
Descriptive studies	Objectives, questions, or none
Correlational studies	Objectives, questions, hypotheses, or none
Quasi-experimental studies	Usually hypotheses
Experimental studies	Hypotheses
Outcomes research	Hypotheses or questions
Intervention research	Hypotheses

characteristics of variables, to examine relationships among variables, or both. Thus, objectives or questions are formulated to direct qualitative and selected quantitative (descriptive and correlational) studies (see Table 8-1). However, some experienced researchers can clearly focus and develop a study without using objectives or questions. In these studies, the research purpose directs the research process.

In some qualitative research, the investigator uses only a problem and purpose to direct the study. The specification of objectives or questions might limit the scope of the study and the methods of data collection and analysis (Munhall, 2012). Discovery is important in qualitative research, and hypotheses are neither necessary nor desirable in qualitative studies.

Researchers often develop hypotheses when the relationships or results of a study can be anticipated or predicted. Hypotheses are typically used in quantitative research to direct predictive correlational, quasi-experimental, and experimental studies and are also important to guide outcomes and intervention studies (Doran, 2011; Forbes, 2009; Shadish et al., 2002).

Identifying and Defining Study Variables

The research purpose and objectives, questions, and hypotheses identify the variables or concepts to be examined in a study. **Variables** are qualities, properties, or characteristics of persons, things, or situations that change or vary in a study. Variables are characterized by degrees, amounts, and differences within a study. Variables are also concepts of various levels of abstraction that are concisely defined so that they can be measured or manipulated within a study (Waltz, Strickland, & Lenz, 2010).

The concepts examined in research can be concrete and directly measurable in practice, such as heart rate, hemoglobin value, and tidal volume of the lung. These concrete concepts are usually referred to as *variables* in a study. Other concepts, such as anxiety, coping, and pain, are more abstract and are indirectly observable in the real world. Thus, the properties of these concepts are inferred from a combination of measurements. For example, one can infer the properties of anxiety by combining information obtained from (1) observing the signs and symptoms of anxiety (frequent movements, sweating, rapid eye movement, lack of eye contact, and verbalization of anxiety), (2) examining completed questionnaires or scales (state and trait anxiety scales), and (3) measuring physiological responses (galvanic skin response). The concept of anxiety might be represented by the variable "reported anxiety" or "perceived level of anxiety" (Waltz et al., 2010).

In many qualitative studies and in some quantitative studies (descriptive and correlational), the focus is abstract concepts, such as grieving, caring, and promoting health (Creswell, 2009; Munhall, 2012). Researchers identify the elements of the study as **concepts**, not variables. In the ethnographic study previously described, Happ et al. (2007) investigated the concept of health-related decision making by critically ill patients during prolonged mechanical ventilation. The concept *health-related decision making* was defined as "choices about initiating, continuing, or discontinuing treatment, diagnostics, or therapeutic care activities" (p. 363). Qualitative studies are often conducted to clarify the definitions of concepts so these definitions are usually presented in the results section of the study. In the results of this study, health-related decision making was described as including the following: "choices about mechanical ventilation and other therapies, such as invasive diagnostic procedures and placement of central lines and nutritional access devices that may or may not require written informed consent, and about discharge placement. Financial or legal decisions, such as appointment of a power of attorney or signing financial documents to enable insurance payment for health care, were considered health-related in the context of prolonged critical illness" (Happ et al., 2007, p. 363).

Types of Variables

Variables have been classified into a variety of types to explain their use in research. Some variables are manipulated; others are controlled. Some variables are identified but not measured; others are measured with refined measurement devices. The different types of variables presented in this section include the following: independent, dependent, research, extraneous, demographic, moderator, and mediator.

Independent and Dependent Variables

The relationship between independent and dependent variables is the basis for formulating hypotheses for predictive correlational, quasi-experimental, and experimental studies. As introduced earlier in this chapter, an **independent variable** is an intervention or treatment manipulated by the researcher to create an effect on the dependent variable. A **dependent variable** is the outcome the researcher wants to predict or explain. Changes measured in the dependent variable are presumed to be caused by the independent variable (Kerlinger & Lee, 2000; Shadish et al., 2002).

Recall the quasi-experimental study by Scott et al. (2011) introduced earlier in this chapter that included independent and dependent variables. These variables were identified in the study's complex, causal, directional research hypothesis that focused on the effect of the FCMPN on sleep duration, sleep quality, daytime sleepiness, drowsiness episodes, risk of auto accident, and actual and near reported work errors. The independent variable that was manipulated in this study was the FCMPN, and the effect of this program was determined by measuring the dependent variables sleep duration, sleep quality, daytime sleepiness, drowsiness episodes, risk of auto accident, and actual and near errors (see the previous figure showing these variables).

Research Variables or Concepts

Qualitative studies and some quantitative (descriptive and correlational) studies involve the investigation of research variables or concepts. **Research variables or concepts** are the qualities, properties, or characteristics identified in the research purpose and objectives or questions that are measured in a study. They are used when the intent of the study is to measure variables as they exist in a natural setting without the implementation of a treatment. Thus, no independent variables are manipulated, and no cause-and-effect relationships are examined.

Qualitative studies often focus on abstract concepts. For example, Hudson et al. (2010) conducted an exploratory-descriptive qualitative study to describe the concept of "health-seeking challenges" among homeless youth. This study, also introduced earlier in the chapter, focused on gaining an understanding of the perceptions of homeless youth regarding their healthcare-seeking behaviors. The study results described the concept of "health-seeking challenges" with a discussion of the young adults' perspectives on the facilitators and barriers to receiving health care.

Extraneous Variables

Extraneous variables exist in all studies and can affect the selection of study participants, implementation of the study intervention, measurement of study variables, and implementation of study procedures. Extraneous variables are of primary concern in quantitative and intervention studies, because they can obscure one's understanding of the relational or causal dynamics within the studies. Extraneous variables are classified as (1) recognized or unrecognized and (2) controlled or uncontrolled.

The extraneous variables that are not recognized until the study is in process or that are recognized before the study is initiated but cannot be controlled are referred to as confounding variables. Sometimes these variables can be measured during the study and controlled statistically during analysis. In other cases, it is not possible to measure a confounding variable, and the variable thus hinders the interpretation of findings. Such extraneous variables must be identified as limitations or areas of study weakness in the discussion section of a research report. As control decreases in quasi-experimental and experimental studies, the potential influence of confounding variables increases.

Researchers attempt to recognize and control as many extraneous variables as possible in quasi-experimental and experimental studies, and specific designs have been developed to control the influence of such variables (see Chapter 11). Youngkin and Lester (2010) conducted a quasi-experimental study to determine the effectiveness of a home self-test system in screening for bacterial vaginosis (BV). The research and null hypotheses developed to direct this study were introduced earlier, in the discussion of the null hypothesis. These researchers controlled some of the extraneous variables in their study by selecting inclusion and exclusion sample criteria to ensure that study participants were similar or homogeneous. The home self-test system for BV was implemented using a detailed protocol to ensure that all participants received consistent, complete implementation of the intervention (Fawcett & Garity, 2009). The intervention was implemented on the basis of the Centers for Disease Control (CDC) 2002 guidelines, which are the same as the Centers for Disease Control and Prevention 2006 guidelines. The researchers used a structured scoring process for determining the incidence of

BV that reduced the potential for measurement error (see Figure 8-3) (Waltz et al., 2010). The design of the study ensured the blinding of researchers to the participants' scores on their home self-test for BV before they determined their own score. The following study excerpts identify the controls the researchers used in their study to decrease the effect of extraneous variables and increase the likelihood that the findings are an accurate reflection of reality and not due to error:

Sample Criteria

"Study eligibility was female participants who were (a) volunteers, (b) aged 18 to 45 years, (c) not pregnant, and (d) able to read and understand English. A prior history of vaginitis or vaginosis was not required for eligibility. Participants came from three clinical sites: a university college of nursing community wellness center, a private family practice, and a university student health service site." (Youngkin & Lester, 2010, p. 5)

Intervention

"The researchers provided the educational component about BV, the BV home self-test system and safe and correct use of the system, interpretation of self-test results and scoring findings, and how to follow up for provider evaluation after self-testing. Visual and verbal instruction methods were employed.... The BV self-test kit was provided free, and all components were reviewed with the specific regimen for use. Researchers selected the kit contents with consideration for cost, future use, and ease of use. Ten applications of self-testing materials and scoring sheets were provided in the kit along with educational materials, a copy of the signed consent form, laminated instructions for kit use, and a listing of contents. Directions for follow-up with the researcher clinicians were on the outside of each kit." (Youngkin & Lester, 2010, p. 5)

Measurement with BV Scoring Sheet

"The women were taught how to safely obtain a vaginal specimen using directions outlined on a card in the kit and to test and score the specimen using the criteria of (a) discharge color and consistency, (b) pH level, and (c) amine odor. The tests and scoring were specific to these three of the four criteria that CDC guidelines (2002) advised for providers to use for clinical diagnosis. Figure 8-3 provides an example of the scoring sheet. The specifics of the scoring

BACTERIAL VAGINOSIS SELF-DIAGNOSIS SCORING SHEET

Please mark the correct item by putting in the points in the blank space beside the item. For instance, if the color of the strip of paper with your discharge is the number 4.5 or a smaller number, please put a "1" in the first column, but if it is a color indicating a higher number, put a 2 in the second column. If the color of the discharge is milky or creamy white or gray, put a 2 in the second colomn. If it is any other color, put a 1 in the first column. If there is no fishy odor, put a 1 in the first column. If there is a fishy odor, put a 2 in the second column.

Remember: don't worry about what you think you have; just put the number that "fits" the characteristic the best in either Column 1 or 2. You should have only one number for the characteristic.

Add the numbers in the two columns up, then, add these two numbers together for the final score. For example, if the total for Column 1 is a 2 and the total for Column 2 is 2, then the total score is 4.

Characterisitic	Column 1 (non BV)	Column 2 (BV)
	Put a 1 in the column beside the correct finding	*Put a 2 in the column beside the correct finding*
Color of paper from dispenser after it is wet from vaginal discharge	4.5 or under _____	5 or higher _____
Color of discharge on cotton of applicator	yellow, green, _____ clumpy white, brown, red	white or gray smooth or creamy or frothy _____
Fishy smell when discharge is mixed with the KOH drop	No fishy smell _____	Fishy smell _____
Scores	Column 1 _____	Column 2 _____

Add the scores from Column 1 and 2 together. The Total Score is _____

If your score is 4, 5, or 6, please make an appointment to see the clinician listed on the front of your BV Self-Diagnosis Kit.

Figure 8-3 Scoring sheet for BV [bacterial vaginosis] home self-test. (From Youngkin, E. Q., & Lester, P. B. [2010]. Promoting self-care and secondary prevention in women's health: A study to test the accuracy of a home self-test system for bacterial vaginosis. *Applied Nursing Research, 23*[1], 6.)

method developed by the researchers and the form for recording the self-test findings were taught as the last component of the BV home self-test system.... Thus, higher total scores would be associated with a greater chance of BV if the woman was accurately testing herself. The provider's scoring would either support or not support the self-test scoring.... The women brought their scored results sheets with them; the researchers did not review these results until after the professional examination was completed and the findings had been scored on separate scoring form." (Youngkin & Lester, 2010, pp. 5-6)

Environmental variables are types of extraneous variables that make up the setting in which the study is conducted. Examples are climate, home, healthcare system, community setting, and governmental organizations. If a researcher is studying humans in an uncontrolled or natural setting, it is impossible and sometimes undesirable to control most of the environmental variables. In qualitative and some quantitative (descriptive and correlational) studies, researchers make little or no attempt to control environmental variables. Their intent is to study subjects in their natural environment without controlling or altering it. The environmental variables in quasi-experimental and experimental research can be controlled through the use of a study protocol and a laboratory setting or a specially constructed research unit in a hospital.

Demographic Variables

Demographic variables are attributes of the subjects that are measured during the study and used to describe the sample. Some common demographic variables examined in nursing research are age, gender, ethnicity, educational level, income, job classification, length of hospital stay, and medical diagnosis. Researchers select demographic variables according to the focus of their study, the demographic variables included in previous studies, and clinical experience. However, age, gender, and ethnicity are essential demographic variables to examine in all types of research. These demographics describe the sample and determine the population for generalization of the findings. More research is needed to improve health care for elderly, women, children, and minorities, and funding agencies often give priority to studies that focus on these individuals.

To obtain data on demographic variables, researchers ask subjects to complete a demographic or information sheet. When the study is completed, the demographic information is analyzed to provide a picture of the sample, which is called the sample characteristics. Sample characteristics are presented in a table and/or discussed in the narrative of the research report. As previously discussed, Scott et al. (2010) implemented the FCMPN intervention to improve staff nurses' sleep duration, sleep quality, daytime sleepiness, drowsiness episodes, risk for auto accident, and actual and near work errors. These researchers summarized their sample characteristics in a table (see Table 8-2) and discussed them in the narrative of their article, as follows:

"Most participants were White (96.8%) and women (96.8%), with an average age of 37.74 years (range = 22-63 years, SD = 11.70 years). Fifty-two (83.9%) of the nurses reported being employed in 12-hour day shifts positions. Although all three work shifts were represented, the nurses worked predominantly 12-hour day shifts (e.g., 7:00 a.m.-7:30 p.m.; n = 25) or night shift (e.g., 7:00 p.m.-7:30 a.m.; n = 29). Only 4 nurses (6.5%) reported working evening shifts. The average length of experience as hospital staff nurses was 9.82 years (range = 1-43 years, SD = 11.83 years). Although the nurses were employed in full-time positions, 4 nurses (6.5%) reported working a second job. No significant differences were noted between participants across the three sites before data aggregation." (Scott et al., 2010, p. 252)

TABLE 8-2	Demographic Summary of Study Participants	
Attribute	**Initial Respondents (n = 62)**	**Intervention Respondents (n = 47)**
Age (years)	37.74 ± 11.70	38.98 ± 12.21
Time as a registered nurse (years)	9.82 ± 10.95	10.95 ± 11.87
Shift length (hours):		
8	9	7
12	52	40
Shift pattern:		
Days	25	17
Evenings	4	2
Nights	29	25
Rotating	0	0
Relationship/marital status:		
Single	15	12
Spouse or significant other	47	35
Additional employment	4 (6.5%)	3 (6.4%)

Note: Frequencies may not match sample size due to missing data.
Adapted from Scott, L. D., Hofmeister, N., Rogness, N., & Rogers, A. E. (2010). An interventional approach for patient and nurse safety: A fatigue countermeasures feasibility study. *Nursing Research, 59*(4), 252.

The demographic variables in this study were ethnicity, gender, age, time as a registered nurse in years, shift length in hours, shift pattern, relationship/marital status, and additional employment (see description of sample and Table 8-2). The participants from three different sites were compared and found to have no differences in demographic variables at the start of the study. These demographic variables seem appropriate to describe the sample of staff nurses for this study. It was important to ensure that the participants from the three different settings were similar at the start of the study so significant differences in the dependent variables might be assumed to be caused by the FCMPN intervention and not due to demographical differences.

Moderator and Mediator Variables

Moderator and mediator variables are examined in intervention effectiveness research to improve our understanding of the effect of the intervention on practice-related outcomes. A moderator variable occurs with the intervention (independent variable) and alters the causal relationship between the intervention and the outcomes. Moderator variables include

TABLE 8-3 Conceptual and Study Variables, Instruments, and Scores or Measurement

Concepts	Variables	Instruments	Possible Scores and Measurement
Sleep loss (deprivation or disruption)	Sleep duration	Logbook (self-report sleep times)	Total sleep duration
	Sleep quality	Pittsburgh Sleep Quality Index	Global score = 0-21
Cognitive-behavioral outcomes	Daytime sleepiness	Epworth Sleepiness Scale	Summative score = 0-24
	Vigilance (inability to remain alert)	Drowsiness and unplanned sleep episodes at work and while driving	Frequencies
	Short-term memory	Logbook (accident or error data)	Frequencies
	Problem solving and coping	Logbook (error description)	Frequencies

From Scott, L. D., Hofmeister, N., Rogness, N., & Rogers, A. E. (2010). An interventional approach for patient and nurse safety: A fatigue countermeasures feasibility study. *Nursing Research, 59*(4), 253.

characteristics of the subjects and of the person implementing the intervention. Mediator variables bring about the effects of the intervention after it has occurred and thus influence the outcomes of the study. The theoretical model that provides the framework for the study usually identifies the relevant moderator and mediator variables to be examined in the study. The design is developed to examine not only the independent (intervention) and dependent (outcomes) variables but also the moderator and mediator variables (see Chapter 14 for a detailed discussion of intervention research).

Operationalizing Variables or Concepts for a Study

Conceptual and Operational Definitions of Variables in Quantitative Studies

Operationalizing a variable or concept in quantitative studies involves developing conceptual and operational definitions. A conceptual definition provides the theoretical meaning of a concept or variable and is derived from a theorist's definition of that concept or is developed through concept analysis. The study framework, which includes concepts and their definitions, provides a basis for conceptually defining the variables. The Scott et al. (2010) study described previously in the sections on causal hypotheses, independent and dependent variables, and demographic variables is presented here as an example of how to operationalize study variables. These researchers implemented the FCMPN intervention with staff nurses to improve the following outcomes: sleep duration, sleep quality, daytime sleepiness, episodes of drowsiness, risk of auto accident, and actual and near work errors. These researchers linked their framework concepts, variables, instruments of measurement, and possible scores and measurement in Table 8-3. Conceptual and operational definitions of the independent variable and three dependent variables in this study are as follows:

Independent Variable: Fatigue Countermeasures Program for Nurses (FCMPN)

Conceptual definition: The FCMPN evolved from the model of impaired sleep by Lee and colleagues (2004). The FCMPN was thought to have the potential to decrease sleep loss and improve sleep quality and their associated cognitive-behavioral responses (Scott et al., 2010).

Operational definition: "Comprehensive program to manage fatigue in work settings usually includes the following six elements: (a) education and training, (b) compliance with hours of service regulations, (c) appropriate scheduling practices, (d) countermeasures that can be instituted in the work setting, (e) design, and (f) research.... The FCMPN used in this study is modeled after the National Aeronautics and Space Administration Ames Research Center's Fatigue Countermeasures Program . . . with additional content obtained from the Sleep, Alertness, and Fatigue Education in Residency Program (American Academy of Sleep Medicine, 2006)." (Scott et al., 2010, pp. 252-253)

Dependent Variables

Sleep Duration

Conceptual definition: Sleep duration is an indication of the sleep loss (deprivation and/or disruption) and fatigue that is experienced by an employee (see Table 8-3 for the link of the model concepts to this study variable).

Operational definition: Sleep duration was measured by self-report in a Logbook that involved the participants completing 15 items about their sleep patterns (Scott et al., 2010).

Daytime Sleepiness

Conceptual definition: Daytime sleepiness is a cognitive-behavior outcome resulting from employees who experience sleep loss or poor quality sleep.

Operational definition: Daytime sleepiness was measured with the Epworth Sleepiness Scale with a summative score equal to 0 through 24.

Episodes of Drowsiness

Conceptual definition: Vigilance is a cognitive-behavioral outcome that focuses on the ability and inability to remain alert at work without drowsiness.

Operational definition: Vigilance was measured by the drowsiness and unplanned sleep episodes at work and while driving. These were part of the self-report items in the participants' Logbook.

The variables in quasi-experimental and experimental quantitative research, outcomes research, and intervention research are narrow and specific in focus and are capable of being quantified (converted to numbers) or manipulated through the use of specified steps. In addition, the variables are objectively defined to reduce researcher bias.

Conceptual Definitions in Qualitative Studies

The concepts in qualitative studies are usually more abstract and broadly defined than the variables in quantitative, outcomes, and intervention studies. Many researchers believe that the concepts in qualitative studies do not have operational definitions because sensitizing or experiencing the real situation rather than operationalizing the concepts is most important. Operational definitions are not appropriate because they are thought to limit the investigation so that a phenomenon, such as pain, or a characteristic of a culture, such as health practices, is not completely experienced or understood. In qualitative research, often the phenomenon being studied is not clearly identified and/or

defined until the results of the study are determined (Marshall & Ross, 2011; Munhall, 2012). Thus, some concepts may not be clearly conceptually defined until late in the conduct of the study. For example, Hudson et al. (2010) developed the following description of the health-seeking challenges among homeless youth during their discussion of study results:

Conceptual Definition of Health-Seeking Challenges among Homeless Youth

"Participants were quite verbal in expressing their perspectives and experiences in order that positive changes could be made. The major themes expressed related to the issues they experienced in accessing health care, followed by barriers that were experienced, as well as a pervasive sense of stigma and discrimination, which was quite telling...

Failing Access to Health Care

"Homeless young adults revealed that accessing health care was challenging due to scarcity of service sites and generally long waiting times for services, yet homeless young adults experienced a number of health problems ranging from chronic conditions such as migraine headaches to more serious conditions of asthma and meningitis. Mental health issues were reported most commonly....

Needing More Help

"Homeless young persons experienced a number of unmet needs.... Despite their hardships, young adults craved for support from family, friends, and homeless peers....

Perceiving Stigma

"The youth were most frustrated by the discrimination they experienced from passersby and law enforcement. Rather than provide resources for homeless youth, youth frequently were confronted with unforgettable comments that were full of judgment....

Making it Work

"Regardless of the challenges experienced, homeless young adults were able to deal with life in the only ways they knew how and were grateful for the help and support of others. For several homeless young adults, they were grateful for the information they received from the more experienced homeless young persons in terms of when services were available and where to go." (Hudson et al., 2010, pp. 215-216)

-------- **KEY POINTS** --------

- Research objectives, questions, and hypotheses are formulated to bridge the gap between the more abstractly stated research problem and purpose and the detailed design and plan for data collection and analysis.
- Research objectives are clear, concise, declarative statements that are expressed in the present tense to provide specific focus to the conduct of a study.
- A research question is a concise, interrogative statement that is worded in the present tense and consists of one or more variables (or concepts).
- A hypothesis is the formal statement of the expected relationships between two or more variables in a selected population.
- Hypotheses can be described in terms of four categories: (1) associative versus causal, (2) simple versus complex, (3) nondirectional versus directional, and (4) null versus research.
- Selecting objectives, questions, or hypotheses for a study is based on (1) the number and quality of relevant studies conducted on a selected problem (existing knowledge base), (2) the framework of the study, (3) the expertise and preference of the researcher, and (4) the type of study to be conducted (quantitative, qualitative, outcomes, and intervention).
- Variables are qualities, properties, or characteristics of persons, things, or situations that change or vary in a study.
- The types of variables discussed in this chapter are independent, dependent, research, extraneous, demographic, moderator, and mediator.
- An independent variable is an intervention or experimental treatment that the researcher manipulates or varies to create an effect on the dependent variable.
- A dependent variable is the outcome, response, or behavior that the researcher wants to predict or explain and is measured in the study.
- Research variables or concepts are the qualities, properties, or characteristics that are measured in selected quantitative studies (descriptive and correlational).
- Demographic variables are attributes of the research participants that are measured in a study to describe the sample. The summary of the data collected on demographic variables is called sample characteristics and is used to describe the sample.
- The variables in quantitative studies require conceptual and operational definitions, and a conceptual definition provides the theoretical meaning of a concept or variable and is derived from a theorist's definition of the concept or is developed through concept analysis.
- An operational definition is derived from a set of procedures or progressive acts that a researcher performs either to manipulate an independent variable or to measure the existence or degree of existence of the dependent variable or research variable.
- Concepts in qualitative research are usually conceptually defined when the results or findings of the study are presented.

REFERENCES

American Academy of Sleep Medicine. (2006). *Sleep Alertness & Fatigue Education in Residency (SAFER)*. Retrieved from http://www.aAmsment.org/.

Bowles, K. H., Pham, J., O'Connor, M., & Horowitz, D. A. 2010. Information deficits in home care: A barrier to evidence-based disease management. *Home Health Care Management and Practice, 22*(4), 278–285.

Brown, S. J. (2009). *Evidence-based nursing: The research-practice connection.* Sudbury, MA: Jones and Bartlett Publishers.

Bucher, C. E. (2008). Toward a needs-based typology of homeless youth. *Journal of Adolescent Health, 42*(6), 549–554.

Centers for Disease Control. (2002). Sexually transmitted diseases treatment guidelines 2002. *Morbidity and Mortality Weekly Report, 52*(RR-6), 42–44.

Centers for Disease Control and Prevention. (2006). Sexually transmitted disease treatment guidelines, 2006. *Morbidity and Mortality Weekly Report, 53*(3), 1–94.

Chinn, P. L., & Kramer, M. K. (2008). *Integrated theory and knowledge development* (7th ed.). St. Louis: Mosby.

Craig, J. V., & Smyth, R. L. (2012). *The evidence-based practice manual for nurses* (3rd ed.). Edinburgh, Scotland: Churchill Livingstone.

Creswell, J. W. (2009). *Research design: Qualitative, quantitative, and mixed methods approaches* (3rd ed.). Los Angeles, CA: Sage.

Delaney, C., Apostolidis, B., Lachapelle, L., & Fortinsky, R. (2011). Home care nurses' knowledge of evidence-based education topics for management of heart failure. *Heart & Lung, 40*(4), 285–292.

Diefenbach, M. A., & Leventhal, H. (1996). The Common-Sense Model of Illness Representation: Theoretical and practical considerations. *Journal of Social Distress and the Homeless, 5*(1), 11–38.

Doran, D. (2011). *Nursing-sensitive outcomes: The state of the science* (2nd ed.). Sudbury, MA: Jones & Bartlett Learning.

Efe, E., & Özer, Z. C. (2007). The use of breast-feeding for pain relief during neonatal immunization injections. *Applied Nursing Research, 20*(1), 10–16.

Fagerhaugh, S. Y., & Strauss, A. (1977). *Politics of pain management.* Menlo Park, CA: Addison-Wesley.

Fawcett, J., & Garity, J. (2009). *Evaluating research for evidence-based nursing practice.* Philadelphia, PA: F. A. Davis.

Forbes, A. (2009). Clinical intervention research in nursing. *International Journal of Nursing Studies*, *46*(4), 557–568.

Happ, M. B., Swigart, V. A., Tate, J. A., Hoffman, L. A., & Arnold, R. M. (2007). Patient involvement in health-related decisions during prolonged critical illness. *Research in Nursing & Health*, *30*(4), 361–372.

Hodges, P. (2009). Heart failure: Epidemiologic update. *Critical Care Nursing Quarterly*, *32*(1), 24–32.

Hudson, A. L., Nyamathi, A., Greengold, B., Slagle, A., Koniak-Griffin, D., Khalilifard, F., et al. (2010). Health-seeking challenges among homeless youth. *Nursing Research*, *59*(3), 212–218.

Hudson, A. L., Nyamathi, A., & Sweat, J. (2008). Homeless youths' interpersonal perspectives of health care providers. *Issues in Mental Health Nursing*, *29*(12), 1277–1289.

Kaplan, A. (1964). *The conduct of inquiry: Methodology for behavioral science*. New York, NY: Harper & Row.

Kerlinger, F. N., & Lee, H. B. (2000). *Foundations of behavioral research* (4th ed.). Fort Worth, TX: Harcourt College Publishers.

Lee, K. A., Landis, C., Chasens, E. R., Dowling, G., Merritt, S., Parker, K. P., et al. (2004). Sleep and chronobiology: Recommendations for nursing education. *Nursing Outlook*, *52*(3), 126–133.

Marshall, C., & Rossman, G. B. (2011). *Designing qualitative research* (5th ed.). Los Angeles, CA: Sage.

Munhall, P. L. (2012). *Nursing research: A qualitative perspective* (5th ed.). Sudbury, MA: Jones & Bartlett Learning.

Orem, D. E. (2001). *Nursing concepts of practice*. St. Louis, MO: Mosby.

Reishtein, J. L. (2005). Relationship between symptoms and functional performance in COPD. *Research in Nursing & Health*, *28*(1), 39–47.

Ross, R., Sawatphanit, W., Mizuno, M., & Takeo, K. (2011). Depressive symptoms among HIV-positive postpartum women in Thailand. *Achieves of Psychiatric Nursing*, *25*(1), 36–42.

Rungruangsiripan, M., Sitthimongkol, Y., Maneesriwongul, W., Talley, S., & Vorapongsathorn, T. (2011). Mediating role of illness representation among social support, therapeutic alliance, experience of medication side effects, and medication adherence in persons with schizophrenia. *Archives of Psychiatric Nursing*, *25*(4), 269–283.

Schulz, P. S., Zimmerman, L., Pozehl, B., Barnason, S., & Nieveen, J. (2011). Symptom management strategies used by elderly patients after coronary artery bypass surgery. *Applied Nursing Research*, *24*(2), 65–73.

Scott, L. D., Hofmeister, N., Rogness, N., & Rogers, A. E. (2010). An interventional approach for patient and nurse safety: A fatigue countermeasures feasibility study. *Nursing Research*, *59*(4), 250–258.

Shadish, W. R., Cook, T. D., & Campbell, D. T. (2002). *Experimental and quasi-experimental designs for generalized causal inference*. Chicago, IL: Rand McNally.

Smith, M. J., & Liehr, P. R. (2008). *Middle range theory for nursing* (2nd ed.). New York, NY: Springer Publishing Company.

Sneller, V. P., Fischbein, D. B., Weinbaum, C. M., Lombard, A., Murray, P., McLaurin, J. A., et al. (2008). Vaccinating adolescents in high-risk settings: Lessons learned from experiences with hepatitis B vaccine. *Pediatrics*, *121*(Suppl. 1), S55–S62.

Tranmer, J. E., & Parry, M. J. (2004). Enhancing postoperative recovery of cardiac surgery patients: A randomized clinical trial of an advanced practice nursing intervention. *Western Journal of Nursing Research*, *26*(5), 515–532.

Vasan, R. S., Beiser, A., D'Agostino, R. B., Levy, D., Selhub, J., Jacques, P. F., et al. (2003). Plasma homocysteine and risk for congestive heart failure in adults without prior myocardial infarction. *Journal of the American Medical Association*, *289*(10), 1251–1257.

Waltz, C. F., Strickland, O. L., & Lenz, E. R. (2010). *Measurement in nursing and health research* (4th ed.). New York, NY: Springer.

Youngkin, E. Q., & Lester, P. B. (2010). Promoting self-care and secondary prevention in women's health: A study to test the accuracy of a home self-test system for bacterial vaginosis. *Applied Nursing Research*, *23*(1), 2–10.

Zimmerman, L., Barnason, S., Nieveen, J., & Schmaderer, M. (2004). Symptom management intervention in elderly coronary artery bypass graft patients. *Outcomes Management*, *8*(1), 5–12.

9

Ethics in Research

Nursing research requires not only expertise and diligence but also honesty and integrity. Conducting research ethically starts with the identification of the study topic and continues through the publication of the study. Over the years, ethical codes and regulations have been developed to provide guidelines for (1) selecting a study purpose, design, and subjects; (2) collecting and analyzing data; (3) interpreting study results; and (4) presenting and publishing a study. One of the more recent regulations, the Health Insurance Portability and Accountability Act (HIPAA), was enacted in 2003 to protect the privacy of an individual's health information. HIPAA has had an important impact on researchers and institutional review boards (IRBs) in universities and healthcare agencies. This chapter provides an overview of this act and the other United States and international regulations that have been developed to promote the ethical conduct of research.

An ethical problem that has received increasing attention since the 1980s is research misconduct. Misconduct has occurred during the conduct, reporting, and publication of studies, and the Office of Research Integrity (ORI, 2012) was developed to manage this problem. Many disciplines, including nursing, have experienced episodes of research misconduct that have affected the quality of research evidence generated and disseminated.

Ethical research is essential to generate a sound evidence-based practice for nursing, but what does the ethical conduct of research involve? This question has been debated for many years by researchers, politicians, philosophers, lawyers, and even research subjects. The debate continues, probably because of the complexity of human rights issues; the focus of research in new, challenging arenas of technology and genetics; the complex ethical codes and regulations governing research; and the various interpretations of these codes and regulations. Even though the phenomenon of the ethical conduct in research defies precise delineation, the historical events, ethical codes, and regulations presented in this chapter provide guidance for nurse researchers. The chapter also discusses the actions essential for conducting research ethically: (1) protecting the rights of human subjects; (2) balancing benefits and risks in a study; (3) obtaining informed consent from study participants; and (4) submitting a research proposal for institutional review. A discussion of current ethical issues related to research misconduct and animals used in research concludes the chapter.

Historical Events Affecting the Development of Ethical Codes and Regulations

The ethical conduct of research has been a focus since the 1940s because of the mistreatment of human subjects in selected studies. Four experimental projects have been highly publicized for their unethical treatment of subjects: (1) Nazi medical experiments; (2) the Tuskegee syphilis study; (3) the Willowbrook study; and (4) the Jewish Chronic Disease Hospital study. Although these were biomedical studies and the primary investigators were physicians, there is evidence that nurses were aware of the research, identified potential subjects, delivered treatments to the subjects, and served as data collectors in these projects. The four projects demonstrate the importance of ethical conduct for anyone reviewing, participating in, and conducting nursing or biomedical research. These four projects and other incidences of unethical treatment of subjects and research misconduct in the development, implementation, and reporting of research have influenced the formulation of ethical codes and regulations that direct research today. In addition, the concern for patient privacy with the electronic storage and exchange of health information has resulted in HIPAA privacy regulations (Olsen, 2003).

Nazi Medical Experiments

From 1933 to 1945, the Third Reich in Europe implemented atrocious, unethical activities (Steinfels & Levine, 1976). The programs of the Nazi regime consisted of sterilization, euthanasia, and numerous medical experiments to produce a population of racially pure Germans, or Aryans, who the Nazis maintained were destined to rule the world. The Nazis encouraged population growth among the Aryans ("good Nazis") and sterilized people they regarded as racial enemies, such as the Jews. They also practiced what they called "euthanasia," which involved killing various groups of people whom they considered racially impure, such as the insane, deformed, and senile. In addition, researchers conducted numerous medical experiments on prisoners of war as well as on racially "valueless" persons who had been confined to concentration camps.

The medical experiments involved exposing subjects to high altitudes, freezing temperatures, malaria, poisons, spotted fever (typhus), and untested drugs and operations, usually without any anesthesia (Steinfels & Levine, 1976). These medical experiments were conducted to generate knowledge about human beings, but the goal often was to destroy certain groups of people. Extensive examination of the records from some of these studies showed that they were poorly designed and conducted. Thus, they generated little if any useful scientific knowledge.

The Nazi experiments violated numerous rights of the research participants. Researchers selected subjects on the basis of their race, demonstrating an unfair selection process. The subjects also had no opportunity to refuse participation; they were prisoners who were coerced or forced to participate. The study participants were frequently killed during the experiments or sustained permanent physical, mental, and social damage (Levine, 1986; Steinfels & Levine, 1976). The mistreatment of human subjects in these Nazi studies led to the development of the Nuremberg Code in 1949.

Nuremberg Code

The people involved in the Nazi experiments were brought to trial before the Nuremberg Tribunals, which publicized their unethical activities. These unethical studies resulted in the **Nuremberg Code** (1949), which was developed with guidelines for (1) subjects' voluntary consent to participate in research; (2) the right of subjects to withdraw from studies; (3) the

protection of subjects from physical and mental suffering, injury, disability, and death during studies; and (4) the balance of benefits and risks in a study. Box 9-1 reproduces the Nuremberg Code, which was formulated mainly to direct the conduct of biomedical research worldwide; however, the rules it contains are essential to research in other sciences, such as nursing, psychology, and sociology.

Declaration of Helsinki

The Nuremberg Code provided the basis for the development of the **Declaration of Helsinki** in 1964 by the World Medical Association (WMA) General Assembly. Over the years, the Declaration of Helsinki has been amended as needed with the final amendment in 2008 (WMA General Assembly). This document differentiates therapeutic research from nontherapeutic research. **Therapeutic research** gives the patient an opportunity to receive an experimental treatment that might have beneficial results. **Nontherapeutic research** is conducted to generate knowledge for a discipline, and the results from the study might benefit future patients but will probably not benefit those acting as research subjects.

The Declaration of Helsinki includes ethical principles for medical research involving human subjects, such as the following: (1) well-being of the individual research subject must take precedence over all other interests; (2) a strong, independent justification must be documented prior to exposing healthy volunteers to risk of harm just to gain new scientific information; (3) investigators must protect the life, health, privacy, and dignity of research subjects; and (4) extreme care must be taken in making use of placebo-controlled trials, which should be used only in the absence of existing proven therapy (WMA General Assembly, 2008). Clinical trials must focus on improving diagnostic, therapeutic, and prophylactic procedures for patients with selected diseases without exposing subjects to any additional risk of serious or irreversible harm. Most institutions worldwide in which clinical research is conducted have adopted the Declaration of Helsinki. However, neither this document nor the Nuremberg Code has prevented some investigators from conducting unethical research (Beecher, 1966; ORI, 2012).

Tuskegee Syphilis Study

In 1932, the U.S. Public Health Service (U.S. PHS) initiated a study of syphilis in black men in the small, rural town of Tuskegee, Alabama (Brandt, 1978; Rothman, 1982). The study, which continued for 40 years, was conducted to determine the natural course

The Nuremberg Code

1. The voluntary consent of the human subject is absolutely essential.
2. The experiment should be such as to yield fruitful results for the good of society, unprocurable by other methods or means of study, and not random and unnecessary in nature.
3. The experiment should be so designed and based on the results of animal experimentation and knowledge of the natural history of the disease or other problem under study that the anticipated results will justify the performance of the experiment.
4. The experiment should be so conducted as to avoid all unnecessary physical and mental suffering and injury.
5. No experiment should be conducted where there is a prior reason to believe that death or disabling injury will occur, except, perhaps, in those experiments where the experimental physicians also serve as subjects.
6. The degree of risk to be taken should never exceed that determined by the humanitarian importance of the problem to be solved by the experiment.
7. Proper preparations should be made and adequate facilities provided to protect the experimental subject against even remote possibilities of injury, disability, or death.
8. The experiment should be conducted only by scientifically qualified persons. The highest degree of skill and care should be required through all stages of the experiment of those who conduct or engage in the experiment.
9. During the course of the experiment the human subject should be at liberty to bring the experiment to an end if he has reached the physical or mental state where continuation of the experiment seems to him to be impossible.
10. During the course of the experiment the scientist in charge must be prepared to terminate the experiment at any stage, if he has probable cause to believe, in the exercise of the good faith, superior skill, and careful judgment required of him, that a continuation of the experiment is likely to result in injury, disability, or death to the experimental subject.

From Nuremberg Code. (1949). *Trials of War Criminals before the Nuremberg Military Tribunals under Control Council Law No. 10, Vol. 2*, pp. 181–182. Washington, D.C.: U.S. Government Printing Office, 1949. Retrieved from http://ohsr.od.nih.gov/guidelines/nuremberg.html/.

of syphilis in the adult black male. The research subjects were organized into two groups: one group consisted of 400 men who had untreated syphilis, and the other was a control group of 200 men without syphilis. Many of the subjects who consented to participate in the study were not informed about the purpose and procedures of the research. Some individuals were unaware that they were subjects in a study.

By 1936, study results indicated that the men with syphilis experienced more health complications than the control group. Ten years later, the death rate of the group with syphilis was twice as high as that of the control group. The subjects were examined periodically but were not treated for syphilis, even after penicillin was determined to be an effective treatment for the disease in the 1940s (Brandt, 1978). Published reports of the Tuskegee syphilis study first started appearing in 1936, and additional papers were published every 4 to 6 years. In 1969, the U.S. Centers for Disease Control (CDC) reviewed the study and decided that it should continue. In 1972, a story describing the study published in the *Washington Star* sparked public outrage. Only then did the U.S. Department of Health, Education, and Welfare (DHEW) stop the study. An investigation of the Tuskegee syphilis study found it to be ethically unjustified.

Willowbrook Study

From the mid-1950s to the early 1970s, Dr. Saul Krugman at Willowbrook, an institution for the mentally retarded, conducted research on hepatitis (Rothman, 1982). The subjects, all children, were deliberately infected with the hepatitis virus. During the 20-year study, Willowbrook closed its doors to new inmates because of overcrowded conditions. However, the research ward continued to admit new inmates. To gain their child's admission to the institution, parents were forced to give permission for the child to be a subject in the study.

From the late 1950s to early 1970s, Krugman's research team published several articles describing the study protocol and findings. Beecher (1966) cited the Willowbrook study as an example of unethical research. The investigators defended injecting the children with the virus by citing their own belief that most of the children would have acquired the infection after admission to the institution. The investigators also stressed the benefits that the subjects received, which were a cleaner environment, better supervision, and a higher nurse-patient ratio on the research ward (Rothman, 1982). Despite the controversy, this unethical study continued until the early 1970s.

Jewish Chronic Disease Hospital Study

Another highly publicized example of unethical research was a study conducted at the Jewish Chronic Disease Hospital in the 1960s. Its purpose was to determine the patients' rejection responses to live cancer cells. Twenty-two patients were injected with a suspension containing live cancer cells that had been generated from human cancer tissue (Levine, 1986).

An extensive investigation of this study revealed that the patients were not informed that they were taking part in research or that the injections they received were live cancer cells. In addition, the Jewish Chronic Disease Hospital's institutional review board never reviewed the study; even the physicians caring for the patients were unaware that the study was being conducted. The physician directing the research was an employee of the Sloan-Kettering Institute for Cancer Research, and there was no indication that this institution had reviewed the research project (Hershey & Miller, 1976). The study was considered unethical and was terminated, with the researcher being in violation of the Nuremberg Code (1949) and the Declaration of Helsinki (WMA General Assembly, 1964). This research had the potential to cause the study participants serious or irreversible harm and possibly death and reinforced the importance of conscientious institutional review and ethical researcher conduct.

U.S. Department of Health, Education, and Welfare Regulations

The continued conduct of harmful, unethical research made additional controls necessary. In 1973, the DHEW published its first set of regulations intended to protect human subjects. Clinical researchers were presented with strict regulations for research involving humans, with additional regulations to protect persons having limited capacities to consent, such as the ill, mentally impaired, and dying (Levine, 1986). All research involving human subjects had to undergo full institutional review, even nursing studies that involved minimal or no risks to study participants. Institutional review improved the protection of subjects' rights; however, reviewing all studies, without regard for the degree of risk involved, overwhelmed the review process and greatly prolonged the time required for study approval. The government recognized the need for additional strategies to manage the problems related to the DHEW regulations.

National Commission for the Protection of Human Subjects of Biomedical and Behavioral Research

Because of the problems related to the DHEW regulations, the National Commission for the Protection of Human Subjects of Biomedical and Behavioral Research (1978) was formed. The goals of the commission were (1) to identify the basic ethical principles that should underlie the conduct of biomedical and behavioral research involving human subjects and (2) to develop guidelines based on these principles. The commission developed The Belmont Report (available online at http://www.fda.gov/). This report identified three **ethical principles** as relevant to research involving human subjects: the principles of respect for persons, beneficence, and justice. The **principle of respect for persons** holds that persons have the right to self-determination and the freedom to participate or not participate in research. The **principle of beneficence** requires the researcher to do good and "above all, do no harm." The **principle of justice** holds that human subjects should be treated fairly. Currently, these ethical principles must be followed when researchers in the United States and internationally conduct studies. The commission developed ethical research guidelines based on these three principles, made recommendations to the U.S. Department of Health and Human Services (U.S. DHHS), and was dissolved in 1978.

In response to the commission's recommendations, the U.S. DHHS developed federal regulations in 1981 to protect human research subjects, which have been revised as needed over the last 30 years. The most current U.S. DHHS (2009) regulations are part of the *Code of Federal Regulations* (CFR), Title 45, Part 46, Protection of Human Subjects (available online at http://www.hhs.gov/ohrp/policy/ohrpregulations .pdf/). These regulations are interpreted by the Office for Human Research Protection (OHRP), an agency within U.S. DHHS (2012), whose functions include: (1) providing guidance and clarification of regulations; (2) developing educational programs and materials; (3) maintaining regulatory oversight of research; and (4) providing advice on ethical and regulatory issues related to biomedical and social-behavior research.

The U.S. DHHS (2009) regulations provide direction for (1) the protection of human subjects in research, with additional protection for pregnant women, human fetuses, neonates, children, and prisoners; (2) the documentation of informed consent; and (3) the implementation of the institutional review board process. These regulations apply to all research involving human subjects in the following areas: (1) studies conducted, supported, or otherwise subject to regulations by any federal department or agency; (2) research conducted in educational and healthcare settings; (3) research involving the use of biophysical measures, educational tests, survey procedures, scales, interview procedures, or observation; and (4) research involving the collection or study of existing data, documents, records, pathological specimens, or diagnostic specimens.

Essentially all the biomedical and behavioral studies conducted in the United States are governed by the U.S. DHHS (2009) Protection of Human Subjects Regulations or the U.S. Food and Drug Administration (U.S. FDA). The FDA, within the U.S. DHHS, manages the CFR Title 21, Food and Drugs, Part 50, Protection of Human Subjects (U.S. FDA, 2010a), and Part 56, Institutional Review Boards (IRBs) (U.S. FDA, 2010b). These regulations apply to studies of drugs for humans, medical devices for human use, biological products for human use, human dietary supplements, and electronic products. The role of the FDA was expanded by the Food and Drug Administration Amendments Act (FDAAA) of 2007 to include increased responsibility for the management of new drugs and medical devices. Physicians and nurses conducting clinical trials to generate new drugs and refine existing drug treatments must comply with these FDA regulations. In summary, these regulations focus on the protection of human subjects' rights, informed consent (U.S. FDA, 2010a), and IRBs (U.S. FDA, 2010b), with content that is consistent with the U.S. DHHS (2009) regulations.

The U.S. DHHS and FDA regulations provide guidelines to protect subjects in federally and privately funded research by ensuring privacy and confidentiality of information obtained through research. However, with the advent of electronic access and transfer, the public was concerned about the potential abuses of the health information of individuals in all circumstances, including research projects. Thus HIPAA was implemented in 2003 to protect an individual's health information. The U.S. DHHS developed regulations titled the Standards for Privacy of Individually Identifiable Health Information, and compliance with these regulations is known as the Privacy Rule (U.S. DHHS, 2003). The HIPAA Privacy Rule established the category of protected health information (PHI), which allows covered entities, such as health plans, healthcare clearinghouses, and healthcare providers that transmit health information, to use or disclose PHI to others only in certain situations. These situations are discussed later in this chapter.

The HIPAA Privacy Rule affects not only the healthcare environment but also the research conducted in this environment (U.S. DHHS, 2010). An individual must provide his or her signed permission, or authorization, before his or her PHI can be used or disclosed for research purposes. To determine how the HIPAA Privacy Rule might impact the informed consent and IRB processes for your study, go to the website at http://privacyruleandresearch.nih.gov/, which was developed to address researchers' questions.

Table 9-1 was developed to clarify the overall objectives and applicability of the HIPAA Privacy Rule, U.S. DHHS Protection of Human Subjects Regulations, and U.S. FDA Protection of Human Subjects Regulations (U.S. DHHS, 2007a). Any study you propose with human subjects must comply with these regulations. Thus, this chapter covers these regulations in the sections on protecting human rights, obtaining informed consent, and institutional review of research.

Protection of Human Rights

Human rights are claims and demands that have been justified in the eyes of an individual or by the consensus of a group of individuals. Having rights is necessary for the self-respect, dignity, and health of an individual (Fry, Veatch, & Taylor, 2011). The American Nurses Association (ANA, 2001) Code of Ethics for Nurses and the American Psychological Association (APA, 2010) Principles of Psychologists and Code of Conduct provide guidelines for protecting the rights of human subjects in biological and behavioral research. Researchers and reviewers of research have an ethical responsibility to protect the rights of

TABLE 9-1 Clarification of the Focus of Federal Regulations and Impact on Research

Area of Distinction	HIPAA Privacy Rule	U.S. DHHS Protection of Human Subjects Regulations Title 45 CFR Part 46	U.S. FDA Protection of Human Subjects Regulations Title 21 CFR Parts 50 and 56
Overall objective	Establishes a federal floor of privacy protections for most individually identifiable health information by establishing conditions for its use and disclosure by certain healthcare providers, health plans, and healthcare clearinghouses.	To protect the rights and welfare of human subjects involved in research conducted or supported by U.S. DHHS. Not specifically a privacy regulation.	To protect the rights, safety, and welfare of subjects involved in clinical investigations regulated by the FDA. Not specifically a privacy regulation.
Applicability	Applies to HIPAA-defined covered entities, regardless of the source of funding.	Applies to human subject research conducted or supported by U.S. DHHS and research with private funding.	Applies to research involving products regulated by the FDA. Federal support is not necessary for FDA regulations to be applicable. When research subject to FDA jurisdiction is federally funded, both the U.S. DHHS Protection of Human Subjects Regulations and FDA Protection of Human Subjects Regulations apply.

CFR, Code of Federal Regulations; *DHHS*, U.S. Department of Health and Human Services; *U.S. FDA*, U.S. Food and Drug Administration; *HIPAA*, Health Insurance Portability and Accountability Act.

From U.S. Department of Health and Human Services. (2007a). *How do other privacy protections interact with the privacy rule?* Retrieved from http://privacyruleandresearch.nih.gov/pr_05.asp/.

human research participants. The human rights that require protection in research are (1) the right to self-determination;, (2) the right to privacy; (3) the right to anonymity and confidentiality; (4) the right to fair treatment or justice; and (5) the right to protection from discomfort and harm (ANA, 2001; APA, 2010; Fry et al., 2011).

Right to Self-Determination

The right to self-determination is based on the ethical principle of respect for persons. This principle holds that because humans are capable of self-determination, or controlling their own destinies, they should be treated as autonomous agents who have the freedom to conduct their lives as they choose without external controls. As a researcher, you treat prospective subjects as autonomous agents by informing them about a proposed study and allowing them to voluntarily choose to participate or not. In addition, subjects have the right to withdraw from a study at any time without a penalty (Fry et al., 2011). Conducting research ethically requires that research subjects' right to self-determination not be violated and that persons with diminished autonomy have additional protection during the conduct of studies (U.S. DHHS, 2009).

Preventing Violation of Research Subjects' Right to Self-Determination

A subject's right to self-determination can be violated through the use of (1) coercion; (2) covert data collection; and (3) deception. Coercion occurs when one person intentionally presents another with an overt threat of harm or the lure of excessive reward to obtain his or her compliance. Some subjects are coerced to participate in research because they fear that they will suffer harm or discomfort if they do not participate. For example, some patients believe that their medical or nursing care will be negatively affected if they do not agree to be research subjects. Sometimes students feel forced to participate in research to protect their grades or prevent negative relationships with the faculty conducting the research. Other subjects are coerced to participate in studies because they believe that they cannot refuse the excessive rewards offered, such as large sums of money, specialized health care, special privileges, and jobs. Most nursing studies do not offer excessive rewards to subjects for participating. Sometimes nursing studies have included a small financial reward of $10 to $30 or support for transportation to increase participation, but this would not be considered coercive (Fawcett & Garity, 2009; Fry et al., 2011).

An individual's right to self-determination can also be violated if he or she becomes a research subject without realizing it. Some researchers have exposed persons to experimental treatments without their knowledge, a prime example being the Jewish Chronic Disease Hospital study. Most of the patients and their physicians were unaware of the study. The subjects were informed that they were receiving an injection of cells, but the word cancer was omitted (Beecher, 1966). With **covert data collection**, subjects are unaware that research data are being collected because the investigator develops a description of the study indicating that it is normal activity or part of health care (Reynolds, 1979). This type of data collection has more commonly been used by psychologists to describe human behavior in a variety of situations, but it has also been used by nursing and other disciplines (APA, 2010). Qualitative researchers have debated this issue, and some believe that certain group and individual behaviors are unobservable within the normal ethical range of research activities, such as the actions of cults or the aggressive or violent behaviors of individuals. Thus, these types of behaviors require study with covert data collection processes. However, covert data collection is considered unethical when research deals with sensitive aspects of an individual's behavior, such as illegal conduct, sexual behavior, and drug use (U.S. DHHS, 2009). With the HIPAA Privacy Rule (U.S. DHHS, 2003), the use of any type of covert data collection would be questionable and illegal if PHI data were being used or disclosed.

The use of **deception** in research can also violate a subject's right to self-determination. Deception is the actual misinforming of subjects for research purposes (Kelman, 1967). A classic example of deception is the Milgram (1963) study, in which the subjects thought they were administering electric shocks to another person. The subjects were unaware that the person was really a professional actor who pretended to feel the shocks. Some subjects experienced severe mental tension, almost to the point of collapse, because of their participation in this study. The use of deception still occurs in some healthcare, social, and psychological investigations, but it is a controversial research activity. If deception is to be used in a study, researchers must determine that there is no other way to gain the essential research data needed and that the subjects will not be harmed. In addition, the subjects must be informed of the deception once the study is completed, provided full disclosure of the study activities that were conducted, (APA, 2010; Fry, 2011; U.S. DHHS, 2009) and given the opportunity to withdraw their data from the study.

Protecting Persons with Diminished Autonomy

Some persons have **diminished autonomy** or are vulnerable and less advantaged because of legal or mental incompetence, terminal illness, or confinement to an institution (Fry et al., 2011). These persons require additional protection of their right to self-determination, because they have a decreased ability, or an inability, to give informed consent. In addition, these persons are vulnerable to coercion and deception. The U.S. DHHS (2009) has identified certain vulnerable groups of individuals, including pregnant women, human fetuses, neonates, children, mentally incompetent persons, and prisoners, who require additional protection in the conduct of research. Researchers need to justify their use of subjects with diminished autonomy in a study, and the need for justification increases as the subjects' risk and vulnerability increase. However, in many situations, the knowledge needed to provide evidence-based care to these vulnerable populations can be gained only by studying them.

Legally and Mentally Incompetent Subjects

Neonates and children (minors), the mentally impaired, and unconscious patients are legally or mentally incompetent to give informed consent. These individuals lack the ability to comprehend information about a study and to make decisions regarding participation in or withdrawal from the study. Their vulnerability ranges from minimal to absolute. The use of persons with diminished autonomy as research subjects is more acceptable if (1) the research is therapeutic, so that the subjects have the potential to benefit directly from the experimental process; (2) the researcher is willing to use both vulnerable and nonvulnerable individuals as subjects; (3) preclinical and clinical studies have been conducted and provide data for assessing potential risks to subjects; and (4) the risk is minimized and the consent process is strictly followed to secure the rights of the prospective subjects (U.S. DHHS, 2009).

Neonates

A *neonate* is defined as a newborn and is identified as either viable or nonviable on delivery. *Viable neonates* are able to survive after delivery, if given the benefit of available medical therapy, and can independently maintain a heartbeat and respiration. A *nonviable neonate* is a newborn who after delivery, although living, is not able to survive (U.S. DHHS, 2009). Neonates are extremely vulnerable and require extra protection to determine their involvement in research. However, research may involve viable neonates, neonates of uncertain viability, and nonviable neonates if the following five conditions are met:

1. The study is scientifically appropriate and the pre-clinical and clinical studies have been conducted and provided data for assessing the potential risks to the neonates.
2. The study provides important biomedical knowledge that cannot be obtained by other means and will not add risk to the neonate.
3. The research has the potential to enhance the probability of survival of the neonate.
4. Both parents are fully informed about the research during the consent process.
5. The research team will have no part in determining the viability of the neonate.

In addition, for the nonviable neonate, the vital functions of the neonate should not be artificially maintained because of the research, and the research should not terminate the heartbeat or respiration of the neonate (U.S. DHHS, 2009).

Children

The unique vulnerability of children makes the decision to use them as research subjects particularly important. To safeguard their interests and protect them from harm, special ethical and regulatory considerations have been put in place for research involving children (U.S. DHHS, 2009). However, the laws defining the minor status of a child are statutory and vary from state to state. Often a child's competency to consent is governed by age, with incompetence being nonrefutable up to age 7 years (Broome, 1999; Fry et al., 2011). Thus, a child younger than 7 years is not believed to be mature enough to assent or consent to research. Developmentally by age 7, a child is capable of concrete operations of thought and can give meaningful assent to participate as a subject in studies (Thompson, 1987). With advancing age and maturity, a child should have a stronger role in the consent process.

To obtain informed consent, federal regulations require both the assent of the children (when capable) and the permission of their parents or guardians (U.S. DHHS, 2009). **Assent** means a child's affirmative agreement to participate in research. **Permission to participate in a study** means the agreement of parents or guardian to the participation of their child or ward in research (U.S. DHHS, 2009). If a child does not assent to participate in the study, he or she should not be included as a subject even if parental permission is obtained.

Using children as research subjects is also influenced by the therapeutic nature of the research and the risks versus the benefits. Thompson (1987) developed a guide for obtaining informed consent that is based on the child's level of competence, the therapeutic nature of the research, and the risks versus the benefits (Table 9-2). Children who are experiencing a developmental delay, cognitive deficit, emotional disorder, or physical illness must be considered individually (Broome, 1999; Broome & Stieglitz, 1992).

A child 7 years or older with normal cognitive development can provide assent or dissent to participation in a study, and the process for obtaining the assent should be included in the research proposal. In the assenting process, the child must be given developmentally appropriate information on the study purpose, expectations, and benefit-risk ratio (discussed later). DVDs, written materials, demonstrations,

TABLE 9-2	Guide to Obtaining Informed Consent Based on the Relationship between a Child's Level of Competence, the Therapeutic Nature of the Research, and Risk versus Benefit				
	Nontherapeutic Research		**Therapeutic Research**	
	MMR-LB	MR-LB	MR-HB	MMR-HB
Child, Incompetent (generally, 0-6 yr)				
Parents' consent	Necessary	Necessary	Sufficient*	Sufficient
Child's assent	Optional†	Optional†	Optional	
Child, Relatively Competent (7 yr and older)				
Parents' consent	Necessary	Necessary	Sufficient‡	Recommended
Child's assent	Necessary	Necessary	Sufficient§	Sufficient

*A parent's refusal can be superseded by the principle that a parent has no power to forbid the saving of a child's life.
†Children making "deliberate objection" would be precluded from participation by most researchers.
‡In cases not involving the privacy rights of a "mature minor."
§In cases involving the privacy rights of a "mature minor."
HB, high benefit; *LB*, low benefit; *MMR*, more than minimal risk; *MR*, minimal risk.
From Thompson, P. J. (1987). Protection of the rights of children as subjects for research. *Journal of Pediatric Nursing, 2*(6), 397.

diagrams, role-modeling, and peer discussions are possible methods for communicating study information. The child also needs an opportunity to sign an assent form and to have a copy of this form. An example assent form is presented in Box 9-2. During the study, the researcher must give the child the opportunity to ask questions and to withdraw from the study if he or she desires (Broome, 1999). Assent becomes more complex if the child is bilingual, because the researchers must determine the most appropriate language to use for the consent process for the child and the parents. Holaday, Gonzales, and Mills (2007) offer a list of seven questions in their article to assist researchers in determining the language for communication during a study.

Rew, Horner, and Fouladi (2010) conducted a study of school-aged children's health behaviors to determine whether they were precursors of adolescents' health-risk behaviors. The sample included Hispanic and non-Hispanic children and their parents. The ethical aspects of the study are described in the following quotation:

"The study took place in a rural setting in central Texas, a state with a rapidly expanding population of Hispanics, primarily of Mexican descent. The non-probability sample was composed of 1,934 children in Grades 4 ($n = 781$), 5 ($n = 621$), and 6 ($n = 532$) who were enrolled in three rural school districts in central Texas and one of their parents....

After study approval was obtained from the university's institutional review board [IRB] and each of the school administrators, a packet was mailed to parents of all the children in Grades 4 through 6 in three rural school districts. The packets included a cover letter from the child's school, an explanatory letter from the researchers, and consent forms. All materials were written in English and Spanish, with forward and backward translations by independent speakers, and were reviewed by bilingual members of the community for translation clarity and accuracy before mailing. Informational meetings were held at the schools after parent-teacher meetings. At those school meetings, the study was explained to the children, questions were answered, and signed permissions were obtained from parents. Data were later collected during school hours using audio (optional) computer-assisted self-interviewing (A-CASI) technology using laptop computers after the children who agreed to participate provided written assent....

The children were oriented to the A-CASI format and were directed to select either the English- or Spanish-language version to complete. For children who had difficulty with reading, audio support was engaged on the laptop computer and the children listened with an earpiece as the items were read to them in their preferred language.... As each child completed the questionnaire, the research assistants saved the data record to a secure Web site." (Rew et al., 2010, pp. 158, 160)

Rew et al. (2010) provided a detailed description of the protection of the children and their parents' rights. The study was described in a language of choice with an offer to answer questions. The parents agreed to their children's participation in the study through signed permissions. The children gave written assent to participating in the study. Other ethical aspects of the study were the IRB approvals from the university and school administrators and the storage of study data in a secure location. All of these activities promoted the ethical conduct of this study according to the U.S. DHHS (2009) regulations. The researchers found that girls have more health-focused behaviors than boys, health behaviors decreased from grades 4 to 6, and the school environment was important for promoting health behaviors.

Pregnant Women

Pregnant women require additional protection in research because of their fetuses. Federal regulations define *pregnancy* as encompassing the period of time from implantation until delivery. "A woman is assumed to be pregnant if she exhibits any of the pertinent presumptive signs of pregnancy, such as missed menses, until the results of a pregnancy test are negative or until delivery" (U.S. DHHS, 2009, 45 CFR Section 46.202). Research conducted with pregnant women should have the potential to directly benefit the woman or the fetus. If your investigation is thought to provide a direct benefit only to the fetus, you must obtain the consent of the pregnant woman and father. In addition, studies with pregnant women should include no inducements to terminate the pregnancy (U.S. DHHS, 2009).

Adults with Diminished Capacity

Certain adults have a diminished capacity for, or are incapable of, giving informed consent because of mental illness (Beebe & Smith, 2010), cognitive impairment, or a comatose state (Simpson, 2010). Persons are said to be incompetent if a qualified clinician judges them to have attributes that designate them

Box 9-2 **Sample Assent Form for Children Ages 6 To 12 Years: Pain Interventions for Children with Cancer**

Oral Explanation

I am a nurse who would like to know whether relaxation, special ways of breathing, and using your mind to think pleasant things help children like you to feel less afraid and feel less hurt when the doctor has to do a bone marrow aspiration or spinal tap. Today, and the next five times you and your mom and/or dad come to the clinic, I would like for you to answer some questions about the things in the clinic that scare you. I would also like you to tell me about how much pain you felt during the bone marrow or spinal tap. In addition, I would like to videotape (take pictures of) you and your mom and/or dad during the tests. The second time you visit the clinic I would like to meet with you and teach you special ways to relax, breathe, and use your mind to imagine pleasant things. You can use the special imagining and breathing during your visits to the clinic. I would ask you and your mom and/or dad to practice the things I teach you at home between your visits to the clinic. At any time you could change your mind and not be in the study anymore.

To Child

1. I want to learn special ways to relax, breathe, and imagine.
2. I want to answer questions about things children may be afraid of when they come to the clinic.
3. I want to tell you how much pain I feel during the tests I have.
4. I will let you videotape me while the doctor does the tests (bone marrow and spinal taps).

If the child says YES, have him/her put an "X" here: _____

If the child says NO, have him/her put an "X" here: _____

Date: _____

Child's signature: _____

From Broome, M. E. (1999). Consent (assent) for research with pediatric patients. *Seminars in Oncology Nursing, 15*(2), 101.

as incompetent (U.S. DHHS, 2009). Incompetence can be temporary (e.g., inebriation), permanent (e.g., advanced senile dementia), or subjective or transitory (e.g., behavior or symptoms of psychosis).

If an individual is judged incompetent and incapable of consent, you must seek approval from the prospective subject and his or her legally authorized representative. A **legally authorized representative** means an individual or other body authorized under law to consent on behalf of a prospective subject to his or her participation in research. However, individuals can be judged incompetent and can still assent to participate in certain minimal-risk research if they have the ability to understand what they are being asked to do, to make reasonably free choices, and to communicate their choices clearly and unambiguously (U.S. DHHS, 2009).

A number of people in intensive care units and nursing homes are experiencing some level of cognitive impairment. These individuals must be assessed for their capacity to give consent to participate in research. The assessment needs to include the following elements: understanding of the study information, developing a belief about the information, reasoning ability, and understanding of a choice. Simpson (2010) reviewed the literature and found that the MacArthur Competency Assessment Tool for Clinical Research (MacCAT-CR) is one of the strongest instruments available for assessing an individual's capacity to give informed consent. Using this instrument or others discussed by Simpson (2010), researchers can make a more sound decision about a subject's ability to consent to research or about whether the legal guardian must be contacted for permission.

Some individuals have become permanently incompetent from the advanced stages of senile dementia of the Alzheimer type (SDAT), and their legal guardians must give permission for their participation in research. Often families or guardians of these patients are reluctant to give consent for their participation in research. However, nursing research is needed to establish evidence-based interventions for comforting and caring for these individuals. Levine (1986) identified two approaches that families, guardians, researchers, or IRBs might use when making decisions on behalf of these incompetent individuals: (1) best interest standard and (2) substituted judgment standard. The **best interest standard** involves doing what is best for the individual on the basis of balancing risks and benefits. The **substituted judgment standard** is concerned with determining the course of action that incompetent individuals would take if they were capable of making a choice (Beattie, 2009).

Jones, Munro, Grap, Kitten, and Edmond (2010) conducted a quasi-experimental study to determine the effect of toothbrushing on bacteremia risk in mechanically ventilated adults. These researchers described their process for obtaining consent from their study participants in the following study excerpt:

> "The study was reviewed and approved by the university's institutional review board. All subjects who met inclusion criteria were assessed for ability to provide informed consent through gesturing or writing. If subjects had medications that impaired cognition or were unable to provide informed consent due to their illness, the legally authorized representative provided informed consent." (Jones et al., 2010, p. S58)

Jones et al. (2010) developed a process for determining the cognitive competence of their potential research participants and obtained appropriate consent on the basis of their assessments. The competent subjects were given the right to self-determination regarding study participation. The researchers found that the toothbrushing intervention did not cause transient bacteremia in this population of ventilated patients.

Terminally Ill Subjects

When conducting research on terminally ill subjects, you should determine (1) who will benefit from the research and (2) whether it is ethical to conduct research on individuals who might not benefit from the study (U.S. DHHS, 2009). Participating in research could have greater risks and minimal or no benefits for these subjects. In addition, the dying subject's condition could affect the study results and lead you to misinterpret the results. However, Hinds, Burghen, and Pritchard (2007) stressed the importance of conducting end-of-life studies in pediatric oncology to generate evidence that will improve the care for terminally ill children and adolescents.

Some terminally ill individuals are willing subjects because they believe that participating in research is a way to contribute to society before they die. Others want to take part in research because they believe that the experimental process will benefit them. For example, individuals with AIDS might want to participate in AIDS research to gain access to experimental drugs and hospitalized care. Researchers studying populations with serious or terminal illnesses are faced with ethical dilemmas as they consider the rights of the subjects and their responsibilities in conducting quality research (Fry et al., 2011; U.S. DHHS, 2009).

Subjects Confined to Institutions

Hospitalized patients have diminished autonomy because they are ill and are confined in settings that are controlled by healthcare personnel (Levine, 1986). Some hospitalized patients feel obliged to be research subjects because they want to assist a particular practitioner (nurse or physician) with his or her research. Others feel coerced to participate because they fear that their care will be adversely affected if they refuse. Some of these hospitalized patients are survivors of trauma (such as auto accidents, gunshot wounds, or physical and sexual abuse) who are very vulnerable and often have decreased decision-making capacities (McClain, Laughon, Steeves, & Parker, 2007). When conducting research with these types of patients, you must pay careful attention to the informed consent process and make every effort to protect these subjects from feelings of coercion and harm (U.S. DHHS, 2009).

In the past, prisoners have experienced diminished autonomy in research projects because of their confinement. They might feel coerced to participate in research because they fear harm if they refuse or because they desire the benefits of early release, special treatment, or monetary gain. Prisoners have been used for drug studies in which there were no health-related benefits and there was possible harm for the prisoners. Current regulations regarding research involving prisoners require that "the risks involved in the research are commensurate with risks that would be accepted by nonprisoner volunteers and procedures for the selection of subjects within the prison are fair to all prisoners and immune from arbitrary intervention by prison authorities or prisoners" (U.S. DHHS, 2009, Section 46.305).

Protecting the rights of subjects with diminished autonomy in research is regulated internationally by the Council for International Organizations of Medical Sciences (CIOMS). CIOMS (2010) developed international ethical guidelines for biomedical research involving human subjects, and the guidelines require protection of vulnerable individuals, groups, communities, and populations during research. Researchers must evaluate each prospective subject's capacity for self-determination and must protect subjects with diminished autonomy during the research process (ANA, 2001, APA, 2010; U.S. DHHS, 2009).

Right to Privacy

Privacy is an individual's right to determine the time, extent, and general circumstances under which personal information will be shared with or withheld from others. This information consists of one's attitudes, beliefs, behaviors, opinions, and records. The Privacy Act of 1974 provided the initial protection of an individual's privacy. Because of this act, data collection methods were to be scrutinized to protect subjects' privacy, and data cannot be gathered from subjects without their knowledge. Individuals also have the right to access their records and to prevent access by others (U.S. DHHS, 2009). The intent of this act was to prevent the **invasion of privacy** that occurs when private information is shared without an individual's knowledge or against his or her will. Invading an individual's privacy might cause loss of dignity, friendships, or employment or create feelings of anxiety, guilt, embarrassment, or shame.

The **HIPAA Privacy Rule** expanded the protection of an individual's privacy, specifically his or her protected individually identifiable health information, and described the ways in which covered entities can use or disclose this information. "**Individually identifiable health information** (IIHI) is information that is a subset of health information, including demographic information collected from an individual, and: (1) is created or received by healthcare provider, health plan, or healthcare clearinghouse; and (2) [is] related to past, present, or future physical or mental health or condition of an individual, the provision of health care to an individual, or the past, present, or future payment for the provision of health care to an individual, and that identifies the individual; or with respect to which there is a reasonable basis to believe that the information can be used to identify the individual" (U.S. DHHS, 2003, 45 CFR, Section 160.103).

According to the HIPAA Privacy Rule, the IIHI is protected health information (PHI) that is transmitted by electronic media, maintained in electronic media, or transmitted or maintained in any other form or medium. Thus, the HIPAA privacy regulations affect nursing research in the following ways: (1) accessing data from a covered entity, such as reviewing a patient's medical record in clinics or hospitals; (2) developing health information, such as the data developed when an intervention is implemented in a study to improve a subject's health; and (3) disclosing data from a study to a colleague in another institution, such as sharing data from a study to facilitate development of an instrument or scale (Olsen, 2003).

The U.S. DHHS developed the following guidelines to help researchers, healthcare organizations, and healthcare providers determine when they can use and disclose IIHI. IIHI can be used or disclosed to a researcher in the following situations:

- The protected health information has been "de-identified" under the HIPAA Privacy Rule.

(De-identifying PHI is defined in the following section.)
- The data are part of a limited data set, and a data use agreement with the researcher(s) is in place.
- The individual who is a potential subject for a study authorizes the researcher to use and disclose his or her PHI.
- A waiver or alteration of the authorization requirement is obtained from an IRB or a privacy board (U.S. DHHS, 2007b) (see http://privacyruleand research.nih.gov/pr_08.asp/).

The first two items are discussed in this section of the chapter. The authorization process is discussed in the section on obtaining informed consent, and the waiver or alteration of authorization requirement is covered in the section on institutional review of research.

De-identifying Protected Health Information under the Privacy Rule

Covered entities, such as healthcare providers and agencies, can allow researchers access to health information if the information has been de-identified. **De-identifying health data** involves removing the 18 elements that could be used to identify an individual or his or her relatives, employer, or household members. The 18 identifying elements are listed in Box 9-3.

An individual's health information can also be de-identified through the use of statistical methods. However, the covered entity and you as the researcher must ensure that the individual subject cannot be identified or that there is a very small risk that the subject could be identified from the information used. The statistical method used for de-identification of the health data must be documented, and you must certify that the 18 elements for identification have been removed or revised to ensure the individual is not identified. You must retain this certification information for 6 years.

Limited Data Set and Data Use Agreement

Covered entities (healthcare provider, health plan, and healthcare clearinghouse) may use and disclose a limited data set to a researcher for a study without an individual subject's authorization or an IRB waiver. However, a limited data set is considered PHI, and the covered entity and the researcher must have a data use agreement. The **data use agreement** limits how the data set may be used and how it will be protected. The HIPAA Privacy Rule requires the data use agreement to do the following (U.S. DHHS, 2003):

1. Specifies the permitted uses and disclosures of the limited data set.
2. Identifies the researcher who is permitted to use or receive the limited data set.
3. Stipulates that the recipient (researcher) will:
   a. Not use or disclose the information other than permitted by the agreement.
   b. Use appropriate safeguards to prevent the use or disclosure of the information, except as provided for in the agreement.
   c. Hold any other person (co-researchers, statisticians, or data collectors) to the standards, restrictions, and conditions stated in the data use agreement with respect to the health information.
   d. Not identify the information or contact the individuals whose data are in the limited data set.

Riegel et al. (2011) conducted a secondary analysis of data from the Heart Failure (HF) Quality of Life Registry database. The purpose of the study was to establish whether confidence and activity status determined the HF patients' self-care performance. The researchers found three levels of self-care performance: (1) novice in self-care with limited confidence and few activity restrictions; (2) inconsistent in self-care abilities; and (3) expert with confidence in self-care abilities. The researchers ensured the PHI of the individuals in the database was ethically managed, as described in the following excerpt:

"By prior consensus of investigators in the HF Quality of Life Registry, study samples are enrolled using comparable inclusion and exclusion criteria, as well as the same variables and measures whenever possible. All data are stored at one site, where one of the investigators has volunteered to integrate newly acquired data. The only identifiers in the data set are site (e.g., Cleveland Clinic) and the specific study name, as more than one study is common at each site. No protected health information [PHI] is included in the database. All requests to use the full database are viewed and approved by the lead investigators. For this analysis, five samples enrolled at three different sites in the United States between 2003 and 2008 were used." (Riegel et al., 2011, p. 133)

Right to Autonomy and Confidentiality

On the basis of the right to privacy, the research subject has the right to anonymity and the right to assume that the data collected will be

---

Box 9-3   **18 Elements that Could Be Used to Identify an Individual to Relatives, Employer, or Household Members**

1. Names.
2. All geographical subdivisions smaller than a state, including street address, city, county, precinct, zip code, and their equivalent geographical codes, depending on size of population according to the current publicly available data from the Bureau of the Census, as follows:
   a. If the geographical unit formed by combining all zip codes with the same three initial digits contains more than 20000 people, the initial three digits of the zip code may be retained.
   b. For all such geographical units containing 20000 or fewer people, the initial three digits of the zip code are changed to 000.
3. All elements of dates (except year) for dates directly related to an individual, including birth date, admission date, discharge date, date of death; and all ages over 89 and all elements of dates (including year) indicative of such age, except that such ages and elements may be aggregated into a single category of age 90 or older.
4. Telephone numbers.
5. Facsimile numbers.
6. Electronic mail (email) addresses.
7. Social security numbers.
8. Medical record numbers.
9. Health plan beneficiary numbers.
10. Account numbers.
11. Certificate/license numbers.
12. Vehicle identifiers and serial numbers, including license plate numbers.
13. Device identifiers and serial numbers.
14. Web universal resource locators (URLs).
15. Internet protocol (IP) address numbers.
16. Biometric identifiers, including fingerprints and voiceprints.
17. Full-face photographic images and any comparable images.
18. Any other unique identifying number, characteristic, or code, unless otherwise permitted by the Privacy Rule for Re-identification (see http://privacyruleand research.nih.gov/pr_08.asp/) (U.S. DHHS, 2007b).

kept confidential. **Anonymity** exists if the subject's identity cannot be linked, even by the researcher, with his or her individual responses (APA, 2010; Fry et al., 2011). For studies that use de-identified health information or data from a limited data set, the subjects are anonymous to the researchers. The researchers are unable to contact these subjects for additional information without special approval, as described in the study by Riegel et al. (2011).

In most studies, researchers desire to know the identity of their subjects and promise that their identity will be kept confidential. **Confidentiality** is the researcher's management of private information shared by a subject that must not be shared with others without the authorization of the subject. Confidentiality is grounded in the following premises: (1) individuals can share personal information to the extent they wish and are entitled to have secrets; (2) one can choose with whom to share personal information; (3) people who accept information in confidence have an obligation to maintain confidentiality; and (4) professionals, such as researchers, have a duty to maintain confidentiality that goes beyond ordinary loyalty (Levine, 1986; U.S. DHHS, 2009).

Breach of Confidentiality

A **breach of confidentiality** can occur when a researcher, by accident or direct action, allows an unauthorized person to gain access to the study raw data. Confidentiality can also be breached in the reporting or publication of a study when a subject's identity is accidentally revealed, violating the subject's right to anonymity (Munhall, 2012a). Breaches of confidentiality can harm subjects psychologically and socially as well as destroy the trust they had in the researchers. Breaches of confidentiality can be especially harmful to a research participant if they involve (1) religious preferences; (2) sexual practices; (3) employment; (4) racial prejudices; (5) drug use; (6) child abuse; or (7) personal attributes, such as intelligence, honesty, and courage. For example, a university researcher conducted a study of nurses' stressful life events and work-related burnout in an acute care hospital. One of the two male participants in the study was a nurse who is being treated for an anxiety disorder. Reporting that one of the male nurses in the study was being treated for an anxiety disorder would violate his confidentiality and potentially cause harm. Nurse administrators might be less likely to promote a nurse who is receiving mental health treatment.

Some nurse researchers have encountered healthcare professionals who believe that they should have access to information about the patients in the hospital and will request to see the data the researchers have collected. Sometimes, family members or close friends would like to see the data collected on specific subjects. Sharing research data in these circumstances is a breach of confidentiality. When requesting permission to conduct a study, you should tell healthcare professionals, family members, and others in the setting that you will not share the raw data. However, you may elect to share the research report, including a summary of the data and findings from the study, with healthcare providers, family members, and other interested parties.

Maintaining Confidentiality

Researchers have a responsibility to protect the anonymity of subjects and to maintain the confidentiality of data collected during a study. You can protect anonymity by giving each subject a code number. Keep a master list of the subjects' names and their code numbers in a locked place; for example, subject Mary Jones might be assigned the code number "001." All of the instruments and forms that Mary completes and the data you collect about her during the study will be identified with the "001" code number, not her name. The master list of subjects' names and code numbers is best kept separate from the data collected to protect subjects' anonymity. You should not staple signed consent forms and authorization documents to instruments or other data collection tools, as this would make it easy for unauthorized persons to readily identify the subjects and their responses. Consent forms are often stored with the master list of subjects' names and code numbers. When entering the data collected into the computer, use the code numbers for identification and ensure that the data are stored in a secure place on a flash drive, in the computer, or on a website. In the study by Rew et al. (2010) that was introduced earlier in this chapter, the school-aged children participating in the study of their health behaviors completed a questionnaire on the computer and their data were saved by the research assistants to a secure website. These actions ensured that each subject's data were kept confidential during and after completion of the study.

Another way to protect your subjects' anonymity is to have subjects or study participants generate their own identification codes (Damrosch, 1986). With this approach, each subject generates an individual code from personal information, such as the first letter of a mother's name, the first letter of a father's name, the number of brothers, the number of sisters, and middle initial. Thus, the code would be composed of three letters and two numbers, such as "BD21M." This code would be used on each form that the subject completes. Using a subject-generated code is especially helpful when the researcher needs to link the subject's data over time. Because of the specific components of the ID number, the subject does not have to remember the code number from one data collection point until the next. Even you as the researcher would not know the subject's identity, only the subject's code. If a qualitative study is being conducted in which extensive, often sensitive data are collected on just a few study participants, researchers might want to use this type of coding system. Qualitative researchers also use the approach of allowing participants to provide pseudonyms by which they want to be known during the study.

Maintaining confidentiality of participants' data in qualitative studies often requires more effort than in quantitative research. The nature of qualitative research requires that the "investigator must be close enough to understand the depth of the question under study, and must present enough direct quotes and detailed description to answer the question" (Ramos, 1989, p. 60). The small number of participants used in a qualitative study and the depth of detail gathered on each participant requires planning to ensure confidentiality. Ford and Reutter (1990) have recommended that to maintain confidentiality, the researcher should (1) use pseudonyms instead of the participants' names and (2) distort certain details in the participants' stories while leaving the contents unchanged. Researchers must respect participants' privacy as they decide how much detail and editing of private information are necessary to publish a study (Munhall, 2012a; Orb, Eisenhauer, & Wynaden, 2001).

Researchers should also take precautions during data collection and analysis to maintain confidentiality in qualitative studies. The interviews conducted with participants are frequently recorded and later transcribed, so the participants' names should not be mentioned during the recording. They have the right to know whether anyone other than you will be transcribing information from the interviews. In addition, participants should be informed on an ongoing basis that they have the right to withhold information. By allowing other researchers to critically appraise the rigor and credibility of a qualitative study, an audit trail is produced. Allowing others to examine the data to confirm the study findings may create a dilemma regarding the confidentiality of participants' data, so you must inform them if other researchers will be examining their data to ensure the credibility of the study findings (Munhall, 2012a; Orb et al., 2001).

Confidentiality of subjects' information can also be ensured during the data analysis process in quantitative research. The data collected should undergo group analysis so that an individual cannot be identified by his or her responses. If the subjects are divided into groups for data analysis and there is only one subject in a group, combine that subject's data with that of another group or delete the data. In writing the research report, you should describe the findings in such a way that an individual or a group of individuals cannot be identified from their responses.

Right to Fair Treatment

The right to fair treatment is based on the ethical principle of justice. This principle holds that each person should be treated fairly and should receive what he or she is due or owed. In research, the selection of subjects and their treatment during the course of a study should be fair.

Fair Selection of Subjects

In the past, injustices in subject selection have resulted from social, cultural, racial, and sexual biases in society. For many years, research was conducted on categories of individuals who were thought to be especially suitable as research subjects, such as the poor, charity patients, prisoners, slaves, peasants, dying persons, and others who were considered undesirable (Reynolds, 1979). Researchers often treated these subjects carelessly and had little regard for the harm and discomfort they experienced. The Nazi medical experiments, Tuskegee syphilis study, and Willowbrook study all exemplify unfair subject selection and treatment.

The selection of a population and the specific subjects to study should be fair, and the risks and benefits of a study should be fairly distributed on the basis of the subject's efforts, needs, and rights. Subjects should be selected for reasons directly related to the problem being studied and not for "their easy availability, their compromised position, or their manipulability" (National Commission for the Protection of Human Subjects of Biomedical and Behavioral Research, 1978, p. 10).

Another concern with subject selection is that some researchers select certain people as subjects because they like them and want them to receive the specific benefits of a study. Other researchers have been swayed by power or money to make certain individuals subjects so that they can receive potentially beneficial treatments. Random selection of subjects can eliminate some of the researcher bias that might influence subject selection.

A current concern in the conduct of research is finding an adequate number of appropriate subjects to take part in certain studies. As a solution to this problem in the past, some biomedical researchers have offered physicians finder's fees for identifying research subjects. For example, investigators studying patients with lung cancer would give a physician a fee for every patient with lung cancer the physician referred to them. However, the HIPAA Privacy Rule requires that individuals give their authorization before PHI can be shared with others. Thus, healthcare providers cannot recommend individuals for studies without their permission. Researchers can obtain a partial waiver from the IRB or privacy board so that they can obtain PHI necessary to recruit potential subjects (U.S. DHHS, 2003). This makes it more difficult for researchers to find subjects for their studies; however, researchers are encouraged to work closely with their IRBs and the personnel in the settings of their studies to enlarge their sample sizes.

Fair Treatment of Subjects

Researchers and subjects should have a specific agreement about what a subject's participation involves and what the role of the researcher will be (APA, 2010). While conducting a study, you should treat the subjects fairly and respect that agreement. If the data collection requires appointments with the subjects, be on time for each appointment and terminate the data collection process at the agreed-on time. You should not change the activities or procedures that a subject is to perform unless you obtain the subject's consent.

The benefits promised the subjects should be provided. For example, if you promise a subject a copy of the study findings, you should deliver on your promise when the study is completed. In addition, subjects who participate in studies should receive equal benefits, regardless of age, race, and socioeconomic status. When possible, the sample should be representative of the study population and should include subjects of various ages, ethnic backgrounds, and socioeconomic status. Treating subjects fairly often facilitates the data collection process and decreases the chances of subjects' withdrawal from a study (Fry et al., 2011; Orb et al., 2001).

Right to Protection from Discomfort and Harm

The right to **protection from discomfort and harm** is based on the ethical principle of beneficence, which holds that one should do good and, above all, do no harm. Therefore, researchers should conduct their studies to protect subjects from discomfort and harm

and try to bring about the greatest possible balance of benefits in comparison with harm. Discomfort and harm can be physiological, emotional, social, and economic in nature. Reynolds (1979) identified the following five categories of studies, which are based on levels of discomfort and harm: (1) no anticipated effects; (2) temporary discomfort; (3) unusual levels of temporary discomfort; (4) risk of permanent damage; and (5) certainty of permanent damage. Each level is defined in the following discussion.

No Anticipated Effects

In some studies, the subjects expect neither positive nor negative effects. For example, studies that involve reviewing patients' records, students' files, pathology reports, or other documents have no anticipated effects on the subjects. In these types of studies, the researcher does not interact directly with the research subjects. Even in these situations, however, there is a potential risk of invading a subject's privacy. The HIPAA Privacy Rule requires that the agency providing the health information de-identify the 18 essential elements (see Box 9-3), which could be used to identify an individual, to promote subjects' privacy during a study.

Temporary Discomfort

Studies that cause temporary discomfort are described as minimal-risk studies, in which the discomfort encountered is similar to what the subject would experience in his or her daily life and ceases with the termination of the study. Many nursing studies require the subjects to complete questionnaires or participate in interviews, which usually involve minimal risk. The physical discomforts might be fatigue, headache, or muscle tension. The emotional and social risks might entail the anxiety or embarrassment associated with responding to certain questions. The economic risks might consist of the time spent participating in the study or travel costs to the study site. Participation in many nursing studies is considered a mere inconvenience for the subject, with no foreseeable risks of harm.

Most clinical nursing studies examining the impact of a treatment involve minimal risk. For example, your study might involve examining the effects of exercise on the blood glucose levels of type 2 diabetics. During the study, you ask the subjects to test their blood glucose level one extra time per day. There is discomfort when the blood is drawn and a risk of physical changes that might occur with exercise. The subjects might also experience anxiety and fear in association with the additional blood testing, and the testing is an added expense. The diabetic subjects in this study would experience similar discomforts in their daily lives, and the discomforts would cease with the termination of the study.

Unusual Levels of Temporary Discomfort

In studies that involve unusual levels of temporary discomfort, the subjects commonly experience discomfort both during the study and after its termination. For example, subjects might experience a deep vein thrombosis (DVT), prolonged muscle weakness, joint pain, and dizziness after participating in a study that required them to be confined to bed for 7 days to determine the effects of immobility. Studies that require subjects to experience failure, extreme fear, or threats to their identity or to act in unnatural ways involve unusual levels of temporary discomfort. In some qualitative studies, participants are asked questions that reopen old emotional wounds or involve reliving traumatic events (Ford & Reutter, 1990; Munhall, 2012a). For example, asking participants to describe their rape experience could precipitate feelings of extreme fear, anger, and sadness. In these types of studies, you should be vigilant about assessing the participants' discomfort and refer them for appropriate professional intervention as necessary.

Risk of Permanent Damage

In some studies, subjects have the potential to suffer permanent damage; this potential is more common in biomedical research than in nursing research. For example, medical studies of new drugs and surgical procedures have the potential to cause subjects permanent physical damage. However, nurses have investigated topics that have the potential to damage subjects permanently, both emotionally and socially. Studies examining sensitive information, such as sexual behavior, child abuse, or drug use, can be risky for subjects. These types of studies have the potential to cause permanent damage to a subject's personality or reputation. There are also potential economic risks, such as reduced job performance or loss of employment.

Certainty of Permanent Damage

In some research, such as the Nazi medical experiments and the Tuskegee syphilis study, the subjects experience permanent damage. Conducting research that will permanently damage subjects is highly questionable, regardless of the benefits gained. Frequently, the benefits are for other people but not for the subjects. Studies causing permanent damage to subjects violate the fifth principle of the Nuremberg Code (1949) (see Box 9-1).

Balancing Benefits and Risks for a Study

Researchers and reviewers of research must examine the balance of benefits and risks in a study. To determine this balance or **benefit-risk ratio**, you must (1) predict the outcome of your study; (2) assess the actual and potential benefits and risks on the basis of this outcome; and then (3) maximize the benefits and minimize the risks (see Figure 9-1). The outcome of a study is predicted on the basis of previous research, clinical experience, and theory.

Assessment of Benefits

The probability and magnitude of a study's potential benefits must be assessed. A **research benefit** is defined as something of health-related, psychosocial, or other value to a subject, or something that will contribute to the acquisition of knowledge for evidence-based practice. Money and other compensations for participation in research are not benefits but, rather, are remuneration for research-related inconveniences (U.S. DHHS, 2009). In most proposals, the

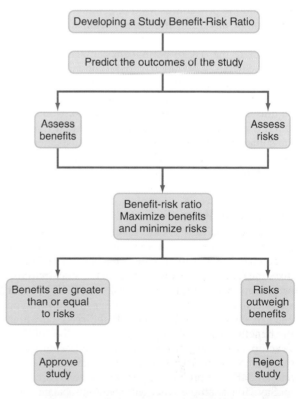

Figure 9-1 Balancing benefits and risks for a study.

research benefits are described for the individual subjects, subjects' families, and society.

The type of research conducted, whether therapeutic or nontherapeutic, affects the potential benefits for the subjects. In therapeutic nursing research, the individual subject has the potential to benefit from the procedures, such as skin care, range of motion, touch, and other nursing interventions, that are implemented in the study. The benefits might include improvement in the subject's physical condition, which could facilitate emotional and social benefits. In addition, the knowledge generated from the research might expand the subjects' and their families' understanding of health. The conduct of nontherapeutic nursing research does not benefit the subject directly but is important to generate and refine nursing knowledge for practice. By participating in research, subjects have the potential to increase their understanding of the research process and an opportunity to know the findings from a particular study (Fry et al., 2011).

Assessment of Risks

You must assess the type, severity, and number of risks that subjects might experience by participating in your study. The risks involved depend on the purpose of the study and the procedures used to conduct it. Research risks can be physical, emotional, social, and economic in nature and can range from no risk or mere inconvenience to the risk of permanent damage (Reynolds, 1979). Studies can have actual (known) risks and potential risks for subjects. In a study of the effects of prolonged bed rest, for example, an actual risk would be muscle weakness and the potential risk would be a DVT. Some studies have actual or potential risks for the subjects' families and society. You must determine the likelihood of the risks and take precautions to protect the rights of subjects when implementing your study.

Benefit-Risk Ratio

The benefit-risk ratio is determined on the basis of the maximized benefits and the minimized risks. The researcher attempts to maximize the benefits and minimize the risks by making changes in the study purpose or procedures or both. If the risks entailed by your study cannot be eliminated or further minimized, you need to justify their existence. If the risks outweigh the benefits, you probably need to revise the study or develop a new one. If the benefits equal or outweigh the risks, you can usually justify conducting the study, and an IRB will probably approve it (see Figure 9-1).

Say, for example, that you want to balance the benefits and risks of a study that would examine the effect of an exercise and diet program on the participants' serum lipid values (serum cholesterol, low-density lipoprotein [LDL], and high-density lipoprotein [HDL]) and cardiovascular (CV) risk level. The benefits to the participants are instruction about exercise and diet and information about their serum lipid values and CV risk level at the start of the program and 1 year later. The potential benefits are improved serum lipid values, lowered CV risk level, and better exercise and dietary habits. The risks consist of the discomfort of having blood specimens drawn twice for serum lipid measurements and the time spent participating in the study (Bruce & Grove, 1994). These discomforts are temporary, are no more than what the subject would experience in his or her daily life, and would cease with the termination of the study. The subjects' time participating in the study can be minimized through organization and precise scheduling of research activities. When you examine the ratio of benefits to risks, you find that (1) the benefits are greater in number and importance than the risks and (2) the risks are temporary and can be minimized. Thus, you could justify conducting this study, and it would probably receive approval from the IRB.

The obligation to balance the benefits and risks of studies is the responsibility of the researcher, health professionals, and society. The researcher must balance the benefits and risks of a particular study and protect the subjects from harm during it. Health professionals participating on IRBs must evaluate the benefit-risk ratio of studies to ensure the conduct of ethical research in their agencies. Society must be concerned with the benefits and risks of the entire enterprise of research and with the protection of all human research subjects from harm.

Obtaining Informed Consent

Obtaining informed consent from human subjects is essential for the conduct of ethical research in the United States (U.S. FDA, 2010a; U.S. DHHS, 2009) and internationally (CIOMS, 2010). *Informing* is the transmission of essential ideas and content from the investigator to the prospective subject. *Consent* is the prospective subject's agreement to participate in a study as a subject, which the subject reaches after assimilating essential information. The phenomenon of **informed consent** was formally defined in the first principle of the Nuremberg Code as follows: "The voluntary consent of the human subject is absolutely essential.... This means that the person involved should have legal capacity to give consent; should be so situated as to be able to exercise free power of choice, without the intervention of any element of force, fraud, deceit, duress, over-reaching or other ulterior form of constraint or coercion; and should have sufficient knowledge and comprehension of the elements of the subject matter involved as to enable him to make an understanding and enlightened decision" (Levine, 1986, p. 425). Prospective subjects, to the degree that they are capable, should have the opportunity to choose whether or not to participate in research. With careful accommodations, the subjects may include persons with cognitive impairment (Simpson, 2010), psychiatric diagnosis (Beebe & Smith, 2010), or dementia (Beattie, 2009).

This definition of informed consent provided a basis for the discussion of consent in all subsequent codes and regulations and has general acceptance in the research community. As the definition indicates, informed consent consists of four elements: (1) disclosure of essential information; (2) comprehension; (3) competence; and (4) voluntarism. This section describes the elements of informed consent and the methods of documenting consent.

Information Essential for Consent

Informed consent requires the researcher to disclose specific information to each prospective subject. The following information has been identified as essential content for informed consent in research by federal regulations (U.S. FDA, 2010a; U.S. DHHS (2009).

Introduction of Research Activities

The introduction of the research must indicate that a study is being conducted and provide key information about the study. Each prospective subject is provided a statement that he or she is being asked to participate in research and a description of the purpose and the expected duration of participation in the study. In clinical nursing research, the patient, serving as a subject, must know which nursing activities are research activities and which are routine nursing interventions. If at any point the prospective subject disagrees with the researchers' goals or the intent of the study, he or she can decline participation or withdraw from the study.

Prospective subjects also need to receive a complete description of the procedures to be followed and identification of any procedures in the study that are experimental (U.S. FDA, 2010a; U.S. DHHS, 2009). Thus, researchers need to describe the research variables and the procedures or mechanisms that will be used to observe, examine, manipulate, or measure these variables. In addition, they must inform prospective subjects about when the study procedures will be implemented, how many times, and in what setting.

Research participants also need to know the funding source(s) of a study and whether the study is sponsored by specific individuals, organizations, or companies. For example, researchers studying the effects of a specific drug must identify any sponsorship by a pharmaceutical company. If the study is being conducted as part of an academic requirement, researchers should also share that information (Fry et al., 2011).

Description of Risks and Discomforts

Prospective subjects need to be informed about any foreseeable risks or discomforts (physical, emotional, social, or economic) that might result from the study (U.S. FDA, 2010b; U.S. DHHS, 2009). They also need to know how the risks of the study were minimized and the benefits were maximized. If the study involves greater than minimal risk, it is a good idea to encourage the prospective subjects to consult another person regarding their participation. A trusted advisor, such as a friend, family member, or another nurse, could serve as a consultant.

Description of Benefits

You should also describe any benefits to the subject or to others that may be expected from the research. The study might benefit the current subjects or might generate knowledge that will provide evidence-based care to patients and families in the future (U.S. FDA, 2010a; U.S. DHHS, 2009).

Disclosure of Alternatives

Study participants must receive a disclosure of alternatives related to their participating in a study. They must be informed about appropriate, alternative procedures or courses of treatment, if any, that might be advantageous to them (U.S. DHHS, 2009). For example, nurse researchers examining the effect of a distraction intervention on the chronic pain of patients with osteoarthritis would need to make potential subjects aware of the other alternatives for pain management.

Assurance of Anonymity and Confidentiality

Prospective subjects must be assured that the confidentiality of their records and PHI will be maintained during and following their study participation (U.S. FDA, 2010a; U.S. DHHS, 2003, 2009). Thus, subjects need to know that their responses and the information obtained from their records during a study will be kept confidential and their identities will remain anonymous in presentations, reports, and publications of the study. Depending on the study design, some participants' identities will be anonymous to the researchers to decrease the potential for bias.

Compensation for Participation in Research

For research involving more than minimal risks, prospective subjects must be given an explanation as to whether any compensation or medical treatments or both are available if injury occurs. If medical treatments are available, you need to describe the type and extent of the treatments. Female prospective subjects need to know whether the study treatment or procedure may involve potential risks to them or their fetuses if they are or may become pregnant during the study (U.S. FDA, 2010a; U.S. DHHS, 2009). Potential subjects also need to know whether they will receive a small financial payment ($10 to $30) to compensate them for their time and effort related to participating in the study.

Offer to Answer Questions

You need to offer to answer any questions that the prospective subjects may have during the consent process. Study participants also need an explanation of whom to contact for answers to questions about the research during the conduct of the study and of whom to contact in the event of a research-related problem or injury as well as how to do so (U.S. FDA, 2010a; U.S. DHHS, 2009).

Noncoercive Disclaimer

A noncoercive disclaimer is a statement that participation is voluntary and refusal to participate will involve no penalty or loss of benefits to which the subject is entitled (U.S. FDA, 2010a; U.S. DHHS, 2009). This statement can facilitate a relationship between you and your prospective subjects, especially if the relationship has a potential for coercion.

Option to Withdraw

Subjects may discontinue participation in or may withdraw from a study at any time without penalty or loss of benefits. However, researchers do have the right to ask subjects whether they think that they will be able to complete the study, to decrease the number of subjects withdrawing early. There may be circumstances under which the subject's participation may be terminated by the researcher without regard to the subject's consent (U.S. DHHS, 2009). For example, if a particular treatment becomes potentially dangerous to a subject, you have an obligation to discontinue the subject's participation in the study. Thus, describe for prospective subjects the circumstances

under which they might be withdrawn from the study, and make a general statement about the circumstances that could lead to the termination of the entire project.

Consent to Incomplete Disclosure

In some studies, subjects are not completely informed of the study purpose because that knowledge would alter the subjects' actions. However, prospective subjects must know that certain information is being withheld deliberately. You must ensure that there are no undisclosed risks to the subjects that are more than minimal and that their questions are truthfully answered regarding the study. Subjects who are exposed to nondisclosure of information must know when and how they will be debriefed about the study. Subjects are debriefed by informing them of the actual purpose of the study and the results that were obtained. At this point, subjects have the option to have their data withdrawn from the study. If the subjects experience adverse effects related to the study, you need to make every attempt to reconcile the effects (APA, 2010; U.S. DHHS, 2009).

Comprehension of Consent Information

Informed consent implies not only the imparting of information by the researcher but also the comprehension of that information by the subject. Studies examining subjects' levels of comprehension of consent information have found their comprehension to be limited (Erlen, 2010). The potential subjects' comprehension of the consent depended on the complexity of the study, the amount of information communicated, and the process for communicating the information. The amount of information to be taught depends on the subjects' knowledge of research and the specific research project proposed. Federal regulations require that the information given to subjects or their representatives must be in a language they can understand (U.S. FDA, 2010a; U.S. DHHS, 2009). Thus, the consent information must be written and verbalized in lay terminology, not professional jargon, and must be presented without the use of biased terms that might coerce a subject into participating in a study. Meade (1999) identified the following tips for promoting the comprehension of a consent document by potential research subjects:

- Introduce the purpose of the study early in the consent form.
- Outline the study treatment with specificity and conciseness.
- Convey the elements of informed consent in an organized fashion.

- Define technical terms, and be consistent in the use of terminology.
- Use clear terminology, and avoid professional jargon.
- Develop the document using headings, uppercase and lowercase letters, and spacing to make it easy to read.
- Use headings for major elements in the consent form, such as "Purpose," "Benefits," and "Risks."
- Use a readable font, that is, a minimum of 12- to 14-point font for text and a 16- to 18-point font for the headers.
- Address the subject directly, using phrases such as, "You are being asked to take part in this study...."

- Estimate the reading level of the document with the use of a computerized readability formula, and revise it to achieve no higher than an eighth grade reading level.

Meade (1999) used these tips to simplify a paragraph from an example consent form, as shown in Box 9-4. Once you have developed the consent document, pilot-test it with patients who are comparable to the proposed subjects for the study. These patients can give feedback on the ease of reading, clarity, and understandability of the consent document. You can then revise the document as needed on the basis of the feedback. These guidelines will help you develop a clear, concise consent document that your study subjects can comprehend.

Box 9-4	**Simplification of Consent Document**

Origin Consent Document

Example A*:
Side effects of the marrow infusion are uncommon and consist primarily of an unusual taste from the preservative, occasional nausea and vomiting, and, rarely, fever and chills. In addition, your chest may feel tight for a while, but that will pass.

Example B†:
The standard approach to treating breast cancer is to give several "cycles" (repeated doses at regularly specified intervals) of a combination of two or more chemotherapy drugs (drugs that kill cancer cells). Recent information suggests that it may be more beneficial to give several cycles of one drug followed by several cycles of another drug. Some researchers think that the second approach may kill more cells that are resistant to chemotherapy. The approach being tested in this study is to administer four cycles of standard chemotherapy (doxorubicin/cyclophosphamide) followed by four cycles of the drug paclitaxel. Researchers hope to show that cancer cells resistant to the doxorubicin/cyclophosphamide chemotherapy may be sensitive to paclitaxel. This may then result in

prolonged patient survival and result in a decrease in the number of patients experiencing a recurrence.

Revised Simplified Consent Document

Example A*:
Side effects of getting stem cells:
- An unusual or funny taste in your mouth
- Mild nausea and vomiting
- Fever and chills (rarely)
- Tightness in chest (rarely)

Example B†:
Why is this study being done?
   The purpose of this research study is to find out whether adding the drug Taxol (paclitaxel) to a commonly used chemotherapy is better than the commonly used chemotherapy by itself at preventing your cancer from coming back. The study also will see what side effects there are from adding Taxol to the commonly used chemotherapy. Taxol has been found to be effective in treating patients with advanced breast cancer. In this study, we want to see whether Taxol will help to treat patients with early stage breast cancer and whether the side effects seem to be worth the possible benefit.

NCI Model Document Sub-Group: Comprehensive Working Group on Informed Consent, 1998.
*Standard doses versus myeloablative therapy for previously untreated symptomatic multiple myeloma. Phase III. SWOG 9321.
†A randomized trial evaluating the worth of paclitaxel (Taxol) following doxorubicin (Adriamycin)/cyclophosphamide (Cytoxan) in breast cancer.
From Broome, M. E. (1999). Consent (assent) for research with pediatric patients. *Seminars in Oncology Nursing, 15*(2), 130.

Researchers can also take steps to determine the prospective subjects' level of comprehension by having them complete a survey or questionnaire examining their understanding of consent information (Cahana & Hurst, 2008). In complex, high-risk studies, it is more difficult for subjects to comprehend consent information, so some researchers might require prospective subjects to pass a test on consent information before becoming research subjects.

In qualitative research, the participants might comprehend their participation in a study at the beginning, but unexpected events or consequences might occur during the study to obscure that understanding. These events might precipitate a change in the focus of the research and the type of participation by the participants. For example, the topics of an interview might change with an increased need for information from the participants to address these topics. Thus, informed consent is an ongoing, evolving process in qualitative research. The researcher must renegotiate the participants' consent and determine their comprehension of that consent as changes occur in the study. By continually informing and determining the comprehension of participants, you will establish trust with them and promote the conduct of an ethical study (Munhall, 2012a).

Competence to Give Consent

Autonomous individuals, who are capable of understanding and weighing the benefits and risks of a proposed study, are competent to give consent. The competence of the subject is often determined by the researcher using an assessment of decisional capacity (Beattie, 2009). Persons with diminished autonomy resulting from legal or mental incompetence, terminal illness, or confinement to an institution might not be legally competent to consent to participate in research (see the earlier discussion of the right to self-determination). However, the researcher makes every effort to present the consent information at a level prospective subjects can understand, so that they can assent to the research. In addition, researchers need to clearly present essential information for consent to the legally authorized representative, such as the parents or guardian, of the prospective subject (U.S. DHHS, 2009).

Voluntary Consent

Voluntary consent means that the prospective subject has decided to take part in a study of his or her own volition without coercion or any undue influence. Voluntary consent is obtained after the prospective subject has been given essential information about the study

and has shown comprehension of this information (U.S. FDA, 2010a; U.S. DHHS, 2009). Some researchers, because of their authority, expertise, or power, have the potential to coerce subjects into participating in research. Researchers need to ensure that their persuasion of prospective subjects is not coercive. Thus, the rewards offered in a study ought to be congruent with the risks taken by the subjects.

Documentation of Informed Consent

The documentation of informed consent depends on (1) the level of risk involved in the study and (2) the discretion of the researcher and those reviewing the study for institutional approval. Most studies require a written consent form, although in some studies, the consent form may be replaced by oral consent or the consent form may be used but the subject's signature is waived.

Written Consent Waived

The requirements for written consent may be waived in research that "presents no more than minimal risk of harm to subjects and involves no procedures for which written consent is normally required outside of the research context" (U.S. DHHS, 2009, 45 CFR Section 46.117c). For example, if you were using questionnaires to collect relatively harmless data, you would not need to obtain a signed consent form from the subjects. The subject's completion of the questionnaire may serve as consent. The top of the questionnaire might contain a statement such as "Your completion of this questionnaire indicates your consent to participate in this study."

Written consent is also waived when the only record linking the subject and the research would be the consent document and the principal risk is the harm that could result from a breach of confidentiality. The subject needs to be given the option of signing a consent form or not and the subject's wishes will govern (U.S. DHHS, 2009). However, the four elements of consent—disclosure, comprehension, competence, and voluntarism—are essential in all studies whether written consent is waived or required.

Written Consent Documents
Short-Form Written Consent Document
The short-form consent document includes the following statement: "The elements of informed consent required by Section 46.116 [see the section on information essential for consent] have been presented orally to the subject or the subject's legally authorized representative" (U.S. DHHS, 2009, 45 CFR Section 46.117b). The researcher must develop a written

summary of what is to be said to the subject in the oral presentation, and the summary must be approved by an IRB. When the oral presentation is made to the subject or to the subject's representative, a witness is required. The subject or representative must sign the short-form consent document. The witness must sign both the short-form and a copy of the summary, and the person actually obtaining consent must sign a copy of the summary. Copies of the summary and short form are given to the subject and the witness; the researcher retains the original documents and must keep these documents for 3 years after the end of the study. The short-form written consent documents might be used in studies that present minimal or moderate risk to the subjects.

Formal Written Consent Document

The written consent document or **consent form** includes the elements of informed consent required by the U.S. DHHS (2009) and U.S. FDA (2010a) regulations (see the previous section on information essential for consent). In addition, a consent form might include other information required by the institution where the study is to be conducted or by the agency funding the study. Most universities provide consent form guidelines for researchers to use. A sample consent form is presented in Figure 9-2 with the common essential consent information. The subject can read the consent form, or the researcher can read it to the subject; however, it is wise also to explain the study to the subject. The subject signs the form, and

---

Study title: The Needs of Family Members of Critically Ill Adults
Investigator: Linda L. Norris, R.N.

Ms. Norris is a registered nurse studying the emotional and social needs of family members of patients in the Intensive Care Units **(research purpose)**. Although the study will not benefit you directly, it will provide information that might enable nurses to identify family members' needs and to assist family members with those needs **(potential benefits)**.

The study and its procedures have been approved by the appropriate people and review boards at The University of Texas at Arlington and X hospital **(IRB approval)**. The study procedures might cause fatigue for you or your family **(potential risks)**. The procedures include: (1) responding to a questionnaire about the needs of family members of critically ill patients and (2) completing a demographic data sheet **(explanation of procedures)**. Participation in this study will take approximately 20 minutes **(time commitment)**. You are free to ask any questions about the study or about being a subject and you may call Ms. Norris at (999) 999-9999 (work) or (999) 999-9999 (home) if you have further questions **(offer to answer questions)**.

Your participation in this study is voluntary; you are under no obligation to participate **(alternative option and voluntary consent)**. You have the right to withdraw at any time and the care of your family member and your relationship with the healthcare team will not be affected **(option to withdraw)**.

The study data will be coded so they will not be linked to your name. Your identity will not be revealed while the study is being conducted or when the study is reported or published. All study data will be collected by Ms. Norris, stored in a secure place, and not shared with any other person without your permission **(assurance of anonymity and confidentiality)**.

I have read this consent form and voluntarily consent to participate in this study.

(If Appropriate)

_____   _____
Subject's Signature   Date   Legal Representative   Date

I have explained this study to the above subject and have sought his/her understanding for informed consent

_____
Investigator's Signature   Date

Figure 9-2 Sample consent form. Words in parentheses and **boldface** identify common essential consent information and would not appear in an actual form.

the investigator or research assistant collecting the data witnesses it. This type of consent can be used for minimal- to moderate-risk studies. All persons signing the consent form must receive a copy of it. The researcher keeps the original consent form for 3 years in a secure location, such as a locked file cabinet in a locked room.

Studies that involve subjects with diminished autonomy require a written consent form. If these prospective subjects have some comprehension of the study and agree to participate as subjects, they must sign the consent form. However, each subject's legally authorized representative also must sign the form. The representative indicates his or her relationship with the subject under the signature (see Figure 9-2).

The written consent form used in a high-risk study often contains the signatures of two witnesses, the researcher, and an additional person. The additional person signing as a witness must observe the informed consent process and must not be otherwise connected with the study. The best witnesses are research or patient advocates who are employed by the institution. Sometimes nurses are asked to sign a consent form as a witness for a biomedical study. They must know the study purpose and procedures and the subject's comprehension of the study before signing the form (Fry et al., 2011). The role of the witness is more important in the consent process if the prospective subject is in awe of the investigator and does not feel free to question the procedures of the study.

Kravits, McAllister-Black, Grant, and Kirk (2010) conducted a study to examine the effect of a psycho-educational intervention on the stress reduction and prevention of burnout in registered nurses (RNs). These researchers provided a detailed description of their consent process in the following quotation. The researchers found that the intervention was useful in reducing the stress and exhaustion of the RNs but recommended additional research on the impact of the intervention.

"Informed Consent

The study was reviewed and approved by the Institutional Review Board. Consent was obtained prior to initiating the intervention. The primary investigator and/or the co-investigator explained the study including risks and benefits to all attendees including community healthcare providers. The potential participants were assured that participation was strictly voluntary and confidential. Consent was obtained by the project director, an RN, and the research assistant after the primary and co-investigators left the room to protect the anonymity of the participants. All instruments and materials were blind coded with an alphanumeric code to further protect participant anonymity. When explaining the study, permission to answer only the questions they were comfortable with was emphasized. All participants, regardless of consent status, then received the psycho-educational intervention." (Kravits et al., 2010, p. 133)

Recording of the Consent Process

A researcher might elect to audio-record or obtain a DVD of the consent process. These methods document what was said to the prospective subject and record the subject's questions and the investigator's answers. Audio-recording and DVD creation are time-consuming and costly, however, and are not appropriate for studies of minimal or moderate risk. If your study is considered high risk, it might be wise to completely document the consent process, because doing so might protect you and your subjects. Both of you would retain a copy of the recording.

Authorization for Research Uses and Disclosure

The HIPAA Privacy Rule provides individuals the right, as research subjects, to authorize covered entities (healthcare provider, health plan, and healthcare clearinghouse) to use or disclose their private health information (PHI) for research purposes. This authorization is regulated by the HIPAA and is separate from the informed consent that is regulated by the U.S. DHHS (2009) and the U.S. FDA (2010a). The authorization focuses on the privacy risks and states how, why, and with whom the PHI will be shared. The authorization form must include the following information:

Authorization Core Elements (see Privacy Rule, 45 CFR Section 164.508[c][1])
- "Description of PHI to be used or disclosed (identifying the information in a specific and meaningful manner).
- The name(s) of person(s) authorized to make the requested use or disclosure.
- The name(s) of person(s) who may use the PHI or to whom the covered entity may make the requested disclosure.
- Description of each purpose of the requested use or disclosure. Researchers should note that this

element must be study specific, not for future unspecified research.

- Authorization expiration date. The terms 'end of the research study' or 'none' may be used for research, including for the creation and maintenance of a research database or repository.
- Signature of the individual and date. If the authorization is signed by an individual's personal representative, a description of the representative's authority to act for the individual must be included." (U.S. DHHS, 2004)

The authorization information can be included as part of the consent form, but it is probably best to have two separate forms (Olsen, 2003). U.S. DHHS (2004) developed a sample authorization form, which is presented in Figure 9-3.

Institutional Review

In institutional review, a committee of the researcher's peers, examines his or her study for ethical concerns. The first federal policy statement on protection of human subjects by institutional review was issued by the U.S. PHS in 1966. The statement required that research involving human subjects must be reviewed by a committee of peers or associates to confirm that (1) the rights and welfare of subjects will be protected, (2) appropriate methods will be used to secure informed consent, and (3) the potential benefits of the investigation are greater than the risks (Levine, 1986). In 1974, DHEW passed the National Research Act, which required that all research involving human subjects undergo institutional review. Currently, the U.S. DHHS (2009, 45 CFR Sections 46.107-46.115) and the U.S. FDA (2010b, 21 CFR Sections 56.101-56.124) have similar regulations for institutional review of research. These regulations describe the membership, functions, and operations of an institutional review board. An institutional review board (IRB) is a committee that reviews research to ensure that the investigator is conducting the research ethically. Universities, hospital corporations, and many managed care centers have IRBs to promote the conduct of ethical research and protect the rights of prospective subjects at these institutions.

Each IRB has at least five members of various backgrounds (cultural, economic, educational, gender, racial) to promote a complete, scholarly, and fair review of research that is commonly conducted in an institution. If an institution regularly reviews studies with vulnerable subjects, such as children, neonates, pregnant women, prisoners, and mentally disabled persons, the IRB should include one or more members with knowledge about and experience in working with these individuals. The members must have sufficient experience and expertise to review a variety of studies, including quantitative, outcomes, intervention, and qualitative research (Munhall, 2012b). The IRB members must not have a conflicting interest related to a study conducted by an institution. Any member having a conflict of interest with a research project being reviewed must excuse himself or herself from the review process, except to provide information requested by the IRB. The IRB also must include other members whose primary concern is nonscientific, such as an ethicist, a lawyer, or a minister. At least one of the IRB members must be someone who is not affiliated with the institution (U.S. FDA, 2010h; U.S. DHHS, 2009). The IRBs in hospitals are often composed of physicians, nurses, lawyers, scientists, clergy, and community laypersons.

In 2009, the U.S. FDA and U.S. DHHS regulations were revised to require all IRBs to register through a system maintained by the DHHS. The registration information includes contact information for the institution with the IRB and the official overseeing the activities performed by the IRB (such as names, addresses, emails, and telephone numbers), the number of active protocols involving federally regulated products reviewed during the preceding 12 months, and a description of the types of products involved in the protocols reviewed (U.S. FDA, 2010b; U.S. DHHS, 2009). The IRB registration requirement was implemented to make it easier for the DHHS to inspect IRBs and communicate information to them. This rule was made effective in July of 2009 and requires each IRB to renew its registration every 3 years.

Levels of Reviews Conducted by Institutional Review Boards

Universities and healthcare agencies have IRBs that function in a similar way to review research following federal regulations (U.S. FDA. 2010b; U.S. DHHS, 2009). Faculty and students must receive IRB approval from their university prior to seeking IRB approval at the agency where the study is to be conducted. The functions and operations of an IRB involve the review of research at three different levels: (1) exempt from review; (2) expedited review; and (3) complete review. We want to stress with students and practicing nurses that the level of the review required for each study is decided by the IRB chairperson and/or committee, not by the researcher.

Studies are usually exempt from review if they pose no apparent risks for the research subjects. The studies that are usually considered exempt from IRB review by the federal regulations are identified in

AUTHORIZATION TO USE OR DISCLOSE (RELEASE) HEALTH INFORMATION
THAT IDENTIFIES YOU FOR A RESEARCH STUDY

REQUIRED ELEMENTS:
If you sign this document, you give permission to [name or other identification of specific healthcare provider(s) or description of classes of persons, e.g., all doctors, all healthcare providers] at [name of covered entity or entities] to use or disclose (release) your health information that identifies you for the research study described below:
[Provide a description of the research study, such as the title and purpose of the research.]

The health information that we may use or disclose (release) for this research includes [complete as appropriate]:
[Provide a description of information to be used or disclosed for the research project. This description may include, for example, all information in a medical record, results of physical examinations, medical history, lab tests, or certain health information indicating or relating to a particular condition.]
The health information listed above may be used by and/or disclosed (released) to:
[Name or class of persons involved in the research; i.e., researchers and their staff**]

[Name of covered entity] is required by law to protect your health information. By signing this document, you authorize [name of covered entity] to use and/or disclose (release) your health information for this research. Those persons who receive your health information may not be required by Federal privacy laws (such as the Privacy Rule) to protect it and may share your information with others without your permission, if permitted by laws governing them.

Please note that [include the appropriate statement]:
- You do not have to sign this Authorization, but if you do not, you may not receive research-related treatment.
  (When the research involves treatment and is conducted by the covered entity or when the covered entity provides health care solely for the purpose of creating protected health information to disclose to a researcher)

- [Name of covered entity] may not condition (withhold or refuse) treating you on whether you sign this Authorization.
  (When the research does not involve research-related treatment by the covered entity or when the covered entity is not providing health care solely for the purpose of creating protected health information to disclose to a researcher)

Please note that [include the appropriate statement]:
- You may change your mind and revoke (take back) this Authorization at any time, except to the extent that [name of covered entity(ies)] has already acted based on this Authorization. To revoke this Authorization, you must write to: [name of the covered entity(ies) and contact information].
  (When the research study is conducted by an entity other than the covered entity)

- You may change your mind and revoke (take back) this Authorization at any time. Even if you revoke this Authorization, [name or class of persons at the covered entity involved in the research] may still use or disclose health information they already have obtained about you as necessary to maintain the integrity or reliability of the current research. To revoke this Authorization, you must write to: [name of the covered entity(ies) and contact information].
  (When the research study is conducted by the covered entity)

_____   _____
Signature of participant or participant's   Date
personal representative

_____   _____
Printed name of participant or participant's   If applicable, a description of the personal
personal representative   representative's authority to sign for the participant

** When a covered entity conducts the research study, the Authorization must list ALL names or other identification, or ALL classes, of persons who will have access through the covered entity to the protected health information (PHI) for the research study (e.g., research collaborators, sponsors, and others who will have access to data that includes PHI). Examples may include, but are not limited to, the following:

- Data coordinating centers that will receive and process PHI;
- Sponsors who want access to PHI or who will actually own the research data; and/or
- Institutional Review Boards or Data Safety and Monitoring Boards.

If the research study is conducted by an entity other than the covered entity, the authorization need only list the name or other identification of the outside researcher (or class of researchers) and any other entity to whom the covered entity is expected to make the disclosure.

Figure 9-3 Sample of authorization language for research uses and disclosures of individually identifiable health information by a covered healthcare provider. Words in parentheses and **boldface** are explanations for the reader and would not appear in an actual form.

| Box 9-5 | Research Qualifying for Exemption from Review |

Unless otherwise required by department or agency heads, research activities in which the only involvement of human subjects will be in one or more of the following categories are exempt from review:

(1) Research conducted in established or commonly accepted educational settings, involving normal educational practices, such as (i) research on regular and special education instructional strategies, or (ii) research on the effectiveness of or the comparison among instructional techniques, curricula, or classroom management methods.

(2) Research involving the use of educational tests (cognitive, diagnostic, aptitude, achievement), survey procedures, interview procedures or observation of public behavior, unless: (i) information obtained is recorded in such a manner that human subjects can be identified, directly or through identifiers linked to the subjects; and (ii) any disclosure of the human subjects' responses outside the research could reasonably place the subjects at risk of criminal or civil liability or be damaging to the subjects' financial standing, employability, or reputation.

(3) Research involving the use of educational tests (cognitive, diagnostic, aptitude, achievement), survey procedures, interview procedures, or observation of public behavior that is not exempt under paragraph (b)(2) of this section, if: (i) the human subjects are elected or appointed public officials or candidates for public office; or (ii) Federal statute(s) require(s) without exception that the confidentiality of the personally identifiable information will be maintained throughout the research and thereafter.

(4) Research involving the collection or study of existing data, documents, records, pathological specimens, or diagnostic specimens if these sources are publicly available or if the information is recorded by the investigator in such a manner that subjects cannot be identified, directly or through identifiers linked to the subjects.

(5) Research and demonstration projects which are conducted by or subject to the approval of Department or Agency heads, and which are designed to study, evaluate, or otherwise examine: (i) Public benefit or service programs; (ii) procedures for obtaining benefits or services under those programs; (iii) possible changes in or alternatives to those programs or procedures; or (iv) possible changes in methods or levels of payment for benefits or services under those programs.

(6) Taste and food quality evaluation and consumer acceptance studies (i) if wholesome foods without additives are consumed or (ii) if a food is consumed that contains a food ingredient at or below the level and for a use found to be safe, or agricultural chemical or environmental contaminant at or below the level found to be safe, by the Food and Drug Administration or approved by the Environmental Protection Agency or the Food Safety and Inspection Service of the U.S. Department of Agriculture.

From U.S. Department of Health and Human Services (U.S. DHHS, 2009). *Protection of human subjects. Code of Federal Regulations, Title 45, Part 46.* Retrieved from http://www.hhs.gov/ohrp/policy/ohrpregulations.pdf/.

Box 9-5. For example, studies by nurses and other health professionals that have no foreseeable risks or are a mere inconvenience for subjects might be identified as exempt from review by the chairperson of the IRB committee. Studies incorporating previously collected data from which PHI has been de-identified are usually exempt as well (U.S. DHHS, 2004).

Studies that have some risks, which are viewed as minimal, are expedited in the review process. **Minimal** **risk** means "that the risks of harm anticipated in the proposed research are not greater, considering probability and magnitude, than those ordinarily encountered in daily life or during the performance of routine physical or psychological examinations or tests" (U.S. DHHS, 2009, 45 CFR Section 46.102). Expedited review procedures can also be used to review minor changes in previously approved research. Under **expedited IRB review** procedures, the review may be

Box 9-6 Research Qualifying for Expedited Institutional Review Board Review

Expedited review (by committee chairpersons or designated members) is authorized for the following research involving no more than minimal risk:

1. Collection of hair and nail clippings, in a nondisfiguring manner; deciduous teeth and permanent teeth if patient care indicates a need for extraction.
2. Collection of excreta and external secretions including sweat, uncannulated saliva, placenta removed at delivery, and amniotic fluid at the time of rupture of the membrane before or during labor.
3. Recording of data from subjects 18 years of age or older using noninvasive procedures routinely employed in clinical practice. This includes the use of physical sensors that are applied either to the surface of the body or at a distance and do not involve input of matter or significant amounts of energy into the subject or an invasion of the subject's privacy. It also includes such procedures as weighing, testing sensory acuity, electrocardiography, electroencephalography, thermography, detection of naturally occurring radioactivity, diagnostic echography, and electroretinography. It does not include exposure to electromagnetic radiation outside the visible range (for example, x-rays, microwaves).
4. Collection of blood samples by venipuncture, in amounts not exceeding 450 mL in an 8-week period and no more than two times per week, from subjects 18 years of age or older and who are in good health and not pregnant.
5. Collection of both supragingival and subgingival dental plaque and calculus, provided the procedure is not more invasive than routine prophylactic scaling of the teeth and the process is accomplished in accordance with accepted prophylactic techniques.
6. Voice recordings made for research purposes such as investigations of speech defects.
7. Moderate exercise by healthy volunteers.
8. The study of existing data, documents, records, pathological specimens, or diagnostic specimens.
9. Research on individual or group behavior or characteristics of individuals, such as studies of perception, cognition, game theory, or test development, where the investigator does not manipulate subjects' behavior and research will not involve stress to subjects.
10. Research on drugs or devices for which an investigational new drug exemption or an investigational device exemption is not required.

From U.S. Department of Health and Human Services (U.S. DHHS, 2009). *Protection of human subjects. Code of Federal Regulations, Title 45, Part 46.* Retrieved from http://www.hhs.gov/ohrp/policy/ohrpregulations.pdf/.

carried out by the IRB chairperson or by one or more experienced reviewers designated by the chairperson from among members of the IRB. In reviewing the research, the reviewers may exercise all of the authorities of the IRB except disapproval of the research. A research proposal may be disapproved only after a complete review by the IRB (U.S. FDA, 2010b; U.S. DHHS, 2009). Box 9-6 identifies research that usually qualifies for expedited review.

A study involving greater than minimal risks to research subjects requires a **complete IRB review**. To obtain IRB approval, researchers must ensure that "(1) risks to subjects are minimized, (2) risks to subjects are reasonable in relation to anticipated benefits, (3) selection of subjects is equitable, (4) informed consent will be sought from each prospective subject or the subject's legally authorized representative, (5) informed consent will be appropriately documented, (6) the research plan makes adequate provision for monitoring data collection for subjects' safety, and (7) adequate provisions are made to protect the privacy of subjects and to maintain the confidentiality of data." (U.S. FDA, 2010b, 21 CFR 56.111; U.S. DHHS, 2009, 45 CFR 46.111).

Every research report must indicate that the study had IRB approval and whether the approval was from a university and/or clinical agency. All the reports used as examples in this chapter indicated the studies had appropriate IRB approval. For example, Riegel et al. (2011) provided the following description of their IRB approval. This study involved a secondary data analysis using a national database of HF patients to determine their levels of self-care performance. These researchers ensured the studies in the database had IRB approval and that they obtained IRB approval from their university.

> "All studies had been approved by local institutional review boards. In each, eligibility was confirmed by a trained nurse research assistant who then explained study requirements and obtained written informed consent. This secondary analysis was approved by the institutional review board of the University of Pennsylvania." (Riegel et al., 2011, p. 134)

Influence of HIPAA Privacy Rule on Institutional Review Boards

Under the 2003 HIPAA Privacy Rule, an IRB or an institutionally established privacy board can act on requests for a waiver or an alteration of the authorization requirement for a research project. If an IRB and a privacy board both exist in an agency, the approval of only one board is required, and it will probably be the IRB for research projects. Researchers can choose to obtain a signed authorization form from potential subjects or can ask for a waiver or an alteration of the authorization requirement. An altered authorization requirement occurs when an IRB approves a request that some but not all of the required 18 elements removed from health information that is to be used in research. The researcher can also request a partial or complete waiver of the authorization requirement from the IRB. For a partial waiver, discussed earlier, the researcher obtains PHI to contact and recruit potential subjects for a study. An IRB can give a researcher a complete waiver of authorization in studies in which the informed consent requirements might also be waived. Thus, a waiver or alteration of the authorization requirement might occur when the following criteria have been met:

- The PHI use or disclosure involves no more than minimal risk to the privacy for research subjects based on (1) an adequate plan presented to the IRB to protect the PHI identifiers from improper use of disclosure; (2) an adequate plan exists to destroy the identifiers at the earliest opportunity; and (3) written assurance the PHI will not be reused or disclosed to any other person.
- The research could not reasonably be conducted without the waiver or alteration of the authorization requirement.
- The research cannot be done without access to and use of the PHI. (U.S. DHHS, 2003)

The healthcare provider, health plan, or healthcare clearinghouse cannot release the PHI to the researcher until the following documentation has been received: (1) the identity of the approving IRB; (2) the date the waiver or alteration was approved; (3) IRB documentation that the criteria for waiver or alteration have been met; (4) a brief description of the PHI to which the researcher has been granted access or use; (5) a statement as to whether the waiver was approved under normal or expedited review procedures; and (6) the signature of the IRB chair or the chair's designee.

The HIPAA Privacy Rule does not change the IRB membership and functions that are designated under the U.S. DHHS and U.S. FDA regulations. For clarification, the responsibilities of the IRB/privacy board for HIPAA (U.S. DHHS, 2007b) and the responsibilities of the IRB under the U.S. DHHS (2009) and U.S. FDA (2010a) are outlined in Table 9-3.

Research Misconduct

The goal of research is to generate sound scientific knowledge, which is possible only through the honest conduct, reporting, and publication of studies. However, since the 1980s, a number of fraudulent studies have been conducted and published in prestigious scientific journals. An example of research misconduct was evident in the publications of Dr. Robert Slutsky, a heart specialist at the University of California, San Diego, School of Medicine, whose study results raised questions of data fabrication (Friedman, 1990). In 6 years, Slutsky published 161 articles, and at one time, he was completing an article every 10 days. Eighteen of the articles were found to be fraudulent and have retraction notations, and 60 articles were judged to be questionable.

Another example of research misconduct is the work of Stephen Breuning, a psychologist at the University of Pittsburgh, who engaged in deceptive and misleading practices in reporting his research on retarded children. He used his fraudulent research to obtain more than $300,000 in federal grants. In 1988, he was criminally charged with research fraud, pleaded guilty, was fined $20,000, and was sentenced to up to 10 years in prison (Garfield & Welljams-Dorof, 1990).

Research misconduct is also evident in nursing as identified by a survey of nurse research directors, coordinators, and deans of nursing programs by Rankin and Esteves (1997). Of the 88 nurses surveyed, 27.2% reported cheating on data collection, 33.2% identified misinterpretations of findings, 65.8% reported protocol violations related to the study site

TABLE 9-3   Comparison of IRB/Privacy Board Responsibilities for HIPAA, U.S. DHHS, and FDA

Area of Distinction	HIPAA Privacy Rule	U.S. DHHS Protection of Human Subjects Regulations Title 45 CFR Part 46	U.S. FDA Protection of Human Subjects Regulations Title 21 CFR Parts 50 and 56
Permissions for research	Authorization	Informed consent and authorization	Informed consent and authorization
IRB/privacy board responsibilities	Requires the covered entity to obtain authorization for research use or disclosure of PHI unless a regulatory permission applies. Because of this, the IRB or privacy board would see only requests to waive or alter the authorization requirement. In exercising privacy rule authority, the IRB or privacy board does not review the authorization form.	Requires the covered entity to obtain authorization for research use or disclosure of PHI unless a regulatory permission applies. Because of this, the IRB or privacy board would see only requests to waive or alter the authorization requirement. In exercising privacy rule authority, the IRB or privacy board does not review the authorization form.	The IRB must ensure that informed consent will be sought from, and documented for, each prospective subject or the subject's legally authorized representative in accordance with, and to the extent required by, FDA regulations. If specified criteria are met, the requirements for either obtaining informed consent or documenting informed consent may be waived. The IRB must review and approve the authorization form if it is combined with the informed consent document. Privacy boards have no authority under the FDA Protection of Human Subjects Regulations.

CFR, Code of Federal Regulations; *DHHS,* U.S. Department of Health and Human Services; *U.S. FDA,* U.S. Food and Drug Administration; *HIPAA,* Health Insurance Portability and Accountability Act; *IRB,* institutional review board; PHI, protected health information.
From U.S. Department of Health and Human Services. (2007b). *How can covered entities use and disclose protected health information for research and comply with the Privacy Rule?* Retrieved from http://privacyruleandresearch.nih.gov/pr_08.asp/.

and subjects, and 49.7% reported an occasional incidence of plagiarism. Habermann, Broome, Pryor, and Ziner (2010) studied 266 research coordinators, predominately RNs, who indicated they had firsthand knowledge of scientific misconduct in the past year. The types and frequencies of research misconduct included: 50% protocol violations, 26.6% consent violations, 13.9% fabrication, 5.2% financial conflict of interest, and 5% falsification.

In response to the increasing incidences of scientific misconduct, the federal government developed the Office of Research Integrity (ORI) in 1989 within the U.S. DHHS. The ORI was to supervise the implementation of the rules and regulations related to research misconduct and to manage any investigations of misconduct. The most current regulations implemented by the ORI (2005) are CFR 42, Parts 50 and 93, Policies of General Applicability, which are discussed in the following section.

Role of the ORI in Promoting the Conduct of Ethical Research

The ORI was responsible for defining important terms used in the identification and management of research

misconduct. **Research misconduct** was defined as "the fabrication, falsification, or plagiarism in processing, performing, or reviewing research, or in reporting research results. It does not include honest error or differences in opinion" (ORI, 2005, 42 CFR Section 93.103). **Fabrication in research** is the making up of results and the recording or reporting of them. **Falsification of research** is manipulating research materials, equipment, or processes or changing or omitting data or results such that the research is not accurately represented in the research record. Fabrication and falsification of research data are two of the most common acts of research misconduct managed by the ORI (2012) over the past 5 years. **Plagiarism** is the appropriation of another person's ideas, processes, results, or words without giving appropriate credit, including those obtained through confidential review of others' research proposals and manuscripts.

Currently, the ORI promotes the integrity of biomedical and behavioral research in approximately 4000 institutions worldwide (ORI, 2011). The office applies federal policies and regulations to protect the integrity of the U.S. PHS's extramural and intramural research programs. The extramural program provides funding to research institutions, and the intramural program provides funding for research conducted within the federal government. The ORI carries out its responsibilities by:

- Developing policies, procedures, and regulations related to the detection, investigation, and prevention of research misconduct and the responsible conduct of research.
- Reviewing and monitoring research misconduct investigations.
- Recommending research misconduct findings and administrative actions to the assistant secretary for health for decision, subject to appeal (ORI, 2012).
- Assisting the Office of the General Counsel (OGC) to present cases before the U.S. DHHS departmental appeals board.
- Providing technical assistance to institutions that respond to allegations of research misconduct.
- Implementing activities and programs to teach responsible conduct of research, promote research integrity, prevent research misconduct, and improve the handling of allegations of research misconduct.
- Conducting policy analyses, evaluations, and research to build the knowledge base in research misconduct, research integrity, and prevention and to improve the DHHS research integrity policies and procedures.
- Administering programs for maintaining institutional assurances, responding to allegations of retaliation against whistleblowers, approving intramural and extramural policies and procedures, and responding to Freedom of Information Act and Privacy Act requests (ORI, 2005).

The ORI classifies research misconduct as (1) an act that involves a significant departure from the acceptable practice of the scientific community for maintaining the integrity of the research record; (2) an act that was committed intentionally; and (3) an allegation that can be proved by a preponderance of evidence. The office has a section on its website titled "Handling Misconduct," which includes a summary of the allegations and investigations managed by its office from 1994 to 2012 (ORI, 2012). The most common sites for the investigations were medical schools (68%), hospitals (11%), and research institutes (10%). The individuals charged with misconduct were primarily males holding a PhD or medical degree (MD) and were mostly associate professors, professors, and postdoctoral fellows. When research misconduct was documented, the actions taken against the researchers or agencies might have included debarment from receiving federal funding for periods ranging from 18 months to 8 years; prohibition from U.S. PHS advisory service; and other actions requiring supervised research, certification of data, certification of sources, and correction or retraction of articles (ORI, 2012).

Role of Journal Editors and Researchers in Preventing Scientific Misconduct

Editors of journals also have a major role in monitoring and preventing research misconduct in the published literature. Friedman (1990, p. 1416) identified criteria for classifying a publication as fraudulent, questionable, or valid and indicated that research articles were "fraudulent if there was documentation or testimony from coauthors that the publication did not reflect what had actually been done." Articles were considered questionable if no coauthor could produce the original data or if no coauthor had personally observed or performed each phase of the research or participated in the research publication. A research article was considered valid if one or more coauthors had personally participated in each aspect of the research and publication.

Preventing the publication of fraudulent research requires the efforts of authors, coauthors, research coordinators, reviewers of research reports for publication, and editors of professional journals (Hansen & Hansen, 1995; Hawley & Jeffers, 1992; Wager, 2007). Authors who are primary investigators for research projects must be responsible in their conduct, reporting, and publication of research. Coauthors and coworkers should question and, if necessary, challenge the integrity of a researcher's claims. Sometimes, well-known scientists' names have been added to a research publication as coauthors to give it credibility. Individuals should not be listed as coauthors unless they were actively involved in the conduct and publication of the research.

Research coordinators in large, funded studies also have a role to promote integrity in research and to identify research misconduct activities. These individuals are often the ones closest to the actual conduct of the study, during which misconduct often occurs. In the Habermann et al. (2010) study introduced earlier, research coordinators were identified as having firsthand experiences with both scientific misconduct and research integrity. Research coordinators often learned of the misconduct firsthand, and the principal investigator was usually identified as the responsible party. The five major categories of misconduct identified were protocol violations, consent violations, fabrication, falsification, and financial conflict of interest. Thus, Habermann et al. recommended that the definition of research misconduct might need to be expanded beyond fabrication, falsification, and plagiarism.

Peer reviewers have a key role in determining the quality and publishability of a manuscript. They are considered experts in the field, and their role is to examine research for inconsistencies and inaccuracies. Editors must monitor the peer review process and must be cautious about publishing manuscripts that are at all questionable. Editors also need procedures for responding to allegations of research misconduct. They must decide what actions to take if their journal contains an article that has proven to be fraudulent. Usually, fraudulent publications require retraction notations and are not to be cited by authors in future publications (ORI, 2005).

The publication of fraudulent research is a major concern in medicine and nursing (Habermann et al., 2010; Njie & Thomas, 2001; Rankin & Esteves, 1997). The smaller pool of funds available for research and the greater emphasis on research publications could lead to a higher incidence of fraudulent publications. However, the ORI (2011; 2012) has made major advances in addressing research misconduct and the management of fraudulent publications by: (1) identifying the administrative actions for acts of research misconduct; (2) developing a process for notifying funding agencies and journals of acts of research misconduct; and (3) providing for public disclosure of the incidents of research misconduct.

Each researcher is responsible for monitoring the integrity of his or her research protocols, results, and publications. In addition, nursing professionals and journal editors must foster a spirit of intellectual inquiry, mentor prospective scientists regarding the norms for good science, and stress quality, not quantity, in publications (Wager, 2007; Wocial, 1995).

Animals as Research Subjects

The use of animals as research subjects is a controversial issue of growing interest to nurse researchers. A small but increasing number of nurse scientists are conducting physiological studies that require the use of animals. Many scientists, especially physicians, believe that the current animal rights' movement could threaten the future of health research. The animal rights groups are active in anti-research campaigns and are often backed by financial resources estimated in the millions of dollars (Pardes, West, & Pincus, 1991). The goal of these groups is to raise the consciousness of researchers and society to ensure that animals are used wisely in the conduct of research and

treated humanely. However, some of these animal rights groups have tried to frighten the public with sometimes distorted stories about inhumane treatment of animals in research. Some of the activist leaders have made broad comparisons between human life and animal life. For example, a major animal rights group called People for the Ethical Treatment of Animals (PETA) has a website that posts videos and blogs about the unethical treatment of animals in research (see http://www.peta.org/tv/videos/investigations-animal-experimentation/). Some of these activists have now progressed to violence, using physical attacks, including real bombs, arson, and vandalism. Even more damage is being done to research through lawsuits that have blocked the conduct of research and the development of new research centers. Medical schools now spend millions of dollars annually for security, public education, and other efforts to defend research.

The use of animals in research is a complicated issue that requires careful consideration by investigators, considering the knowledge that is needed to manage healthcare problems. Two important questions must be addressed: Should animals be used as subjects in research, and, if animals are used in research, what mechanisms ensure that they are treated humanely? In regard to the first question, the type of research project developed influences the selection of subjects. Animals are just one of a variety of types of subjects used in research; others are human beings, plants, and computer data sets. Most researchers use nonanimal subjects in their studies because they are generally less expensive for the type of study being conducted. In studies that are low risk, which most nursing studies are, human beings are commonly used as subjects.

Some studies, however, require the use of animals to answer the research question. Animals are more commonly used in laboratory studies that involve investigation of high-risk physiological variables. Approximately 17 to 22 million animals are used in research each year, and 90% of them are rodents, with the combined percentage of dogs and cats being only 1% to 2% (Goodwin & Morrison, 2000). Studies using animals account for about one eighth of the published studies (Osborne, Payne, & Newman, 2009). Because animals are deemed valuable subjects for selected research projects, the second question, concerning their humane treatment, must also be answered. At least five separate types of regulations exist to protect research animals from mistreatment. The federal government, state governments, independent accreditation organizations, professional societies, and individual institutions work to ensure that research animals are used only when necessary and only under humane conditions. At the federal level, animal research is conducted according to the guidelines of U.S. PHS Policy on Humane Care and Use of Laboratory Animals, which was adopted in 1986, reprinted essentially unchanged in 1996, and is available on the Office of Laboratory Animal Welfare (OLAW, 2008) website (http://grants.nih.gov/grants/olaw/olaw.htm/).

The Humane Care and Use of Laboratory Animals Regulations define *animal* as any live, vertebrate animal used or intended for use in research, research training, experimentation, or biological testing or for related purposes. Any institution proposing research involving animals must have a written Animal Welfare Assurance statement acceptable to the U.S. PHS that documents compliance with the U.S. PHS policy. Every assurance statement is evaluated by the National Institutes of Health's Office for Protection from Research Risks (OPRR) to determine the adequacy of the institution's proposed program for the care and use of animals in activities conducted or supported by the U.S. PHS (OLAW, 2011). The studies including animals require an animal-use protocol that describes the following elements: (1) research project; (2) rationale for animal use and consideration of alternatives; (3) justification for the choice of species and numbers of animals; (4) research procedures involving animals; (5) procedures to minimize pain and distress; (6) animal living conditions and veterinary care; (7) names and qualifications of personnel who will perform work with animals; (8) method of euthanasia; and (9) endpoint criteria. OLAW (2011) website includes guidelines for the care and use of animals in research (http://grants.nih.gov/grants/olaw/Investiga torsNeed2Know.pdf/).

Institutions' assurance statements about compliance with the U.S. PHS policy have promoted the humane care and treatment of animals in research. In addition, more than 700 institutions conducting health-related research have sought accreditation by the American Association for Accreditation of Laboratory Animal Care (AAALAC), which was developed to ensure the humane treatment of animals in research (OLAW, 2011). In conducting research, each investigator must carefully select the type of subject needed; if animals are used as subjects, they require humane treatment. Osborne et al. (2009) conducted a study to determine the journal editorial policies regarding use of animals in research. These researchers found that journals need clear polices on the essential information to be included in a research report to reflect the fair treatment of animals in studies.

KEY POINTS

- The ethical conduct of research starts with the identification of the study topic and continues through the publication of the study if quality research evidence is going to be developed for practice.
- The debate about ethics and research must continue probably because of (1) the complexity of human rights issues; (2) the focus of research in new, challenging arenas of technology and genetics; (3) the complex ethical codes and regulations governing research; and (4) the variety of interpretations of these codes and regulations.
- Two historical documents that have had a strong impact on the conduct of research are the Nuremberg Code and the Declaration of Helsinki. More recently, the U.S. Department of Health and Human Services (U.S. DHHS, 2009) and the U.S. Food and Drug Administration (U.S. FDA, 2010a, 2010b) have promulgated regulations that direct the ethical conduct of research. These regulations include (1) general requirements for informed consent; (2) documentation of informed consent; (3) institutional review board (IRB) review of research; (4) exempt and expedited review procedures for certain kinds of research; and (5) criteria for IRB approval of research.
- The Council for International Organizations of Medical Sciences revises and updates ethical guidelines for biomedical research conducted internationally.
- Public Law 104-191, the Health Insurance Portability and Accountability Act (HIPAA), was enacted in 1996 and implemented in 2003 to protect an individual's health information.
- Conducting research ethically requires protection of the human rights of subjects. Human rights are claims and demands that have been justified in the eyes of an individual or by the consensus of a group of individuals. The human rights that require protection in research are (1) self-determination; (2) privacy; (3) anonymity and confidentiality; (4) fair treatment; and (5) protection from discomfort and harm.
- The rights of research subjects can be protected by balancing benefits and risks of a study, securing informed consent, and submitting the research for institutional review.
- To balance the benefits and risks of a study, the type, level, and number of risks are examined, and the potential benefits are identified. If possible, the risks must be minimized and the benefits

maximized to achieve the best possible benefit-risk ratio.

- Informed consent involves the transmission of essential information, comprehension of that information, competence to give consent, and voluntary consent of the prospective subject.

- In institutional review, a committee of peers called an institutional review board (IRB) examines each study for ethical concerns. The IRB conducts three levels of review: exempt, expedited, and complete. The process for accessing protected health information according to the HIPAA Privacy Rule is also detailed.

- Research misconduct includes fabrication, falsification, and plagiarism during the conduct, reporting, or publication of research. The Office of Research Integrity (ORI) was developed to investigate and manage incidents of research misconduct to protect the integrity of research in all disciplines.

- Another current ethical concern in research is the use of animals as subjects. Two important questions are addressed: Should animals be used as research subjects? and If animals are used in research, what mechanisms ensure that they are treated humanely? The U.S. Public Health Service Policy on Humane Care and Use of Laboratory Animals provides direction for the conduct of research with animals as subjects.

REFERENCES

American Nurses Association (ANA, 2001). *Code of ethics for nurses with interpretive statements.* Washington, DC: American Nurses Association.

American Psychological Association (APA, 2010). *Ethical principles of psychologists and code of conduct.* Washington, DC: American Psychological Association. Retrieved June 20, 2011, from http://www.apa.org/ethics/code/index.aspx/.

Beattie, E. (2009). Research participation of individuals with dementia: Decisional capacity, informed consent, and considerations for nurse investigators. *Research in Gerontological Nursing, 2*(2), 94–102.

Beebe, L. H. & Smith, K. (2010). Informed consent to research in persons with schizophrenia spectrum disorders. *Nursing Ethics, 17*(4), 425–434.

Beecher, H. K. (1966). Ethics and clinical research. *New England Journal of Medicine, 274*(24), 1354–1360.

Brandt, A. M. (1978). Racism and research: The case of the Tuskegee Syphilis Study. *Hastings Center Report, 8*(6), 21–29.

Broome, M. E. (1999). Consent (assent) for research with pediatric patients. *Seminars in Oncology Nursing, 15*(2), 96–103.

Broome, M. E. & Stieglitz, K. A. (1992). The consent process and children. *Research in Nursing & Health, 15*(2), 147–152.

Bruce, S. L. & Grove, S. K. (1994). The effect of a coronary artery risk evaluation program on serum lipid values and cardiovascular risk levels. *Applied Nursing Research, 7*(2), 67–74.

Cahana, A. & Hurst, S. A. (2008). Voluntary informed consent in research and clinical care: An update. *Pain Practice, 8*(6), 446–451.

Council for International Organizations of Medical Sciences (CIOMS, 2010). *CIOMS: About us.* Retrieved from http://www.cioms.ch/about/frame_about.htm/.

Damrosch, S. P. (1986). Ensuring anonymity by use of subject-generated identification codes. *Research in Nursing & Health, 9*(1), 61–63.

Erlen, J. A. (2010). Informed consent: Revisiting the issues. *Orthopaedic Nursing, 29*(4), 276–280.

Fawcett, J. & Garity, J. (2009). *Evaluation research for evidence-based practice.* Philadelphia, PA: F. A. Davis.

Ford, J. S. & Reutter, L. I. (1990). Ethical dilemmas associated with small samples. *Journal of Advanced Nursing, 15*(2), 187–191.

Friedman, P. J. (1990). Correcting the literature following fraudulent publication. *JAMA, 263*(10), 1416–1419.

Fry, S. T., Veatch, R. M. & Taylor, C. (2011). *Case studies in nursing ethics* (4th ed.). Sudbury, MA: Jones & Bartlett Learning.

Garfield, E. & Welljams-Dorof, A. (1990). The impact of fraudulent research on the scientific literature: The Stephen E. Breuning case. *JAMA, 263*(10), 1424–1426.

Goodwin, F. K. & Morrison, A. R. (2000). Science and self-doubt. *Reason, 32*(5), 22–28.

Habermann, B., Broome, M., Pryor, E. R., & Ziner, K. W. (2010). Research coordinators' experiences with scientific misconduct and research integrity. *Nursing Research, 59*(1), 51–57.

Hansen, B. C. & Hansen, K. D. (1995). Academic and scientific misconduct: Issues for nursing educators. *Journal of Professional Nursing, 11*(1), 31–39.

Hawley, D. J. & Jeffers, J. M. (1992). Scientific misconduct as a dilemma for nursing. *Image—Journal of Nursing Scholarship, 24*(1), 51–55.

Hershey, N. & Miller, R. D. (1976). *Human experimentation and the law.* Germantown, MD: Aspen.

Hinds, P. S., Burghen, E. A., & Pritchard, M. (2007). Conducting end-of-life studies in pediatric oncology. *Western Journal of Nursing Research, 29*(4), 448–465.

Holaday, B., Gonzales, O., & Mills, D. (2007). Assent of school-age bilingual children. *Western Journal of Nursing Research, 29*(4), 466–485.

Jones, D. J., Munro, C. L., Grap, M. J., Kitten, T., & Edmond, M. (2010). Oral care and bacteremia risk in mechanically ventilated adults. *Heart & Lung, 39*(6S) S57–S65.

Kelman, H. C. (1967). Human use of human subjects: The problem of deception in social psychological experiments. *Psychological Bulletin, 67*(1), 1–11.

Kravits, K., McAllister-Black, R., Grant, M., & Kirk, C. (2010). Self-care strategies for nurses: A psycho-educational intervention for stress reduction and the prevention of burnout. *Applied Nursing Research, 23*(3), 130–138.

Levine, R. J. (1986). *Ethics and regulation of clinical research* (2nd ed.). Baltimore-Munich: Urban & Schwarzenberg.

McClain, N., Laughon, K., Steeves, R., & Parker, B. (2007). Balancing the needs of scientist and the subject in trauma research. *Western Journal of Nursing Research, 29*(1), 121–128.

Meade, C. D. (1999). Improving understanding of the informed consent process and document. *Seminars in Oncology Nursing, 15*(2), 124–137.

Milgram, S. (1963). Behavioral study of obedience. *Journal of Abnormal and Social Psychology, 67*(4), 371–378.

Munhall, P. L. (2012a). Ethical considerations in qualitative research. In P. L. Munhall (Ed.), *Nursing research: A qualitative perspective* (5th ed.) (pp. 491–502). Sudbury, MA: Jones & Bartlett Learning.

Munhall, P. L. (2012b). Institutional review of qualitative research proposals: A task of no small consequence. In P. L. Munhall (Ed.), *Nursing research: A qualitative perspective* (5th ed.) (pp. 503–515). Sudbury, MA: Jones & Bartlett Learning.

National Commission for the Protection of Human Subjects of Biomedical and Behavioral Research. (1978). *Belmont report: Ethical principles and guidelines for research involving human subjects (DHEW Publication No. [05] 78-0012).* Washington, DC: U.S. Government Printing Office.

Njie, V. P. S. & Thomas, A. C. (2001. Quality issues in clinical research and the implications on health policy (QICHRHP). *Journal of Professional Nursing, 17*(5), 233–242.

Nuremberg Code. (1949). *Trials of War Criminals before the Nuremberg Military Tribunals under Control Council Law No. 10, Vol. 2* (pp. 181–182) Washington, D.C.: U.S. Government Printing Office, 1949. Retrieved from http://ohsr.od.nih.gov/guidelines/nuremberg.html/.

Office of Laboratory Animal Welfare (OLAW, 2008). *Policy and guidance: Policy and guidance for the care and use of animals.* Retrieved from http://grants.nih.gov/grants/olaw/olaw.htm/.

Office of Laboratory Animal Welfare (OLAW, 2011). *For researchers and institutions. Good animal care and good science go hand-in-hand.* Retrieved from http://grants.nih.gov/grants/policy/air/researchers_institutions.htm/.

Office of Research Integrity (ORI, 2005). *Public Health Service Policies on Research Misconduct.* Code of Federal Regulations, Title 42, Parts 50 and 93, Policies of General Applicability. Retrieved from http://ori.dhhs.gov/documents/FR_Doc_05–9643.shtml.

Office of Research Integrity (ORI, 2011). *About ORI—History.* Retrieved from http://ori.dhhs.gov/about/history.shtml/.

Office of Research Integrity (ORI, 2012). *Handling misconduct—Case summaries.* Retrieved from http://ori.dhhs.gov/misconduct/cases/.

Olsen, D. P. (2003). Methods: HIPAA privacy regulations and nursing research. *Nursing Research, 52*(5), 344–348.

Orb, A., Eisenhauer, L., & Wynaden, D. (2001). Ethics in qualitative research. *Journal of Nursing Scholarship, 33*(1), 93–96.

Osborne, N. J., Payne, D., & Newman, M. L. (2009). Journal editorial policies, animal welfare, and the 3 Rs. *The American Journal of Bioethics, 9*(12), 55–59.

Pardes, H., West, A., & Pincus, H. A. (1991). Physicians and the animal-rights movement. *New England Journal of Medicine, 324*(23), 1640–1643.

Ramos, M. C. (1989). Some ethical implications of qualitative research. *Research in Nursing & Health, 12*(1), 57–63.

Rankin, M. & Esteves, M. D. (1997). Perceptions of scientific misconduct in nursing. *Nursing Research, 46*(5), 270–275.

Rew, L., Horner, S. D., & Fouladi, R. T. (2010). Factors associated with health behaviors in middle childhood. *Journal of Pediatric Nursing, 25*(3), 157–166.

Reynolds, P. D. (1979). *Ethical dilemmas and social science research.* San Francisco, CA: Jossey-Bass.

Riegel, B., Lee, C. S., Albert, N., Lennie, T., Chang, M., Song, E. K., Bentley, B., et al. (2011). From novice to expert: Confidence and activity status determine heart failure self-care performance. *Nursing Research, 60*(2), 132–138.

Rothman, D. J. (1982). Were Tuskegee and Willowbrook "studies in nature"? *Hastings Center Report, 12*(2), 5–7.

Simpson, C. (2010). Decision-making capacity and informed consent to participate in research by cognitively impaired individuals. *Applied Nursing Research, 23*(4), 221–226.

Steinfels, P. & Levine, C. (1976). Biomedical ethics and the shadow of Naziism. *Hastings Center Report, 6*(4), 1–20.

Thompson, P. J. (1987). Protection of the rights of children as subjects for research. *Journal of Pediatric Nursing, 2*(6), 392–399.

U.S. Department of Health and Human Services (U.S. DHHS, 1981, January 26). *Final regulations amending basic HHS policy for the protection of human research subjects.* Code of Federal Regulations, Title 45, Part 46.

U.S. Department of Health and Human Services (U.S. DHHS, 2003). *Health information privacy: Summary of the HIPAA Privacy Rule.* Retrieved from http://www.hhs.gov/ocr/privacy/hipaa/understanding/summary/index.html/.

U.S. Department of Health and Human Services (U.S. DHHS, 2004). *Institutional review boards and the HIPAA Privacy Rule.* Retrieved from http://privacyruleandresearch.nih.gov/irbandprivacyrule.asp/.

U.S. Department of Health and Human Services (U.S. DHHS, 2007a). *How do other privacy protections interact with the privacy rule?* Retrieved from http://privacyruleandresearch.nih.gov/pr_05.asp/.

U.S. Department of Health and Human Services (U.S. DHHS, 2007b). *How can covered entities use and disclose protected health information for research and comply with the Privacy Rule?* Retrieved from http://privacyruleandresearch.nih.gov/pr_08.asp/.

U.S. Department of Health and Human Services (U.S. DHHS, 2009). *Protection of human subjects.* Code of Federal Regulations, Title 45, Part 46. Retrieved from http://www.hhs.gov/ohrp/policy/ohrpregulations.pdf/.

U.S. Department of Health and Human Services (U.S. DHHS, 2010). *HIPAA Privacy Rule Information for researchers: Overview.* Retrieved from http://privacyruleandresearch.nih.gov/.

U.S. Department of Health and Human Services (U.S. DHHS, 2012). *Office for Human Research Protections (OHRP).* Retrieved from http://www.hhs.gov/ohrp/.

U.S. Food and Drug Administration (U.S. FDA, 2007). *Regulatory information: Food and Drug Administration Amendments Act (FDAAA) of 2007.* Public Law 110-185. Retrieved from http://www.fda.gov/RegulatoryInformation/Legislation/FederalFoodDrugandCosmeticActFDCAct/SignificantAmendmentstotheFDCAct/FoodandDrugAdministrationAmendmentsActof2007/FullTextofFDAAALaw/default.htm/.

U.S. Food and Drug Administration (FDA, 2010a). *Protection of human subjects (informed consent)*. Code of Federal Regulations, Title 21, Part 50. Retrieved from http://www.accessdata.fda.gov/scripts/cdrh/cfdocs/cfcfr/CFRsearch.cfm?CFRPart=50/.

U.S. Food and Drug Administration (FDA, 2010b). *Institutional review boards*. Code of Federal Regulations, Title 21, Part 56. Retrieved from http://www.accessdata.fda.gov/scripts/cdrh/cfdocs/cfcfr/CFRsearch.cfm?CFRPart=56/.

Wager, E. (2007). What do journal editors do when they suspect research misconduct? *Medicine & Law, 26*(3), 535–544.

Wocial, L. D. (1995). The role of mentors in promoting integrity and preventing scientific misconduct in nursing research. *Journal of Professional Nursing, 11*(5), 276–280.

World Medical Association (WMA) General Assembly. (1964). *Declaration of Helsinki (1964)*. Helsinki, Finland: Author. Retrieved June 20, 2011, from http://www.cirp.org/library/ethics/helsinki/.

World Medical Association (WMA) General Assembly. (2008). *World Medical Association Declaration of Helsinki: Ethical principles for medical research involving human subjects*. Seoul, Korea: Author. Retrieved from http://www.wma.net/en/30publications/10policies/b3/.

Understanding Quantitative Research Design

A research design is the blueprint for conducting a study. It maximizes control over factors that could interfere with the validity of the study findings. Being able to identify the study design and to evaluate design flaws that might threaten the validity of findings is an important part of critically appraising studies. When you are conducting a study, the research design guides you in planning and implementing the study in a way to achieve accurate results. The control achieved through the quantitative study design increases the probability that your study findings are an accurate reflection of reality.

The term *research design* is used in two ways in the nursing literature. Some consider research design to be the entire strategy for the study, from identification of the problem to final plans for data collection. Others limit design to clearly defined structures within which the study is implemented. In this text, the first definition refers to the **research methodology** and the second is a definition of the research design. The research design of a study is the end result of a series of decisions you will make concerning how best to implement your study. The design is closely associated with the framework of the study. As a blueprint, the design is not specific to a particular study but rather is a broad pattern or guide that can be applied to many studies (see Chapter 11 for different types of quantitative research designs). Just as the blueprint for a house must be individualized to the house being built, so the design must be made specific to a study. Using the problem statement, framework, research questions, and clearly defined variables, you can map out the design to achieve a detailed research plan for collecting and analyzing data.

This chapter gives you a background for understanding the elements of a design and critically appraising the designs in published quantitative studies. You are introduced to (1) the concepts important to design; (2) design validity; and (3) the elements of a good design. You are also provided questions to assist you in selecting and implementing a design in a study. The chapter concludes with a discussion of mixed methods, which are relatively recent approaches used in nursing that combine quantitative and qualitative research designs.

Concepts Important to Design

Many terms used in discussing research design have special meanings within this context. An understanding of these concepts is essential for recognizing the purpose of a specific design. Some of the major concepts used in relation to research design are causality, bias, manipulation, control, and validity.

Causality

The first assumption you must make in examining causality is that causes lead to effects. Some of the ideas related to causation emerged from the logical positivist philosophical tradition. Hume, a positivist, proposed that the following three conditions must be met to establish **causality** (1) there must be a strong relationship between the proposed cause and the effect; (2) the proposed cause must precede the effect in time; and (3) the cause has to be present whenever the effect occurs. Cause, according to Hume, is not directly observable but must be inferred (Kerlinger & Lee, 2000; Shadish, Cook, & Campbell, 2002).

A philosophical group known as essentialists proposed that two concepts must be considered in determining causality: necessary and sufficient. The proposed cause must be *necessary* for the effect to occur. (The effect cannot occur unless the cause first occurs.) The proposed cause must also be *sufficient* (requiring no other factors) for the effect to occur. This leaves no room for a variable that may sometimes, but not always, serves as the cause of an effect. John Stuart Mill, another philosopher, added a third idea related to causation. He suggested that, in addition to the preceding criteria for causation, there must be no *alternative explanations* for why a change in one variable seems to lead to a change in a second variable (Campbell & Stanley, 1963).

Causes are frequently expressed within the propositions of a theory. Testing the accuracy of these theoretical statements indicates the usefulness of the theory (Fawcett & Garity, 2009). A theoretical understanding of causation is considered important because it improves our ability to predict and, in some cases, to control events in the real world. The purpose of an experimental design is to examine cause and effect. The independent variable in a study is expected to be the cause, and the dependent variable is expected to reflect the effect of the independent variable.

Multicausality

Multicausality, the recognition that a number of interrelating variables can be involved in causing a particular effect, is a more recent idea related to causality. Because of the complexity of causal relationships, a theory is unlikely to identify every variable involved in causing a particular phenomenon. A study is unlikely to include every component influencing a particular change or effect.

Cook and Campbell (1979) have suggested three levels of causal assertions that one must consider in establishing causality. Molar causal laws relate to large and complex objects. Intermediate mediation considers causal factors operating between molar and micro levels. Micromediation examines causal connections at the level of small particles, such as atoms. Cook and Campbell (1979) used the example of turning on a light switch, which causes the light to come on (molar). An electrician would tend to explain the cause of the light coming on in terms of wires and electrical current (intermediate mediation). However, the physicist would explain the cause of the light coming on in terms of ions, atoms, and subparticles (micromediation).

The essentialists' ideas of necessary and sufficient do not hold up well when one views a phenomenon from the perspective of multiple causation. The light switch may not be necessary to turn on the light if the insulation has worn off the electrical wires. Additionally, even though the switch is turned on, the light will not come on if the light bulb is burned out. Although this is a concrete example, it is easy to relate it to common situations in nursing.

Few phenomena in nursing can be clearly reduced to a single cause and a single effect. However, the greater the proportion of causal factors that can be

identified and explored, the clearer the understanding of the phenomenon. This greater understanding improves our ability to predict and control. For example, currently nurses have a limited understanding of patients' preoperative attitudes, knowledge, and behaviors and their effects on postoperative attitudes and behaviors. Nurses assume that high preoperative anxiety leads to less healthy postoperative responses and that providing information before surgery improves healthy responses in the postoperative period. Many nursing studies have examined this particular phenomenon. However, the causal factors involved are complex and have not been clearly delineated. The research evidence needed to reduce patients' anxiety and improve their postoperative recovery is still evolving.

Probability

The original criteria for causation required that a variable should have an identified effect each time the cause occurred. Although this criterion may apply in the basic sciences, such as chemistry or physics, it is unlikely to apply in the health sciences or social sciences. Because of the complexity of the nursing field, nurses deal in probabilities. Probability addresses relative, rather than absolute, causality. From the perspective of probability, a cause will not produce a specific effect each time that particular cause occurs.

Reasoning changes when one thinks in terms of probabilities. The researcher investigates the probability that an effect will occur under specific circumstances. Rather than seeking to prove that A causes B, a researcher would state that if A occurs, there is a 50% probability that B will occur. The reasoning behind probability is more in keeping with the complexity of multicausality. In the example about preoperative attitudes and postoperative outcomes, nurses could seek to predict the probability of unhealthy postoperative patient outcomes when preoperative anxiety levels are high.

Causality and Nursing Philosophy

Traditional theories of prediction and control are built on theories of causality. The first research designs were also based on causality theory. Nursing science must be built within a philosophical framework of multicausality and probability. The strict senses of single causality and of "necessary and sufficient" are not in keeping with the progressively complex, holistic philosophy of nursing. To understand multicausality and increase the probability of being able to predict and control the occurrence of an effect, researchers need to comprehend both wholes and parts (Fawcett & Garity, 2009; Shadish et al., 2002).

Practicing nurses must be aware of the molar, intermediate mediational, and micromediational aspects of a particular phenomenon. A variety of differing approaches, reflecting both qualitative and quantitative research, are necessary to develop a knowledge base for nursing. Some see explanation and causality as different and perhaps opposing forms of knowledge. Nevertheless, the nurse must join these forms of knowledge, sometimes within the design of a single study, to acquire the knowledge needed for nursing practice (Creswell, 2009; Marshall & Rossman, 2011).

Bias

The term bias means to slant away from the true or expected. A biased opinion has failed to include both sides of the question. A biased witness is one who is strongly for or against one side of the situation. A biased scale is one that does not provide a valid measurement of a concept.

Bias is of great concern in research because of the potential effect on the meaning of the study findings. Any component of the study that deviates or causes a deviation from true measure leads to error and distorted findings. Many factors related to research can be biased: the researcher, the measurement methods, the individual subjects, the sample, the data, and the statistics (Grove, 2007; Thompson, 2002; Waltz, Strickland, & Lenz, 2010). In critically appraising a study, you need to look for possible biases in these areas. An important concern in designing a study is to identify possible sources of bias and eliminate or avoid them. If they cannot be avoided, you need to design your study to control them. Designs, in fact, are developed to reduce the possibilities of bias (Shadish et al., 2002).

Manipulation

Manipulation tends to have a negative connotation and is associated with one person underhandedly maneuvering a second person so that he or she behaves or thinks in the way the first person desires. Denotatively, to manipulate means to move around or to control the movement of something, such as manipulating a syringe to give an injection. The major role of nurses is to implement interventions that involve manipulation of events related to patients and their environment to improve their health. Manipulation has a specific meaning when used in experimental or quasi-experimental research because it is the manipulation or implementation of the study treatment or intervention. The experimental group receives the treatment or intervention during a study and the control group does not. For example, in a study on preoperative care, preoperative relaxation therapy might be manipulated so that the experimental group receives the treatment and the control group does not. In a study on oral care, the frequency of care might be manipulated to determine its effect on patient outcomes (Doran, 2011).

In nursing research, when experimental designs are used to explore causal relationships, the nurse must be free to manipulate the variables under study. For example, in a study of pain management, if the freedom to manipulate pain control measures is under the control of someone else, a bias is introduced into the study. In qualitative, descriptive, and correlational studies, the researcher does not attempt to manipulate variables. Instead, the purpose is to describe a situation as it exists (Marshall & Rossman, 2011; Munhall, 2012).

Control

Control means having the power to direct or manipulate factors to achieve a desired outcome. In a study of pain management, one must be able to control interventions to relieve pain. The idea of control is important in research, particularly in experimental and quasi-experimental studies. The more control the researcher has over the features of the study, the more credible the study findings. The purpose of research designs is to maximize control factors in the study (Shadish et al., 2002).

Study Validity

Study validity, a measure of the truth or accuracy of a claim, is an important concern throughout the research process. Study validity is central to building sound evidence for practice. Questions of validity refer back to the propositions from which the study was developed and address their approximate truth or falsity. Is the theoretical proposition from the study framework an accurate reflection of reality? Was the study designed to provide a valid test of the proposition? Validity is a complex idea that is important to the researcher and to those who read the study report and consider using the findings in their practice. Critical appraisal of research requires that we think through threats to validity and make judgments about how seriously these threats affect the integrity of the findings. Validity provides a major basis for making decisions about which findings are sufficiently valid to add to the evidence base for practice.

Shadish et al. (2002) have described four types of validity: statistical conclusion validity, internal validity, construct validity, and external validity. These types of design validity need to be critically appraised for strengths and possible threats in published studies. When conducting a study, you will be confronted with major decisions about the four types of design validity. To make these decisions, you must address a variety of questions, such as the following:

1. Is there a relationship between the two variables? (*statistical conclusion validity*)
2. Given that there is a relationship, is it possibly causal from the independent variable to the dependent variable, or would the same relationship have been obtained in the absence of any treatment or intervention? (*internal validity*)
3. Given that the relationship is probably causal and is reasonably known to be from one variable to another, what are the particular cause-and-effect constructs involved in the relationship? (*construct validity*)
4. Given that there is probably a causal relationship from construct A to construct B, can this relationship be generalized across persons, settings, and times? (*external validity*) (Cook & Campbell, 1979; Shadish et al., 2002)

Statistical Conclusion Validity

The first step in inferring cause is to determine whether the independent and dependent variables are related. You can determine this relationship (covariation) through statistical analysis. Statistical conclusion validity is concerned with whether the conclusions about relationships or differences drawn from statistical analysis are an accurate reflection of the real world. The second step is to identify differences between groups. There are reasons why false conclusions can be drawn about the presence or absence of a relationship or difference. The reasons for the false conclusions are called threats to statistical conclusion validity. These threats are described in the following section.

Low Statistical Power

Low statistical power increases the probability of concluding that there is no significant difference between samples when actually there is a difference (Type II error, failing to reject a false null) (see Chapter 8 for discussion of the null hypothesis). A Type II error is most likely to occur when the sample size is small or when the power of the statistical test to determine differences is low (Aberson, 2010). The concept of statistical power and strategies to improve it are discussed in Chapters 15 and 21.

Violated Assumptions of Statistical Tests

Most statistical tests have assumptions about the data collected, such as the following: (1) the data are at least at the interval level; (2) the sample was randomly obtained; and (3) the distribution of scores was normal. If these assumptions are violated, the statistical analysis may provide inaccurate results (Corty, 2007; Grove, 2007). The assumptions of statistical tests commonly conducted in nursing studies are provided in Chapters 23, 24, and 25.

Fishing and the Error Rate Problem

A serious concern in research is incorrectly concluding that a relationship or difference exists when it does not (Type I error, rejecting a true null). The risk of Type I error increases when the researcher conducts multiple statistical analyses of relationships or differences; this procedure is referred to as fishing. When fishing is used, a given portion of the analyses shows significant relationships or differences simply by chance. For example, the *t*-test is commonly used to make multiple statistical comparisons of mean differences in a single sample (Kerlinger & Lee, 2000). This procedure increases the risk of a Type I error because some of the differences found in the sample occurred by chance and are not actually present in the population. Multivariate statistical techniques have been developed to deal with this error rate problem (Goodwin, 1984). Fishing and error rate problems are discussed in Chapter 21.

Reliability of Measures

The technique of measuring variables must be reliable to reveal true differences. A measure is a reliable measure if it gives the same result each time the same situation or factor is measured. If a scale is used to measure anxiety, it should give the same score (be reliable) if repeatedly given to the same person in a short time (unless, of course, repeatedly taking the same test causes anxiety to increase or decrease) (Waltz et al., 2010). Physiological measurement methods that consistently measure physiological variables are considered precise (Ryan-Wenger, 2010). For example, a thermometer would be precise if it showed the same temperature reading when tested repeatedly on the same patient within a limited time (see Chapter 16).

Reliability of Intervention Implementation

Intervention reliability ensures that the research treatment is standardized and applied consistently each time it is administered in a study. In some studies, the consistent implementation of the treatment is referred to as intervention fidelity. Intervention fidelity often includes a protocol to standardize the elements of the treatment and a plan for training to ensure consistent implementation of the treatment protocol (Forbes, 2009; Santacroce, Maccarelli, & Grey, 2004). If the method of administering a research intervention varies from one person to another, the chance of detecting a true difference decreases. During the planning and implementation phases, researchers must ensure that the study intervention is provided in exactly the same way each time it is administered to prevent a threat to statistical conclusion design validity. Chapter 14 provides a detailed discussion of types of interventions, intervention development, and intervention fidelity.

Random Irrelevancies in the Experimental Setting

Environmental extraneous variables in complex field settings (e.g., a clinical unit) can influence scores on the dependent variable. These variables increase the difficulty of detecting differences. Consider the activities occurring on a nursing unit. The numbers and variety of staff, patients, crises, and work patterns merge into a complex arena for the implementation of a study. Any of the dynamics of the unit can influence manipulation of the independent variable or measurement of the dependent variable.

Random Heterogeneity of Respondents

Subjects in a treatment or intervention group can differ in ways that correlate with the dependent variable, a situation referred to as random heterogeneity. This difference can influence the outcome of the intervention and prevent detection of a true relationship between the independent variable and the dependent variable. For example, subjects may have a variety of responses to preoperative interventions to lower anxiety because of unique characteristics of patients associated with their differing levels of anxiety.

Internal Validity

Internal validity is the extent to which the effects detected in the study are a true reflection of reality rather than the result of extraneous variables. Although internal validity should be a concern in all studies, it is addressed more commonly in relation to studies examining causality than in other studies. When examining causality, the researcher must determine whether the independent and dependent variables may have been affected by a third, often unmeasured, variable (an extraneous variable). Chapter 8 describes the different types of extraneous variables. The possibility of an alternative explanation of cause is sometimes referred to as a rival hypothesis (Shadish et al.,

2002). Any study can contain threats to internal design validity, and these validity threats can lead to false-positive or false-negative conclusions. The researcher must ask, "Is there another reasonable (valid) explanation (rival hypothesis) for the finding other than the one I have proposed?" Threats to internal validity are described here.

Controlling the Environment

History effect results when an event that is not related to the planned study occurs during the time of the study and creates an effect on the study outcome. History could influence a subject's response to the treatment and alter the measurements obtained on the dependent variables. For example, if you are studying the effect of an emotional support intervention on subjects' completion of their cardiac rehabilitation program and several of the nurses quit their jobs in the rehabilitation center during your study, this event could influence the subjects' rehabilitation program completion rate in your study.

Maturation

In research, maturation is defined as growing older, wiser, stronger, hungrier, more tired, or more experienced during the study. Such unplanned and unrecognized changes are a threat to the study internal design validity and can influence the findings of the study.

Testing Effect

Sometimes, the effect being measured (referred to as the *testing effect*) can be due to the number of times the subject's responses have been tested. The subject may remember earlier, inaccurate responses and then modify them, thus altering the outcome of the study. The test itself may influence the subject to change attitudes or may increase the subject's knowledge.

Instrumentation

Effects can be due to changes in measurement instruments (instrumentation) between the pretest and the posttest rather than a result of the treatment. For example, a weight scale that was accurate when the study began (pretest) could now show subjects to weigh 2 lbs less than they actually weigh (posttest). Instrumentation is also involved when people serving as observers or data collectors become more experienced between the pretest and the posttest, thus altering in some way the data they collect.

Selection

Selection addresses the process by which subjects are chosen to take part in a study and how subjects are grouped within a study. A selection threat is more likely to occur in studies in which randomization is not possible (Kerlinger & Lee, 2000; Thompson 2002). In some studies, people selected for the study may differ in some important way from people not selected for the study. In other studies, the threat is due to differences in subjects selected for study groups. For example, people assigned to the control group could be different in some important way from people assigned to the experimental group. This difference in selection could cause the two groups to react differently to the treatment; in this case, the treatment would not have caused the differences in group responses.

Subject Attrition

The **subject attrition** threat is due to subjects who drop out of a study before completion. Participants' attrition becomes a threat when (1) those who drop out of a study are different types of people from those who remain in the study or (2) there is a difference between the kinds of people who drop out of the experimental group and the people who drop out of the control or comparison group (see Chapter 15).

Interactions with Selection

The aforementioned threats can interact with selection to further complicate the validity of the study. The threats most likely to interact with selection are history effect, maturation, and instrumentation. For example, if the control group you selected for your study has a different history from that of the experimental group, responses to the treatment may be due to this difference rather than to the treatment.

Diffusion or Imitation of Treatments

The control group may gain access to the treatment intended for the experimental group (diffusion) or a similar treatment available from another source (imitation). For example, suppose your study examined the effect of teaching specific information to hypertensive patients as a treatment and then measured the effect of the teaching on blood pressure readings and adherence to treatment protocols. Suppose that the experimental group patients shared the teaching information with the control patients (**treatment diffusion**). This sharing changed the behavior of the control group. The control group patients' responses to the outcome measures may show no differences from those of the experimental group even though the teaching actually did make a difference (Type II error; fail to reject a false null).

Compensatory Equalization of Treatments

When the experimental group receives a treatment seen as desirable, such as a new treatment for AIDS, administrative people and other health professionals may not tolerate the difference and may insist that the control group also receive the treatment. The researcher therefore no longer has a control group and cannot document the effectiveness of the treatment through the study. In health care, both giving treatment and withholding treatment have ethical implications.

Resentful Demoralization of Respondents Receiving Less Desirable Treatments

If control group subjects believe that they are receiving less desirable treatment, they may withdraw, give up, or become angry. Changes in behavior resulting from this reaction rather than from the treatment can lead to differences that cannot be attributed to the treatment.

Construct Validity

Construct validity examines the fit between the conceptual definitions and operational definitions of variables. Theoretical constructs or concepts are defined within the study framework (conceptual definitions). These conceptual definitions provide the basis for the operational definitions of the variables. Operational definitions (methods of measurement) must validly reflect the theoretical constructs. (Theoretical constructs are discussed in Chapter 7; conceptual and operational definitions of concepts and variables are discussed in Chapter 8.)

Is use of the measure a valid inference about the construct? By examining construct validity, we can determine whether the instrument actually measures the theoretical construct it purports to measure. The process of developing construct validity for an instrument often requires years of scientific work. When selecting methods of measurement, the researcher must determine the previous development of instrument construct validity (DeVon et al., 2007; Waltz et al., 2010). The threats to construct validity are related both to previous instrument development and to the development of measurement techniques as part of the methodology of a particular study. Threats to construct validity are described here.

Inadequate Preoperational Clarification of Constructs

Measurement of a construct stems logically from a concept analysis of the construct, either by the theorist who developed the construct or by the researcher. The conceptual definition should emerge from the concept analysis, and the method of measurement (operational definition) should clearly reflect both. A deficiency in the conceptual or operational definition leads to low construct validity.

Mono-Operation Bias

Mono-operation bias occurs when only one method of measurement is used to assess a construct. When only one method of measurement is used, fewer dimensions of the construct are measured. Construct validity greatly improves if the researcher uses more than one instrument (Waltz et al., 2010). For example, if anxiety were a dependent variable, more than one measure of anxiety could be used. It is often possible to apply more than one measurement of the dependent variable with little increase in time, effort, or cost.

Monomethod Bias

In monomethod bias, the researcher uses more than one measure of a variable, but all the measures use the same method of recording. Attitude measures, for example, may all be paper and pencil scales. Attitudes that are personal and private, however, may not be detected through the use of paper and pencil tools. Paper and pencil tools may be influenced by feelings of nonaccountability for responses, acquiescence, or social desirability. For example, construct validity would improve if anxiety were measured by a paper and pencil test, verbal messages of anxiety, the galvanic skin response, and the observer's recording of incidence and frequency of behaviors that have been validly linked with anxiety.

Hypothesis Guessing within Experimental Conditions

Hypothesis guessing occurs when subjects within a study guess the hypotheses of the researcher. The validity concern relates to behavioral changes that may occur in the subjects as a consequence of knowing the hypothesis. The extent to which this issue modifies study findings is not currently known.

Evaluation Apprehension

Subjects want researchers to see them in a favorable light. They want to be seen as competent and psychologically healthy. Evaluation apprehension occurs when the subject's responses in the experiment are due to this desire rather than the effects of the independent variable.

Experimenter Expectancies (Rosenthal Effect)

The expectancies of the researcher can bias the data. For example, experimenter expectancy occurs if a researcher expects a particular intervention to relieve pain. The data he or she collects may be biased to reflect this expectation. If another researcher who does not believe the intervention would be effective had collected the data, results could have been different. The extent to which this effect actually influences studies is not known. Because of their concern about experimenter expectancy, some researchers are not involved in the data collection process. In other studies, data collectors do not know which subjects are assigned to treatment and control groups.

Another way to control this threat is to design the study so that the various data collectors have different expectations. If the sample size is large enough, the researcher could compare data gathered by the different data collectors. Failing to determine differences in the data collected by the collectors would give evidence that the construct is valid.

Confounding Constructs and Levels of Constructs

When developing the methodology of a study, you must decide about the intensity of the variable that will be measured or provided as a treatment. This intensity influences the level of the construct that will be reflected in the study. These decisions can affect validity, because the method of measuring the variable influences the outcome of the study and the understanding of the constructs in the study framework.

For example, in reviewing your research, you might find that variable A does not affect variable B when, in fact, it does, but either not at the level of A that was manipulated or not at the level of B that was measured. This issue is a particular problem when A is not linearly related to B or when the effect being studied is weak. To control this threat, you will need to include several levels of A in the design and will have to measure many levels of B. For example, in a study in which A is preoperative teaching and B is anxiety, (1) the instrument being used to measure anxiety measures only high levels of anxiety or (2) the preoperative teaching is provided for 15 minutes but 30 minutes or an hour of teaching is required to cause significant changes in anxiety.

In some cases, confounding of variables occurs, leading to mistaken conclusions. Few measures of a construct are pure measures. Rather, a selected method of measuring a construct can measure a portion of the construct as well as other related constructs. Thus, the measure can lead to confusing results, because the variable measured does not accurately reflect the construct.

Interaction of Different Treatments

The interaction of different treatments is a threat to construct validity if subjects receive more than one treatment in a study. For example, your study might examine the effectiveness of pain relief measures, and subjects might receive medication, massage, distraction, and relaxation strategies. In this case, each one of the treatments interacts with the others, and the effect of any single treatment on pain relief would be impossible to extract. Your study findings could not be generalized to any situation in which patients did not receive all four pain treatments. Chapter 14 provides direction in preventing and managing interactions of treatments.

Interaction of Testing and Treatment

In some studies, pretesting the subject is thought to modify the effect of the treatment. In this case, the findings can be generalized only to subjects who have been pretested. Although there is some evidence that pretest sensitivity does not have the impact that was once feared, it must be considered when the validity of the study is examined. The Solomon four-group design (discussed in Chapter 11) tests this threat to validity. Repeated posttests can also lead to an interaction of testing and treatment.

External Validity

External validity is concerned with the extent to which study findings can be generalized beyond the sample used in the study. With the most serious threat, the findings would be meaningful only for the group being studied. To some extent, the significance of the study depends on the number of types of people and situations to which the findings can be applied. Sometimes, the factors influencing external validity are subtle and may not be reported in research reports; however, the researcher must be responsible for these factors. Generalization is usually narrower for a single study than for multiple replications of a study using different samples, perhaps from different populations in different settings. The threats to the ability to generalize the findings (external validity) in terms of study design are described here.

Interaction of Selection and Treatment

Seeking subjects who are willing to participate in a study can be difficult, particularly if the study requires extensive amounts of time or other investments by subjects. If a large number of the persons approached to participate in a study decline to participate, the sample actually selected will be limited in ways that might not be evident at first glance. For example, the researcher knows the subjects well and probably why they consented to participate in the study. Subjects might be volunteers, "do-gooders," or people with nothing better to do. In this case, generalizing the findings to all members of a population, such as all nurses, all hospitalized patients, or all persons experiencing diabetes, is not easy to justify.

The study must be planned to limit the investment demands on subjects and thereby improve participation. The researcher must report the number of persons who were approached and refused to participate in the study (refusal rate) so that those who are examining the study can judge any threats to external validity. As the percentage of those who decline to participate increases, external design validity decreases. Sufficient data need to be collected on the subjects to allow the researcher to be familiar with the characteristics of subjects and, to the extent possible, the characteristics of those who decline to participate.

Interaction of Setting and Treatment

Bias exists in types of settings and organizations that agree to participate in studies. This bias has been particularly evident in nursing studies. For example, some hospitals welcome nursing studies and encourage employed nurses to conduct studies. Others are resistant to the conduct of nursing research. These two types of hospitals may be different in important ways; thus, there might be an interaction of setting and treatment that limits the generalizability of the findings. As a researcher, you must consider this factor when making statements about the population to which your findings can be generalized.

Interaction of History and Treatment

The circumstances in which a study was conducted (history) influence the treatment and thus the generalizability of the findings. Logically, one can never generalize to the future; however, replicating the study during various periods strengthens the usefulness of findings over time. In critically appraising studies, you must always consider the period of history during which the study was conducted and the effect of nursing practice and societal events during that period on the reported findings (see Chapter 14 for more details on research with interventions).

Elements of a Good Design

The purpose of design is to set up a situation that maximizes the possibilities of obtaining accurate responses to objectives, questions, or hypotheses. Select a design that is (1) appropriate to the purpose of the study; (2) feasible given realistic constraints; and (3) effective in reducing threats to design validity.

In most studies, comparisons are the basis of obtaining valid answers. A good design provides the subjects, the setting, and the protocol within which those comparisons can be clearly examined. The comparisons may focus on differences or relationships or both. The study may require that comparisons be made between or among individuals, groups, or variables. A comparison may also be made of measures taken before a treatment (pretest) and measures taken after a treatment (posttest). After these comparisons have been made, you can compare the sample values with statistical tables reflecting population values. In some cases, the study may involve comparing group values with population values.

Designs were developed to reduce threats that might invalidate the comparisons. However, some designs are more effective in reducing threats than others. It may be necessary to modify the design to reduce a particular threat. Before selecting a design, you must identify the design validity threats that are most likely to invalidate your study.

Strategies for reducing threats to design validity are sometimes addressed in terms of control. Selecting a design involves decisions related to control of the environment, sample, treatment, and measurement. Increasing control (to reduce threats to validity) will require you to carefully think through every facet of your design. An excellent description of one research team's efforts to develop a good design and control threats to validity is offered by McGuire et al. (2000) in their study, "Maintaining Study Validity in a Changing Clinical Environment."

Controlling the Environment

The study environment has a major effect on research outcomes. An uncontrolled environment introduces many extraneous variables into the study situation. Therefore, the study design may include strategies for controlling that environment. In many studies, it is important that the environment be consistent for all subjects. Elements in the environment that may influence the application of a treatment or the measurement of variables must be identified and, when possible, controlled.

Controlling Equivalence of Subjects and Groups

When comparisons are made, it is assumed that the individual units of the comparison are relatively equivalent except for the variables being measured. The researcher does not want to be comparing "apples and oranges." To establish equivalence, the researcher defines sampling criteria. Deviation from this equivalence is a threat to internal design validity. Deviation

occurs when sampling criteria have not been adequately defined or when unidentified extraneous variables increase variation in the group.

The most effective strategy for achieving equivalence consists of random sampling followed by random assignment to groups. However, this strategy does not guarantee equivalence. Even when randomization has been used, the researcher must examine the extent of equivalence by measuring and comparing characteristics for which the groups must be equivalent. This comparison is usually reported in the description of the sample (Shadish et al., 2002).

Contrary to the aforementioned need for equivalence, groups must be as different as possible in relation to the research variables. Small differences or relationships are more difficult to distinguish than large differences. These differences are often addressed in terms of effect size. Although sample size plays an important role, effect size is maximized by a good design. Effect size is greatest when variance within groups is small.

Control and Comparison Groups

If the study involves an experimental treatment, the design usually calls for a comparison. Outcome measures for individuals who receive the experimental treatment are compared with outcome measures for those who do not receive the experimental treatment. This comparison requires a control group, subjects who do not receive the experimental treatment. However, in nursing studies, all patients require care and those who do not receive the study intervention receive standard or usual care. Nurse researchers often refer to the group receiving standard care, but no treatment, as the comparison group rather than the control group.

One threat to validity is the lack of equivalence between the experimental and control groups. This threat is best controlled by random assignment to groups. Another strategy is for the subjects to serve as their own controls. With this design strategy, pretest and posttest measures are taken of the subjects in the absence of a treatment, as well as before and after the treatment. In this case, the timing of measures must be comparable between control and treatment conditions.

Controlling the Treatment

In a well-designed experimental study, the researcher has complete control of any treatment provided. The first step in achieving control is to develop a detailed description of the treatment, such as an intervention protocol, to ensure standardization of the treatment. The next step is to use strategies to ensure consistency in implementing the treatment. Consistency may involve elements of the treatment such as equipment, time, intensity, sequencing, and staff skill. This process is referred to as *intervention fidelity* and is discussed in more detail in Chapter 14.

Variations in the treatment reduce the effect size. It is likely that subjects who receive fewer optimal applications of the treatment will have a smaller response, resulting in more variance in posttest measures for the experimental group. To avoid this problem, the treatment is administered to each subject in exactly the same way. This consideration requires the researcher to think carefully through every element of the treatment to reduce variation wherever possible (Morrison et al., 2009; Santacroce et al., 2004). For example, if information is being provided as part of the treatment, some researchers record the information, present it to each subject in the same environment, and attempt to decrease variation in the subject's experience before and during the viewing of the DVD content. Variations include elements such as time of day, mood, anxiety, experience of pain, interactions with others, and amount of time spent waiting. Yamada, Stevens, Sidani, Watt-Watson, and Silva (2010) provide a detailed discussion of the process they used to measure intervention implementation fidelity in their study.

In many nursing studies, the researcher does not have complete control of the treatment. It may be costly to control the treatment carefully; it may be difficult to persuade staff to be consistent in the treatment, or the time required to implement a carefully controlled treatment may seem prohibitive. In some cases, the researcher may be studying causal outcomes of an event occurring naturally in the environment. Regardless of the reason for the researcher's decision, internal design validity is reduced when the treatment is inconsistently applied. The risk of a Type II error is higher owing to greater variance and a smaller effect size. Thus, studies with uncontrolled treatments need larger samples to reduce the risk of a Type II error. External validity may improve if the treatment is studied as it typically occurs clinically. If the study does not reveal a statistically significant difference, then perhaps the typical clinical application of the treatment does not have an important effect on patient outcomes. The question then becomes whether a difference might have been found if the treatment had been consistently applied.

Counterbalancing

In some studies, each subject receives several different treatments sequentially (e.g., relaxation, distraction, and visual imagery) or various levels of the same treatment (e.g., different doses of a drug or varying lengths of relaxation time). Sometimes the application of one treatment can influence the response to later treatments, a phenomenon referred to as a **carryover effect**. If a carryover effect is known to occur, it is not advisable for a researcher to use this design strategy for the study. However, even when no carryover effect is known, the researcher may take precautions against the possibility that this effect will influence outcomes. In one such precaution, known as **counterbalancing**, the various treatments are administered in random order rather than being provided consistently in the same sequence.

Controlling Measurement

Measurement methods play a key role in the validity of a study. Instruments such as scales must have documented validity and reliability, and physiological measures require accuracy and precision (Ryan-Wenger, 2010; Waltz et al., 2010). When measurement is crude or inconsistent, variance within groups is high, and it is more difficult to detect differences or relationships among groups. Thus, the study does not provide a valid test of the hypotheses. However, the consistent implementation of measurements enhances validity. For example, each subject must receive the same instructions about completing a pain scale. Data collectors must be trained and observed for consistency. Designs define the timing of measures (e.g., pretest, posttest). Sometimes, the design calls for multiple measures over time. The researcher must specify the points in time during which measures will be taken. The research report must include a rationale for the timing of measures.

Controlling Extraneous Variables

When designing a study, you must identify variables not included in the design (extraneous variables) that could explain some of the variance that occurs when the study variables are measured. In a good design, the effect of these variables on variance is controlled. The extraneous variables commonly encountered in nursing studies are age, education, gender, social class, severity of illness, level of health, functional status, and attitudes. For a specific study, you must think carefully through the variables that could have an impact on that study.

Design strategies used to control extraneous variables include random sampling, random assignment to groups, selecting subjects who are homogeneous in terms of a particular extraneous variable, selecting a heterogeneous sample, blocking, stratification,

TABLE 10-1 Studies Using Control Strategies for Good Design	
Design Strategy	**Example Studies**
Control group	McCorkle, R., Jeon, S., Ercolano, E., & Schwartz, P. (2011). Healthcare utilization in women after abdominal surgery for ovarian cancer. *Nursing Research, 60*(1), 47–57.
	Chen, K., Fan, J., Wang, H., Wu, S., Li, C., & Lin, H. (2010). Silver yoga exercises improved physical fitness of transitional frail elders. *Nursing Research, 59*(5), 364–370.
Counterbalancing	Cacciola, J. S., Alterman, A. I., McLellan, A. T., Lin, Y., & Lynch, K. G. (2007). Initial evidence for the reliability and validity of a "Lite" version of the Addiction Severity Index. *Drug and Alcohol Dependence, 87*(2–3), 297–302.
	Ivarsson, B., Larsson, S., Lührs, C., & Sjöberg, T. (2007). Patients' perceptions of information about risks at cardiac surgery. *Patient Education and Counseling, 67*(1–2), 32–38.
Random sampling	Laschinger, H. K. S., Finegan, J., & Wilk, P. (2011). Situational and dispositional influences on nurses' workplace well-being: The role of empowering unit leadership. *Nursing Research, 60*(2), 124–131.
	Simons, S. R., Stark, R. B., & DeMarco, R. F. (2011). A new, four-item instrument to measure workplace bullying. *Research in Nursing & Health, 34*(2), 132–140.
Random assignment	Jones, D., Duffy, M. E., & Flanagan, J. (2011). Randomized clinical trial testing efficacy of a nurse-coached intervention in arthroscopy patients. *Nursing Research, 60*(2), 92–99.
	Lee, K. A., & Gay, C. L. (2011). Can modifications to the bedroom environment improve sleep of new parents? Two randomized controlled trials. *Research in Nursing & Health, 34*(1), 7–19.
Homogeneity	Hodgin, R. F., Chandra, A., & Weaver, C. (2010). Correlates to long-term-care nurse turnover: Survey results from the State of West Virginia. *Hospital Topics, 88*(4), 91–97.
	Estok, P. J., Sedlak, C. A., Doheny, M. O., & Hall, R. (2007). Structural model for osteoporosis preventing behavior in postmenopausal women. *Nursing Research, 56*(3), 148–158.
Heterogeneity	Kwok, C. S., Loke, Y. K., Hale, R., Potter, J. F., & Myint, P. K. (2011). Atrial fibrillation and incidence of dementia: A systematic review and meta-analysis. *Neurology, 76*(10), 914–922.
	Neufeld, A., & Harrison, M. J. (2003). Unfulfilled expectations and negative interactions: Nonsupport in the relationships of women caregivers. *Journal of Advanced Nursing, 41*(4), 323–331.
Blocking	Rousaud, A., Blanch, J., Hautzinger, M., De Lazzari, E., Peri, J. M., Puig, O., et al. (2007). Improvement of psychosocial adjustment to HIV-1 infection through a cognitive-behavioral oriented group psychotherapy program: A pilot study. *AIDS Patient Care and STDs, 21*(3), 212–222.
	Tsay, S. L., Wang, J. C., Lin, K. C., & Chung, U. L. (2005). Effects of acupressure therapy for patients having prolonged mechanical ventilation support. *Journal of Advanced Nursing, 52*(2), 142–150.
Stratification	Botticello, A. L., Chen, Y., Cao, Y., & Tulsky, D. S. (2011). Do communities matter after rehabilitation? The effect of socioeconomic and urban stratification on well-being after spinal cord injury. *Archives of Physical Medicine & Rehabilitation, 92*(3), 464–471.
	Carey, T. A. (2006). Estimating treatment duration for psychotherapy in primary care. *Journal of Public Mental Health, 5*(3), 23–28.
Matching	Mehta, S., Chen, H., Johnson, M. L., & Aparasu, R. R. (2010). Risk of falls and fractures in older adults using antipsychotic agents: A propensity-matched retrospective cohort study. *Drugs & Aging, 27*(10), 815–829.
	Trevisanuto, D., Micaglio, M., Pitton, M., Magarotto, M., Piva, D., & Zanardo, V. (2006). Laryngeal mask airway: Is the management of neonates requiring positive pressure ventilation at birth changing? *Journal of Neonatal Nursing, 12*(5), 185–192.
Statistical control (partialing out)	Griffin-Blake, C. S., & DeJoy, D. M. (2006). Evaluation of social-cognitive versus stage-matched, self-help physical activity interventions at the workplace. *American Journal of Health Promotion, 20*(3), 200–209.
	Roberts, J. E., Burchinal, M. R., & Zeisel, S. A. (2002). Otitis media in early childhood in relation to children's school-age language and academic skills. *Pediatrics, 110*(4), 696–706.

matching subjects between groups in relation to a particular variable, and statistical control. Table 10-1 identifies some nursing studies and the various strategies they have used to control extraneous variables.

Random Sampling

Random sampling increases the probability that subjects with various levels of an extraneous variable are included and are randomly dispersed throughout the groups within the study (Thompson, 2002).

This strategy is particularly important for controlling unidentified extraneous variables. Whenever possible, however, extraneous variables must be identified, measured, and reported in the description of the sample.

Random Assignment

Random assignment enhances the probability that subjects with various levels of extraneous variables are equally dispersed in treatment and control or comparison groups. When subjects are randomly assigned to groups, these groups are considered independent. Independent groups exist when the selection and assignment of subjects to one group, such as the experimental group, are unrelated to the subjects selected and assigned to the control group. Whenever possible, however, this dispersion must be evaluated rather than assumed.

Homogeneity

Homogeneity is a more extreme form of equivalence in which the researcher limits the subjects to only one level of an extraneous variable to reduce its impact on the study findings. To use this strategy, you must have previously identified the extraneous variables. You might choose to include subjects with only one level of an extraneous variable in the study. For example, only subjects between the ages of 20 and 30 years may be included in a study, or only subjects with a particular level of education. The study may include only breast cancer patients who have been diagnosed within 1 month, are at a particular stage of disease, and are receiving a specific treatment for cancer. The difficulty with this strategy is that it limits generalization to the types of subjects included in the study. Findings could not justifiably be generalized to types of people excluded from the study.

Heterogeneity

In studies using nonrandom sampling methods, the researcher may attempt to obtain subjects with a wide variety of characteristics (or who are heterogeneous) to reduce the risk of biases. When using the strategy of heterogeneity, you may seek subjects from multiple diverse sources. The strategy is designed to increase generalizability of the study findings. Characteristics of the sample must be described in the research report to indicate the heterogeneity of the sample.

Blocking

In blocking, the researcher includes subjects with various levels of an extraneous variable in the sample but controls the numbers of subjects at each level of the variable and their random assignment to groups within the study. Designs using blocking are referred to as randomized block designs (see Chapter 11). The extraneous variable is then used as an independent variable in the data analysis. Therefore, the extraneous variable must be included in the framework and the study hypotheses.

Using this strategy, you might randomly assign equal numbers of subjects in three age categories (younger than 18 years, 18 to 60 years of age, and older than 60 years) to each group in the study. You could use blocking for several extraneous variables. For example, you could block the study in relation to both age and ethnic background (African American, Hispanic, Caucasian, and Asian). Table 10-2 summarizes an example of this approach.

During data analysis for the randomized block design, each cell in the analysis is treated as a group.

TABLE 10-2 Example of Blocking Using Age and Ethnic Background

Age	Ethnic Group		Experimental	Control
Younger than 18 years ($n = 160$)	African American	$n = 40$	$n = 20$	$n = 20$
	Hispanic, nonwhite	$n = 40$	$n = 20$	$n = 20$
	White, non-Hispanic	$n = 40$	$n = 20$	$n = 20$
	Asian	$n = 40$	$n = 20$	$n = 20$
19 to 60 years of age ($n = 160$)	African American	$n = 40$	$n = 20$	$n = 20$
	Hispanic, nonwhite	$n = 40$	$n = 20$	$n = 20$
	White, non-Hispanic	$n = 40$	$n = 20$	$n = 20$
	Asian	$n = 40$	$n = 20$	$n = 20$
Older than 60 years ($n = 160$)	African American	$n = 40$	$n = 20$	$n = 20$
	Hispanic, nonwhite	$n = 40$	$n = 20$	$n = 20$
	White, non-Hispanic	$n = 40$	$n = 20$	$n = 20$
	Asian	$n = 40$	$n = 20$	$n = 20$

Therefore, you must evaluate the cell sample size and the effect size to ensure adequate power to detect differences in the study. A minimum of 20 subjects per group is recommended but the final group size is best determined by power analysis (Aberson, 2010). Thus, the example described for Table 10-2 would require a minimal sample of 480 subjects. Using randomized block designs usually require very large sample sizes to implement.

Stratification

Stratification involves the distribution of subjects throughout the sample, using sampling techniques similar to those used in blocking, but the purpose of the procedure is even distribution throughout the sample. The extraneous variable is not included in the data analysis. Distribution of the extraneous variable is included in the description of the sample.

Matching

To ensure that subjects in the control or comparison group are equivalent to subjects in the experimental group, some studies are designed to match subjects in the two groups. Matching is used when a subject in the experimental group is randomly selected and then a subject similar in relation to important extraneous variables is randomly selected for the control group. This matching of subjects on selected characteristics to be included in both the experimental and control groups results in dependent groups. For example, subjects in the experimental and control groups might be matched for age, gender, severity of illness, or number of chronic illnesses. Clearly, the pool of available subjects would have to be large to accomplish this goal. In quasi-experimental studies, matching may be performed without randomization (Cook & Campbell, 1979).

Statistical Control

In some studies, it is not considered feasible to control extraneous variables through the design. However, the researcher recognizes the possible impact of extraneous variables on variance and effect size. Therefore, measures are obtained for the identified extraneous variables. Data analysis strategies that have the capacity to remove (*partial out*) the variance explained by the extraneous variable are performed before the analysis of differences or relationships between or among the variables of interest in the study. One statistical procedure commonly used for this purpose is analysis of covariance (Corty, 2007). Although statistical control seems to be a quick and easy solution to the problem of extraneous variables, its results are not as satisfactory as those of the various methods of design control.

Questions to Direct Design Development and Implementation in a Study

Developing and implementing a study design requires the researcher to consider multiple details such as those discussed in the sections on design validity and elements of a good design. The more carefully thought out these details are, the stronger the design. Strong research designs are essential to generate valid research evidence for nursing (Brown, 2009; Melnyk & Fineout-Overholt, 2011). The elements central to the study design include the presence or absence of a treatment, the number of groups in the sample, the number and timing of measurements, the sampling method, the time frame for data collection, planned comparisons, and the control of extraneous variables. Finding answers to the following questions will help you to develop a study design:

1. Is the primary purpose of the study to describe variables and groups within the study situation, to examine relationships, or to examine causality within the study situation? (Kerlinger & Lee, 2000; Shadish et al., 2002)
2. Will a treatment or intervention be implemented in the study? (Forbes, 2009)
3. If an intervention is implemented, will the researcher control the intervention? (Forbes, 2009; Morrison et al., 2009; Santacroce et al., 2004)
4. Will the sample be pretested before the intervention?
5. Will the sample be randomly or nonrandomly selected?
6. What sampling method is used to obtain study participants? (Thompson, 2002)
7. Will the sample be studied as a single group or divided into groups? (Fawcett & Garity, 2009)
8. How many groups will there be?
9. What will be the size of each group? (Aberson, 2010)
10. Will there be a control group, or will a comparison group or standard care group be compared with the experimental group?
11. Will the study participants be randomly assigned to the groups? If the participants are randomly assigned, how is this assignment accomplished?
12. What instruments will be used to measure the variables? (Bialocerkowski, Klupp, & Bragge, 2010; Waltz et al., 2010)

13. Are the measurement methods valid and reliable or precise and accurate? (DeVon et al., 2007)
14. Will the variables be measured more than once?
15. Will the data be collected cross-sectionally or over time?
16. Have extraneous variables been identified?
17. Are data being collected on extraneous variables?
18. What strategies are being used to control for extraneous variables?
19. What strategies are being used to compare variables or groups?
20. Will data be collected at a single site or at multiple sites?
21. What strategies are used to ensure consistent collection of data? (Creswell, 2009; Fawcett & Garity, 2009; Shadish et al., 2002)

Mixed Methods

There is controversy among researchers about the relative validity of various approaches to research. Designing quantitative experimental studies with rigorous controls may provide strong external validity but questionable or limited internal validity. Qualitative studies may have strong internal validity but questionable external validity. A single approach to measuring a concept may be inadequate to justify a claim that it is a valid measure of a theoretical concept. Testing a single theory may leave the results open to the challenge of rival hypotheses from other theories (Creswell, 2009).

As research methodologies continue to evolve, **mixed-methods approaches** offer investigators the ability to utilize the strengths of both qualitative and quantitative research designs. Mixed-methods research is characterized as research that contains elements of both qualitative and quantitative approaches (Coward, 1990; Creswell, 2009; Duffy, 1987; Marshall & Rossman, 2011; Mitchell, 1986; Morse, 1991; Myers & Haase, 1989; Patton, 2002; Porter, 1989). The philosophical underpinnings of mixed-methods research and what paradigms best fit these research methods are still evolving. It is recognized that all researchers bring assumptions to their studies, consciously or unconsciously, and investigators decide whether they are going to view their study from a post-positivist (quantitative) or constructivist (qualitative) perspective, or through an "advocacy lens," such as feminism (Fawcett & Garity, 2009; Munhall, 2012).

Over the last few years, many researchers have departed from the idea that one paradigm or one research strategy is right and have taken the perspective that the search for the truth requires the use of all available strategies. To capitalize on the representativeness and generalizability of quantitative research and the in-depth, contextual nature of qualitative research, several methods are combined in a single research study (Creswell, 2009).

The idea of using mixed-methods approaches to conduct studies has a long history. More than 50 years ago, quantitative researchers Campbell and Fiske (1959) recommended mixed methods to more accurately measure a psychological trait. The multi-trait–multi-method matrix was designed to rule out method effects to allow researchers to attribute individual variation to the personality trait itself (Rocco, Bliss, Gallagher, & Perez-Prado, 2003). This mixed methodology was later expanded into what Denzin (1989) identified as "triangulation." Denzin (1989) believed that combining multiple theories, methods, observers, and data sources can help researchers overcome the intrinsic bias that comes from single-theory, single-methods, and single-observer studies. Triangulation evolved to include using multiple data collection and analysis methods, multiple data sources, multiple analysts, and multiple theories or perspectives (Patton, 2002). The concept of triangulation has now been replaced by the idea of mixed-methods approaches (Creswell, 2009).

Because phenomena are complex, combining qualitative and quantitative methods enables researchers to be more likely to capture the essence of the phenomenon. There are selected techniques or strategies associated with conducting mixed-methods studies. Strategies frequently associated with the mixed-methods approaches include the following:

Sequential procedures are those in which the researcher investigates a phenomenon so that findings of one method may elaborate on or elucidate the findings of another method. This may involve beginning with a qualitative method to explore and then following up with a quantitative method using a large sample so that results can be generalized to a population. Alternatively, the study may begin with a quantitative method so that theories or propositions can be tested, followed by a qualitative method using in-depth interviews with study participants to expand a theory (Creswell, 2009).

Concurrent procedures is an approach in which the researcher merges quantitative and qualitative data in order to present an all-inclusive analysis of the research problem. Collection of quantitative and qualitative data is done concurrently during the study. Then the investigator assimilates the results obtained from both methods in order to interpret the overall findings. The researcher may nest one form of data within another larger data collection to analyze different questions (Creswell, 2009).

Transformative procedure is one in which the researcher uses a "theoretical lens" in order to encompass a broad perspective within a design that contains both quantitative and qualitative data. This broad perspective is based on a theoretical framework and provides methods for data collection and anticipated outcomes from the study. This method usually serves a larger purpose to advocate for minority or marginalized groups. Data could be sequential or concurrent (Creswell, 2009).

In each of these three strategies, both quantitative and qualitative data are collected and the researcher may integrate the data at different stages of the research process. The priority may be given to one type of data over the other (i.e., quantitative over qualitative or vice versa), or they can be equal (concurrent). If the sequential approach is implemented and qualitative data are collected first, then qualitative data are the priority, and integration of the two data sets occurs during data interpretation and is then explicated in the discussion. If quantitative data are collected first, then these data are the priority, and qualitative data are used to augment the quantitative data. Data integration is completed during analysis and interpretation and is expressed in the discussion. With the concurrent approach, data are considered equal and therefore are collected at the same time, or concurrently. Integration of the data occurs during data collection.

Creswell (2009) identifies six types of mixed-methods approaches, expanding the three strategies previously introduced. The four approaches usually implemented in nursing research are: (1) sequential explanatory strategy; (2) sequential exploratory strategy; (3) sequential transformative strategy; and (4) concurrent triangulation strategy. Models of these mixed-methods approaches and examples are provided to expand your understanding of these designs.

Sequential Explanatory Strategy

With the sequential explanatory strategy, the researcher collects and analyzes quantitative data and then collects and analyzes qualitative data. Integration of the data occurs during the interpretation phase. The purpose of this approach is to assist in explaining and interpreting quantitative data (see Figure 10-1). It is useful when unexpected quantitative results are revealed. Qualitative examination of the phenomenon facilitates a fuller understanding and is well suited to explaining and interpreting relationships. There may or may not be a theoretical perspective to the study. This approach is easy to implement because the steps fall in sequential stages; however the two-stage approach extends the time involved in data collection and is seen as a weakness of the design.

This type of methodology was used in a study by Carr (2009), who examined the experience of postoperative pain. Women undergoing surgery completed questionnaires to measure pain, anxiety, and depression (quantitative data). Follow-up telephone interviews explored their pain experiences (qualitative data). Using a second series of patients, Carr once again looked at the frequency and patterns of anxiety in the immediate preoperative and postoperative periods, followed by semi-structured telephone interviews. During the interviews, patients identified events/situations occurring during their hospitalization that contributed to their anxiety.

As indicated by the use of sequential explanatory strategy, priority was given to the quantitative data.

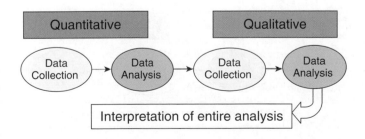

Figure 10-1 Sequential explanatory strategy. (Adapted from Creswell, J. W. [2009]. *Research design: Qualitative, quantitative, and mixed methods approaches* [3rd ed.]. Los Angeles, CA: Sage; and Hanson, W. E., Creswell, J. W., Plano Clark, V. L., Petska, K. S., & Creswell, J. D. [2005]. Mixed methods research designs in counseling psychology. *Journal of Counseling Psychology, 52*[2], 224–235.)

Quantitative   Qualitative

Data Collection → Data Analysis → Data Collection → Data Analysis

Interpretation of entire analysis

- Purpose is to use qualitative results to assist in explaining and interpreting the findings of a primarily quantitative study.
- Easy to implement, describe and report.
- Weakness is the length of time involved in data collection, with the two separate phases.

However, during interpretation, the qualitative data seemed to indicate that lack of knowledge about the operative procedure, which is traditionally thought to be a contributor to anxiety, was not as contributory to patient anxiety as expected. By interpreting both quantitative and qualitative data in the same study, the investigator was able to broaden the understanding of the pain and anxiety of postoperative patients. Carr (2009) also noted that some of the events that led to patients' anxiety and pain were amenable to nursing interventions and not solely due to lack of knowledge.

Sequential Exploratory Strategy

Sequential exploratory strategy is very similar to the sequential explanatory strategy except the collection and analysis of qualitative data precedes the collection of quantitative data. Integration of the data occurs during the interpretation phase, and the quantitative data are used to understand the qualitative data (see Figure 10-2). There may or may not be a theoretical perspective to the study. The purpose of this approach is to: (1) explore a phenomenon's distribution within a population; (2) test elements of an emerging theory; or (3) develop and test new measurement instruments. The sequential exploratory strategy is also easy to implement because of the staged approach, but the length of time required for data collection is considered a weakness.

An example of sequential exploratory strategy is the research by Choi and Harwood (2004), who conducted a qualitative study to explore the themes of Korean women's response to domestic violence. Five themes emerged centered on intolerance to abusive husbands and were the basis for the development of a quantitative scale to explore each item. A pilot study was conducted to examine the women's intolerance to physical abuse by their husbands, and a third phase of the study was conducted to establish construct validity of the scale (Choi, Phillips, Figueredo, Insel, & Min, 2008).

Sequential Transformative Strategy

When the sequential transformative strategy is employed, qualitative or quantitative data collection and analysis can come first. The results are integrated during the interpretation phase. But unlike the prior two approaches, sequential transformative strategy is guided by a theory or through the advocacy lens. The purpose of this approach is to employ methods that will best serve the theoretical perspective. The theoretical perspective drives the entire research process from the introduction of the problem to the directional research question, which generates a sensitive approach to data collection and ends with an appeal to act (see Figure 10-3). Using this strategy, researchers may have the opportunity to speak out about different perspectives, serve as an advocate for study participants, or better understand a phenomenon that is changing as a result of being studied. The staging inherent in the design is a strength, but once again, this approach extends the length of time required to collect data. There is little written on this approach, so there is little guidance on how to use the "transformative vision" to guide the methods.

The sequential transformative strategy was used by Park, Knapp, and Shin (2009) in the conduct of their mixed-methods study of social engagement in assisted living communities. These researchers used a framework of social relationships and support among older

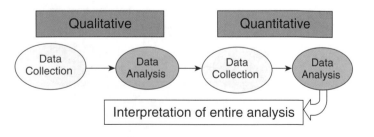

Figure 10-2 Sequential exploratory strategy. (Adapted from Creswell, J. W. [2009]. *Research design: Qualitative, quantitative, and mixed methods approaches* [3rd ed.]. Los Angeles, CA: Sage; and Hanson, W. E., Creswell, J. W., Plano Clark, V. L., Petska, K. S., & Creswell, J. D. [2005]. Mixed methods research designs in counseling psychology. *Journal of Counseling Psychology, 52*[2], 224–235.)

- Purpose is to use quantitative data and results to assist in the interpretation of qualitative findings.
- Primary focus of this model is to explore a phenomenon.
- Weakness is the length of time involved in data collection, with the two separate phases.

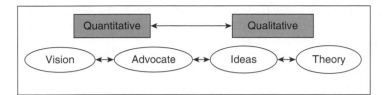

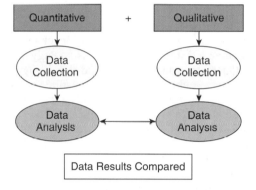

Figure 10-3 Sequential transformative strategy. (Adapted from Creswell, J. W. [2009]. *Research design: Qualitative, quantitative, and mixed methods approaches* [3rd ed.]. Los Angeles, CA: Sage; and Hanson, W. E., Creswell, J. W., Plano Clark, V. L., Petska, K. S., & Creswell, J. D. [2005]. Mixed methods research designs in counseling psychology. *Journal of Counseling Psychology, 52*[2], 224–235.)

adults to guide the research design. Although there was substantial information on female older adults in assisted living communities, a review of the literature revealed that little was known about how social engagement is experienced by men in later life. Using a quantitative approach followed by a qualitative approach, the researchers were able to examine gender differences in social engagement and psychological well-being among residents in assisted living communities. In addition, they explored experiences and challenges concerning social relationships for older men. Their findings suggested that older men are less likely to be satisfied with their lives in an assisted living community because they feel that their social worlds are limited. The most striking finding was that assisted living communities are not well designed for men's emotional or social needs. These researchers gave a "voice" to older men and a call for assisted living administrators, social workers, and staff to be aware of the specialized social and emotional needs of male residents (Park et al., 2009).

Concurrent Triangulation Strategy

Concurrent triangulation strategy is a more familiar approach to researchers. This model is selected when a researcher wishes to use quantitative and qualitative methods in an attempt to confirm, cross-validate, or corroborate findings within a single study. This model generally uses separate quantitative and qualitative methods as a mechanism to compensate for the weaknesses intrinsic in one method with the strengths of the other method. Therefore, the quantitative and qualitative data collection processes are conducted concurrently. This strategy usually integrates the results of the two methods during the interpretation phase; and convergence strengthens the knowledge claims or explains lack of convergence (see Figure 10-4). Great researcher effort and expertise are needed to study a phenomenon with two methods. Because of the different methods, researchers are challenged with the

Figure 10-4 Concurrent triangulation strategy. (Adapted from Creswell, J. W. [2009]. *Research design: Qualitative, quantitative, and mixed methods approaches* [3rd ed.]. Los Angeles, CA: Sage; and Hanson, W. E., Creswell, J. W., Plano Clark, V. L., Petska, K. S., & Creswell, J. D. [2005]. Mixed methods research designs in counseling psychology. *Journal of Counseling Psychology, 52*[2], 224–235.)

difficulty of comparing the study results and determining the study findings. It is still unclear how to best resolve discrepancies in findings between methods (Creswell, 2009).

An example of the concurrent mixed-methods or triangulation approach is the study by Manuel et al. (2007). These researchers concurrently conducted quantitative and qualitative approaches to examine the coping strategies used by young women diagnosed with breast cancer. The modified Ways of Coping–Cancer Version (WOC-CA) scale was used to collect quantitative data. After the WOC-CA scale, participants were asked two open-ended questions (qualitative) because studies have consistently found that younger women show greater psychological distress in response to breast cancer than older women. The researchers thought the open-ended responses would be particularly important because they provided the opportunity to explore whether existing scales adequately cover the strategies used by younger women to cope with breast cancer. In the discussion section of their report, the researchers indicated that the data did not converge to confirm current knowledge. The qualitative data provided useful insights about coping in the population of younger women. For example, although quantitative data revealed that "wishful thinking" was commonly used in dealing with the cancer, responses of the younger women to the open-ended items indicated this strategy was not used. Qualitative analysis revealed that being physically active, seeking information, resting, and using medications and complementary and alternative therapies were the most effective strategies used by younger women. However, these items are not included in either the WOC-CA or other commonly used cancer coping scales. These findings suggest that researchers and healthcare professionals should be aware that frequently used coping scales may not include significant strategies used by younger women dealing with the diagnosis of breast cancer.

KEY POINTS

- Research design is a blueprint for the conduct of a study that maximizes the researcher's control over factors that could interfere with the desired outcomes.
- Before selecting a design, the researcher must understand certain concepts: causality, multicausality, probability, bias, manipulation, and control.
- The purpose of design is to set up a situation that maximizes the possibilities of obtaining valid answers to research questions or testing hypotheses.
- Study validity is a measure of the truth or accuracy of the research findings and is an important concern throughout the research process.
- The four types of study design validity requiring examination in a study are (1) statistical conclusion validity; (2) internal validity; (3) construct validity; and (4) external validity.
- Statistical conclusion validity is concerned with whether the conclusions about relationships or differences drawn from statistical analyses are an accurate reflection of the real world. Several potential threats to statistical conclusion design validity are addressed.
- Internal validity is the extent to which the effects detected in the study are a true reflection of reality rather than the result of extraneous variables, and potential threats to internal validity are discussed.
- Construct validity examines the fit between the conceptual and operational definitions of a variable, and threats to this type of design validity are discussed.
- External validity is concerned with the extent to which study findings can be generalized beyond the sample used in the study. The potential threats to external design validity are identified.
- A good design provides the subjects, the setting, and the protocol within which these comparisons can be clearly examined.
- Designs are developed to reduce threats to the validity of the comparisons. However, some designs are more effective in reducing threats than others.
- The elements of a good design include control of (1) the environment; (2) equivalence of subjects and groups; (3) treatment; (4) measurement; and (5) extraneous variables.
- In designing the study, the researcher must identify extraneous variables that could explain some of the variance in measurement of the study variables.
- Questions are provided to direct the reader in developing and implementing a study design.
- Mixed-methods approaches include the combined use of quantitative and qualitative research methods. Data are collected either sequentially or concurrently, and theory may or may not be used in conducting the study. Merging of data occurs at different points of the study depending on how the qualitative and quantitative methods are implemented.
- The four mixed-methods approaches usually implemented in nursing research are (1) sequential explanatory strategy; (2) sequential exploratory strategy; (3) sequential transformative strategy; and (4) concurrent triangulation strategy.

REFERENCES

Aberson, C. L. (2010). *Applied power analysis for the behavioral sciences.* New York, NY: Routledge Taylor & Francis Group.

Bialocerkowski, A., Klupp, N., & Bragge, P. (2010). Research methodology series: How to read and critically appraise a reliability article. *International Journal of Therapy and Rehabilitation, 17*(3), 114–120.

Brown, S.J. (2009). *Evidence-based nursing: The research-practice connection.* Boston, MA: Jones & Bartlett.

Campbell, D. T., & Fiske, D. W. (1959). Convergent and discriminate validation by the multitrait-multimethod matrix. *Psychological Bulletin, 56*(2), 81–105.

Campbell, D. T., & Stanley, J. C. (1963). *Experimental and quasi-experimental designs for research*. Chicago, IL: Rand McNally.

Carr, E. C. (2009). Understanding inadequate pain management in the clinical setting: The value of the sequential explanatory mixed method study. *Journal of Clinical Nursing, 18*(1), 124–131.

Choi, M., & Harwood, J. (2004). A hypothesized Model of Korean Women's Responses to Abuse. *Journal of Transcultural Nursing, 15*(3), 207–216.

Choi, M., Phillips, L. R., Figueredo, A. J., Insel, K., & Min, S. K. (2008). Construct validity of the Korean Women's Abuse Intolerance Scale. *Nursing Research, 57*(1), 40–50.

Cook, T. D., & Campbell, D. T. (1979). *Quasi-experimentation: Design and analysis issues for field settings*. Chicago, IL. Rand McNally.

Corty, E. W. (2007). *Using and interpreting statistics: A practical text for the health, behavioral, and social sciences*. St. Louis, MO: Mosby Elsevier.

Coward, D. D. (1990). Critical multiplism: A research strategy for nursing science. *Image—Journal of Nursing Scholarship, 22*(3), 163–167.

Creswell, J. W. (2009). *Research design: Qualitative, quantitative, and mixed methods approaches* (3rd ed.). Los Angeles, CA: Sage.

Denzin, N. K. (1989). *The research act: A theoretical introduction to sociological methods* (3rd ed.). New York: McGraw-Hill.

DeVon, H. A., Block, M. E., Moyle-Wright, P., Ernst, D. M., Hayden, S. J., Lazzara, D. J., et al. (2007). A psychometric toolbox for testing validity and reliability. *Journal of Nursing Scholarship, 39*(2), 155–164.

Doran, D. M. (2011). *Nursing outcomes: The state of the science* (2nd ed.). Sudbury, MA: Jones & Bartlett Learning.

Duffy, M. E. (1987). Methodological triangulation: A vehicle for merging quantitative and qualitative research methods. *Image—Journal of Nursing Scholarship, 19*(3), 130–133.

Fawcett, J., & Garity, J. (2009). *Evaluating research for evidence-based nursing practice*. Philadelphia, PA: F. A. Davis.

Forbes, A. (2009). Clinical intervention research in nursing. *International Journal of Nursing Studies, 46*(4), 557–568.

Goodwin, L. D. (1984). Increasing efficiency and precision of data analysis: Multivariate vs. univariate statistical techniques. *Nursing Research, 33*(4), 247–249.

Grove, S. K. (2007). *Statistics for health care research: A practical workbook*. Philadelphia, PA: Saunders Elsevier.

Hanson, W. E., Creswell, J. W., Plano Clark, V. L., Petska, K. S., & Creswell, J. D. (2005). Mixed methods research designs in counseling psychology. *Journal of Counseling Psychology, 52*(2), 224–235.

Kerlinger, F. N., & Lee, H. B. (2000). *Foundations of behavioral research* (4th ed.). Fort Worth, TX: Harcourt College Publishers.

Manuel, J. C., Burwell, S. R., Crawford, S. L., Lawrence, R. H., Farmer, D. F., Hege, A., et al. (2007). Younger women's perceptions of coping with breast cancer. *Cancer Nursing, 30*(2), 85–94.

McGuire, D. B., DeLoney, V. G., Yeager, K. A., Owen, D. C., Peterson, D. E., Lin, L. S., et al. (2000). Maintaining study validity in a changing clinical environment. *Nursing Research, 49*(4), 231–235.

Marshall, C., & Rossman, G. B. (2011). *Designing qualitative research* (5th ed.). Thousand Oaks, CA: Sage.

Melnyk, B. M., & Fineout-Overholt, E. (2011). *Evidence-based practice in nursing & healthcare: A guide to best practice* (2nd ed.). Philadelphia, PA: Lippincott Williams, & Wilkins.

Mitchell, E. S. (1986). Multiple triangulation: A methodology for nursing science. *Advances in Nursing Science, 8*(3), 18–26.

Morrison, D. M., Hoppe, M. J., Gillmore, M. R., Kluver, C., Higa, D., & Wells, E. A. (2009). Replicating an intervention: The tension between fidelity and adaptation. *AIDS Education and Prevention, 21*(2), 128–140.

Morse, J. M. (1991). Approaches to qualitative-quantitative methodological triangulation. *Nursing Research, 40*(1), 120–123.

Munhall, P. L. (2012). *Nursing research: A qualitative perspective* (5th ed.). Miami: Jones & Bartlett.

Myers, S. T., & Haase, J. E. (1989). Guidelines for integration of quantitative and qualitative approaches. *Nursing Research, 38*(5), 299–301.

Park N. S., Knapp, M. A., & Shin, H. J. (2009). Mixed methods study of social engagement in assisted living communities: Challenges. *Journal of Gerontological Social Work, 52*(8), 767–783.

Patton, M. Q. (2002). *Qualitative research and evaluation methods* (3rd ed.). Thousand Oaks, CA: Sage.

Porter, E. J. (1989). The qualitative-quantitative dualism. *Image—Journal of Nursing Scholarship, 21*(2), 98–102.

Rocco, T. S., Bliss, L. A., Gallagher, S., & Perez-Prado, A. (2003). Taking the next step: Mixed methods research in organizational systems. *Information Technology, Learning, and Performance Journal, 21*(1), 19–29.

Ryan-Wenger, N. A. (2010). Evaluation of measurement precision, accuracy, and error in biophysical data for clinical research and practice. In C. F. Waltz, O. L. Strickland, & E. R. Lenz (Eds.), *Measurement in nursing and health research* (4th ed.) (pp. 371–383). New York, NY: Springer Publishing Company.

Santacroce, S. J., Maccarelli, L. M., & Grey, M. (2004). Methods: Intervention fidelity. *Nursing Research, 53*(1), 63–66.

Shadish, W. R., Cook, T. D., & Campbell, D. T. (2002). *Experimental and quasi-experimental designs for generalized causal inference*. Chicago, IL: Rand McNally.

Thompson, S. K. (2002). *Sampling* (2nd ed.). New York, NY: John Wiley & Sons.

Waltz, C. F., Strickland, O. L., & Lenz, E. R. (2010). *Measurement in nursing and health research* (4th ed.). New York, NY: Springer Publishing Company.

Yamada, J., Stevens, B., Sidani, S., Watt-Watson, J., & De Silva, N. (2010). Content validity of a process evaluation checklist to measure intervention implementation fidelity of the EPIC intervention. *Worldviews of Evidence-Based Nursing, 7*(3), 158–164.

11

CHAPTER

Selecting a Quantitative Research Design

A design is the blueprint for conducting a study that maximizes control over factors that could interfere with the validity of the findings. A research design gives you greater control and thus improves the validity of your study. To select an appropriate research design, you will need to integrate many elements. Chapter 10 began with questions that will help you select a design or identify by name the design of a study you are critically appraising. Identifying the design of a published study is not always easy, because many published studies do not identify the design used. Determining the design may require you to put together bits of information from various parts of the research report.

This chapter describes the designs most commonly used in nursing research, using the study categories described in Chapter 3: descriptive, correlational, quasi-experimental, and experimental. Descriptive and correlational designs examine variables in natural environments, such as home, and do not include researcher-designed treatments or interventions. Quasi-experimental and experimental designs examine the effects of an intervention by comparing differences between groups that have received the intervention and those that have not received the intervention. As you review each design, note the threats to validity that are controlled by the design, keeping in mind that uncontrolled threats in the design you choose may weaken the validity of your study. Box 11-1 lists the designs discussed in this chapter. Each of the designs is briefly described, and a model is provided so you can see the different elements of the designs. After the descriptions of the designs, we provide a series of decision trees or algorithms that will help you to select the appropriate design for your study or to identify the design used in a published study.

Investigators have always developed designs to meet emerging research needs. In the 1930s, Sir Ronald A. Fisher (1935) developed the first experimental designs that were published in a book titled *The Design of Experiments*. However, most work on design has been conducted since the 1970s, and the designs of the last 20 years have become much more sophisticated and varied. There is no universal standard for categorizing designs. Names of designs change as various writers discuss them. Researchers sometimes merge elements of several designs to meet the research needs of a particular study. From these developments, new designs sometimes emerge.

Originally, only experimental designs were considered of value. In addition, many believed that the only setting in which an experiment can be conducted is a laboratory, where stricter controls can be maintained than in a field or natural setting. This approach is appropriate for the natural sciences but not for the social sciences. From the social sciences have emerged additional quantitative designs (descriptive, correlational, and quasi-experimental), methodological designs, and qualitative designs (Cook & Campbell, 1979; Creswell, 2009; Fawcett & Garity, 2009). The epidemiology, public health, and community health fields have presented time-series designs, health promotion designs, and prevention designs.

Currently, most nurse researchers are using designs developed in other disciplines, such as psychology, medicine, sociology, epidemiology, and education, that meet the needs of those disciplines. Will these designs be effective in adding to the knowledge base required for nursing? These designs are a useful starting point, but nurse scientists must go beyond them to develop designs that will more appropriately meet the needs of the nursing community. To go beyond current designs, nurse scientists must have a working knowledge of available designs and of the logic on which they are based. Designs created to meet nursing needs should be congruent with nursing philosophy. They must provide a means for nurses to examine dimensions of nursing within a holistic framework and to review those dimensions over time. Designs must be developed that can seek answers to important nursing questions rather than answering only questions that can be examined by existing designs.

Innovative design strategies are beginning to appear within nursing research. One example is the intervention research design described in Chapter 14. Developing designs to study the outcomes of nursing actions is also important. The emerging field of outcomes research in nursing is described in Chapter 13. Nurse researchers must see themselves as credible scientists before they will dare to develop new design strategies to explore little-understood aspects of nursing. To develop a new design, the researcher must carefully consider possible threats to validity and ways to diminish them. Nurses must also be willing to risk the temporary failures that are always inherent in the development of something new.

Descriptive Study Designs

Descriptive study designs (see Box 11-1) are crafted to gain more information about characteristics within a particular field of study. Their purpose is to provide a picture of situations as they naturally happen. In many aspects of nursing, a phenomenon must be clearly delineated before prediction or causality can be examined. A descriptive design may be used to develop theory, identify problems with current practice, justify current practice, make judgments, or determine what others in similar situations are doing. Variables are not manipulated, and there is no treatment or intervention. Dependent and independent variables are not appropriate for use within a descriptive design, because the design involves no attempt to establish causality.

Descriptive designs vary in levels of complexity. Some contain only two variables, whereas others may have multiple variables. The relationships among variables present an overall picture of the phenomenon being examined, but examination of types and degrees of relationships is not the primary purpose of a descriptive study. Protection against bias (or threat to the validity) in a descriptive design is achieved through (1) links between conceptual and operational definitions of variables (Fawcett & Garity, 2009); (2) sample selection and size (Aberson, 2010; Thompson, 2002); (3) the use of valid and reliable instruments (Waltz,

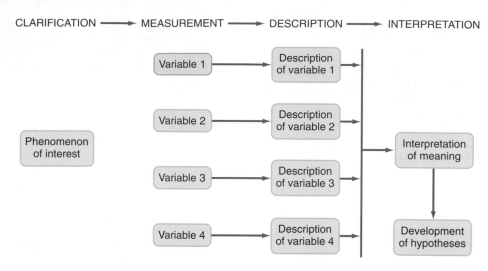

CLARIFICATION ⟶ MEASUREMENT ⟶ DESCRIPTION ⟶ INTERPRETATION

Figure 11-1 Typical descriptive study design.

Strickland, & Lenz, 2010) or accurate and precise biophysical measures (Ryan-Wenger, 2010); and (4) data collection procedures that achieve some environmental control (Bialocerkowski, Klupp, & Bragge, 2010; Creswell, 2009; DeVon et al., 2007; Kerlinger & Lee, 2000).

Typical Descriptive Study Designs

Figure 11-1 presents the commonly used descriptive study design that examines characteristics of a single sample. The design identifies a phenomenon of interest and the variables within the phenomenon, develops conceptual and operational definitions of the variables, and describes the variables. The description of the variables leads to an interpretation of the theoretical meaning of the findings and provides knowledge of the variables and the study population that can be used for future research in the area.

Most studies contain descriptive components; however, the methodology of some studies is confined to the typical descriptive design. This is a critically important design for acquiring knowledge in an area in which little research has been conducted. Peterson, Schwab, van Oostrom, Gravenstein, and Caruso (2010) implemented a descriptive study design to examine the effects of various patient positions on the development of pressure in common areas such as the sacrum and hips. Minimizing skin–support surface interface pressure is important in preventing and controlling pressure ulcers, but the effects of standard patient repositioning on skin interface pressure has not been clearly described. The study design and key results are presented in the abstract, which is reprinted in full:

"*Aim:* This paper is a report of a study of the effects of lateral turning on skin-bed interface pressures in the sacral, trochanteric and buttock regions, and its effectiveness in unloading at-risk tissue.

Design: This was a *descriptive, observational study.* Data were collected from 15 healthy adults from a university-affiliated hospital. Mapped 24-inch × 24-inch (2304 half-inch sensors) interface pressure profiles were obtained in the supine position, followed by lateral turning with pillow or wedge support and subsequent head-of-bed elevation to 30°." (Peterson et al., 2010, pp. 1557-1558)

"*Results:* Raising the head-of-bed to 30° in the lateral position statistically significantly increased peak interface pressures and total area $\geq$ 32 mm Hg. Comparing areas $\geq$ 32 mm Hg from all positions, 93% of participants had skin areas with interface pressures $\geq$ 32 mm Hg throughout all positions (60 ± 54 cm^2), termed 'triple jeopardy areas'. The triple jeopardy area increased statistically significantly with wedges as compared to pillows (153 ± 99 cm^2 vs. 48 ± 47 cm^2, $p < 0.05$).

Conclusions: Standard turning by experienced intensive care unit nurses does not reliably relieve elevated skin-bed interface pressures as intended. These areas of the body remain at risk for skin breakdown, and help to explain why pressure ulcers occur despite the implementation of standard preventive measures. Support materials for maintaining lateral turned positions can also influence tissue unloading and triple jeopardy areas." (Peterson et al., 2010, p. 1556)

A descriptive research design is appropriate when the current practice (that is, routine turning of patients) does not seem sufficient to alleviate the problem (risk for pressure ulcers). To discover why traditional nursing interventions have failed to eliminate the pressure ulcers on three at-risk areas of the body, Peterson et al. (2010) decided to explore the currently used techniques (pillows versus wedges) and objectively measure and describe the pressures that participants experienced using digital pressure sensors. This study involved no treatment and had one study group of participants who were measured for pressures in the at-risk areas.

Some descriptive studies use questionnaires (surveys) to describe an identified area of concern. For example, Strand and Lindgren (2010) used a descriptive design to study nurses' knowledge, attitude, and barriers regarding preventing pressure ulcers in patients in intensive care units (ICUs). The following excerpt from the abstract describes the design of their study:

Background: "Pressure ulcer incidence varies between 1 and 56% in intensive care and prevention is an important quest for nursing staff. Critically ill patients that develop pressure ulcers suffer from increased morbidity and mortality and also require prolonged intensive care.

Purpose: The aim of this study was to investigate registered nurses' and enrolled nurses' (1) attitudes, (2) knowledge, and (3) perceived barriers to opportunities towards pressure ulcer prevention, in an ICU setting. These are important aspects in the Theory of Planned Behaviour, a conceptual framework when trying to predict, understand, and change specific behaviours.

Method: The study is descriptive. Questionnaires were distributed to registered nurses and enrolled nurses in four ICUs in a Swedish hospital.

Results: The mean score regarding attitude was 34 ± 4. Correct categorization of pressure ulcers was made by 46.8% of the nursing staff.... Pressure relief (97.3%) and nutritional support (36.1%) were the most frequently reported preventive measures. Reported barriers were lack of time (57.8%) and severely ill patients (28.9%); opportunities were knowledge (38%) and access to pressure relieving equipment (35.5%)." (Strand & Lindgren, 2010, p. 335)

The results of this descriptive study indicated that nurses are lacking in comprehensive knowledge of pressure ulcers; additionally, time, acuity of the patient's condition, and the availability of supportive equipment were barriers to the prevention of pressure ulcers. The study focused on surveying nurses' knowledge of, attitudes toward, and perceived barriers to opportunities for pressure ulcer prevention using a questionnaire. A descriptive design was appropriate for identifying variables that might influence nursing care of patients at risk for pressure ulcers in ICU settings.

Some descriptive studies obtain data from retrospective chart review. For example, Kline and Edwards (2007) conducted a chart review to describe the effectiveness of intrapartum intravenous (IV) insulin on antepartum and intrapartum control of the mother's diabetes and on the occurrence and severity of hypoglycemia in the neonate. Researchers measured and described the variables of intrapartum IV insulin, antepartum diabetic control, intrapartum diabetic control, and hypoglycemia in the neonate.

It is not uncommon for researchers using a descriptive design to combine quantitative descriptive methods and qualitative methods (mixed methods) (Creswell, 2009). Chapter 10 includes a discussion of different types of mixed-methods approaches. To use this strategy, consult with a researcher experienced in using qualitative methods or include this person as a research partner to appropriately collect, analyze, and interpret qualitative data.

Meghani and Keane (2007) used quantitative and qualitative methods in their study of preference for analgesic treatment in African-American cancer patients. The investigators used demographic data, the Brief Pain Inventory, and in-depth semi-structured interviews. Their sample of 35 patients was taken from three outpatient oncology clinics. Their study identified the major sources of anxiety described by this sample. The goal of this study was to improve our understanding of patients' needs and assist in the development of specific interventions that might alleviate their problems.

Comparative Descriptive Designs

The comparative descriptive design (Figure 11-2) examines and describes differences in variables in two or more groups that occur naturally in the setting. Descriptive statistics and inferential statistical analyses may be used to examine differences between or among groups. Commonly, the results obtained from these analyses are not generalized to a population because the description is for a very specific sample and would not necessarily apply to a larger population. An example of this design is the study by Cramer,

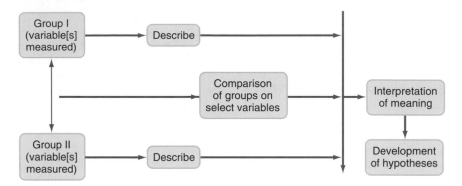

Figure 11-2 Comparative descriptive design.

Chen, Roberts, and Clute (2007) of the social and economic impact of community-based prenatal care. The abstract for this study, which is reprinted in full, describes the focus, design, and major findings:

"Objective: This article describes the evaluation and findings of a community-based prenatal care program, Omaha Healthy Start (OHS), designed to reduce local racial disparities in birth outcome.

Design: This evaluative study used a comparative descriptive design, and Targeting Outcomes of Programs was the conceptual framework for evaluation. Sample: The evaluation followed 3 groups for 2 years: OHS birth mothers (N = 79; N = 157); non-OHS participant birth mothers (N = 746; N = 774); and Douglas County birth mothers (N = 7,962; N = 7,987).

Measurement: OHS provided case management, home visits, screening, referral, transportation, and health education to participants. Program outcome measures included low birth weight, infant mortality, adequacy of care, trimester of care, and costs of care.

Results: OHS birth outcomes improved during year 2, and there was a 31% cost saving in the average hospital expenditure compared with the nonparticipant groups. Preliminary evaluative analysis indicates that prenatal case management and community outreach can improve birth outcomes for minority women, while producing cost savings.

Conclusions: Further prospective study is needed to document trends over a longer period of time regarding the relationship between community-based case management programs for minority populations, birth outcomes, and costs of care." (Cramer et al., 2007, p. 329)

Using a comparative descriptive design, Cramer and colleagues (2007) described the variables incidence of case management, home visits, screening, referral, transportation, and health education, as well as the outcomes low birth weight, infant mortality, adequacy of care, trimester of care, and costs of care in three groups (OHS birth mothers, non-OHS birth mothers, and Douglas County birth mothers) yearly for 3 years. The results of the study were comparisons across the 3 years and among the three groups.

Time-Dimensional Designs

Time-dimensional designs were developed within the discipline of epidemiology, a field that studies the occurrence and distribution of disease among populations. These designs examine trends over time, growth, or sequences and patterns of change. The dimension of time, then, becomes an important factor. Within the field of epidemiology, the samples in time-dimensional studies are called **cohorts**. Originally, cohorts were age categories; however, the concept has been expanded to apply to groups distinguished by many other variables. Other means of classifying populations that have relevance in relation to time are time of diagnosis, point of entry into a treatment protocol, point of entry into a new lifestyle, and age at which the subject started smoking. An understanding of temporal sequencing is an important prerequisite to examining causality between variables. Thus, the results of these designs lead to description of trends, processes, patterns, and changes over time as well as the development of hypotheses, and are often forerunners of experimental designs (Fawcett & Garity, 2009).

Epidemiological studies that use time-dimensional designs determine the risk factors or causal factors of illness states. Cause determined in this manner is called *inferred causality* (Kerlinger & Lee, 2000).

Time 1	Time 2	Time 3	Time 4	Time..n
measure variables	measure variables	measure variables	measure variables	measure variables
Sample 1	Sample 1	Sample 1	Sample 1	Sample 1

Figure 11-3 Longitudinal design.

These studies also examine trends, patterns, and changes over time. The best-known studies in this area are those on smoking and cancer. Because of the strength of studies that have undergone multiple repetitions, the causal link is strong. The strategy is not as powerful as experimental designs in supporting causality; however, in this situation, as in many nursing contexts, one can never ethically conduct a true experiment. A true experiment requires that there be an experimental group (who would not smoke) and a control group (who smoke). The participants must be randomly assigned to one of these groups. Therefore, without being provided a choice, some individuals would be required to smoke and others would be required to abstain from smoking over a long period.

Epidemiologists use two strategies to examine changes over time: retrospective studies and prospective studies. The norm in epidemiological studies is to use the word *cohorts* to refer to groups of subjects in prospective studies, but the term is generally not used in **retrospective studies**. In retrospective studies, both the proposed cause and the proposed effect have already occurred. For example, the subjects could have a specific type of cancer, and the researcher could be searching for commonalities among subjects that may have led to the development of that type of cancer. In a **prospective cohort study**, causes may have occurred, but the proposed effect has not.

The Framingham study is the best-known example of a prospective study (U.S. Department of Health and Human Services, 1968). In this study, researchers monitored members of a community for 20 years and examined variables such as dietary patterns, exercise, weight, and blood lipid levels. As the subjects experienced illnesses, such as heart disease, hypertension, and lung disease, their illnesses could be related to previously identified variables.

Prospective studies are considered more powerful than retrospective studies in inferring causality, because the researcher can demonstrate that the risk factors occurred before the illness and are positively related to the illness. Both designs are important for use in nursing studies, because a person's responses to health situations are patterns that developed long before the health situation occurred. These patterns then influence the person's responses to nursing interventions. Several designs are used to conduct time-dimensional studies: longitudinal, cross-sectional, trend, and event or treatment partitioning. These designs are discussed in the following sections.

Longitudinal Designs

Longitudinal designs examine changes in the same subjects over time. They are sometimes called panel designs (Figure 11-3). Longitudinal designs are expensive and require a long period of researcher and subject commitment. The area to be studied, the variables, and their measurement must be clearly identified before data collection begins. Measurement must be carefully planned and implemented because the measures will be used repeatedly over time. If children are being studied, the measures must be valid for all the ages being studied. To use this design, researchers must be familiar with how the construct being measured changes and its patterns and trends over time. In addition, they need to provide a clear rationale for the points of time they have selected for measurement. There is often a bias in selection of subjects because of the requirement for a long-term commitment. Individuals participating in a study conducted over long periods might differ in some important ways from the target population. In addition, attrition or loss of subjects from the study can be high and can decrease the validity of findings.

The sample size calculated with power analysis needs to take into consideration the potential attrition rate when determining the final number of subjects to recruit. As a researcher, you must invest considerable energy in developing effective strategies to maintain the sample (see Chapter 15). The period during which subjects will be recruited into the study must be carefully planned, and a timeline depicting data collection points for each subject must be developed to enable planning for the numbers and availability of data collectors. If this issue is not carefully thought out, data collectors may be confronted with the need to recruit new subjects while they are attempting to collect data scheduled for subjects recruited earlier. You must also decide whether you will use a single data collector to obtain all data from a particular subject or whether you will use a different data collector at each point to ensure that data are collected blindly.

Because of the large volumes of data acquired in a longitudinal study, you must give careful attention to strategies for managing the data. The repetition of measures requires that data analysis be carefully thought through. Analyses commonly used are repeated measures analyses of variance, multivariate analyses of variance (MANOVA), regression analysis, cluster analysis, and time-series analysis (see Chapters 24 and 25) (Corty, 2007; Munro, 2005).

Lee, Chaboyer, and Wallis (2010) conducted a descriptive study using a longitudinal cohort design. This study was conducted to describe the perceptions and physical manifestations of injury and illness of patients with traumatic injury and to examine the changes they experienced over time. The following abstract from the study demonstrates the background, longitudinal design, key results, conclusions, and implications for practice:

"*Background:* Traumatic injury has attracted global concern because it is the major reason for death and disability in people under 45 years old. One model, the Common Sense Model of Illness Representation (CSMIR), has the potential to help individuals adjust to changes in health status such as traumatic injury.

Design: Longitudinal study design.

Methods: This study was conducted using data collected prior to hospital discharge and at three and six months after hospital discharge. One individual question form and the Chinese Illness Perception Questionnaire Revised (IPQ-R) (Trauma) were used to collect demographic data, clinical data, and illness representations.

Results: A total of 114 participants completed the survey three times. The overall response rate was 79.7%. Six subscales of the Chinese IPQ-R (Trauma)... identity, emotional representations, consequences, controllability, illness coherence, and causes... changed significantly over time. Two subscales, Timeline (acute/chronic) and Timeline Cyclical, did not change significantly.

Conclusions: Based on these findings, there may be a window of opportunity to provide appropriate interventions to individuals with traumatic injury at each time point. The results of this study have implications for nursing practice and further nursing research.

Relevance to Clinical Practice: Understanding illness representation in patients with traumatic injury may help nurses to provide anticipatory guidance and to design nursing interventions before and after hospital discharge, ultimately to improve health outcomes of those patients." (Lee et al., 2010, p. 556)

Cross-Sectional Designs

Cross-sectional designs examine groups of subjects in various stages of development, trends, patterns, and changes simultaneously with the intent to describe changes in the phenomenon across stages (see Figure 11-4). The assumption is that the stages are part of a

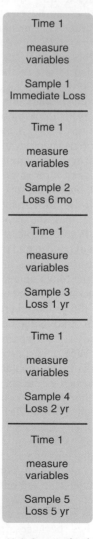

Figure 11-4 Cross-sectional design.

process that will progress over time. Selecting subjects at various points in the process provides important information about the totality of the process, even though the same subjects are not monitored through the entire process. The processes of development selected for the study might be related to age, position in an educational system, growth pattern, or stages of maturation or personal growth (if they could be clearly enough defined that criteria could be developed for inclusion within differentiated groups or disease stages). Subjects are then categorized by group, and data on the selected variables are collected at a single point in time.

For example, suppose you wish to study grief reactions at various periods after the death of a spouse. With a cross-sectional design, you could study a group of individuals whose spouses had died 1 week ago, another group composed of individuals whose losses occurred 6 months ago, and other groups whose losses occurred 1 year, 2 years, and 5 years ago (see Figure 11-4). You could study all of these groups during one period of time, but you could describe a pattern of grief reactions over a 5-year period. The design is not as strong as the longitudinal design, in which the same participants continue in the study over time, thus eliminating some variance, but it allows some understanding of the phenomenon over time when time allowed for the study is limited.

Sidani et al. (2007) conducted a cross-sectional study titled "Outcomes of Nurse Practitioners in Acute Care: An Exploration." The following abstract describes the design of their study:

"The purpose of this study was to compare the outcomes achieved by adult patients who did ($n = 78$) and did not ($n = 45$) receive care by acute care nurse practitioners (ACNPs), within one week following discharge. A comparative, cross-sectional design was used. Consenting patients completed the outcome measures within one week following discharge. The outcomes included satisfaction with care, functional status, symptom resolution, and sense of well-being, which were measured with established instruments. The two groups of patients were equivalent in terms of their demographic profile and severity of condition. The results indicated that patients who received ACNP care, as compared to those who did not, reported higher levels of satisfaction with care and of physical, psychological, and social functioning. These findings provide preliminary evidence supporting the contribution of ACNPs to high quality care. However, the small sample size limits the generalizability of the study findings." (Sidani et al., 2007, p. 1)

Trend Designs

Trend designs examine changes in the general population in relation to a particular phenomenon (see Figure 11-5). The researchers select different samples of subjects from the same population at preset intervals of time, and at each selected time, they collect data from that particular sample. Researchers need to be able to justify generalizing from the samples to the population under study. Analysis involves strategies to predict future trends by examining past trends. Harris, Gordon-Larsen, Chantala, and Udry (2006, p. 74) used a trend design to describe "longitudinal trends in race/ethnic disparities in 20 leading health indicators from Healthy People 2010 [U.S. Department of Health and Human Services, 2000] across multiple domains from adolescence to young adulthood." These researchers examined the study trends in an ethnically diverse, national database, and their study design is described in the following excerpt.

"*Design, Setting, and Participants*: Nationally representative data for more than 14,000 adolescents enrolled in wave I (1994-1995) or wave II (1996) of the National Longitudinal Study of Adolescent Health

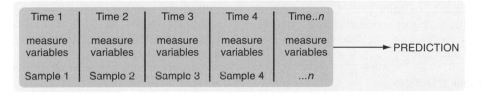

Time 1	Time 2	Time 3	Time 4	Time..n	
measure variables	measure variables	measure variables	measure variables	measure variables	→ PREDICTION
Sample 1	Sample 2	Sample 3	Sample 4	...n	

Figure 11-5 Trend design.

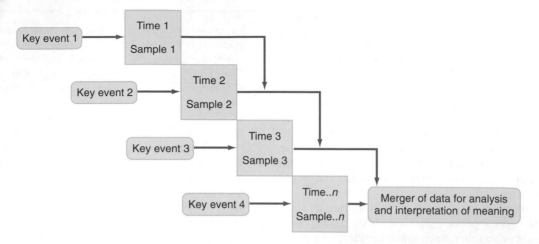

Figure 11-6 Cross-sectional study with treatment partitioning.

(Add Health) were followed up into adulthood (wave III; 2001-2002). We fit longitudinal regression models to assess and contrast the trend in health indicators among racial/ethnic groups of adolescents as they transition into adulthood....

Results: Diet, inactivity, obesity, health care access, substance use, and reproductive health worsened with age. Perceived health, mental health, and exposure to violence improved with age. On most health indicators, white and Asian subjects were at the lowest risk and Native American subjects at the highest risk. Although white subjects had more favorable health in adolescence, they experienced the greatest declines by young adulthood. No single race/ethnic group consistently leads or falters in health across all indicators." (Harris et al., 2006, p. 74)

Harris et al. (2006) found the trend design to be an effective way to examine health indicators of Americans over time. They noted for 15 of 20 indicators that the health risk increased and access to health care decreased from teen to adult years for most Americans. The health indicators varied over time by gender and race/ethnicity, causing the health disparities to fluctuate over time.

Event-Partitioning Designs

A merger of the cross-sectional or longitudinal and trend designs, the **event-partitioning design**, is used in some cases to enlarge sample size and to avoid the effects of history on the validity of findings. Cook and Campbell (1979) referred to these as cohort designs with treatment partitioning. Figure 11-6 shows a model of the cross-sectional study design with treatment partitioning, and Figure 11-7 provides the model of a longitudinal design with treatment partitioning. The term treatment is used loosely here to mean a key event that is thought to lead to change. In a descriptive study, the researcher would not cause or manipulate the key event but rather would clearly define it so that when it occurred naturally, it would be recognized.

For example, you could use the event-partitioning design to study subjects who have completed programs to stop smoking. Smoking behaviors and incidence of smoking-related diseases might be measured at intervals of 1 year for a 5-year period. However, the number of subjects available at one time might be insufficient for you to adequately analyze findings. Therefore, you could use subjects from several programs offered at different times. You would examine the data in terms of the relative time since the subjects' completion of the stop-smoking program, not the absolute length of time. Data would be assumed to be comparable, and a larger sample size would be available for analysis of changes over time.

Sutton's (2007) dissertation described a study to examine the relationship of preoperative education for the aging adult and anxiety. Most individuals experience anxiety in anticipation of surgery, and they expect education and support to help alleviate their anxiety prior to entering the operating room. Because a growing number of surgical procedures are being

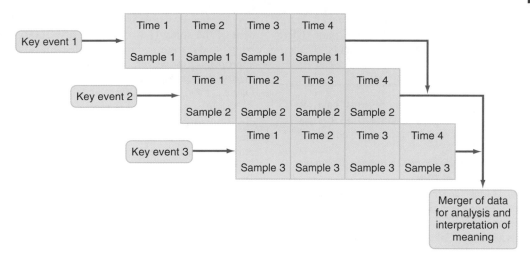

Figure 11-7 Longitudinal design with treatment partitioning.

conducted on an outpatient basis (day surgery), there is limited time for healthcare personnel to provide psychological preparation of patients for the perioperative process. Sutton used an event-partitioning design and correlational analysis to examine the relationship between education and the state anxiety experienced by aging adults in the preoperative setting. Quantitative data were collected using the Visual Analog Scale (VAS) to measure state anxiety in a pretest and post-test format, with treatment consisting of a scripted preoperative educational presentation.

Patients scheduled for general anesthesia for a surgical procedure in two acute care facilities in southern West Virginia were asked to participate in this study over a 4-week time frame. The sample included 52 pre-surgical patients, ages 65 to 94 years, who were asked to participate in the study. Participants were asked to score their state anxiety on the VAS prior to the scripted educational presentation to establish a baseline anxiety level. *State anxiety* is the emotion a person experiences in a particular situation, versus *trait anxiety,* which is the innate anxiety of a person. Upon completion of this presentation, the participants were given an opportunity to ask questions and receive answers. They were then asked to indicate their state anxiety on the VAS. The study results indicated that 75% of the study participants reported a decrease in their state anxiety levels following the preoperative educational presentation. This intervention requires further testing using a quasi-experimental study design but has the potential to reduce state anxiety in individuals experiencing day surgery (Sutton, 2007).

Case Study Designs

The **case study design** involves an intensive exploration of a single unit of study, such as a person, family, group, community, or institution, or of a small number of subjects. Although the number of subjects tends to be small, the number of variables involved is usually large. In fact, it is important to examine all variables that might have an impact on the situation being studied.

Case studies were commonly used in nursing research in the 1970s. Their use then declined, but they are beginning to appear in the literature more frequently today. Well-designed case studies are good sources of descriptive information and can be used as evidence for or against theories. Case studies can use a mixed-methods approach, incorporating both quantitative and qualitative methods (Creswell, 2009; Fawcett & Garity, 2009). Sterling and McNally (1992) recommended single-subject case studies for examining process-based nursing practice. This strategy allows the researcher to investigate daily observations and interventions that are a common aspect of nursing practice.

Case studies also can demonstrate the effectiveness of specific therapeutic techniques. In fact, by reporting a case study, the researcher introduces the technique to other practitioners. The case study design also has potential for revealing important findings that can generate new hypotheses for testing. Thus, the case study can lead to the design of large sample studies to examine factors identified through the case study. For example, Sprague and Chang (2011) used a single subject case study design to examine the effect of acupuncture on the treatment of chronic pain. Their study abstract identifies the key elements of their study:

"Background: Chronic complex regional pain syndrome (CRPS) is a chronic pain conduction that leads to sympathetic nervous system involvement and trophic changes.

Objective: This study describes the use of acupuncture in a case study of CRPS.

Design, Setting, and Patient: This is a single case report of a 34-year-old patient diagnosed with CRPS.

Intervention: Acupuncture treatment including acupoints along the Gallbladder, Liver, Spleen, Heart, and Kidney meridians. Self-treatment plan included a laser acupuncture pen device and disposable press needles.

Main Outcome Measures: Beck Depression Inventory (BDI), McGill Pain Questionnaire, and Sheehan Disability Scale (SDS).

Results: The patient reported a decrease in pain levels, depression, and an improved quality of life. Pretreatment SDS score of 17, a 12 on the BDI, and a 67 on the McGill Pain Questionnaire. Post-treatment SDS decreased to 4, her BDI went to 0, and her McGill Pain Questionnaire decreased to a 10." (Sprague & Change, 2011, p. 67)

Sprague and Chang (2011) noted that this patient had dramatic improvements in depression, disability, and pain scores over the 6 months of the study. Thus, this case study justifies conducting further clinical studies to determine the effectiveness of acupuncture in the management of patients with CRPS. They recommended conducting studies with larger samples and randomized controlled treatment designs.

How you design a case study depends on the circumstances of the case but usually includes an element of time. History and previous behavior patterns are usually explored in detail. As the case study proceeds, you may become aware of components important to the phenomenon being examined that were not originally built into the study. A case study is likely to have both quantitative and qualitative elements; and if the study incorporates both of these components, the study design must clearly present this fact (Creswell, 2009). Methods used to analyze and interpret qualitative data need to be carefully planned. Consultation with a qualitative researcher can strengthen the study. Large volumes of data are generally obtained during a case study. Organizing the findings of a case study

into a coherent whole is a difficult but critical component of the study (Fawcett & Garity, 2009). Generalizing study findings in the statistical sense is not appropriate; however, generalizing the findings to theory is appropriate and important (Crombie & Davies, 1996; Gray, 1998; Sandelowski, 1996).

Not all case studies are research. Many of the articles referring to case studies are clinical practice articles, in which a clinical situation is reported for the purpose of illustrating clinical practice, problems in clinical practice, or changes that need to be made in clinical practice. These articles do not use research methods but, rather, describe events out of the patient record or the writer's personal experience.

Surveys

The term survey is used in two ways within scientific thought. It is used in a broad sense to mean any descriptive or correlational study; in this sense, *survey* tends to mean nonexperimental (Kerlinger & Lee, 2000). In a narrower sense, the term is used to describe a data collection technique in which the researcher uses questionnaires (collected by email, by mail, or in person) or personal interviews to gather data about an identified population.

Surveys, in the narrower definition, are used to gather data that can be acquired through self-report. Because of this limitation in data, some researchers view surveys as rather shallow and as contributing in a limited way to scientific knowledge. This belief has led to a bias in the scientific community against survey research. In this context, the term survey is used derisively. However, surveys can be an extremely important source of data. In this text, we use the term **survey** to designate a data collection technique, not a design. Surveys can be used within many designs, including descriptive, correlational, and quasi-experimental studies.

Correlational Study Designs

Correlational study designs examine relationships among variables. The examination can occur at several levels of the independent variable. The researcher can seek to describe a relationship, predict relationships among variables, or test the relationships proposed by a theoretical proposition or a model. In any correlational study, a representative sample must be selected for the study. That sample reflects the full range of values possible on the variables being measured. Thus, large samples are required. In correlational designs, a large variance in the variable values is necessary to determine the existence of a relationship. Therefore, correlational designs are unlike experimental designs, in which variance in variable scores is controlled by controlling such design elements as the study setting, sampling criteria, and sampling method (Kerlinger & Lee, 2000).

In correlational designs, if the range of scores is truncated, the obtained correlational value will be artificially depressed. Truncated means that the lowest values and the highest values for a variable either are not measured or are condensed and merged with less extreme values. For example, if an attitude scale were scored from a low score of 1 to a high score of 50, truncated scores might indicate only scores in the range 10 to 40. More extreme scores would be combined with scores within the designated range. If truncation is performed, the researcher may not find a correlation when the variables are actually correlated.

Neophyte researchers tend to make two serious errors with correlational studies. First, they often attempt to establish causality by correlation, reasoning that if two variables are related, one must cause the other. Second, they confuse studies in which differences are examined with studies in which relationships are examined. Although the existence of a difference assumes the existence of a relationship, the design and statistical analysis of studies examining differences are not the same as those of studies examining relationships. If your study examines two or more groups in terms of one or more variables, then you are exploring differences between or among groups as reflected in scores on the identified variables. If your study examines a single group in terms of two or more variables, then you are exploring relationships between or among variables. In a correlational study, the relationship examined is between or among two or more research variables within an identified situation. Thus, the sample is not separated into groups. Analyses examine variable values in the entire sample. In a correlational design, data from the entire sample are analyzed as a single group (Grove, 2007; Kerlinger & Lee, 2000).

Descriptive Correlational Designs

A descriptive correlational design examines the relationships that exist in a situation. Using this design facilitates the identification of many interrelationships in a situation in a short time. Although the descriptive design discussed earlier may reveal relationships among variables, the descriptive correlational design focuses specifically on relationships among study variables. Descriptive correlational studies may lead to hypotheses for later studies. Figure 11-8 provides a model of a typical descriptive correlational design for examining a relationship between two research variables. This design can be expanded to include examination of relationships among several study variables.

A descriptive correlational study may examine variables in a situation that has already occurred or is currently occurring. No attempt is made to control or manipulate the situation. As with descriptive studies, variables must be clearly identified and defined. An example of a descriptive correlational design is the study by Bailey, Sabbagh, Loiselle, Boileau, and McVey (2010, p. 114) titled "Supporting families in the ICU: A descriptive correlational study of informational support, anxiety, and satisfaction with care." The researchers conducted this study to describe family members' perceptions of informational support,

MEASUREMENT

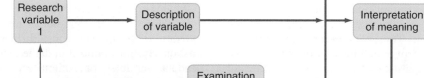

Figure 11-8 Descriptive correlational design.

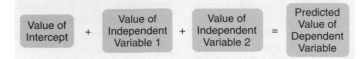

Figure 11-9 **Predictive design.**

anxiety, and satisfaction with care and to examine the relationships among these variables. The design for this study is described in the following excerpt from its abstract:

"Methodology/Design: This cross-sectional descriptive correlational pilot study collected data from a convenience sample of 29 family members using self-report questionnaires.

Setting: 22-bed medical-surgical intensive care unit of 659-bed University affiliated teaching hospital in Montreal, Quebec, Canada.

Results: Mean informational support, assessed with a modified version of the CCFNI [Critical Family Needs Inventory]..., was 55.41 (*SD* = 13.28; theoretical range of 20-80). Mean anxiety, assessed with the State Anxiety Scale (Spielberger et al., 1983) was 45.41 (*SD* = 15.27; theoretical range 20-80). Mean satisfaction with care... was 83.09 (*SD* = 15.49; theoretical range 24-96). A significant positive correlation was found between informational support and satisfaction with care ($r = 0.741$, $p < 0.001$). No significant relationships were noted between informational support and anxiety or between satisfaction with care and anxiety." (Bailey et al., 2010, p. 114)

By implementing a descriptive, correlational research design, Bailey et al. (2010) were able to describe their study variables and determine relationships among them. The ultimate objective of the researchers was to further refine a local informational support initiative for families with members in the intensive care unit. Thus, this research provided the basis for development of an intervention that might be tested in future quasi-experimental or experimental studies.

This study had a descriptive correlational design, as evidenced by the single study group, the absence of treatment, and the use of descriptive and correlational statistical techniques to analyze study data. The study variables informational support, anxiety, and satisfaction with care were described with means, standard deviations, and ranges (see Chapter 22). The

relationships among these three variables were determined using Pearson's product moment correlational coefficient (see Chapter 23).

Predictive Designs

Predictive designs are used to predict the value of one variable on the basis of values obtained from another variable or variables. Prediction is one approach you can use to examine causal relationships between or among variables. Because causal phenomena are being examined, the terms dependent and independent are used to describe the variables. One variable (the one to be predicted) is classified as the dependent variable, and all other variables (those that are predictors) are classified as independent variables.

The aim of a predictive design is to predict the level of the dependent variable from the independent variables. Figure 11-9 is a model of a predictive design with two independent variables used to predict the dependent variable. Independent variables most effective in prediction are highly correlated with the dependent variable but not highly correlated with other independent variables used in the study. Predictive designs require you to develop a theory-based mathematical hypothesis proposing the independent variables that are expected to predict the dependent variable effectively. You can then test the hypothesis using regression analysis (see Chapter 24) (Corty, 2007; Munro, 2005). Predictive studies are also used to establish the predictive validity of measurement scales.

Mancuso (2010) conducted a correlational study with a cross-sectional predictive correlational design to examine the impact of health literacy and patient trust on glycemic control in diabetic adults. The independent variables of patient trust, health literacy, knowledge of diabetes, performance of self-care activities, and depression were used to predict the dependent variable of glycosylated hemoglobin concentration (HbA1c). Regression analysis was conducted to determine how effective the independent variables were in predicting the dependent variable of HbA1c. The following except from the abstract describes the study design, results, and conclusions:

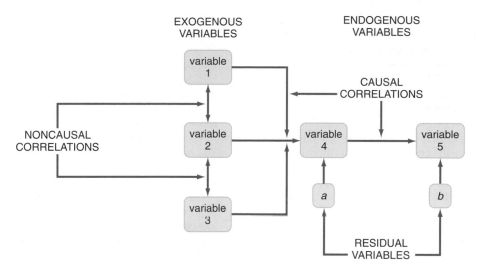

EXOGENOUS VARIABLES

ENDOGENOUS VARIABLES

Figure 11-10 Model-testing design.

"A quantitative study was conducted that examined health literacy and patient trust as predictors of glycemic control. The related factors of demographic, socioeconomic status, diabetes knowledge, self-care activities, and depression were also considered. Implementing a cross-sectional, predictive design, a convenience sample of 102 patients with diabetes was recruited from two urban primary care clinics in the USA. A simultaneous multiple regression was conducted. The regression analysis was significant, with patient trust and depression accounting for 28.5% of the variance in HbA1c." (Mancuso, 2010, p. 94)

Mancuso (2010) reported that patient trust and depression were important factors that significantly predicted HbA1c ($R^2 = 0.320$; $R^2_{adj} = 0.285$; $F(5, 96) = 9.047$; $p < 0.05$). However, knowledge of diabetes, health literacy, and self-care activities was not a significant predictor of glycemic control. She recommended further research examining depression and patient trust as predictors of glycemic control and additional studies to explore other influences on or barriers to glycemic control. Mancuso's implementation of a predictive correlational design and conduct of regression analysis were appropriate to address the study purpose and research questions.

Model-Testing Designs

Some studies are designed specifically to test the accuracy of a hypothesized causal model. The **model-testing design** requires that all variables relevant to the model be measured. A large, heterogeneous sample

is required. All the paths expressing relationships between concepts are identified, and a conceptual map is developed (see Figure 11-10). The analysis determines whether or not the data are consistent with the model. For some studies, you might set aside data from half of the subjects and not include them in the initial path analysis. You might use these data from the second half of the subjects to test the fit of the paths defined by the initial analysis.

Variables are classified into three categories: exogenous variables, endogenous variables, and residual variables. **Exogenous variables** are within the theoretical model but are caused by factors outside this model. **Endogenous variables** are those whose variation is explained within the theoretical model. Exogenous variables influence the variation of endogenous variables. **Residual variables** indicate the effect of unmeasured variables not included in the model. These variables explain some of the variance found in the data but not the variance within the model (Mason-Hawkes & Holm, 1989; Norris, 2005a).

In Figure 11-10, the illustration of a model-testing design, paths are drawn to demonstrate directions of cause and effect. The arrows (paths) from the exogenous variables 1, 2, and 3 lead to the endogenous variable 4, indicating that variable 4 is theoretically proposed to be caused by variables 1, 2, and 3. The arrow (path) from endogenous variable 4 to endogenous variable 5 indicates that variable 4 theoretically causes variable 5.

To measure exogenous and endogenous variables, you would collect data from the subjects and analyze the accuracy of the proposed paths. Historically, these analysis procedures were performed with a series of regression analyses. Researchers now conduct statistical procedures that have been developed specifically for path analysis using the computer programs LISREL and EQS (Norris, 2005a). Structural equation modeling is a commonly used statistical procedure (Norris, 2005b). Path coefficients are calculated that indicate the effect that one variable has on another. The amount of variance explained by the model, as well as the fit between the path coefficients and the theoretical model, indicates the accuracy of the theory. Variance that is not accounted for in the statistical analysis is attributed to residual variables (variables a and b) not included in the analyses (Mason-Hawkes & Holm, 1989; Norris, 2005a).

An example of this design is the Cummings, Estabrooks, Midodzi, Wallin, and Hayduk (2007) study testing a model of the influence of organizational characteristics and context on research utilization in nursing. The following study abstract identifies the study purpose, design, results, and conclusions:

"*Background:* Despite three decades of empirical investigation into research utilization and a renewed emphasis on evidence-based medicine and evidence-based practice in the past decade, understanding of factors influencing research uptake in nursing remains limited. There is, however, increased awareness that organizational influences are important.

Objectives: To develop and test a theoretical model of organizational influences that predict research utilization by nurses and to assess the influence of varying degrees of context, based on the Promoting Action on Research Implementation in Health Services (PARIHS) framework, on research utilization and other variables.

Methods: The study sample was drawn from a census of registered nurses working in acute care hospitals in Alberta, Canada, accessed through their professional licensing body (n = 6,526 nurses; 52.8% response rate). Three variables that measured PARIHS dimensions of context (culture, leadership, and evaluation) were used to sort cases into one of four mutually exclusive data sets that reflected less positive to more positive context. Then, a theoretical model of hospital- and unit-level influences on research utilization was developed and tested, using structural equation modeling, and 300 cases were randomly selected from each of the four data sets.

Results: Hospital characteristics that positively influenced research utilization by nurses were staff development, opportunity for nurse-to-nurse collaboration, and staffing and support services. Increased emotional exhaustion led to less reported research utilization and higher rates of patient and nurse adverse events. Nurses working in contexts with more positive culture, leadership, and evaluation also reported significantly more research utilization, staff development, and lower rates of patient and staff adverse events than did nurses working in less positive contexts (i.e., those that lacked positive culture, leadership, or evaluation).

Conclusion: The findings highlight the combined importance of culture, leadership, and evaluation to increase research utilization and improve patient safety. The findings may serve to strengthen the PARIHS framework and to suggest that, although it is not fully developed, the framework is an appropriate guide to implement research into practice." (Cummings et al., 2007, S24)

Defining Therapeutic Nursing Interventions

In quasi-experimental and experimental studies, an intervention (or protocol) is developed that is expected to result in differences in posttest measures of the treatment and control or comparison groups. This intervention may be physiological, psychosocial, educational, or a combination of these and should be designed to maximize the differences between the groups. Thus, it should be the best intervention possible in the circumstances of the study and should be expected to improve the outcomes of the experimental group (Egan, Snyder, & Burns, 1992; Forbes, 2009; Santacroce, Maccarelli, & Grey, 2004).

Over the last 5 years, the nursing literature has included a growing number of publications focused on the methodology for designing interventions for nursing studies (Morrison et al., 2009; Wyatt, Sikorskii, Rahbar, Victorson, & Adams, 2010; Yamada, Stevens, Sidani, Watt-Watson, & Silva, 2010). In addition, descriptions of nursing interventions in published studies have more detail and specificity but still not at the level given to describing measurement instruments (Fawcett & Garity, 2009; Waltz et al., 2010). Thus, nurse researchers provide detailed information about measurement but often do not provide sufficient detail to allow a nurse to implement a nursing intervention as it was used in a published nursing study. To some extent, this situation may reflect the state of knowledge in the nursing field regarding the provision of nursing interventions in clinical practice. Many clinical nursing interventions are not well defined; thus, each nurse may use her or his own terminology to describe a particular intervention. In addition, an intervention tends to be applied differently in each case by a single nurse and even less consistently by different nurses. However, the quality of nursing interventions has been greatly enhanced with the development of the Nursing Interventions Classification by a team of nurses at the University of Iowa.

The Nursing Interventions Classification

The Nursing Interventions Classification (NIC) is a standardized language used to describe interventions or treatments performed by nurses in research and practice. Each intervention consists of a label, a definition, and a set of activities performed by nurses carrying out the intervention. The NIC was initiated by the University of Iowa in Iowa City, IA, in 1987 (NIC, 2011). The intervention labels developed over the last 20 years were derived from nursing education and practice. The research to develop the NIC was initiated in 1987 and progressed through four phases that overlapped in time: "Phase I: Construction of the Classification (1987-1992); Phase II: Construction of the Taxonomy (1990-1995); Phase III: Clinical Testing and Refinement (1993-1997); and Phase IV: Use and Maintenance (1996-ongoing)" (Bulechek, Butcher, & Dochterman, 2008, p. 5). The research methods used to develop the classification included content analysis, surveys, focus groups, similarity analysis, and hierarchical clustering. The NIC Taxonomy contained seven domains: Domain 1: Physiological: Basic; Domain 2: Physiological: Complex; Domain 3: Behavioral; Domain 4: Safety; Domain 5: Family; Domain 6: Health System; and Domain 7: Community. There are a total of 30 classes under the seven domains (Bowles & Naylor, 1996; Bulechek et al., 2008).

Tripp-Reimer, Woodworth, McCloskey, and Bulechek (1996), in their analysis of the structure of the NIC interventions, identified three dimensions: intensity of care, focus of care, and complexity of care. A high intensity of care is associated with the physiological illness level of the patient and the emergency nature of the illness. The dimension of intensity of care includes indicators of (1) intensity (or acuity) and (2) whether the care is typical or novel. The dimension of focus of care addresses (1) the target of the intervention, ranging from the individual to the system; (2) whether the care action is direct or on behalf of the patient; and (3) the continuum of practice from independent to collaborative actions. The dimension of complexity of care encompasses a range of knowledge, skill, and urgency of the interventions (Bulechek et al., 2008).

The interventions in the NIC have been subjected to multiple studies examining the effects on different populations and the effects of varying degrees of intensity. The 5th edition of the Nursing Interventions Classification, developed by faculty at the University of Iowa, included 542 research-based interventions (Bulechek et al., 2008). NIC development continues through the Center for Nursing Classification & Clinical Effectiveness located at the University of Iowa, and you can email them with questions (classification-center@uIowa.edu/; see Chapter 14 for more details on NIC).

Currently, studies are being conducted to determine the outcomes of each intervention and to establish links between the intervention and outcomes at varying points in time after the intervention has been implemented. Outcomes that occur immediately following the intervention are easiest to determine. However, the most important outcomes may be those that occur after a client has been discharged or several weeks or months after the intervention. Table 11-1 provides some of the most current examples of the research related to the NIC and the Nursing Outcomes Classification (NOC) being conducted nationally and internationally. This information is critical for ensuring the quality of care provided by nurses and justifying nursing actions in a cost-conscious market (Doran, 2011). For a more extensive discussion of the importance of linking interventions with outcomes measures, see Chapter 13.

Designing an Intervention for a Nursing Study

The therapeutic nursing intervention implemented in a nursing study needs to be carefully designed, clearly described, and well linked to the outcomes (dependent variables) to be measured in the study. Each of these dimensions must be considered to develop consistency in the intervention. The intervention needs to be provided consistently to all subjects. Thus, a published study should document intervention fidelity, which includes the detailed description of the essential elements of the intervention and the consistent implementation of the intervention during the study (Forbes, 2009; Morrison et al., 2009; Santacroce et al., 2004). In some studies, you may need to develop a step-by-step protocol in order to ensure the detail and control the consistency of the study intervention. Educational treatments or educational components of treatments might be audio or video recorded for consistency.

TABLE 11-1	Work in Nursing Related to the NIC and the Nursing Outcomes Classification (NOC)
Year	**Source**
2011	Lee, E., Park, H., Nam, M., & Whyte, J. (2011). Identification and comparison of interventions performed by Korean school nurses and U.S. school nurses using the Nursing Interventions Classification (NIC). *Journal of School Nursing, 27*(2), 93–101.
2011	Scherb, C. A., Head, B. J., Maas, M. L., Swanson, E. A., Moorhead, S., Reed, D., & Kozel, M. (2011). Most frequent nursing diagnoses, nursing interventions, and nursing-sensitive patient outcomes of hospitalized older adults with heart failure: Part 1. *International Journal of Nursing Terminologies & Classifications, 22*(1), 13–22.
2010	de Cordova, P., Lucero, R. J., Hyun, S., Quinlan, P., Price, K., & Stone, P. W. (2010). Using the Nursing Interventions Classification as a potential measure of nurse workload. *Journal of Nursing Care Quality, 25*(1), 39–45.
2010	Lunney, M., McGuire, M., Endozo, N., & McIntosh-Waddy, D. (2010). Consensus-validation study identifies relevant nursing diagnoses, nursing interventions, and health outcomes for people with traumatic brain injuries. *Rehabilitation Nursing, 35*(4), 161–166.
2010	Smith, K. J., & Craft-Rosenberg, M. (2010). Using NANDA, NIC, and NOC in an undergraduate nursing practicum. *Nurse Educator, 35*(4), 162–166.
2010	Solari-Twadell, P., & Hackbarth, D. P. (2010). Evidence for a new paradigm of the ministry of parish nursing practice using the nursing intervention classification system. *Nursing Outlook, 58*(2), 69–75.
2009	Scherb, C. A., & Weydt, A. P. (2009). Work complexity assessment, nursing interventions classification, and nursing outcomes classification: Making connections. *Creative Nursing, 15*(1), 16–22.
2009	Schneider, J. S., & Slowik, L. H. (2009). The use of the Nursing Interventions Classification (NIC) with cardiac patients receiving home health care. *International Journal of Nursing Terminologies & Classifications, 20*(3), 132–140.
2009	Wong, E. (2009). Novel nursing terminologies for the rapid response system. *International Journal of Nursing Terminologies & Classifications, 20*(2), 53–63.
2009	Wong, E., Scott, L. M., Briseno, J. R., Crawford, C. L., & Hsu, J. Y. (2009). Determining critical incident nursing interventions for the critical care setting: A pilot study. *International Journal of Nursing Terminologies & Classifications, 20*(3), 110–121.
2008	Schneider, J. S., Barkauskas, V., & Keenan, G. (2008). Evaluating home health care nursing outcomes with OASIS and NOC. *Journal of Nursing Scholarship, 40*(1), 76–82.
2008	Sheerin, F. K. (2008). Diagnoses and interventions pertinent to intellectual disability nursing. *International Journal of Nursing Terminologies & Classifications, 19*(4), 140–149.

The first step in designing an intervention should be a thorough review of the clinical and research literature related to the intervention. Because of the scarcity of information in the literature on selected nursing interventions, you may need to rely on your personal knowledge emerging from expertise in clinical practice. The nursing actions that are included in the intervention must be spelled out sequentially so that other nurses are able to follow the description and provide the intervention in a consistent manner. The intervention implemented in a study must be consistent in areas such as (1) content, (2) intensity, and (3) length of time. You need to review the interventions that are provided in the NIC text to help you develop an intervention protocol for a study (Bulechek et al., 2008). This text provides details for numerous interventions that have been implemented in previous studies. You might find an intervention to implement in your study with a different population, or you might use the format to develop a detailed new intervention to be implemented in your study. Also visit the NIC website for additional information on interventions (http://www.nursing.uiowa.edu/excellence/nursing_knowledge/clinical_effectiveness/nic.htm/) (NIC, 2011).

The person or persons designated to implement the study intervention must be trained for this process. These individuals need to be trained in a precise way to ensure that they are 90% to 100% consistent and accurate in their implementation of the study treatment. Often during the study, the implementation of the treatment is evaluated with a protocol checklist to ensure consistent implementation throughout the study. If an intervention is complex, you may need to employ a pilot study to refine the intervention so that it can be applied consistently (Wyatt et al., 2010; Yamada et al., 2010).

Pierce et al. (2011) provided a detailed discussion of the intervention they implemented in their quasi-experimental study to raise stroke awareness among people in rural areas. The intervention they implemented was the Facts for Action to Stroke Treatment (FAST) educational intervention program to improve 402 participants' knowledge about stroke. The FAST intervention was chosen because of its success in teaching people to identify stroke symptoms. The following excerpt from the study describes the intervention content and implementation process:

"The FAST educational program consisted of a 43-slide PowerPoint presentation developed from materials from AHA [American Heart Association], the ASA [American Stroke Association], a review of the literature, and the CPSS [Cincinnati Prehospital Stroke Scale]. FAST team members presenting the program were registered nurse faculty members or graduate students at the School of Nursing who used a printed script to ensure the programs were equal in content. The CPSS test highlighted in the presentation takes 1 minute to perform and is appropriate for teaching to the public. CPSS includes looking for asymmetry of the face when a person is instructed to smile, arm drift when asked to raise both arms with eyes closed for 10 seconds, and slurred or inappropriate speech when asked to repeat a familiar saying. The saying used in this program was 'You can't teach an old dog new tricks.' To help individuals remember the components of the CPSS, this program made the connection to the acronym FAST by pointing out they should look at the Face, Arm, Speech, and if there were abnormalities in any of these areas it was Time to call 911 (see FAST components below).

F − Face, check for droop or asymmetry
A = Arm, look for drift or lack of movement
S = Speech, use common saying / listen for
    slurred or garbled speech
T = Time to call 911 if any of these signs are
    abnormal." (Pierce et al., 2011, p. 85)

Pierce et al. (2011) selected a strong intervention (FAST Educational Program) that had been used in previous research and implemented it with a relative new population of rural adults. The content of the intervention was detailed and based on current research and national organizations' (AHA and ASA) materials. The intervention was implemented consistently using PowerPoint slides and a script. The study would have been strengthened by a description of the training of the faculty and students who implemented the intervention. The researchers concluded that the FAST-based program was an effective intervention for teaching rural adults to recognize stroke symptoms. Chapter 14 provides a detailed discussion of the development and implementation of interventions and the conduct of intervention research.

Quasi-experimental Study Designs

Quasi-experimental and experimental designs examine causality. The power of the design to accomplish this purpose depends on the extent to which the actual effects of the experimental treatment (the independent variable) can be detected by measuring the dependent variable. Obtaining an understanding of the true effects of an experimental treatment or intervention requires action to control threats to the validity of the findings. Threats to design validity are controlled through selection of subjects, control of the environment, manipulation of the treatment, and reliable and valid measurement of the dependent variables. These design validity threats are described in Chapter 10.

Experimental study designs, with their strict control of variance, are the most powerful method of examining causality. For many reasons, both ethical and practical, however, experimental designs cannot always be used in social science research. Quasi-experimental study designs were developed to provide alternative means of examining causality in situations not conducive to experimental controls. Campbell and Stanley first described quasi-experimental designs as a group in 1963, when only experimental designs were considered of any worth. Cook and Campbell expanded this description in 1979 and Shadish, Cook, and Campbell (2002) provide the most current discussion of quasi-experimental and experimental designs. Quasi-experimental designs facilitate the search for knowledge and examination of causality in situations in which complete control of a study design is not possible. These designs have been developed to control as many threats to validity as possible in a situation in which at least one of the three components of true experimental design (randomization, comparison groups, and controlled manipulation of the treatment) is lacking.

There are differences of opinion in nursing about the classification of a particular study as quasi-experimental or experimental. The experimental designs emerged from a logical positivist perspective with the purpose of determining cause and effect. The focus is to determine differences between or among groups using statistical analyses on the basis of decision theory. The true experimental design (from a logical positivist view) requires the use of random sampling to obtain subjects, random assignment to control and experimental groups, rigorous control of the treatment, a highly controlled study environment, and designs that control threats to validity (Shadish et al., 2002).

A less rigorous type of experimental design is referred to as the **comparative experimental design**. Researchers in both nursing and medicine are using it for clinical situations in which the expectation of random sampling is difficult, if not impossible, to achieve. These studies use convenience samples with random assignment to groups. For example, randomized controlled trials (RCT) usually do not use randomly obtained samples but tend to be considered experimental in nature. These studies are classified as experimental because they have internal validity if the two groups (experimental and control) are comparable on variables important to the study, even though there are biases in the original sample. However, these designs do not address threats to statistical conclusion validity and threats to external validity by the nonrandom sample. Threats to external validity have not, in the past, been considered a serious concern because they affect not the claim that the treatment caused a difference but rather the ability to generalize the findings. The importance of external validity, although discounted in the past, is taking on greater importance in the current political and health policy climate. Chapter 13, on outcomes research, explores the concerns some researchers and clinicians have about the validity of RCTs.

Random Assignment to Groups

Random assignment to groups is a procedure used to assign subjects to treatment or control groups randomly. Random assignment is most commonly used in nursing and medicine to assign subjects obtained through convenience sampling methods to groups for purposes of comparison. Random assignment used without random sampling is purported to decrease the risk of bias in the selection of groups. However, Ottenbacher (1992) performed a meta-analysis to examine the effect of random assignment versus nonrandom assignment on outcomes. The results failed to reveal significant differences in these two sampling techniques. He suggested that previous assumptions about design strategies should be empirically tested. The term RCT usually means that the study used random assignment of subjects to groups, not that the sample was obtained through random sampling methods.

Traditional approaches to random assignment involve using a random numbers table or flipping an unbiased coin to determine group assignment. However, these procedures can lead to unequal group sizes and thus a decrease in power. Hjelm-Karlsson (1991) suggested using what is referred to as a **biased coin design** to randomly assign subjects to groups. With this technique, selection of the group to which a particular subject will be assigned is biased in favor of groups that have smaller sample sizes at the point of the assignment of that subject. This strategy is particularly useful when assignment is being made to more than two groups. The researcher can complete calculations for the sequencing of assignment to groups before collecting data, thus freeing the researcher for other activities during this critical period. Hjelm-Karlsson (1991) suggested using cards to make group assignments. The subject numbers and random group assignments are written on cards. As each subject agrees to participate in the study, the next card is drawn from the stack, indicating that subject's number and group assignment. These activities could also be accomplished with the computer.

Stout, Wirtz, Carbonari, and Del Boca (1994) suggested a similar strategy they referred to as urn randomization, which they described as follows:

"One would begin the study with two urns, each urn containing a red marble and a blue marble. There is one urn for each level of the stratifying variable; that is, in this example there is an urn for severely ill patients and another urn for the less severe[ly ill] patients. When a subject is ready for randomization, we determine whether or not he/she is severely ill and consult the corresponding urn. From this urn (say, for the severely ill group) we randomly select one marble and note its color. If the marble is red we assign the patient to Treatment A. Then we drop that marble back into the urn and put a blue marble into the urn as well. This leaves the 'severely ill' urn with one red and two blue marbles. The next time a severely ill patient shows up, the probability that he/she will be assigned to Group B will be 2/3 rather than 2, thus biasing the selection process toward balance. A similar procedure is followed every time a severely ill subject presents for randomization. After each subject is assigned, the marble chosen from the urn is replaced together with a marble of the opposite color. The urn for the less severely ill group is not affected. If a low-severity patient presents for the study, that patient's probability of assignment to either treatment is not affected by the assignment of patients in the other stratum. To some extent, urn randomization can be tailored to maximize balancing or to maximize randomization." (Stout et al., 1994, p. 72)

Stout and colleagues (1994) also provided strategies for balancing several variables simultaneously during random assignment.

Matthews, Cook, and Terada (2010) tested the ability of urn randomization versus simple random assignment to groups in producing balanced groups with small sample sizes. They conducted simulated randomizations 10 times, developing "sample size scenarios of 20, 40, 60 (group sizes of 10, 20, and 30, respectively), for 30 trials in total. For groups of 20-30, urn surpassed simple randomization in the equal distribution of confounding variables between groups, leading to effects of these variables that were both smaller on average and more consistently close to zero over multiple trials" (Matthews et al., 2010, p. 243). These researchers concluded that the urn method was easy to implement and has the advantages of unpredictability in assignment of participants to groups and decreased potential for investigator bias. This article includes an illustration of the urn method to facilitate your understanding of the process for assigning study participants to groups (see Figure 1 in Matthews et al., 2010, p. 248).

Schlairet and Pollock (2010) used random assignment of participants to groups in their study of undergraduate nursing students' knowledge obtained with traditional versus simulated clinical experiences. The following excerpt from the study describes the design with participant group assignment:

"This intervention study used a 2x2 crossover design and equivalence testing to explore the effects of simulated clinical experiences on undergraduate students' (n = 74) knowledge acquisition in a fundamentals of nursing course. Following random assignment, students participated in laboratory-based simulated clinical experiences with high-fidelity human patient simulators and traditional clinical experiences and completed knowledge pretests and posttests." (Schlairet & Pollock, 2010, p. 43)

These researchers administered the knowledge pretest to establish equivalence between the groups. After the simulated clinical experience and traditional clinical experience, the students were administered a posttest. Analysis revealed a significant knowledge gained associated with both simulated and traditional clinical experiences, with the groups' knowledge scores being statistically significantly equivalent. Thus, the researchers concluded that the simulated clinical experience was as effective as the traditional clinical experience in this study. The description of the study design would have been strengthened by a discussion of how random assignment of participants to groups was accomplished.

Each of the quasi-experimental designs described in this section involves threats to validity owing to constraints in controlling variance. Some achieve greater amounts of control than others. When choosing a design for a study, you must select the design that offers the greatest amount of control possible within your study situation (Shadish et al., 2002). Even the first designs described in this section, which have low power in terms of establishing causality, can provide useful information from which to design later studies.

Control and Comparison Groups

Quasi-experimental and experimental studies include an experimental or intervention group that receives the treatment or intervention and a control that receives no treatment. Control groups, traditionally used in experimental studies, are selected randomly from the same population as the experimental group and receive no treatment. Use of a control group increases the ability of the researcher to detect differences between groups in the real world. Thus, control groups reduce the risk of error. Control groups are rarely used in nursing or medical studies because of requirements related to consent, ethical issues regarding withholding treatment, and the difficulty of acquiring sufficient potential subjects from which to select a sample (Shadish et al., 2002).

Comparison groups are usually selected through the use of convenience sampling rather than random sampling methods. There are four types of **comparison groups**: (1) groups that receive no treatment; (2) groups that receive a placebo treatment; (3) groups that receive the "usual treatment" or standard care; and (4) groups that receive a second experimental treatment or a different treatment dose for comparison with the first experimental treatment (e.g., clinical trials of drug effectiveness). As a researcher, you should clarify the type of comparison group you are using.

When a study uses a comparison group that receives no treatment, demonstrating statistical significance is easier because there is less variation in the treatment and a greater difference between the two groups. Placebo treatments provide consistency in the comparison group, provide less difference between groups than in no-treatment comparison groups, and would be unethical in some nursing studies. "Usual treatment" is the care routinely provided by the healthcare system. However, usual treatment is uneven and thus is often not standardized for all patients. Thus, provision of care may vary from one patient to another depending on the availability of nursing staff and the intensity of care demands being made on nurses at the time the care is provided. Some patients may receive little or no care, whereas others may receive considerably more or better care. There will likely be a greater amount of difference between patients who received little or no care and patients in the experimental group, and less difference between patients in the "usual care group" who received considerably more care and the experimental group. This wide variation reduces the effect size of the experimental treatment, increases the variance, and decreases the possibility of obtaining a significant difference between groups. The researcher should carefully spell out "usual or standard care" and the degree of variation in the care in the facility in which the study is being conducted.

Nonequivalent Comparison Group Designs

A comparison group is one in which the groups are not selected by random means. Some groups are more nonequivalent than others, and some quasi-experimental designs involve using groups (comparison and treatment or intervention) that have evolved naturally rather than being developed randomly. For example, the treatment group might include students registered for an 8:00 AM class in a university, and the comparison group might be students registered for a 7:00 PM class. These groups cannot be considered equivalent because the individuals in the comparison group may be different from individuals in the treatment group. Allowing individuals to select the group they will be in (treatment or comparison) rather than being randomly assigned by the researcher also increases the threat to design validity. For example, allowing subjects to select either the treatment group that receives an exercise program or the comparison group that has no exercise program threatens the validity of the study. The subjects selecting the treatment of the exercise program are different from those selecting no exercise program.

The approach to statistical analysis is problematic in quasi-experimental designs. Although many researchers use the same approaches to analysis as are used for experimental studies, the selection bias inherent in nonequivalent comparison groups makes this practice questionable. Reichardt (1979) recommended using additional statistical analyses to examine the data from various perspectives and to compare levels of significance obtained from each analysis. As a researcher, you must carefully assess the potential threats to validity in interpreting statistical results, because statistical analysis cannot control for threats to validity (Munro, 2005; Shadish et al., 2002). The following sections describe examples of nonequivalent comparison group designs.

One-Group Posttest-Only Design

The one-group posttest-only design is referred to as pre-experimental rather than quasi-experimental because of its weaknesses and the numerous threats to validity it involves. It is inadequate for making causal inferences (see Figure 11-11). Usually in this design, no attempt is made to control the selection of subjects who receive the treatment (the experimental group). It is difficult to justify generalizing findings beyond those tested. The group is not pretested; therefore, there is no direct way to measure change. The researcher cannot claim that posttest scores were a consequence (effect) of the treatment if scores before the treatment are unknown. Because there is no comparison group, one does not know whether groups not receiving the treatment would have similar scores on the dependent variable. The one-group posttest-only design is used more commonly in evaluation than in research.

Cook and Campbell (1979) suggested situations in which the one-group posttest-only design can be appropriate and adequate for inferring causality. For example, the design could be used to determine that a single factory's use of vinyl chloride is causing an increase in the rate of neighborhood and employee cancers. The incidence of cancer in the community at large is known. The fact that vinyl chloride causes cancer and the types of cancer it causes are also known. These norms would then take the place of the pretest and the comparison group. Thus, to use this design intelligently, one must know a great deal about the causal factors interacting within the situation (Shadish et al., 2002). This is not the usual situation in nursing studies.

Posttest-Only Design with a Comparison Group

Although the posttest-only design with a comparison group offers an improvement on the previous design because of the addition of a nonequivalent comparison group, it is still referred to as pre-experimental (see Figure 11-12). The addition of a comparison group can lead to a false confidence in the validity of the findings. Selection threats are a problem with both groups. The lack of a pretest remains a serious impediment to defining change. Differences in posttest scores between groups may be caused by the treatment or by differential selection processes (Shadish et al., 2002).

One-Group Pretest-Posttest Design

Another pre-experimental design, the one-group pretest-posttest design, is one of the more commonly used designs. However, it has such serious weaknesses that findings are often uninterruptable

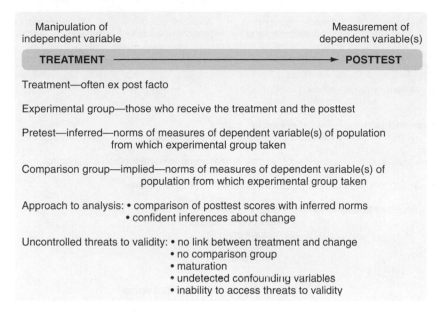

Figure 11-11 One-group posttest-only design.

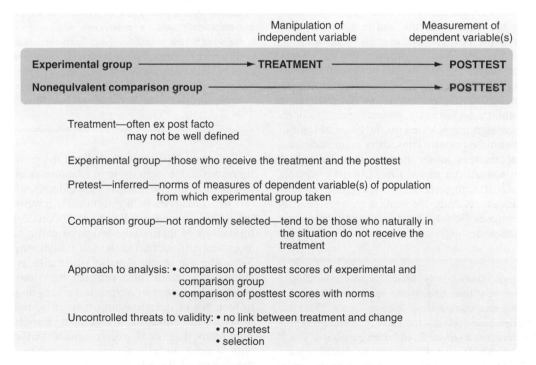

Figure 11-12 Posttest-only design with a comparison group.

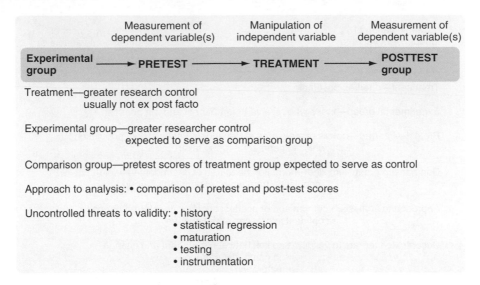

Figure 11-13 One-group pretest-posttest design.

(see Figure 11-13). Pretest scores cannot adequately serve the same function as a comparison group. Events can occur between the pretest and posttest that alter responses to the posttest. These events then serve as alternative hypotheses to the proposal that the change in posttest scores is due to the treatment. Posttest scores might be altered by (1) maturation processes; (2) administration of the pretest; and (3) changes in instrumentation. Additionally, subjects in many studies using this design are selected on the basis of high or low scores on the pretest. Thus, there is an additional threat that changes in the posttest may be due to regression toward the mean. Lim, Chiu, Dohrmann, and Tan (2010) implemented a one-group pretest-posttest design to study medication management by registered nurses (RNs). The following study excerpt describes their design:

"This exploratory study used a non-randomized pre- and post-test one group quasi-experimental design without comparators. It comprised a 23-item knowledge-based test questionnaire, one-hour teaching session, and a self-directed learning package. The volunteer sample was RNs from residential aged care facilities, involved in medication management. Participants sat a pre-test immediately before the education, and post-test 4 weeks later (same questionnaire).... Pre-test sample $n = 58$, post-test $n = 40$, attrition rate of 31%.... Descriptive statistical data analysis of overall pre- and post-test incorrect responses showed: pre-test proportion of incorrect responses = 0.40; post-test proportion of incorrect responses = 0.27; Z-test comparing pre- and post-tests scores of incorrect responses = 6.55 and one-sided p-value = 2.8E-11 ($p < 0.001$)." (Lim et al., 2010, p. 98)

Lim et al. (2010) concluded that the pretest identified knowledge deficits in medication management and adverse drug reactions in the elderly and the posttest indicated statistically significant improvement in the RNs' knowledge. The researchers recognized the limitations of their study design by calling it exploratory and also identified the fairly high attrition rate, 31%. The use of the same questionnaire as a pretest and posttest could also threaten the study validity because the change in the posttest scores might be due to memory of questionnaire items in addition to the effect of the educational treatment. Based on these limitations, Lim et al. recommended further studies with larger samples and stronger design to determine the impact of the educational treatment on the RNs' knowledge of medication management. The addition of a nonequivalent comparison group, as described in the next design, can greatly strengthen the validity of the findings.

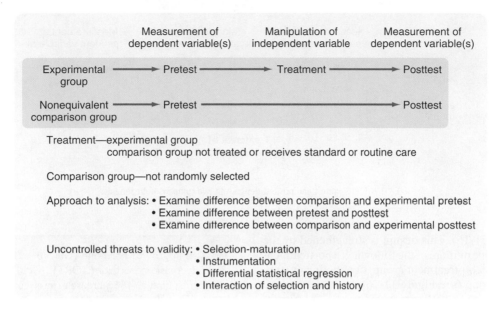

	Measurement of dependent variable(s)	Manipulation of independent variable	Measurement of dependent variable(s)
Experimental group	⟶ Pretest ⟶	Treatment ⟶	Posttest
Nonequivalent comparison group	⟶ Pretest ⟶		Posttest

Treatment—experimental group
           comparison group not treated or receives standard or routine care

Comparison group—not randomly selected

Approach to analysis: • Examine difference between comparison and experimental pretest
                       • Examine difference between pretest and posttest
                       • Examine difference between comparison and experimental posttest

Uncontrolled threats to validity: • Selection-maturation
                           • Instrumentation
                           • Differential statistical regression
                           • Interaction of selection and history

Figure 11-14 Pretest and posttest design with a comparison group.

Pretest and Posttest Design with a Comparison Group

The **pretest and posttest design with a comparison group** is the most commonly used design in social science research (see Figure 11-14). This quasi-experimental design is the first design discussed here that is generally interpretable. The uncontrolled threats to validity are primarily due to the absence of randomization and, in some studies, the inability of the researcher to manipulate the treatment. Cook and Campbell (1979) offered a detailed discussion of the effects of these threats on interpreting study findings.

Variations in this design include the use of (1) proxy pretest measures (a different pretest that correlates with the posttest); (2) separate pretest and posttest samples; and (3) pretest measures at more than one time interval. The first two variations weaken the design, but the last variation greatly strengthens it. In some studies, the comparison group consists of patients cared for before a new treatment was initiated. Data on this comparison group are obtained through chart audit or from electronic databases owned by the facility. Obviously there is no opportunity to control the quality of the data obtained through chart audit. Thus, this strategy weakens the design.

Costanzo, Walker, Yates, McCabe, and Berg (2006) used a pretest-posttest comparison group design in their study of physical activity counseling for older women. They described their design as follows:

"Physical inactivity is a major factor in increasing women's risk for chronic disease, disability, and premature mortality. This study compared the effectiveness of five behavioral counseling (BC) sessions with a comparison group receiving one BC session based on the five A's (ask, advise, assist, arrange, and agree) to increase moderate-intensity physical activity, muscle strengthening, and stretching activity. The health promotion model provided the framework for the intervention. A pretest/posttest comparison group design was used, with random assignment of 46 women recruited from an urban Midwestern community. A significant group interaction was found only for cardiorespiratory fitness ($p < 0.001$). Significant time effects were found ($p < 0.001$) for both groups in increasing handgrip, leg strength, and flexibility. BC is a promising intervention to achieve physical activity behavior change with older women." (Costanzo et al., 2006, p. 786)

Pretest and Posttest Design with Two Comparison Treatments

The two-treatment design is used when two experimental treatments are being compared to determine which is the more effective. In most cases, this design is used when one treatment is the currently identified treatment of choice and the researcher has identified a treatment that might lead to even better outcomes

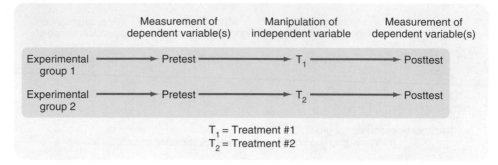

Figure 11-15 Pretest and posttest design with two comparison treatments.

(see Figure 11-15). This design is strengthened by the addition of one or more of the following: a no-treatment group, a placebo-treatment group, or a routine or standard care group (see Figure 11-16).

Dudgeon et al. (2010) conducted a quasi-experiment study of HIV-infected men using a pretest and posttest design with two comparison treatment groups and a control group (see Figure 11-16). The two treatment groups participated in moderate- and low-intensity exercise interventions, and the control group participated in no activity. This study had a strong design, and the moderate-intensity exercise was found to be the most effective in improving circulating hormones and cytokines in the HIV-infected men. The researchers provided a clear discussion of their study design that is presented in the following excerpt:

"Exercise has the potential to impact disease by altering circulating anabolic and catabolic factors. It was the goal of this study to determine if two different regimes of low-intensity and moderate-intensity exercise affected circulating levels of anabolic and catabolic factors in HIV-infected men. Exercise-naïve, HIV-infected men, medically cleared for study participation, were randomized into one of the following groups: a moderate-intensity group (MOD), who completed 30 minutes of moderate-intensity aerobic training followed by 30 minutes of moderate-intensity resistance training; a low-intensity group (LOW), who completed 60 minutes of treadmill walking; or a control group (CON), who attended the clinic but participated in no activity. Blood and saliva samples were collected at selected time points before, during, and after each of the 3 required sessions. Compared with baseline, the MOD group ($n = 14$) had a 135%

increase in growth hormone (GH) ($p < 0.05$) and a 34% decrease in cortisol (CORT) ($p < 0.05$) at the post time point, a 31% increase in interleukin-6 (IL-6) ($p < 0.05$) at 30 minutes post exercise, a 23% increase in IL-6 ($p < 0.05$), and a 13% decrease in soluble tumor necrosis factor receptor 2 (sTNFrII) ($p < 0.05$) at 60 minutes post exercise. The LOW ($n = 11$) group had a 3.5% decrease in sTNFrII ($p < 0.05$) at 30 minutes post exercise compared with baseline and 49% decrease ($p < 0.05$) in GH at 60-minutes post exercise. The CON group ($n = 13$) had a decrease in GH at 30-minutes (62%, $p < 0.05$) and 60-minute (61%, $p < 0.05$) post exercise [group participated in no exercise] compared with baseline. The increase in GH from baseline to post was greater in the MOD group ($p < 0.05$) than the other groups and the decrease in CORT from pre to post was greater in the MOD group ($p < 0.05$) than in the other groups. These data suggest that individual sessions of both low-intensity and moderate-intensity exercise can alter circulating anabolic and catabolic factors in HIV-infected men. The changes in the MOD group present potential mechanisms for the increases in lean tissue mass seen with resistance exercise training." (Dudgeon et al., 2010, p. 560)

Pretest and Posttest Design with a Removed Treatment

In some cases, gaining access to a comparison group is not possible. The removed-treatment design with pretest and posttest creates conditions that approximate the conceptual requirements of a control group receiving no treatment. The design is basically a one-group pretest-posttest design. However, after a delay, a third measure of the dependent variable is taken, followed by an interval in which the treatment is

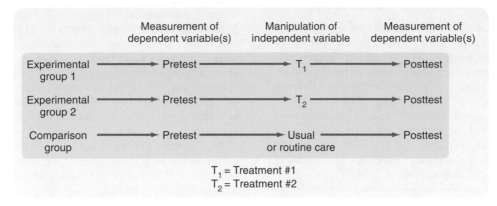

Figure 11-16 Pretest and posttest design with two comparison treatments and a usual or routine care group used as a comparison group.

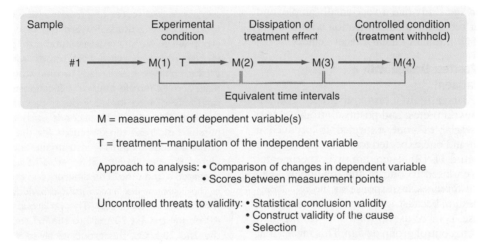

Figure 11-17 Pretest and posttest design with a removed treatment. M(1), pretest; M(2), posttest; M(3), pretest of controlled condition; M(4), posttest of controlled condition.

removed, followed by a fourth measure of the dependent variable (see Figure 11-17). The periods between measures must be equivalent. In nursing situations, the researcher must consider the ethics of removing an effective treatment. Even if doing so is ethically acceptable, the response of subjects to the removal may make interpreting changes difficult.

It is difficult in CINAHL (*Cumulative Index to Nursing and Allied Health Literature*) and MEDLINE to locate examples of studies using removed-treatment designs because of the search process required. A search in PsychInfo located one study: Schneider (1998) described a study of the effects of virtual reality on symptom distress in children receiving cancer chemotherapy, as shown in the following excerpt:

"An interrupted time series design with removed treatment was used to answer the following research questions: (1) Is virtual reality an effective distraction intervention for reducing chemotherapy related symptom distress in children? And (2) Does virtual reality in children have a lasting effect? Hypotheses: (1) There will be differences in measures of symptom distress in a single group of children with cancer who receive a virtual reality distraction intervention during the second chemotherapy treatment and who receive no virtual reality intervention during the first and third chemotherapy treatments. The convenience sample consisted of 11 children receiving outpatient chemotherapy at a clinical cancer center. Measures of symptom distress were obtained at nine time points during three consecutive chemotherapy treatments. Four indicators were used to measure the dependent variable of symptom distress. The Symptom Distress Scale (SDS) (McCorkle & Young, 1978) was considered a general indicator. Specific indicators of symptom distress included the State-Trait Anxiety Inventory for Children (STAIC C-1) (Spielberger et al., 1978) and single item indicators for nausea and vomiting." (Schneider, 1998, p. 2126)

Schneider (1998) found that the use of a virtual reality distraction intervention did decrease symptom distress in children receiving outpatient chemotherapy. However, the study had a very small sample, and the researcher recommended replication with a larger sample using additional clinical cancer centers.

Pretest and Posttest Design with a Reversed Treatment

The **reversed-treatment nonequivalent control group design** with pretest and posttest introduces two independent variables—one expected to produce a positive effect and one expected to produce a negative effect (see Figure 11-18). There are two experimental groups, each exposed to one of the treatments. The design tests differences in response to the two treatments. This design, because of its high construct validity of the cause, is more useful for theory testing than the no-treatment control group design. This means that there are strong theoretical sources proposing that specific treatments cause specific effects. The theoretical

causal variable must be rigorously defined to allow differential predictions of directions of effect. To be maximally interpretable, the following two groups must be added: (1) a placebo control group in which the treatment is not expected to affect the dependent variable and (2) a no-treatment control group to provide a baseline. This design is not commonly used in nursing, so an older study is presented as an example.

McConnell (1976) used a reversed-treatment design to test how knowledge of the results affected a subject's attitude toward a motor learning task, as described in the following excerpt:

The study "tested the hypotheses that a group which has the greatest number of gains in performance in successive trial scores of a motor task will develop a more positive attitude toward the task, and that a group which has the greatest number of gains in performance in successive trial scores will show the greatest change in an already formed attitude. Twelve male and 12 female physical education majors were randomly divided into 2 groups. Each subject performed 20 trials of 15 seconds each on a rotary pursuit task, read the directions for the completion of the attitude measuring instrument, and then completed the instrument. This series of activities was repeated a 2nd time. The difference in the treatment of the 2 groups occurred in the knowledge of results (KR: i.e., time on target). The 1st group received its KR during the 1st 20 trials to the full second; during the 2nd 20 trials, this group received its KR to .01 second. The other group received the reverse

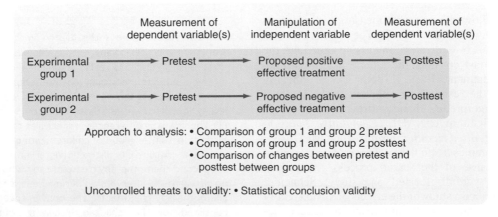

Figure 11-18 Pretest and posttest design with a reversed treatment.

treatment. The difference in treatment caused the subjects in the group being given KR to .01th of a second to achieve more gains in performance than those whose KR was to the full second. Further analyses supported both hypotheses." (McConnell, 1976, p. 394)

Interrupted Time-Series Designs

The **interrupted time-series designs** are similar to descriptive time designs except that a treatment is applied at some point in the observations. Time-series analyses have some advantages over other quasi-experimental designs. First, repeated pretest observations can assess trends in maturation before the treatment. Second, the repeated pretest observations allow measures of trends in scores before the treatment, decreasing the risk of statistical regression, which would lead to misinterpretation of findings. If you keep records of events that could influence subjects in your study, you can determine whether historical factors that could modify responses to the treatment were in operation between the last pretest and the first posttest.

Some threats, however, are particularly problematic in time-series designs. Record-keeping procedures and definitions of constructs used for data collection tend to change over time. Thus, maintaining consistency can be a problem. The treatment can result in attrition so that the sample before treatment may be different in important ways from the post-treatment group. Seasonal variation or other cyclical influences can be interpreted as treatment effects. Therefore, identifying cyclical patterns and controlling for them are critical to the analysis of study findings (Shadish et al., 2002).

McCain and McCleary (1979) have suggested using the autoregressive integrated moving average (ARIMA) statistical model to analyze time-series data. The ARIMA is a statistical model that has some distinct advantages over regression analysis techniques. For adequate statistical analysis, at least 50 measurement points are needed; however, Cook and Campbell (1979) believe that ARIMA with even small numbers of measurement points can provide better information than that obtained in cross-sectional studies. The numbers of measurements of the dependent variables (M) shown in the designs illustrated in Figures 11-19 through 11-21 are limited by space.

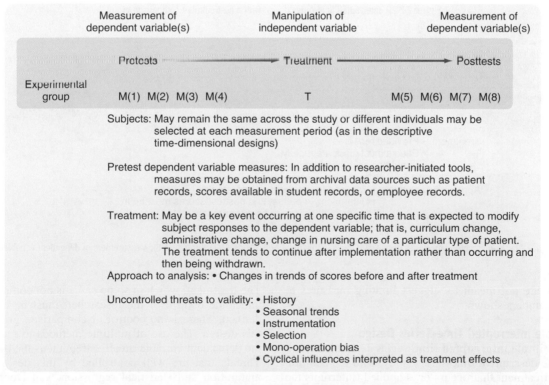

Figure 11-19 Simple interrupted time-series design. M(1) through M(8), Measurement of dependent variable(s).

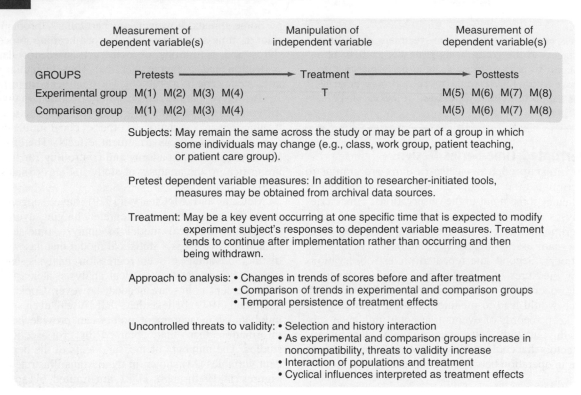

Figure 11-20 Interrupted time-series design with a no-treatment comparison group.

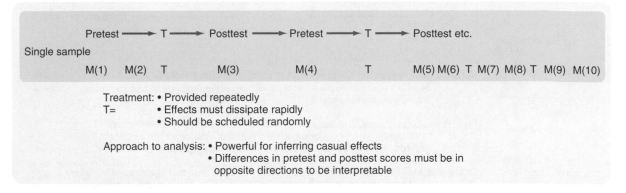

Figure 11-21 Interrupted time-series design with multiple treatment replications. M(1) through M(8), Measurement of dependent variable(s).

They are not meant to suggest limiting measures to the numbers shown.

Simple Interrupted Time-Series Design

The **simple interrupted time-series design** is similar to the descriptive time-series study, with the addition of a treatment that occurs or is applied (interrupts the time series) at a given point in time (see Figure 11-19).

The treatment, which in some cases is not completely under the control of the researcher, must be clearly defined. There is no control or comparison group in this design. The use of multiple methods to measure the dependent variable greatly strengthens the design. Threats that are well controlled by this design are maturation and statistical regression. van Doormaal et al. (2009) implemented an interrupted time-series design to determine the effect of a Computerized Physician Order Entry system with basic Clinical Decision Support (CPOE/CDSS) on the incidence of medication errors (MEs) and preventable adverse drug events (PADEs). The outcome measurements included percentage of medication orders with one or more MEs and the percentage of patients with one or more PADEs. The following study excerpt describes the study design:

Design

"The study was set up as an interrupted time series that is characterized by a series of measurements over time interrupted by an intervention. In this study the intervention was the implementation of a Computerized Physician Order Entry system in combination with a basic Clinical Decision Support System (CPOE/CDSS). Data collection took place during a 5-month pre-implementation period (during which the hand-written medication order system continued to be used) and during a 5-month post-implementations period (when the CPOE/CDSS system continued to be used.) The post-implementation data collection period started 8 weeks after finishing the implementation process in order to make sure that initial problems were solved." (van Doormaal et al., 2009, p. 817)

These researchers found that 55% of the medication orders contained at least one ME prior to the implementation of the CPOE/CDSS, and 17% post intervention. Thus, the implementation of the CPOE/CDSS led to a significant immediate reduction of 40.3% in medication orders with one or more errors. Pre-implementation, the mean percentage of admitted patients experiencing at least one PADE was 15.5%, as opposed to 7.3% post implementation. However, when the use of interrupted time-series design is considered, the immediate change was not significant (−0.42%; 95% CI: −15.52%, 14.68%) because of the observed underlying negative trend and could not be attributed to the introduction of CPOE/CDSS. van Doormaal et al. (2009, p. 816) concluded that the "CPOE/CDSS reduces the incidence of medication errors. However, a direct effect on actual patient harm (PADEs) was not demonstrated."

Interrupted Time-Series Design with a No-Treatment Comparison Group

The addition of a comparison group to the interrupted time-series design greatly strengthens the validity of the findings. The comparison group allows the researcher to examine the differences in trends between groups after the treatment and the persistence of treatment effects over time (see Figure 11-20). Although the treatment may continue (e.g., a change in nursing management practices or patient teaching strategies), the initial response to the change may differ from later responses.

Zhang, Adams, Ross-Degnan, Zhang, and Soumerai (2009, p. 520) implemented an interrupted time-series design with a comparison group to determine the impact of a prior-authorization policy in Maine on the ordering of second-generation antipsychotic and anticonvulsant for patients with bipolar disorder, how often they were discontinued, and pharmacy costs among Medicaid beneficiaries." The excerpt from the study abstract describes the study design, key results, and conclusions:

"*Methods*: Using Medicaid and Medicare utilization data for 2001-2004, the authors identified 5,336 patients with bipolar disorder in Maine (study group) and 1,376 in New Hampshire (comparison group). With an interrupted time-series and comparison group design, longitudinal changes were measured in second-generation antipsychotic and anticonvulsant use; survival analysis was used to examine treatment discontinuations and rates of switching medications.

Results: The prior-authorization policy resulted in an 8-percentage point reduction in the prevalence of use of nonpreferred second-generation antipsychotic and anticonvulsant medications (those requiring prior authorization) but did not increase use of preferred agents (no prior authorization) or rates of switching. The prior-authorization policy reduced total pharmacy reimbursements for bipolar disorder by $27 per patient during the eight-month policy period. However, the hazard rate of treatment discontinuation (all bipolar drugs) while the policy was in effect was 2.28 (95% confidence interval = 1.36-4.33) higher than during the pre-policy period, with adjustment for trends in the comparison state.

Conclusion: The small reduction in pharmacy spending for bipolar treatment per patient after the policy was implemented may have resulted from higher rates of medication discontinuation rather than switching. The findings indicate that the prior-authorization policy may have increased patient risk without appreciable cost savings." (Zhang et al., 2009, p. 520)

Interrupted Time-Series Design with Multiple Treatment Replications

The **interrupted time-series design with multiple treatment replications** is a powerful design for inferring causality (see Figure 11-21). It requires greater researcher control than is usually possible in social science research outside closed institutional settings, such as laboratories or research units. The studies that led researchers to adopt behavior modification techniques used this design. For significant differences to be interpretable, the pretest and posttest scores must be in different directions with the introduction and removal of the treatment. Within this design, treatments can be modified by substituting one treatment for another or combining two treatments and examining interaction effects (Shadish et al., 2002).

Experimental Study Designs

Experimental study designs provide the greatest amount of control possible to examine causality more closely. To examine cause, one must eliminate all factors influencing the dependent variable other than the cause (independent variable) being studied. Other factors are eliminated by being controlled. The study is designed to prevent any other element from intruding into observation of the specific cause and effect that the researcher wishes to examine.

The three essential elements of experimental research are (1) randomization; (2) researcher-controlled manipulation of the independent variable; and (3) researcher control of the experimental situation, including a control or comparison group. Experimental designs exert much effort to control variance. Sample criteria are explicit, the independent variable or intervention is provided in a precisely defined way, the dependent variables are carefully operationalized, and the situation in which the study is conducted is highly controlled to prevent the interference of unstudied factors from modifying the dynamics of the process being studied (Shadish et al., 2002).

Table 11-2 was developed so you might compare the four major types of designs: descriptive, correlational, quasi-experimental, and experimental. The key focus of each type of design is identified with an example study. Interventions are implemented only in quasi-experimental and experimental study designs.

TABLE **11-2** Comparison of Four Major Types of Design			
Type of Design	**Key Focus**	**Sample Purpose Statement**	**Intervention?**
Descriptive	Describes "what is"	The purpose of this study was to (a) "determine practice and differences in practices between registered nurses and respiratory therapists in managing patients receiving mechanical ventilation" (Kjonegaard, Fields, & King, 2010, p. 168).	No
Correlational	Examines relationships among study variables	"The purpose of this study was to examine Jordanian mental health nurses' experiences of providing mental health care, their work-related stress, and organizational support received "(Hamdan-Mansour, Al-Gamal, Puskar, Yacoub, & Marini, 2011, p. 86).	No
Quasi-experimental	Tests causality with suboptimal control	"The aim of the study was to investigate the outcome of nursing assessment, pain assessment and nurse-initiated intravenous opioid analgesic compared to standard procedure for patients seeking emergency care for abdominal pain. Outcome measures were: (a) pain intensity, (b) frequency of received analgesic, (c) time to analgesic, (d) transit time, and (e) patients' perceptions of the quality of care in pain management" (Muntlin, Carlsson, Safwenberg, & Gunningberg, 2011, p. 13).	Yes
Experimental	Tests causality with optimal control	The purpose of this "experimental study was to examine the effects of a moderate-intensity aerobic exercise program on pain-like behavior and neurotrophin-3 (NT-3) in female mice. The rationale for conducting this study was that the literature and clinical practice have supported the use of aerobic exercise in reducing pain and improving function in people with chronic pain but the molecular basis for these positive actions are poorly understood" (Sharma, Ryals, Gajewski, & Wright, 2010, p. 714).	Yes

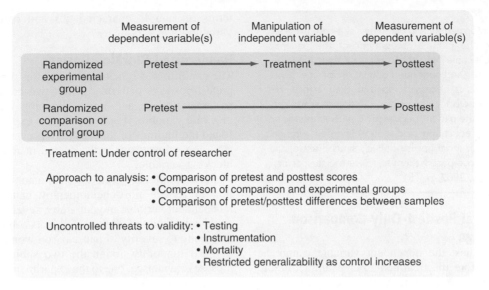

	Measurement of dependent variable(s)	Manipulation of independent variable	Measurement of dependent variable(s)
Randomized experimental group	Pretest ⟶	Treatment ⟶	Posttest
Randomized comparison or control group	Pretest ⟶		Posttest

Treatment: Under control of researcher

Approach to analysis: • Comparison of pretest and posttest scores
                    • Comparison of comparison and experimental groups
                    • Comparison of pretest/posttest differences between samples

Uncontrolled threats to validity: • Testing
                        • Instrumentation
                        • Mortality
                        • Restricted generalizability as control increases

Figure 11 22 **The classic experimental design; pretest-posttest control group design.**

Classic Experimental Design

The original, or **classic, experimental design**, or **pretest-posttest control group design**, is still the most commonly used experimental design (see Figure 11-22). There are two randomized groups, one receiving the experimental treatment and one receiving no treatment, a placebo treatment, or the routine or standard care. By comparing pretest scores and the groups' demographic characteristics, one can evaluate the effectiveness of randomization in providing equivalent groups. The researcher implements the treatment or independent variable under very controlled conditions. The dependent variable is measured twice, before and after the manipulation of the independent variable (Shadish et al., 2002). As in all well-designed studies, the dependent and independent variables are conceptually linked, conceptually defined, and operationalized. Instruments used to measure the dependent variable clearly reflect the conceptual meaning of the variable and have good evidence of reliability and validity. Often, more than one means of measuring the dependent variable is advisable to avoid mono-operation and mono-method biases (Waltz et al., 2010).

Most other experimental designs are variations of the classic experimental design. Multiple groups (both experimental and comparison) can be used to great advantage in the pretest-posttest design and the posttest-only design. For example, the researcher could withhold treatment from one comparison group and treat another comparison group with a placebo. Multiple experimental groups could receive varying levels of the treatments, such as differing frequency, intensity, or duration of nursing care interventions. These additions greatly increase the generalizability of the study findings.

Malm, Karlsson, and Fridlund (2007) conducted an experimental study of the effects of a self-care program on health-related quality of life (HRQoL) for pacemaker patients. The abstract describes their study as follows:

"An experimental, multi-centre, randomized study with a nurse-led intervention was conducted with the aim of evaluating the effects on HRQoL of a 10-month self-care program for pacemaker patients. In the present study, there were no significant differences in HRQoL when comparisons were made between the experimental group and the control group. Results show two main findings for patients in the self-care program ($n = 97$; mean age 71 years): a significantly better HRQoL in terms of experiencing the symptoms that were the reason for pacemaker implantation, as having decreased or disappeared, and a higher level of perceived exertion in a 1 1/2-minute stair test compared with patients who had standard checkups ($n = 115$; mean age 73 years). It is important to actively include pacemaker patients in a self-care program while still in the acute phase in the hospital. Healthcare professionals should support the patient in a kind and professional manner by providing clear, relevant information, and planning a self-care program based on the nurse's assessment of the patient's needs. To enable patients to manage their life situations, training and continued education for healthcare professionals is necessary so that their efforts are based on a holistic approach to nursing care and recognition of the patient perspective, with emphasis on developing education and counseling for women, patients with atrial fibrillation/sick sinus disease, and patients whose pacemakers have ventricular pacing." (Malm et al., 2007, p. 15)

Experimental Posttest-Only Comparison Group Design

In some studies, the dependent variable cannot be measured before the treatment. For example, before the beginning of treatment, it is not possible to measure, in a meaningful way, a subject's responses to interventions designed to control nausea from chemotherapy or postoperative pain. Additionally, in some cases, subjects' responses to the posttest can be due, in part, to learning from or having a subjective reaction to the pretest (pretest sensitization). If this issue is a concern in your study, you may eliminate the pretest and use an experimental posttest-only design with a comparison group (see Figure 11-23). However, you then will not be able to use many powerful statistical analysis techniques within the study. Additionally, the effectiveness of randomization in obtaining equivalent experimental and comparison groups cannot be evaluated in terms of the study variables. Nevertheless, the groups can be evaluated in terms of sample characteristics and other relevant variables.

Randomized Blocking Designs

The randomized blocking design uses the two-group pretest-posttest pattern or the two-group posttest pattern with one addition: a blocking variable. The blocking variable, if uncontrolled, is expected to confound the findings of the study. To prevent this confusion, the subjects are rank ordered in relation to the blocking variable.

For example, if effectiveness of a nursing intervention to relieve post-chemotherapy nausea was the independent variable in your study, severity of nausea could confound the findings. Subjects could be ranked according to severity of nausea. You would then identify and randomly assign the two subjects with the most severe nausea, one to the experimental group and one to the comparison group. You then would identify and randomly assign the two subjects next in rank. You would follow this pattern until the entire sample was randomly assigned as matched pairs. This procedure ensures that the experimental group and the comparison group are equal in relation to the potentially confounding variable.

The effect of blocking can also be accomplished statistically (through the use of analysis of covariance) without categorizing the confounding variable into discrete components. However, for this analysis to be accurate, one must be careful not to violate the assumptions of the statistical procedure (Shadish et al., 2002; Spector, 1981).

Santana-Sosa, Barriopedro, Lopez-Mojares, Perez, and Lucia (2009) implemented a randomized block

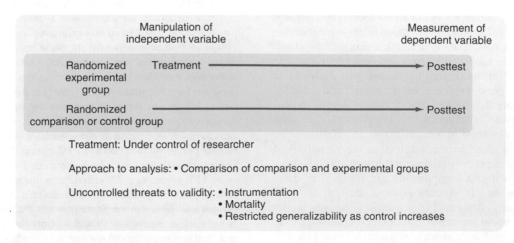

Figure 11-23 Experimental posttest-only comparison group design.

design in their study of the effect of exercise training on patients with Alzheimer's disease (AD). The purpose of this study was to determine the effects of a 12-week training program for patients with AD using the Senior Fitness test on their (1) overall functional capacity and (2) ability to perform activities of daily living. With use of a randomized block design, 16 patients (8 control; 8 experimental) were assigned to a training group (mean age 76 ± 4 years) or a control group (73 ± 4 years). The results showed significant improvements after training ($p < 0.05$) in upper and lower body muscle strength and flexibility; agility and dynamic balance; and endurance, fitness, gait, and balance abilities in performing activities of daily living (ADLs) independently. No changes were found in the control group over the 12-week period. The researchers indicated that exercise training should be included in the nursing care for patients with AD.

Factorial Design

In a factorial design, two or more different characteristics, treatments, or events are independently varied within a single study. This design is a logical approach to examining multicausality. The simplest arrangement is one in which two treatments or factors are involved and, within each factor, two levels are manipulated (for example, the presence or absence of the treatment); this is referred to as a 2×2 factorial design. This design is illustrated in Figure 11-24, in which the two independent variables are relaxation and distraction as means of relieving pain.

A 2×2 factorial design produces a study with four cells (A through D). Each cell must contain an approximately equivalent number of subjects. Cells B and C allow the researcher to examine each intervention separately. Cell D subjects receive no treatment and serve as a control group. Cell A allows the researcher to examine the interaction between the two independent variables. This design can be used, as in the randomized block design, to control for confounding variables. The confounding variable is included as an independent variable, and interactions between it and the other independent variable are examined (Shadish et al., 2002; Spector, 1981).

Extensions of the factorial design to more than two levels of variables are referred to as $M \times N$ factorial designs. Within this design, independent variables can have any number of levels within practical limits. Note that a 3×3 design involves 9 cells and requires a much larger sample size. A 4×4 design would require 16 cells. A 4×4 design would allow relaxation to be provided at four levels of intensity, such as no relaxation, relaxation for 10 minutes twice a day, relaxation for 15 minutes three times a day, and relaxation for 20 minutes four times a day. Distraction would be provided at similar levels.

Factorial designs are not limited to two independent variables; however, interpretation of larger numbers becomes more complex and requires greater knowledge of statistical analysis. Factorial designs do allow the examination of theoretically proposed interrelationships between multiple independent variables. However, very large samples are required (Shadish et al., 2002).

Winzer et al. (2010) conducted a clinical trial using a factorial design to examine the effects of radiotherapy and tamoxifen on the breast cancer recurrence rates of patients after breast-conserving surgery (BCS). The following excerpt from this study's abstract describes the design and key outcomes of the study.

"Between 1991 and 1998, 361 patients... were randomised to radiotherapy (yes/no) and tamoxifen for 2 years (yes/no) in a 2 x 2-factorial design; the exclusion of 7 centers (14 patients) left 347 patients for the analysis. First results after a median follow-up of 5.9 years were published. Herein we present updated results after a median follow-up of about 10 years. One hundred and eleven events concerning event-free survivals (EFS) have been observed. Since a strong interactive effect between radiotherapy and tamoxifen has been established, the results are presented in terms of the treatment effects for all four treatment groups separately. Mainly due to the presence of local recurrences, the event rate was much higher in the group with BCS only than in the other three groups. No significant difference could be established between the four treatment groups for distant disease-free survival rates (DDFS). Updated results give further evidence that even in patients with a favorable prognosis, the avoidance of radiotherapy and tamoxifen after BCS increases the rate of local

Level of Relaxation	Level of Distraction	
	Distraction	No Distraction
Relaxation	A	B
No Relaxation	C	D

Figure 11-24 **Example of factorial design.**

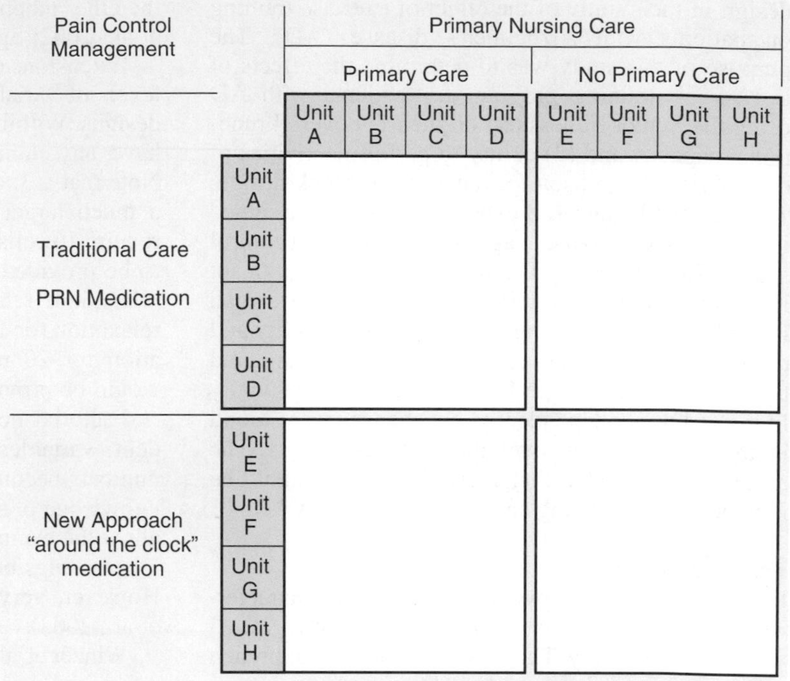

Pain Control Management		Primary Nursing Care							
		Primary Care				No Primary Care			
		Unit A	Unit B	Unit C	Unit D	Unit E	Unit F	Unit G	Unit H
Traditional Care PRN Medication	Unit A								
	Unit B								
	Unit C								
	Unit D								
New Approach "around the clock" medication	Unit E								
	Unit F								
	Unit G								
	Unit H								

Figure 11-25 Nested design.

recurrences substantially. Rates are about three times higher in the BCS only group. For the two outcomes, EFS and DDFS, no important difference could be seen between the three groups with an additional treatment. However, because of the limited sample size with corresponding low power, the strength of evidence for such a comparison is weak." (Winzer et al., 2010, p. 95)

Nested Designs

In some experimental situations, you may wish to consider the effect of variables that are found only at some levels of the independent variables being studied. Variables found only at certain levels of the independent variable are called **nested variables** and are best investigated with **nested designs** (Shadish et al., 2002). Possible nested variables are gender, race, socioeconomic status, and education. A nested variable may also be the patients who are cared for on specific nursing units or at different hospitals; the statistical analysis in this case would be conducted as though the unit or hospital were the subject rather than the individual patient. Figure 11-25 illustrates the nested design. In actual practice, nursing units used in this manner would have to be much larger in number than those illustrated, because each unit would be

considered a subject and would be randomly assigned to a treatment.

Sawyer, Deatrick, Kuna, and Weaver (2010) explored patients with obstructive sleep apnea and their perceptions of their disease and treatment with continuous positive airway pressure by implementing a nested design. A picture of this study design is presented in Figure 11-26. The following study excerpts describe its design and key findings:

Background: "Obstructive sleep apnea (OSA) patients' consistent use of continuous positive airway pressure (CPAP) therapy is critical to realizing improved functional outcomes and reducing untoward health risks associated with OSA.

Methods: We conducted a mixed methods, concurrent, nested study to explore OSA patients' beliefs and perceptions of the diagnosis and CPAP treatment that differentiate adherent from nonadherent patients prior to and after the first week of treatment, when the pattern of CPAP use is established [see Figure 11-26]. Guided by social cognitive theory, themes were derived from 30 interviews conducted post-diagnosis and after 1 week of CPAP use. Directed content analysis, followed by categorization of participants as adherent/nonadherent from

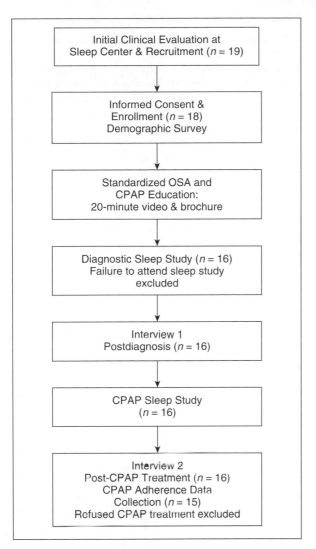

Figure 11-26 Nested study design. (From Sawyer, A. M., Deatrick, J. A., Kuna, S. T., & Weaver, T. E. [2010]. Differences in perceptions of the diagnosis and treatment of obstructive sleep apnea and continuous positive airway pressure therapy among adherers and nonadherers. *Qualitative Health Research, 20*[7], 876.)

objectively measured CPAP use, preceded across-case analysis among 15 participants with severe OSA. Beliefs and perceptions that differed between adherers and nonadherers included OSA risk perception, symptom recognition, self-efficacy, outcome expectations, treatment goals, and treatment facilitators/barriers. Our findings suggest opportunities for developing and testing tailored interventions to promote CPAP use." (Sawyer et al., 2010, p. 373)

Crossover or Counterbalanced Designs

In some studies, more than one treatment is administered to each subject. The treatments are provided sequentially rather than concurrently. Comparisons are then made of the effects of the different treatments on the same subject. For example, two different methods known to achieve relaxation might be used as the two treatments. One difficulty with this type of study is that exposure to one treatment may result in effects (called **carryover effects**) that persist and influence responses of the subject to later treatments. Also, subjects can improve as they become more familiar with the experimental protocol, a situation called a **practice effect**. They may become tired or bored with the study, a development called a **fatigue effect**. The direct interaction of one treatment with another, such as the use of two drugs, can confound differences in the two treatments.

Crossover, or *counterbalancing,* is a strategy designed to guard against possible erroneous conclusions resulting from carryover effects. With **crossover or counterbalancing design**, subjects are randomly assigned to a specific sequencing of treatment conditions. This approach distributes the carryover effects equally throughout all the conditions of the study, thus canceling them out. To prevent an effect related to time, the same amount of time must be allotted to each treatment, and the crossover point must be related to time, not to the condition of the subject (Shadish et al., 2002).

In addition, the design must allow for an adequate interval between treatments to dissipate the effects of the first treatment; this interval is referred to as a *washout period.* For example, the design would specify that each treatment would last 6 days and that on the eighth day, each subject would cross over to the alternative treatment after a 2-day washout period.

The researcher also must be alert to the possibility that changes may be due to factors such as disease progression, the healing process, or the effects of treatment of the disease rather than the study treatment. The process of counterbalancing can become complicated when more than two treatments are involved. Counterbalancing is effective only if the carryover effect is essentially the same from treatment A to treatment B as it is from treatment B to treatment A. If one treatment is more fatiguing than the other or more likely to modify response to the other treatment, counterbalancing will not be effective. You can use the crossover design to control variance in your study and thus allow the sample size to be smaller. The sample size required to detect a significant effect is considerably smaller because the subjects serve as their own controls. Because the data collection period is longer, however, the rate of subject dropout may increase (Beck, 1989).

An example of this design is the Chang, Lin, Lin, and Lin (2007) study of feeding premature infants using either single-hole or cross-cut nipple units. They described their study as follows:

"The purpose of this study was to compare the amount of total milk intake, feeding time, sucking efficiency, heart rate (HR), respiratory rate (RR), and oxygen saturation (SpO2) of premature infants when fed with either single-hole or cross-cut nipple units. Twenty stable infants admitted to a level II nursery in a tertiary care center with gestational ages averaging 32.2 +/- 3.2 wks were enrolled. Subjects had an average postmenstrual age of 34.1 +/- 1.6 wks, and average body weight of 1996 +/- 112 gm. A crossover design was used and infants were observed for two consecutive meals separated by a four-hour interval. They were bottle fed with equal feeding amounts using a single-hole and cross-cut nipple administered in random order. Results showed that infants fed with single-hole nipple units took more milk (57.5 +/- 8.3 ml vs. 51.6 +/- 9.5 ml, $p = 0.011$), had a shorter feeding time per meal (11.5 +/- 4.9 min vs. 20.9 +/- 5.0 min, $p < 0.001$), and sucked more efficiently (5.8 +/- 2.5 ml/min vs. 2.7 +/- 1.0 ml/min, $p < 0.001$) compared to those fed through cross-cut nipples. Infants using cross-cut nipple units had a higher RR (44.4 +/- 4.6 breaths/minutes vs. 40.8 +/- 4.9 breaths/minutes, $p = 0.002$) and SpO2 (96.1 +/- 1.4% vs. 94.6 +/- 3.2%, $p = 0.044$) than those using single-hole nipples. Oxygen desaturation (SpO2 < 90% and lasting for longer than 20 sec) and bradycardia were not recorded in either group of infants during feeding. Compared to using cross-cut nipple units, premature infants using single-hole nipple units take more milk and tend to tolerate feedings better. A single-hole nipple may be a choice for physiologically stable bottle-fed premature infants." (Chang et al., 2007, p. 215)

Clinical Trials

Clinical trials have been used in medicine since 1945. Wooding (1994) described the strategies that were used to introduce new medical therapies before that time:

"Until very recently, the genesis and use of new treatments came about by means having little to do with the scientific method. For millennia, the majority of therapies appear to have evolved by one of three methods: accidental discovery of treatments with unmistakable efficacy; the use of hypotheses alone, without any experimentation; or the utilization of experimentation without controls, randomization, blinding,… or adequate sample sizes. Treatments originating by one of the latter two routes frequently persisted for a very long time despite a lack of unbiased evidence of their efficacy. Bloodletting, purging, and the use of homeopathic dosages of drugs are examples. Failure of a treatment in any particular case was usually attributed by its practitioners to its misuse, to poor diagnosis, or to complicating factors." (Wooding, 1994, p. 26)

Over the years, the methodology for clinical trials has evolved in medicine, resulting in less bias in sampling, treatment implementation, and data collection (Meinert & Tonascia, 1986; Piantadosi, 1997; Pocock, 1996; Whitehead, 1992; Wooding, 1994). Meinert and Tonascia (1986) defined a **clinical trial** as a planned experiment designed to determine the efficacy of a treatment or independent variable in a study in which the experimental group receives the treatment and the control group does not. The experimental group and the control group are usually established through random assignment, and the study outcomes or dependent variables are compared for the two groups. In clinical trials, the patients in both groups are enrolled, treated, and followed over the same time. The outcome measures are usually clinical events, laboratory tests, or mortality.

The phase I, II, III, and IV clinical trial categories were developed specifically for testing experimental drug therapy (Meinert & Tonascia, 1986; Whitehead, 1992). Phase I, the initial testing of a new drug, focuses on determining the best drug dose and identifying safety effects. Phase II trials seek preliminary evidence of efficacy and side effects of the drug dose determined by the phase I trial. Sometimes in Phase II, the experimental group receiving the drug is compared with a placebo group.

Phase III trials are comparative definitive studies in which the new drug's effects are compared with those of the drug considered standard therapy. Phase III trials are sometimes referred to as "full-scale definitive clinical trials," suggesting that a decision is made on the basis of the findings as to whether the experimental drug is more effective than standard treatment. In some phase III clinical trials, the sample size is not determined before initiation of data collection. Rather, data are analyzed at intervals to test for significant differences between groups. If a significant difference is found, data collection may be discontinued. Otherwise, the data collection will continue and retesting is initiated after accrual of additional subjects (Meinert & Tonascia, 1986; Whitehead, 1992). Phase IV trials occur after regulatory approval of the drug and are designed to monitor patients over time to determine drug safety, uncommon side effects, and long-term consequences in a larger population. Phase IV trials might also focus on testing marketing strategies and examining cost-effectiveness for the drug (Piantadosi, 1997; Wooding, 1994).

Piantadosi (1997) recommended redefining these stages to be broader and applicable to more types of trials. He suggested using the following terminology: early development, middle development, comparative studies, and late development. In early development trials, researchers would develop and test the treatment mechanism (thus, they could also be called TM trials). Middle development studies would focus on clinical outcomes and treatment "tolerability." Tolerability would have three components: feasibility, safety, and efficacy; thus, Piantadosi (1997) referred to middle development studies as safety and efficacy trials, or SE trials. In this phase, the researcher would estimate the probability that patients would benefit from the treatment (or experience side effects from it). Performance criteria such as success rate might be used.

Comparative studies, according to Piantadosi (1997), would have defined clinical end points and would address comparative treatment efficacy (so could be called CTE trials). These studies would include a concurrent control group that receive the standard treatment and an experimental group that receives the experimental treatment. These studies might also include a placebo group, which receives a faux treatment to determine the psychological response to receiving a treatment. Late development studies would be designed to identify uncommon side effects, interactions with other treatments, and unusual complications. They would be developed as expanded safety trials, or ES trials, conducted overtime with larger samples. Over the years, researchers have increased the control in the development and implementation of healthcare clinical trials and these trials are usually referred to as randomized controlled trials (RCTs) in the research literature.

Randomized Controlled Trials

Currently in medicine and nursing, the **randomized controlled trial (RCT) design** is noted to be the strongest methodology for testing the effectiveness of a treatment because of the elements of the design that limit the potential for bias. Subjects are randomly assigned to the treatment and control groups to reduce selection bias (Shadish et al., 2002). Biases developing from participant attrition from studies are managed with intention-to-treat analyses (Polit, Gillespie, & Griffin, 2011). In addition, blinding or withholding of study information from data collectors, participants, and their healthcare providers can reduce the potential for bias. Thus, RCTs when appropriately conducted are considered the gold standard for determining the effectiveness of healthcare interventions.

However, there were serious criticisms of the inconsistencies and biases identified in the clinical trials conducted. Thus, in 1993, a panel of 30 experts—clinical trial researchers, medical journal editors, epidemiologists, and methodologists—met in Ottawa, Canada, to develop a scale to assess the quality of RCTs reports. This group initiated the Standardized Reporting of Trials (SORT) statement (CONSORT, 2011). This statement included a checklist and flow diagram that investigators were encouraged to follow when conducting and reporting RCTs. The initial work of this group was revised in 2001 and became the Consolidated Standards for Reporting Trials (CONSORT). This guideline was updated with the CONSORT 2010 Statement published by Schultz, Altman, and Moher (2010) as representatives of the CONSORT Group. Figure 11-27 provides a flow diagram of the progression through the phases of an RCT—enrollment, intervention allocation, follow-up, and data analysis—for two randomized parallel groups. This diagram was included in the CONSORT 2010 Statement to facilitate the conduct of quality RCTs nationally and internationally (Schulz et al., 2010). The CONSORT 2010 Statement also offers a checklist of information that researchers need to supply when reporting a RCT; it can be found in Chapter 19, the Schulz et al. (2010) publication, or online (http://www.consort-statement.org/consort-statement/) (CONSORT, 2012).

Only in the past 10 years has the term RCT been used to describe studies conducted in nursing. When implementing these clinical trials in nursing, the methodology needs to be redefined to fit the knowledge-building needs of nursing and also conform to the CONSORT standards. Thus, an RCT conducted in nursing needs to meet the following expectations:

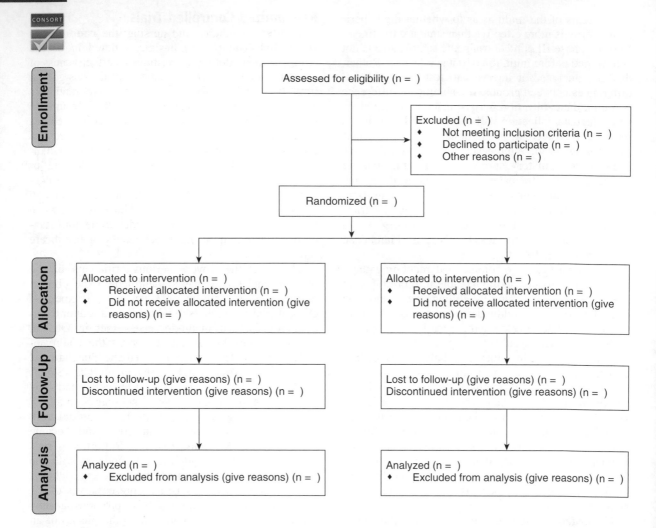

Figure 11-27 2010 Statement flow diagram of the progress through the phases of a parallel randomized trial of two groups (that is, enrollment, intervention allocation, follow-up, and data analysis). (From CONSORT. [2012]. The CONSORT Statement. Retrieved from http://www.consort-statement.org/consort-statement/; Schulz, K. F., Altman, D. G., Moher, D., for the CONSORT Group [2010]. CONSORT 2010 Statement: Updated guidelines for reporting parallel group randomised trials. *British Medical Journal,* 340, c332.)

1. The study is designed to be a definitive test of the hypothesis that the intervention causes the defined effects or outcomes.
2. Previous studies have provided evidence that the intervention causes the desired outcome.
3. The intervention is clearly defined, and a protocol has been established for its clinical application ensuring intervention fidelity (Santacroce et al., 2004; Yamada et al., 2010).
4. The study is conducted in a clinical setting, not in a laboratory.
5. The design meets the criteria of an experimental study (Schulz et al., 2010).
6. Subjects are drawn from a reference population through the use of clearly defined criteria. Baseline states are comparable in all groups included in the study. Selected subjects are then randomly assigned to treatment and comparison groups—thus, the term randomized clinical trial (CONSORT, 2012; Schulz et al., 2010).
7. Subjects are accrued individually over time as they enter the clinical area, are identified as

meeting the study criteria, and agree to participate in the study.

8. The study has high internal validity. The design is rigorous and involves a high level of control of potential sources of bias that will rule out possible alternative causes of the effect (Shadish et al., 2002). The design may include blinding to accomplish this purpose. **Blinding** means that the patient, those providing care to the patient, and/or the data collectors do not know whether the patient is in the experimental group or the control group. The CONSORT 2010 Statement recommends that the researchers clearly designate who is blinded in the research plan, conduct the study as planned, and designate who was blinded in the final report (Polit et al., 2011; Schulz et al., 2010).

9. The treatment or independent variable is equal and consistently applied to all subjects in the experimental group (CONSORT, 2012).

10. Dependent variables or outcomes are measured consistently with quality measurement methods (Waltz et al., 2010).

11. The proposed study has been externally reviewed by expert researchers who have approved the design.

12. The study has received external funding sufficient to allow a rigorous design with a sample size adequate to provide a definitive test of the intervention.

13. The research report covers the items on the CONSORT 2010 Statement checklist (CONSORT, 2012).

14. If the clinical trial results indicate a significant effect of the intervention, the evidence is sufficient to warrant application of the findings in clinical practice (Melnyk & Fineout-Overholt, 2011).

15. The intervention is defined in sufficient detail so that clinical application can be achieved (Bulechek et al., 2008; Polit et al., 2011; Schulz et al., 2010).

Elwood (1998) suggested that clinical trial methodology could be used for prevention intervention studies as well as testing treatments. Murray (1998) proposed methods of randomizing groups rather than subjects in prevention studies and explored issues related to community-based trials such as sample mortality.

Clinical trials may be carried out simultaneously in multiple geographical locations to increase sample size and resources and to obtain a more representative sample (Schulz et al., 2010). In this case, the primary researcher must coordinate activities at all the sites. Meinert and Tonascia (1986) indicated that the costs

per patient per year of the study are less for multicenter studies than for single-center trials. If you plan to use this technique in your research, you must confront several problems. Coordination of a project of this type requires much time and effort. Keeping up with subjects is critical but may be difficult. Communication with and cooperation of staff assisting with the study in the various geographical locations are essential but sometimes challenging. You may encounter attempts to ignore the protocol and provide traditional care (Fetter et al., 1989; Gilliss & Kulkin, 1991; Schulz et al., 2010; Tyzenhouse, 1981). Meinert and Tonascia (1986) recommended the development of a coordinating center for multisite clinical trials that will be responsible for receiving, editing, processing, analyzing, and storing data generated in the study. Nurse researchers need to follow the CONSORT 2010 Statement recommendations in the conduct of RCTs and in their reporting (CONSORT, 2012; Schulz et al., 2010).

Jones, Duffy, and Flanagan (2011) conducted an RCT to test the efficacy of a nurse-coached intervention (NCI) on the outcomes of patients undergoing ambulatory arthroscopy surgery. The NCI was developed to improve the postoperative experiences of patients and families following ambulatory surgery. This study was funded by the National Institute of Nursing Research. The following study excerpt identifies the study hypothesis, design and major findings:

"This study was conducted to test the hypothesis that ambulatory arthroscopic surgery patients who receive a nurse-coached telephone intervention will have significantly less symptom distress and better functional health status than a comparable group who receive usual practice....

The study sample in this randomized clinical trial with repeated measures was 102 participants (52 in the intervention group and 50 in the usual practice group) drawn from a large academic medical center in the Northeast United States. Symptom distress was measured using the Symptom Distress Scale, and functional health was measured using the Medical Outcomes Study 36-Item Short-Form Health Survey General Health Perceptions and Mental Health subscales." (Jones et al., 2011, p. 92)

Jones et al. (2011) detailed their study intervention and the steps taken by the researchers to promote fidelity in the implementation of the NCI. The nurses were trained in the delivery of the NCI by the study team using a video. Each nurse coach was given a packet of guidelines for management of the participants' symptoms:

> "The guidelines addressed common patient problems associated with postoperative recovery after arthroscopy with general anesthesia (e.g., nausea, vomiting, pain, immobility). The guidelines contained five areas to evaluate: (a) assessment (self-report), (b) current management of symptoms, (c) evaluation by the coach of the adequacy of the intervention, (d) additional intervention strategies to address the presenting symptoms, and (e) proposed outcome (self-report)." Jones et al., 2011, p. 95)

The sample criteria were detailed to identify the target population. Once the patients consented to be in the study, they were randomly assigned to the NCI group or the usual care group with use of the sealed-envelope method (Maxwell & Delaney, 2004). The researchers found that the NCI delivered by telephone postoperatively to patients undergoing arthroscopic surgery significantly reduced their symptom distress and improved their physical and mental health. The steps of this study followed the steps outlined in the CONSORT flow diagram in Figure 11-27. More details for conducting RCTs can be found in Chapter 14.

Studies That Do Not Use Traditional Research Designs

In some approaches to research, the research designs described in this chapter cannot be used. These studies tend to be in highly specialized areas that require unique design strategies to accomplish their purposes. Designs for primary prevention and health promotion, secondary analysis, and methodological studies are described here.

Primary Prevention and Health Promotion Studies

To study primary prevention and health promotion as a nurse researcher, you must apply a treatment of primary prevention (the cause) and then attempt to measure the effect (an event that does not occur if the treatment was effective). **Primary prevention studies**, then, attempt to measure things that do not happen. One cannot select a sample to study, apply a treatment, and then measure an effect. The sample must be the community. The design involves examining changes

in the community, and the variables are called *indicators*. A change in an identified indicator is inferred to be a consequence of the effectiveness of the prevention program (treatment).

Specific indicators would depend on the focus of prevention. For example, nurses in Canada identified oral mucositis as a recurring issue in oncology clinical practice and developed an oral care guide. They used the University Health Network Nursing Research Utilization Model and the Neuman Systems Model as conceptual frameworks (Salvador, 2006). The following excerpt describes their study:

> "A flowchart was developed to ensure a coordinated and continuous provision of oral care. Educational presentations were conducted to familiarize nurses and members of the multidisciplinary team of the practice changes. The introduction of the oral care regimen as primary prevention, plus systematic oral assessment and monitoring had the potential to reduce the occurrence and severity of oral mucositis in patients undergoing autologous stem cell transplantation." (Salvador, 2006 p. 18)

How might you study the effectiveness of this primary prevention strategy? Because one indicator alone would be insufficient to infer effect, multiple indicators and statistical analyses appropriate for these indicators must be used. For example, you might measure the color of the oral mucosa, moistness in the mouth, severity of oral mucositis, and amount of pain expressed by the patient when eating.

Secondary Analyses

Secondary analysis design involves studying data previously collected in another study. Data are reexamined with the use of different subsets of the data or variables and different statistical analyses from those previously used. The design involves analyzing data to validate the reported findings, examine dimensions previously unexamined, or redirect the focus of the data to allow comparison with data from other studies (Gleit & Graham, 1989; Windle, 2010).

Secondary analysis studies may use data collected by state and national governments. For example, Chertok, Luo, and Anderson (2011) analyzed over 17 years of West Virginia's birth certificate data to answer a research question about associations between changes in prenatal smoking habits and subsequent infant birth weights. Cipher, Hooker, and Guerra (2006) compared the prescribing trends of nurse practitioners, physician assistants, and physicians using data in the National Ambulatory Medical Care Survey (NAMCS) database. They found that for 70% of the visits, the three clinician types were likely to write at least one prescription, and that PAs were more likely than NPs or physicians to prescribe controlled substances.

Because data collected for some national databases may have used oversampling of underrepresented groups, researchers using these databases must carefully examine the inclusion and exclusion sampling criteria used by the original research team. Providing substantive information about the challenges presented by large database research is beyond the scope of this book. Researchers interested in using large databases for secondary analysis should consult a reference book on the topic (Kiecolt & Nathan, 1985; Trzesniewski, Donnellan, & Lucas, 2011; Vartanian, 2011).

Data accumulated during the research programs of groups of faculty provide opportunities for secondary data analysis as well. This approach allows the investigators to examine questions related to the data that were not originally posed. These data sets may provide opportunities for junior faculty members or graduate students to become involved in a research program. This type of secondary data analysis requires thoughtful, honest consideration to avoid violation of professional standards, as Aaronson (1994) recommends:

> "Fundamentally, each paper written from the same study or the same dataset must make a distinct and significant scientific contribution. Presumably this is not only the major overriding criterion used by reviewers, but also the author's intent when writing the paper. When a particular paper is one of several from the same study, project, or dataset, the author's responsibility to identify the source of the data is that much greater. To lead readers to think a report is from a new study or a different dataset than that used in the authors' previous work is dishonest, particularly if the second paper purports to substantiate findings of the first one.... Apart from the overriding concern about 'milking the data,' the most common objection to multiple articles from a single study is concern about the age of the data.... Concerns in nursing about the number of papers generated from a single study may reflect the emerging status of secondary analysis as a legitimate approach to nursing research....

> All of the reasons offered for using secondary analysis—answering new questions with existing data, applying new methods to answer old questions, the real exigencies of cost and feasibility—serve equally to justify the continued use of data collected years ago, by the original investigator of a large project, as well as by others.... The issue remains one of sound science. The question that must be asked is: Does this particular paper make a meaningful and distinct contribution to the scientific literature?" (Aaronson, 1994, pp. 61-62)

An example of secondary analysis is Koci and Strickland's (2007) study of the relationship of adolescent physical and sexual abuse with perimenstrual syndrome (PMS) in adulthood. Data analyzed in this study were from a longitudinal study of a community sample of 568 women in a database called Nursing Assessment of PMS: Neurometric Indices. A study such as this yields an enormous amount of data that are not examined in the original study. Koci and Strickland (2007) posed a different research question that could be examined using the data from the longitudinal study. They found that "a history of both adolescent physical abuse and sexual abuse was significantly associated with PMS in adulthood. Women with a history of adolescent physical and sexual abuse had significantly more severe PMS patterns with more dysphoria than women without abuse" (Koci & Strickland, 2007, p. 75).

Methodological Designs

Methodological designs are used to develop the validity and reliability of instruments to measure constructs used as variables in research. The process is lengthy and complex. The average researcher time required to develop a research tool to the point of appropriate use in a study is 5 years (Waltz et al., 2010). Methodological studies include assessment of content validity, evaluation of the conceptual structure of a scale, construct validity, and assessment of reliability.

Simons, Stark, and DeMarco (2011) conducted a methodological study to develop a new, four-item instrument to measure bullying of nurses in the workplace. These researchers described their process for developing a valid and reliable questionnaire for measuring workplace bullying and provided direction for further research to support continued development of this instrument. The key ideas of this study are presented in the following abstract:

"Studies on workplace bullying either in the U.S. or internationally rarely include nurses. We tested the concurrent validity of the Negative Acts Questionnaire-Revised (22 items) with a sample of nurses. Five hundred eleven registered nurses (RNs) responded to a mailed survey. Factor, reliability, and regression analyses tested dimensionality, reliability, and construct and criterion validity. Workplace bullying is best seen as a one-dimensional construct. A subset of four items was found to be both valid and reliable in measuring bullying in this sample. Findings support use of a one-dimensional, four-item questionnaire to measure perceived bullying in nursing populations. Using a four-item questionnaire decreases participant and researcher burden and makes available an outcome measure for future descriptive and predictive interventional research." (Simons et al., 2011, p. 132)

Algorithms for Selecting Research Designs

To select a research design, the investigator must follow paths of logical reasoning. You need a calculating mind to explore all the possible consequences of using a particular design in a study. In some ways, selecting a design is like thinking through the moves in a chess game. You must carefully think through the consequences of each option. The research design organizes all the components of the study in a way that is most likely to lead to valid answers to the questions that have been posed. Studies with high-quality research designs implemented over time have a strong influence on the research evidence generated for practice (Brown, 2009; Fawcett & Garity, 2009; Melnyk & Fineout-Overholt, 2011).

To help you select the most appropriate design for your study, we encourage you to use the algorithms, or decision trees, provided at the end of this chapter. The first algorithm (see Figure 11-28) will help you identify the type of study you plan to conduct or to determine the type of study in a publication. The next four algorithms (see Figures 11-29 through 11-32) will assist you in identifying designs in published studies and in selecting a specific design for a study you plan to conduct. Figure 11-29 is an algorithm of commonly conducted descriptive study designs, and Figure 11-30 includes common correlational study designs. Figure 11-31 is an algorithm for identifying common quasi-experimental designs, and Figure 11-32 includes experimental designs. Most of the designs identified in these figures have been discussed in this chapter. Selecting a design is not a rigid, rule-guided task. As a researcher, you have considerable flexibility in choosing a design. The pathways within the algorithms arc not absolute and are to be used as guides. Sometimes researchers combine different types of designs to address their study purpose and their research objectives, questions, or hypotheses.

KEY POINTS

- Researchers have developed designs to meet unique research needs as they emerge.
- At present, most nurse researchers are using designs developed by other disciplines, which are a useful starting point, but nurse scientists need to go beyond them to develop designs that will more appropriately meet the needs of the knowledge base in nursing.
- Descriptive studies are designed to gain more information about variables within a particular field of study.
- Correlational studies examine relationships between variables but do not provide information on causality.
- Quasi-experimental and experimental designs examine causality. The power of the design to accomplish this purpose depends on the degree to which the actual effects of the experimental treatment (the independent variable) can be detected by measuring the dependent or outcome variable.
- Obtaining an understanding of the true effects of an experimental treatment requires action to control threats to the validity of the findings.
- Threats to validity are controlled through selection of subjects, manipulation of the treatment, and measurement of variables.
- Currently in medicine and nursing, the randomized controlled trial (RCT) design is noted to be the strongest methodology for testing the effectiveness of a treatment because of the elements of the design that limit the potential for bias. The CONSORT 2010 Statement clarifies the steps for conducting and reporting an RCT.
- Studying primary prevention and health promotion involves applying a treatment of primary prevention (the cause) and then attempting to measure the effect (an event that does not occur if the treatment was effective).

Text continued on p. 261

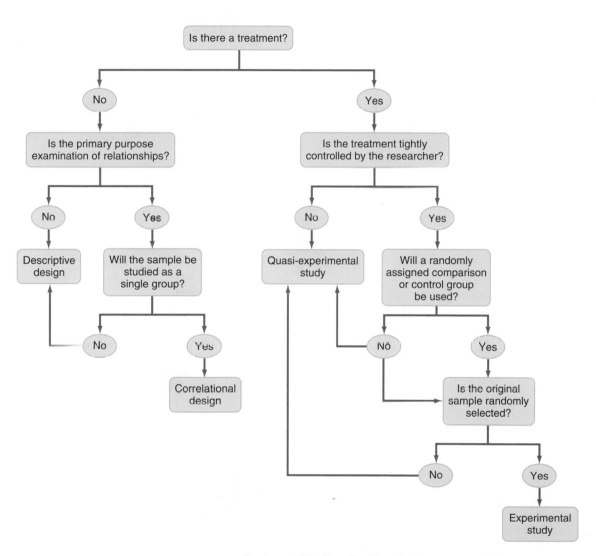

Figure 11-28 Type of study.

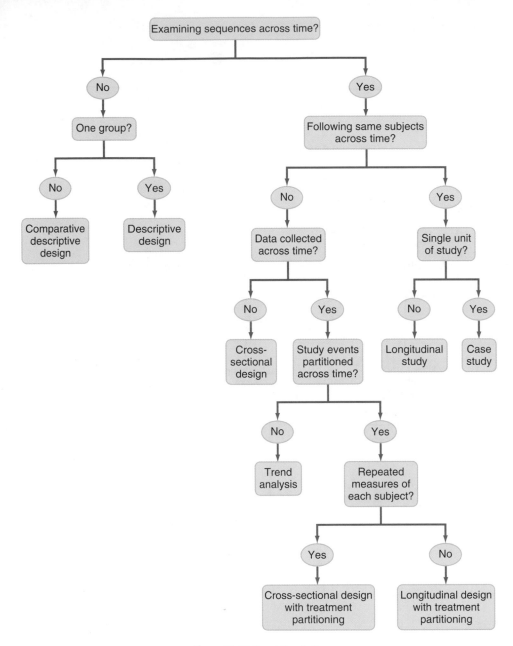

Figure 11-29 **Descriptive studies.**

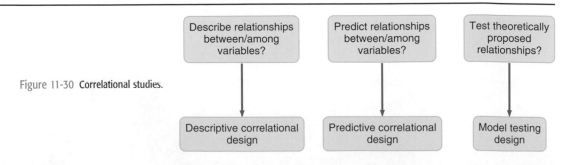

Figure 11-30 **Correlational studies.**

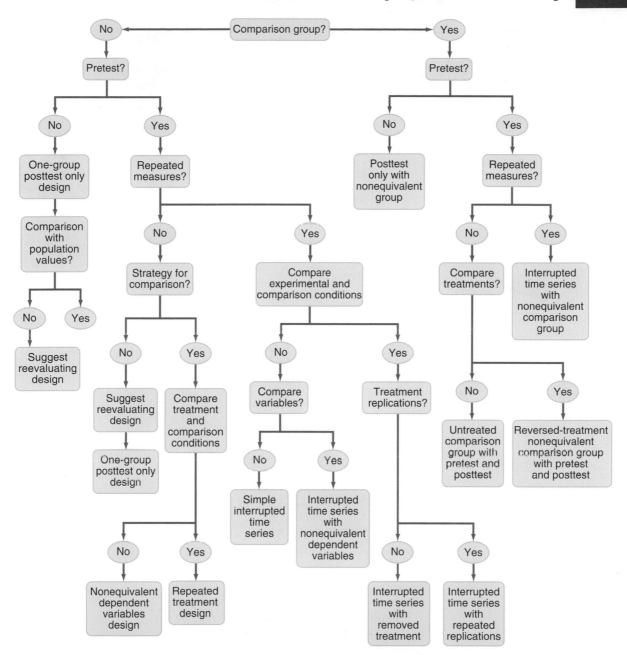

Figure 11-31 Quasi-experimental studies.

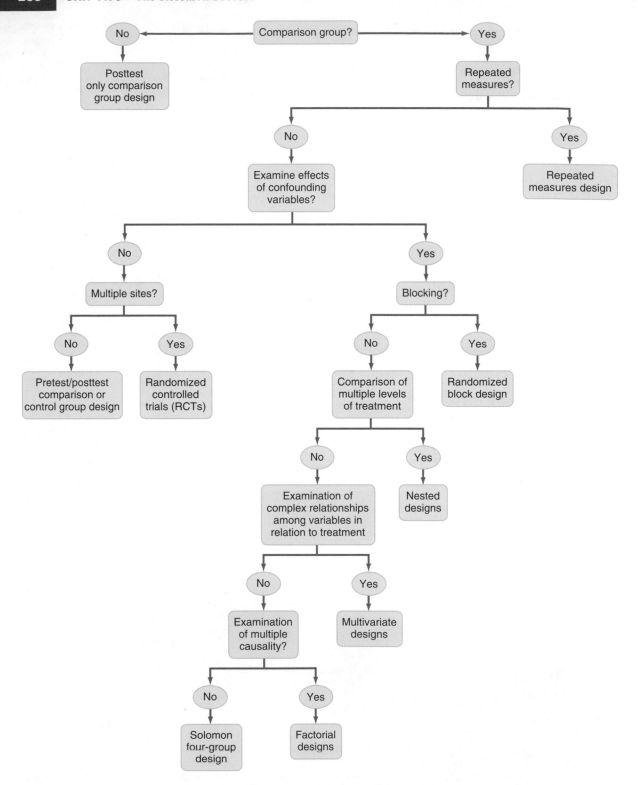

Figure 11-32 Experimental studies.

- Secondary analysis is the study of data previously collected in another study or for a non-research purpose.
- Methodological studies are designed to develop the validity and reliability of instruments to measure constructs used as variables in research.
- Algorithms for design identification and selection are provided in Figures 11-29 to 11-32.

REFERENCES

Aaronson, L. S. (1994). Milking data or meeting commitments: How many papers from one study? *Nursing Research*, *43*(1), 60–62.

Aberson, C. L. (2010). *Applied power analysis for the behavioral sciences*. New York, NY: Routledge Taylor & Francis Group.

Bailey J. J., Sabbagh M., Loiselle C. G., Boileau J., & McVey L. (2010). Supporting families in the ICU: A descriptive correlational study of informational support, anxiety, and satisfaction with care. *Intensive & Critical Care Nursing*, *26*(2), 114–122.

Beck, S. L. (1989). The crossover design in clinical nursing research. *Nursing Research*, *38*(5), 291–293.

Bialocerkowski, A., Klupp, N., & Bragge, P. (2010). Research methodology series: How to read and critically appraise a reliability article. *International Journal of Therapy and Rehabilitation*, *17*(3), 114–120.

Bowles, K.H., & Naylor, M.D. (1996). Nursing intervention classification systems. *Journal of Nursing Scholarship*, *28*(4), 303–308.

Brown, S.J. (2009). *Evidence-based nursing: The research-practice connection*. Boston, MA: Jones and Bartlett.

Bulechek, G. M., Butcher, H. K., & Dochterman, J. M. (2008). *Nursing Interventions Classification (NIC)* (5th ed.). St. Louis, MO: Mosby Elsevier.

Campbell, D. T., & Stanley, J. C. (1963). *Experimental and quasi-experimental designs for research*. Chicago, IL: Rand McNally.

Chang, Y. J., Lin, C. P., Lin, Y. J., & Lin, C. H. (2007). Effects of single-hole and cross-cut nipple units on feeding efficiency and physiological parameters in premature infants. *Journal of Nursing Research*, *15*(3), 215–223.

Chertok, I. R. A., Luo, J., & Anderson, R. H. (2011). Association between changes in smoking habits in subsequent pregnancy and infant birth weight in West Virginia. *Maternal and Child Health Journal*, *15*(2), 249–254.

Cipher, D. J., Hooker, R. S., & Guerra, P. (2006). Prescribing trends by nurse practitioners and physician assistants in the United States. *Journal of the American Academy of Nurse Practitioners*, *18*(6), 291–291.

CONSORT. (2011). *How CONSORT began*. Retrieved, from http://www.consort-statement.org/about-consort/history/.

CONSORT. (2012). *The CONSORT Statement*. Retrieved from http://www.consort-statement.org/consort-statement/.

Cook, T. D., & Campbell, D. T. (1979). *Quasi-experimentation: Design and analysis issues for field settings*. Chicago, IL: Rand McNally.

Corty, E. W. (2007). *Using and interpreting statistics: A practical text for the health, behavioral, and social sciences*. St. Louis, MO: Mosby Elsevier.

Costanzo, C., Walker, S. M., Yates, B. C., McCabe, B., & Berg, K. (2006). Physical activity counseling for older women. *Western Journal of Nursing Research*, *28*(7), 786–810.

Cramer, M. E., Chen, L. W., Roberts, S., & Clute, D. (2007). Evaluating the social and economic impact of community-based prenatal care. *Public Health Nursing*, *24*(4), 329–336.

Creswell, J. W. (2009). *Research design: Qualitative, quantitative, and mixed methods approaches* (3rd ed.). Los Angeles, CA: Sage.

Crombie, I. K., & Davies, H. T. O. (1996). *Research in health care: Design, conduct and interpretation of health services research*. New York, NY: Wiley.

Cummings, G. G., Estabrooks, C. A., Midodzi, W. K., Wallin, L., & Hayduk, L. (2007). Influence of organizational characteristics and context on research utilization. *Nursing Research*, *56*(4 Suppl), S24–S39.

DeVon, H. A., Block, M. E., Moyle-Wright, P., Ernst, D. M., Hayden, S. J., Lazzara, D. J., et al. (2007). A psychometric toolbox for testing validity and reliability. *Journal of Nursing Scholarship*, *39*(2), 155–164.

Doran, D. M. (2011). *Nursing outcomes: The state of the science* (2nd ed.). Sudbury, MA: Jones & Bartlett Learning.

Dudgeon, W. D., Phillips, K. D., Durstine, J. L., Burgess, S. E., Lyerly, G. L. W., Davis, J. M., et al. (2010). Individual exercise sessions alter circulating hormones and cytokines in HIV-infected men. *Applied Physiology, Nutrition & Metabolism*, *35*(4), 560–568.

Egan, E. C., Snyder, M., & Burns, K. R. (1992). Intervention studies in nursing: Is the effect due to the independent variable? *Nursing Outlook*, *40*(4), 187–190.

Elwood, J. M. (1998). *Critical appraisal of epidemiological studies and clinical trials*. New York: Oxford University Press.

Fawcett, J., & Garity, J. (2009). *Evaluating research for evidence based nursing practice*. Philadelphia, PA: F. A. Davis.

Fetter, M. S., Fettham, S. L., D'Apolito, K., Chaze, B. A., Fink, A., Frink, B. B., et al. (1989). Randomized clinical trials: Issues for researchers. *Nursing Research*, *38*(2), 117–120.

Fisher, R. A. (1935). *The design of experiments*. New York, NY: Hafner.

Forbes, A. (2009). Clinical intervention research in nursing. *International Journal of Nursing Studies*, *46*(4), 557–568.

Gilliss, C. L., & Kulkin, I. L. (1991). Monitoring nursing interventions and data collection in a randomized clinical trial. *Western Journal of Nursing Research*, *13*(3), 416–422.

Gleit, C., & Graham, B. (1989). Secondary data analysis: A valuable resource. *Nursing Research*, *38*(6), 380–381.

Gray, M. (1998). Introducing single case study research design: An overview. *Nurse Researcher*, *5*(4), 15–24.

Grove, S. K. (2007). *Statistics for health care research: A practical workbook*. St. Louis, MO: Saunders Elsevier.

Hamdan-Mansour, A. M., Al-Gamal, E., Puskar, K., Yacoub, M., & Marini, A. (2011). Mental health nursing in Jordan: An investigation into experience, work stress and organizational support. *International Journal of Mental Health Nursing*, *20*(2), 86–94.

Harris, K. M., Gordon-Larsen, P., Chantala, K., & Udry, J. R., R. (2006). Longitudinal trends in race/ethnic disparities in leading health indicators from adolescence to young adulthood. *Archives of Pediatric & Adolescent Medicine*, *160*(4), 74–81.

Hjelm-Karlsson, K. (1991). Using the biased coin design for randomization in health care research. *Western Journal of Nursing Research*, *13*(2), 284–288.

Jones, D., Duffy, M. E., & Flanagan, J. (2011). Randomized clinical trial testing efficacy of a nurse-coached intervention in arthroscopy patients. *Nursing Research*, *60*(2), 92–99.

Kerlinger, F. N., & Lee, H. B. (2000). *Foundations of behavioral research* (4th ed.). Fort Worth, TX: Harcourt College Publishers.

Kiecolt, J. K., & Nathan, L. E. (1985). *Secondary data analysis of survey data*. Beverly Hills, CA: Sage Publications.

Kjonegaard, R., Fields, R., & King, M. L. (2010). Current practice in airway management: A descriptive evaluation. *American Journal of Critical Care*, *19*(2), 168–174.

Kline, G.A., & Edwards, A. (2007). Antepartum and intra-partum insulin management of type 1 and type 2 diabetic women: Impact on clinically significant neonatal hypoglycemia. *Diabetes Research & Clinical Practice*, *7*(22), 223–230.

Koci, A., & Strickland, O. (2007). Relationship of adolescent physical and sexual abuse to perimenstrual symptoms (PMS) in adulthood. *Issues in Mental Health Nursing*, *28*(1), 75–87.

Lee, B. O., Chaboyer, W., & Wallis, M. (2010). Illness representations in patients with traumatic injury: A longitudinal study. *Journal of Clinical Nursing*, *19*(3-4), 556–563.

Lim, L. M., Chiu, L. H., Dohrmann, J., & Tan, K. L. (2010). Registered nurses' medication management of the elderly in aged care facilities. *International Nursing Review*, *57*(1), 98–106.

Malm, D., Karlsson, J. E., & Fridlund, B. (2007). Effects of a self-care program on the health-related quality of life of pacemaker patients: A nursing intervention study. *Canadian Journal of Cardiovascular Nursing*, *17*(1), 15–26.

Mancuso, J. M. (2010). Impact of health literacy and patient trust on glycemic control in an urban USA population. *Nursing and Health Sciences*, *12*(1), 94–104.

Mason-Hawkes, J., & Holm, K. (1989). Casual modeling: A comparison of path analysis and LISREL. *Nursing Research*, *38*(5), 312–314.

Matthews, E. E., Cook, P. F., & Terada, M. (2010). Randomizing research participants: Promoting balance and concealment in small samples. *Research in Nursing & Health*, *33*(3), 243–253.

Maxwell, S. E., & Delaney, H. D. (2004). *Designing experiments and analyzing data: A model comparison perspective* (2nd ed.). Mahway, NJ: Lawrence Erlbaum Associates.

McCain, L.J., & McCleary, R. (1979). The statistical analysis of the simple interrupted time-series quasi-experiment. In T. D. Cook & D. T. Campbell (Eds.), *Quasi-experimentation: Design and analysis issues for field settings* (pp. 233–293). Chicago, IL: Rand McNally.

McConnell, A. (1976). Effect of knowledge of results on attitude formed toward a motor learning task. *Research Quarterly in Exercise & Sport*, *47*(3), 394–399.

McCorkle, R., & Young, K. (1978). Development of a symptom distress scale. *Cancer Nursing*, *1*(5). 373–378.

Meghani, S. H., & Keane, A. (2007). Preference for analgesic treatment for cancer pain among African Americans. *Journal of Pain & Symptom Management*, *34*(2), 136–147.

Meinert, C. L., & Tonascia, S. (1986). *Clinical trials: Design, conduct, and analysis*. New York, NY: Oxford University Press.

Melnyk, B. M., & Fineout-Overholt, E. (2011). *Evidence-based practice in nursing & healthcare: A guide to best practice* (2nd ed.). Philadelphia, PA: Lippincott Williams, & Wilkins.

Morrison, D. M., Hoppe, M. J., Gillmore, M. R., Kluver, C., Higa, D., & Wells, E. A. (2009). Replicating an intervention: The tension between fidelity and adaptation. *AIDS Education and Prevention*, *21*(2), 128–140.

Munro, B. H. (2005). *Statistical methods for health care research* (5th ed.). Philadelphia, PA: Lippincott Williams & Wilkins.

Muntlin, Å., Carlsson, M., Säfwenberg, U., & Gunningberg, L. (2011). Outcomes of a nurse-initiated intravenous analgesic protocol for abdominal pain in an emergency department: A quasi-experimental study. *International Journal of Nursing Studies*, *48*(1), 13–23.

Murray, D. M. (1998). *Design and analysis of group-randomized trials*. New York, NY: Oxford University Press.

Norris, A. E. (2005a). Path analysis. In B. H. Munro (Ed.), *Statistical methods for health care research* (5th ed.) (pp. 377–403). Philadelphia, PA: Lippincott Williams, & Wilkins.

Norris, A. E. (2005b). Structural equation modeling. In B. H. Munro (Ed.), *Statistical methods for health care research* (5th ed.) (pp. 405–434). Philadelphia, PA: Lippincott Williams, & Wilkins.

Nursing Interventions Classification (NIC, 2011). *Overview: Nursing interventions classification (NIC)*. Retrieved from http://www.nursing.uiowa.edu/cncce/nursing-interventions-classification-overview/.

Ottenbacher, K. (1992). Impact of random assignment on study outcome: An empirical examination. *Controlled Clinical Trials*, *13*(1), 50–61.

Peterson, M. J., Schwab, W., van Oostrom, J. H., Gravenstein, N., & Caruso, L. J. (2010). Effects of turning on skin-bed interface pressures in healthy adults. *Journal of Advanced Nursing*, *66*(7), 1556–1564.

Piantadosi, S. (1997). *Clinical trials: A methodologic perspective*. New York, NY: Wiley.

Pierce, C., Fahs, P. S., Dura, A., Fronczek, A., Morgan, L. L., Leppert, T., et al. (2011). Raising stroke awareness among rural dwellers with a Facts for Action to Stroke Treatment-based Educational Program. *Applied Nursing Research*, *24*(2), 82–87.

Pocock, S. J. (1996). *Clinical trials: A practical approach*. New York, NY: Wiley.

Polit, D. F., Gillespie, B. M., & Griffin, R. (2011). Deliberate ignorance: A systematic review of blinding in nursing clinical trials. *Nursing Research*, *60*(1), 9–16.

Reichardt, C. S. (1979). The statistical analysis of data from nonequivalent group designs. In T. D. Cook & D. T. Campbell (Eds.), *Quasi-experimentation: Design and analysis issues for field settings* (pp. 147–206). Chicago, IL: Rand McNally.

Ryan-Wenger, N. A. (2010). Evaluation of measurement precision, accuracy, and error in biophysical data for clinical research and practice. In C. F. Waltz, O. L. Strickland, & E. R. Lenz (Eds.), *Measurement in nursing and health research* (4th ed.) (pp. 371–383). New York, NY: Springer Publishing Company.

Salvador, P. T. (2006). Development of an oral care guide for patients undergoing autologous stem cell transplantation. *Canadian Oncology Nursing Journal*, *16*(1), 18–20.

Sandelowski, M. (1996). One is the liveliest number: The case orientation of qualitative research. *Research in Nursing & Health*, *19*(6), 525–529.

Santacroce, S. J., Maccarelli, L. M., & Grey, M. (2004). Methods: Intervention fidelity. *Nursing Research, 53*(1), 63–66.

Santana-Sosa, E., Barriopedro, M. I., López-Mojares, L. M., Pérez, M., & Lucia, A. (2009). Exercise training is beneficial for Alzheimer's patients. *International Journal of Sports Medicine, 29*(10), 845–850.

Sawyer, A. M., Deatrick, J. A., Kuna, S. T., & Weaver, T. E. (2010). Differences in perceptions of the diagnosis and treatment of obstructive sleep apnea and continuous positive airway pressure therapy among adherers and nonadherers. *Qualitative Health Research, 20*(7), 873–892.

Schlairet, M. C., & Pollock, J. W. (2010). Equivalence testing of traditional and simulated clinical experiences: Undergraduate nursing students' knowledge acquisition. *Journal of Nursing Education, 49*(1), 43–47.

Schneider, S. M. (1998). Effects of virtual reality on symptom distress in children receiving cancer chemotherapy. *Dissertation Abstracts International: Section B: The Sciences & Engineering, 59*(5-B), 2126.

Schulz, K. F., Altman, D. G., & Moher, D. (2010). CONSORT 2010 Statement: Updated guidelines for reporting parallel group randomized trials. *Annals of Internal Medicine, 152*(11), 726–733.

Shadish, W. R., Cook, T. D., & Campbell, D. T. (2002). *Experimental and quasi-experimental designs for generalized causal inference.* Boston, MA: Houghton Mifflin.

Sharma, N. K., Ryals, J. M., Gajewski, B. J., & Wrights, D. E. (2010). Aerobic exercise alters analgesia and neurotrophin-3 synthesis in an animal model of chronic widespread pain. *Physical Therapy, 90*(5), 714–725.

Sidani, S., Doran, D., Porter, H., LeFort, S., O'Brien-Pallas, L. L., Zahn, C., et al. (2007). Outcomes of nurse practitioners in acute care: An exploration. *Internet Journal of Advanced Nursing Practice, 8*(1), 15.

Simons, S. R., Stark, R. B., & DeMarco, R. F. (2011). A new, four-item instrument to measure workplace bullying. *Research in Nursing & Health, 34*(2), 132–140.

Spector, P. E. (1981). *Research designs.* Beverly Hills, CA: Sage.

Spielberger, C. D., Edwards, C. D., Lushene, R. E., et al. (1978). *Manual for the State-Trait Anxiety Inventory.* Palo Alto, CA: Consulting Psychologist Press.

Spielberger, C. D., Gorsuch, R. L., Lushene, R., Vagg, P. R., & Jacobs, G. A. (1983). *Manual for the State-Trait Anxiety Inventory for Children.* Palo Alto, CA: Consulting Psychologist Press.

Sprague, M., & Chang, J. C. (2011). Integrative approach focusing on acupuncture in the treatment of chronic complex regional pain syndrome. *The Journal of Alternative and Complementary Medicine, 17*(1), 67–70.

Sterling, Y. M., & McNally, J. A. (1992). Single-subject research for nursing practice. *Clinical Nurse Specialist, 6*(1), 21–26.

Stout, R. L., Wirtz, P. W., Carbonari, J. P., & Del Boca, F. K. (1994). Ensuring balanced distribution of prognostic factors in treatment outcome research. *Journal of Studies in Alcoholism, 12*(Suppl.), 70–75.

Strand, T. & Lindgren, M. (2010). Knowledge, attitudes and barriers towards prevention of pressure ulcers in intensive care units: A descriptive cross-sectional study. *Intensive and Critical Care Nursing, 26*(6), 335–342.

Sutton, T. R. (2007). Anxiety and preoperative education in the senescent patient (Doctoral dissertation, Mountain State University). Retrieved from ProQuest Dissertations and Theses database. (Document ID 1446895).

Thompson, S. K. (2002). *Sampling* (2nd ed.). New York, NY: John Wiley & Sons.

Tripp-Reimer, T., Woodworth, G., McCloskey, J. C., & Bulechek, G. (1996). The dimensional structure of nursing interventions. *Nursing Research, 45*(1), 10–17.

Trzesniewski, K. H., Donnellan, M. B., & Lucas, R. E. (Eds.) (2011). *Secondary data analysis: An introduction for psychologists.* Washington, DC: American Psychological Association.

Tyzenhouse, P.S. (1981). Technical notes: The nursing clinical trial. *Western Journal of Nursing Research, 3*(1), 102–109.

U.S. Department of Health and Human Services (U.S. DHHS) (1968). *The Framingham study: An epidemiological investigation of cardiovascular disease (USDHHS Publication No. RC667F813).* Bethesda, MD: Author.

U.S. Department of Health and Human Services (U.S. DHHS) (2000). *Healthy People 2010: With understanding and improving health and objectives for improving health.* Retrieved from www.healthypeople.gov/Publications/.

van Doormaal J. E., van den Bemt P. M., Zaal R. J., Egberts A. C., Lenderink B. W., Kosterink J. G., et al. (2009). The influence that electronic prescribing has on medication errors and preventable adverse drug events: An interrupted time-series study. *Journal of the American Medical Informatics Association, 16*(6), 816–825.

Vartanian, J. P. (2011). *Secondary data analysis.* New York, NY: Oxford University Press.

Waltz, C. F., Strickland, O. L., & Lenz, E. R. (2010). *Measurement in nursing and health research* (4th ed.). New York, NY: Springer.

Whitehead, J. (1992). *The design and analysis of sequential clinical trials.* New York, NY: Ellis Horwood.

Windle, P. E. (2010). Secondary data analysis: Is it useful and valid? *Journal of PeriAnesthesia Nursing, 25* (5), 323–324.

Winzer, K., Sauerbrei, W., Braun, M., Liersch, T., Dunst, J., Guski, H., & Schumacher, M. (2010). Radiation therapy and tamoxifen after breast-conserving surgery: Updated results of a 2 x 2 randomized clinical trial in patients with low risk of recurrence. German Breast Cancer Study Group (GBSG). *European Journal of Cancer, 46*(1), 95–101.

Wooding, W. M. (1994). *Planning pharmaceutical clinical trials: Basic statistical principles.* New York, NY: Wiley.

Wyatt, G., Sikorskii, A., Rahbar, M. H., Victorson, D., & Adams, L. (2010). Intervention fidelity: Aspects of complementary and alternative medicine research. *Cancer Nursing, 33*(5), 331–342.

Yamada, J., Stevens, B., Sidani, S., Watt-Watson, J., & De Silva, N. (2010). Content validity of a process evaluation checklist to measure intervention implementation fidelity of the EPIC Intervention. *Worldviews of Evidence-Based Nursing, 7*(3), 158–164.

Zhang Y., Adams A. S., Ross-Degnan D., Zhang F., & Soumerai S.B. (2009). Effects of prior authorization on medication discontinuation among Medicaid beneficiaries with bipolar disorder. *Psychiatric Services, 60*(4), 520–527.

12

Qualitative Research Methodology

Qualitative researchers begin the research process with reviewing the literature and identifying a research problem. Depending on the research problem and type of knowledge that is needed, the qualitative researcher develops objectives or questions and determines which philosophical approach will be used to guide the study (see Chapter 4). The early steps of the qualitative research process, which is similar to the quantitative research process, are explored in Chapters 5 and 6. Other steps in the research process are implemented differently in or are unique to qualitative studies. In this chapter, information about qualitative methodology will be provided so that you can understand the process and envision what the experience will be like if you conduct a qualitative study.

Qualitative analysis techniques use words rather than numbers as the basis of analysis. In qualitative analysis, reasoning flows from the images, documents, or words provided by the participant toward more abstract concepts and themes. This reasoning process, inductive thinking, guides the organizing, reducing, and clustering of the data. To achieve the goal of describing and understanding participant perspectives, qualitative methods of sampling, data gathering, and analyses allow for more flexibility than the methods of the quantitative paradigm. Because data analysis begins as data are gathered, insights from early data may suggest additional questions that need to be asked or other modifications to the study methods. For example, suppose a researcher was conducting a grounded theory study about personal identity after losing a limb during military combat. During the interviews, a participant mentions feeling he is an imposter when others treat him as a war hero. Although the planned interview questions did not include a question about feelings related to the reactions of others to military service, the researcher may choose to add such a question for subsequent interviews. The researcher may adapt the data collection or analysis strategies during the study; however, changes are not impulsive and must be supported with clear rationale. These changes are documented as part of maintaining rigor.

Maintaining rigor in the context of flexibility can be difficult. Therefore, we suggest that you seek primary and additional sources of guidance for understanding the philosophical base you plan to use, as well as the process of collecting and analyzing qualitative data. A research mentor, especially a researcher with more experience with the methods you are using, can be invaluable. By sharing their personal experiences with the mentees, research mentors can guide less experienced researchers in application of research principles in qualitative studies (Kostovich, Saban, & Collins, 2010).

This chapter provides examples of qualitative methods used to gather, analyze, and interpret data. Literature reviews, theoretical frameworks, study purposes, and research questions or objectives are described in the context of qualitative methods, because these are steps in the research process that are implemented somewhat differently in qualitative studies. The chapter also includes qualitative sampling and the data collection methods of observation, interviews, focus groups, and electronically mediated data. Data analysis strategies are described, and examples are provided. The chapter ends with a presentation of methods specific to different philosophical approaches.

Clinical Context and Research Problems

Qualitative studies are motivated by the desire to know more about a phenomenon, a social process, or a culture from the perspectives of the people who are experiencing the phenomenon, involved in the social process, or living in the culture (Creswell, 2007). The motivation may be that nurses realize that patient teaching is not effective with a specific group. A new project may be planned for low-income teenage mothers, but all those implementing the project are more than 40 years of age and have above average incomes. A hurricane ravages a community, and disaster relief efforts are not well received by the community. Persons with sickle cell anemia are living past age 60 years, and previous studies are focused on younger persons who are being diagnosed with the disease. Any of these situations may indicate the need for understanding the insider's perspective that could be addressed by a qualitative study.

For example, Lesniak (2010) established the need for her phenomenological study by defining the phenomenon of self-injury from the literature, indicating the problem of uncaring treatment, and identifying the nurses who could most benefit from the information:

"Self-Injury behavior is the nonsuicidal, deliberate infliction of a wound to oneself in an attempt to seek expression. Self-injury is more prevalent in the adolescent population, and often emergency and advanced practice nurses are the health professionals who encounter this phenomenon.... [M]any of these adolescents have reported receiving less than caring treatment in those emergency departments. Emergency nurses are on the frontline in many emergencies involving adolescents; therefore, a working knowledge of self-injury behavior would impact their practice. It would benefit them to be provided information concerning the characteristics of adolescents who are self-injuring, how the behavior is expressive in nature, and the repeating emotional patterns of those who self-injure (Lesniak, 2008)." (Lesniak, 2010, pp. 137-138)

Swanlund (2010) provided the rationale for her exploratory descriptive study by describing the research findings related to medication management in older adults. She noted that other researchers had focused on medication management for a single illness, instead of the more realistic situation of taking medications for multiple chronic illnesses. "Additionally, the research questions for these studies were derived from the healthcare providers' perspectives. These studies have left many questions unanswered regarding the reasons for nonadherence from the perspective of the older adult" (Swanlund, 2010, p. 23). On the basis of this reasoning, Swanlund asked 27 adults older than 74 years to describe situations that helped or hindered their ability to manage their cardiovascular medications.

Literature Review for Qualitative Studies

Both Lesniak (2010) and Swanlund (2010) conducted a review of the literature and referred to the conclusions of their review, which confirmed a lack of evidence about their topics. However, some qualitative researchers defer the literature review until after data collection and analysis to avoid biasing their analysis and interpretation of the data (Walls, Parahoo, & Fleming, 2010). Most often, qualitative researchers review the literature at the beginning of the process to establish the need for the study and to provide guidance for the development of data collection methods. A more thorough review of published research findings and theories may occur during data analysis and interpretation to "place the findings of the study in the context of what is already known about the phenomena" (Speziale & Carpenter, 2007).

Theoretical Frameworks

Most qualitative researchers do not identify specific theoretical frameworks during the design of their studies, as is expected for quantitative studies. The concern of most qualitative researchers is that designing a study in the context of a theory will influence the researcher's thinking and result in findings that are meaningful in the theoretical context but may not be true to the participants' perspectives on the topic. However, the philosophical bases for the various approaches to qualitative studies provide theoretical grounding for qualitative studies without predisposing the data analysis to a single interpretation.

Theory is an explicit component in some qualitative research designs. The expectation of grounded theory researchers is that qualitative research is inductive in nature and that theory will emerge from the data (Speziale & Carpenter, 2007; Walls et al., 2010). Parse's (2001) research methodology begins with selecting phenomena to study that are universal human experiences, move through analysis using Parse's theoretical principles as a guide, and end with evaluating the findings for their contribution to her theory. Researchers who used Parse's research methodology usually present their findings using language from Parse's theory. Chen (2010) used Parse's research method to study the lived experiences of persons with spinal cord injuries. From the stories told by the participants, Chen stated the structure of the experience in one sentence: "The lived experience of moving forward is confronting difficulties, going on and finding self-value and confidence to affirm oneself while co-creating successes amid opportunities and restrictions" (p.1138). Chen further transformed the structure through conceptual integration into the conclusion that "moving forward is transforming the valuing of originating 'enabling-limiting'" (p. 1138).

Exploratory qualitative study design may benefit from making explicit the researcher's theoretical perspective on the research problem. Scott and Wilson (2011) used the ecology theory for their qualitative study of African Americans living in the South in the United States. The ecology theory was consistent with their research objective, "identifying potential social determinants of health among African Americans in a rural community in the Deep South, from the perspectives of African American community members" (p. 3). In Singapore, researchers Cheng, Qin, and Tee (2009) interviewed patients with hematological disorders about their experiences in isolation. They noted that Maslow's (1987) hierarchy of needs theory and Roy's Adaptation Theory (1976) guided the development of the interview questions and the data analysis. Qualitative researchers who use frameworks during study development must maintain intellectual honesty to prevent the theoretical perspective from obscuring the perspectives of the participants. Your decision about whether to identify a theoretical perspective should be consistent with the research approach you have chosen. If a theoretical perspective has shaped your views of a research problem, you should acknowledge that influence and indicate explicitly the components of the study guided by the theory.

Purposes

The purpose should clearly identify the goal or aim of the study that has emerged from the research problem and literature review. The purpose of qualitative studies should include the phenomenon of interest, the population, and the setting (see Chapter 5). Ask yourself, "Can I achieve this purpose with a qualitative study?" Study purposes such as testing an intervention and determining the effectiveness of a program are not consistent with qualitative approaches. However, a qualitative researcher could address the participants' experiences with the intervention or their perceptions about a program. The purpose of qualitative studies will vary slightly depending on the qualitative approach that is being used. For example, note in Table 12-1 that the phenomenological study focused

TABLE 12-1	Selected Examples of Purpose Statements in Qualitative Studies
Qualitative Approach	**Purpose Statement**
Phenomenological research	"[E]xplore patients' lifeworld and way of managing life with advanced PD [Parkinson's disease] prior to DBS [deep brain stimulation] and to illuminate what they expect from life following DBS" (Haahr, Kirkevold, Hall, & Ostergaard, 2010, p. 410).
Grounded theory research	"[D]escribe the processes that patients in palliative home care use to maintain hope" (Ollson, Ostlund, Strang, Grassman, & Friedrichsen, 2010, p. 607).
Ethnographic research	"[U]nderstand the culture care value and beliefs of women during addiction and recovery" (Lange, 2007, p. 74).
Exploratory qualitative research	"[D]etermine the situations or variables that influence successful cardiovascular medication management, as perceived by community-dwelling adults over age 74" (Swanlund, 2010, p. 23).
Historical research	"[C]harts the international travels of four especially mobile nurses... tells these nurses' stories and analyzes their ideologies of development and progress" (Irwin, 2011, p. 78).

on life-world of the participants and the grounded theory study focused on the processes used to maintain hope. The purposes listed in Table 12-1 are consistent with the study's identified philosophical approach.

Research Objectives or Questions

Hypotheses are not appropriate for qualitative studies because hypotheses specify outcomes of studies and variables that are to be manipulated or measured, actions that are not consistent with the philosophical orientation of qualitative research. Qualitative researchers may identify research objectives or questions to connect the purpose of the study to the plan for data collection and analysis. Because qualitative research is more open-ended and the focus is on the participants' perspectives, qualitative researchers may not specify research objectives or research questions in order to avoid prematurely narrowing the topic. In their study of the occupational stress of children's palliative care nurses, McCloskey and Taggart (2010) identified two research objectives:

> "Two objectives were set. Firstly, to explore the experiences of occupational stress within nurses working in three distinct young people's palliative care services (i.e., hospice care, hospital care and community care) and secondly, to examine the consequences of such stress upon the nurses' lives." (McCloskey & Taggart, 2010, p. 234)

These objectives clearly stated and did not limit what the researcher might find. These are ideal characteristics of objectives for a qualitative study. McCloskey and Taggart (2010) found four themes that described the experiences of the nurses: work demands, relationships, maintaining control, and support and roles. The theme of relationships was seen as particularly challenging because of emotional demands and ethical conflicts.

A research question establishes "the perimeters of the project and suggest the methods to be used for data gathering and analysis" (Corbin & Strauss, 2008, p. 19). Research questions may be broadly stated or may be based on a theoretical framework if the researcher has identified a framework. Schumacher (2010) identified Leininger's (1985) theory of culture care diversity and universality as the conceptual guide for her ethnographic study with persons in rural Dominican Republic. Schumacher identified four comprehensive research questions based on the theory. Questions 2 and 4 are provided as examples:

> "Research Question 2: In what ways do technological, religious, philosophical, kinship and social, cultural, political and legal, economic, and educational factors influence care meanings, beliefs, and practices of Dominicans?...
>
> "Research Question 4: In what ways can Leininger's care modes of preservation/maintenance, accommodation/negotiation, and repatterning/restructuring be used to plan nursing care that is culturally congruent for rural Dominicans?" (Schumacher, 2010, p. 94)

Schumacher (2010) developed research questions that were congruent with Leininger's theory. When a researcher identifies a conceptual framework or guiding theory for a study, the research questions

should be congruent with the theory. Schumacher clearly stated appropriately broad questions that included the study's sample (rural Dominicans) and desired outcome (plan culturally congruent nursing care). The following three themes were identified, each consistent with Leininger's theory: "(a) family presence is essential for meaningful care experiences and care practices, (b) respect and attention are central to the meaning of care, and (c) rural Dominicans both value and use generic (folk) and professional care practices" (Schumacher, 2010, p. 97).

Obtaining Research Participants

The goal of sampling for quantitative studies is to obtain data from a subgroup of a population that is statistically representative of the population with the intent of being able to generalize the findings to the population (see Chapter 15). Qualitative researchers seek participants who have experienced the phenomenon of interest (Speziale & Carpenter, 2007) and are thus deemed to be "information-rich cases for in-depth study" (Liamputtong & Ezzy, 2005, p. 46). For ethnographic studies, the participants may also include key informants who are knowledgeable of the culture being studied. The selection of participants is nonrandom and may not be totally specified before the study begins.

Depending on the research question and the aims of the study, the researcher may use more than one sampling strategy during the study. For example, a researcher who is studying the experience of reacting to a diagnosis of breast cancer may choose to select only women who have not previously been diagnosed with cancer, have not had a family member die from breast cancer, and have been diagnosed within the last 6 weeks. This approach to sampling is called criterion sampling. Similar logic can be applied to identify participants for a focus group, when it is desirable to have participants who can identify with each other's experiences. When used for focus groups, this sampling method is called *homogeneous group sampling* (Liamputtong & Ezzy, 2005). Table 12-2 provides definitions and references for sampling strategies that are frequently used by qualitative researchers. These sampling strategies are not mutually exclusive and may be labeled differently by various researchers.

The sample for a rigorous qualitative study is not as large as the sample for a rigorous quantitative study. The researcher stops collecting data when enough rich, meaningful data have been obtained to achieve the study aims. For new researchers, this answer to "How big should my sample be?" is totally unsatisfactory. When applying for human subjects' approval, the

TABLE 12-2	Sampling Strategies used by Qualitative Researchers
Sampling	**Definition**
Convenience sampling	Inviting participants from a location or group because of ease and efficiency.
Snowball sampling	Researcher asks participants to refer others who have had similar experiences to participate in the study; also called chain sampling or network sampling.
Historical sampling	Exhaustive search for all relevant, surviving primary and secondary sources about an event or phenomenon that occurred in the past (Lundy, 2012).
Purposive sampling	Recruitment of participants as sources of data that can provide and expand upon the data needed to achieve the study aims.
Theoretical sampling*	Recruitment of participants who are considered to be best sources of data related to the study (Wuest, 2012); additional participants may be recruited to validate or expand upon emerging concepts; associated with grounded theory approaches.
Criterion sampling*	Recruitment of participants who do or do not have certain characteristics deemed to affect the phenomena being studied (Liamputtong & Ezzy, 2005).
Maximum variation sampling*	Recruitment of participants who represent potentially different experiences related to the domain of interest (Seidman, 2006).
Critical case sampling*	Recruitment of participants whose experiences with the research topic are expected to be very different.
Deviant case sampling*	Recruitment of participants who may be outliers or represent extreme cases of the domain of interest.

*Considered by some authors to be subtypes of purposive sampling.

researcher will be asked the maximum sample size. Giving a generous range of 12 to 25 can be a way to answer this question but will depend on the study design. Researchers who use focus groups often have larger samples. The actual number depends on when data saturation is achieved. **Data saturation** is the point when new data begins to repeat what has already been found. Patterns emerge in the data. The researcher has the data needed to answer the research question and remain true to the principles of the study design. Marshall and Rossman (2011) indicate that a better term is *theoretical sufficiency*, because one can never completely know all there is to know about a topic. Chapter 15 also provides some detailed ideas about sampling methods and sample size in qualitative studies.

Researcher-Participant Relationships

One of the important differences between quantitative research and qualitative research is the nature of relationships between the researcher and the individuals being studied. The nature of these relationships has an impact on the data collected and their interpretation. In varying degrees, the researcher influences the individuals being studied and, in turn, is influenced by them. The mere presence of the researcher may alter behavior in the setting. The researcher desires to connect at the human level with the participant (Corbin & Strauss, 2008). Although this involvement is considered a source of bias in quantitative research, qualitative researchers consider it to be a natural and necessary element of the research process. Shorter and Stayt (2010, p. 161) noted that "the research findings are thus a product of a co-constructive process between researcher and participant."

The researcher's personality is a key factor in qualitative research, in which skills in empathy and intuition are cultivated. You will need to become closely involved in the subject's experience to interpret it. Participants need to feel safe and to be able to trust the researcher prior to sharing their deepest experiences with the researcher. It is necessary for you to be open to the perceptions of the participants rather than attaching your own meaning to the experience. To do this, you need to be aware of personal experiences and potential biases related to the phenomenon being studied. It is helpful to document these experiences and potential biases before and during the study in a reflective journal, to be able to set them aside or bracket them. For example, a researcher who plans to interview women undergoing irradiation for breast cancer would need to acknowledge that his/her own mother died from complications of breast cancer. This awareness and ability to be involved with the participants and yet be able to analyze the data abstractly with intellectual honesty is called **reflexivity**. Reflexivity consists of the ability to be aware of your biases and past experiences that might influence how you would respond to a participant or interpret the data. This ability is critical in qualitative studies because data emerge from a relationship with the participant and are analyzed in the mind of the researcher, rather than through a statistical program (Wolf, 2012).

Data Collection Methods

Because data collection occurs simultaneously with data analysis in qualitative studies, the process is complex. Collecting data is not a mechanical process that can be completely planned before it is initiated. The researcher as a whole person is completely involved—perceiving, reacting, interacting, reflecting, attaching meaning, and recording. For a particular study, the researcher may need to address data collection issues related to relationships between the researcher and the participants, reflect on the meanings obtained from the data, and organize management and reduction of large volumes of data. Qualitative researchers are not limited to a single type of data or collection method during a study. For example, one research team used interviews and focus groups in their study of fall prevention for older people in the community (Dickinson, Machen, Horton, Jain, & Maddex, 2011). Lopez (2009) used data from semi-structured interviews, nonparticipant observation, and informal conversational interviews to describe the processes used to make decisions about the care of nursing home residents who become acutely ill. Quali tative data collection may also be combined in a study with the collection of quantitative data. These mixed-methods studies are described in detail in Chapter 10.

Observations, interviews, and focus groups are the most common methods of gathering qualitative data, and each is described in detail, followed by an example from the literature. Electronic means of qualitative data collection, such as photographs, videos, and blogs, are briefly described as well. Following the general types of data collection, methods specific to each qualitative approach are discussed.

Observations

In many qualitative studies, the researcher observes social behavior and may participate in social interactions with those being studied. **Observation** is collecting data through listening, smelling, touching, and seeing, with an emphasis on what is seen. Even when other data collection methods are being used, such as interviews, you want to stay aware of your surroundings and attend to the nonverbal communication that occurs between the participant and others in the immediate surroundings (Marshall & Rossman, 2011). **Unstructured observation** involves spontaneously observing and recording what one sees. Although unstructured observations give the observer freedom, there is a risk that the observer may lose objectivity or may not remember all of the details of the event. The most complete way to collect observation data is to video-record the situation being studied, but doing so may alter the behavior of those being observed or may not be possible because of confidentiality concerns. If video recording is not possible, then the researcher may take notes during the observation

periods. If taking notes is a problem, then the researcher needs to record the observations as soon as possible afterwards.

Collecting data through unstructured observation may evolve into more structured observations. The researcher may begin with few predetermined ideas about what will be observed. As the study progresses, the researcher clarifies the situations or areas of focus that are most relevant to the research questions and begins to structure the observation. A researcher observing parent behavior in an ambulatory pediatric care clinic may initially focus on the interaction of parents with their children in the waiting area and in the room with the provider. During data collection, the researcher begins to notice common nurturing behaviors of the parents and, from these observations, develops a checklist to use while observing. In this way, the researcher has structured the observations that might be the focus of future studies. Other researchers may enter the setting with a checklist or tool for documenting observations and revise the tool as needed. The notes made during and immediately following the observations are called **field notes** (Speziale & Carpenter, 2007). Recording observations can be as simple as using a pad and writing utensil in a public place or as sophisticated as producing an electronic diagram of the locations of nurses by having them wear positioning devices. Observations may be supplemented by taking photographs in the setting or video recording an observation. After the observation, the diagrams of the nurses' positions, the photographs, or the videos may serve to remind the observer of specific elements of the situation. In addition, the researcher may analyze the video by viewing short segments and making notes about each. By reflecting on the photographs and videos, the researcher may identify details that were not captured in the actual observation. The field notes, notes about the electronic records made during the observation, and the researcher's memories of and reflections about being in the setting are the data that are analyzed.

The researcher, by virtue of being in the setting, becomes a participant to some degree. The balance between participation and observation has been described in four ways. The first is **complete participation**. The people in the situation may not be aware that the participant is a researcher (Speziale & Carpenter, 2007). In public settings, a researcher can ethically observe people and interactions without obtaining permission (Liamputtong & Ezzy, 2005). In less public settings, the researcher may observe others who learn later that he or she is a researcher. When the researcher's role is unknown to the study participants, they need to have consented to incomplete disclosure before the study is conducted. After the study, they must be debriefed regarding the undisclosed aspects of the study (see Chapter 9). The participants have the option as to whether the data the researcher collected about them is included or not in the study. When the researcher is in the **participant as observer** role, participants are aware of the dual roles of the researcher from the beginning of the study. Full engagement in the situation may interfere with the researcher's ability to note important details and move within the setting to follow an evolving situation. In these situations, the role of **observer as participant** may be more appropriate. As the term indicates, the researcher's observer role takes priority and is the focus of the data collection. **Complete observation** occurs when the researcher remains passive and has no direct social interaction in the situation.

When the researcher is observing for the purposes of data collection, multiple types of information should be noted. The observer may gather data on the physical setting, the people in the setting, and their activities and interactions. Activities and interactions can be described in terms of their frequency, duration, precipitating factors, and organization. Hall, Pedersen, and Fairley (2010) observed the activities and interactions of nurses during their work on medical and surgical units in three hospitals. The data from 480 hours of observations were analyzed to produce a framework to describe interruptions by source, type, cause, the activity that was interrupted, and the outcomes of the interruptions. In addition to interviewing nurses in a burn intensive care unit, Zengerle-Levy (2006) observed them for 134 hours as they cared for pediatric patients. Through observation, the researcher was able to "uncover common practices that were not articulated" about how they cared for children in the unit in which parents were absent (p.227). Hall et al. (2010) used observation as the primary source of data. Zengerle-Levy (2006) used observations to supplement the data collected during the interview. In both cases, the researchers clearly described the purpose of the observations and details such as total time spent and types of activities observed. This information indicates that observations were effectively used and the study was rigorous.

Example Study Using Observation

Lauzon Clabo (2008) studied pain assessment on two postoperative units in a teaching hospital. During the first phase of the study, her primary method of data collection was observation. Note the emphasis placed on gaining access to the setting.

> "[T]he focus was on gaining entry to the hospital and simultaneously to each unit, establishing the researcher's role, developing relationships with the nursing staff, becoming familiar with the general routines and rhythms of practice, as well as beginning to map out the social context of each unit. During this phase, the primary method was participant observation. The researcher (LLC) [one of the authors] was present on the unit through the course of normal care primarily for the purpose of observation, but also interacted informally with staff in hallway conversations. Data were recorded and analysed on an ongoing basis using field notes that included a daily event log and a series of observational, theoretical and methodological notes." (Lauzon Clabo, 2008, p. 533)

Lauzon Clabo (2008) followed the initial phase of data collection with observations of individual nurses on the day shift. Each of these observations was followed by an interview with the nurse.

> "The observations provided an overall sense of how any one nurse went about conducting a pain assessment, while the semi-structured interviews captured more detail regarding the nurse's actual thinking, especially in regard to the approaches used to assess each client's pain." (Lauzon Clabo, 2008, p. 533)

The final phase of the study was a focus group on each unit, during which Lauzon Clabo (2008) presented a rough draft of the findings for that unit. On Unit A, the nurses had similar expectations for level and type of pain for specific surgical procedures. They found caring for patients whose pain did not follow the usual trajectory to be challenging because of the need to contact the physician frequently and the desire to keep the physician happy. On Unit B, the nurses focused on the patient's description of his or her pain and supplemented it with objective and subjective data, such as the use of pain medications. Lauzon Clabo (2008) concluded that pain assessment was a synthesis of the patient's narrative, evidence from behaviors and medication usage, and expectations based on experience. This study had rigorous methodology as evidenced by the researcher's going back to the nurses as individuals (interviews) and as a group (focus group) to supplement and validate the initial findings. This rigor gives the reader of the study confidence to view the results as credible. The clinical implications are that nurses must allow the patient's narrative to take precedence over behaviors, medication usage, and the nurses' expectations in the assessment of postoperative pain.

Interviews

Interviews are interactions between the participant and the qualitative researcher that produce data as words. The researcher as an interviewer seeks information from a number of individuals, whereas the focus group strategy is designed to obtain the perspective of the normative group, not individual perspectives. Interviews may also be conducted in quantitative studies to assist subjects in the completion of a survey or questionnaire. This assistance may include reading the questions to subjects with limited literacy and documenting their responses to the questions in person or over the phone. The focus of this section is interviewing in qualitative studies.

Depending on the research question, the qualitative researcher may conduct multiple interviews with each participant or may follow an initial interview with another during which the participant can review the researcher's description of the first interview. Seidman (2006) recommends that the researcher interview each participant three times for phenomenological studies. The first interview is focused on a life history, the second on details of the phenomenon, and the third on reflection on the experience. Using multiple interviews allows the relationship between the researcher and the participant to develop. Over time, the participant may learn to trust the researcher more and reveal insights about his or her experiences that contribute to the study's findings. Follow-up interviews may be used to share the results of the ongoing data analysis with participants and ask additional questions for clarification. Multiple interviews may be required to study an ongoing process. For a grounded theory study of women undergoing coronary artery bypass graft surgery, Banner (2010a) interviewed the women preoperatively and at 6 weeks and 6 months after surgery.

In addition to determining how many times each participant will be interviewed, the researcher will need to plan the interview location, format, and method of documenting the interview. Interviews might be conducted in a room in a public library, a fast-food restaurant at an off-peak time, an exam room in a clinic, or the participant's home. The location should be selected as a neutral place that has

private areas, is convenient for the participant (Speziale & Carpenter, 2007), and considers the safety of those involved. Accessibility and confidentiality should also be considerations. An exam room may not be a neutral site for a study exploring the patient-provider relationship. During a community-based study, the researcher's appearance may become associated with a stigmatized topic, such as HIV infection, substance use, or domestic violence. A public place may not protect the participant's identity and confidentiality. A participant's home may not be safe for the researcher to come to at certain times of day. A participant's home, however, can offer a sense of comfort and familiarity for the participant and provide the researcher insight into the participant's experience. Gharaibeh and Owels (2009) conducted a qualitative study of Jordanian women who stayed in abusive relationships ($N = 28$). They allowed participants to "choose the place of the interview in order to make them feel comfortable and secure" (p. 379). All participants chose to be interviewed in their homes when the husband or other relatives were not present.

The format of the interview can be unstructured, semistructured, or structured. **Unstructured interviews** are informal and conversational and may be useful during an ethnographical study or the early stages of a study. Most qualitative interviews are **semistructured**, or organized around a set of open-ended questions. Some experts call these *topical* or *guided interviews* (Marshall & Rossman, 2011). The degree of guidance may be as minimal as having one initial abstract question or prompt or as structured as multiple predefined questions to narrow the interview to specific aspects of the phenomenon being studied. In either case, the researcher remains open to how the participant responds and carefully words follow-up questions or prompts to allow the **emic view**, the participant's perspective, to emerge. **Structured interviews** are organized with narrower questions in a specific order. The questions may be asked without follow-up questions, and the researcher responses may be scripted in a structured interview (Marshall & Rossman, 2011). Having this level of structure may decrease the anxiety of less experienced interviewers but may result in findings that reflect the **etic**, or outsider's, **view**.

The words spoken and the nonverbal communication during an interview are the data. Some researchers prefer to audio-record or video-record the interview and focus on the interaction and relationship with the participant during the interview (Banner, 2010b). A recording of the interview results in a "transportable, repeatable resource that allows multiple hearings or viewings as well as access to other readers" (Nikander, 2008, p. 229). The participant must be aware that the interview is being electronically recorded, but the less obtrusive the equipment, the more quickly the participant will forget its presence, relax, and speak more freely. Logistically, the researcher needs to plan ahead to have the power cords or batteries needed for the recording device (Banner, 2010b). Using batteries may make the device less obtrusive. A sensitive microphone will allow you to pick up even faint or distorted voices, thereby increasing your ability to make an accurate transcription later. If tapes are being used, ensure that the lengths of the tapes are adequate to record the entire interview with few interruptions to change the tape. More likely, the recording will be made on a digital device that can be saved on a computer for transcription. In some situations, recording devices may not be appropriate or the participant may prefer that the interview not be recorded. During the unrecorded interviews, the researcher may take notes and set aside time immediately following the interview to document the interview with as much detail as possible.

Learning to Interview

Preparing to interview is critical because interviewing is a skill that directly affects the quality of the data produced (Marshall & Rossman, 2011). Researchers must give themselves the opportunity to develop this skill before they start interviewing study participants. A skilled interviewer can elicit higher-quality data than an inexperienced interviewer by allowing for silence or asking a probing follow-up question without alienating the participant. Unskilled interviewers may not know how or when to intervene, when to encourage the participant to continue to elaborate, or when to divert to another subject. The interviewer must know how to handle intrusive questions. For practice, conduct interviews with colleagues with experience in interviewing (Munhall, 2012). These rehearsals will help you identify problems before initiating the study (Banner, 2010b). You may want to conduct one or more trial interviews with individuals who meet the sampling criteria to allow you to try out the proposed questions. Practice sessions and pilot interviews also allow you to determine a realistic time estimate for the interviews. Researchers often underestimate the time needed for an interview. Allow yourself enough time so that you can conduct the interview without feeling rushed. Be sensitive to time-related concerns of the participants, however, and offer the option of stopping if an interview is going longer than expected.

Participants may need to be able to catch a bus to get home, pick up children from child care, or stop to take a dose of medication.

Establishing a Positive Environment for an Interview

When preparing for an interview, establish an environment that encourages an open, relaxed conversation. Be sensitive to the physical surroundings. Sit in comfortable chairs so that neither you nor the participant is facing windows with direct sunlight. Sitting at a table may be more comfortable and provides a surface for the participant to sign the consent form or complete a demographic form. You may want to offer water or other beverage as a way to provide time for a social connection prior to beginning the interview. When dressing for an interview, the researcher needs to consider how the participant is likely to be dressed. Dressing in formal business attire or a nursing uniform may emphasize the power differences in the relationship. Dressing too casually may be viewed as an indication that the interaction is not important to the researcher. Power issues may affect the effectiveness of the interview.

Conducting an Effective Interview

As the researcher, you have the power to shape the interview agenda. Participants have the power to choose the level of responses they will provide. You might begin the interview with a broad request such as "Describe for me your experience with…" or "Tell me about…." Ideally, the participant will respond as though she or he is telling a story. You respond nonverbally with a nod or eye contact to convey your interest in what is being said. Try to avoid agreeing or disagreeing with what the participant is saying. Being nonjudgmental allows the participants to share their experiences more freely. When it seems appropriate, encourage your subject to elaborate further on a particular dimension of the topic. Use of nonthreatening but thought-provoking questions is often called **probing**. Participants may need validation that they are providing the needed information. Some participants may give short answers, so you may have to encourage them to elaborate. When the participant stops talking, ask a follow-up question that reflects back on what you have heard. Interviewer responses should be encouraging and supportive without being leading. Listening more and talking less is a key principle of effective interviews (Seidman, 2006). That includes tolerating silence. If the participant is not talking but seems to be thinking or considering the topic, stay quiet. Silence can be a powerful invitation that allows the participant to show deeper emotions and thoughts.

Problems during Interviews

Difficulties can occur during interviews. Common problems include interruptions such as telephone calls or text messages, "stage fright" that often arises when the participant realizes he or she is being recorded, failure to establish a rapport with your subject, verbose participants, and those who tend to wander off the subject. Turn off or silence your cell phone at the beginning of the interview, and ask the participant to do the same. If a participant seems paralyzed by the presence of the recording device, move the device out of his or her line of sight if possible. Ask demographic questions or factual questions to ease into the interview. When the participant moves to a subject that you think is unrelated to the focus of the study, you may want to ask how this new subject is related to previous comments on the topic of interest. You may be surprised to learn that what you perceived to be unrelated is associated with the topic in the participant's perspective. You may also need to tactfully guide the interview back to the topic. Remind participants that they can decline answering any question and can end the interview at any time.

The physical, mental, and emotional condition of the participant may cause difficulties during the interview. The data you obtain are affected by characteristics of the person being interviewed. These include age, ethnicity, gender, professional background, educational level, and relative status of interviewer and interviewee as well as impairments in vision or hearing, speech impediments, fatigue, pain, poor memory, disorientation, emotional state, and language difficulties. Although institutional review boards tend to view interviews as noninvasive, interviews are an invasion of the psyche. For some participants, the experience may be therapeutic. However, an interview is capable of producing risks to the health of the participant. Therefore, the interviewer must always avoid inflicting unnecessary harm upon the participant. Participants with fatigue or pain related to illness or treatments should be offered the opportunity to stop, take a break, or schedule a second interview for another day.

In a phenomenological study of persons hospitalized for depression, Moyle (2002) noted challenges with obtaining rich data due to the flattened emotions and slowed cognition that may result from severe depression. During the study, some of the participants underwent electroconvulsive therapy that led to some memory loss. The participants in Moyle's study had health professionals readily available because they were hospitalized. In other settings, the researcher needs to prepare to refer the participant if necessary. Emotional expression during an interview may be expected, depending on the topic. When the participant becomes distressed or overcome with emotion, however, you may choose to turn off the recording device and stop the interview completely or for a few minutes. You may be able to continue if the participant is able to become composed. Stay with the individual, offer a tissue, and move closer to the participant. Recognize topics that are more likely to be distressing, and have a plan developed for emergency assistance if needed or a list of mental professionals available if support or a referral is needed. For example, you might schedule interviews in collaboration with the chaplain or psychiatric mental health nurse practitioner to ensure that one of them is available for consultation when you will be interviewing family members whose spouses are receiving hospice care. Recognize that you, the researcher, may also need emotional and psychological support. The researcher may be strongly affected by the stories of the participants. Arrange to have a mentor or trusted friend available to talk with before or after interviews. The researcher may need to rest following an interview, because the experience requires heightened focus for an extended period, which can result in fatigue (Creswell, 2007).

Example Study Using Interviews

Greco, Nail, Kendall, Cartwright, and Messecar (2010), in the report of their grounded theory study on mammography decision making among older women ($N = 23$), limited the sample to women who were 55 years or older and had at least one relative who had been diagnosed with breast cancer. They clearly described the rationale for the study, the selection of participants, and collection of data in the following excerpt:

"[D]ecision-making studies of women with a breast cancer family history have largely focused on younger women who have undergone genetic testing for breast cancer disposition.... In this study, older woman are defined as 55 years of age and older since 65% of the breast cancers occur in this age group.... Women who met the study criteria and agreed to participate were interviewed in person at a private place of their choosing. Recruitment was discontinued when the analysis provided no new information contributing to the development of the theory. The

> researcher conducted open-ended interviews using a semi-structured interview guide. For the purpose of describing the participants, demographic data were collected at the end of the interview. Field notes were maintained to describe the environmental and emotional context of the interviews. Interviews were recorded and transcribed verbatim, with all personally identifying information deleted." (Greco et al., 2010, p. 349-350)

Greco et al. (2010) used a collaborative process to come to consensus during the data collection and analysis process. In addition, some participants were interviewed a second time to assist in refining the theory. These actions strengthened the data collection and analysis process and improved the credibility of the findings. The researchers produced a theory they called "guarding against cancer" (p. 351). Study limitations included an all-white sample and the use of self-report for mammograms. Implications for practice are that health professionals recommending that a woman obtain a mammogram was a strong motivator. Another was that older women may believe they no longer need to be screened and so may stop obtaining mammograms.

Focus Groups

Focus groups were designed to obtain the participants' perceptions in a focused area in a setting that is permissive and nonthreatening. One of the assumptions underlying the use of focus groups is that interactions among people can help them to express and clarify their views in ways that are less likely to occur in a one-on-one interview (Gray, 2009). People in a focus group who are alike in some characteristic may feel safer or less anxious when talking about difficult experiences. Many different communication forms occur in focus groups, including teasing, arguing, joking, anecdotes, and nonverbal clues, such as gesturing, facial expressions, and other body language.

Focus groups as a means of data collection serve a variety of purposes in nursing research. Focus groups have been used to understand the experiences of people who are receiving care or may need care. Researchers have used focus groups to explore the fatigue of patients following a stroke (Finn & Stube, 2010) and the social support needs of older African Americans who have survived cancer (Hamilton, Moore, Powe, Agarwai, & Martin, 2010). The use of prescription medications without medical care of

Latino immigrants (Coffman, Shobe, & O'Connell, 2008) and the excessive drinking of college students (Dodd, Glassman, Arthur, Webb, & Miller, 2010) have also been studied by means of focus groups. Using focus groups, researchers have explored nurses' experiences such as the stress of providing palliative care for children (McCloskey & Taggart, 2010) and the strategies used in critical care units to prevent and correct medical errors (Henneman et al., 2010). Focus groups of nurses have also been the data collection method for studies of the barriers school nurses encounter when talking to parents about their children's weight (Steele et al., 2011) and teamwork as experienced by nurses in the neonatal intensive care units and emergency departments (Simmons & Sherwood, 2010).

Instrument development and refinement are frequently based on the data collected during focus groups. An example of instrument development was the study conducted by Anatchkova and Bjorner (2010). They conducted focus groups to identify key elements of role functioning as a part of health. The roles identified were to be used to develop items for research instruments measuring quality of life. An example of instrument refinement was the study conducted by Owen-Smith, Sterk, McCarty, Hankeson-Dyson, and DiClemente (2010). Their sample consisted of persons diagnosed with AIDS who used complementary and alternative medicine (CAM) therapies. During two focus groups, the researchers provided the copy of an existing measure of CAM use and asked each participant to complete the instrument. Following completion of the instrument, the participants were asked to identify the strengths and limitations of the instrument. The third and fourth focus groups were not given the CAM instrument but were asked to describe what CAM meant to them. By combining the data from the focus groups, the researchers developed a revised CAM instrument. They validated their findings by having participants in a fifth focus group complete a computer-based version of the revised instrument and provide feedback. This rigorous process produced a revised instrument that will be appropriate for use with the persons diagnosed with AIDS.

The effective use of focus groups requires careful planning. The location needs to be carefully selected to ensure privacy, comfort, and safety. Meeting rooms in public facilities such as schools, libraries, or churches may be appropriate community locations for focus groups, depending on the research question and the study aims. For focus groups with specific populations, the facility used for support services may have a quiet room that is accessible and known to participants. Nurses or other health professionals may participate in focus groups in the healthcare facility but might be more forthcoming in a location away from the facility. For a focus group with Hispanic persons who were infected with HIV, a hospital meeting room was selected. When the research team approached the reception desk in a hospital waiting area to ask the location of the room, the staff person stated the location of the "AIDS focus group" in a loud voice heard by the waiting visitors (Gray, 2009). In this case, the researchers' schedule for travel to the out-of-town focus group did not allow for previewing the location so they did not have the opportunity to inform the reception staff of the name being used for the focus group meeting. If a focus group is planned for a sensitive topic, indicate on the invitation and any materials the name by which the group will be identified. For example, instead of identifying the group as the "Testicular Cancer Study," a better name might be the "Men's Health Study."

Other logistics include the expected length of the meeting, recruiting subjects, and recording the group interaction. Focus groups typically last from 45 minutes to $1\frac{1}{2}$ hours. Liamputtong and Ezzy (2005) indicate that a group might go as long as 3 hours but that participants will begin to tire before 2 hours have passed. Be clear on the recruitment materials about the expected duration of the focus group. Allow for the time it will take to complete consent and demographic forms in determining the length of the data collection process. Provide a reasonable estimate of the time needed, recognizing that whether people attend may be affected by how long the group is expected to last.

Recruiting appropriate participants for each of the focus groups is critical, because recruitment is the most common source of failure. Each focus group should consist of 4 to 12 participants (Marshall & Rossman, 2011). If there are fewer participants, the discussion tends to be inadequate. In most cases, participants are expected to be unknown to one another. However, for a focus group targeting professional groups such as clinical nurses or nurse educators, such anonymity usually is not possible. You may use purposive sampling to seek out individuals known to have the desired expertise (see Chapter 15). In other cases, you may look for participants through the media, posters, or advertisements. A single contact with an individual who agrees to attend a focus group does not ensure that this person will attend the group session. You will need to make repeated phone calls and remind the candidates by mail. You may need to offer compensation for their time and effort in the form of cash, phone card, gift card, or bus token incentives. Cash payments are, of course, the most effective if the resources are available through funding. Other incentives include refreshments at the focus group meeting, T-shirts, coffee mugs, gift certificates, and coupons. Over-recruiting may be necessary; a good rule is to invite two more potential participants than you need for the group.

Recruiting participants with common social and cultural experiences creates more homogeneous groups (Liamputtong & Ezzy, 2005). Selecting participants who are similar to one another in lifestyle or experiences, views, and characteristics is believed to facilitate open discussion and interaction. These characteristics might be age, gender, social class, income level, ethnicity, culture, lifestyle, or health status. For example, for a study of barriers to implementing HIV/AIDS clinical trials in low-income minority communities, focus groups might be organized by race/ethnicity and gender. In heterogeneous groups, communication patterns, roles, relationships, and traditions might interfere with the interactions within the focus group. Be cautious about bringing together participants with considerable variation in social standing, education, or authority, because some group members may hesitate to participate fully, whereas others may discount the input of those with perceived lower standing.

Establish a setting for your focus group that is relaxed. There should be space for participants to sit comfortably in a circle or U shape and maintain eye contact with one another. Ensure that the acoustics of the room will allow you to obtain a quality audio-recording of the sessions. As with the one-on-one interview discussed earlier, place your audio or video recorders unobtrusively. Use a highly sensitive microphone. Hiring a court reporter to do a real-time transcription may have advantages over recording the interaction for transcription later (Scott et al., 2009). Inaudible voices on the recording or overlapping voices can pose challenges to later transcription.

The facilitator is critical to the success of a focus group. Select a facilitator when possible who reflects the age, gender, and race/ethnicity of the group. The researcher may be the facilitator of the group or may train another person for the role. Training of the facilitator should be thorough and allow time for practice (Gray, 2009). The facilitator, sometime called the moderator, needs to deeply understand the aims of the focus groups and to communicate these aims to the participants before the group session. Instruct participants that all points of view are valid and helpful and that speakers should not be asked to defend their positions. Make clear to the group that the facilitator's role is to moderate the discussion, not to contribute. In addition to the moderator, you may want to have an observer or assistant moderator who takes notes, especially of facial expressions or interactions not captured by the recording (Liamputtong & Ezzy, 2005). Making notes on the dynamics of the group is also useful. Note how group members interact with one another.

Carefully plan the questions that are to be asked during the focus group and, if time permits, pilot-test them. Limit the number of questions to those most essential to allow adequate time for discussion. You may elect to give participants some of the questions before the group meeting to enable them to give careful thought to their responses. Questions should be posed in such a way that group members can build on the responses of others in the group, raise their own questions, and question one another. Probes can be used to elicit richer details, by means of questions such as "How would that make a difference?" or responses such as "Tell us more about that situation." Avoid pushing participants toward taking a stand and defending it. Once rapport has been established, you may be able to question or challenge ideas and increase group interaction.

The researcher and/or facilitator may come to the focus groups with preconceived ideas about the topic. Early in the session, provide opportunities for participants to express their views on the topic of discussion. Use probes or questions if the discussion wanders too far from the focus of the study. A good facilitator will weave questions into the discussion naturally. The facilitator's role is to clarify, paraphrase, and reflect back what group members have said. These discussions tend to express group norms, and individual voices of dissent may be stifled. However, when a sensitive topic is being discussed, the group may actively facilitate the discussion because less inhibited members break the ice for those who are more reticent. Participants may also provide group support for expressing feelings, opinions, or experiences. Late in the session, the facilitator may encourage group members to go beyond the current discussion or debate and reflect on inconsistencies among the views of participants and within their own thinking.

Example Study Using Focus Groups

Taylor and Burch (2011) conducted focus groups to evaluate an enhanced recovery protocol (ERP) that was developed for patients undergoing colorectal surgery. The following excerpt gives further details:

"Patients who had entered onto the ERP between 1 September 2008 and 28 February 2009, and lived locally (i.e., within 1 hour's drive from the hospital) were included. Fifty patients who met these criteria were identified from the ERP database. They were contacted by post, inviting them to participate and explaining what the focus groups would involve and how their participation could help. If willing to participate, patients completed a detachable slip at the bottom of the letter stating their availability for one of three planned focus group sessions. It was hoped that 4-6 people would participate in each session.

"A quiet non-clinical room was arranged which had a circular table allowing participants to maintain eye contact with each other. Refreshments were offered, enabling informal interaction before the focus groups began. The focus groups commenced with an introduction by the facilitators (CT and JB) explaining the purpose and how the session would run. Written consent was obtained using a specifically developed participant information sheet. Initial ground rules were generated to ensure everyone's opinions were respected and heard without interruption, and confidentiality would be maintained." (Taylor & Burch, 2011, p. 287)

The researchers invited 50 participants, but only 10 patients and 3 relatives participated in the three focus groups. One group had two patients; the second had four patients and two relatives; and the third had four patients and one relative. The low response rate and the small sample may have limited the data that were collected. The data reflected those who participated but may not have accurately reflected other patients in the enhanced recovery protocol program. The researchers could have been clearer about whether the invited participants were continuing to receive care from the hospital. If so, some participants may have hesitated to participate, especially if their perceptions of the program were less than satisfactory. The data from the focus groups revealed that environmental details such as hot meals and available washing facilities for family members were as important as the clinical aspects of the care they received.

Electronically Mediated Data

Images created by still and video photography and Internet communication are newer methods of qualitative data collection that are being used by health-related researchers. Each is described briefly, and an example provided. Prior to using one of these forms of data, the reader is encouraged to study in greater depth the technology used and the ethical issues due to potential loss of confidentiality and breach of the privacy of participants' protected health information (see Chapter 9).

Anthropologists and historical researchers have included photographs as data in their studies for many years. However, creating photographic images as part of data collection is emerging as a viable scientific method in different types of qualitative and quantitative studies the past few years. The ubiquitous nature of digital photography is likely to speed the acceptance of the method. When used as research data, photographs and videos may be made by participants, researchers, or a combination of the two. **Photovoice** is the idea of "recording and reflecting on the strengths and concerns" of one's community and is most often used in participatory research studies (Findholt, Michael, & Davis, 2011, p. 186). Caroline Wang and her colleagues are credited with guiding the first health-related study during which rural Chinese women were given cameras to photograph their lives and especially their health needs (Wang, Burris, & Ping, 1996). Wang called this practice *photo novella,* but others since have used the term photovoice. Nurse researchers have used photovoice in studies with rural adolescents to increase awareness of childhood obesity and the need for prevention (Findholt et al., 2011) and with siblings in families with children who have Down syndrome (Rampton et al., 2007). Other health-related studies conducted by non-nurses have included studies with older adults who experience chronic pain (Baker & Wang, 2006) and with African American men in rural and urban communities to explore their perceptions of social and cultural factors that affect individual and community health (Ornelas et al., 2009).

Photovoice is a creative way to facilitate communication across cultures. Cooper and Yarborough (2010) first conducted a focus group with 20 traditional birth attendants or comodronas in rural Guatemala. They defined *comodronas* as "generally older women who have become recognized for their knowledge and experience in caring for pregnant women, delivering babies, and caring for the neonate and the mother post delivery" (p. 646). After the focus group, six participants were given disposable 35-mm cameras and asked to take photographs of positive and negative aspects of health in their communities. The researchers asked the comodronas to obtain written consent from any persons in the photographs and not to take any photographs that would put themselves at risk for

harm. These cameras were collected and the photographs processed by the local research assistant using research funds. Four months later, the researchers returned to Guatemala and each of the photographs was discussed with the photographers in a second focus group. The researchers noted the differences in the focus group discussions. "Although the first phase produced specific and concrete ideas and concerns, such as specific illnesses and environmental problems, the second phase elicited, for the most part, a 'peeling back' of health issues" (p. 649). For example, a picture of a basin of water and a dipper took on new meaning when the photographer explained that this represented the entire daily water supply for the family. One of the strengths of this study was the researchers' procedures that protected the rights of the participants and those photographed. Another strength was the unique combination of data collection methods that produced a rich picture of health in these rural communities. The researchers identified limitations of the study to be that the health ministry nurse was present during the focus groups and that the photographers were younger participants.

Photovoice can often generate a deeper understanding of stigmatizing conditions. Fleming, Mahoney, Carlson, and Engebretson (2009) examined images in a photovoice exhibit on mental illness. They identified their data as the "renderings of the artist's observations and firsthand narrative accounts of persons living with mental illness" (p. 18). They selected 15 photographs with narratives that were available in the museum exhibit, in the online exhibit, and in the printed brochure. This choice allowed the researchers to encounter the data in different formats and strengthened the analysis process. The researchers developed the themes of suffering and stigma. A loss of identity was an overarching theme linking the other two themes. The analysis process was rigorous with notes made on each case that resulted in a three-page interpretive statement for each. The thematic analysis was validated through repeated meetings of the researchers to debrief and compare within-case studies with the original data for logic, coherence, and fittingness" (p. 19). The researchers provided details about the analysis process and their conclusions that support the quality of the study and the credibility of the findings.

Photovoice may pose unique ethical considerations because people in photographs can be identified and may not have consented to participating in the study. Researchers who are considering photovoice as a research methodology are urged to read primary sources and consult with researchers experienced in the methodology. The rights of the research participants must be protected during the conduct and reporting of the research.

Internet communication provides a way to collect data from persons separated by distance. Quantitative researchers are regularly using World Wide Web–based surveys and instruments to gather data, but qualitative researchers are also using Web-based communities such as online forums and blogs for research purposes. The number of participants available for Internet-based research is extensive but does have the limitation that the sample include only those who can read and write, are comfortable using a computer, and have access to the Internet (Marshall & Rossman, 2011). A nurse leader using Internet communication for data collection is Eun-Ok Im. Im has used mixed-methods studies with quantitative and qualitative phases. The focus here is on the qualitative phases. Im, Chee, Lim, Liu, and Kim (2008) used an online forum created for their study to gather data about physical activity of middle-aged women. The month-long online forum was completed by 15 of the 30 women who started. The researchers posted 17 topics for discussion with three or four introduced each week. The topics were about physical activity and cultural influences on physical activity. The participants used pseudonyms when posting to the forum to protect anonymity. The text of the discussions was converted into transcripts for analysis. As themes were identified, the researchers shared them with participants and asked for feedback. Im's program of research using online forums includes 11 studies. As examples, her team has completed studies on ethnic differences in cancer pain (Im et al., 2009), ethnic commonalities and differences in the experience of menopause (Im, Lee, Chee, Domire, & Brown, 2010), black women's experiences with menopause (Im, Seoung Hee Lee, & Chee, 2010), Asian Americans' perspectives on Internet cancer support groups (Im, Bokim Lee, & Chee, 2010), and white women's attitudes toward physical activity (Im, Lee, Chee, Stuifbergen, and the eMAPA Research Team, 2011). Im and other colleagues noted in these studies that one of the limitations was that the data represent only those who have Internet access and were comfortable describing personal experiences in the online forum.

The literature on using Internet communication for collecting data, or Internet-mediated research, is growing. Whitehead (2007) produced an integrated review of the literature on issues of quantitative and qualitative Internet-mediated research. On the basis of her review of 46 papers, she concluded that three major themes affect the credibility of the findings of Internet-mediated studies. The first is sample bias. This concern is diminishing as access to the Internet continues to increase. A researcher could minimize concerns about sample bias by comparing the demographic characteristics of the online sample with those of samples in traditional studies on the same topic. Whitehead (2007) identified the second concern to be ethical issues such as seeking consent, assuring anonymity of the participants, and protecting the security of the site. The third concern was the reliability and validity of the data collected because the researcher cannot verify whether participants meet the inclusion criteria for the study and has no control over distractions that may occur during data collection. Despite these issues, studies will continue to be conducted using the Internet and researchers aware of these issues can develop studies to minimize the concerns. Researchers considering this methodology may benefit from reading the research reports of Im's teams, which contain how they addressed issues of confidentiality and security.

Transcribing Recorded Data

Transcription of verbal data into written data is almost an assumption in qualitative research. Transcripts present the data in a form that allows the researcher to share the data with team members for analysis and validation. Data collected during a qualitative study may be narrative descriptions of observations, transcripts from audio recordings of interviews, entries in the researcher's diary reflecting on the dynamics of the setting, or notes taken while reading written documents. Audio-recorded interviews are generally transcribed verbatim with different punctuation marks used to indicate laughter, changes in voice tone, or other nuances. Verbatim transcripts contribute to the expense and time required for qualitative research and may not always be needed to answer the research question (Halcomb & Davidson, 2006). For example, in qualitative studies used to evaluate a program and mixed-methods studies, interviews may be used with structured questions that may not require word-for-word transcription.

Transcription may require 4 to 6 hours for each 1 hour of interview or focus group time, depending on the equipment used and the transcriber's skill. Hiring a professional transcriptionist may decrease the time but may be too expensive, depending on the study's budget. When hiring a transcriptionist, indicate the details that you want included and whether you want the transcript to be verbatim (Davidson, 2009).

Transcribing the recordings yourself has the advantage of immediately immersing you in the data. A pedal-operated recorder allows you to listen, stop, and start the recording without removing your hands from the computer or word processor keyboard. Even when you hire another person to transcribe the recordings, you want to check the transcription by listening to the recording while reviewing the transcript. Voice recognition programs may be of some benefit but require time for the software to "learn" the voice of the interviewee (Alcock & Iphofen, 2007). For transcription of focus group recordings, voice recognition software is not likely to be effective. Other software may allow conversion of audio recording to digital formats ready for analysis within computer analysis software. You also may code the actual recording, negating the need for a word transcription. Hutchinson (2005) developed an innovative method of data analysis that uses audio-editing software to save selected audio bytes from digital audio recordings. The data are never transcribed but remain in audio form. A database is used to code and manage the linked audio files and generate detailed and summary reports. Although the system is time consuming to set up, it negates the need for expensive and time-intensive transcription of recorded data.

Video recordings are maintained in their original format. However, the researcher may make notes on sequential segments of the recording, creating a type of field notes. The researcher may also code the recordings directly. Video recordings can be used for quantitative studies, but the recordings are coded and assigned a numerical value.

Data Management

Because data are collected simultaneously with data analysis, the study manager, who may be the researcher, needs to have a plan developed for how to organize and store data. Label electronic files consistently. For example, the digital files from recordings can be labeled with the date and the code number or pseudonym of the participant. Make copies of all original files on a second computer or external storage device. Similarly, scan or copy all handwritten notes, field notes, or memos and, if possible, store originals in a waterproof and fireproof storage box. Any electronic files containing personally identifiable information (family member, hospital name, addresses, doctor's name) should be encrypted prior to being sent electronically to a transcriptionist or team member. You may want to keep a Word document or Excel file listing all files by date, file name, and type such as

observational memo, transcript, analysis record, or field note. The study manager may also want to keep records of who is currently working on that file and whether it is being transcribed, analyzed, or reviewed by a team member.

Some researchers may prefer to make notes, mark text, and label (code) sections of data on a hard copy of a transcript or field note using colored markers, pencil, or pen. If hard copies are to be used, ensure that each page is clearly identified with the file name in the header or footer of the document. You may want to format the document with large right-hand margins to allow more space for coding and notes. It is recommended that you also include line numbers, not for each page, but for the entire document continuously. Having line numbers allows the researcher to note the source of a code by line number within a specific document.

Other researchers prefer to work on electronic files within a software program, using tools ranging from as simple as highlight or comment functions in a document within a word processing file to as complex as analysis of visual images, transcripts, field notes, and memos within one of several specialized computer programs. The program does not analyze the data but records the analysis performed in the mind of the researcher (Banner & Albarran, 2009; Leech & Onwuegbuzie, 2011). It can also allow links to be made between codes, facilitate retrieval of similar text, or produce diagrams of relationships among codes.

Computer-assisted qualitative data analysis software (CAQDAS) can maintain a file directory, allow for annotation of coding decisions, and retrieve sections of text that the researcher has identified with the same code (Banner & Albarran, 2009; Garcia-Horta & Guerra-Ramos, 2009; Hoover & Koerber, 2011). Hoover and Koerber (2011) summarize the advantages of CAQDAS to be efficiency, transparency, and multiplicity. Table 12-3 provides a more detailed list of the advantages and disadvantages of using CAQDAS, and Table 12-4 contains descriptions and suppliers of a selected group of CAQDAS programs.

Data Analysis

Qualitative data analysis is "a process of examining and interpreting data in order to elicit meaning, gain understanding, and develop empirical knowledge" (Corbin & Strauss, 2008, p. 1). Qualitative data analysis is creative, challenging, time consuming, and, consequently, expensive (Jirwe, 2011). Less experienced

TABLE 12-3	Advantages and Disadvantages of Computer-Assisted Qualitative Data Analysis Software (CAQDAS)
Advantages	Store and organize data files
	Provide documentation of coding and analysis
	Click and drag to merge codes
	Search for related codes and quotations efficiently
	Send coded data files to others
	Link memos to text
	Generate a list of all codes
	Minimize clerical tasks to allow focus on actual analysis
	Support and integrate the work of multiple team members
	Decrease paper usage
Disadvantages	Cost of software
	Need to allow time and expend energy to learn the software and its functions
	Potential that technical/functional aspects will overwhelm thinking about the analysis
	Potential for computer problems interfering with the software and causing data and analysis to be lost

TABLE 12-4	Examples of Computer-Assisted Qualitative Data Analysis Software (CAQDAS)	
Software	**Description and Website**	
ATLAS/ti 6.2	Robust CAQDAS functions; large searchable data storage including media files; multiple users allowed; facilitates theory building; flexible; supports use of PDF files. http://www.atlasti.com/	
Ethnograph v6	Originally developed for use by ethnographers; import and code data files; sort and sift codes; retrieve data and files. http://www.qualisresearch.com/	
FrameWork	Textual analysis tools plus summarization tool and ability to analyze using a matrix format. http://www.framework-natcen.co.uk/	
HyperRESEARCH	Code and retrieval functions; theory building features added on; handles media files; compatible with Macintosh computers. http://www.researchware.com/	
MAXQDA 10	Robust CAQDAS functions, but less powerful search tool; allows integration of quantitative and qualitative analysis; color-based filing; supports different types of text analysis. http://www.maxqda.com/products	
NVivo 9 (combined with NUD*IST)	Robust CAQDAS functions including several types of queries; familiar format of file organization system; handles multimedia files; latest version includes compatibility with quantitative analysis and bibliographic software. http://www.qsrinternational.com/#tab_you/	
Weft QDA	Free software that provides most commonly used CAQDAS functions. http://www.pressure.to/qda/	

Synthesized from Davis and Meyer (2009), Hoover and Koerber (2011), Speziale and Carpenter (2007), and websites of suppliers and professional organizations.

researchers may feel uncertain about how to proceed because the process feels ambiguous (Speziale & Carpenter, 2007). Data analysis in qualitative research occurs concurrently with data collection. Analysis of an interview's data may result in the asking of an additional question in subsequent interviews to confirm or not confirm an initial interpretation of the data. The process of **interpretation** occurs in the mind of the reader. Corbin and Strauss (2008) describe interpretation as translating the words and actions of participants into meanings that readers and consumers can understand. The virtual text grows in size and complexity as the researcher reads and rereads the transcripts. Throughout the process of analysis, the virtual text develops and evolves. Although multiple valid interpretations may occur if different researchers examine the text, all findings must remain trustworthy to the data. This trustworthiness applies to the unspoken meanings emerging from the totality of the data, not just the written words of the text. The first step in data analysis is to be familiar with the data.

Immersion in the Data

Becoming familiar with the data involves reading and rereading notes and transcripts, recalling observations and experiences, listening to audio recordings and viewing videotapes until you have become **immersed in the data**. Being immersed means that you are fully invested in the data and are spending extensive amounts of time reading and thinking about the data. Recordings contain more than words; they contain feeling, emphasis, and nonverbal communications. These aspects are at least as important to the communication as the words are. As you listen to recordings, look at photographs, or read transcripts, you relive the experiences described and become very familiar with the phrases that different participants used or the images that were especially poignant. In phenomenology, this immersion in the data has been referred to as **dwelling with the data** (Munhall, 2012). Byers and France (2008) designed a phenomenological study using van Manen's (1984) approach to phenomenology. They examined the experiences of registered nurses who cared for dementia patients in acute care settings. Byers and France described dwelling with the data in the following excerpt:

> "Staying true to phenomenology as philosophy and method, data collection and analysis occurred simultaneously and the researchers maintained a stance of sensitive attunement and openness to the possibilities of meaning to reach self-reflection, bracketing, and phenomenological reduction. Following each interview, the researchers transcribed the interview and dwelt with the data, continually writing and rewriting, and reading and re-reading the transcript, eventually formulating judgments about the recurring patterns and emerging themes of the parts within the whole staying true to van Manen's phenomenology." (Byers & France, 2008, p. 45)

Coding

Because of the volumes of data acquired in a qualitative study, initial efforts at analysis focus on reducing the volume of data so that the researcher can more effectively examine them. The reduction of the data occurs as you attach meaning to elements in your data and document that meaning with a word, symbol, or phrase known as a code. **Coding** is a means of naming and labeling. A **code** is a symbol or abbreviation used to label words or phrases in the data. Through coding, the researcher explores the phenomenon of the study. Therefore, it is important that the codes be consistent with the philosophical base of the study. Organization of data, selection of specific elements of the data for categories, and naming of these categories all reflect the philosophical basis of the study. Later in the study, coding may progress to the development of a taxonomy or a theoretical framework. For example, you might develop a taxonomy of types of pain, types of patients, or types of patient education. Initial categories should be as broad as possible with minimal

overlap. As data analysis proceeds, the codes may be merged and relabeled at a higher level of abstraction. In a study of medication adherence, the initial codes might be "paying attention to time," "counting and recounting," and "remembering to get prescription." These codes might be grouped later into the more abstract code "attending to logistics." The first level of coding is descriptive and uses participant phrases as the label for the code. The label for the merged codes is interpretive and might be called a **theme** if repeatedly identified in the data.

Trimm and Sanford (2010) studied the experiences of people waiting while a family member undergoes surgery. Their grounded theory study resulted in a middle-range theory that they called "maintaining balance during the wait" (p. 441). Their analysis yielded 56 open codes that they transformed into six axial codes. Further analysis resulted in four domains that comprise the theory: "focusing on the patient, passing the time, interplay of thoughts and feelings, and giving and/or receiving support" (p. 440). Table 12-5 contains excerpts from quotations of participants with their corresponding codes for one of the substantive domains, focusing on the patient. Trimm and Sanford (2010) provided extensive detail about their analysis and validated their findings with some of the participants. These actions indicate that the study was rigorously implemented and lend credibility to the findings.

The type and level of coding vary somewhat according to the qualitative approach being used. Table 12-6 displays types of codes described in the social science literature. The terms can be confusing, because different writers have given different names to similar codes.

Content Analysis

Content analysis is designed to classify the words in a text into categories. The researcher is looking for repeated ideas or patterns of thought. In exploratory-descriptive qualitative studies, researchers may analyze the content of the text using concepts from a guiding theory, if one was selected during planning for the study. During historical studies, the researcher analyzes documents and photographs to describe their content related to the focus of the study.

Garwick, Seppelt, and Riesgraf (2010) used a participatory qualitative study design to explore the challenges of managing asthma of children in urban Head Start programs at multiple sites. They conducted focus groups with teachers and managers of Head Start Centers and transcribed the data, as described in the following excerpt:

TABLE 12-5 Example of Participants' Quotations and Codes for the Substantive Domain of Focusing on the Patient

Participants' Quotations	Code
From the wife of a patient having back surgery on why they spent the night before surgery in a hotel: "Because we live a long way . . . we had kind of a rough night ... because I know he's nervous." (p. 443)	Driving/admitting the patient
"I just wanted to go back there [holding area] and reassure him that I loved him and boost him up a little bit. I definitely wanted to see him before surgery, 'cause it could have been the last time." (p. 443)	Reassure/comfort the patient
"I was better when I got here last night, just to see dad and that he was really okay ... just wondering if he was okay. Like if he *really* [italics added] was okay, if he really could talk well and didn't have any physical disabilities or so and he was fine." (p. 443)	Getting information first hand
"I love you. I'll see you in a few minutes." (p. 444) "I never say goodbye, because it feels so final." (p. 444) "We'll be right here in the waiting room." (p. 444)	'See you soon'
Description of family behavior, not a participant quotation: "When the family entered the waiting area, they would look at the room's arrangement and select a place to sit. Once seated, the conversations and actions focused on how the patient looked, when they would hear information, and what activity should be done first." (p. 445)	Entering the waiting room
"I was thinking about [spouse's name] and I know exactly what they are doing in that surgery, because he's had it done before. So I pictured the saw. I pictured the hammer. I mean I have a wild imagination, so I was just crying and thinking of all those things. I can picture the surgery happening and the position that he's in and it just made me feel so emotional and that's why I was crying." (p. 445)	Thinking about the surgical procedure
"This time the surgery will either result in her being able to continue her life or she's going to have to remain an invalid ... we're banking on everything on this move. There's the potential that she would be permanently paralyzed from below the waist. Everything hinges on this operation, because none of her plans can go forwards unless this works." (p. 446)	Worried about the outcome

From Trimm, D. R., & Sanford, J. T. (2010). The process of family waiting during surgery. *Journal of Family Nursing*, *16*(4), 435–461.

"Descriptive content analytic techniques (Neuendorf, 2002) were used to identify and categorize asthma management issues and action plan strategies. First, the [principal investigator] PI and research associate (RA) read and reread each focus group transcript in its entirety to understand the context of the focus group discussions. Next, each independently read the responses in the verbatim transcripts on a line-by-line basis to identify types of asthma management issues within and across the focus groups. Then they met to confirm, through a consensus process, common themes that participants emphasized in all three of the teacher focus groups. After the RA systematically organized the findings by theme and ID number, the PI validated the categorization of findings. Exemplars of each of the common themes or challenges are included in the findings." (Garwick et al., 2010, p. 331)

The credibility of the findings was increased through checking the accuracy of the transcription, assessing consistency between two data coders, and validating the findings with participants. The Head Start teachers and managers noted helpful and challenging interactions with parents of children with asthma and the complexity of the treatment plans that must be implemented with no additional staff and limited equipment.

Narrative Analysis

Narrative inquiry is a qualitative approach that uses stories as its data (Duffy, 2012). Through a series of life experiences, people create their identities in the historical and social context in which they live. As a philosophical approach to qualitative research, narrative inquiry was not included in this textbook (see Duffy, 2012, for additional information on the method). Data analysis, however, may yield stories, and researchers using other philosophical approaches may tell a participant's story in their analysis and presentation of findings. In addition to being organized chronologically, you might analyze a story as one would a published book during a literature course, looking for characters, setting, plot, conflict, and resolution. Historical researchers may compare participants' stories to present a broader picture of an event. Lesniak (2010), in her phenomenological study of adolescents who injure themselves (mentioned earlier in this chapter), did not indicate that she used narrative analysis. She presented, however, rich descriptions of the

TABLE 12-6 Types of Coding for Qualitative Data Analysis*	
Type	**Description**
Axial coding	Finding and labeling connections between concepts; assigning codes to categories; also may be called Level II coding in grounded theory studies
Descriptive coding	Classifying elements of data using terms that are close to the participant's words, usually early in the analysis
Explanatory coding	Connecting coded data to an emerging theory; describing coded data as patterns, themes, and links
Interpretive coding	Labeling coded data into more abstract terms that represent merged codes
In-vivo coding	"Concepts using actual words of research participants rather than being named by analyst" (Corbin & Strauss, 2008, p. 65)
Open coding	"Breaking data apart and delineating concepts to stand for blocks of raw data" (Corbin & Strauss, 2008, p. 195); also called Level I coding in grounded theory studies
Process coding	Incorporating previously assigned codes into an overall basic social process that is the core of the phenomenon of interest; used in grounded theory studies (Speziale & Carpenter, 2007)
Selecting coding	"Building a 'story' that connects the categories" (Creswell, 2007). The researcher may generate propositions or statements that bridge the categories.
Substantive coding	Includes in-vivo coding (using words of participants) and implicit coding, in which the unspoken codes are constructed by researchers

*These terms are not mutually exclusive, because different writers have used different labels for similar analytical processes.

lived experiences of the adolescents as stories. She then extracted themes from the stories. This is an excerpt of one of the stories:

> "Emma had just turned 17 years old when she agreed to be interviewed.... Emma cut as a means to gain a sense of control over her life. She could not control her parents' divorce or the loneliness she experienced during her childhood. She had no friends and her parents began dating other people, which further isolated Emma. Cutting was there for her and did not abandon her. It was a dependable variable in her life. Emma felt she did not fit in with other girls at school, becoming a target of their jokes and cruelty. After the first time she cut, Emma felt immediate relief from her pent-up emotions, and she was able to sleep. She stated that before she cut, she would feel numb inside and after she cut, the emotional pain became tangible through the physical pain of cutting. Cutting made Emma not want to die; instead, she cut to feel alive. The wound became a tangible and visible external representation of the pain she felt internally. It also gave her a location upon which to focus as the scars became a reminder of everything she had gone through; it was the story of her life. She stated that cutting was her expression, but on her skin. It became, in other words, her voice." (Lesniak, 2010, p. 143)

Stories may produce an emotional link between the research consumer and the participant beyond that achieved through discussion of codes and themes.

Lesniak (2010) gave the readers insight into the lives of the participants by presenting the descriptions as stories. When one goal of a study is to influence policy makers or promote behavior change, stories can be a powerful tool to generate support for the advocated message. Table 12-7 provides definitions of additional types of qualitative data analysis.

Memoing

The researcher develops a memo to record insights or ideas related to notes, transcripts, or codes. Memos move the researcher toward theorizing and are conceptual rather than factual. They may link pieces of data together or use a specific piece of data as an example of a conceptual idea. The memo may be written to someone else involved in the study or may be just a note to yourself. The important thing is to value your ideas and document them quickly. Initially you might feel that the idea is so clear in your mind that you can write or record it later. However, you may soon forget the thought and be unable to retrieve it. As you become immersed in the data, these ideas will occur at odd times, such as when you are sleeping, walking, or driving (Schiellerup, 2008). Whenever an idea emerges, even if it is vague and not well thought out, develop the habit of writing it down immediately or recording it on a hand-held device such as a cell phone.

Findings and Conclusions

Qualitative findings reflect the study's philosophical roots and the data that were collected. Unlike in quantitative research, conclusions are formed throughout

TABLE 12-7 Types of Qualitative Data Analysis

Data Analysis	Description
Chronological analysis	Identifying and organizing major elements in a time-ordered description as events and epiphanies
Componential analysis	Identifying units of meaning that are cultural attributes; process allows ethnographer to identify gaps in observations and selectively collect additional data
Constant comparison	Analyzing new data for similarities to and differences from existing data
Direct interpretation	Identifying a single instance of the phenomenon or topic and drawing out its meaning without comparing to other instances
Domain analysis	Focusing on specific aspects of a social situation such as people involved; used in ethnography
Narrative analysis	Looking for the story in the data; identifying the characters, setting, plot, conflict, and resolution as an exemplar of the phenomenon being studied
Taxonomic analysis	Identifying categories with a domain (see domain analysis); used in ethnography
Thematic analysis	Finding within the data three to six overriding abstract ideas that summarize the phenomenon of interest
Theoretical comparison	Thinking about the properties and characteristics of categories; linking to existing theories and models
Three-dimensional analysis	Thinking about and identifying continuity, interactions, and situations within a story

Synthesized from Corbin and Strauss (2008) and Creswell (2007).

the data analysis process in qualitative research. Conclusions are intertwined with the findings in a qualitative study. For a phenomenological study, the findings are presented as an exhaustive description (Speziale & Carpenter, 2007). The findings of a focused ethnographic study would include a description of the culture that achieved the study objectives or answered the research questions. In grounded theory studies, the researcher's aim is to produce a text or graphic description of social processes. As the description is refined, a theoretical structure or framework emerges that might be considered a tentative theory (Fawcett & Garity, 2009; Marshall & Rossman, 2011; Munhall, 2012).

Reporting Results

In any qualitative study, the first section of a research report should be a detailed description of the participants. The ethnography report will also include details about the setting and the environment in which the data were gathered. The results of the data analysis may be displayed in the form of a table with the themes in the first column of a table and exemplar quotations in the second column. Using tables in this way increases the transparency of the analysis and interpretation. Other writers incorporate supporting or disconfirming evidence from the literature within the results section of the report. How the results are presented depends on the philosophical approach upon which the study was developed. As previously mentioned, phenomenologists provide a thick, rich, and exhaustive description of the phenomenon that was studied. Ground theorists present their tentative

theory. Exploratory-descriptive qualitative studies are reported by addressing each research question and providing the pertinent findings. The report of a historical study may have limited information about the methods; rather, the report is the story of the events or series of events that were studied.

Methods Specific to Qualitative Approaches

Phenomenological Research Methods

Phenomenological researchers have several choices about methods that are related to their specific philosophical views on phenomenology. In Chapter 4, differences in Husserl's and Heidegger's views on phenomenology were discussed. Researchers subscribing to Husserl's views would use bracketing, which is consciously identifying, documenting, and choosing to set aside one's own views on the phenomenon (Dowling, 2007). Heidegger's view was that researchers could not separate their own perspectives from that of the participants' during the collection, analysis, and interpretation of the data. In phenomenology, additional philosophical approaches to the analysis and interpretation of data are available, such as those advocated by van Kaam (1966), Giorgi (1970), Colaizzi (1978), and van Manen (1984). Munhall (2012) calls these men "second-generation phenomenologists" (p. 126). Prior to selecting an approach, you are encouraged to read the primary sources listed in the references. Shorter and Stayt

(2010) conducted a phenomenology study according to Heidegger's philosophy. They emphasized the importance of co-creating the data, as follows:

> "A key tenet of Heideggerian phenomenology is co-construction of knowledge between researcher and participant, which assumes that both contribute to understanding the topic. Adequate participant contribution to the construction of knowledge was ensured in the present study by providing each participant with an annotated version of their interview transcription, detailing subject themes that had been identified. They were offered the opportunity to clarify meaning and comment on identified themes." (Shorter & Stayt, 2010, p. 161)

Shorter and Stayt (2010) concluded with the following paragraph:

> "Confronting death and dying is unavoidable in critical care settings. End-of-life care is therefore an important aspect of critical care nursing. This study has revealed a complex web of predisposing factors and occurrences that can shape both the nature of care for the dying and critical care nurses' subsequent grief experiences." (Shorter & Stayt, 2010, p. 165)

This study was congruent with the Heideggerian philosophy as evidenced by the validation of the analysis with the participants. From their findings, the researchers indicated several areas needing additional study, such as the informal support structures that allow critical care nurses to deal with patient deaths. The inferred clinical implications are that nurses involved in end-of-life care in acute care settings experience patients' deaths in complex ways and use multiple ways to deal with the grief. Nurses and managers in critical care units need to be aware of the diversity of grief responses and coping methods.

Grounded Theory Methodology

Philosophical discussions of grounded theory methodology center on the nuances of the different approaches (Cooney, 2010). Sociologists Glaser and Strauss (1967) worked together during their early years, but eventually their philosophies resulted in at least two variations of grounded theory. The original works provided little detail on data analysis methods, so Corbin and Strauss (2008) described a structured method of data analysis (Cooney, 2010). In Table 12-5, substantive and theoretical codes are attributed to Glaser, and open, axial, and selective are attributed to Strauss (Cooney, 2010). Researchers considering grounded theory methodology will want to read the primary sources on the different methods and choose the one that is most compatible with the researchers' beliefs. During grounded theory studies, data analysis formally begins with the first interview or focus group. The researchers review the transcript and code each line, constantly comparing the meaning of one line with the meanings in the lines that preceded it. Concepts as abstract representations of processes or entities are named. As the data analysis continues, relationships between concepts are hypothesized and then tested for validity (Wuest, 2012). Researchers are looking for a core category that explains the underlying social process in the experience. Existing theory and literature are reviewed for contributions to the researcher's understanding of the core category.

Banner (2010a) conducted a grounded theory study of women ($N = 30$) undergoing coronary-artery bypass graft (CABG) surgery. She explicitly described the methodological principles guiding the study, as follows:

> "Key principles of the grounded theory methodology are the following: (1) recursive data collection and analysis to the explore merging data, (2) construction of codes and categories, (3) theoretical sampling techniques to achieve conceptual density, (4) constant comparison, (5) generation of substantive theory as opposed to pure analytical description, (6) use of theoretical memos to track emerging data and theory and (7) deferred literature review until after analysis is complete to encourage analytical sensitivity (Charmaz 2006)." (Banner, 2010a, p. 3125)

Using Strauss and Corbin's (1998) approach to data analysis, Banner (2010a) found six categories in the pre-operative experiences of women scheduled for CABG surgery: "help seeking, diagnosis and referral, conceptualizing surgery, living with coronary heart disease, and waiting for surgery" (p. 3123). Banner reported quotations that exemplified each category and then compared the categories with the findings of other studies. The underlying social process was described as "the public-private dialogue around maintaining and renegotiating normality" (Banner, 2010a, p. 3123). Banner did not develop a graphic representation of the relationships among the categories and with the overall social process, but provided a description of the theoretical structure. The theoretical structure could be further refined by Banner or other investigators on this topic. The clinical implications are that nurses who read the study report may be sensitized to the significant life disruption and challenges faced by women through CABG surgery into recovery. Because several of the participants did not see themselves as being at risk for coronary artery disease, they may have delayed seeking care. Nurses must teach women how the symptoms of coronary artery disease may be different in women and that the women need to seek care when they experience symptoms.

Ethnographical Methodology

Ethnography is unique among the qualitative approaches because of its cultural focus. Thus, ethnography requires field work, which is spending time in the selected culture to learn by being present, observing, and asking questions. Wolf (2012) defines field work as a "disciplined mode of inquiry that engages the ethnographer firsthand in data collection over extended periods of time" (p. 302). Field work allows the researcher to participate in a wide range of activities. The observations of the researcher typically focus on objects, communication patterns, and behaviors to understand how values are socially constructed and transmitted (Wolf, 2012). The researcher looks below the surface to identify the shared meaning and values expressed through everyday actions, language, and rituals (Creswell, 2007). Meanings and values may reveal power differences, gender issues, optimism, or views of diversity.

One difficulty in planning an ethnographic study is knowing how much time is needed and actually what will be observed. Enough time in the field is needed to achieve some degree of cultural immersion (Speziale & Carpenter, 2007). The length of an ethnographic study is usually limited by the resources—money and time—that the researcher has allotted for the project. When one is studying a different culture, the time might extend to months or even a year. When studying the culture of a nursing unit or waiting area, the researcher will not live on the unit, but would identify a tentative plan for observing on the unit at different times during the day and night and on different days of the week. The researcher may want to observe unit meetings, change-of-shift reports, or other unit rituals, such as holiday meals. Initial acceptance into a culture may lead to resistance later if the researcher's presence extends beyond the community's expectations or the ethnographer is perceived as prying or violating the community's privacy. The researcher needs to blend into the culture but remain in an outsider role. A researcher who over-identifies with the culture being studied and becomes an insider is said to be going native. In going native, the researcher becomes a part of the culture and loses all objectivity—and with it the ability to observe clearly. Negotiating relationships and roles is a critical skill for ethnographers, who must possess self-awareness and social acumen.

Gatekeepers and Informants

Gatekeepers are people who can provide access to the culture, facilitate the collection of data, and increase the legitimacy of the researcher (Wolf, 2012). A gatekeeper may be a formal leader, such as a mayor, village leader, or nurse manager, or an informal leader, such as the head of the women's club, the village midwife, or the nurse who is considered the unit's clinical expert. The support of people who are accepted in the culture is key to gaining the access needed to understand the culture. In addition to gatekeepers, you may seek out other individuals who are willing to interpret the culture for you. These other individuals may be informants, insiders in the community who can provide their perspective on what the researcher has observed (Wolf, 2012). Not only will the informants answer questions, but they may also help you to formulate the questions because they understand the culture better than you do.

Gathering and Analyzing Data

During field work, the researcher will make extensive notes about what is observed and thoughts on possible interpretations. The researcher may seek input on the possible interpretations with an informant or a person being interviewed. Data analysis is coding field notes and interviews for common ideas to allow patterns to emerge. Data may also be subjected to content analysis. The notes themselves may be superficial. However, during the process of analysis, you will clarify, extend, and interpret those notes. Abstract thought processes such as intuition and reasoning are involved in analysis. The data are then formed into categories and relationships developed between categories. From these categories and relationships, the ethnographer describes patterns of behavior and supports the patterns with specific examples.

The analysis process in ethnography provides detailed descriptions of cultures. The descriptions may be presented as cultural themes or a cultural inventory (Speziale & Carpenter, 2007). These descriptions may be applied to existing theories of cultures. In some cases, the findings may lead to the development of hypotheses, theories, or both. The results may be useful to nurses when members of the community that was studied interact with the health system. The results may be tested by whether another ethnographer, using the findings of the first ethnographical study, can accurately anticipate human behavior in the studied culture.

McGibbon, Peter, and Gallop (2010) conducted an institutional ethnography of nurses' stress, a specific type of ethnography, as the following excerpt explains:

> "Institutional ethnography is a framework that describes how people's activities are socially organized in a particular way as they go about the routine activities of their daily lives.... Institutional ethnography provides a specific method to link nurses' everyday work with institutional structures that shape practice. Although ethnographic practice in general provides a framework for rich description of the contexts of everyday life, the aim of institutional ethnography is not thick description; rather, the aim is to expose the articulation of the activities of everyday life with institutional power relations." (McGibbon et al., 2010, p. 1356)

The researchers collected and analyzed data from numerous sources, as described here:

> "Data collection included tape-recorded interviews at a time and place that was convenient for the nurses, participant observation in the pediatric ICU (PICU) for a 3-month period, focus groups with participating nurses, field notes that incorporated a researcher journal, and the examination of selected nonconfidential texts related to the nurses' everyday work.... The focus of data analysis was explicating the forms of stress in nurses' everyday PICU work and their social organization. Data analysis initially consisted of coding for the forms of stress in nurses' work, particularly given the absence of much of nurses' experiences in current formulations of nurses' stress.... The purpose of attending to thematic codes in the data was not necessarily to arrive at any unifying description of the nurses' experiences across individual accounts; rather, thematic coding helped to identify aspects of the nurses' experiences related to the research questions and the social relations inherent in their work." (McGibbon et al., 2010, pp. 1356, 1357)

McGibbon et al. (2010) found six forms of nurses' stress, "including emotional distress; constancy of presence; burden of responsibility; negotiating hierarchical power; engaging in bodily caring; and being mothers, daughters, aunts, and sisters" (p. 1357).

> "Prolongation of life and active caring for those declared dead were socially organized and textually mediated processes that obscured nurses' emotional suffering through their scientific and rational character.... Nurses were uniquely situated temporally and spatially in the PICU. Their presence for 12 hours for almost any given shift and for consecutive shifts meant that their temporal connection with patients was markedly different than that of any of the other clinicians." (McGibbon et al., 2010, p. 1359)

The study was rigorous, as evidenced by the use of multiple sources of data and thorough analysis by the team. The researchers conclude that nurses' stress was increased and perpetrated by the organizational structures that de-emphasized the centrality of nurses to the work of hospitals. The study's findings substantiated the complexity of nurses' stress in the workplace and the need for nurses to develop effective stress management strategies.

Exploratory-Descriptive Qualitative Methodology

Researchers often design exploratory-descriptive qualitative studies to address a specific research question. For example, Mahoney and Ladd (2010) conducted focus groups at a national meeting of gerontological nurse practitioners (GNPs) to fill a specific gap in the literature, the lack of knowledge about the influence of pharmaceutical marketing on GNP prescribing practices. The 15 GNPs who participated were not asked to describe all aspects of their practice: "This study was undertaken to explore NP participants' prescriptive decision-making issues related to older adult patients with specific inquiry about the influence of pharmaceutical marketing" (Mahoney & Ladd, p. 18). Kaddoura (2010) designed a study with a slightly broader focus, as described in this excerpt:

> "This study explored new graduate nurses' perceptions of factors that helped to develop their critical thinking skills throughout their critical care orientation program. The study attempted to answer the following research question: How do new graduate

> nurses characterize the role of the ECCO [Essential of Critical Care Orientation] program in influencing the critical thinking of new critical care nurses educated by this program?" (Kaddoura, 2010, p. 426)

Data analysis for exploratory-descriptive qualitative studies is often content analysis, with or without a guiding theoretical framework. Kaddoura (2010) did not identify a guiding theory and described her data analysis in this way.

> "Data were analyzed by the qualitative content analysis approach to identify key points that described graduate nurses' perceptions of how their critical thinking skills were developed throughout the critical care orientation program. Four key codes or themes emerged as the participants verbalized their perceptions and experiences with the ECCO program. The major themes were related to knowledge and its application in the development of new graduates' critical thinking skills as well as the graduates' perceptions of the merits and concerns related to the ECCO program presentation. These primary themes included gathering knowledge, application of knowledge, benefits of the ECCO program, and concerns about the ECCO program in relation to the new graduate nurses' critical thinking skills." (Kaddoura, 2010, p. 426)

Kaddoura's (2010) study provided helpful information to use in evaluating the orientation program. Nurse educators designing orientation programs for new graduates may find the study's results applicable to their work. Other than this group, the study has limited applicability. Kaddoura does provide an exploratory design that would be helpful in evaluating programs, especially when combined with quantitative data in a mixed design study.

Exploratory-descriptive qualitative studies may be designed using a theoretical framework. In their qualitative study with low-income young fathers ($N =17$), Devault et al. (2008) examined the participants' life stories in the context of the Belsky (1984) model of parental behavior. From Belsky's model, Devault et al. (2008) developed a conceptual framework in which the concepts of individual history, coparental history, and professional history influenced fathering. Fathering influenced meaning and involvement in parenting. Although the researchers indicated that they were interested in the life stories, they did not use narrative data analysis. They selected interview questions that reflected the different components of Belsky's model and then used the components as a structure for content analysis of the transcripts, as described in the following excerpt:

> "The life story method is used to understand the subjective experience of individuals within a given group (here, vulnerable fathers). Being told by the person who experienced it, the life story's purpose is not only to get factual information but also to understand the meaning given to events. This enables the researcher to compare different life stories and discover common themes that emerge within the identified group. Thus, data collection was essentially intended to encourage fathers to tell us about their lives. The participants' life stories were examined from a variety of angles that correspond with those identified in our conceptual framework." (Devault, 2008, p. 231)

The researchers presented their conclusions in the context of the conceptual framework, as follows:

> "Returning to our conceptual framework, our study suggests that the mother of origin plays an important role in the individual history of vulnerable fathers.... In regards to the co-parental relationship, we found that a positive co-parental relationship is manifested by frequent contacts, shared activities, and mutual support.... The influence of work on fatherhood was less clear. In fact, we found that it is the other way around: becoming a father seems to have an influence on work. Most fathers try to overcome their professional instability in order to meet the family needs. Finally, we found that fatherhood had a very important meaning to vulnerable fathers and that it pushes them to better themselves and become more responsible. Involvement can take different forms but we found that the most involved fathers were active in every aspect of their child's life; they formed a stronger commitment to the father role and status, and were more centered on their children than on themselves." (Devault et al., 2008, p. 242)

Devault et al. (2008) are not nurses but they conducted a study of interest to nurses working with families, especially child-bearing families. The researchers clearly described their analysis process and recognized the limitations of their study. Their methods lend credibility to their results.

Historical Research Methodology

The methodology of **historical research** consists of (1) identifying a question or study topic; (2) identifying, inventorying, and evaluating sources; and (3) writing the historical narrative. Whether motivated by curiosity, personal factors, or professional reasons, the researcher's interest in a specific topic needs to be explainable to others (Lundy, 2012). One way to do this is for the researcher to develop a clear, concise statement of the topic. The topic may be narrowed to be manageable with available resources. Although the historical researcher may be interested in the effect of World War II on nursing science, the researcher may need to narrow the study to one or a few nurse theorists who were nurses during the war or the nurse scientists educated at one university. The statement of the topic may evolve into a title for the study, which includes the period being addressed. Prior to determining the years to be studied, you must have knowledge of the broader social, political, and economic factors that would have an impact on the topic. Using this knowledge, you can identify the questions you will examine during the research process.

Sources

Sources in a historical study may be documents such as books, letters, newspaper clippings, professional journals, and diaries. Sources may also be people who were alive during the time being studied or who heard stories from older relatives. Review the literature that is available on the topic you have selected, and start a bibliography or inventory of materials you want to review. Library searches identify published materials and may have some archives, unpublished materials purchased or donated for their historical value (Speziale & Carpenter, 2007). Pay attention to the organizations and institutions with which the person was affiliated. These organizations and affiliations provide clues to the location of primary sources (Lundy, 2012). **Primary sources** are "firsthand accounts of the person's experience, an institution, or an event and may lack critical analysis" (Speziale & Carpenter, 2007, p. 263). For example, historical researchers interested in Martha Rogers and the effect of World War II on her theory would note that Rogers was the Dean of New York University, increasing the likelihood that the university has documents written by her. In the case of Rogers, however, an Internet search

reveals that many of her materials are housed in Boston University's Howard Gotlieb Archival Research Center. Accessing these documents would include obtaining permission to review the documents, traveling to Boston, and making notes about or images of the documents.

Secondary sources are those written about the time or the people involved, but not by the person of interest. Secondary sources are also examined because they may validate or corroborate primary sources or present additional information or opinions (Lundy, 2012; Speziale & Carpenter, 2007). In fact, validation and corroboration are important for determining whether sources are genuine and authentic. **External criticism** determines the "genuineness of primary sources" (Lundy, 2012, p. 265). The researcher needs to know where, when, why, and by whom a document was written, which may involve verifying the handwriting or determining the age of the paper on which it was written. **Internal criticism** involves establishing the authenticity of the document. The researcher may ask whether the document's content is consistent with what was known at the time the document was written. Are dates, locations, and other details consistent across sources? The researcher remains open to the views presented in the documents or other sources but remains somewhat skeptical until sources are verified.

Historical Data Analysis

Data gathering and analysis occur simultaneously as the researcher samples documents, seeking descriptions, conflicting records, or contextual details. As with other qualitative approaches, historical researchers become immersed in the data. Content analysis yields data that the researcher will use to develop a description of the topic. The connections made among documents, opinions, and stories constitute the interpretation of the data that are essential to an unfolding, deep understanding of the topic. Figuring out when to stop examining sources may be one of the major challenges faced by historical researchers. Like phenomenological researchers, who stop interviewing participants when redundancy in the data is confirmed, historical researchers decide to stop gathering data when new data are no longer being found. The researcher may return to data gathering if gaps or questions emerge as the findings are being written.

Writing the Historical Narrative

The historical researcher keeps extensive records of the source of each fact, event, and story that is extracted. The extracted data may be organized as a chronology or attached to an outline. The chronology or outline will become the skeleton of the narrative that will be written. The historical narrative may take the form of a case study, a rich narrative, or a biography. The links made by the historical researcher from the past to the present give historical research its significance to nursing (Lundy, 2012).

Irwin (2011) conducted a historical study but gave few details of the methods, a situation that is common with this qualitative research approach. Historical researchers focus on the final product, which may be a book, a documentary, or an essay. Early in her essay of findings, Irwin indicates her purpose in conducting the study:

"The archives, sources, and figures that are central to the field [nursing] provide a ready means to trace the spread of U.S. global influence in the early twentieth century. The discipline should not be relegated to the peripheries of U.S. international history, therefore, but must be made central in any historical consideration of the United States in the world.... To demonstrate how the history of nursing can inform the study of both U.S. international history and the broader history of medicine, this essay traces the careers of four nurses during World War I and the following decade." (Irwin, 2011, p. 80)

The four nurses who Irwin highlighted were selected because of their service with the American Red Cross, as described in this excerpt:

"Pansy V. Besom, Helen L. Bridge, Kathleen D'Olier, and Alice L. Fitzgerald were among nearly 20,000 nurses from the United States who volunteered for overseas service with the American Red Cross (ARC) in World War I and the 1920s. These women graduated from U.S. hospital training schools during the first decade of the twentieth century and went to work as nurses in U.S. urban centers." (Irwin, 2011, p. 80)

A review of Irwin's reference list makes it clear that she used personal letters, press releases, and organizational documents from the National Archives, College Park, Maryland. Each citation includes the box number and the file from which data were extracted. In addition, Irwin listed more than 100 books as references.

Irwin (2011) intertwines the career of each nurse with the concurrent events of that era. She concludes as follows, with support for a fresh view of the United States' role in international health:

"Taking the histories of U.S. nurses into account and highlighting their centrality to the study of U.S. international history invites a reconsideration of the history of U.S. foreign relations in new and vital ways. These nurses—Besom, Bridge, D'Olier, Fitzgerald, and many others—are our U.S. international history, for they were the actual, physical embodiments of the United States in the world. Their letters, writings, and biographies are an invaluable archive for scholars interested in examining the on-the-ground workings of U.S. influence and soft power." (Irwin, 2011, p. 96)

This is a rigorous study with extensive archive and literature support. The study could have been strengthened, however, if Irwin had provided more information about how she integrated the facts from various documents into a coherent whole.

KEY POINTS

- Qualitative methods are more flexible than quantitative methods to ensure that the participant's voice is heard.
- Qualitative data collection and data analysis occur simultaneously.
- Researchers and participants in qualitative studies co-create the data that will be analyzed.
- Qualitative methods of data collection are observation, interviews, focus groups, images, and electronically mediated communication.
- Recordings and notes are transcribed into data files prior to analysis.
- Qualitative researchers select coding and analysis strategies consistent with the philosophical approach of their studies.
- Phenomenological methods may include bracketing and interviewing to elicit rich descriptions of lived experiences.
- Methods specific to grounded theory studies are coding, describing concepts, and identifying links between the concepts for the purpose of developing a theory.
- Ethnographic methods are characterized by extensive field work that includes observations and interviews for the purpose of describing aspects of the culture being studied.

- Exploratory qualitative studies may use a theoretical perspective on the research topic as the basis for data analysis.
- Historical researchers extract the meaning from primary and secondary source documents to describe and analyze the context and chronology of past events.
- Rigorous qualitative researchers are reflexive, a characteristic that requires the ability to be aware of nuances of the research situation and one's own biases.

REFERENCES

Alcock, J. & Iphofen, R. (2007). Computer assisted software transcription of qualitative interviews. *Nurse Researcher*, 15(1), 16–26.

Anatchkova, M. D. & Bjorner, J. B. (2010). Health and role functioning: The use of focus groups in the development of an item bank. *Quality of Life Research*, 19(1), 111–123.

Baker, T. A. & Wang, C. C. (2006). Photovoice: Use of a participatory action research method to explore the chronic pain experience of older adults. *Qualitative Health Research*, 16(10), 1405–1413.

Banner, D. (2010a). Becoming a coronary artery bypass graft surgery patient: A grounded theory study of women's experiences. *Journal of Clinical Nursing*, 19(21/22), 3123–3133.

Banner, D. (2010b). Qualitative interviewing: Preparation for practice. *Canadian Journal of Cardiovascular Nursing*, 20(2), 27–30.

Banner, D. & Albarran, J. W. (2009). Computer-assisted qualitative data analysis software: A review. *Canadian Journal of Cardiovascular Nursing*, 19(3), 24–27.

Belsky, J. (1984). The determinants of parenting: A process model. *Child Development*, 55(1), 83–96.

Byers, D. C. & France, N. E. M. (2008). The lived experience of registered nurses providing care for patients with dementia in the acute care setting: A phenomenological study. *International Journal for Human Caring*, 12(4), 44–49.

Charmaz, K. (2006) *Constructing grounded theory: A practical guide through qualitative analysis*. London, England: Sage Publications.

Chen, H.-Y. (2010). The lived experience of moving forward for clients with spinal cord injury: A Parse research method study. *Journal of Advanced Nursing*, 66(5), 1132–1141.

Cheng, H. C., Qin, L. X., & Tee, H. K. (2009). An exploratory study on the isolation experiences of patients with haematological disorders. *Singapore Nursing Journal*, 35(1), 15–23.

Coffman, M. J., Shobe, M. A., O'Connell, B. (2008). Self-prescription practices in recent Latino immigrants. *Public Health Nursing*, 25(3), 203–211.

Colaizzi, P. (1978). Psychological research as the phenomenologist views it. In R.S. Valle, M. King (Eds.), *Existential phenomenological alternatives for psychology* (pp. 48–71). New York, NY: Oxford University Press.

Cooney, A. (2010). Choosing between Glaser and Strauss: An example. *Nurse Researcher*, 17(4), 18–28.

Cooper, C. M. & Yarborough, S. P. (2010). Tell me-show me: Using combined focus group and photovoice methods to gain understanding of health issues in rural Guatemala. *Qualitative Health Research*, 20(5), 644–653.

Corbin, J. & Strauss, A. (2008). *Basics of qualitative research: Techniques and procedures for developing grounded theory* (3rd ed.). Thousand Oaks, CA: Sage Publications.

Creswell, J. W. (2007). *Qualitative inquiry and research design: Choosing among five approaches* (2nd ed.). Thousand Oaks, CA: Sage Publications.

Davidson, C. (2009). Transcription: Imperative for qualitative research. *International Journal of Qualitative Methods*, 8(1), 36–52.

Devault, A., Milcent, M.-P., Ouellet, F., Laurin, I., Jauron, M., & Lacharite, C. (2008). Life stories of young fathers in the contexts of vulnerability. *Fathering*, 6(3), 226–248.

Dickinson, A., Machan, I., Horton, K., Jain, D., & Maddex, J. (2011). Fall prevention in the community: What older people say they need. *British Journal of Community Nursing*, 16(4), 174–180.

Dodd, V., Glassman, T., Arthur, A., Webb, M., & Miller, M. (2010). Why underage college students drink in excess: Qualitative research findings. *American Journal of Health Education*, 41(2), 93–101.

Dowling, M. (2007). From Husserl to van Manen: A review of different phenomenological approaches. *International Journal of Nursing Studies*, 44(1), 131–142.

Duffy, M. (2012). Narrative inquiry: The method. In P. L. Munhall (Ed.), *Nursing research: A qualitative perspective* (5th ed.) (pp. 421–440). Sudbury, MA: Jones & Bartlett.

Fawcett, J. & Garity, J. (2009). *Evaluating research for evidence-based nursing practice*. Philadelphia, PA: F. A. Davis.

Findholt, N. E., Michael, Y. L., & Davis, M. M. (2011). Photovoice engages rural youth in childhood obesity prevention. *Public Health Nursing*, 28(2), 186–192.

Finn, N. A. & Stube, J. E. (2010). Post stroke fatigue: Qualitative study of three focus groups. *Occupational Therapy International*, 17(2), 81–91.

Fleming, J., Mahoney, J., Carlson, E., & Engebretson, J. (2009). An ethnographic approach to interpreting a mental illness photovoice exhibit. *Archives of Psychiatric Nursing*, 23(1), 16–24.

Garcia-Horton, J. B. & Guerra-Ramos, M. T. (2009). The use of CADQDAS in educational research: Some advantages, limitations, and potential risks. *International Journal of Research & Method in Education*, 32(2), 151–165.

Garwick, A. W., Seppelt, A., & Riesgraf, M. (2010). Addressing asthma management challenges in multisite, urban Head Start Program. *Public Health Nursing*, 27(4), 329–336.

Gharaibeh, M. & Owels, A. (2009). Why do Jordanian women stay in an abusive relationship: Implications for health and social well-being. *Journal of Nursing Scholarship*, 41(4), 376–384.

Giorgi, A. (1970). *Psychology as a human science: A phenomenologically based approach*. New York, NY: Harper & Row.

Glaser, B. G. & Strauss, A. (1967). *The discovery of grounded theory: Strategies for qualitative research*. Chicago, IL: Aldine.

Gray, J. (2009). Rooms, recording, and responsibilities: The logistics of focus groups. *Southern Online Journal of Nursing Research*, 9(1), Article 5. Available from http://snrs.org/publications/SOJNR_articles2/Vol09Num01Art05.html.

Greco, K. E., Nail, L. M., Kendall, J., Cartwright, J., & Messacar, D. C. (2010). Mammography decision making in older women with a breast cancer family history. *Journal of Nursing Scholarship, 42*(3), 348–356.

Haahr, A., Kirkevold, M., Hall, E. O. C., & Ostergaard, K. (2010). Living with advanced Parkinson's disease: A constant struggle with unpredictability. *Journal of Advanced Nursing, 67*(2), 408–417.

Halcomb, E. J. & Davidson, P. M. (2006). Is verbatim transcription of interview data always necessary? *Applied Nursing Research, 19*(1), 38–42.

Hall, L. M., Pedersen, C., & Fairley, L. (2010). Losing the moment: Understanding interruptions to nurses' work. *Journal of Nursing Administration, 40*(4), 169–176.

Hamilton, J. B., Moore, C. E., Powe, B. D., Agarwai, M., & Martin, P. (2010). Perceptions of support among older African American cancer survivors. *Oncology Nurse Forum, 37*(4), 484–493.

Henneman, E. A., Gawlinski, A., Blank, F. S., Henneman, P. L., Jordan, D., & McKenzie, J. B. (2010). Strategies used by critical care nurses to identify, interrupt, and correct medical errors. *American Journal of Critical Care, 19*(6), 500–509.

Hoover, R. S. & Koerber, A. L. (2011). Using NVivo to answer the challenges of qualitative research in professional communication: Benefits and best practices. *IEEE Transations on Professional Communication, 54*(1), 68–82.

Hutchinson, A. (2005). Analysing audio-recorded data: Using computer software applications. *Nurse Researcher, 12*(3), 20–31.

Im, E.-O., Chee, W., Lim, H.-J., Liu, Y., & Kim, H. K. (2008). Midlife women's attitudes toward physical activity. *Journal of Obstetric, Gynecologic and Neonatal Nursing, 37*(2), 203–213.

Im, E.-O., Lee, B., & Chee, W. (2010). Shielded from the real world: Perspectives on Internet cancer support groups by Asian Americans. *Cancer Nursing, 33*(3), E10–E20.

Im, E.-O., Lee, B., Chee, W., Domire, S., & Brown, A. (2010). A national multiethnic online forum study on menopausal symptom experience. *Nursing Research, 59*(1), 26–33.

Im, E.-O., Lee, B., Chee, W., Stuifbergen, A. and the eMAPA Research Team. (2011). Attitudes toward physical activity of white midlife women. *Journal of Obstetric, Gynecologic and Neonatal Nursing, 40*(3), 312–321.

Im, E.-O., Lee, S. H., Liu, Y., Lim, H.-J., Guevara, E., & Chee, W. (2009). A national online forum on ethnic differences in cancer pain experiences. *Nursing Research, 58*(2), 86–91.

Im, E.-O., Lee, S. H., & Chee, W. (2010). Black women in menopausal transition. *Journal of Obstetric, Gynecologic and Neonatal Nursing, 39*(4), 435–443.

Irwin, J. F. (2011). Nurses without borders: The history of nursing as U.S. international history. *Nursing Historical Review, 19*(1), 78–102.

Jirwe, M. (2011). Analysing qualitative data. *Nurse Researcher, 18*(3), 4–5.

Kaddoura, M. A. (2010). New graduate nurses' perceptions of the effects of clinical simulation on their critical thinking, learning, and Confidence. *The Journal of Continuing Education in Nursing, 41*(11), 506–516.

Kostovich, C., Saban, K., & Collins, E. (2010). Becoming a nurse researcher: The importance of mentorship. *Nursing Science Quarterly, 23*(4), 281–286.

Lange, B. (2007). The prescriptive power of caring for self: Women in recovery from substance use disorders. *International Journal of Human Caring, 11*(2), 74–80.

Lauzon Clabo, L. M. (2008). An ethnography of pain assessment and the role of social context on two postoperative units. *Journal of Advanced Nursing, 61*(5), 531–539.

Leech, N. L. & Onwuegbuzie, A. J. (2011). Beyond constant comparison qualitative data analysis: Using NVivo. *School Psychology Quarterly, 26*(1), 70–84.

Leininger, M. M. (1985). Transcultural care diversity and universality: A theory of nursing. *Nursing and Health Care, 6*(4), 208–212.

Lesniak., R. G. (2008). The lived experience of adolescent females who self-injure by cutting (Doctoral dissertation). *Dissertation Abstracts International*, B60 (05). (UMI No. 9932285).

Lesniak, R. G. (2010). The lived experience of adolescent females who self-injure by cutting. *Advanced Emergency Nursing Journal, 32*(2), 137–147.

Liamputtong, P. & Ezzy, D. (2005). *Qualitative research methods* (2nd ed.). Victoria, Australia: Oxford University Press.

Lopez, R. P. (2009). Decision-making for acutely ill nursing home residents: Nurses in the middle. *Journal of Advanced Nursing, 65*(5), 1001–1009.

Lundy, K. S. (2012). Historical research. In P. L. Munhall (Ed.), *Nursing research: A qualitative perspective* (5th ed.) (pp. 381–397). Sudbury, MA: Jones & Bartlett.

Mahoney, D. F. & Ladd, E. (2010). More than a prescriber: Gerontological nurse practitioners' perspectives on prescribing and pharmaceutical marketing. *Geriatric Nursing, 31*(1), 17–27.

Maslow., A. H. (1987). *Motivation and personality* (3rd ed.). New York City, NY: Harper & Row Publishers.

Marshall, C. & Rossman, G. B. (2011). *Designing qualitative research* (5th ed.). Los Angeles, CA: Sage.

McCloskey, S. & Taggart, L. (2010). How much compassion have I left? An exploration of occupational stress among children's palliative care nurses. *International Journal of Palliative Care, 16*(5), 233–240.

McGibbon, E., Peter, E. & Gallop, R., (2010) An Institutional Ethnography of Nurses' Stress. *Qualitative Health Research*, DOI: 10.1177/1049732310375435.

Moyle, W. (2002). Unstructured interviews: Challenges when participants have major depressive illness. *Journal of Advanced Nursing, 39*(3), 266–273.

Munhall, P. L. (2012). *Nursing research: A qualitative perspective* (5th ed.). Sudbury, MA: Jones & Bartlett.

Neuendorf, K. A. (2002). *The content analytic guidebook*. Newbury Park, CA: Sage.

Nikander, P. (2008). Working with transcripts and translated data. *Qualitative Research in Psychology, 5*(3), 225–231.

Ollson, L., Ostlund, G., Strang, P., Grassman, E. J., & Friedrichsen, M. (2010). Maintaining hope when close to death: Insight from cancer patients in palliative home care. *International Journal of Palliative Nursing, 16*(12), 607–612.

Ornelas, I. J., Amell, J., Tran, A. N., Royster, M., Armstrong-Brown, J., & Eng, E. (2009). Understanding African American men's perceptions of racism, male gender socialization, and social capital through photovoice. *Qualitative Health Research, 19*(4), 552–565.

Owen-Smith, A., Sterk, C., McCarty, F., Hankerson-Dyson, D., & DiClemente, R. (2010). Development and evaluation of a complementary and alternative medicine use survey in African-Americans with acquired immune deficiency syndrome. *Journal of Alternative & Complementary Medicine*, *16*(5), 569–577.

Parse, R. R. (2001). *Qualitative inquiry: The path of sciencing.* Boston, MA: Jones and Bartlett Publishers.

Rampton, T. B., Rosemann, J. L., Latta, A. L., Mandleco, B. L., Roper, S. O., & Dyches, T. T. (2007). Images of life: Siblings of children with Downsyndrome. *Journal of Family Nursing*, *13*(4), 420–442.

Richards, K. M. (2008). RAP Project: An instrument development study to determine common attributes for pain assessment among men and women who represent multiple pain-related diagnoses. *Pain Management Nursing*, *9*(1), 33–43.

Roy, C. (1976). *Introduction to nursing: An adaptation model.* Englewood Cliffs, NJ: Prentice-Hall.

Schiellerup, P. (2008). Stop making sense: The trials and tribulations of qualitative data analysis. *Area*, *40*(2), 161–171.

Schumacher, G. (2010). Culture care meanings, beliefs, and practices in rural Dominican Republic. *Journal of Transcultural Nursing*, *21*(2), 93–103.

Scott, A. J. & Wilson, R. F. (2011). Social determinants of health among African Americans in a rural community in the Deep South: An ecological study. *Rural and Remote Health*, *11*, 1634 (Online). Available from http://www.rrh.org.au.

Scott, D., Sharpe, H., O'Leary, K., Dehaeck, U., Hindmarsh, K., Moore, J. G., & Osmond, M. H. (2009). Court reporters: A viable solution for the challenges of focus group data collection? *Qualitative Health Research*, *19*(1), 140–146.

Seidman, I. (2006). *Interviewing as qualitative research: A guide for researchers in education and the social sciences.* New York City, NY: Teachers College Press

Shorter, M. & Stayt, L. C. (2010) Critical care nurses' experiences of grief in an adult intensive care unit. *Journal of Advanced Nursing*, *66*(1), 159–167.

Simmons, D. & Sherwood, G. (2010). Self-prescription practices in recent Latino immigrants. *Critical Care Nursing Clinics of North America*, *22*(2), 253–260.

Speziale, H. J. S. & Carpenter, D. R. (2007). *Qualitative research in nursing: Advancing the humanistic perspective* (4th ed.). Philadelphia. PA: Lippincott Williams & Wilkins.

Steele, R. G., Wu, Y. P., Jensen, C. D., Pankey, S., Davis, A. M., & Aylward, B. S. (2011). School nurses' perceived barriers to discussing weight with children and their families: A qualitative approach. *Journal of School Health*, *81*(3), 128–137.

Strauss, A. & Corbin, J. (1998). *Basics of qualitative research: Techniques and procedures for developing grounded theory* (2nd ed.). Thousand Oaks, CA: Sage Publications.

Swanlund, S. L. (2010). Successful medication management processes as perceived by community-dwelling adults over age 74. *Applied Nursing Research*, *23*(1), 22–29.

Taylor, C. & Burch, J. (2011). Feedback on an enhanced recovery programme for colorectal surgery. *British Journal of Nursing*, *20*(5), 286–290.

Trimm, D. R. & Sanford, J. T. (2010). The process of family waiting during surgery. *Journal of Family Nursing*, *16*(4), 435–461.

van Kaam, A. (1966). *Existential foundations of psychology*. Pittsburgh, PA: Duquesne University Press.

van Manen, M. (1984). *"Doing" phenomenological research and writing*. Alberta, Canada: University of Alberta Press.

Walls, P., Parahoo, K., & Fleming, P. (2010). The role and place of knowledge and literature in grounded theory. *Nurse Researcher*, *17*(4), 8–17.

Wang, C., Burris, M. A., & Ping, X. Y. (1996). Chinese village women as visual anthropologists: A participatory approach to reaching policymakers. *Social Science & Medicine*, *42*(10), 1391–1400.

Whitehead, L. C. (2007). Methodological and ethical issues in Internet-mediated research in the field of health: An integrated review of the literature. *Social Science & Medicine*, *65*(4), 782–791.

Wolf, Z. E. (2012). Ethnography: The method. In P. L. Munhall (Ed.), *Nursing research: A qualitative perspective* (5th ed.) (pp. 285–338). Sudbury, MA: Jones & Bartlett.

Wuest, J. (2012). Grounded theory: The method. In P. L. Munhall (Ed.), *Nursing research: A qualitative perspective* (5th ed.) (pp. 225–256). Sudbury, MA: Jones & Bartlett.

Zengerle-Levy, K. (2006). Nursing the child who is alone in the hospital. *Pediatric Nursing*, *32*(3), 226–231, 237.

13
CHAPTER

Outcomes Research

O utcomes research, now an established field of health research, focuses on the end results of patient care. Numerous studies have been conducted by nursing and medicine over the last three decades in the United States (Aiken, Clarke, Sloane, Lake, & Cheney, 2008; Bakker et al., 2011; Stone et al., 2007), Canada (Tourangeau, 2003; Tourangeau et al., 2007), and internationally (Van den Heede et al., 2009) that explore the relationships among nursing interventions and patient outcomes. Nursing-related interventions and variables that have been studied include skill mix and configuration of nursing personnel; staffing levels; assignment patterns (primary, functional, or team); shift patterns; levels of nursing education, experience, and expertise; ratios of full-time to part-time nurses; level and type of nursing leadership available centrally and on units; cohesion and communication among the nursing staff and between nurses and physicians; the implementation of clinical care maps for patients with selected diagnoses; and the interrelationships of these factors.

The momentum propelling outcomes research comes primarily from policy makers, insurers, and the public. There is a growing demand for data from providers that justify interventions and costs and for systems of care that demonstrate improved patient outcomes. By linking the care people receive to the outcomes they experience, outcomes research has become the key to developing better ways to monitor and improve the quality of care. There has been a major shift in published nursing studies as the number of studies using traditional quantitative or qualitative methods is dwarfed by the number of outcomes studies.

This chapter describes the theoretical basis of outcomes research, provides a brief history of the emerging endeavors to examine outcomes, explains the importance of outcomes research designed to examine nursing practice, and highlights methodologies used

in outcomes research. A broad base of literature from a variety of disciplines was used to develop the content for this chapter, in keeping with the multidisciplinary perspective of outcomes research.

Theoretical Basis of Outcomes Research

The theory on which outcomes research is based emerged from evaluation research (Structure-Process-Outcomes Framework). The theorist Avedis Donabedian (1976, 1978, 1980, 1982, 2005) proposed a theory of quality health care and the process of evaluating it. Quality is the overriding construct of the theory; however, Donabedian never defined this concept himself (Mark, 1995). He noted that quality of care is a "remarkably difficult notion to define and is a reflection of the values and goals current in the medical care system and in the larger society of which it is a part" (Donabedian, 2005, p. 692). The World Health Organization (2009, p. 13) defined quality of care as the "degree to which health services for individuals and populations increase the likelihood of desired health outcomes and are consistent with current professional knowledge."

The cube shown in Figure 13-1 explains the elements of quality health care. The three dimensions of the cube are health, subjects of care, and providers of care. The concept *health* has many aspects; three are shown on the cube: physical-physiological function, psychological function, and social function. Donabedian (1987, p. 4) proposed that "the manner in which we conceive of health and of our responsibility for it, makes a fundamental difference to the concept of quality and, as a result, to the methods that we use to assess and assure the quality of care."

The concept subjects of care has two primary aspects: patient and person. A patient is defined as

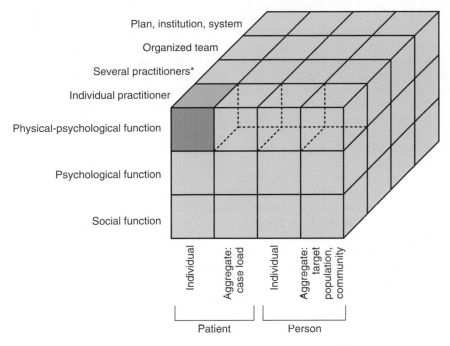

Figure 13-1 Level and scope of concern as factors in the definition of quality.

someone who has already gained access to some care, and a **person** as someone who may or may not have gained access to care. Each of these concepts is further categorized by the concepts *individual* and *aggregate.* Within patient, the aggregate is a caseload; within person, the aggregate is a target population or a community.

The concept **providers of care** shows levels of aggregation and organization of providers. The first level is the individual practitioner. At this level, consideration is given to the individual provider rather than others who might be involved in the subject's care, whether individual or aggregate. As the levels progress, providers of care include several practitioners, who might be of the same profession or different professions and "who may be providing care concurrently, as individuals, or jointly, as a team" (Donabedian, 1987, p. 5). At higher levels of aggregation, the provider of care is institutions, programs, or the healthcare system as a whole.

Donabedian theorized that the dimensions of health are defined by the subjects of care, not by the providers of care, and are based on "what consumers expect, want, or are willing to accept" (Donabedian, 1987, p. 5). Thus, practitioners cannot unilaterally enlarge the definition of *health* to include other aspects; this action

requires social consensus that "the scope of professional competence and responsibility embraces these areas of function" (Donabedian, 1987, p. 5). Donabedian indicated, however, that providers of care may make efforts to persuade subjects of care to expand their definition of the dimensions of health.

The essence of Donabedian's framework is the physical-physiological function of the individual patient being cared for by the individual practitioner. Examining quality at this level is relatively simple. As one moves outward to include more of the cubical structure, the notions of quality and its assessment become increasingly difficult (see Figure 13-1). When more than one practitioner is involved, both individual and joint contributions to quality must be evaluated. Concepts such as coordination and teamwork must be conceptually and operationally defined. When a person is the subject of care, an important attribute is access. When an aggregate is the subject of care, an important attribute is resource allocation. Access and resource allocation are interrelated, because they each define who gets care, the kind of care received, and how much care is received.

As more elements of the cube are included, conflicts among competing objectives emerge. The chief conflict is between the practitioner's responsibilities to the individual and to the aggregate. The practitioner is expected to have an exclusive commitment to each patient, yet the aggregate demands a commitment to the well-being of society, a situation that may lead to ethical dilemmas for the practitioner. Spending more time with an individual patient decreases access for other patients. Society's demand to reduce costs for an overall financing program may require raising costs to the individual. From an examination of the cube, logic would suggest that one could build up quality beginning with the primordial, or elemental, cell and increase by increments with the assumption that each increment would contribute positively to a greater total quality (see Figure 13-1). However, the conflicts among competing objectives may preclude this possibility and lead instead to moral dilemmas.

Donabedian (1987) identified three objects to evaluate when appraising quality: structure, process, and outcome. A complete quality assessment program requires the simultaneous use of all three constructs and an examination of the relationships among the three. However, researchers have had little success in accomplishing this theoretical goal. Studies designed to examine all three constructs would require sufficiently large samples of various structures, each with the various processes being compared and large samples of subjects who have experienced the outcomes of those processes. The funding and the cooperation necessary to accomplish this goal have not yet been realized; however, examples of nursing research in which two or more aspects have been evaluated are provided in this chapter.

Evaluating Outcomes

The goal of outcomes research is the evaluation of outcomes as defined by Donabedian. However, this goal is not as simple as it might immediately appear. Donabedian's theory requires that identified outcomes be clearly linked with the process that caused the outcome. Researchers need to define the process and justify the causal links with the selected outcomes. The identification of desirable outcomes of care requires dialogue between the subjects of care and the providers of care. Although the providers of care may delineate what is achievable, the subjects of care must clarify what is desirable. The outcomes must also be relevant to the goals of the health professionals, the healthcare system of which the professionals are a part, and society.

Outcomes are time dependent. Some outcomes may not be apparent for a long period after the process that is purported to cause them, whereas others may be apparent immediately. Some outcomes are temporary, and others are permanent. Thus, an appropriate time frame for determining the selected outcomes must be established.

A final obstacle to outcomes evaluation is determining attribution. This requires assigning the place and degree of responsibility for the outcomes observed. Many factors other than health care may influence outcomes, and precautions must be taken to hold all significant factors other than health care constant or account for their effect if valid conclusions can be drawn from outcomes research. A particular outcome is often influenced by a multiplicity of factors. Patient factors, such as compliance, predisposition to disease, age, propensity to use resources, high-risk behaviors (e.g., smoking, poor dietary habits, and drug abuse), and lifestyle, must be taken into account. Environmental factors such as air quality, public policies related to smoking, and occupational hazards must be included. The responsibility for outcomes may be distributed among providers, patients, employers, insurers, the community, and the government.

There is as yet little scientific basis for judging the precise relationship between each of these factors and the selected outcome. Many of the influencing factors may be outside the jurisdiction or influence of the healthcare system or of the providers within it. One solution to this problem of identifying relevant outcomes is to define a set of proximate outcomes specific to the condition for which care is being provided. Critical pathways and care maps may help the researcher to define at least proximate outcomes. However, proximate outcomes do not provide the level of evidence that examining the desired outcomes does. In addition, researchers must be ever vigilant not to confound causality and correlation, because an association or relationships between or among factors cannot imply that certain factors caused particular outcomes.

Evaluating Process

Clinical management has been, for most health professionals, an art rather than a science. Understanding the process sufficiently to study it must begin with much careful reflection, dialogue, and observation. There are multiple components of clinical management, many of which have not yet been clearly defined or tested. Three components of process that are of particular interest to Donabedian are standards of care, practice styles, and costs of care.

Standards of Care

A standard of care is a norm on which quality of care is judged. Clinical guidelines, critical paths, and care maps define standards of care for particular situations. According to Donabedian (1987), a practitioner has legitimate responsibility to apply available knowledge when managing a dysfunction or disease state. This management consists of (1) identifying or diagnosing the dysfunction; (2) deciding whether or not to intervene; (3) choosing intervention objectives; (4) selecting methods and techniques to achieve the objectives; and (5) skillfully executing the selected techniques or interventions.

Donabedian (1987) recommended the development of criteria to be used as a basis for judging the quality of care. These criteria may take the form of clinical guidelines or care maps based on prior validation that the care contributed to the desired outcomes. The clinical guidelines published by the Agency for Healthcare Research and Quality (AHRQ, 2011) establish norms or standards against which the validity of clinical management can be judged. These norms are now established through clinical practice guidelines available through the National Guideline Clearinghouse within the AHRQ (see http://www.guideline.gov/). However, the core of the problem, from Donabedian's perspective, is clinical judgment. Analysis of the process of making diagnoses and therapeutic decisions is critical to the evaluation of the quality of care. The emergence of decision trees and algorithms is a response to Donabedian's concerns and provides a means of evaluating the adequacy of clinical judgments.

Practice Styles

The style of practitioners' practice is another dimension of the process of care that influences quality; however, it is problematic to judge what constitutes "goodness" in style and to justify the decisions regarding it. Donabedian (1987) identified the following problem-solving styles: (1) routine approaches to care versus flexibility; (2) parsimony versus redundancy; (3) variations in degree of tolerance of uncertainty; (4) propensity to take risks; and (5) preference for Type I errors versus Type II errors. There are also diverse styles of interpersonal relationships. Westert and Groenewegen (1999, p. 174) suggest that "differences in practice styles are a result of differences in opportunities, incentives, and influences." They suggest that "there is an (often implicit) idea of what should be done and how, and this shared (local) standard influences the choices made by individual practitioners." This alternative originates in the borders between economics and sociology and it can be characterized as the social production function approach. The Medical Outcomes Study, described later in this chapter, was designed to determine whether variations in patient outcomes are explained by differences in system of care, clinician specialty, and clinicians' technical and interpersonal styles (Tarlov et al., 1989).

Practice pattern is a concept closely related to practice style. Although practice style represents variation in *how* care is provided, practice pattern represents variation in *what* care is provided. Small area analysis is an example of research that attempts to describe variation in practice patterns. Researchers of variations in practice patterns have found that such variation is not totally explained by patients' clinical conditions. For example, previous researchers have found that prescribing practices differ by region of the country and are influenced in part by drug company resources and marketing practices. The research methodology involved in small area analysis is described later in this chapter, under the term *geographical analysis*.

Evidence-based practice (EBP) is another dimension of the process of care that is considered a critical aspect of professional practice (Stetler & Caramanica, 2007). The ultimate goals of EBP are improved patient health status and quality of care (Graham, Bick, Tetroe, Strause, & Harrison, 2011). Thus, the impact of EBP should be assessed through measurement of patient outcomes. Graham et al. (2011) suggest that when planning evaluation of EBP, evaluators should begin by defining a clear question to guide their evaluation. They use the *PICO* question as a framework for structuring their evaluation question (Straus, Tetroe, Graham, Zwarenstein, & Bhattacharyya, 2009). *P* refers to the population of interest, which could be the public or a specific patient population. *I* refers to the implementation of a knowledge translation (KT) intervention. *C* refers to a comparison or control group who did not receive the intervention, and *O* refers to the outcome of interest. For instance, the outcome could be improvement in health status. Very few empirical studies have assessed the impact of evidence-based nursing practice on patient outcomes. Davies, Edwards, Ploeg, and Virani (2008) found implementation of best practice guidelines in nursing resulted in improved outcomes in diverse settings, but there was considerable variability in the indicators evaluated, suggesting the need for more research in this area. Chapter 19 provides more details on the synthesis of research evidence and the implementation of EBP in nursing.

Costs of Care

A third dimension of the examination of the process of care is cost. There are cost consequences to maintaining a specified level of quality of care. Providing more and better care is likely to raise costs but is also likely to produce savings. Economic benefits (savings) result from preventing illness, preventing complications, maintaining a higher quality of life, and prolonging productive life. The Institute for Healthcare Improvement has identified the following simple framework for identifying the return on investment for quality initiatives (Sadler, Joseph, Keller, & Rostenberg, 2009):

Step 1: Identify your improvement goal.
Step 2: Estimate improvement costs.
Step 3: Calculate revenue improvement through cost avoidance.
Step 4: Calculate the return on investment.

Schifalacqua, Mamula, and Mason (2011) used this framework in their development of a cost of care calculator for evaluating an EBP program. The goal was to compare the costs of care before and after implementation of an EBP program. The cost of care analysis focused on potential cost savings realized through the prevention of serious adverse events, such as healthcare-associated infections, pressure ulcers, and falls. Many challenges were revealed in identifying costs that were comparable among healthcare facilities participating in the implementation of the EBP program for preventing serious adverse events. Baseline costs associated with each adverse event were estimated on the basis of U.S. published studies and refined using organizational event data.

A related issue is who bears the costs of care. Some measures purported to reduce costs have instead simply shifted costs to another party. For example, a hospital might reduce its costs by discharging a particular type of patient early, but total costs could increase if the necessary community-based health care raised costs above those incurred by keeping the patient hospitalized longer or if complications resulted in rehospitalization. In this case, the third-party provider could experience higher costs. In many cases, the costs are shifted from the healthcare system to the family as **out-of-pocket costs** or costs that are not covered by healthcare reimbursement systems. Studies examining changes in costs of care should consider total costs, which include out-of-pocket costs. Table 13-1 provides a few examples of studies that examine the direct and indirect costs of care.

Evaluating Structure

Structures of care are the elements of organization and administration, as well as provider and patient characteristics, that guide the processes of care. The first step in evaluating structure is to identify and describe the elements of the structure. Various administration and management theories could be used to identify the elements of the structure. These elements might be leadership, tolerance of innovativeness,

TABLE **13-1**	**Studies Examining Costs of Care**
Year	**Source**
2011	Madsen, L. B., Christiansen, T., Kirkegaard, P., & Pedersen, E. B. (2011). Economic evaluation of home blood pressure telemonitoring: A randomized controlled trial. *Blood Pressure, 20*(2), 117–125.
2010	Spekle, E. M., Heinrich, J., Hoozemans, M. J., Blatter, B. M., van der Beek, A. J., van Dieen et al. (2010). The cost-effectiveness of the RSI QuickScan program for computer workers: Results of an economic evaluation alongside a randomized controlled trial. *BMC Musculoskeletal Disorders, 11*, 259–271.
2010	Van Oostrom, S. H., Heymans, M. W., de Vet, H. C., van Tulder, M. W., van Mechelen, W., & Anema, J. R. (2010). Economic evaluation of a workplace intervention for sick-listed employees with distress. *Occupational & Environmental Medicine, 67*(9), 603–610.
2009	Marchetti, A., & Rossiter, R. (2009). Managing acute acetaminophen poisoning with oral versus intravenous N-acetylcysteine: A provider-perspective cost analysis. *Journal of Medical Economics, 12*(4), 384–391.
2007	Griffiths, P. D., Edwards, M. H., Forbes, A., Harris, R. L., & Ritchie, G. (2007). Effectiveness of intermediate care in nursing-led inpatient units. *Cochrane Database of Systematic Reviews,* (2), CD002214.
2006	Phibbs, C. S., Holty, J. C., Goldstein, M. K., Garber, A. M., Wang, Y., Feussner, J.R., et al. (2006). The effect of geriatrics evaluation and management on nursing home use and health care costs: Results from a randomized trial. *Medical Care, 44*(1), 91–95.
2005	Harris, R., Richardson, G., Griffiths, P., Hallett, N., & Wilson-Barnett, J. (2005). Economic evaluation of a nursing-led inpatient unit: The impact of findings on management decisions of service utility and sustainability. *Journal of Nursing Management, 13*(5), 428–438.
2004	Altimier, L. B., Eichel, M., Warner, B., Tedeschi, L., & Brown, B. (2004). Developmental care: Changing the NICU physically and behaviorally to promote patient outcomes and contain costs. *Neonatal Intensive Care, 17*(2), 35–39.

TABLE 13-2 **Studies Investigating the Relationship between Structural Variables and Outcomes**

Year	Source
2011	McHugh, M. D., Shang, J., Sloane, D. M., & Aiken, L. H. (2011). Risk factors for hospital-acquired 'poor glycemic control': A case control study. *International Journal for Quality in Health Care, 23*(1), 44–51.
2011	Trinkoff, A. M., Johantgen, M., Storr, C. L., Gurses, A. P., Liang, Y., & Han, K. (2011). Nurses' work schedule characteristics, nurse staffing, and patient mortality. *Nursing Research, 60*(1), 1–8.
2010	Flynn, L., Liang, Y., Dickson, G. L., & Aiken, L. H. (2010). Effects of nursing practice environments on quality outcomes in nursing homes. *Journal of the American Geriatrics Society, 58*(12), 2401–2406.
2010	Fries, C. R., Earle, C. C., & Silber, J. H. (2010). Hospital characteristics, clinical severity, and outcomes for surgical oncology patients. *Surgery, 147*(5), 602–609.
2010	Cummings, G. G., Midodzi, W. K., Wong, C. A., & Estabrooks, C. A. (2010). The contribution of hospital nursing leadership styles to 30-day patient mortality. *Nursing Research, 59*(5), 331–339.
2009	Silber, J. H., Rosenbaum, P. R., Romano, P. S., Rosen, A. K., Wang, Y., Teng, Y., et al. (2009). Hospital teaching intensity, patient race, and surgical outcomes. *Archives of Surgery, 144*(2), 113–120.
2008	Kutney-Lee, A., & Aiken, L. H. (2008). Effect of nurse staffing and education on the outcomes of surgical patients with comorbid serious mental illness. *Psychiatric Services, 59*(12), 1466–1469.
2007	Castle, N. G., & Engberg, J. (2007). The influence of staffing characteristics on quality of care in nursing homes. *Health Services Research, 42*(5), 1822–1847.
2007	Goldman, L. E., Vittinghoff, E., & Dudley, R. A. (2007). Quality of care in hospitals with a high percent of Medicaid patients. *Medical Care, 45*(6), 579–583.
2007	Standing, M. (2007). Clinical decision-making skills on the developmental journal from student to registered nurse: A longitudinal inquiry. *Journal of Advanced Nursing, 60*(3), 257–269.
2006	Mor, V. (2006). Defining and measuring quality outcomes in long term care. *Journal of the American Medical Directors Association, 7*(8), 532–538.
2006	Rubin, F. H., Williams, J. T., Lescisin, D. A., Mook, W. J., Hassan, S., & Innouye, S. K. (2006). Replicating the Hospital Elder Life Program in a community hospital and demonstrating effectiveness using quality improvement methodology. *Journal of the American Geriatrics Society, 54*(6), 969–974.
2005	Donaldson, N., Brown, D. S., Aydin, C. E., Bolton, M. L., & Rutledge, D. N. (2005). Leveraging nurse-related dashboard benchmarks to expedite performance improvement and document excellence. *Journal of Nursing Administration, 35*(4), 163–172.
2005	Kleinpell, R., & Gawlinski, A. (2005). Assessing outcomes in advanced practice nursing practice: The use of quality indicators and evidence-based practice. *AACN Clinical Issues, 16*(1), 43–57.
2005	Wilson, I. B., Landon, B. E., Hirschhorn, L. R., McInnes, K., Ding, L., Marsden, P. V., et al. (2005). Quality of HIV care provided by nurse practitioners, physician assistants, and physicians. *Annals of Internal Medicine, 143*(10), 729–736.

organizational hierarchy, decision-making processes, distribution of power, financial management, and administrative decision-making processes. Nurse researchers investigating the influence of structural variables on quality of care and outcomes have studied factors such as nurse staffing, nursing education, nursing work environment, hospital characteristics, and organization of care delivery (Table 13-2).

The second step is to evaluate the impact of various structure elements on the process of care and on outcomes. This evaluation requires comparing different structures that provide the same processes of care. In evaluating structures, the unit of measure is the structure. The evaluation requires access to a sufficiently large sample of "like" structures with similar processes and outcomes, which can then be compared with a sample of another structure providing the same processes and examining the same outcomes. For example, in your research you might want to compare various structures providing primary health care, such as the private physician office, the health maintenance organization (HMO), the rural health clinic, the community-oriented primary care clinic, and the nurse-managed center. You might examine surgical care provided within the structures of a private outpatient surgical clinic, a private hospital, a county hospital, and a teaching hospital associated with a health science center. Within each of these examples, the focus of your study would be the impact of structure on processes and outcomes of care. Table 13-2 lists some current outcomes studies that examined the impact of structure of care and process of care on patient outcomes.

The federal government requires nursing homes, home healthcare agencies, and hospitals to collect and report specifically measured quality variables to the government. The mandate was established because of considerable variation in the quality of care in these structures. Various government agencies analyze the quality of these structures so that they can adequately oversee the quality of care provided to the American public. These data are made available to the general public so that individuals can make their own determination of the quality of care provided by various nursing homes, home healthcare agencies, or hospitals. Researchers can also access these data for studies of the quality of various structures. To access these data on the Internet, you can search using the phrases *nursing home compare, home health compare,* and *hospital compare.* In addition to being able to select a specific hospital, nursing home, or home healthcare agency, you can access considerable general information about quality related to these structures of health care. You can also do a search for Magnet hospitals on the American Nurses Credentialing Center website (http://www.nursecredentialing.org/Magnet/Finda MagnetFacility.aspx/) to check the status of a particular hospital regarding its recognition for excellence in nursing care.

Federal Government Involvement in Outcomes Research

Agency for Healthcare Research and Quality

Nurses participated in the initial federal involvement in studying the quality of health care. In 1959, two National Institutes of Health (NIH) study sections, the Hospital and Medical Facilities Study Section and the Nursing Study Section, met to discuss concerns about the adequacy and appropriateness of medical care, patient care, and hospital and medical facilities. As a result of their dialogue, a Health Services Research Study Section was initiated. This study section eventually became the Agency for Health Services Research (AHSR), and subsequently the Agency for Health Care Policy and Research (AHCPR). With a growing budget and strong political support, proponents of the AHCPR were becoming a powerful force. They insisted on a change in health care because of the demand for healthcare reform that existed throughout the government and among the public. A reauthorization act changed the name of the AHCPR to the Agency for Healthcare Research and

Quality (AHRQ). The AHRQ is designated as a scientific research agency. The term *policy* was removed from the agency name to avoid the perception that the agency determined federal healthcare policies and regulations. The word *quality* was added to the agency's name, establishing the AHRQ as the lead federal agency on quality of care research, with a new responsibility to coordinate all federal quality improvement efforts and health services research. The new legislation eliminated the requirement that the AHRQ develop clinical practice guidelines. However, the AHRQ (2011) still supports these efforts through EBP centers and the dissemination of evidence-based guidelines through its National Guideline Clearinghouse (see Chapter 19 for a more detailed discussion of EBP guidelines).

The AHRQ, as a part of the U.S. Department of Health and Human Services (DHHS), supports research designed to improve the outcomes and quality of health care, reduce its costs, address patient safety and medical errors, and broaden access to effective services. The AHRQ website (at http://www.ahrq.gov/) is a valuable source of information about outcomes research, funding opportunities, and results of recently completed research, including nursing research. In 2010, AHRQ awarded $25 million in funding to support efforts by states and health systems to implement and evaluate patient safety approaches and medical liability reform models. In addition, AHRQ invested $17 million to expand projects to help prevent healthcare-associated infections (HAIs), the most common complication of hospital care. The AHRQ initiated several major research efforts to examine medical outcomes and improve quality of care. One of the latest, which is described in the next section, is their comparative effectiveness research.

American Recovery and Reinvestment Act

Funding from the American Recovery and Reinvestment Act (Recovery Act), signed into law in February 2009, allowed AHRQ to expand its work in support of comparative effectiveness research, including enhancing the Effective Health Care Program. A total of $473 million was designated for funding patient-centered outcomes research (AHRQ, 2010). This AHRQ program provides patients, clinicians, and others with evidence-based information to make informed decisions about health care, through activities such as comparative effectiveness reviews conducted through AHRQ's Evidence-based Practice Center (EPC) (see Chapter 19). The AHRQ has a broad research portfolio that touches on nearly every aspect of health care, including:

- Clinical practice
- Outcomes and effectiveness of care
- Evidence-based practice
- Primary care and care for priority populations
- Healthcare quality
- Patient safety/medical errors
- Organization and delivery of care and use of healthcare resources
- Healthcare costs and financing
- Health information technology
- Knowledge transfer

The United States is not the only country demanding improvements in quality of care and reductions in healthcare costs. Many countries are experiencing similar concerns and addressing them in relation to their particular government structures. Thus, the movement into outcomes research and the approaches described in this chapter are a worldwide phenomenon.

Medical Outcomes Study

The Medical Outcomes Study (MOS) was the first large-scale study in the United States to examine factors influencing patient outcomes. The study was designed to identify elements of physician care associated with favorable patient outcomes. Figure 13-2 shows the conceptual framework for the MOS. The following describes the MOS:

"The Medical Outcomes Study was designed to (1) determine whether variations in patient outcomes are explained by differences in system of care, clinician specialty, and clinicians' technical and interpersonal styles and (2) develop more practical tools for the routine monitoring of patient outcomes in medical practice. Outcomes included clinical end points; physical, social, and role functioning in everyday living; patients' perceptions of their general health and well-being; and satisfaction with treatment. Populations of clinicians ($n = 523$) were randomly sampled from different healthcare settings in Boston, MA; Chicago, IL; and Los Angeles, CA. In the cross-sectional study, adult patients ($n = 22,462$) evaluated their health status and treatment. A sample of these patients ($n = 2349$) with diabetes, hypertension, coronary heart disease, and/or depression were selected for the longitudinal study. Their hospitalizations and other treatments were monitored and they periodically reported outcomes of care. At the beginning and end of the longitudinal study, Medical Outcomes Study staff performed physical examinations and laboratory tests. Results [were] reported serially, primarily in the [*Journal of the American Medical Association*]." (Tarlov et al., 1989, p. 925)

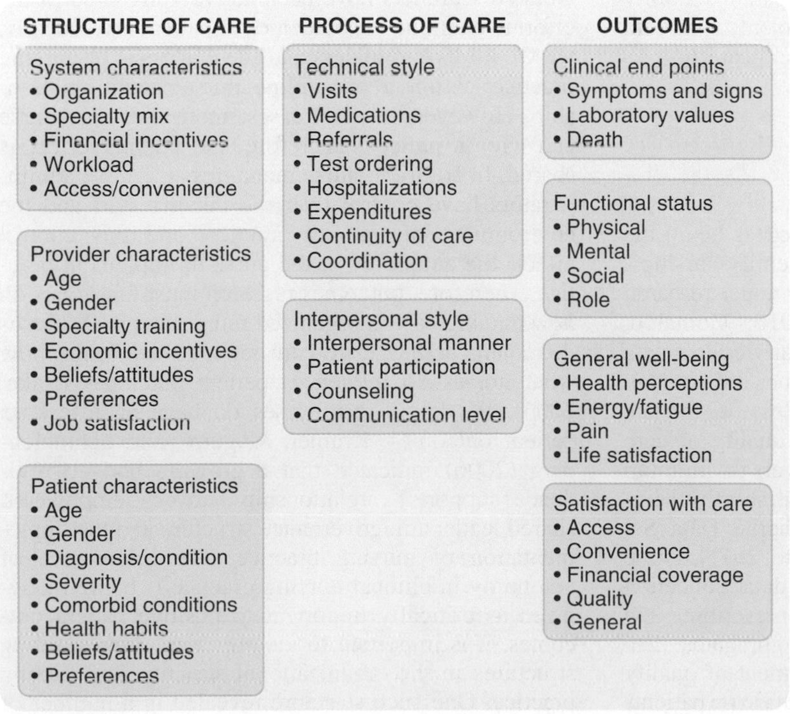

STRUCTURE OF CARE	PROCESS OF CARE	OUTCOMES
System characteristics • Organization • Specialty mix • Financial incentives • Workload • Access/convenience	Technical style • Visits • Medications • Referrals • Test ordering • Hospitalizations • Expenditures • Continuity of care • Coordination	Clinical end points • Symptoms and signs • Laboratory values • Death
Provider characteristics • Age • Gender • Specialty training • Economic incentives • Beliefs/attitudes • Preferences • Job satisfaction	Interpersonal style • Interpersonal manner • Patient participation • Counseling • Communication level	Functional status • Physical • Mental • Social • Role
Patient characteristics • Age • Gender • Diagnosis/condition • Severity • Comorbid conditions • Health habits • Beliefs/attitudes • Preferences		General well-being • Health perceptions • Energy/fatigue • Pain • Life satisfaction
		Satisfaction with care • Access • Convenience • Financial coverage • Quality • General

Figure 13-2 Conceptual framework of the Medical Outcomes Study.

MOS failed to control for the effects of nursing interventions, staffing patterns, and nursing practice delivery models on medical outcomes. Coordination of care, counseling, and referral activities, which are more commonly performed by nurses than physicians, were inappropriately considered in the MOS to be components of medical practice. Kelly, Huber, Johnson, McCloskey, and Maas (1994) suggested modifications to the MOS framework that would represent the collaboration among physicians, nurses, and allied health practitioners and the influence of their interactions on patient outcomes. These researchers also suggested adding the domain of societal outcomes to include such outcome variables as cost. They noted that "the MOS outcomes framework incorporated areas in which nursing science contributed to health and medical care effectiveness. It also includes structure, process, and outcome variables in which nursing practice overlaps with that of other health professionals" (p. 213). Kelly et al. (1994) further observed that "client outcome categories of the MOS framework that go beyond the scope of physician treatment and intervention alone include functional status, general well-being, and satisfaction with care" (p. 213). A review of the state of the science on nursing-sensitive outcomes published in 2011 confirmed the relevance of these outcomes to nursing practice and suggested several more, including self-care; therapeutic self-care, defined as patients' ability to manage their disease and its treatment; symptom control; psychosocial functioning; healthcare utilization; and mortality (Doran, 2011).

Origins of Outcomes/Performance Monitoring

Florence Nightingale has been credited as being the first nurse to collect data in order to identify nursing's contribution to quality care and to conduct research into patient outcomes (Magnello, 2010; Montalvo, 2007). However, efforts to systematically collect data to assess outcomes in more modern times did not gain widespread attention in the United States until the late 1970s. At that time, concerns about quality of care prompted the development of the "Universal Minimum Health Data Set," which was followed shortly thereafter by the Uniform Hospital Discharge Data Set (Kleib, Sales, Doran, Mallette, & White, 2011). These data sets facilitated consistency in data collection among healthcare organizations by prescribing the data elements to be gathered. The aggregated data were then used to perform the assessment of quality of care in hospitals and provide information on patients discharged from hospitals.

Over time other countries developed similar data sets. In Canada, "Standards for Management Information Systems" (MIS) were developed in the 1980s. Upon the establishment of the Canadian Institute for Health Information (CIHI) in 1994, the MIS became a set of national standards used to collect and report financial and statistical data from health service organizations' daily operations (Canadian Institute for Health Information, 2012). Simultaneously, CIHI implemented a national Discharge Abstract Database (DAD), which has become a key resource. However, as was the case with the Medical Outcomes Study discussed earlier, these data sets did not include information about nursing care delivered to patients in the hospital (Kleib et al., 2011). Without this information, the contribution of nursing care to patient, organizational, and system outcomes was rendered invisible. This major gap in information was addressed by the development of nursing minimum data sets in the Unites States, Canada, and other countries around the world.

Outcomes Research and Nursing Practice

Outcome studies provide rich opportunities to build a stronger scientific underpinning for nursing practice. Nurse researchers have been actively involved in the effort to examine the outcomes of patient care. Ideally, we would like to understand the outcomes of nursing practice within a one-to-one nurse/patient relationship. However, in most cases, more than one nurse cares for a patient. Therefore, the nursing effect is shared. In addition, nurse managers and nurse administrators have control over the nursing staff and the environment of nursing practice, and this control affects the autonomy of the nurse to implement practice. Therefore, outcomes research must first focus on *how* nursing care is organized rather than *what* nurses do. Then, perhaps, we can begin to determine how what nurses do influences patient outcomes (Lake, 2006). We know that nurses do have an effect on patient outcomes. Kramer, Maguire, and Schmalenberg (2006) indicated that a growing body of evidence supports a relationship between empowered shared leadership/governance structure and the implementation of nursing practice. The importance of autonomy in clinical nursing practice is being recognized as critically important to positive patient outcomes. It is important to identify autonomy-enabling structures in the organizational structures of nursing practice. One such structure revealed in a number of nursing studies is the Magnet hospital designation, which represents excellence in nursing in the agency with this designation.

Nursing-Sensitive Patient Outcomes

A **nursing-sensitive patient outcome (NSPO)** is "sensitive" because it is influenced by nursing care decisions and actions. It may not be caused by nursing but is associated with nursing. In various situations, "nursing" might be the individual nurse, nurses as a working group, the approach to nursing practice, the nursing unit, or the institution that determines numbers of nurses, salaries, educational levels of nurses, assignments of nurses, workload of nurses, management of nurses, and policies related to nurses and nursing practice. It might even include the architecture of the nursing unit. In whatever form, nursing actions have a role in the outcome, even though acts of other professionals, organizational acts, and patient characteristics and behaviors often are involved in the outcome. What patient outcomes can you think of that might be nursing-sensitive?

Nursing-sensitive outcomes have become an issue because of national concerns related to the quality of care. The demand for professional accountability regarding patient outcomes dictates that nurses be able to identify and document outcomes influenced by nursing care. Efforts to study nursing-sensitive outcomes were initiated by the American Nurses Association (ANA). In 1994, the ANA, in collaboration with the American Academy of Nursing Expert Panel on Quality Health Care, launched a plan to identify indicators of quality nursing practice and to collect and analyze data using these indicators throughout the United States (Mitchell, Ferketich, & Jennings, 1998). The goal was to identify and/or develop nursing-sensitive quality measures. Donabedian's theory was used as the framework for the project. Together, these indicators were referred to as the ANA **Nursing Care Report Card**, which could facilitate benchmarking, or setting a desired standard that would allow comparisons of hospitals in terms of their nursing care quality.

No one knew empirically what indicators were sensitive to nursing care provided to patients or what the relationships were between nursing inputs and patient outcomes. Every hospital had a different way of measuring the indicators that the ANA had selected. Persuading them to change to a standardized measure of the indicators for consistency among hospitals was a major endeavor (Jennings, Loan, DePaul, Brosch, & Hildreth, 2001; Rowell, 2001). Multiple pilot studies were conducted as nurse researchers and cooperating hospitals put in place the mechanisms required for data collection. These pilot studies identified multiple problems that had to be resolved before the project could go forward. Researchers learned that not only must the indicators be measured consistently but data collection must also be standardized. As studies continued, indicators were amplified and continue to be tested.

The ANA proposed that all hospitals collect and report on the nursing-sensitive quality indicators. To encourage researchers to collect these indicators, the ANA accredited organizations and the federal government helped by sharing the data with key groups. The ANA also encouraged state nurses' associations to lobby state legislatures to include the nursing-sensitive quality indicators in regulations or state law.

In 1998, the ANA provided funding to develop a national database to house data collected using nursing-sensitive quality indicators. This became the National Database of Nursing Quality Indicators (NDNQI). Currently, NDNQI has more than 1500 participating organizations. Participation in NDNQI meets requirements for the Magnet Recognition Program®, and 20% of database members participate for that reason. The remaining 80% of the members participate voluntarily to support their evaluation and improvement of nursing care quality and outcomes (Montalvo, 2007).

Detailed guidelines for data collection, including definitions and decision guides, are provided by NDNQI (2010). Healthcare organizations submit data electronically via the internet. Statistical methods such as hierarchical mixed models are used to examine the correlation between the nursing workforce characteristics and outcomes (Montalvo, 2007). Quarterly and annual reports of structure, process, and outcome indicators are available 6 weeks after the close of each reporting period. The database is housed at the Midwest Research Institute (MRI), Kansas City, Missouri, and is managed by MRI in partnership with the University of Kansas School of Nursing (Alexander, 2007). The NDNQI nursing sensitive indicators are as follows:

1. Patient falls/injury falls
2. Pressure ulcers (hospital acquired, unit acquired)
3. Physical/sexual assault
4. Pain assessment/intervention/reassessment cycle
5. Peripheral intravenous (IV) infiltration
6. Physical restraints
7. Registered Nurse (RN) survey: Job satisfaction; Practice Environment Scale
8. Healthcare associated infections:
   (a) Catheter-associated urinary tract infections (UTI)
   (b) Central line–associated bloodstream infection
   (c) Ventilator-associated pneumonia

9. Staff mix (RN; Licensed Practical Nurse [LPN]/ Licensed Vocational Nurse [LVN]/Unlicensed Assistive Personnel [UAP])
10. Nursing care hours provided per patient day
11. Nurse turnover (total, adapted National Quality Forum voluntary, Magnet controllable)
12. RN education/certification
13. RN survey:
    (a) Practice Environment Scales
    (b) Job Satisfaction Scales (option)
    (c) Job Satisfaction Scales–Short Form (option)

Other organizations currently involved in efforts to study nursing-sensitive outcomes include the National Quality Forum (NQF), Collaborative Alliance for Nursing Outcomes California Database, Veterans Affairs Nursing Outcomes Database, the Center for Medicare and Medicaid Services' (CMS) Hospital Quality Initiative, the American Hospital Association, the Federation of American Hospitals, The Joint Commission, and the AHRQ. A description of the Collaborative Alliance for Nursing Outcomes California Database project follows.

The Collaborative Alliance for Nursing Outcomes California Database Project

California Nursing Outcomes Coalition (CalNOC) was a statewide nursing quality report card pilot project launched in 1996. CalNOC was a joint venture of the ANA/California and the Association of California Nurse Leaders that was funded by ANA. Membership is voluntary and is composed of approximately 300 hospitals from the United States, with pilot work in Sweden, England, and Australia. As its membership grew nationally, CalNOC was renamed the Collaborative Alliance for Nursing Outcomes (CALNOC, 2010). It is a not-for-profit corporation, and member hospitals pay a size-based annual data management fee to participate and access CALNOC industry Web-based benchmarking reporting system.

Hospital-generated unit-level acute nurse staffing and workforce characteristics and processes of care data as well as key endorsed nursing-sensitive outcomes measures are submitted electronically via the Web. In addition, the CALNOC database includes unique measures such as its Medication Administration Accuracy metric, which helps in tracking medication errors. CALNOC data are stratified by unit type and hospital characteristics, and reports can be aggregated to division, hospital, and system/group/geographical levels. The following list of nursing-sensitive indicators has been extracted from Nurse Minimum Data Sets and CALNOC:

Structure indicators:

1. Hours per patient-day (RN, LPN, UAP)
2. Skill mix
3. Nurse/patient ratios
4. Percentage of contracted staff utilization (hours)
5. Staff voluntary turnover rate
6. Workload intensity (admissions, discharges, transfers)
7. Sitter hours as percentage of total care hours
8. RN characteristics (education, certification, years of experience)

Process indicators:

1. Risk assessment for pressure ulcers (Braden Scale)
2. Time since last risk assessment
3. Risk score (pressure ulcers)
4. Risk status (pressure ulcers, falls)
5. Prevention protocols in place (pressure ulcers, falls)
6. Medication administration accuracy: observed prevalence of 6 key safe practices
7. Peripherally inserted central catheter (PICC): line insertion practices (who inserted, where, presence of a dedicated team)
8. Restraint use: type and clinical justification

Outcome measures:

1. Community-acquired pressure ulcer prevalence
2. Hospital-acquired pressure ulcer prevalence stages 1-4
3. Patient fall rate per 1000 patient-days and consequences (injury fall rate)
4. Restraint prevalence
5. Central line–associated bloodstream infections (CABSIs) in PICC lines
6. Medication administration error rates

For further information on these outcome initiatives, you can review Doran, Mildon, and Clarke's (2011) knowledge synthesis of the state of science on nursing outcomes measurement and international nursing report card initiatives. The knowledge synthesis was a review of nursing-sensitive outcome and report card initiatives in the United States, Canada, the United Kingdom, and Belgium.

National Quality Forum

The National Quality Forum was created in 1999 as a national standard-setting organization for healthcare performance measures (NQF, 2011). The NQF portfolio of voluntary consensus standards includes performance measures, serious reportable events, and preferred practices (i.e., safe practices). A complete list of measures included in the NQF portfolio can be found online (www.qualityforum.org/Measures_List.aspx/). Approximately one third of the measures in NQF's portfolio are measures of patient outcomes. Examples are mortality, readmissions, health functioning, depression, and experience of care (NQF, 2011).

The NQF includes in their performance measurement portfolio several nursing-sensitive measures. Those that were submitted by the ANA under the NDNQI include the following:

- Nursing staff skill mix
- Nursing hours per patient-day
- Catheter-associated urinary tract infection (UTI) rate
- Central line–associated bloodstream infection rate
- Fall/injury rates
- Hospital/unit-acquired pressure ulcer rates
- Nurse turnover rate
- RN practice environment scale
- Ventilator-associated pneumonia rate

These indicators are the first nationally standardized performance measures of nursing-sensitive outcomes in acute care hospitals, and they are designed to assess healthcare quality, patient safety, and a professional and safe work environment. Although most measures currently used focus on the failure to meet the expected standards, the NQF believes that quality is as much about influencing positive outcomes as about avoiding negative outcomes. Thus, the NQF is interested in developing measures that reflect the positive effects of nursing care. Priority areas for indicators include assessment, patient education, and care coordination (Naylor, 2007).

Oncology Nursing Society

The Oncology Nursing Society (ONS) is a professional organization of more than 35,000 RNs and other healthcare providers dedicated to excellence in patient care, education, research, and administration in oncology nursing (ONS, 2012). The ONS has taken a leadership role among specialty nursing organizations in developing an EBP resource area on its website (http://www.ons.org/ClinicalResources/). The site provides nurses with a guide to identify, critically appraise, and use evidence to solve clinical problems. The ONS website also assists nurses—especially advanced practice nurses—who are helping others develop EBP protocols. The outcomes resource area helps nurses to achieve desired outcomes for people with cancer by providing outcome measures, resource cards, and evidence tables.

Advanced Practice Nursing Outcomes Research

Studies of outcomes of advanced practice nurses (APNs) are now appearing in the literature. APNs are RNs educationally prepared at the master's or doctoral level. These practitioners have expertise in a particular area of clinical practice and provide direct patient care. The ANA recognizes four types of APNs: certified registered nurse anesthetists (CRNAs), certified nurse midwives (CNMs), clinical nurse specialists (CNSs), and nurse practitioners (NPs). Studying APNs requires determining what happens during the process of APN care. This care involves a set of activities within, among, and between practitioners and patients and includes both technical and interpersonal elements. This process of care is complex and somewhat mysterious. However, clearly describing what occurs during this process of care is essential to developing a comprehensive understanding of how APNs affect outcomes. Although researchers have provided descriptions of APN care, considerable detailed work must still be done to more thoroughly describe the activities and interactions that occur between APNs and patients during the process of care (Cunningham, 2004).

The next step is to establish the relationship between APN interventions and outcomes. The outcomes must be clearly defined and measurable or observable. Outcomes may require risk adjustments for factors that may confound the results, such as comorbidity, stage of illness, severity of illness, and demographic characteristics. Failure to use rigor in measurement will limit your ability to interpret study findings meaningfully. It is important for variables to be measured using the same measurement methods across studies so that results are more readily compared. Understanding which outcomes are sensitive to APN interventions is critical to building knowledge in this area. We need a classification of outcomes of APN practice. Ingersoll, McIntosh, and Williams (2000) generated a beginning list of 27 relevant outcome indicators of APN practice. The nine highest outcomes are as follows:

- Satisfaction with care delivered
- Symptom resolution or reduction
- Perception of being well cared for
- Compliance with or adherence to treatment plan
- Knowledge of patients and families
- Trust of care provider
- Collaboration among care providers
- Frequency and type of procedures ordered
- Quality of life

Doran, Sidani, and DiPietro (2010) conducted a systematic review of the empirical evidence on outcomes of CNS practice. CNSs are licensed registered professional nurses with graduate preparation demonstrated in an earned master's or doctorate degree (National Association of Clinical Nurse Specialists

[NACNS], 2004). CNS-sensitive outcomes are those that can be theoretically linked to the activities of CNSs and observed in the three domains of CNS practice: patient and patient care, nurse and nursing practice, and organization and system (NACNS, 2004). Examples of CNS-sensitive outcomes are disease-specific patient outcomes, physical and psychosocial patient outcomes, nurse outcomes (job satisfaction), and system outcomes (costs of care) (Doran et al., 2010).

Methodologies for Outcomes Studies

Outcomes research methodologies have been developed to link the care people receive to the results they experience, thereby providing better ways to monitor and improve the quality of care (Clancy & Eisenberg, 1998). This section describes some of the current methodologies used in conducting outcomes research, including sampling methods, research strategies or designs, measurement processes, and statistical approaches. These descriptions are not sufficient to guide you in using the approaches described; rather they provide a broad overview of the variety of methodologies being used. This knowledge will help you understand and critically appraise the methodologies used in published outcomes studies. For additional information, you can refer to the citations in each section. Outcomes studies cross a variety of disciplines; thus, the emerging methodologies are being enriched by a cross-pollination of ideas, some of which are new to nursing research.

Samples and Sampling

The preferred methods of obtaining samples are different in outcomes studies; random sampling is not considered desirable and is seldom used. Heterogeneous, rather than homogeneous, samples are obtained. Rather than using sampling criteria—which restrict subjects included in the study to decrease possible biases and also reduce the variance and increase the possibility of identifying a statistically significant difference—outcomes researchers seek large heterogeneous samples that reflect, as much as possible, all patients who would be receiving care in the real world. For example, samples need to include patients with various comorbidities and patients with varying levels of health status. In addition, persons should be identified who do not receive treatment for their condition.

Devising ways to evaluate the representativeness of such samples is problematic. As noted in Chapter 15 of this text, for a sample to be representative it must be as much like the target population as possible, particularly in relation to the variables being studied. Because the target population in outcomes research is often heterogeneous, there are a large number of variables for which sample representativeness needs to be determined. Another challenge in outcomes research is developing strategies to locate untreated individuals and include them in follow-up studies. To address some of these challenges, outcomes researchers have used large databases as sample sources in observational research designs.

Large Databases as Sample Sources

One source of samples for outcomes studies is large databases. Two broad categories of databases emerge from patient care encounters: clinical databases and administrative databases, as illustrated by Figure 13-3 (Waltz, Strickland, & Lenz, 2010). **Clinical databases** are created by providers such as hospitals, HMOs, and healthcare professionals. The clinical data are generated either as a result of routine documentation of care or in relation to a research protocol. Some databases

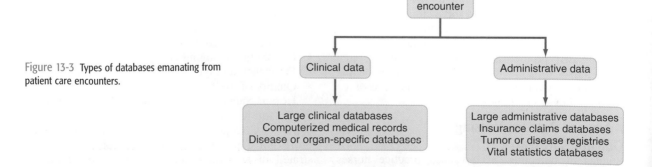

Figure 13-3 Types of databases emanating from patient care encounters.

are data registries that have been developed to gather data related to a particular disease, such as heart disease or cancer (Lee & Goldman, 1989). With a clinical database, you can link observations made by many practitioners over long periods. Links can be made between the process of care and outcomes (Mitchell et al., 1994; Moses, 1995).

Administrative databases are created by insurance companies, government agencies, and others not directly involved in providing patient care. Administrative databases have standardized sets of data for enormous numbers of patients and providers (Deyo et al., 1994; McDonald & Hui, 1991). An example is the Medicare database managed by the Centers for Medicare & Medicaid Services. These databases can be used to determine the incidence or prevalence of disease, geographical variations in medical care utilization, characteristics of medical care, outcomes of care, and complementarity with clinical trials. Wray et al. (1995) cautioned, however, that analyses should be restricted to outcomes specific to a particular subgroup of patients rather than to one adverse outcome of all disease states. Examples of large database indicators used to assess the quality of care are provided in Table 13-3.

Large databases are used in outcomes studies to examine patient care outcomes. The outcomes that can be examined are limited to those recorded in the database and thus tend to be general. Existing databases can be used for analyses such as (1) assessing nursing care delivery models; (2) varying nursing practices; or (3) evaluating patients' risk of hospital-acquired

TABLE 13-3 Examples of Large Database Indicators Used to Monitor Nursing Structural, Process, and Outcome Indicators

Type of Indicator	Indicator	Source
Structural	Nursing (e.g., RN, LPN, UAP) hours per patient day	National Database Nursing Quality Indicators (NDNQI, 2010)
		Collaborative Alliance for Nursing Outcomes (CALNOC, 2010)
		National Quality Forum (NQF, 2011)
	Staff mix (RN, LPN, LVN, UAP)	NDNQI (2010)
		CALNOC (2010)
		NQF (2011)
	Nurse turnover	NDNQI (2010)
		CALNOC (2010)
		NQF (2011)
	RN Practice Environment	NDNQI (2010)
		NQF (2011)
Process	Risk assessment for pressure ulcers	CALNOC (2010)
	Physical restraints	NDNQI (2010)
		CALNOC (2010)
	Prevention protocols in place	CALNOC (2010)
		B-NMDS (Belgian nursing minimum data set) (Van den Heede, et al., 2009; Sermeus, Delesie, Van den Heede, Diya, & Lesaffre, 2008)
	Medication administration accuracy	CALNOC
Outcome	Patient falls/injury falls	NDNQI (2010)
		CALNOC (2010)
		NQF (2011)
	Catheter-associated urinary tract infection rate	NDNQI (2010)
		NQF (2011)
	Hospital-acquired pressure ulcer	NDNQI (2010)
		CALNOC (2010)
		NQF (2011)
	Central line–associated bloodstream infection rate	NDNQI (2010)
		CALNOC (2010)
		NQF (2011)

LPN, licensed practical nurse; *LVN,* licensed vocational nurse; *RN,* registered nurse; *UAP,* unlicensed assistive personnel.

infection, hospital-acquired pressure ulcer, or falls. To examine these questions, nurses must develop the statistical and methodological skills needed for working with large databases. Large databases contain patient and institutional information from huge numbers of patients. They exist in computer-readable form, require special statistical methods and computer techniques, and can be used by researchers who were not involved in the creation of the database.

Initiatives such as CALNOC (2010), NDNQI (2010; Montalvo, 2007), and the Veterans Affairs Nursing Outcome Database (Alexander, 2007) are making nursing data more accessible for large database research. The following nursing classification schemes have been used in national databases:

- The North American Nursing Diagnosis Association (NANDA) Classification
- The Omaha System: Applications for Community Health Nursing Classification
- The Home Health Care Classification
- The Nursing Interventions Classification (NIC)
- The Nursing Outcomes Classification (NOC)

Research Strategies for Outcomes Studies

Outcomes research programs usually consist of studies with a mix of strategies carried out sequentially. Although these strategies could be referred to as designs, for some the term *design* as used in Chapters 10 and 11 is inconsistent with the strategies used in outcomes studies. Research strategies for outcomes studies have emerged from a variety of disciplines, and innovative new strategies continue to appear in the literature. Strategies for outcomes studies tend to employ fewer controls than traditional research designs and cannot be as easily categorized. The research strategies described in this section are only a sampling from the outcomes research literature and include consensus knowledge building, practice pattern profiling, prospective cohort studies, retrospective cohort studies, population-based studies, geographical analyses, economic studies, and ethical studies.

Consensus Knowledge Building

Consensus knowledge building is usually performed by a multidisciplinary group representing a variety of constituencies. Initially, the group conducts an extensive international search of the literature on the topic of concern, including unpublished studies, studies in progress, dissertations, and theses. Several separate reviews may be performed, focusing on specific questions about the outcomes of care, diagnosis, prevention, or prognosis. The results are dispersed to researchers and clinical experts in the field, who are asked to carefully examine the material and then participate in a consensus conference. The consensus conference yields clinical guidelines, which are published and widely distributed to clinicians. The clinical guidelines are also used as practice norms to study process and outcomes in that field. Gaps in the knowledge base are identified and research priorities determined by the consensus group.

Preliminary steps in this process might include conducting extensive integrative reviews and seeking consensus from a multidisciplinary research team and locally available clinicians. A review could be accomplished by establishing a website and conducting dialogue with experts via the internet. The review could be published in Sigma Theta Tau's online journal, *Knowledge Synthesis in Nursing,* and then dialogue related to the review could be conducted over the internet. The Delphi method has also been used to seek consensus (Tork, Dassen, & Lohrmann, 2008). Described as a group process to obtain judgments from a panel of experts, the Delphi method involves a series of questionnaires or rounds until a predetermined level of group consensus is reached (see Chapter 17). The experts are questioned individually, and a summary of the individual judgments is distributed to panel members, with subsequent questionnaires to influence the panel members through group feedback (Keeney, Hasson, & McKenna, 2011).

Practice Pattern Profiling

Practice pattern profiling is an epidemiological technique that focuses on patterns of care rather than individual occurrences of care. Researchers use large database analysis to identify a provider's pattern of practice and compare it with that of similar providers or with an accepted standard of practice. The technique has been used to determine overutilization and underutilization of services, to examine costs associated with a particular provider's care, to uncover problems related to efficiency and quality of care, and to assess provider performance. The provider being profiled could be an individual practitioner, a group of practitioners, or a healthcare organization such as a hospital or an HMO. The provider's pattern is expressed as a rate aggregated over time for a defined population of patients under the provider's care. For example, using data on the universe of deliveries in Florida and New York over a 15-year period, Epstein and Nicholson (2009) examined why treatment styles differ among obstetricians at a point in time and why styles change over time. They found that variation in cesarean section rates among physicians within a market is about twice as large as variation between markets.

Profiling can be used when the data contain hierarchical groupings: Patients could be grouped by nurse, nurses by unit, and units by larger organizations. The analysis uses regression equations to examine the relationship of an outcome to the characteristics of the various groupings. To be effective, the analysis must include data on the different sources of variability that might contribute to a given outcome.

The structure of the analysis reflects the structure of the data. For example, patient characteristics could be data on disease severity, comorbidity, emergent or developing status, behavioral characteristics, socioeconomic status, and demographics. Nurse characteristics might consist of level of education, specialty status, years of practice, age, gender, and certifications. Unit characteristics could comprise number of beds, nursing management style used on the unit, ratio of patients to nurses, and the proportion of staff who are RNs (Doran et al., 2006). Profiles are designed to generate some type of action, such as to inform the provider that his or her rates of patient improvement are high or too low in comparison with the norm. By examining aggregate patterns of practice, profiling can be used to compare the care provided by different organizations or received by different populations of patients. Critical pathways or care maps can then be used to determine the proportion of patients who diverged from the pathway for a particular nurse, group of nurses, or group of nursing units. Profiling can be used to improve quality, assess provider performance, and review utilization patterns.

Profiling does not address methods of improving outcomes, although this process can identify problem areas. It can be used to determine how performance should be changed to improve outcomes and who should make those changes. Profiling can also identify outliers, allowing more detailed examination of these individuals and their practice. To date, most of the profiling research has been about medical practice. The development of nursing-sensitive structure, process, and outcome indicators that are assessed and benchmarked over time, as is being done with NDNQI (Montalvo, 2007; NDNQI, 2010) will enable profiling of nursing practice.

Prospective Cohort Studies

A **prospective cohort study** is an epidemiological study in which the researcher identifies a group of people who are at risk for experiencing a particular event. Sample sizes for these studies often must be very large, particularly if only a small portion of the at-risk group will experience the event. The entire group is followed over time to determine the point at which the event occurs, the variables associated with the event, and the outcomes for those who experienced the event in comparison with those who did not.

The Harvard Nurses' Health Study is an example of a prospective cohort study. This study recruited 100,000 nurses to determine the long-term consequences of the use of birth control pills. Every 2 years or more often, nurses complete a questionnaire about their health and health behaviors. The study has now been in progress for more than 20 years. Multiple studies reported in the literature have used the large data set yielded by the study. The following summary describes a prospective cohort study on smoking and risk of psoriasis in women, using the Nurses' Health Study II, a second study using a younger population than the Harvard study (Setty, Curhan, & Choi, 2007). These researchers were able to obtain an extremely large, heterogeneous sample for their study by using data from the Nurses' Health Study.

Background: Psoriasis is a common, chronic, inflammatory skin disorder. Smoking may increase the risk of psoriasis.

Methods: Over a 14-year time period from 1991 to 2005, the relation between smoking status, duration, intensity, cessation, exposure to second-hand smoke, and incident of psoriasis was prospectively examined in 78,532 women from the Nurses Health Study II. The primary outcome was incident, self-reported, physician-diagnosed psoriasis.

Results: Eight hundred eighty-seven incident cases of psoriasis were documented. The multivariate relative risk (RR) of psoriasis was 1.78 (95% confidence interval [CI], 1.46 to 2.16) for current smokers and 1.37 (95% CI, 1.17 to 1.59) for past smokers in comparison with persons who had never smoked. The multivariate RR of psoriasis was 1.60 (95% CI, 1.31 to 1.97) for those who had smoked 11 to 20 pack-years and 2.05 (95% CI, 1.66 to 2.53) for those who had smoked 21 or more pack-years in comparison with nonsmokers. The multivariate RR of psoriasis was 1.61 (95% CI, 1.30 to 2.00) for those who quit smoking less than 10 years ago, 1.31 (95% CI, 1.05 to 1.64) for those who had quit 10 to 19 years ago, and 1.15 (95% CI, 0.88 to 1.51) for those who had quit 20 or more years ago in comparison with persons who had never smoked. An increased risk of psoriasis was associated with prenatal and childhood exposure to passive smoke.

Conclusions: The prospective analysis suggests that current and past smoking, and cumulative measures of smoking, were associated with the incidence of psoriasis. After 20 years of smoking cessation, the risk of the incident psoriasis among ex-smokers decreases nearly to that of persons who have never smoked. (Setty et al., 2007, p. 953)

Retrospective Cohort Studies

A retrospective cohort study is an epidemiological study in which the researcher identifies a group of people who have experienced a particular event. This is a common research technique used in the field of epidemiology to study occupational exposure to chemicals. Events of interest to nursing that could be studied in this manner include a procedure, an episode of care, a nursing intervention, and a diagnosis. Nurses might use a retrospective cohort study to follow a cohort of women who had received a mastectomy for breast cancer or of patients in whom a urinary bladder catheter was placed during and after surgery. The cohort is evaluated after the event to determine the occurrence of changes in health status, usually the development of a particular disease or death. Nurses might be interested in the pattern of recovery after an event or, in the case of catheterization, the incidence of bladder infections in the months after surgery.

On the basis of the study findings, epidemiologists calculate the relative risk of the identified change in health for the group. For example, if death were the occurrence of interest, the expected number of deaths would be determined. The observed number of deaths divided by the expected number of deaths and multiplied by 100 yields a standardized mortality ratio (SMR), which is regarded as a measure of the relative risk of the studied group to die of a particular condition. In nursing studies, patients might be followed over time after discharge from a healthcare facility to determine complication rates and the SMR (Swaen & Meijers, 1988).

In retrospective studies, researchers commonly ask patients to recall information relevant to their previous health status. This information is often used to determine the amount of change occurring before and after an intervention. Recall can easily be distorted, thereby misleading researchers in determining outcomes. Thus, recall should be used with caution. Herrmann (1995) identified three sources of distortion in recall: (1) the question posed to the subject may be conceived or expressed incorrectly; (2) the recall process may be in error; and (3) the research design used to measure recall can result in the recall's appearing to be different from what actually occurred. Herrmann (1995, p. AS90) also identified four bases of recall:

Direct recall: The subject "accesses the memory without having to think or search memory," resulting in correct information.

Indirect recall: The subject "accesses the memory after thinking or searching memory," resulting in correct information.

Limited recall: "Access to the memory does not occur but information that suggests the contents of the memory is accessed," resulting in an educated guess.

No recall: "Neither the memory nor information relevant to the memory may be accessed, resulting in a wild guess."

The following abstract developed by Rozen, Ugoni, and Sheehan (2011), on their study of vaginal birth after cesarean section, is presented as an example of a retrospective cohort study:

"Background: Previous studies assessing the safety of vaginal birth after caesarean section (VBAC) have compared VBAC to elective repeat caesarean section (ERCS), despite the fact that the risks posed by each are considerably different. Explaining the complications of VBAC in a way that is meaningful to women can be challenging, and thus a comparison to a similar group of women who have also not undergone previous vaginal delivery may be a more relevant comparison.

Research Question: When counseling women undergoing planned VBAC, should a comparison of outcomes be made to women undergoing ERCS, or is a comparison to other nulliparous women undergoing vaginal birth a more valid comparison in terms of risk outcomes?

Participants and Methods: A retrospective cohort study was undertaken comprising a consecutive cohort of 21,389 women who delivered, stratified by Robson's criteria into Robson groups 1-5. Those in Robson groups 6-10 were not included. Demographic data and maternal/neonatal outcomes were reviewed, with main outcome measures comprising uterine rupture, post-partum hemorrhage (PPH), 3rd/4th degree tears, and neonatal morbidity.

Results: There was no increase in PPH, vaginal tears, or neonatal complications in the VBAC group when compared to Robson groups 1 and 2 (nulliparous women in spontaneous or induced labour, respectively). Uterine rupture rates were low in all groups, with no correlation identified.

Discussion: The maternal and neonatal morbidity associated with VBAC is comparable to primiparous women undergoing a vaginal birth.

Conclusion: In demonstrating the low relative morbidity in this comparison, these outcomes may aid in counseling women faced with the choice of VBAC versus ERCS." (Rozen et al., 2011, p. 3)

Population-Based Studies

Population-based studies are also important in outcomes research. Conditions must be studied in the context of the patient's community rather than of the medical system. With this method, all cases of a condition occurring in the defined population are included, rather than only patients treated at a particular healthcare facility, because the latter could introduce a selection bias. The researcher might make efforts to include individuals with the condition who had not received treatment.

Community-based norms of tests and survey instruments obtained in this manner provide a clearer picture of the range of values than the limited spectrum of patients seen in specialty clinics. Estimates of instrument sensitivity and specificity are more accurate. This method enables researchers to understand the natural history of a condition or of the long-term risks and benefits of a particular intervention (Guess et al., 1995). Bakker et al. (2011) conducted a study examining the differences in birth outcomes related to maternal age. The following is an abstract of their study:

"*Background*: Previous studies have shown that birth weight and preterm birth are strong predictors of neonatal morbidity and mortality. Maternal age might be a modifiable determinant of weight and gestational age at birth. In most Western countries the age of mothers having their first child is increasing due to prolonged education, professional commitment, delayed marriage, and other personal reasons. It has been suggested that older maternal age is associated with increased risks of pregnancy complications, such as gestational hypertension or diabetes, preterm delivery, fetal malformations, and fetal death.

Methods: This is a population-based prospective cohort study with 8,568 mothers and their children based in Rotterdam, Netherlands. Maternal age, sociodemographic, lifestyle-related determinants, and birth outcomes were obtained from questionnaires and hospital records. The main outcome measures were birth weight, preterm delivery, small-for-gestational-age, and large-for-gestational-age babies. Multivariate linear and logistic regression analyses were used to analyze study data.

Results: In this study, mothers aged 30-34.9 years had no differences in risk of preterm delivery. Mothers <20 years had the highest risk of delivering small-for-gestational-age babies (OR 1.6, 95% CI: 1.1-2.5); however, after adjustment for sociodemographic and lifestyle-related determinants this increased risk was not present. Mothers >40 years had the highest risk of delivering large-for-gestational-age babies (OR 1.3, 95% CI: 0.8-2.4); however no associations of maternal age with the risks of delivering large-for-gestational-age babies could be explained by sociodemographic and lifestyle-related determinants.

Conclusions: Younger mothers have an increased risk of small-for-gestational age babies, whereas older mothers have an increased risk of large-for-gestational-age babies when compared with mothers aged 30-34.9 years. Sociodemographic and lifestyle-related determinants cannot entirely explain these differences." (Bakker et al., 2011, p. 500)

Geographical Analyses

Geographical analyses examine variations in health status, health services, patterns of care, or patterns of use by geographical area and are sometimes referred to as small area analyses. Variations may be associated with sociodemographic, economic, medical, cultural, or behavioral characteristics. Locality-specific factors of a healthcare system, such as capacity, access, and convenience, may play a role in explaining variations. The social setting, environment, living conditions, and community may also be important factors.

The interactions between the characteristics of a locality and of its inhabitants are complex. The characteristics of the total community may transcend the characteristics of individuals within the community and may influence subgroup behavior. High educational levels in the community are commonly associated with greater access to information and receptiveness to ideas from outside the community.

Regression analyses are commonly used to develop models using all the risk factors and the characteristics of the community. Results are often displayed through the use of maps (Kieffer, Alexander, & Mor, 1992). After the analysis, the researcher must determine whether differences in rates are due to chance alone and whether high rates are too high. From a more theoretical perspective, the researcher must then explain the geographical variation uncovered by the analysis (Volinn, Diehr, Ciol, & Loeser, 1994).

Geographical information systems (GISs) can provide an important tool for performing geographical analyses. A GIS uses relational databases to facilitate processing of spatial information. The software tools in a GIS can be used for mapping, data summaries, and analysis of spatial relationships. GISs have the capability of modeling data flows so that the effect of proposed changes in interventions applied to individuals or communities on outcomes can be modeled. Dunn, Anderson, and Bierman (2009) conducted a study of temporal and regional trends in intrauterine device (IUD) insertion. Their study abstract is reprinted here:

"*Background:* In Canada, intrauterine device (IUD) use is low and declined between 1985 and 1995. This study examines temporal and regional trends in IUD insertion in Ontario, Canada, from 1996 to 2006.

Study Design: Physician billing data was used to determine annual age-adjusted IUD insertion rates for women aged 15-55 years and proportions inserted by gynecologists and family physicians (FPs). Small area variation statistics were used to analyze variation in rates across the province.

Results: Annual insertion rates followed a U-shaped distribution and were lowest in 2001 and highest in 2006. From 1996 to 2006, the proportion inserted by FPs fell from 38.2% to 31.6% (*p*<0.001). In 2006, women in regions with the highest rates were twice as likely to have an IUD inserted as those in the lowest-rate regions.

Conclusions: IUD insertion rate began to increase in 2001, the year of introduction of levonorgestrel-releasing intrauterine system. Regional variation in rates suggests that access is not equal across the province and that strategies to support FPs to insert IUDs may be important to ensure sufficient access." (Dunn et al., 2009, p. 469)

Economic Studies

Many of the problems studied in health services research address concerns related to the efficient use of scarce resources and, thus, to economics. Health economists are concerned with the costs and benefits of alternative treatments or ways of identifying the most efficient means of care. The economist's definition of *efficiency* is the least expensive method of achieving a desired end while obtaining the maximum

benefit from available resources. If available resources must be shared with other programs or other types of patients, an economic study can determine whether changing the distribution of resources will increase total benefit or welfare.

Economic evaluation is a "set of formal, quantitative methods used to compare two or more treatments, programs, or strategies with respect to their resource use and their expected outcomes" (Guyatt, Rennie, Meade, & Cook, 2008, p. 781). In 1993, the U.S. Public Health Service established the Panel on Cost-Effectiveness in Health and Medicine to address the Public Health System's growing need for evaluating techniques that could guide decision-making processes in an era of rising cost restrictions (Gold, 1996). The Panel was charged with the development of recommendations for addressing the (1) poor quality of many economic analyses; (2) lack of comparability across cost-effectiveness analyses (CEAs) of different interventions or types of illness; and (3) lack of data on the costs and effects of interventions (Gold, 1996). Cost-effectiveness analysis, rather than cost-benefit analysis, was identified as the appropriate tool for economic analysis for the purpose of public health uses because of the former's focus on health rather than economic outcomes. The recommendations of the Panel are summarized here.

CEAs compare different ways of accomplishing a clinical goal, such as diagnosing a condition, treating an illness, or providing a service. The alternative approaches are compared in terms of costs and benefits. The purpose is to identify the strategy that provides the most value for the money. There are always tradeoffs between costs and benefits. When making decisions for patient groups, clinicians need to consider whether the benefits of providing treatment are worth the healthcare costs. It is also important to indicate whose perspective the analysis will consider, for example, that of patients, providers, insurers, or the broader society. The Panel on Cost-Effectiveness in Health and Medicine assumed a societal perspective. The Panel's recommendations fell into the following eight categories (Weinstein, Siegel, Gold, Kamlet, & Russell, 1996):

1. The nature and limits of CEA and of the reference case for the analysis.
2. Components (variables) belonging in the numerator and denominator of a cost/effectiveness ratio.
3. Measuring terms in the numerator (i.e., costs).
4. Valuing the health consequences in the denominator.
5. Estimating effectiveness of the intervention.
6. Time preference and discounting.

7. Handling uncertainty in CEA.
8. Reporting guidelines.

With regard to category #1, the Panel chose the societal perspective for the reference case they considered in their analysis, because it does not represent the viewpoint of any specific group and provides a benchmark against which to assess results from other perspectives. "The reference case is defined by a standard set of methods and assumptions. It includes a set of standard results: the reference case results" (Russell, Gold, Siegel, Daniels, & Weinstein, 1996, p. 1173). As to category #2, the "results of CEA are summarized in cost-effectiveness ratios that demonstrate the cost of achieving a unit of health effect (e.g., cost per year of life gained) for diverse types of patients and for variations of the intervention" (Russell et al., 1996, p. 1173). Changes in health due to the intervention are captured in the denominator, and changes in resource use due to the intervention are captured in the numerator. The societal perspective dictates that all important effects on human health (e.g., social and physical function, quality of life, years of life) and on resources must be included in the analysis. Therefore the panel recommended that the denominator of the C/E ratio be reserved for the improvement in health associated with an intervention (Weinstein et al., 1996). With regard to category #3, there were several recommendations related to what to include in the numeration of the C/E ratio, which reflects the change in costs or use of resources caused by a health intervention. For example, the Panel recommended that costs be measured in constant dollars, an approach that requires adjusting dollars for different years because of inflation. Valuing the health consequences in the denominator (category #4) requires a measurement of adjusted life-years expressed in an interval scale so that the ratio of differences between values is meaningful. Acceptable data for estimating effectiveness of the intervention, which is category #5, may come from a variety of sources such as randomized controlled trials, observational studies, uncontrolled experiments, or descriptive series (Weinstein et al., 1996). As to category #6, on time preference and discounting, the Panel recommended that costs and health outcomes occurring during different time periods should be discounted to their present value and that they should be discounted at the same rate. The Panel recommended a discount rate of 3%. It is important to address uncertainty in conclusions of CEA (category #7) because CEA conclusions might change with changes in assumptions or values (e.g., discount rate). Uncertainty is addressed by varying the values/assumptions in the analysis and assessing whether the

conclusions still hold. For the last category, reporting guidelines, the Panel developed a set of recommendations for reporting CEA that addressed how to report the background to the problem, data and methods, results, and discussion (Siegel, Weinstein, Russell, & Gold, 1996). Building on these recommendations, Stone (1998) described the methodology for conducting and reporting cost-effectiveness analyses in nursing.

Costs can vary hugely across jurisdictions, because hospitals may have different success in negotiating with suppliers for drugs and equipment (Drummond, Groeree, Moayyedi, & Levine, 2008). Costs also depend on how care is organized. "The same service may be delivered by a physician or a nurse practitioner, in the outpatient setting or in the hospital, and with or without administrative costs related to the adjudication of patient eligibility to receive the service" (Drummond et al., 2008, p. 623). It is time for nurses to take a more active role in conducting cost-effectiveness research. Nurses are well positioned to evaluate healthcare practices and have the incentive to conduct the studies. However, nursing practice is seldom a subject of cost-effectiveness analyses. The knowledge gained from this effort could enable nurses to refine their practice by substituting interventions that maximize nurses' time (a cost variable) to the best advantage of patient outcomes.

Fraher, Collins, Bourke, Phelan, and Lynch (2009) conducted an economic analysis of employing a total parenteral nutrition surveillance nurse for the prevention of catheter-related bloodstream infections. The following is an abstract of that study.

Background: "The cost of catheter-related bloodstream infection (CRBSI) is substantial in terms of morbidity, mortality, and financial resources. Total parenteral nutrition (TPN) is a recognized risk factor for CRBSI. In 1997, an intravenous nutrition nurse was promoted to TPN surveillance clinical nurse manager (CNM) and quarterly infection audit meetings were introduced to monitor trends in CRBSI."

Methods: "Data were prospectively collected over a 15-year period using specific TPN records in a 535-bed tertiary acute university hospital. A total of 20,439 CVC-days and 307 CRBSIs were recorded. Mean number of infections before, and after, the introduction of a dedicated TPN surveillance CNM were compared."

Results: "Mean CRBSI per 1000 catheter-days ± SD was $20.5 + 6.34$ prior to 1997 and 14.64 ± 7.81 after

1997, representing a mean reduction of 5.84 CRBSIs per 1000 catheter-days (95% CI: −4.92 to 16.60; $p=0.05$). Mean number of CRBSIs per year $\pm$ SD was 28.3 ± 4.93 prior to 1997 and 18.5 ± 7.37 after 1997, representing a mean decrease of 9.8 infections per year (95% CI: 0.01 to 19.66; $p<0.05$). The savings made by preventing 9.8 infections per year were calculated from data on bed-days obtained from the hospital finance office. The cost in hospital days saved per annum was € 135,000."

Conclusions: "Introduction of the TPN surveillance CNM saved the hospital at least € 78,300 per annum and led to a significant decrease in CRBSIs in TPN patients." (Fraher et al., 2009, p. 129)

Ethical Studies

Outcomes studies often lead to policies for allocating scarce resources. Ethicists take the position that moral principles, such as justice, constrain the use of costs and benefits to choose treatments that might maximize the benefit per unit cost. Value commitments are inherent in choices about research methods and about the selection and interpretation of outcome variables, and researchers should acknowledge these commitments. "The choices researchers make should be documented and the reasons for those choices should be given explicitly in publications and presentations so that readers and other users of the information are enabled and expected to bear more responsibility for interpreting and applying the findings appropriately" (Lynn & Virnig, 1995, p. AS292). Veatch (1993) proposed that by analyzing the implications of rationing decisions in terms of the principles of justice and autonomy, we would establish more acceptable criteria than we would by using outcomes predictors alone. As an example, Veatch performed an ethical analysis of the use of outcome predictors in decisions related to the early withdrawal of life support. Ethical studies need to play an important role in outcomes programs of research.

Sperling and Simon (2010) investigated physician attitudes and policies regarding access to fertility care and assisted reproductive technologies in Israel. The abstract of that study follows:

"Despite the high profile of fertility care and assisted reproductive technologies, their social and regulatory contexts remain largely unexplored. Yet, studies reveal a practice of candidate screening on a somewhat arbitrary basis. Examining the above issues is of special importance to Israel, given its high fertility rates. To this end, this study conducted a survey of physicians' attitudes regarding access to fertility care and treatment. An anonymous questionnaire was distributed among IVF [in vitro fertilization] providers in all fertility clinics in Israel during 2008-2009. A total of 46 physicians (> 40%) responded. Although all agree that every person has a right to procreate, 15.25% believe it is important to screen candidates and 55.6% believe they should consider non-medical criteria when providing care. Only 47.8% of physicians acknowledge the existence of guidelines in their units, but where they exist, 22.5% state they do not follow them. Furthermore, between 24.4-63.0% of physicians are willing to perform controversial procedures if backed by official guidelines. In conclusion, existing guidelines are often vague or ignored. Contrary to the USA, IVF providers in Israel are shaped by the pro-natalist [an attitude or policy that encourages childbearing] approach highly encouraged by the state and they act less as trustees and gatekeepers to the future child." (Sperling & Simon, 2010, p. 854)

Measurement Methods

The selection of appropriate outcome variables is critical to the success of a study (Bernstein & Hilborne, 1993). As in any study, the researcher must evaluate the evidence of validity and the reliability of the measurement methods. Outcomes selected for nursing studies should be those most consistent with nursing practice and theory (Harris & Warren, 1995). In some studies, rather than selecting the final outcome of care, which may not occur for months or years, researchers use measures of intermediate end points. **Intermediate end points** are events or markers that act as precursors to the final outcome. It is important, however, to document the validity of the intermediate end point in predicting the outcome (Freedman & Schatzkin, 1992). In early outcomes studies, researchers selected outcome measures that they could easily obtain rather than those most desirable for outcomes studies. Later outcome studies have selected outcome measures from secondary data sources (e.g., Aiken et al., 2008; Cummings, Midodzi, Wong, & Estabrooks, 2010). Secondary analysis is "any reanalysis of data or information collected by another researcher or organization, including analysis of data sets collected from a variety of sources to create time-series or area-based data sets" (Shi, 2008, p. 129). Outcomes researchers have used secondary data from sources such as hospital discharge data (Aiken et al., 2008; Cummings et al., 2010). Data collected through NDNQI or CALNOC can also be utilized in nursing outcomes research.

Table 13-4 identifies characteristics important to evaluate in selecting methods of measuring outcomes. In evaluating a particular outcome measure, the researcher should consult the literature for previous studies that have used that particular method of measurement, including the publication describing development of the method of measurement. This approach was used by Doran et al. (2011) when they reviewed the state of the science on nursing-sensitive outcomes. For each outcome concept (e.g., functional status, pain, pressure ulcer, self-care), the empirical literature investigating the concept in nursing research was reviewed. The approach to measurement of the outcome concept was identified, and the reliability, sensitivity, and validity of the measurement tools were appraised and summarized in tabular form. Sensitivity to change is an important measurement property to consider in outcomes research because researchers are often interested in evaluating how outcomes change in response to healthcare interventions. As the sensitivity of a measure increases, statistical power increases, allowing smaller sample sizes to detect significant differences. For a full discussion of reliability and validity of scales and questionnaires, precision and accuracy of physiological measures, and sensitivity and specificity of diagnostic tools, refer to Chapter 16 of this text.

Statistical Methods for Outcomes Studies

Although outcomes researchers test for the statistical significance of their findings, this evaluation is not considered sufficient to judge the findings as important. Their focus is the clinical importance of study findings (see Chapter 21 for more information on clinical importance). In analyzing data, outcomes researchers have moved away from statistical analyses that use the mean to test for group differences. They place greater importance on analyzing change scores and use exploratory methods for examining the data to identify outliers.

Analysis of Change

With the focus on outcomes studies has come a renewed interest in methods of analyzing change. Gottman and Rushe (1993) reported that the first book addressing change in research, *Problems in Measuring Change*, edited by Harris (1967), is the basis for most of the current approaches to analyzing change. However, some new ideas have emerged regarding the analysis of change, such as the studies by Tracy et al.

(2006) and Bettger, Coster, Latham, and Keysor (2008).

For some outcomes, the changes may be nonlinear or may go up and down rather than always increasing. Thus, it is as important to uncover patterns of change as it is to test for statistically significant differences at various time points. Some changes may occur in relation to stages of recovery or improvement. These changes may occur over weeks, months, or even years. A more complete picture of the process of recovery can be obtained by examining the process in greater detail and over a broader range. With this approach, the examiner can develop a recovery curve, which provides a model of the recovery process that can then be tested (Boz et al., 2004; Hernandez, Fernandez, Luzon, Cuena, & Montejo, 2007; McCauley, Hannay, & Swank, 2001).

Analysis of Improvement

In addition to reporting the mean improvement score for all patients treated, it is important to report what percentage of patients improved. Do all patients improve slightly, or is there a divergence among patients, with some improving greatly and others not improving at all? This divergence may best be illustrated by plotting the data. Researchers studying a particular treatment or approach to care might develop a standard or index of varying degrees of improvement that might occur. The index would allow better comparisons of the effectiveness of various treatments. Characteristics of patients who experience varying degrees of improvement should be described, and outliers should be carefully examined. This step requires that the study design include baseline measures of patient status, such as demographic characteristics, functional status, and disease severity measures. An analysis of improvement allows better judgments of the appropriate use of various treatments (Fasting & Gisvold, 2003).

Variance Analysis

Variance analysis is used to track individual and group variance from a specific critical pathway. The goal is to decrease preventable variance in process, thus helping patients and their families achieve optimal outcomes. Some of the variance is due to comorbidities. You may find that keeping a patient with comorbidities on the desired pathway may require you to utilize more resources early in the patient's care. Thus, it is important to track both variance and comorbidities. Studies examining variations from pathways may make it easier for healthcare providers to tailor existing critical pathways for specific comorbidities.

TABLE 13-4 Characteristics of Outcomes Assessment Instruments*

Characteristic	Considerations in Patient Outcomes Evaluation	References
Applicability	Consider purpose of instruments Discriminate between subjects at a point in time Predict future outcomes Evaluate changes within subjects over time Screen for problems Provide case-mix adjustment Assess quality of care Consider whether norms are established for clinical population of interest Instrument format is compatible with assessment approach (e.g., observer-rated versus self-administered) Setting in which instrument was developed	Deyo & Carter, 1992 Stewart et al., 1989 Guyatt, Walter, & Norman, 1987 Feinstein, Josephy, & Wells, 1986 Deyo, 1984
Practicality (clinical utility)	The Instrument: Includes outcomes important to the patient Is short and easy to administer (low respondent burden) includes questions that are easy to understand and acceptable to patients and interviewers Has scores that reflect condition severity and condition-specific features, and discriminate those with conditions from those without Is easily scored and has readily understandable scores Uses a level of measurement that allows a change score to be determined Provides information that is clinically useful Is performance or capacity based Includes patient rating of magnitude of effort and support needed for performance of physical tasks	Leidy, 1991 Nelson, Landgraf, Hays, Wasson, & Kirk, 1990 Stewart et al., 1989 Lohr, 1988 Bombardier & Tugwell, 1987 Feinstein et al., 1986 Kirshner & Guyatt, 1985 Deyo, 1984
Comprehensiveness	Generic measures are designed to summarize a spectrum of concepts applied to different impairments, illnesses, patients, and populations Disease-specific measures are designed to assess specific patients with specific conditions or diagnoses Dimensions of the instrument; a core set of physical, mental, and role functions-desirable	Nelson et al., 1990 Patrick & Deyo, 1989 Deyo, 1984
Reliability	Can be influenced by day-to-day variations in patients, differences between observers, items in the scale, mode of administration Is the critical determinant of usefulness of an instrument Is designed for discriminative purpose	Nelson et al., 1990 Spitzer, 1987 Guyatt et al., 1987 Deyo, 1984
Validity	No consensus of what are scientifically admissible criteria for many indices No "gold standard" exists for establishing criterion validity for many indices	Spitzer, 1987 Deyo, 1984
Responsiveness	Not yet indexed for virtually any evaluative measures Coarse scale rating may not detect changes Aggregated scores may obscure changes in subscales Useful for determining sample size and statistical power Reliable instruments are likely to be responsive, but reliability not adequate as sole index of consistent results over time Detail in scaling should be considered As baseline variability of score changes within stable subjects, larger treatment effects may be needed to demonstrate efficacy Temporal relationship between intervention and outcome should be considered	Stewart & Archbold, 1992 Leidy, 1991 Jaeschke, Singer, & Guyatt, 1989 Bombardier & Tugwell, 1987 Guyatt et al., 1987 Deyo & Centor, 1986 Deyo, 1984

*Examples are illustrative; for complete list of structural, process, and outcome indicators, refer to original sources cited in the table.
Modified from Harris M. R., & Warren, J. J. (1995). Patient outcomes: Assessment issues for the CNS. *Clinical Nurse Specialist, 9*(2), 82.

Variance analysis can also be used to identify at-risk patients who might benefit from the services of a case manager. Variance analysis tracking is expressed through the use of graphics, with the expected pathway plotted on a graph. The care providers plot deviations (negative variance) on the graph, allowing immediate comparison with the expected pathway. Deviations may be related to the patient, system, or provider (Okita et al., 2009; Olive & Solomonides, 2009; Tidwell, 1993).

Latent Transition Analysis

Latent transition analysis (LTA) is used in situations in which stages or categories of recovery have been defined and transitions between stages can be identified. To use this analysis method, the researchers assign each member of the population to a single category or stage for a given point of time. However, stage membership changes over time. The analysis tests stage membership to provide a realistic picture of development.

Roberts and Ward (2011) described an example of latent transition analysis (LTA) for nursing research by presenting a case example, using secondary analysis. The secondary analysis involved a psychoeducational intervention for cancer pain management in which LTA was used to describe for whom and in what direction the tailored intervention resulted in change with respect to attitudinal barriers and pain symptoms. The study sample consisted of 791 participants from the original study. Participants' response patterns to the Barriers Questionnaire II (Ward, Wang, Serlin, Peterson, & Marray, 2009) were used to determine latent classes for the LTA, as described here:

"The LTA model was specified using a four-step process. ... Specifically, these steps were (a) defining latent class structure using latent class analysis, (b) predicting class membership by adding demographic predictors to the latent class model at Time 1, (c) testing distal pain outcomes across latent classes at Time 2, and (d) modeling and testing transition probabilities for change in class membership over time." (Roberts & Ward, 2011, p. 75)

Roberts and Ward (2011) found that the older, less educated individuals in the study were more likely to be in the High Barriers class at Time 1. For those individuals who transitioned across classes, those who received the intervention were more likely to move in a favorable direction (to the Low Barriers class). The results from LTA provided useful information about for whom and in what direction the intervention resulted in change. In addition, LTA is a useful procedure for nurse researchers because it collapses large arrays of categorical data into meaningful patterns (Roberts & Ward, 2011). For example, Cain, Epler, Steinley, and Sher (2010) used LTA to examine change in patterns of concerns related to eating, weight, and shape in young adult women.

Multilevel Analysis

Multilevel analysis is a statistical technique that is useful when data exist at several different levels, for example, if data are nested or if a study has several different units of analysis. It has been used in epidemiology to study how environmental factors (aggregate-level characteristics) and individual attributes and behaviors (individual-level characteristics) interact to influence individual-level health behaviors and disease risks. Growing numbers of nursing studies have used multilevel analysis as a statistical technique to study phenomena measured at different units of analysis. One such example is the study by Simon, Muller, and Hasselhorn (2010), who used multilevel analysis to determine which variables were associated with nurses' intention to leave the profession and which were associated with their intention to leave the organization. As described in the following excerpt from the abstract, data existed at individual, departmental, and hospital levels:

"A secondary data analysis of the German sample of the European Nurses' Early Exit-Study was performed, using a generalized linear mixed-model approach... Data from 2119 Registered Nurses in 71 departments of 16 hospitals from 2003 were analyzed. Models for intentions to leave the profession explained more variance ($R^2 = 0.46$) than models for intentions to leave the organization ($R^2 = 0.28$). Both leaving intentions were associated with age, professional commitment, and job satisfaction. Intentions to leave the profession were strongly associated with variables related to the personal background and the work/home interface whereas intentions to leave the organization were related to organizational leadership and the local context." (Simon et al., 2010, p. 616)

In this example, the multilevel analysis was a useful technique for differentiating the determinants of nurses' intention to leave, demonstrating that departmental level variables (e.g., leadership) had an influence on intention to leave the organization whereas individual level variables (e.g., personal background) had an influence on intention to leave the profession. In another nursing study, Tak, Sweeney, Alterman, Baron, and Calvert (2010) examined determinants of workplace assaults on nursing assistants in U.S. nursing homes. Data from the National Nursing Assistant Survey (individual level) were linked to facility information (organizational level). The investigators found that mandatory overtime and not having enough time to assist residents with their activities of daily living (i.e., workload) were associated with experiencing injuries from assault as well as working in a facility with Alzheimer care units.

Disseminating Outcomes Research Findings

Once you have completed fieldwork and data analysis and have documented your findings, you need to ensure that your research findings are disseminated. Often funding agencies have particular requirements about the dissemination of research findings, which involves the communication of studies through presentations and publications. This means that the first step in deciding the format of your reporting is to understand the responsibilities that you have to funders and others. Including plans for the dissemination of findings is an essential component of a program of research. Strategies for the dissemination of research findings need to be carefully planned and need to include at least the following:

- Decide on the objectives of dissemination.
- Identify the audience for your material.
- Ascertain whether you will be preparing a written or oral report (usually both).
- Identify other methods for disseminating results.
- Identify timelines for each section of the reporting strategy.

The audiences for your research could include (1) the clinicians, who will apply the knowledge to practice; (2) the public, who may make healthcare decisions on the basis of the information; (3) healthcare institutions, which must evaluate care in their facilities on the basis of the information; (4) health policy makers, who may set standards on the basis of the information; and (5) researchers, who may use the information in designing new studies. Disseminating information to these various constituencies through presentations at meetings and publications in a variety of journals, as well as releasing the information to the news media, requires careful planning (see Chapter 27, Disseminating Research Findings).

KEY POINTS

- Outcomes research examines the end results of patient care.
- The scientific approaches used in outcomes studies differ in some important ways from those used in traditional research.
- Donabedian (1987, 2005) developed the theory on which outcomes research is based.
- Quality is the overriding construct of the theory, although Donabedian never defined this term.
- The three major concepts of the theory are health, subjects of care, and providers of care.
- Donabedian identified three objects of evaluation in appraising quality: structure, process, and outcome.
- The goal of outcomes research is to evaluate outcomes as defined by Donabedian, whose theory requires that identified outcomes be clearly linked with the process that caused the outcome.
- Clinical guideline panels are developed to incorporate available evidence on health outcomes.
- Outcome studies provide rich opportunities to build a stronger scientific underpinning for nursing practice.
- A nursing-sensitive patient outcome is "sensitive" because it is influenced by nursing.
- Organizations currently involved in efforts to study nursing-sensitive outcomes include the American Nurses Association, the National Quality Forum, the Collaborative Alliance for Nursing Outcomes, the Veterans Affairs Nursing Outcomes Database, the Center for Medicare and Medicaid Services' Hospital Quality Initiative, the American Hospital Association, the Federation of American Hospitals, The Joint Commission, and the Agency of Healthcare Research and Quality.
- Another area of interest in terms of outcomes research is the process of care delivered by advanced practice nurses (nurse practitioners, nurse midwives, nurse anesthetists, and clinical nurse specialists).
- Outcome design strategies tend to have less control than traditional research designs and, except for the clinical trial, seldom use random samples; rather, they use large representative samples.
- Statistical approaches used in outcomes studies include new approaches to examining measurement reliability, strategies to analyze change, the

analysis of improvement, variance analysis, latent transition analysis, and multilevel analysis.

- Dissemination is an important part of the outcomes research process to ensure the study results have an impact on patients, providers, and healthcare organizations.

REFERENCES

Agency for Healthcare Research and Quality (AHRQ, 2010). *HHS awards $437 million in patient-centered outcomes research funding.* Retrieved from http://www.ahrq.gov/news/press/pr2010/recoveryawpr.htm/.

Agency for Healthcare Research and Quality (AHRQ, 2011). *National Guideline Clearinghouse.* Retrieved from http://www.guideline.gov/.

Aiken, L. H., Clarke, S. P., Sloane, D. M., Lake, E. T., & Cheney, T. (2008). Effects of hospital care environment on patient mortality and nurse outcomes. *Journal of Nursing Administration, 38*(5), 223–229.

Alexander, G. R. (2007). Nursing sensitive databases: Their existence, challenges and importance. *Medical Care Research and Review, 64*(2), 44S–63S.

Bakker, R., Steegers, E., Biharie, A., Mackenbach, J., Hofman, A., & Jaddoe, V. (2011). Explaining differences in birth outcomes in relation to maternal age: The Generation R Study. *BJOG: An International Journal of Obstetrics and Gynaecology, 118*(4), 500–509.

Bernstein, S. J., & Hilborne, L. H. (1993). Clinical indicators: The road to quality care? *Joint Commission Journal on Quality Improvement, 19*(11), 501–509.

Bettger, J. A., Coster, W. J., Latham, N. K., & Keysor, J. J. (2008). Analyzing change in recovery patterns in the year after acute hospitalization. *Achieves of Physical Medicine & Rehabilitation, 89*(7), 1267–1275.

Bombardier, C., & Tugwell, P. (1987). Methodological considerations in functional assessment. *Journal of Rheumatology, 14*(Suppl. 15), 7–10.

Boz, C., Ozmenoglu, M., Alioglu, Z., Velioglu, S., Altunayoglu, V., & Gazioglu, S. (2004). Local cold effect on the excitability recovery curve of the sympathetic skin response. *Electromyography & Clinical Neurophysiology, 44*(8), 497–501.

Cain, A. S., Epler, A. J., Steinley, D., & Sher, K. J. (2010). Stability and change in patterns of concerns related to eating, weight, and shape in young adult women: A latent transition analysis. *Journal of Abnormal Psychology, 119*(2), 255–267.

Canadian Institute for Health Information. (2012). *Frequently-asked questions about the MIS Standards.* Ottawa, Canada: Author. Retrieved from http://www.cihi.ca/cihi-ext-portal/internet/en/document/standards+and+data+submission/standards/mis+standards/mis_faq/.

Clancy, C. M., & Eisenberg, J. M. (1998). Outcomes research: Measuring the end results of health care. *Science, 282*(5387), 245–246.

Collaborative Alliance for Nursing Outcomes (CALNOC, 2010). *CALNOC: About us.* Retrieved from https://www.calnoc.org/globalPages/mainpage.aspx/.

Cummings, G. G., Midodzi, W. K., Wong, C. A., & Estabrooks, C. A. (2010). The contribution of hospital nursing leadership styles to 30-day patient mortality. *Nursing Research, 59*(5), 331–339.

Cunningham, R. S. (2004). Advanced practice nursing outcomes: A review of selected empirical literature. *Oncology Nursing Forum, 31*(2), 219–230.

Davies, B., Edwards, N., Ploeg, J., & Virani, T. (2008). Insights about the process and impact of implementing nursing guidelines on delivery of care in hospitals and community settings. *BMC Health Services Research, 8,* 29.

Deyo, R. A. (1984). Measuring functional outcomes in therapeutic trials for chronic disease. *Controlled Clinical Trials, 5*(3), 223–240.

Deyo, R. A., & Carter, W. B. (1992). Strategies for improving and expanding the application of health status measures in clinical settings. *Medical Care, 30*(5 suppl), MS176–MS186.

Deyo, R. A., & Centor, R. M. (1986). Assessing the responsiveness of functional scales to clinical change: An analogy to diagnostic test performance. *Journal of Chronic Disease, 39*(11), 897–906.

Deyo, R. A., Taylor, V. M., Diehr, P., Conrad, D., Cherkin, D. C., Ciol, M., et al. (1994). Analysis of automated administrative and survey databases to study patterns and outcomes of care. *Spine, 19*(18), 2083S–2091S.

Donabedian, A. (1976). *Benefits in medical care programs.* Cambridge, MA: Harvard University Press.

Donabedian, A. (1978). *Needed research in quality assessment and monitoring.* Hyattsville, MD: U.S. Department of Health, Education, and Welfare, Public Health Service: National Center for Health Services Research.

Donabedian, A. (1980). *Explorations in quality assessment and monitoring.* Ann Arbor, MI: Health Administration Press.

Donabedian, A. (1982). *The criteria and standards of quality.* Ann Arbor, MI: Health Administration Press.

Donabedian, A. (1987). Some basic issues in evaluating the quality of health care. In: L. T. Rinke (Ed.), *Outcome measures in home care* (p. 338) (Vol. I). New York, NY: National League for Nursing. (Original work published 1976.)

Donabedian, A. (2005). Evaluating the quality of medical care. *The Milbank Quarterly, 83*(4), 691–729.

Doran, D. M. (Ed.) (2011). *Nursing outcomes: The state of the science* (2nd ed.). Sudbury, MA: Jones & Bartlett.

Doran, D. M., Mildon, B. & Clarke, S. (2011). Toward a national report card in nursing: A knowledge synthesis. *Canadian Journal of Nursing Leadership, 24*(2), 38–57.

Doran, D. M., Sidani, S., & Di Pietro, T. (2010). Nursing sensitive outcomes. In J. S. Fulton, B. Lyon, & K. Goudreau (Eds.), *Foundations of Clinical Nurse Specialist Practices* (pp. 35–37), New York, NY: Springer.

Doran, D., Harrison, M. B., Laschinger, H., Hirdes, J., Rukholm, E., Sidani, S., et al. (2006). Relationship between nursing interventions and outcome achievement in acute care settings. *Research in Nursing & Health, 29*(1), 61–70.

Drummond, M., Goeree, R., Moayyedi, P., & Levine, M. (2008). Economic analysis. In G. Guyatt, D. Rennie, M. O. Meade, & D. J. Cook (Eds.), *Users' guides to the medical literature: A manual for evidence-based practice* (2nd ed.) (pp. 619–641). New York, NY: McGraw-Hill Medical.

Dunn, S., Anderson, G. M., & Bierman, A. S. (2009). Temporal and regional trends in IUD insertion: A population-based study in Ontario, Canada. *Contraception, 80*(5), 469–473.

Epstein, A. J., & Nicholson, S. (2009). The formation and evolution of physician treatment styles: An application to cesarean sections. *Journal of Health Economics, 28*(6), 1126–1140.

Fasting, S., & Gisvold, S. E. (2003). Statistical process control methods allow the analysis and improvement of anesthesia care. *Canadian Journal of Anesthesia, 50*(8), 767–774.

Feinstein, A. R., Josephy, B. R., & Wells, C. K. (1986). Scientific and clinical problems in indexes of functional disability. *Annals of Internal Medicine, 105*(3), 413–420.

Fraher, M. H., Collins, C. J., Bourke, J., Phelan, D., & Lynch, M. (2009). Cost-effectiveness of employing a total parenteral nutrition surveillance nurse for the prevention of catheter-related bloodstream infections. *Journal of Hospital Infection, 73*(2), 129–134.

Freedman, L. S., & Schatzkin, A. (1992). Sample size for studying intermediate endpoints within intervention trials or observational studies. *American Journal of Epidemiology, 136*(9), 1148–1159.

Gold, M. (1996). Panel on cost-effectiveness in health and medicine. *Medical Care, 34*(12), DS197–DS199.

Gottman, J. M., & Rushe, R. H. (1993). The analysis of change: Issues, fallacies, and new ideas. *Journal of Consulting and Clinical Psychology, 61*(6), 907–910.

Graham, I. D., Bick, D., Tetroe, J., Straus, S. E., & Harrison, M. B. (2011). Measuring outcomes of evidence-based practice: Distinguishing between knowledge use and its impact. In D. Bick & I. D. Graham (Eds.), *Evaluating the impact of implementing evidence-based practice* (pp. 18–37). Oxford, United Kingdom: Wiley-Blackwell.

Guess, H. A., Jacobsen, S. J., Girman, C. J., Oesterling, J. E., Chute, C. G., & Panser, L. A., et al. (1995). The role of community-based longitudinal studies in evaluating treatment effects. Example: Benign prostatic hyperplasia. *Medical Care, 33*(Suppl. 4), AS26–AS35.

Guyatt, G., Rennie, D., Meade, M. O., & Cook, D. J. (2008). *Users' guides to the medical literature: A manual for evidence-based practice* (2nd ed.). New York, NY: McGraw-Hill Medical.

Guyatt, G., Walter, S., & Norman, G. (1987). Measuring change over time: Assessing the usefulness of evaluative instruments. *Journal of Chronic Disease, 40*(2), 171–178.

Harris, C. W. (1967). *Problems in measuring change.* Madison, WI: University of Wisconsin Press.

Harris, M. R., & Warren, J. J. (1995). Patient outcomes: Assessment issues for the CNS. *Clinical Nurse Specialist, 9*(2), 82–86.

Hernandez, G., Fernandez, R., Luzon, E., Cuena, R., & Montejo, J. C. (2007). The early phase of the minute ventilation recovery curve predicts extubation failure better than the minute ventilation recovery time. *Chest, 131*(5), 1315–1322.

Herrmann, D. (1995). Reporting current, past, and changed health status: What we know about distortion. *Medical Care, 33*(Suppl. 4), AS89–AS94.

Ingersoll, G. L., McIntosh, E., & Williams, M. (2000). Nurse-sensitive outcomes of advanced practice. *Journal of Advanced Nursing, 32*(5), 1272–1282.

Jaeschke, R., Singer, J., & Guyatt, G. H. (1989). Measurement of health status: Ascertaining the minimal clinically important difference. *Controlled Clinical Trials, 10*(4), 407–415.

Jennings, B. M., Loan, L. A., DePaul, D., Brosch, L. R., & Hildreth, P. (2001). Lessons learned while collecting ANA indicator data. *Journal of Nursing Administration, 31*(3), 121–129.

Keeney, S., Hasson, F., & McKenna, H. P. (2011). *The Delphi technique in nursing and health research.* Oxford, United Kingdom: Wiley-Blackwell.

Kelly, K. C., Huber, D. G., Johnson, M., McCloskey, J. C., & Maas, M. (1994). The Medical Outcomes Study: A nursing perspective. *Journal of Professional Nursing, 10*(4), 209–216.

Kieffer, E., Alexander, G. R., & Mor, J. (1992). Area-level predictors of use of prenatal care in diverse populations. *Public Health Reports, 107*(6), 653–658.

Kirshner, B., & Guyatt, G. (1985). A methodological framework for assessing health indices. *Journal of Chronic Diseases, 38*(1), 27–36.

Kleib, M., Sales, A., Doran, D. M., Malette, C. & White, D. (2011). Nursing minimum data sets. In D. M. Doran (Ed.), *Nursing outcomes: The state of the science* (2nd ed.) (pp. 487–512). Sudbury, MA: Jones & Bartlett.

Kramer, M., Maguire, P., & Schmalenberg, C. (2006). Excellence through evidence: The what, when, and where of clinical autonomy. *Journal of Nursing Administration, 36*(10), 479–491.

Lake, E. T. (2006). Multilevel models in health outcomes research Part I: Theory, design, and measurement. *Applied Nursing Research, 19*(1), 51–53.

Lee, T. H., & Goldman, L. (1989). Development and analysis of observational data bases. *Journal of the American College of Cardiology, 14*(Suppl. 3A), 44A–47A.

Leidy, N. K. (1991). Survey measures of functional ability and disability of pulmonary patients. In: B. L. Metzger (Ed.), *Synthesis conference on altered functioning: Impairment and disability* (pp. 52–79). Indianapolis, IN: Nursing Center Press of Sigma Theta Tau International.

Lohr, K. N. (1988). Outcome measurement: Concepts and questions. *Inquiry, 25*(1), 37–50.

Lynn, J., & Virnig, B. A. (1995). Assessing the significance of treatment effects: Comments from the perspective of ethics. *Medical Care, 33*(4), AS292–AS298.

Magnello, M. E. (2010). The passionate statistician. In S. Nelson & A. M. Rafferty (Eds.), *Notes on Nightingale: The influence and legacy of a nursing icon* (pp. 115–129). Ithaca, NY: Cornell University.

Mark, B. A. (1995). The black box of patient outcomes research. *Image: Journal of Nursing Scholarship, 27*(1), 42.

McCauley, S. R., Hannay, H. J., & Swank, P. R. (2001). Use of the disability rating scale recovery curve as a predictor of psychosocial outcome following closed-headed injury. *Journal of the International Neuropsychology Society, 7*(4), 457–467.

McDonald, C. J., & Hui, S. L. (1991). The analysis of humongous databases: Problems and promises. *Statistics in Medicine, 10*(4), 511–518.

Mitchell, J. B., Bubolz, T., Pail, J. E., Pashos, C. L., Escarce, J. J., Muhlbaier, L. H., et al. (1994). Using Medicare claims for outcomes research. *Medical Care, 32*(Suppl. 7), JS38–JS51.

Mitchell, P. H., Ferketich, S., & Jennings, B. M. (1998). American Academy of Nursing Expert Panel on Quality Health Care 1998 Quality Health Outcomes Model. *Image—Journal of Nursing Scholarship, 30*(1), 43–46.

Montalvo, I. (2007). The national database of nursing quality indicators (NDNQI). *The Online Journal of Issues in Nursing, 12*(3). Retrieved from http://www.nursingworld.org/ojin.

Moses, L. E. (1995). Measuring effects without randomized trials? Options, problems, challenges. *Medical Care, 33*(4), AS8–AS14.

National Association of Clinical Nurse Specialists. (NACNS, 2004). *Statement on clinical nurse specialist practice and education* (2nd ed.). Harrisburg, PA: Author.

National Database of Nursing Quality Indicators. (NDNQI, 2010). *ANA's NQF-endorsed measure specifications: Guidelines for data collection on the American Nurses Association's national quality forum endorsed measures: Nursing care hours per patient day; skill mix; falls and falls with injury.* Kansas City, KS: Author. Retrieved from home page link https://www.nursingquality.org/Default.aspx/.

National Quality Forum. (NQF, 2011). *NQF Advancing performance measurement.* Report to the Congress and the Secretary of the U.S. Department of Health and Human Services, covering the period of January 14, 2010–January 13, 2011. Retrieved from http://www.qualityforum.org/About_NQF/HHS_Performance_Measurement.aspx/.

Naylor, M. D. (2007). Advancing the science in the measurement of health care quality influenced by nurses. *Medical Care Research & Review, 64*(Suppl. 4), 144S–169S.

Nelson, E. C., Landgraf, J. M., Hays, R. D., Wasson, J. H., & Kirk, J. W. (1990). The functional status of patients: How can it be measured in physicians' offices? *Medical Care, 28*(12), 1111–1126.

Okita, A., Yamashita, M., Abe, K., Nagel, C., Matsumoto, A., Akehi, M., et al. (2009). Variance analysis of a clinical pathway of video-assisted single lobectomy for lung cancer. *Surgery Today, 39*(2), 104–109.

Olive, M., & Solomonides, T. (2009). Variance analysis as practice-based evidence. *Studies in Health Technology & Informatics, 147,* 190–198.

Oncology Nursing Society (ONS, 2012). *About the ONS.* Retrieved from http://www.ons.org/about/.

Patrick, D. L., & Deyo, R. A. (1989). Generic and disease-specific measures in assessing health status and quality of life. *Medical Care, 27*(Suppl. 3), S217–S232.

Roberts, T. J., & Ward, S. E. (2011). Using latent transition analysis in nursing research to explore change over time. *Nursing Research, 60*(1), 73–79.

Rowell, P. (2001). Lessons learned while collecting ANA indicator data: The American Nurses Association responds. *Journal of Nursing Administration, 31*(3), 130–131.

Rozen, G., Ugoni, A. M. & Sheehan, P. M. (2011). A new perspective on VBAC: A retrospective cohort study. *Women and Birth, 24*(1), 3–9.

Russell, L. B., Gold, M. R., Siegel, J. E., Daniels, N., & Weinstein, M. C. (1996). The role of cost-effectiveness analysis in health and medicine. Panel on Cost-Effectiveness in Health and Medicine. *Journal of the American Medical Association, 276*(14), 1172–1177.

Sadler, B. L., Joseph, A., Keller, A., & Rostenberg, B. (2009). *Using evidence-based environmental design to enhance safety and quality. Institute for Healthcare Improvement (IHI): Innovation series white paper.* Cambridge, MA: IHI. Retrieved from http://www.IHI.org/.

Schifalacqua, M. M., Mamula, J., & Mason, A. R. (2011). Return on investment imperative: The cost of care calculator for an evidence-based practice program. *Nursing Administration Quarterly, 35*(1), 15–20.

Sermeus, W., Delesie, L., Van den Heede, K., Diya, L., & Lesaffre, E. (2008). Measuring the intensity of nursing care: Making use of the Belgian nursing minimum data set. *International Journal of Nursing Studies, 45*(7), 1011–1021.

Setty, A. R., Curhan, G. & Choi, H. K. (2007). Smoking and the risk of psoriasis in women: Nurses' Health Study II. *American Journal of Medicine, 120*(11), 953–959.

Shi, L. (2008). *Health services research methods* (2nd ed.). Clifton Park, NY: Delmar Cengage Learning.

Siegel, J. E., Weinstein, M. C., Russell, L. B., & Gold, M. R. (1996). Recommendations for reporting cost-effectiveness analyses. Panel on Cost-Effectiveness in Health and Medicine. *Journal of the American Medical Association, 276*(16), 1339–1341.

Simon, M., Muller, B. H., & Hasselhorn, H. M. (2010). Leaving the organization or the profession—a multilevel analysis of nurses' intentions. *Journal of Advanced Nursing, 66*(3), 616–626.

Sperling, D., & Simon, Y. (2010). Attitudes and policies regarding access to fertility care and assisted reproductive technologies in Israel. *Reproductive Biomedicine Online, 21*(7), 854–861.

Spitzer, W. O. (1987). State of science 1986: Quality of life and functional status as target variables for research. *Journal of Chronic Disease, 40*(6), 465–471.

Stetler, C. B., & Caramanica, B. (2007). Evaluation of an evidence-based practice initiative: Outcomes, strengths, and limitations of a retrospective conceptually based approach. *Worldviews on Evidence-Based Nursing, 4*(4), 187–199.

Stewart, A. L., Greenfield, S., Hays, R. D., Wells, K., Rogers, W. H., Berry, S. D., et al. (1989). Functional status and well-being of patients with chronic conditions. *JAMA, 262*(7), 907–913.

Stewart, B. J., & Archbold, P. G. (1992). Nursing intervention studies require outcome measures that are sensitive to change: Part 2. *Research in Nursing & Health, 16*(1), 77–81.

Stone, D. W. (1998). Methods for conducting and reporting cost-effectiveness analysis in nursing. *Image—Journal of Nursing Scholarship, 30*(3), 229–234.

Stone, P. W., Mooney-Kane, C., Larson, E. L., Horan, T., Glance, L. G., Zwanziger, J., & Dick, A. W. (2007). Nurse working conditions and patient safety outcomes. *Medical Care, 45*(6), 571–578.

Straus, S., Tetroe, J., Graham, I. D., Zwarenstein, M., & Bhattacharyya, O. (2009). Monitoring and evaluating knowledge. In: S. Straus, J. Tetroe, & I. D. Graham (Eds.), *Knowledge translation in health care* (pp. 151–159). Oxford, UK: Wiley-Blackwell.

Swaen, G. M., & Meijers, J. M. (1988). Influence of design characteristics on the outcomes of retrospective cohort studies. *British Journal of Industrial Medicine, 45*(9), 624–629.

Tak, S., Sweeney, M. H., Alterman, T., Baron, S., & Calvert, G. M. (2010). Workplace assaults on nursing assistants in U.S. nursing homes: A multilevel analysis. *American Journal of Public Health*, *100*(10), 1938–1945.

Tarlov, A. R., Ware, J. E., Jr., Greenfield, S., Nelson, E. C., Perrin, E., & Zubkoff, M. (1989). The Medical Outcomes Study: An application of methods for monitoring the results of medical care. *JAMA*, *262*(7), 925–930.

Tidwell, S. L. (1993). A graphic tool for tracking variance and comorbidities in cardiac surgery case management. *Progress in Cardiovascular Nursing*, *8*(2), 6–19.

Tork, H. K., Dassen, T., & Lohrmann, C. (2008). Care dependency of children in Egypt. *Journal of Clinical Nursing*, *17*(3), 287–295.

Tourangeau, A. E. (2003). Modeling the determinants of mortality for hospitalized patients. *International Nursing Perspectives*, *3*(1), 37–48.

Tourangeau, A. E., Doran, D. M., Hall, L. M., O'Brien Pallas, L., Pringle, D., Tu, J. V., et al (2007). Impact of hospital nursing care on 30-day mortality for acute medical patients. *Journal of Advanced Nursing 57*(1), 32–44.

Tracy, S., Schinco, M. A., Griffen, M. M., Kerwin, A. J., Devin, T., & Tepas, J. J. (2006). Urgent airway intervention: Does outcome change with personnel performing the procedure? *Journal of Trauma*, *61*(5), 1162–1165.

Van den Heede, K., Sermeus, W., Diya, L., Clarke, S. P., Lesaffre, E., Vleugels, A., et al (2009). Nurse staffing and patient outcomes in Belgian acute hospitals: Cross-sectional analysis of administrative data. *International Journal of Nursing Studies*, *46*(7), 928–939.

Veatch, R. (1993). Justice and outcomes research: The ethical limits. *Journal of Clinical Ethics*, *4*(3), 258–261.

Volinn, E., Diehr, P., Ciol, M. A., & Loeser, J. D. (1994). Why does geographic variation in health care practices matter (and seven questions to ask in evaluating studies on geographic variation)? *Spine*, *19*(18S), 2092S–2100S.

Waltz, C. F., Strickland, O. L., & Lenz, E. R. (2010). *Measurement in nursing and health research* (4th ed.). New York, NY: Springer.

Ward, S. E., Wang, K. K., Serlin, R. C., Peterson, S. L., & Murray, M. E. (2009). A randomized trial of a tailored barriers intervention for cancer information service (CIS) callers in pain. *Pain*, *144*(1–2), 49–56.

Weinstein, M. C., Siegel, J. E., Gold, M. R., Kamlet, M. S., & Russell, L. B. (1996). Recommendations of the Panel on Cost-Effectiveness in Health and Medicine. *Journal of the American Medical Association*, *276*(15), 1253–1258.

Westert, G. P., & Groenewegen, P. P. (1999). Medical practice variations: Changing the theoretical approach. *Scandinavian Journal of Public Health*, *27*(3), 173–180.

World Health Organization. (2009). *The Conceptual Framework for the International Classification for Patient Safety, Version 1.0, 2007-2008*. Geneva, Switzerland: Author. Retrieved from http://www.who.int/patientsafety/taxonomy/en/.

Wray, N. P., Ashton, C. M., Kuykendall, D. H., Petersen, N. J., Souchek, J., & Hollingsworth, J. C. (1995). Selecting disease-outcome pairs for monitoring the quality of hospital care. *Medical Care*, *33*(1), 75–89.

14
CHAPTER

Intervention-Based Research

Investigations of interventions that address problems or issues of concern to patients, nurses, and healthcare organizations are vitally important to expanding the scientific basis for nursing practice. Intervention-based research verifies the efficacy, effectiveness, and efficiency of interventions needed for the development of evidence-based nursing practice. This type of research requires careful decision making regarding the optimal study design, controlled implementation of the treatment protocol and procedures, use of quality outcome measure(s), and appropriate analysis of data to ensure the best conditions for testing a selected intervention. A rigorously developed and implemented intervention study improves the likelihood of detecting statistically significant differences between the experimental and comparison groups on specified outcomes. The ability to find a statistical difference with an intervention is also based on having enough statistical power from an adequately sized sample and controlling sources of error and bias that can obscure study findings. Error and bias introduced into a study create threats to the validity of the study and limit the ability of drawing definitive conclusions about the effects of the intervention.

This chapter examines approaches to intervention-based research and describes various aspects of the research process that are unique to the study of interventions. The focus is on highlighting those distinct features of intervention-oriented research and explaining designs and methods to accomplish such research. Because the methods employed in testing interventions can be complex and rigorous, additional guidelines are provided for critically appraising these studies. The ability to critically appraise intervention-based research has wide-spread implications for examining the scientific merit of studies and translating findings into practice. This chapter also covers essential information for nurses conducting intervention studies.

Intervention-Based Research Conducted by Nurses

Thousands of intervention-based studies conducted by nurses have contributed to the scientific foundations for nursing practice. Nurse scientists, such as PhD-prepared nurses, not only have conducted individual studies but also have summarized the state of the science in selected areas with meta-analyses and systematic reviews. This high level of synthesis of research findings through meta-analyses and systematic reviews has enabled the pooling of data from multiple studies to formulate statistical and evaluative conclusions about the strength of evidence for interventions. Data compiled from intervention-based studies have guided the development and application of evidence-based practice approaches to care and, in some instances, have contributed to the development of national evidence-based guidelines. One of the most influential meta-analyses that forever changed nursing practice demonstrated that saline was just as effective as heparin flush solution in maintaining the patency of peripheral intravenous locks in adults (Goode et al., 1991). Investigators pooled data from 15 studies involving a total of 3490 patients to draw this conclusion. This would not have been possible without the individual studies conducted to examine the efficacy and effectiveness of a very common nursing intervention.

Summaries of intervention-based research are also valuable in determining how strong an intervention might be by gauging its effectiveness among multiple studies. For example, it is vitally important to understand what health promotion interventions work best and under what conditions. To address this issue, Conn, Hafdahl, and Mehr (2011) conducted a meta-analysis of studies focused on physical activity interventions in adults. They found that behavioral approaches were more effective than cognitive ones in improving adults' activity outcomes. Face-to-face delivery of the intervention, instead of telephone or mail, and individualized-focused interventions, rather than targeting of communities, were more effective in promoting physical activities. Systematic review, meta-analysis, meta-synthesis, and mixed-methods systematic review techniques in the evaluation of interventions across multiple studies provide much stronger evidence for implementing them in practice than one isolated investigation (see Chapter 19 for conducting these research syntheses).

This chapter introduces you to approaches to inquiry, ways of interpreting outcomes, and the evaluative aspects of research aimed at testing nursing interventions and plans of care. You will learn to examine components of intervention studies and to appreciate the scientific approaches that are relevant to the study of interventions. Few investigators do research alone, and intervention research is no exception. More often than not, research teams are required to accomplish studies using interventions. These research teams are composed of nurse scientists and sometimes investigators from other disciplines, such as medicine, pharmacy, psychology, and sociology. Interprofessional and/or interdisciplinary studies include additional intellectual perspectives, collective efforts among scientists, and additional resources that promote quality research. Whether interventions are unique to nursing or have implications for other disciplines, intervention-based research involves similar processes consisting of thoughtful planning, theory- or literature-driven rationales, appropriate designs for testing the intervention, systematic and consistent methods of implementing the intervention and collecting data, data analyses using parametric or nonparametric statistics, and dissemination of results. Examples of these steps in carrying out intervention research are described and illustrated with examples from published nursing studies.

Nursing Interventions

The term **intervention-based research** encompasses a broad range of investigations that examines the effects of any *intervention* or treatment having relevance to nursing. **Nursing interventions** are defined as "deliberative cognitive, physical, or verbal activities performed with, or on behalf of, individuals and their families [that] are directed toward accomplishing particular therapeutic objectives relative to individuals' health and well-being" (Grobe, 1996, p. 50). An expansion of this definition includes nursing

interventions that are performed with, or on behalf of, communities. Sidani and Braden (1998, p. 8) view **interventions** as "treatments, therapies, procedures, or actions implemented by health professionals to and with clients, in a particular situation, to move the clients' condition toward desired health outcomes that are beneficial to the clients." Nursing interventions are nurse-initiated and based on nursing classifications of interventions unique to clinical problems or issues addressed by nurses (Bulechek, Butcher, & Dochterman, 2008; Forbes, 2009).

Historically, nursing interventions have tended to be viewed as discrete actions, such as "positioning a limb with pillows," "raising the head of the bed 30 degrees," and "assessing a patient's pain." Interventions can be described more broadly as all of the actions required to address a particular nursing problem or issue. But there is little agreement regarding the conceptualization of interventions and how these discrete actions fit together (McCloskey & Bulechek, 2000). Frameworks have been proposed in moving from isolated action-oriented interventions to more integrative approaches to care. For example, dance therapy might be used as part of a falls reduction initiative (Krampe et al., 2010). In addition, **care bundles**, which are combinations of interrelated nursing actions, might be the basis for comprehensive approaches to care (Deacon & Fairhurst, 2008; Quigley et al., 2009). These variations in interventions are discussed in the following section.

Variations in Nursing Interventions

Nursing intervention research involves quite a few variations in how the intervention is conceived, delivered, and evaluated. An intervention can be: (1) a treatment, protocol, or clinical tools to improve patient care processes and outcomes; (2) an educational program to provide support for the patient; (3) an educational program targeting nurses or other healthcare providers (e.g., a continuing education program); or (4) a leadership practice to change staffing patterns or improve the workplace environment.

Sequencing of interventions is also an important consideration when one is designing and conducting intervention-based research. A single intervention can be delivered and studied at one point in time. This approach is typically reserved for interventions that require limited exposure to produce a response, such as a one-time educational intervention of preoperative teaching on the study participants' knowledge. A single intervention might also be delivered over a series of time points. These interventions include those that have to be repeated for their maximum benefits, such as exercise programs, counseling sessions, pain reduction strategies, and medication adherence teaching. The effects of two or more separate interventions might be examined in the context of a study at just one point in time or delivered over multiple time points. Interventions can be combined and administered together to determine the collective impact that they may have on outcomes. Thus, researchers can deliver different variations of interventions and examine outcomes at one time point or across time points.

Stage-based interventions are tailored to a specific phase of recovery, response to treatment, or change in behavior. These interventions can be delivered to: (1) study participants as they progress into different phases along a continuum or recovery trajectory over time that require different approaches or (2) discrete or selected samples in various settings at various points in recovery or along a continuum, as with a cross-sectional design, when the intervention is tailored to this stage. Stage-based interventions are used in studies such as testing of smoking cessation techniques when the intervention strategies differ according to whether a person is contemplating quitting smoking, has just quit smoking, or has remained free of smoking (Cahill, Lancaster, & Green, 2010). As a novice researcher, you might want to implement a specific intervention and measure a selected outcome at one point in time. Students are also encouraged to join research teams to examine the effects of interventions.

Nursing Intervention Taxonomies

An intervention taxonomy is an organized categorization of the interventions performed by nurses. A number of classifications of nursing diagnoses and interventions have been developed, which include the following:

* The Nursing Interventions Classification (NIC), containing 542 direct and indirect care interventions, each of which has an assigned numerical code and that are categorized in seven domains including a new community domain (McCloskey & Bulechek, 2000; Bulechek et al., 2008). The Center for Nursing Classification & Clinical Effectiveness is housed at the University of Iowa College of Nursing and can be accessed online (http://www.nursing.uiowa.edu/excellence/nursing_knowledge/clinical_effectiveness/nic.htm/).
* NANDA International (NANDA-I; formerly North American Nursing Diagnosis Association) compiles nursing diagnoses and classifications (http://www.nanda.org/Home.aspx/). NANDA-I publishes the *International Journal of Nursing Terminologies and Classifications (IJNTC)* quarterly, which is distributed internationally.
* Home Health Care Classification System (HHCC) has two taxonomies with 20 Care Components used as a standardized framework to code, index, and classify home health nursing practice (Saba, 2002).
* The Omaha System provides a list of diagnoses and an Intervention Scheme designed to describe and communicate multidisciplinary practice intended to prevent illness, improve or restore health, decrease deterioration, and/or provide comfort before death. There are 75 targets or objects of action (Martin, 2005). Martin and Bowles (2008) address the link between practice and research that is predicated on the Omaha System.
* The Nursing Intervention Lexicon and Taxonomy (NILT) (Grobe, 1996). Grobe (1996, p. 50) suggested that "theoretically, a validated taxonomy that describes and categorizes nursing interventions can represent the essence of nursing knowledge about care phenomena and their relationship to one another and to the overall concept of care."

Although taxonomies may contain brief definitions of interventions, they do not provide sufficient detail to allow one to implement an intervention. The actions identified in taxonomies may be too discrete for testing and may not be linked to the resolution of a particular patient problem. Populations and settings for which nursing interventions are intended are not elucidated through nursing intervention taxonomies, making them somewhat ambiguous for guiding studies (Sidani & Braden, 1998; Forbes, 2009).

Problems Examined by Intervention Studies

Interventions are developed to address problems or issues in practice. The researcher must make a careful analysis of the situational or contextual aspects of a problem or issue prior to designing an intervention. Box 14-1 outlines a list of questions that researchers often ask to focus their attention on who, what, where, and how in designing and implementing an intervention in a study. Upon answering many of these questions, researchers gain a better idea of the planning process needed before undertaking an intervention-based study. Moreover, plans for a grand-scale study may need to be executed in phases, depending on the resources, commitment, support, and feasibility of the study.

Box 14-1	Problem Analysis Questions

1. Who?
   a. For whom is the situation, condition, or circumstance a problem (e.g., patients, families, nurses, other healthcare professionals)?
   b. Who (if anyone) would benefit from a change as it is now?
   c. Who should share the responsibility for "solving" the problem?
   d. Who are stakeholders having an invested interest and stake in wanting positive resolution to the problem?
   e. Who might support change?
   f. Who might function as champions for change?
   g. Who should be involved in designing the intervention?
2. What?
   a. What are the negative consequences of the problem for the affected individuals?
   b. What are the negative consequences of the problem for the community (healthcare providers or the healthcare system or agency)?
   c. What barriers exist to implementing an intervention?
   d. What has to occur for the problem to be considered solved?

   e. What conditions must change to establish or support a resolution of the problem?
   f. What is an acceptable and realistic level of change that needs to occur?
   g. What does each stakeholder have invested in the status quo?
3. Where?
   a. Where would the greatest impact for the greatest numbers occur?
   b. Where would it be easiest to bring about change (technically, financially, and politically)?
   c. Where are the most resources available?
   d. Where are the individuals who would be most willing to participate in change?
4. How?
   a. How should the problem be addressed (e.g., small scale or large scale)?
   b. How will the complexity of the problem require multilevel actions to have the greatest impact for change?
   c. How should stakeholders be involved and at what points in development and execution of a study might they be best used?
   d. How long might it take to accomplish the goals of the research?

Questions adapted from Fawcett, S. B., Suarez-Belcazar, Y., Belcazar, F. E., White, G. W., Paine, A. L., Blanchard, K. A., et al. (1994). Conducting intervention research: The design and development process. In J. Rothman & E. J. Thomas (Eds.), *Intervention research: Design and development for human service* (pp. 25–54). New York, NY: Haworth Press.

Programs of Nursing Intervention Research

It is becoming increasingly clear that the design and testing of a nursing intervention require an extensive program of research rather than a single well-designed study (Forbes, 2009; Sidani & Braden, 1998). As the discipline of nursing advances its mission to accumulate a strong practice science, it is apparent that a larger portion of nursing studies must focus on designing and testing interventions. Moreover, intervention research is central to the role of nurses in practice, education, and leadership. Vallerand, Musto, and Polomano (2011), in an extensive review of nurses' roles in pain management, depict intervention-based research as an integral component of advocacy, quality care, and innovation in patient care (see Figure 14-1).

Equally important in advancing nursing science are replication studies, which mimic the design and procedures of interventions tested in previous research. Despite the recognized importance of replicating intervention studies, few have been repeated to validate and verify their results.

Intervention research is a methodology that holds great promise as a more effective way of testing interventions. It shifts the focus from causal connection to causal explanation. In causal connection, the focus of a study is to provide evidence that the intervention contributes to the outcome. In causal explanation, in addition to demonstrating that the intervention causes the outcome, the researcher must provide scientific evidence to explain why the intervention contributes to changes in outcomes and how it does so. Causal explanation is theory based. Thus, research focused on

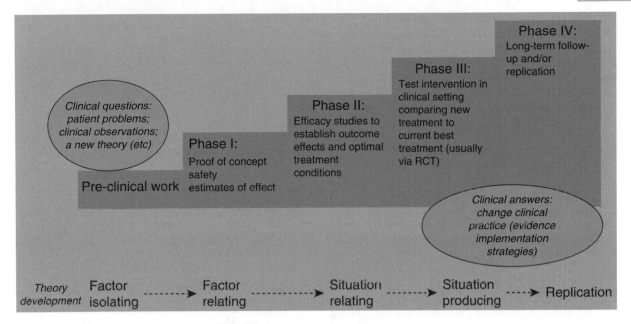

Figure 14-1 Model of the integral components of the role of nurses in pain management.
Note: *RCT,* randomized controlled trial. Adapted from Vallerand, A. H., Musto, S., & Polomano, R. C. (2011). Nursing's role in cancer pain management. *Current Pain and Headache Reports, 15*(4), 250–562; Vallerand, A. H., Musto, S., & Polomano, R. C. (2011). Nursing's role in cancer pain management. *Current Pain and Headache Reports, 15*(4), 250–562.

causal explanation is guided by theory, and the findings are expressed theoretically. Researchers employ a broad base of methodologies, including qualitative studies, to examine the effectiveness of an intervention. Qualitative approaches offer substantial value to the development, feasibility, and validation of nursing interventions. For example, Van Hecke et al. (2011) used qualitative research in the development and validation of their nursing intervention for promoting lifestyle changes in patients with leg ulcers.

Theory-based Interventions

Knowledge obtained through a synthesis of collected information can be used to develop a middle-range intervention theory. An **intervention theory** is explanatory and combines characteristics of descriptive, middle-range theories and prescriptive, practice theories. A **descriptive theory** describes the causal processes that are occurring. A **prescriptive theory** specifies what must be done to achieve the desired effects, including (1) the components, intensity, and duration required; (2) the human and material resources needed; and (3) the procedures to be followed to produce the desired outcomes.

A theory or model can be used to guide the development of an intervention as well as provide direction in the design of the study and testing procedures. The theory itself should contain conceptual definitions, propositions linked to hypotheses, and any empirical generalizations available from previous studies (Rothman & Thomas, 1994; Sidani & Braden, 1998). Theoretical constructs serve as frameworks for many nursing intervention studies, for example, risk reductions strategies for cardiovascular disease (Gholizadeh, Davidson, Salamonson, & Worrall-Carter, 2010), improving quality of life with pressure ulcers (Gorecki et al., 2010), and goal-directed therapies for rehabilitative care (Scobbie, Wyke, & Dixon, 2009). Kolanowski, Litaker, Buettner, Moeller, and Costa (2011) derived their activity interventions for nursing home residents with dementia from the Need-Driven Dementia–Compromised Behavior Model for responding to behavioral symptoms. Their randomized double-blind controlled trial involving cognitively impaired residents also linked theory-based underpinnings to the behavioral outcome measures for the study.

Not all interventions are examined in the context of theories and theoretical propositions, but some researchers contend that they should, especially when frameworks can be used to help refine interventions and select outcomes (Li, Melnyk, & McCann, 2004).

Master's and doctoral nursing students working in collaboration with faculty researchers or project teams should recognize the value of theory-driven interventions in providing greater clarity to their studies and contributing to the science of intervention theory.

Deciding on the best theory to guide intervention research requires: (1) a thorough and thoughtful review and synthesis of the literature (see Chapters 6 and 19); (2) scholarly papers that discuss appropriate theory-based interventions in areas of research interest; (3) interactive discussions among faculty, students, and other nurses about options for an optimal theory to guide interventions; and (4) once a theory has been selected, conversations with the project team to determine its application to the study.

Theory-based interventions can be developed for broad populations of patients, such as those with chronic illnesses, and then be more specifically applied to patients with diabetes. For example, Kazer, Bailey, and Whittemore (2010) used a theory-based intervention for self-management of the uncertainty associated with active surveillance for prostate cancer. These researchers discussed an uncertainty management intervention from a theory-based perspective to formulate approaches to care for men with prostate cancer. *Research and Theory for Nursing Practice* is a specific journal that seeks intervention-based research derived from theoretical frameworks and perspectives.

An intervention theory must include a careful description of the problem the intervention will address, the intermediate actions that must be implemented to address the problem, moderator variables that might change the impact of the intervention, mediator variables that might alter the effect of the intervention, and expected outcomes of the intervention. Box 14-2 lists the elements of an intervention theory that are applied to research processes. Models of theories or frameworks help explain the relationships of concepts, interventions, and outcomes. When critically appraising intervention research, students need to keep in mind that a major threat to construct study validity arises if a framework or model used to guide a study and its intervention has no clear link to the development and implementation of the intervention and the interpretation of study findings. Evidence as to how the framework has guided the study needs to be threaded throughout the research report (see Chapter 7 for understanding the inclusion of frameworks in studies).

Scientific Rationale for Interventions

Not all interventions need to be derived from theory or conceptual frameworks. Interventions can be based

Box 14-2	**Elements of Intervention Theory**

Problem or Issue

Nature of the problem or issue
Manifestations
Causative factors
Level of severity
Variation in different patient populations
Variation in different conditions

Critical Inputs

Activities to be performed
Procedures to be followed
Amounts of the intervention elements (intensity)
Frequency of the intervention
Duration of the intervention

Mediating Processes

Stages of change that occur after the intervention
Mediating variables that bring about treatment effects
Hypothesized relations among mediating variables

Expected Outcomes

Aspects of health status affected
Biopsychosocial (physical, psychological, social, and spiritual)
Timing and pattern of changes
Hypothesized interrelationships among outcomes

Extraneous Factors

Contextual factors
Environmental factors
Patient characteristics

Treatment Delivery System Resources

Setting
Equipment
Intervener characteristics

solely on empirical evidence from existing literature that provides scientific perspectives for different interventions. A thorough review and synthesis of prior research should let researchers know the basis for an intervention and justify the study design. Several peer-reviewed nursing journals publish studies without theoretical underpinnings or models depicting the relationships of interventions to outcomes. In such cases, clarity in the scientific basis for the intervention must be presented throughout the research report.

Some interventions might evolve from experiential knowledge in clinical practice, nursing education, and administrative leadership. These interventions might not have a strong scientific foundation to support their use. Investigators conducting studies on these types of interventions need to make a case for the importance of their research. These types of studies can be important in formulating study methodologies, establishing relevant outcomes for novel interventions, and advancing nursing science.

An example of an intervention with minimal scientific rationale is evident in the early work of Schmelzer and Wright (1993). These gastroenterology nurses began a series of studies that examined the procedures for administering an enema. At that time, they found no research in the nursing or medical literature that tested the effectiveness of various enema procedures. Without scientific evidence to justify the use of various procedures for administering enemas—such as the amount of solution, temperature of solution, speed of administration, content of the solution (soap suds, normal saline, or water), positioning of the patient, or measurement of expected outcomes or possible complications—they were faced with relying on the tradition of practice and clinical experience. Their first study involved telephone interviews with nurses across the country in an effort to identify patterns in the methods used to administer enemas; however, this study was unsuccessful in helping Schmelzer and Wright (1996) validate any commonly used techniques to establish guidelines for enema interventions.

In their next study, these researchers developed their own protocol for enemas and pilot-tested it on hospitalized patients awaiting liver transplantation. In their subsequent study with a sample of liver transplant patients, these researchers tested for differences in the effects of various enema solutions (Schmelzer, Case, Chappell, & Wright, 2000). Schmelzer (1999-2001) then conducted a study funded by the National Institute for Nursing Research to compare the effects of three enema solutions on the bowel mucosa. Healthy subjects were paid $100 for each of three enemas, after which a small biopsy specimen was collected. These researchers' experiences illustrate how the lack of scientific evidence for an intervention requires a series of studies before a large-scale study can be launched to answer important research questions.

Eventually, these programs of intervention-based research with enemas led to a safety and effectiveness study involving healthy volunteers that showed that enemas using soap suds and tap water produced greater return in bowel evacuation but were more uncomfortable than those using a polyethylene glycol electrolyte solution (Schmelzer, Schiller, Meyer, Rugari, & Case, 2004). Although the two former interventions resulted in a more effective response, a higher degree of surface epithelium loss in the bowel was confirmed on biopsy. These investigators concluded that the risks and benefits of selecting an enema solution must be balanced with the desire to produce a better response versus safety concerns, for example, the resultant effects on the bowel and the patient.

Terminology for Intervention-Based Research

Specific research terms and concepts have importance to intervention-based research, and it is necessary to understand these when critically appraising and conducting this type of research. Master's and Doctor of Nursing Practice (DNP) students need to be able to critically appraise individual intervention studies and those synthesized in meta-analyses and systematic reviews. PhD students have the preparation to be principal investigators for various types of studies, including intervention-based research. Thus, this section discusses relevant terms to increase nurses' expertise in critically appraising and conducting intervention research.

Efficacy versus Effectiveness

Fundamental terms that are often mistakenly interchanged with intervention-based research are *efficacy* and *effectiveness*. Both words are used to describe an effect of a treatment or intervention; however, these terms are different and should not be used synonymously. **Efficacy** refers to the ability to produce a desired, beneficial, or therapeutic effect, and it can be determined only in controlled experimental research trials in which study criteria are stringent. **Randomized controlled trials** (RCTs) involving the testing of drugs or procedures are most often efficacy studies designed to demonstrate, under optimal conditions, the desired outcomes that a drug or procedure produces (Compher, 2010). Efficacy studies require strict control of as many potentially confounding variables as possible to allow measures of efficacy to be quantified. A treatment that is deemed "efficacious" is one that produces good outcomes when subjected to highly controlled, experimental conditions. Randomized, placebo-controlled trials are required in drug development before the U.S. Federal Drug Administration (U.S. FDA) can approve the new drug.

TABLE 14-1 Comparison of Characteristics for Efficacy vs. Effectiveness Studies

Criteria	Efficacy	Effectiveness
Purpose	Test a question	Assess effectiveness
Sample size	Smallest adequate sample size	Large sample size
Study cohort	Homogeneous	Heterogeneous
Population	Study population in tertiary care setting	Study population in initial care setting
Eligibility criteria	Stringent or strict	Minimally restrictive or relaxed
Outcomes	Single or minimal outcomes	Multiple outcomes
Duration	Short study duration	Long study duration
Adverse event recording	Minimal	Comprehensive
Focus of inference	Internal validity	External validity
Analysis	Completer-only analysis	Intent-to-treat analysis

Adapted from Piantadosi, S. (2005). *Clinical trials: A methodologic perspective* (2nd ed) (p. 323). Hoboken, NJ: John Wiley & Sons; and Gartlehner, G., Hansen, R. A., Nissman, D., Lohr, K. N., & Carey, T. S. (2006). *Criteria for distinguishing effectiveness from efficacy trials in systematic reviews. Technical Review, Agency for Healthcare Research and Quality.* (AHRQ Publication No. 06-0046.) Rockville, MD: U.S. Department of Health and Human Services.

Effectiveness of a treatment or intervention indicates that it is capable of producing positive results in a usual or routine care condition. This term is generally reserved for interventions studied in situations in which stringent controls on group assignment are not possible or the study might not include a placebo, control, or comparison group. With effectiveness studies, the new intervention may be compared with the existing standard of care to ascertain whether the new treatment is better, worse, or the same as the existing intervention. These studies still require controls in the design and execution of the interventions but are not nearly as stringent as occurs in RCTs. Effectiveness studies most often use real-world clinicians and patients available to researchers. Table 14-1 contrasts the characteristics of efficacy and effectiveness.

Treatment Effect Size

The treatment **effect size** (*ES*) refers to the magnitude of effect produced by the intervention. Cohen (1988) and Aberson (2010) provide parameters for qualifying and quantifying the *ES* but caution that there are inherent risks in applying *ES* parameters across diverse fields of study because interpretations of *ES*s can vary. Cohen (1988) identifies a small ES as 0.2, a medium *ES* as 0.5, and a large *ES* as 0.8. A small *ES* of 0.20 for an intervention means a 20% difference can be expected between the intervention and comparison groups. Likewise, a 0.5 ES represents a 50% difference attributed to the intervention. Knowledge of the *ES* for any intervention is helpful and often necessary for calculations of the sample size needed to provide sufficient statistical power to detect a treatment difference. The nature of the *ES* also varies from one statistical procedure to the next; it could be the difference in cure rates, a standardized mean difference, or a correlation coefficient. However, the *ES* function in conducting a power analysis is the same in all procedures (Aberson, 2010; see Chapter 15 for a more detailed discussion of *ES* and power analysis).

Placebo and Sham Interventions

A **placebo** is an intervention intended to have no effect. However, a placebo generally looks, tastes, smells, and/or feels like the test intervention or is experienced like the real study intervention. The purpose of a placebo is to account for how study participants would respond without actually receiving the active intervention. **Sham** interventions are often used with procedures, and are a variation of a "fake" intervention that omits the essential therapeutic element of the intervention. A "sham" intervention also attempts to control for the placebo effect. Rates for placebo responses do differ depending on the types of interventions and populations studied. For example, the rate for a placebo response with symptom management research can be as high as 90% (Kwekkeboom, 1997). Very complex psychobiological responses occur in the brain, called the real placebo effect, even when an intervention is perceived to be inert or of no known therapeutic value (Benedetti, Carlino, & Pollo, 2011). It is important to note that designs using placebo or sham interventions are typically carefully evaluated by institutional review boards (IRBs) to ensure that patients' rights are not violated.

The placebo effect is extremely complex and often attributed to multiple variables. These might include attention that a participant receives in a study even if there is no structured intervention or documented therapeutic value. The influence of the nurse or physician demeanor, patient factors such as motivations to do better, and the patient-provider relationship can have a placebo effect. Other factors, such as co-interventions that cannot be controlled, expectations of a treatment effect, the context in which an intervention is delivered, relief associated with receiving some treatment, and spontaneous improvement of problem during a study, are also likely explanations for placebo effects.

A placebo or sham intervention is intended to specifically blind study participants and/or research personnel to the treatment conditions in intervention trials. Placebos also blind healthcare providers taking care of or interacting with study participants, who might introduce bias into the study if study conditions are known. Placebos are most frequently used with RCTs involving drug testing.

Sham procedures are often used in research focused on interventions such as healing touch, relaxation therapy, acupuncture, cognitive and behavioral therapy, or any treatment that might produce an effect just from the intervener/participant interactions. To account for the benefits of paying attention to participants or doing something to them that might in and of itself lead to a positive response, researchers sometimes use sham techniques to control for the confounding effects of a treatment. For example, Baird, Murawski, and Wu (2010) studied the efficacy of guided imagery and relaxation on pain reduction, improvements in mobility, and decreased over-the-counter medication use in older adults with osteoarthritis. These investigators provided a sham condition with planned relaxation provided to the comparison group to control for any positive influence on outcomes that might be caused by simply engaging patients in a study. With this type of design, the investigators were able to detect the true effects of the experimental condition under investigation, guided imagery and relaxation. It is always important that the design of a sham technique be similar in many respects to the experimental treatment, such as the circumstances surrounding the encounter with the researcher or intervener, duration of the encounter, and implementation of procedural steps or sequencing of the mock treatment.

Blinding versus Open Label

The term blinding refers to preventing disclosure of group assignment while a study is being conducted to avoid bias or undesirable influence in the ways participants respond and researchers perform. According to the CONSORT (CONsolidated Standards of Reporting Trials, 2011) Transparency Reporting of Trials statement, the term "blinding" or "masking," which is gaining greater acceptance as the more appropriate designation, "refers to withholding information about the assigned interventions from people involved in the trial who may potentially be influenced by this

knowledge." Procedures for blinding or masking in the conduct of clinical trials are of utmost importance to the validity of findings and estimates of treatment effects. One reason is that participants may respond differently on study outcomes if they have knowledge of their exposure to a treatment condition. Along these same lines, investigators and data collectors can unknowingly or knowingly encourage certain responses from participants in favor of one treatment over another if they are aware of a patient's treatment group assignment. Those caring for patients in studies could inadvertently share information about treatments that might bias participant performance on outcome measures. Some study conditions even stipulate that knowledge of group assignment be kept from data analysts or statisticians to safeguard against bias in the analysis and interpretation of data.

Blinding or masking occurs at various levels. Although this procedure helps to reduce bias in favor of one intervention over another, only 33% of 199 published RCTs from 2007 to 2009 published in 16 nursing journals reported using blinding procedures (Polit, Gillespie, & Griffin, 2011). With single-blinded studies, there are two variations. Study participants are not aware of their treatment assignment, but investigators and research staff may have knowledge of who is in what group. The reverse may be used when participants have knowledge of their treatment group assignment, but this information is not available to the investigators and research staff. For example, children involved in research comparing the calming effects of music alone with those of music with mother's voice delivered by audiotaped recordings would recognize the contents of the tape if they were alert. Researchers and data collectors may not be told of participant group assignment. Double-blinded studies keep knowledge of study conditions from study participants, investigators, and research staff. When a study is triple-blinded, the participants, researchers, and those involved in data management are unaware of group assignment.

Open-label extension is a term that usually applies to RCTs or other clinical trials whereby participants in the active treatment group are offered an opportunity to continue treatment and those in the placebo or control group are given the option to transition to the active treatment at the conclusion of the intervention period. This phase of a clinical trial is often used in drug studies as a continuation phase to obtain safety data about the frequency of adverse events or side effects over an extended period. This aspect of the study is required by the FDA for approval of new drugs. Participants are closely monitored by research coordinators and study personnel, and data are often still collected on the study primary end points to demonstrate whether treatment effectiveness continues. Important attention needs to be paid to the side effect profile of the drug that develops over time. Other treatment trials may use open-label extensions to accumulate more data about the treatment and its effect on study outcomes.

Treatment Fidelity

Treatment fidelity has to do with the accuracy, consistency, and thoroughness of how an intervention is delivered according to the specified protocol, treatment program, or intervention model. Strict adherence to treatment specifications must be evaluated on an ongoing basis during the course of a study. Thus, intervention fidelity is "the adherent and competent delivery of an intervention by the interventionist as set forth in the research plan" (Santacroce, Maccarelli, & Grey, 2004, p. 63), and this fidelity is of utmost importance to the inference of the study's internal validity in intervention-based research. Stringent controls for implementation of study procedures are critical to the study's integrity. Methodological approaches to treatment fidelity include education and training of all persons implementing the treatment, periodic monitoring or surveillance of the implementation of the treatment or fidelity checks (either conspicuous or inconspicuous observation), and retraining and reevaluation of study research staff if deviations from the prescribed protocol for study procedures are found. Gearing et al. (2011) propose a scientific guide to treatment fidelity and discuss implications at all phases of the treatment, including: (1) implementing the design; (2) training the research staff; and (3) monitoring the delivery and receipt of the intervention.

Treatment fidelity is important in the conduct of all intervention-based research, but it is especially critical for complex interventions such as those involving information dissemination, social support, counseling, and other interventions intended to bring about changes in health behaviors and psychosocial outcomes. Radziewicz et al. (2009) reported their experiences maintaining treatment fidelity in a study testing a communication support by telephone intervention for older adults with advanced cancer and their family caregivers. These researchers contended that fidelity was maximized by the following: ensuring that the intervention is congruent with relevant theory, standardizing the training, using stringent criteria for conducting fidelity checks to determine interventionist competence, monitoring the delivery of the intervention, and carefully documenting findings. "The degree

to which internal validity can be established affects the conclusions' accuracy drawn from the intervention" (Radziewicz et al., p. 194).

Best practices in constructing treatment fidelity criteria and executing sound methodological procedures have been summarized for behavioral research (Bellg et al., 2004; Borrelli et al., 2005). According to Bellg et al. (2004), specific goals should direct fidelity checks. The goals include: (1) ensuring same treatment dose within conditions; (2) ensuring equivalent dose across conditions; and (3) planning for implementation setbacks. Investigators should make provisions to accomplish these goals while formulating criteria by which fidelity or adherence to treatment protocols can be assessed. Often a sampling parameter is set prior to initiation of the study that a certain percentage of study intervention episodes will be evaluated. Manipulation checks are also a critical part of ensuring the integrity of study procedures. These types of checks are valuable in gathering information about circumstances and study conditions that might interfere with or impede implementation of the study intervention. Box 14-3 shows an example of a manipulation check used by interventionists in a study of activity interventions for nursing home residents with dementia (Kolanowski et al., 2011). This type of checklist is also useful to investigators in determining intervention frequency, dose intensity, and protocol deviations. This information not only is critical in recording adherence to the study intervention but also might be included in the analyses of data to separate out or account for variations in exposures to the intervention.

Dose-Intensity of the Intervention

The exposure to an intervention can influence the response to it; therefore, the dose-intensity of the intervention must be carefully monitored and tracked. Dose-intensity refers to the amount of the intervention delivered in terms of the (1) components of the intervention; (2) duration of a single session for the intervention; (3) the frequency with which the intervention is delivered (e.g., daily, times per week, times per month); and (4) cumulative intervention intensity (number of treatments received and duration). The latter is the product of dose × dose frequency × total intervention duration (Breit-Smith, Justice, McGinty, & Kaderavek, 2009). The ability to capture, quantify, and report the exposure to an intervention in the context of a single study enhances the ability to draw conclusions about how effective an intervention might be on the basis of the quantity delivered. Reed et al. (2007) provide a comprehensive review of ways to measure the dose of nursing interventions and offer

Box 14-3	Example of a Manipulation Check for a Study of an Activity Intervention for Nursing Home Residents with Dementia

Subject Code: _____   Facility: _____

Date: _____   Time: _____

Interventionist: _____

At the completion of each activity session, please evaluate the extent to which the activity was implemented by answering the following questions:

1. Was today's activity the one selected for this condition?

   a. Yes ___

   b. No ____

   Explain:

2. Were there any extraneous circumstances that influenced the delivery of the activity?

   _____ a. Inability to form group activity.

   Explain:

   _____ b. Inability of study participant to stay by himself or herself for independent activity.

   Explain:
   _____

_____ c. Interference from staff, other residents, visitors, etc.

Explain:

_____ d. Subject uncooperative.

Explain:

_____ e. Subject ill.

Explain:

_____ f. Subject engaged in another activity.

Explain:

_____ g. Subject not available.

Explain:

_____ h. Interventionist not available.

Explain:

Kolanowski, A., Buettner, L., & Moeller, J. (2006). Treatment fidelity plan for an activity intervention designed for persons with dementia. *American Journal of Alzheimer's Disease and Other Dementias, 21*(5), 326–332.

formulas for calculating intervention exposure in terms of metrics for frequency and duration of the intervention.

For repeated measures designs involving interventions delivered over time, research staff must maintain accurate records of all intervention sessions for all study participants, including completed sessions (the full intervention was delivered), partial sessions (only a part or parts of the intervention were administered), and missed sessions (the intervention was not administered at the appropriate time point in the study). Field notes should be kept to explain reasons for the inability to deliver the total intervention. Maintaining detailed information regarding dose-intensity is essential for determining the treatment effect. If known, varying levels of the exposure to the intervention can be handled in the statistical analyses to separate out the magnitude of benefits on the outcome(s) if participants received full exposure to the intervention or only partial exposure.

Numbers Needed to Treat

Numbers needed to treat (NNT) is a metric that is defined as the number of patients who would need to be treated with the new intervention to avoid one event that might have occurred with standard treatment. It is necessary that NNT be estimated in context of those deriving a benefit or those who might be harmed by the intervention (Day, 2007). Intuitively, it is an easy concept to grasp because it is expressed in a numeric value. For example, if the NNT is 4 for a benefit from an intervention, then a prescriber of an intervention could expect that 1 out of 4 patients treated with the intervention would derive a positive outcome. The NNT is determined by an analysis of the data following the completion of a study that is adequately powered (i.e., the sample size is adequate) to detect treatment differences. The researcher establishes criteria for the primary outcome measure for the study that is indicative of a positive or undesirable response, and the NNT is expressed in terms of either outcome. Researchers are often required to calculate the NNT for clinical trials prior to submitting a manuscript for publication to influential research journals. NNT values are often pooled and analyzed in meta-analyses and systematic reviews of studies. Moreover, the NNT is a meaningful parameter for practice because it informs clinicians of the overall effectiveness of the intervention and of the expected response when prescribing an intervention.

When one is interpreting NNT, it is important to determine whether the NNT value is for a single administration of the intervention, at a single time point, or overall across multiple time points. For example, Hatfield, Gusic, Dyer, and Polomano (2008) conducted a blinded, placebo-controlled trial of oral sucrose administration for pain associated with immunizations in infants 2 and 4 months of age. With use of a repeated measures design, infants receiving 24% oral sucrose ($n = 38$) or sterile water (placebo) ($n = 45$) via a pacifier were assessed for pain at baseline and 2, 5, 7 and 9 minutes after a series of vaccine injections. Pain was measured using the University of Wisconsin Children's Hospital (UWCH) Pain Scale (0 denoting the absence of any pain response to 5 reflecting the highest degree of the pain response). These investigators assigned a pain score of 2 or less as the desirable criterion for a favorable response to the treatment. At 2 minutes the NNT was 4, and at 9 minutes, the end of the study, it was 2. This can be interpreted that at 9 minutes after administration of oral sucrose with a sequence of vaccine injections, 1 in 2 infants (50%) received a beneficial response to the therapy; whereas earlier, at 2 minutes, the intervention was not as effective with only 1 in 4 infants (25%) achieving the desired level of response.

Analysis of Intention-to-Treat

Intention-to-treat (ITT) is an analysis based on the principle that participant data are analyzed according to the groups into which they were randomly assigned regardless of what happens to them in the study. In other words, if a participant drops out or changes therapy after randomization, this individual would be retained in the data set and in the group to which he or she was randomly assigned in the analysis. If any participants are not included in the analysis, then the equalization of the treatment groups is no longer maintained, possibly introducing bias into the results. Nurses need to understand the concept of intention to treat, especially because this analysis strategy is widely used by healthcare researchers.

There are several ways to account for the missing data for subjects who leave a study earlier than expected. It is important, however, to understand that all methods of imputing data values create "made-up" data. The ideal clinical trial or intervention-based study must be designed to minimize participant dropout and missed interventions to limit as much missing data as possible. There are many ways to impute data. They have a variety of advantages and disadvantages, which have been well described in a National Academy of Science report (National

Research Council, 2010). Two of the more commonly used methods are baseline observation carried forward (BOCF) and last observation carried forward (LOCF). BOCF populates the missing data points for an outcome following the last data collection value obtained with the baseline value obtained for that participant. Use of this procedure assumes that the participant would have returned to baseline without further treatment. LOCF, on the other hand, assumes that the last value obtained for a particular outcome for a participant would continue for the rest of the study. A variation on these techniques is termed the worst observation carried forward (WOCF), which takes the worst value for the participant no longer in the study and carries this value forward for all the missing data collection points for the study outcomes. Sometimes the preferred method(s) for observation carried forward in drug development studies is stipulated by the FDA drug approval section. For example, the FDA guidance for studies of pain stipulates that the more conservative BOCF analysis be used for all regulatory submissions for drug approval (National Research Council, 2010). There are no known guidelines for nursing research studies using intention-to-treat designs.

A review of 71 clinical trials published in high-impact medical journals in the late 1990s found that 63 (89%) had incomplete data sets owing to missing data, and for 13 of these trials, outcomes data were missing for more than 20% of participants (Wood, White, & Thompson, 2004). In 37 trials using repeated measures to obtain outcome measurements over time, 46% performed the analysis after excluding those with only some follow-up data, 19% of the trials used LOCF, and 11% imputed missing data with the worst case value (WOCF). LOCF is less conservative, assuming that participants who drop out may have had some benefit before dropping out, and has been favored as an analytical strategy for missing data; however, in studies of pharmacotherapy for chronic pain, for example, there are circumstances in which BOCF may be more appropriate and scientifically justified (Dworkin, et al., 2009). The imputation of missing data allows the application of intention-to-treat analysis for clinical trials. It is vital that the method selected as the strategy of handling missing data be determined and specified a priori (before the study is initiated) to maximize the likelihood of obtaining a valid conclusion from the data analysis.

Responder Analysis

Responder analysis is an additional technique to identify variables associated with a beneficial response to an intervention or to determine outcomes of potential importance to the treatment. This technique can be performed when one is analyzing the effect of the intervention or during a secondary analysis of study data after the primary data have been reported. A responder analysis can also be conducted on more than one study using pooled data from investigations with similar designs and outcomes. This type of analysis informs researchers and clinicians about the significant variables contributing to participants' response or lack of response to a particular intervention. Responder analyses provide useful information about sample characteristics and conditions likely to lead to significant results for researchers conducting similar future studies. Criterion-based parameters on outcome measures can also be determined to define what is considered to be a positive or beneficial response to a treatment.

Clinicians often relish these types of studies to guide practice in selecting those individuals who might benefit most from an intervention and to quantify levels of responses on specific instruments. Weaver, Chasens, and Arora (2009) conducted a responder analysis with two randomized, double-blind, placebo-controlled studies examining the efficacy of modafinil, a drug used to treat excessive sleepiness in individuals with sleep disorders. The response to treatment with modafinil in these two previous studies was measured with the Functional Outcomes of Sleep Questionnaire (FOSQ). The FOSQ was administered to patients with obstructive sleep apnea who were experiencing residual excessive sleepiness with continuous positive airway pressure (CPAP) use. A secondary data analysis using a covariance model showed that a greater proportion of responders were in the active drug arm, and functional outcomes indicative of a beneficial response were characterized on the basis of improvements for certain items and domains on the FOSQ. These findings will help both researchers and clinicians better understand the items and subscales on the FOSQ that are most important in capturing improvements with modafinil in this patient population.

Types of Research Designs

Experimental or quasi-experimental research designs are required if investigators want to test the efficacy or effectiveness of nursing interventions. The effects of interventions can also be examined, evaluated, described, or observed in the context of nonexperimental designs such as descriptive, correlational, or observational research designs. Models and descriptions of both experimental and nonexperimental quantitative research designs are presented in Chapter 11. A qualitative research design may be used if a researcher is in the initial phase of developing a model or prototype for an intervention. This type of research methodology might also be used in later phases, when the intervention is implemented and the experiences encountered with the intervention from the perspectives of those who receive or deliver it are of interest (see Chapter 12, which is focused on qualitative research). Mixed-methods studies that combine both quantitative and qualitative research methods are of great value when the interventions are complex or various aspects of the interventions must be validated (Brady et al., 2011; Creswell & Zhang, 2009). Chapter 10 explains different types of mixed-method designs.

In the context of interventional research, one way of examining research designs is to focus on the types of clinical trials and the design strategies used to test interventions. From a generic view, a clinical trial involves the systematic study of the effects of a treatment in human subjects (Day, 2007). There are many types of clinical trials, and many levels of scientific rigor are applied in studying treatment effects. Duffy (2006) provides a basic overview for types of clinical trial designs and also emphasizes the growing use of these designs in nursing research. Some of the clinical trial designs discussed here are gaining greater acceptance for studying nursing interventions. Additionally, nonexperimental approaches can be used to observe and describe outcomes that result from nursing interventions, and these also need to be considered as part of intervention research.

Experimental and Quasi-experimental Designs

Parallel Group Randomized Controlled Trials

Parallel group RCTs represent the most common or standard type of RCTs. Subjects are randomly assigned to receive either one or two or more concurrently administered treatments (Piantadosi, 2005). This design is experimental in nature and offers a high degree of scientific rigor in determining the efficacy (if placebo control is used) of a treatment or the effectiveness if the comparison group includes another treatment and/or a control group receiving no treatment, just routine care. RCTs can be costly and difficult to conduct because of the complexity of the design and stringent controls that must be in place to ensure the validity of results. An integrative review of published nurse-led RCTs revealed several challenges encountered by nurse researchers. They included: (1)

difficulties with sufficient patient recruitment; (2) non-adherence to research protocols; and (3) economic and organizational barriers to conducting these trials (Vedelø & Lomborg, 2011). Nonetheless, RCTs are vitally important to advancing nursing science and evidence-based practice because they yield the strongest level of evidence for single studies. When possible, both nurses in clinical practice and students need to participate in nurse-led RCTs as co-investigators and research assistants.

Crossover Randomized Controlled Trials

A crossover randomized controlled trial exposes each subject to both treatment conditions, which can be a placebo and an active intervention or two active interventions. This type of design is used to determine how each subject responds to both study conditions, and it enables investigators to examine each subject's responses under these study conditions. As such, participants serve as their own controls. This design maximizes enrollment because fewer subjects are needed in crossover than in parallel RCTs. This design is typically executed using a repeated measures design, whereby time is the variable under which within-subject variability is examined. Study conditions need to be delivered in random order so that the influence of sequence of exposure to the intervention is controlled and does not result in a confounding variable. This approach lessens the likelihood that exposure to one study condition first would influence the response to the second condition, and vice versa.

A washout period (or time) is incorporated into crossover designs, which occurs between exposures to study conditions. The purpose of this interval is to provide ample time for any effects of first exposure to the active intervention or placebo to dissipate. Consequently, each study condition can be examined separately with little risk that diffusion of their effects may contaminate the outcomes. During this washout period, subjects do not receive any intervention; however, they remain in the study and may also be monitored or asked to complete study outcome measures. Overall, crossover designs are thought to offer greater precision in conducting comparisons of treatments (Matthews, 2000). A major disadvantage is that subjects are often required to stay in the study longer and are exposed to two and not just one study condition.

Cluster Randomized Controlled Trials

Intervention-based research can often be costly, and gaining access to representative samples in multiple study sites can be time consuming and difficult. Further, interventions that may be highly influenced by existing clinical practices, which cannot be controlled, are challenging to study. Cluster randomized controlled trials or group randomized trials employ a randomized sampling method to more efficiently test interventions using representative groups of samples randomized to study conditions rather than individuals. In this design, the unit of analysis is the research site, and investigators randomly select research settings from a sampling frame of eligible and willing sites, which would then be assigned to serve as test sites receiving either the experimental intervention or the control condition. This type of random selection involving clinical settings can more efficiently accomplish participant accrual, control for confounding variables introduced by site-specific practice variations, and ensure more representative groups or clusters. For example, Pellfolk, Gustafson, Bucht, and Karlsson (2010) selected 40 group dwelling units of individuals with dementia to examine the impact of a 6-month educational program in restraint reduction offered to the nursing staff. Because their study involved both nurses and patients, nursing units were randomized for nursing staff members either to receive a 6-month educational intervention or to serve as the controls. Nurses working on these units participated in the study, and outcomes from their patients were collected and analyzed. Knowledge and attitudes regarding restraint practices improved for the educational intervention group, and this improvement translated into a reduction in restraint use in comparison with practices by the staff in the control group.

Preference Clinical Trials

With most clinical trials, participants are randomly assigned to treatment or control conditions. However, in some situations, patient preference takes precedence over randomization to maximize enrollment. Understandably, preference for treatment conditions plays an important role prior to randomization and has significant implications for outcomes. A meta-analysis of clinical trials for musculoskeletal conditions demonstrated that patients who were randomly assigned to their preferred treatment had a standardized *ES* of the treatment that was greater than those who were indifferent to their group assignment (Preference Collaborative Review Group, 2009). Although not found to be statistically significant in this study, a trend emerged showing that those who received their preferred treatment did better on outcome measures than participants not assigned to their preferred treatment. Outcomes were similar for participants allocated to their undesired treatment and those who were indifferent to the treatment arm.

One way to handle participant preference or partiality for treatment conditions is through the use of preference designs that allow an option for patients to receive the treatment of their choice (Day, 2007). These types of designs include Wennberg's design and Zelen's randomized consent design. In the latter, patients are randomly assigned to treatment conditions and informed of the group assignment prior to consent to participate. If they decline, patients are offered the alternative treatment option(s) of their choice. This procedure is used to prevent the biasing of the results of clinical trial associated with "resentful demoralization" (unhappiness with the group assignment) and the Hawthorne effect (responses that result when study participants change their behavior because they are being observed and are not a true reflection of the intervention) (Adamson, Cockayne, Puffer, & Torgerson, 2006). Thus, in preference clinical trials, rather than being randomly assigned to subject groups, patients choose among all treatments available. With preference clinical trials, researchers blend both experimental and quasi-experimental design strategies in the context of a single study.

Treatment Matching Designs

Treatment matching or **client treatment matching** (CTM) compares the relative effectiveness of various treatments. Treatment matching designs are used when the following conditions are met: (1) there is no clearly superior treatment for all individuals with a given problem; (2) a number of treatments with some proven efficacy have comparable effectiveness for undifferentiated groups of subjects; and (3) there is evidence of differential outcomes, either within or among treatments, for defined subtypes of patients (Donovan & Mattson, 1994; Donovan et al., 1994).

Unlike sample matching techniques to ensure equal distribution of sample characteristics across treatment groups, treatment matching designs align interventions with predetermined criteria that will ensure the best possible benefit to subjects. Thus far, CTM intervention studies have been successful, albeit limited to studies involving treatment approaches for substance abuse and addiction (Melnick, De Leon, Thomas, & Kressel, 2001). Faul et al. (2011) have suggested that this strategy be used in studies of exercise therapy for patients with cancer in order to consider pre-intervention activity levels as criteria for matching patients to the most appropriate type of exercise programs to improve participants' functionality and overall quality of life.

Open-Label Designs

Open-label designs refers to the absence of any blinding or masking procedures for the intervention. For obvious reasons, open-label clinical trials, or other intervention-based designs in which the intervention groups are known, must be used when it is impossible to blind or mask the intervention. In such cases, researchers, research participants, and healthcare professionals caring for research participants have knowledge of the intervention. Research participants can still be randomly assigned to groups of intact cohorts receiving an intervention as part of routine clinical care. Regardless of the design, it is critical for researchers to take measures to ensure that investigator or participant bias does not interfere with the validity or credibility of the results. Safeguards to control for bias and improve internal validity of the study include: (1) clear specifications for the implementation of the study protocol or treatment; (2) education and training of research assistants or nurses implementing the interventions; (3) establishing interrater reliability for the implementation of study procedures and interobserver reliability for measurement of the study outcome(s); and (4) separation of study participants to avoid experimental diffusion of the treatment effect, which may occur when study participants interact with one another. As with all intervention-based research, any violations in execution of study procedures or data collection should be immediately communicated to the investigators, however minor these may be.

Nonexperimental Designs

Observational Studies

The effects of nursing interventions can be studied through observation. Although observation is also used in experimental research designs, nonexperimental observational designs can be used to assess patient responses and outcomes to the implementation of new or existing nursing practices; new technology or equipment; or specific prevention protocols to reduce, for example, occurrences of falls, hospital-acquired pressure ulcers, and catheter-associated bloodstream infections. Observational studies are generally carried out in the naturalistic setting in the course of routine clinical care. Methods for data collection might include surveillance, extraction of clinical data from electronic health information systems or paper health records, compliance monitoring by observers, and data storage or output from monitoring technology or devices.

For example, Shever (2011) conducted an observational study of the impact of nursing surveillance on failure to rescue, a nursing-sensitive indicator related to surgical death from preventable complications. Data were extracted from various electronic clinical information repositories and a nursing documentation system based on the Nursing Interventions Classification (NIC). A high level of nursing surveillance of patients was quantified as an average of 12 times per day or more. Patients receiving low and high nursing surveillance were evaluated, and when nursing surveillance was high, there was a significant decrease ($p = 0.006$) in the likelihood of experiencing failure to rescue.

Retrospective Descriptive Studies

Not all interventions occur in prospective studies, so retrospective designs are employed to examine the effects of interventions. In a retrospective study of nursing practice across three community nursing sites, Schoneman (2002) compiled data on nursing interventions using the computerized Omaha Classification System (OCS) to examine "surveillance" as a nursing intervention. The practice of surveillance was identified as a significant nursing intervention accounting for 27.1% of all nursing interventions. Of the 1506 clients studied, those most likely to receive surveillance were more than 40 years of age ($p = 0.001$) and female ($p = 0.001$). The primary reasons for this intervention were to promote health and prevent disease. Specifically, subjects with a nursing diagnosis of circulation and nutrition deficits seemed to be assessed more frequently with surveillance nursing practices.

Planning Intervention Research

Project Planning

Because an intervention research project often involves a study extended over a long time, sometimes years, nurse researchers are advised to give careful thought to the composition of their research teams. Researchers need to determine (1) who will be included on the project team; (2) what level of expertise is required for team members; (3) how team members will function together; and (4) the roles team members will assume.

Forming a Project Team

Because of the nature of intervention research, you may need to gather a multidisciplinary project team to facilitate distribution of the work and a broader generation of ideas. If both quantitative and qualitative data will be gathered during the research project, your team should include members experienced in various qualitative and quantitative data collection and analysis approaches. Including a team member with marketing expertise will be beneficial, because the final step of the project will be to market the intervention. Teams are enhanced by the inclusion of undergraduate, master's, and doctoral nursing students.

Recruiting colleagues located in other areas of the country or the world for the research team can add an important dimension by permitting multisite intervention studies. To achieve this goal, investigators need to: (1) contact researchers with similar interests; (2) attend specialty conferences related to the research area, during which they can speak with researchers and possibly extend an invitation to participate in the project; (3) invite colleagues to join the project after presentations at a professional meeting; (4) develop a project website that invites other researchers to participate; and (5) develop or participate in an internet mailing list (Listserv) or a blog related to the topic. The process of developing a team is dynamic rather than static, with changes occurring as development of the research program continues.

Work of the Project Team

There is almost always a core group in a project team that carries on most of the work, maintains group activities, and encourages the achievement of tasks. However, other people can contribute in lesser ways to benefit the project. For example, you may want to establish liaison groups from the clinical facilities in which the intervention will be studied. In some cases, the addition of other advisory groups can be helpful.

The initial focus of the team is to clarify the problem or issue of interest. In analyzing identified problems or issues, the team should answer the questions listed in Box 14-1. Considering these questions may provide new insights that redefine the problem or issue and may lead to a more effective intervention. Sidani and Braden (1998) have cautioned the project team to be alert to the risk of making a Type III error. A **Type III error** is the risk of asking the wrong question—a question that does not address the problem of concern. This error is most likely to occur when the researchers do not thoroughly analyze the problem and, as a result, have a fuzzy or inaccurate understanding of the issue of concern. The solution, then, does not fit the problem. A study conducted on the basis of a Type III error provides the right answer to the wrong question, leading to the incorrect conclusion that the newly designed intervention will resolve the problem.

Once the problem or issue to be examined is clarified, you must establish your goals and objectives. Project team tasks include: (1) gathering information;

(2) developing an intervention theory; (3) designing the intervention; (4) establishing an observation system;, (5) testing the intervention; (6) collecting and analyzing data; and (7) disseminating the intervention. Seeking funding for the various studies of the project will be an ongoing effort.

Gathering Information

Once a clinical problem or issue has been identified, the investigators and members of the research team can begin by conducting an extensive search for information related to the project. This search is considerably more focused and encompassing than the traditional literature review. Box 14-4 lends some organization and clarity to topics that need to be addressed as the basis for developing a plan for intervention research. Several sources of information can be accessed to gain knowledge of existing nursing interventions, extant research conducted on these interventions, and evidence-based practice guidelines that incorporate these interventions and guide their application to practice (Box 14-5). It is important to keep in mind that researchers should not "reinvent the wheel." For many nursing interventions, prescriptive procedures are already published in credible scientific sources that can be adapted for the purposes of intervention testing. Undergraduate, master's, and doctoral nursing students as well as clinicians working with the project team can be very helpful in retrieving literature and resources and assisting with synthesizing information.

Design and Testing of Interventions

Researchers either develop their own procedures for implementing an intervention or replicate an intervention and its protocol from an existing study. As mentioned earlier, theory-driven intervention research is conceived from theoretical or conceptual perspectives that form the basis of the intervention and its perceived effectiveness or benefit. Theory-based intervention research can begin with a concept analysis of the problem or the intervention intended to address it. By dissecting the components of problems and plausible solutions, investigators can gain clarity of the issues at hand. At the other end of the spectrum are replication studies that involve similar intervention designs, approaches, and outcomes used by other investigators. These types of studies are especially important to validate or refute results from published research. Replication studies add to the strength of

---

Box 14-4	Topics for Information Gathering

Nature of the Problem (Actual or Potential) or Issue

Manifestations
Causative factors
Level of severity
Variation in different patient populations
Variation in different conditions

Intervention

How people who have actually experienced the problem or issue have addressed it
Previous interventions designed to address the problem or issue
Unsuccessful interventions
Value to target population
Sensitivity to cultural diversity
Biases or prejudices
Processes underlying the intervention effects
Intervention actions
Components
Mode of delivery
Strength of dosage
Amount
Frequency
Duration

Mediating Processes

Patient characteristics
Setting characteristics
Intervener characteristics

Expected Outcomes

Contextual factors
Environmental factors
Patient characteristics
Provider factors
Healthcare system factors

---

using specific interventions in selected populations and settings.

A study by Forbes (2009) provides an excellent model of the four phases of testing clinical interventions. The model in Figure 14-2 reflects the testing of interventions on a continuum from preclinical work to the final phase of study replication. This model is particularly useful in guiding students through the phases of intervention-based research. Initially, ideas for interventions and the need for intervention research

Box 14-5   Sources of Information about Interventions

Peer-reviewed journal articles on nursing interventions

Nursing intervention taxonomies

Computerized databases containing data on nursing interventions

Nursing textbooks

Previous intervention studies (theses, dissertations, and other publications)

Clinical guidelines: http://www.guidelines.gov (see Chapter 19 for additional websites)

Critical pathways

Intervention protocols

Interviews with patients who have experienced the problem and related interventions

Interviews with providers who have addressed the problem

Interviews with researchers who have tested previous interventions

Probing of personal experiences

Observations of care provided to patients with the problem

begin with problems and questions that arise in practice. You might be involved in any of these four phases of intervention research as an investigator, consultant, or research assistant (see Figure 14-2).

Designing the Intervention

An intervention to be tested must be carefully developed and well thought out to accomplish the purpose of the study. The study framework should guide the identification of the research hypotheses and the development of the study design and intervention. Investigators may need to consult other researchers who have designed and tested similar interventions, the research project team who will carry out the research, and clinical experts who might use the intervention in practice. Aranda (2008) recommends taking a similar approach to that used in pharmacological research, which is illustrated by a progressive path from phase I to phase IV studies in determining safety, efficacy, and effectiveness.

During the design period, and guided by the intervention theory, the project team specifies the procedural elements of the intervention and develops an observation system (Fawcett et al., 1994). The intervention may be (1) a strategy; (2) a technique; (3) a program; (4) informational or training materials; (5) environmental design variables; (6) a motivational system; or (7) a new or modified policy. The intervention must be specified in sufficient detail to allow interveners to implement it consistently.

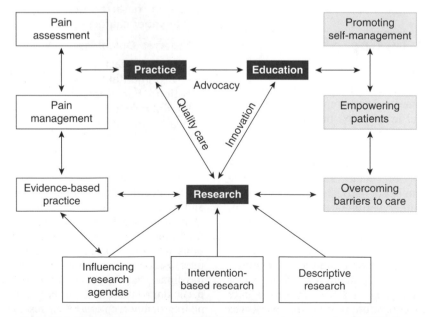

Figure 14-2 Phases of intervention-based research from theory development to study replication.

Box 14-6	Criteria for Intervention Design

1. The intervention is effective.
2. The intervention is replicable by typical interveners.
3. The intervention is simple to use.
4. The intervention is practical.
5. The intervention is adaptable to various contexts and settings.
6. The intervention is compatible with patient preferences and values.

Adapted from Fawcett, S. B., Suarez-Belcazar, Y., Belcazar, F. E., White, G. W., Paine, A .L., Blanchard, K. A., et al. (1994). Conducting intervention research: The design and development process. In J. Rothman & E. J. Thomas (Eds.), *Intervention research: Design and development for human service* (pp. 25–54). New York: Haworth Press.

During the design process, the intervention emerges in stages as it is repeatedly tested, redesigned, and retested. Training materials and programs for interveners also must be developed and repeatedly tested and revised. Design criteria are established to evaluate the implementation of the intervention and outcomes (Box 14-6). In addition to the detailed development of the intervention, an operational development of the design guided by the theory should include the following actions:

- Define the target population.
- List acceptable strategies for selecting a sample.
- Identify subgroups that might show differential effects of the intervention.
- Specify essential characteristics of interventionists.
- Determine study variables.
- Indicate appropriate measures of variables.
- Specify the appropriate time or times to measure outcomes.
- Indicate what analyses to perform and what relationships to test on the basis of the relationships among the treatment and the mediating and outcome variables specified by the intervention theory guiding the study.

Study Outcomes

Outcomes are determined by the problem and purpose of the intervention and reflect the various effects of the intervention. Selecting study endpoints to capture the outcomes of an intervention must reflect changes that occur as a consequence of the intervention.

Typically, in an experimental or quasi-experimental study in which intervention efficacy and effectiveness are determined, there is a primary end point or outcome of greatest interest to investigators and secondary outcomes that add value to the impact of the intervention. Regardless of whether they are primary or secondary, outcome measures have to represent the concept or concepts within the measurement domain(s) for the study and must be sensitive and specific to the desired effects brought about by the intervention.

Outcomes can be obtained using self-reported questionnaires, survey instruments, or scales administered by the investigators or research personnel. These outcome measures can be related to experiences categorized as physical, psychological, social, spiritual, or any combination of these types. Physiological outcomes can be measured by specialized equipment that records patients' physical status, such as heart rate, blood pressure, respiratory rate, and oxygen saturation. Outcomes can also be measured by criteria-based observational instruments or scales that capture observed phenomena relevant to the intervention. Box 14-7 lists the steps of the observation process for intervention research. For example, a study of an intervention to reduce hospital-acquired pressure ulcers would require a grading scale to assess the presence and severity of pressure ulcers that can only be determined by a rater. Study outcomes can be clinical indicators relating to events, sequences of care, and resultant effects of care. Length of hospitalization, transfer to a critical care unit, rates of complications, and disposition at discharge as defined by the need for home health care, long-term care, or rehabilitative therapy all represent clinical indicators of care.

The timing and expected pattern of changes must also be considered and specified for the frequency and sequencing of collecting outcome measures. Timing is the point in time after the intervention that a change is expected to occur. Some changes occur immediately after an intervention, whereas others may not appear for some time. The sequencing of data collection on outcomes should be done at the early and most optimal points in which that intervention may show an effect. However, the selected outcomes measures must be able to demonstrate these changes at the particular time points. For example, studies involving interventions focused on quality of life need to allow ample time during and following the intervention to detect improvements in quality of life. Changes in symptoms, on the other hand, may occur more rapidly with an intervention, so more frequent surveillance of these outcomes is often warranted. Interventions that have

Steps of the Observation Process

1. Determine elements that must be observed on the basis of the intervention theory.
2. Develop methods of measuring essential elements.
3. Develop criteria for determining whether or not the event to be observed has occurred.
4. Select observers.
5. Train observers.
6. Develop scoring instructions to guide recording of desired behaviors or outcomes.
7. Develop a schedule of observations to include the following:
   a. What is happening before the intervention is implemented?
   b. What is happening during the intervention?
   c. What changes occur after the intervention?
8. Perform preliminary analysis of pre-intervention data.
9. Apply preliminary analysis results to further develop the intervention.
10. Analyze changes in environment and behaviors before, during, and after the intervention.
11. Refine intervention theory.

no anticipated or appreciable carry-over effect following implementation do require study outcomes collected at the time or shortly after the intervention. Typically, the literature and psychometric properties of instruments and scales can be used to guide schedules for collection of outcomes.

If theory-guided intervention research is used, there may be mediating variables, referred to in some studies as **intermediate outcomes,** that have relevance to understanding the intervention. Hypothesized interrelationships among the outcomes must be indicated in the theory and must be represented in the study through either controlling for these variables in the design and sampling procedures, or measuring them as part of the study in order to manage them in the analysis and interpretations of results.

Extraneous Factors

Extraneous factors or variables are elements of the environment or characteristics of the patient that significantly affect the problem, the treatment process, or the outcomes. Unlike mediator variables, extraneous factors tend not to be well understood and may not be identified until a study has been initiated. They are seldom included in explanations of the causal links between intervention and outcomes. Thus, they are extraneous to existing theoretical explanations of cause. They are sometimes referred to as **confounding variables.** If the researcher recognizes their potential effect, extraneous factors may be held constant or measured so that they can be statistically controlled during analysis. Careful analyses may indicate that some variables defined as extraneous are actually moderator or mediator variables. (For additional information on types of variables refer to Chapter 8.)

Process of Testing the Intervention

Intervention Validation

For some interventions, before the pilot test, it is useful to test prototypes in situations and environments that are similar to those planned for the actual study. Van Meijel, Gamel, van Swieten-Duijfjes, and Grypdonck (2004) contend that too little time is spent on the development of an intervention, since more time is spent in the actual testing of the intervention. Before one proceeds with a formal study, an intervention should be examined in the setting in which the problem occurs or in a situation resembling the natural setting. This examination helps investigators and research staff, as well as nurses caring for study participants, to experience how an intervention may play out under actual study conditions. Logistical aspects of the intervention may not be fully developed or foreseeable until a "real world" trial can be realized, and the problems addressed. This method of preliminary validation of the intervention is quite helpful for studies involving sensitive issues, such as sexual abuse, alcohol abuse, and drug use. Intervention validation is important when there is uncertainty about how research staff will perform and/or participants will react. It helps researchers determine the feasibility of the intervention and its components as well as how accepting nurses and potential participants might be to the intervention.

Another strategy is to conduct intervention validation under simulated conditions. Conducting simulation exercises in an artificial environment close to the natural study environment might identify issues in delivering the intervention that can be corrected before the study is conducted. Role-playing techniques are often used to deliver the intervention. Members of the project team, staff from the settings to be used for the project, or nursing students might perform the roles. Simulation scenarios are constructed following the exact steps prescribed by the intervention protocol. Video recording may be used to allow investigators to carefully examine any issues or procedures that require modifications prior to implementing the pilot or final study. Observers also make notes during the testing of the intervention to identify missing elements, gain insights, or develop questions the project team must explore. Some degree of inference is gleaned from validating an intervention in an artificial environment and being proactive in refining study procedures and measurement outcomes on the basis of simulated experiences.

Pilot Testing of an Intervention

For multiple reasons, pilot or field testing of an intervention is recommended. In some cases, pilot testing is required when a researcher is applying for grant funding, seeking approval from an IRB, or garnering support from an institution to conduct the study. Feeley et al. (2009) underscore the importance of pilot testing in developing RCTs for the following reasons: (1) to assess the feasibility and acceptability of the intervention; (2) to determine the feasibility and acceptability of the design and procedures; and (3) to facilitate the determination of treatment ES to use in power analysis calculations of sample size. In general, pilot studies are very useful to:

1. Determine whether the intervention as a prototype will work and whether it is feasible.
2. Guide the refinement of the intervention and to work out any problems or issues with implementing it in clinical or research settings. Pilot studies are especially valuable when interventions are delivered in the context of usual or routine clinical care. Investigators can determine any barriers to as well as facilitators for the execution of study procedures, and seek support and resources to administer the intervention in the manner intended.
3. Test and refine instructions, manuals, or training programs to ensure that study procedures are understandable and the preparation of study staff is adequate.
4. Estimate how long it takes to recruit the study population, implement the intervention, and collect the desired data.
5. Assess whether the intervention has been described in sufficient detail to allow clinicians and other researchers to replicate the work. During

pilot tests, clinicians and research staff should continually question any concerns or issues that arise.
6. Verify whether there are problems in gaining access to study participants and how participants are reacting to study conditions and procedures.
7. Ensure that study participants understand what is required of the study and can interpret and complete outcome measures.
8. Test the feasibility of the design.
9. Obtain reliability and validity estimates for measurement methods in the target population.
10. Ascertain whether there are any unanticipated effects that may be of concern for participants or detrimental to the internal and external validity of the study.

Importantly, pilot testing allows the generation of data or point estimates (such as means and standard deviations) for the study outcomes. These estimates can be used to calculate sufficient statistical power in terms of study sample size needed to detect a statistically significant treatment effect. Pilot data are often a prerequisite for determining adequate sample sizes when there are no available studies to calculate the ES for the intervention. Typically, only 10 to 20 participants are needed to obtain estimates of variance in the primary outcome measure(s) needed to determine intervention ES (Hertzog, 2008; see Chapter 15 for calculation of ESs for interventions).

Pilot studies should be conducted with the target population and in settings similar to those planned for the proposed study. These studies must also be approved by the organization's IRB in compliance with all regulations and mandates for acceptable conduct of research and protection of human subjects. The manner in which all study procedures are implemented must also be exactly the same as described in the study proposal. Strict adherence to study procedures enables investigators to use pilot data as the starting point for the study if no amendments or changes are made. The pilot testing phase can move right into the larger-scale study if this is a condition stipulated in the approved IRB application.

Often pilot studies are separate studies, and investigators may alter protocols on the basis of the experience of the pilot study. Keeping field notes is particularly useful during pilot studies so relevant issues can be addressed prior to implementing the larger-scale study. Pilot data may be published, although with controlled trials, findings must be meaningful to the body of research (Watson, Atkinson, & Rose, 2007). Thus, pilot studies need to be published if they provide estimates of variance in the outcomes, help determine the quality of the intervention protocol, and/or identify issues relevant to future studies. However, it is imperative that researchers avoid any inference to hypothesis testing using pilot studies. Some researchers have cautioned that problems remain in the interpretation of pilot studies' findings in publications (Arain, Campbell, Cooper, & Lancaster, 2010).With the limited sample sizes, researchers run the risk of misinterpreting any significant or nonsignificant results. Type II errors are common when the sample size is insufficient to provide acceptable statistical power to detect differences from interventions. Pilot samples are nonrepresentative of the target population, and data tend to be nonnormally distributed. Assumptions of normally distributed data are often violated if parametric statistical tests were used in the analyses of pilot data. Nonparametric statistics are more appropriate for conducting group comparisons with pilot data and should be considered. Sometimes only descriptive statistics (frequencies, means, standard deviations, ranges, scatter plots or diagrams, and medians) are most appropriate in reporting the results from pilot studies.

Graduate students should consider opportunities to work on pilot studies because they are generally of short duration and instructive about the research process. Investigators often try to recruit graduate students for their studies because they have knowledge of research and can provide useful feedback about the experience as well as flexible daytime schedules to accommodate the work.

Formal Testing of an Intervention

The most desirable formal test of an intervention is a conventional experimental design to determine whether the intervention causes the intended effects. The design should be as rigorous as possible. Researchers need to conduct a power analysis to determine a sample size sufficient to avoid a Type II error (see Chapter 15 for discussion of power analysis). Analyses must be performed to ensure that the treatment and control groups are comparable on important demographic variables. The measurement methods used in studies must have documented reliability and validity (see Chapter 16). The ES for each outcome needs to be examined and reported. The observation system established before the initiation of testing must be continued, and patient characteristics, intervener characteristics, and setting characteristics need to be measured and described (Sidani & Braden, 1998). Researchers also must develop plans for statistical analyses to detect differences between the intervention and comparison groups (see Chapter 25).

Advanced Testing

Advanced testing of the intervention occurs after sufficient evidence is available that the intervention is effective in achieving the desired outcomes. The model proposed by Forbes (2009) places this type of testing in phases III and IV, during which the intervention is compared with standard of care interventions, followed by replication studies with long-term follow-up of the intervention's effectiveness (see Chapter 11 for discussion of phases I to IV of clinical trials). Phase III of intervention testing might involve a single, well-designed study that indicates a satisfactory ES for an intervention, but often an intervention requires modification through additional studies. Replication studies ensure that an intervention is refined to create the desired effect in practice. Sidani and Braden (1998) emphasize that the advanced testing phase must include variations in the studies conducted to ensure the intervention is ready for delivery in practice to a variety of patients.

Testing Variations in Effectiveness Based on Variations in Patient Characteristics

Intervention effects that have been determined through the use of a sample of only white, middle-class Americans may not have the same effect with other groups. The intervention should be tested among various ethnic groups and vulnerable populations, such as the socioeconomically and educationally disadvantaged. Pilot tests may reveal a need to refine the intervention to make it more culturally appropriate and adaptive to diverse groups. Minority and disadvantaged populations may respond differently to interventions because they: (1) have different views of health and preventive behaviors; (2) do not fully understand the purpose of the study and their role in participation; (3) are more vulnerable to persuasion from researchers and healthcare professionals; and (4) encounter difficulties in comprehending patient-reported outcome measures used in the study. For these reasons, researchers need to design studies and select outcomes that are tailored to diverse patients or screen potential participants for variables that might interfere with study participation. However, eliminating diversity as a requisite for a study can limit the generalizability of findings and hamper efforts to better understand and reduce healthcare disparities.

Studies also must be conducted to examine the effect of an intervention on patients with comorbidities or differing levels of illness severity. Other variations in patient characteristics, such as age, gender, and diagnosis, must be examined. Characteristics specific to the intervention may be identified as important for determining differential effects. When sufficiently large samples are obtained in initial studies, these patient characteristics can be examined in secondary analyses of available data.

Testing Variations in Effectiveness Based on Setting

If the research setting is similar for the testing of an intervention with similar circumstances, conditions, and subjects, then the effects of a different setting can potentially confound the treatment effects. Therefore, one component of testing the intervention is to set up multisite projects, in which the settings are varied and the effects of the settings on outcomes are examined (Sidani & Braden, 1998).

Testing Variations in Effectiveness Based on Variations in Intervener Characteristics

The initial study examining the effectiveness of an intervention is usually conducted under ideal conditions. Ideal conditions involve the selection of highly educated interveners judged to be experts in the field of practice related to the intervention. However, after the intervention is found to be effective, questions arise regarding the use of less well-prepared

interveners to provide the intervention. Studies need to be conducted to determine variations in the effectiveness of the intervention based on the competencies of interveners.

Testing Variations in Effectiveness Based on Strength of an Intervention

The strategy of testing the variations of an intervention's strength is used to determine the amount of treatment needed to achieve the desired outcome in practice. To test this issue, the researcher must provide varying doses of the intervention. Researchers might vary the intensity of the intervention, the length of time of a single treatment, the frequency of an intervention, and/or the span of time over which the intervention is continued or repeated.

Data Collection

Data collection in intervention research consists of not only accurate collection and recording of study outcomes but also accurate documentation of the study intervention. Researchers need to document the timing of the intervention, dose-intensity of the intervention,

---

Box 14-8	Factors Affecting the Integrity of an Intervention and Study Validity

Lack of Stringent Study Controls

Poorly defined study intervention

Lack of attention to detail in planning the intervention(s)

Lack of or inadequate use of written guidelines and protocols for the intervention(s)

Unreported protocol violations or deviations from standardized procedures

Inadequate supervision and guidance during study from the principal investigator and/or research coordinator

Variations in dose intensity of study intervention(s) across study participants

Lack of reliable and valid outcome measures

Complexity of Intervention Procedures

Level of complexity of the intervention(s)

Variation in elements of intervention provided

Difficulties in implementing intervention activities

Number of sites involved in implementing the intervention

Study Intervener and Staff Variables

Too many individuals delivering the intervention(s)

Level of education and research experience of study staff

Failure to obtain intraobserver and interobserver reliability

Lack of initial and ongoing preparation and competency verification assessments

Level of compliance of staff with treatment protocol

Competing priorities and responsibilities of study staff

Turnover of study staff during the investigation

Level of staff interest and commitment to the intervention

Study Site Variables

Lack of human, professional, and financial resources to support the study

Changes in organizational policies, procedures, and practices after initiation of study

Adoption of new technology or equipment as part of the intervention

Box 14-9 **Step by Step Approach to Critically Apprising Intervention-Based Research: A Focus on the Intervention**

Step 1: Background and Review of Literature

Examine the scientific basis for the study intervention:
- Is the scientific rationale for the intervention supported by the study literature review?
- Do authors cite variations in ways the intervention has been studied?
- Has the intervention been tested in different study populations?
- Is the magnitude or effect size of the intervention provided from previous studies?

Step 2: Theoretical Framework

Establish whether the intervention is theory-based or conceptually derived and the level to which theory drives the intervention:
- Does the intervention evolve from a theory or conceptual framework?
- How has the intervention been developed using a theory?
- Are the relationships of the study framework to the intervention explicit?
- Is the intervention represented in a model of the study framework?

Step 3: Design

Determine the appropriateness of the design to test the intervention:
- Is the design appropriate to test study hypotheses?
- Are confounding variables controlled by the design?
- Is an experimental design with a control, placebo, or standard care group used to test the efficacy or effectiveness of an intervention?
- In a study with a quasi-experimental design, is a comparison group used in testing the intervention?

Step 4: Sample

Examine the appropriateness of the sample and sampling process:
- Is the sample representative of the population that might benefit most from the intervention?
- How are subjects allocated to treatment and, if appropriate, control or comparison groups?
- Was a power analysis performed to determine an adequate sample size to yield sufficient statistical power to detect statistically significant differences between or among study treatment conditions?
- Do inclusion and exclusion sample criteria control for sample characteristics that might influence the outcomes?
- To what extent does the sample allow for generalizations to similar populations, thereby improving the study's external validity?

Step 5: Study Outcomes

Evaluate the study outcomes:
- Are reliability and validity (psychometric properties) of all instruments and outcome measures reported, and are they acceptable?
- Do investigators plan to conduct psychometric testing of instruments or outcomes measures if existing ones are applied to different populations or if new ones are designed by the investigators for the purpose of the study?
- Has interrater or intrarater reliability been established for data collectors if observational methods are used to obtain outcome measurements?
- What limitations are evident for the outcome measures, and are these addressed?

Step 6: Study Procedures

Evaluate the integrity for the implementation of the intervention:
- Are the study procedures clearly explained to the degree that other researchers might be able to replicate the study?
- How were study personnel or clinical staff prepared to execute study procedures?
- Were fidelity or manipulation checks conducted during training or in the course of the study?
- Was information collected on protocol deviations and dose intensity of the intervention?

Step 7: Statistical Analyses

Assess the appropriateness of statistical methods:
- Are appropriate statistical methods applied given the level of measurement for outcome variables?

Box 14-9	Step by Step Approach to Critically Apprising Intervention-Based Research: A Focus on the Intervention—cont'd

• Have the investigators violated any statistical assumptions in the selection of analytical procedures raising statistical conclusion validity issues?	• Did the intervention show a statistically significant difference in the study outcomes? • Were the study results clinically important?

subject responses to the intervention, missed treatments, and any protocol deviations that occur even if these are beyond the intervener's control. Investigators also must keep track of any unexpected circumstances that occur in the implementation of the study intervention or at the time the outcomes are measured. These types of field notes can be vital to the interpretation of study participants' responses during data analysis and the development of findings (see Chapter 20 for more details on the data collection process).

Threats to Study Validity

Like other types of research, intervention research is subject to threats to validity. Box 14-8 summarizes aspects of the research design, intervention, and analyses that need to be examined for threats to validity. Determining threats to internal validity in the execution of a study is critically important to examining study results and interpreting findings. Studies must be evaluated for sources of bias from systematic error that might occur with problems of treatment fidelity and uncontrolled confounding variables. Researchers also need to evaluate the bias and possible threats to design validity occurring from random error introduced by low statistical power, imprecise instruments, and inappropriate statistical methods (Gerhard, 2008; Shadish, Cook, & Campbell, 2002; see Chapter 10).

Critical Appraisal of Intervention-Based Research

Criteria for critically appraising intervention-based research are very similar to those for the appraisal of any type of study. However, a more thorough and systematic evaluation of the integrity of the intervention, study procedures for implementing the intervention, and outcomes for measuring its efficacy or effectiveness is required. The validity of research findings involving interventions depends on sound methodological practices including accuracy, precision, and consistency in the delivery of a study intervention.

Equally important are controls to reduce bias and error that pose threats to study validity. Many of these issues have been discussed previously. Guidelines for evaluating components of the intervention are outlined in Box 14-9. Important questions are posed to help nurses identify aspects of studies specific to the intervention and to assist them in critically appraising the intervention and its implementation in a study.

KEY POINTS

- Intervention research holds great promise for designing and testing nursing interventions and advancing nursing science.
- Nursing interventions are defined as "deliberative cognitive, physical, or verbal activities performed with, or on behalf of, individuals and their families that are directed toward accomplishing particular therapeutic objectives relative to individuals' health and well-being" (Grobe, 1996, p. 50).
- Nursing interventions are nurse-initiated and can be based on nursing classifications of interventions unique to clinical problems addressed by nurses.
- Intervention research programs consist of multiple studies conducted over a period of years by a project team that may include undergraduate and graduate nursing students.
- Some teams use a participatory research method that involves community groups.
- An intervention theory must include: (1) a careful description of the problem to be addressed; (2) the intervening actions that must be implemented to address the problem; (3) moderator variables that might change the impact of the intervention; (4) mediator variables that might alter the effect of the intervention; and (5) expected outcomes of the intervention.
- The intervention theory guides the design and development of an intervention, which is then extensively tested, refined, and retested using quantitative, qualitative, and mixed-methods research designs.

- Experimental and quasi-experimental research designs are particularly useful in determining intervention effectiveness through the use of such methods as parallel groups, crossover, cluster, preference, client treatment matching, and open-label designs.
- Advanced testing of the intervention occurs after sufficient evidence is available to determine that the intervention is effective in achieving desired outcomes.
- When the intervention is sufficiently refined and evidence of effectiveness has been determined, the intervention is field-tested to ensure that it can be effectively implemented in clinical settings.
- An observation system is developed for use throughout the intervention design and development process. This system allows the researchers to observe events related to the intervention naturalistically and to analyze these observations.
- Dissemination efforts are more extensive than in traditional experimental studies and involve choosing a brand name, establishing a price, and setting standards for the intervention's use.
- As with any study, intervention-based research needs to be critically appraised to ascertain the integrity of the intervention, its implementation fidelity, and reported outcomes.

REFERENCES

Aberson, C. L. (2010). *Applied power analysis for the behavioral sciences.* New York, NY: Routledge Taylor & Francis Group.

Adamson, J., Cockayne, S., Puffer, S., & Torgerson, D. J. (2006). Review of randomised trials using the post-randomised consent (Zelen's) design. *Contemporary Clinical Trials, 27*(4), 305–319.

Arain, M., Campbell, M. J., Cooper, C. L., & Lancaster, G. A. (2010). What is a pilot or feasibility study? A review of current practice and editorial policy. *BMC Medical Research Methodology, 10,* 67.

Aranda, S. (2008). Designing nursing interventions. *Collegian, 15*(1), 19–25.

Baird, C. L., Murawski, M. M., & Wu, J. (2010). Efficacy of guided imagery with relaxation for osteoarthritis symptoms and medication intake. *Pain Management Nursing, 11*(1), 56–65.

Bellg, A. J., Borrelli, B., Resnick, B., Hecht, J., Minicucci, D. S., Ory, M., et al.; Treatment Fidelity Workgroup of the NIH Behavior Change Consortium. (2004). Enhancing treatment fidelity in health behavior change studies: Best practices and recommendations from the NIH Behavior Change Consortium. *Health Psychology, 23*(5), 443–451.

Benedetti, F., Carlino, E., & Pollo, A. (2011). How placebos change the patient's brain. *Neuropsychopharmacology, 36*(1), 339–354.

Borrelli, B., Sepinwall, D., Ernst, D., Bellg, A. J., Czajkowski, S., Breger, R., et al. (2005). A new tool to assess treatment fidelity and evaluation of treatment fidelity across 10 years of health behavior research. *Journal of Consulting and Clinical Psychology, 73*(5), 852–860.

Brady, M. C., Stott, D. J., Norrie, J., Chalmers, C., St. George, B., Sweeney, P. M., et al. (2011). Developing and evaluating the implementation of a complex intervention: Using mixed methods to inform the design of a randomised controlled trial of an oral healthcare intervention after stroke. *Trials, 12,* 168.

Breit-Smith, A., Justice, L. M., McGinty, A., & Kaderavek, J. (2009). How often and how much? Intensity of print referencing intervention. *Topics in Language Disorders, 29*(4), 360–369.

Bulechek, G., Butcher, H., & Dochterman, J. (2008). *Nursing interventions classification (NIC)* (5th ed.). St. Louis, MO: Elsevier.

Cahill, K., Lancaster, T., & Green, N. (2010). Stage-based interventions for smoking cessation. *Cochrane Database Systematic Review, 11,* CD004492.

Cohen, J. (1988). *Statistical power analysis for the behavioral sciences* (2nd ed.). Hillsdale, NJ: Lawrence Earlbaum Associates.

Compher, C. (2010). Efficacy vs. effectiveness. *Journal of Parenteral and Enteral Nutrition, 34*(6), 598–599.

Conn, V. S., Hafdahl, A. R., & Mehr, D. R. (2011). Interventions to increase physical activity among healthy adults: Meta-analysis of outcomes. *American Journal of Public Health, 101*(4), 751–758.

Consolidated Standards of Reporting Trials (CONSORT, 2011). *Transparency reporting of trials.* Retrieved from http://www.consort-statement.org/consort-statement/3-12-methods/item11a_blinding/.

Creswell, J. W. & Zhang, W. (2009). The application of mixed methods designs to trauma research. *Journal of Traumatic Stress, 22*(6), 612–621.

Day, S. (2007). *Dictionary for clinical trials* (2nd ed.). Hoboken, NJ: John Wiley & Sons.

Deacon, M. & Fairhurst, E. (2008). The real-life practice of acute inpatient mental health nurses: An analysis of "eight interrelated bundles of activity." *Nursing Inquiry, 15*(4), 330–340.

Donovan, D. M. & Mattson, M. E. (1994). Alcoholism treatment matching research: Methodological and clinical issues. *Journal of Studies of Alcohol, 12*(Suppl), 5–14.

Donovan, D. M., Kadden, R. M., DiClemente, C. C., Carroll, K. M., Longabaugh, R., Zweben, A., et al. (1994). Issues in the selection and development of therapies in alcoholism treatment matching research. *Journal of Studies of Alcohol, 12*(Suppl), 138–148.

Duffy, M. (2006). The randomized controlled trial: Basic considerations. *Clinical Nurse Specialist, 20*(2), 62–64.

Dworkin, R. H., Turk, D. C., McDermott, M. P., Peirce-Sandner, S., Burke, L. B., Cowan, P., et al. (2009). Interpreting the clinical importance of group differences in chronic pain clinical trials: IMMPACT recommendations. *Pain, 146*(3), 238–244.

Faul, L. A., Jim, H. S., Minton, S., Fishman, M., Tanvetyanon, T., & Jacobsen, P. B. (2011). Relationship of exercise to quality of life in cancer patients beginning chemotherapy. *Journal of Pain & Symptom Management, 41*(5), 859–869.

Fawcett, S. B., Suarez-Belcazar, Y., Balcazar, F. E., White, G. W., Paine, A. L., Blanchard, K. A., et al. (1994). Conducting intervention research: The design and development process. In: J. Rothman & E. J. Thomas (Eds.), *Intervention research: Design and development for human service* (pp. 25–54). New York, NY: Haworth Press.

Feeley, N., Cossette, S., Côté, J., Héon, M., Stremler, R., Martorella, G., et al. (2009). The importance of piloting an RCT intervention. *Canadian Journal of Nursing Research*, *41*(2), 85–99.

Forbes, A. (2009). Clinical intervention research in nursing. *International Journal of Nursing Studies*, *46*(4), 557–568.

Gartlehner, G., Hansen, R. A., Nissman, D., Lohr, K. N., & Carey, T. S. (2006). *Criteria for distinguishing effectiveness from efficacy trials in systematic reviews. Technical Review, Agency for Healthcare Research and Quality*. (AHRQ Publication No. 06-0046.) Rockville, MD: U.S. Department of Health and Human Services.

Gearing, R. E., El-Bassel, N., Ghesquiere, A., Baldwin, S., Gillies, J., & Ngeow, E. (2011). Major ingredients of fidelity: A review and scientific guide to improving quality of intervention research implementation. *Clinical Psychological Reviews*, *31*(1), 79–88.

Gerhard, T. (2008). Bias: Considerations for research practice. *American Journal of Health System Pharmacists*, *65*(22), 2159–2168.

Gholizadeh, L., Davidson, P., Salamonson, Y., & Worrall-Carter, L. (2010). Theoretical considerations in reducing risk for cardiovascular disease: Implications for nursing practice. *Journal of Clinical Nursing*, *19*(15-16), 2137–2145.

Goode, C. J., Titler, M., Rakel, B., Ones, D. S., Kleiber, C., Small, S., et al. (1991). A meta-analysis of effects of heparin flush and saline flush: Quality and cost implications. *Nursing Research*, *40*(6), 324–330.

Gorecki, C., Lamping, D. L., Brown, J. M., Madill, A., Firth, J., & Nixon, J. (2010). Development of a conceptual framework of health-related quality of life in pressure ulcers: A patient-focused approach. *International Journal of Nursing Studies*, *47*(12), 1525–1534.

Grobe, S. J. (1996). The nursing intervention lexicon and taxonomy: Implications for representing nursing care data in automated patient records. *Holistic Nursing Practice*, *11*(1), 48–63.

Hatfield, L. A., Gusic, M. E., Dyer, A. M., & Polomano, R. C. (2008). Analgesic properties of oral sucrose during routine immunizations at 2 and 4 months of age. *Pediatrics*, *121*(2), e327–e334.

Hertzog, M. A. (2008). Considerations in determining sample size for pilot studies. *Research in Nursing & Health*, *31*(2), 180–191.

Kazer, M. W., Bailey, D. E. Jr., & Whittemore, R. (2010). Out of the black box: Expansion of a theory-based intervention to self-manage the uncertainty associated with active surveillance (AS) for prostate cancer. *Research & Theory in Nursing Practice*, *24*(2), 101–112.

Kolanowski, A., Buettner, L., & Moeller, J. (2006). Treatment fidelity plan for an activity intervention designed for persons with dementia. *American Journal of Alzheimer's Disease and Other Dementias*, *21*(5), 326–332.

Kolanowski, A., Litaker, M., Buettner, L., Moeller, J., & Costa, P. T. Jr. (2011). A randomized clinical trial of theory-based activities for the behavioral symptoms of dementia in nursing home residents. *Journal of the American Geriatric Society*, *59*(6), 1032–1041.

Krampe, J., Rantz, M. J., Dowell, L., Schamp, R., Skubic, M., & Abbott, C. (2010). Dance-based therapy in a program of all-inclusive care for the elderly: An integrative approach to decrease fall risk. *Nursing Administrative Quarterly*, *34*(2), 156–161.

Kwekkeboom, K. L. (1997). The placebo effect in symptom management. *Oncology Nursing Forum*, *24*(8), 1393–1399.

Li, H., Melnyk, B. M., & McCann, R. (2004). Review of intervention studies of families with hospitalized elderly relatives. *Journal of Nursing Scholarship*, *36*(1), 54–59.

Martin, K. S. (2005). *The Omaha System: A key to practice, documentation, and information management* (2nd ed.). Omaha, NE: Health Connections Press.

Martin, K. S. & Bowles, K. H. (2008). Using a standardized language to increase collaboration between research and practice. *Nursing Outlook*, *56*(3), 138–139.

Matthews, J. N. S. (2000). *An introduction to randomized controlled clinical trials*. London, England: Arnold, Hodder Headline Group.

McCloskey, J. C. & Bulechek, G. M. (2000). *Nursing interventions Classification (NIC)* (3rd ed.). St. Louis: Mosby-Year.

Melnick, G., De Leon, G., Thomas, G., & Kressel, D. (2001). A client-treatment matching protocol for therapeutic communities: First report. *Journal of Substance Abuse and Treatment*, *21*(3), 119–128.

National Research Council. (2010). *The prevention and treatment of missing data in clinical trials*. Panel on Handling Missing Data in Clinical Trials. Committee on National Statistics, Division of Behavioral and Social Sciences and Education. Washington, DC: The National Academies Press.

Pellfolk, T. J., Gustafson, Y., Bucht, G., & Karlsson, S. (2010). Effects of a restraint minimization program on staff knowledge, attitudes, and practice: A cluster randomized trial. *Journal of the American Geriatric Society*, *58*(1), 62–69.

Piantadosi, S. (2005). *Clinical trials: A methodologic perspective* (2nd ed.). Hoboken, NJ: John Wiley & Sons.

Polit, D. F., Gillespie, B. M., & Griffin, R. (2011). Deliberate ignorance: A systematic review of blinding in nursing clinical trials. *Nursing Research*, *60*(1), 9–16.

Preference Collaborative Review Group. (2009). Patients' preferences within randomised trials: Systematic review and patient level meta-analysis. *BMJ*, *337*, a1864.

Quigley, P. A., Hahm, B., Collazo, S., Gibson, W., Janzen, S., Powell-Cope, G., et al. (2009). Reducing serious injury from falls in two veterans' hospital medical-surgical units. *Journal of Nursing Care Quality*, *24*(1), 33–41.

Radziewicz, R. M., Rose, J. H., Bowman, K. F., Berila, R. A., O'Toole, E. E., & Given, B. (2009). Establishing treatment fidelity in a coping and communication support telephone intervention for aging patients with advanced cancer and their family caregivers. *Cancer Nursing*, *32*(3), 193–202.

Reed, D., Titler, M. G., Dochterman, J. M., Shever, L. L., Kanak, M., & Picone, D. M. (2007). Measuring the dose of nursing intervention. *International Journal of Nursing Terminology Classification*, *18*(4), 121–130.

Rothman, J., & Thomas, E. J. (1994). *Intervention research: Design and development for human service*. New York, NY: Haworth Press.

Saba, V. (2002). Nursing classifications: Home Health Care Classification System (HHCC): An overview. *Online Journal of Issues in Nursing*, *7*(3), 9. Retrieved from http://www.nursingworld.org/MainMenuCategories/ANAMarketplace/ANAPeriodicals/OJIN/

TableofContents/Volume72002/No3Sept2002/ArticlesPrevious Topic/HHCCAnOverview.asp/.

Santacroce, S. J., Maccarelli, L. M., & Grey, M. (2004). Intervention fidelity. *Nursing Research*, *53*(1), 63–66.

Schmelzer, M. (1999-2001). Safety and effectiveness of large volume enema solutions. (Unpublished paper.) National Institutes of Health Research Enhancement Award (AREA) NIH grant number R15NR04867-01.

Schmelzer, M. & Wright, K. (1993). Risky enemas: What's the ideal solution? *American Journal of Nursing*, *93*(7), 16.

Schmelzer, M. & Wright, K. (1996). Enema administration techniques used by experienced registered nurses. *Gastroenterology Nursing*, *19*(5), 171–175.

Schmelzer, M., Case, P., Chappell, S., & Wright, K. (2000). Colonic cleansing, fluid absorption, and discomfort following tap water and soapsuds enemas. *Applied Nursing Research*, *13*(2), 83–91.

Schmelzer, M., Schiller, L. R., Meyer, R., Rugari, S. M., & Case, P. (2004). Safety and effectiveness of large-volume enema solutions. *Applied Nursing Research*, *17*(4), 265–274.

Schoneman, D. (2002). The intervention of surveillance across classification systems. *International Journal of Nursing Terminology in Classification*, *13*(4), 137–147.

Scobbie, L., Wyke, S., & Dixon, D. (2009). Identifying and applying psychological theory to setting and achieving rehabilitation goals. *Clinical Rehabilitation*, *23*(4), 321–333.

Shadish, W. R., Cook, T. D., & Campbell, D. T. (2002). *Experimental and quasi-experimental designs for generalized causal inference*. Boston, MA: Houghton Mifflin.

Shever, L. L. (2011). The impact of nursing surveillance on failure to rescue. *Research & Theory in Nursing Practice*, *25*(2), 107–126.

Sidani, S. & Braden, C. J. (1998). *Evaluating nursing interventions: A theory-driven approach*. Thousand Oaks, CA: Sage.

Vallerand, A. H., Musto, S., & Polomano, R. C. (2011). Nursing's role in cancer pain management. *Current Pain and Headache Reports*, *15*(4), 250–562.

Van Hecke, A., Verhaeghe, S., Grypdonck, M., Beele, H., Flour, M., & Defloor, T. (2011). Systematic development and validation of a nursing intervention: The case of lifestyle adherence promotion in patients with leg ulcers. *Journal of Advanced Nursing*, *67*(3), 662–676.

van Meijel, B., Gamel, C., van Swieten-Duijfjes, B., & Grypdonck, M. H. (2004). The development of evidence-based nursing interventions: Methodological considerations. *Journal of Advanced Nursing*, *48*(1), 84–92.

Vedelø, T. W. & Lomborg, K. (2011). Reported challenges in nurse-led randomised controlled trials: An integrative review of the literature. *Scandinavian Journal of Caring Science*, *25*(1), 194–200.

Watson, R., Atkinson, I., & Rose, K. (2007). Pilot studies: To publish or not? *Journal of Clinical Nursing*, *16*(4), 619–620.

Weaver, T. E., Chasens, E. R., & Arora, S. (2009). Modafinil improves functional outcomes in patients with residual excessive sleepiness associated with CPAP treatment. *Journal of Clinical Sleep Medicine*, *5*(6), 499–505.

Wood, A. M., White, I. R., & Thompson, S. G. (2004). Are missing outcome data adequately handled? A review of published randomized controlled trials in major medical journals. *Clinical Trials*, *1*(4), 368–376.

15
CHAPTER

Sampling

Many of us have preconceived notions about samples and sampling, which we acquired from television commercials, polls of public opinion, market researchers, and newspaper reports of research findings. The advertiser boasts that four of five doctors recommend its product; the newscaster announces that John Jones is predicted to win the senate election by a margin of 3 to 1; the newspaper reports that scientists' studies have found that taking a statin drug, such as atorvastatin (Lipitor), significantly reduces the risk of coronary artery disease.

All of these examples use sampling techniques. However, some of the outcomes are more valid than others, partly because of the sampling techniques used. In most instances, television, newspapers, and advertisements do not explain their sampling techniques. You may hold opinions about the adequacy of these techniques, but there is not enough information to make a judgment.

The sampling component is an important part of the research process that needs to be carefully thought out and clearly described. To achieve these goals, researchers need to understand the techniques of sampling and the reasoning behind them. With this knowledge, you can make intelligent judgments about sampling when you are critically appraising studies or developing a sampling plan for your own study. This chapter examines sampling theory and concepts; sampling plans; probability and nonprobability sampling methods for quantitative, qualitative, outcomes, and intervention research; sample size; and settings for conducting studies. The chapter concludes with a discussion of the process for recruiting and retaining subjects or participants for study samples in various settings.

Sampling Theory

Sampling involves selecting a group of people, events, behaviors, or other elements with which to conduct a study. A **sampling plan** defines the process of making the sample selections; **sample** denotes the selected group of people or elements included in a study. Sampling decisions have a major impact on the meaning and generalizability of the findings.

Sampling theory was developed to determine mathematically the most effective way to acquire a sample that would accurately reflect the population under study. The theoretical, mathematical rationale for decisions related to sampling emerged from survey research, although the techniques were first applied to experimental research by agricultural scientists. One of the most important surveys that stimulated improvements in sampling techniques was the U.S. census. Researchers have adopted the assumptions of sampling theory identified for the census surveys and incorporated them within the research process (Thompson, 2002).

Key concepts of sampling theory are (1) populations, (2) elements, (3) sampling criteria, (4) representativeness, (5) sampling errors, (6) randomization, (7) sampling frames, and (8) sampling plans. The following sections explain these concepts; later in the chapter, these concepts are used to explain various sampling methods.

Populations and Elements

The **population** is a particular group of people, such as people who have had a myocardial infarction, or type of element, such as nasogastric tubes, that is the focus of the research. The **target population** is the entire set of individuals or elements who meet the sampling criteria, such as women who have experienced a myocardial infarction in the past year. Figure 15-1 shows the relationships among the population, target population, and accessible populations. An **accessible population** is the portion of the target population to which the researchers have reasonable access. The accessible population might be elements

351

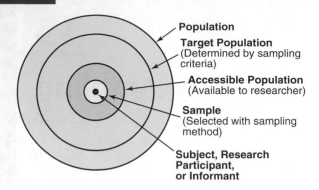

Population

Target Population
(Determined by sampling criteria)

Accessible Population
(Available to researcher)

Sample
(Selected with sampling method)

Subject, Research Participant, or Informant

Figure 15-1 Population, sample, and subject selected for a study.

within a country, state, city, hospital, nursing unit, or clinic, such as the adults with diabetes in a primary care clinic in Fort Worth, Texas. The sample is obtained from the accessible population by a particular sampling method, such as simple random sampling. The individual units of the population and sample are called **elements**. An element can be a person, event, behavior, or any other single unit of study. When elements are persons, they are usually referred to as **subjects** or **research participants** or **informants** (see Figure 15-1). The term used by researchers depends of the philosophical paradigm that is reflected in the study and the design. The term *subject,* and sometimes *research participant,* is used within the context of the postpositivist paradigm of quantitative research (see Chapter 2). The term *study* or *research participant* or *informant* is used in the context of the naturalistic paradigm of qualitative research (Fawcett & Garity, 2009; Munhall, 2012). In quantitative, intervention, and outcomes research, the findings from a study are generalized first to the accessible population and then, if appropriate, more abstractly to the target population.

Generalizing means that the findings can be applied to more than just the sample under study because the sample is representative of the target population. Because of the importance of generalizing, there are risks to defining the accessible population too narrowly. For example, a narrow definition of the accessible population reduces the ability to generalize from the study sample to the target population and diminishes the meaningfulness of the findings. Biases may be introduced that make generalization to the broader target population difficult to defend. If the accessible population is defined as individuals in a white, upper-middle-class setting, one cannot generalize to nonwhite or lower income populations. These

biases are similar to biases that may be encountered in a nonrandom sample (Thompson, 2002).

In some studies, the entire population is the target of the study. These studies are referred to as **population studies** (Barhyte, Redman, & Neill, 1990). Many of these studies use data available in large databases, such as the census data or other government-maintained databases. Epidemiologists sometimes use entire populations for their large database studies. In other studies, the entire population of interest in the study is small and well defined. For example, one could conduct a study in which the defined population was all living recipients of heart and lung transplants.

In some cases, a hypothetical population is defined for a study. A **hypothetical population** assumes the presence of a population that cannot be defined according to sampling theory rules, which require a list of all members of the population. For example, individuals who successfully lose weight would be a hypothetical population. The number of individuals in the population, who they are, how much weight they have lost, how long they have kept the weight off, and how they achieved the weight loss are unknown. Some populations are elusive and constantly changing. For example, identifying all women in active labor in the United States, all people grieving the loss of a loved one, or all people coming into an emergency department would be impossible.

Sampling or Eligibility Criteria

Sampling criteria, also referred to as **eligibility criteria**, include a list of characteristics essential for membership or eligibility in the target population. The criteria are developed from the research problem, the purpose, a review of literature, the conceptual and operational definitions of the study variables, and the design. The sampling criteria determine the target population, and the sample is selected from the accessible population within the target population (see Figure 15-1). When the study is complete, the findings are generalized from the sample to the accessible population and then to the target population if the study has a representative sample (see the next section).

You might identify broad sampling criteria for a study, such as all adults older than 18 years of age able to read and write English. These criteria ensure a large target population of **heterogeneous** or diverse potential subjects. A heterogeneous sample increases your ability to generalize the findings to a larger target population. In descriptive or correlational studies, the sampling criteria may be defined to ensure a heterogeneous population with a broad range of values for the variables being studied. However, in quasi-experimental or experimental studies, the primary purpose of sampling criteria is to limit the effect of extraneous variables on the particular interaction between the independent and dependent variables. In these types of studies, the sampling criteria need to be specific and designed to make the population as homogeneous or similar as possible to control for the extraneous variables. Subjects are selected to maximize the effects of the independent variable and minimize the effects of variation in other extraneous variables so that they have a limited impact on the dependent variable scores.

Sampling criteria may include characteristics such as the ability to read, to write responses on the data collection instruments or forms, and to comprehend and communicate using the English language. Age limitations are often specified, such as adults 18 years and older. Subjects may be limited to individuals who are not participating in any other study. Persons who are able to participate fully in the procedure for obtaining informed consent are often selected as subjects. If potential subjects have diminished autonomy or are unable to give informed consent, consent must be obtained from their legal representatives. Thus, persons who are legally or mentally incompetent, terminally ill, or confined to an institution are more difficult to access as subjects (see Chapter 9). However, sampling criteria should not become so restrictive that the researcher cannot find an adequate number of study participants.

A study might have inclusion or exclusion sampling criteria (or both). Inclusion sampling criteria are characteristics that a subject or element must possess to be part of the target population. Exclusion sampling criteria are characteristics that can cause a person or element to be excluded from the target population. Researchers need to provide logical reasons for their inclusion and exclusion sampling criteria, and certain groups should not be excluded without justification. In the past, some groups, such as women, ethnic minorities, elderly adults, and poor people, were unnecessarily excluded from studies (Larson, 1994). Today, federal funding for research is strongly linked to including these populations in studies. Exclusion criteria limit the generalization of the study findings and should be carefully considered before being used in a study.

Twiss et al. (2009) conducted a quasi-experimental study to examine the effects of strength and weight training (ST) exercises on muscle strength, balance, and falls of breast cancer survivors (BCSs) with bone loss (population). This study included clearly identified inclusion and exclusion sampling or eligibility criteria that are presented in the following excerpt.

"Women were included if they were 35-77 years of age, had a history of stage 0 (in situ), I, or II breast cancer, a BMD [bone mineral density] T-score of −1.0 or less at any of three sites (hip, spine, forearm), were at least 6 months post breast-cancer treatment and 12 months postmenopausal, resided within 100 miles of one of four research sites (Omaha, Lincoln, Kearney, and Scottsbluff, NE), and had their physicians' permission to participate [inclusion sampling criteria]. Women were excluded if they (a) had a recurrence of breast cancer; (b) were currently taking hormone therapy, bisphosphonates, glucocorticosteroids, or other drugs affecting bone; (c) were currently engaging in ST exercises; (d) had a body mass index (BMI) of 35 or greater; (e) had serum calcium, creatinine, or thyroid stimulating hormone (if on thyroid therapy) outside normal limits; or (f) had active gastrointestinal problems or other conditions that prohibited ST exercises, risedronate, calcium, or vitamin D intake [exclusion sampling criteria]." (Twiss et al., 2009, p. 72)

Twiss et al. (2009) identified specific inclusion and exclusion sampling criteria to designate the subjects in the target population precisely. These sampling criteria probably were narrowly defined by the researchers to promote the selection of a homogeneous sample of postmenopausal BCSs with bone loss. These inclusion and exclusion sampling criteria were appropriate for the study to reduce the effect of possible extraneous variables that might have an impact on the treatment (ST exercises) and the measurement of the dependent variables (muscle strength, balance, and falls). Because this is a quasi-experimental study that examined the impact of the treatment on the dependent or outcome variables, the increased controls imposed by the sampling criteria strengthened the likelihood that the study outcomes were caused by the treatment and not by extraneous variables. Twiss et al. (2009) found significant improvement in muscle strength and balance for the treatment group but no significant difference in the number of falls between the treatment and comparison groups.

Sample Representativeness

For a sample to be representative, it must be similar to the target population in as many ways as possible. It is especially important that the sample be representative in relation to the variables you are studying and to other factors that may influence the study variables. For example, if your study examines attitudes toward acquired immunodeficiency syndrome (AIDS), the sample should represent the distribution of attitudes toward AIDS that exists in the specified population. In addition, a sample must represent the demographic characteristics, such as age, gender, ethnicity, income, and education, which often influence study variables.

The accessible population must be representative of the target population. If the accessible population is limited to a particular setting or type of setting, the individuals seeking care at that setting may be different from the individuals who would seek care for the same problem in other settings or from individuals who self-manage their problems. Studies conducted in private hospitals usually exclude poor patients, and other settings could exclude elderly or undereducated patients. People who do not have access to care are usually excluded from health-focused studies. Subjects and the care they receive in research centers are different from patients and the care they receive in community clinics, public hospitals, veterans' hospitals, and rural health clinics. Obese individuals who choose to enter a program to lose weight may differ from obese individuals who do not enter a program. All of these factors limit representativeness and limit our understanding of the phenomena important in practice.

Representativeness is usually evaluated by comparing the numerical values of the sample (a **statistic** such as the mean) with the same values from the target population. A numerical value of a population is called a **parameter**. We can estimate the **population parameter** by identifying the values obtained in previous studies examining the same variables. The accuracy with which the population parameters have been estimated within a study is referred to as **precision**. Precision in estimating parameters requires well-developed methods of measurement that are used repeatedly in several studies. You can define parameters by conducting a series of descriptive and correlational studies, each of which examines a different segment of the target population; then perform a meta-analysis to estimate the population parameter (Thompson, 2002).

Sampling Error

The difference between a sample statistic and a population parameter is called the **sampling error** (Figure 15-2). A large sampling error means that the sample is not providing a precise picture of the population; it is not representative. Sampling error is usually larger

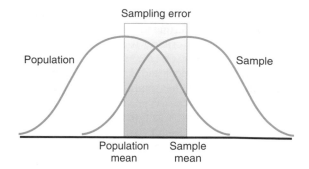

Figure 15-2 **Sampling error.**

with small samples and decreases as the sample size increases. Sampling error reduces the **power** of a study, or the ability of the statistical analyses conducted to detect differences between groups or to describe the relationships among variables (Aberson, 2010; Cohen, 1988). Sampling error occurs as a result of random variation and systematic variation.

Random Variation

Random variation is the expected difference in values that occurs when one examines different subjects from the same sample. If the mean is used to describe the sample, the values of individuals in that sample will not all be exactly the same as the sample mean. Values of individual subjects vary from the value of the sample mean. The difference is random because the value of each subject is likely to vary in a different direction. Some values are higher and others are lower than the sample mean. The values are randomly scattered around the mean. As the sample size becomes larger, overall variation in sample values decreases, with more values being close to the sample mean. As the sample size increases, the sample mean is also more likely to have a value similar to that of the population mean.

Systematic Variation

Systematic variation, or **systematic bias**, is a consequence of selecting subjects whose measurement values are different, or vary, in some specific way from the population. Because the subjects have something in common, their values tend to be similar to the values of others in the sample but different in some way from the values of the population as a whole. These values do not vary randomly around the population mean. Most of the variation from the mean is in the same direction; it is systematic. All the values in the sample may tend to be higher or lower than the mean of the population (Thompson, 2002).

For example, if all the subjects in a study examining some type of healthcare knowledge have an intelligence quotient (IQ) higher than 120, many of their scores will likely be higher than the mean of a population that includes individuals with a wide variation in IQ, such as IQs that range from 90 to 130. The IQs of the subjects have introduced a systematic bias. This situation could occur, for example, if all the subjects were college students, which has been the case in the development of many measurement methods in psychology.

Because of systematic variance, the sample mean is different from the population mean. The extent of the difference is the sampling error (see Figure 15-2). Exclusion criteria tend to increase the systematic bias in the sample and increase the sampling error. An extreme example of this problem is the highly restrictive sampling criteria used in some experimental studies that result in a large sampling error and greatly diminished representativeness.

If the method of selecting subjects produces a sample with a systematic bias, increasing the sample size would not decrease the sampling error. When a systematic bias occurs in an experimental study, it can lead the researcher to believe that a treatment has made a difference when, in actuality, the values would be different even without the treatment. This situation usually occurs because of an interaction of the systematic bias with the treatment.

Refusal and Acceptance Rates in Studies

Systematic variation or bias is most likely to occur when the sampling process is not random. However, even in a random sample, systematic variation can occur if potential subjects decline participation. Systematic bias increases as the subjects' refusal rate increases. A refusal rate is the number and percentage of subjects who declined to participate in the study. High refusal rates to participate in a study have been linked to individuals with serious physical and emotional illnesses, low socioeconomic status, and weak social networks (Neumark, Stommel, Given, & Given, 2001). The higher the refusal rate, the less the sample is representative of the target population. The refusal rate is calculated by dividing the number of potential subjects refusing to participate by the number of potential subjects meeting sampling criteria and multiplying the results by 100%.

Refusal rate formula = number potential subjects refusing to participate ÷ number potential subjects meeting sample criteria × 100%

For example, if 200 potential subjects met the sampling criteria, and 40 refused to participate in the study, the refusal rate would be 20%.

Refusal rate = 40 (number refusing) ÷ 200 (number meeting sampling criteria) = $0.2 \times 100\% = 20\%$

Sometimes researchers provide an acceptance rate, or the number and percentage of the subjects who agree to participate in a study, rather than a refusal rate. The acceptance rate is calculated by dividing the number of potential subjects who agree to participate in a study by the number of potential subjects who meet sampling criteria and multiplying the result by 100%.

Acceptance rate formula = number potential subjects agreeing to participate ÷ number potential subjects meeting sample criteria × 100%

If you know the refusal rate, you can also subtract the refusal rate from 100% to obtain the acceptance rate. Usually researchers report either the acceptance rate or the refusal rate but not both. In the example mentioned earlier, 200 potential subjects met the sampling criteria; 160 agreed to participate in the study, and 40 refused.

Acceptance rate = 160 (number accepting) ÷ 200 (number meeting sampling criteria) = $0.8 \times 100\% = 80\%$

Acceptance rate = 100% − refusal rate or 100% − 20% = 80%

Sample Attrition and Retention Rates in Studies

Systematic variation can also occur in studies with high sample attrition. Sample attrition is the withdrawal or loss of subjects from a study. Systematic variation is greatest when a high number of subjects withdraw from the study before the data have been collected or when a large number of subjects withdraw from one group but not the other in the study (Kerlinger & Lee, 2000; Thompson, 2002). In studies involving a treatment, subjects in the control group who do not receive the treatment may be more likely to withdraw from the study. Sample attrition should be reported in the published study to determine if the final sample represents the target population. Researchers also need to provide a rationale for subjects withdrawing from the study and to determine if they are different from the subjects who complete the study. The sample is most like the target population if the attrition rate is low (<10% to 20%) and the subjects withdrawing from the study are similar to the subjects completing the study. Sample attrition rate is calculated by dividing the number of subjects withdrawing from a study by the sample size and multiplying the results by 100%.

Sample attrition rate formula = number subjects withdrawing ÷ sample size × 100%

For example, if a study had a sample size of 160, and 40 people withdrew from the study, the attrition rate would be 25%.

Attrition rate = 40 (number withdrawing) ÷ 160 (sample size) = 0.25 × 100% = 25%

The opposite of the attrition rate is the retention rate, or the number and percentage of subjects completing the study. The higher the retention rate, the more representative the sample is of the target population, and the more likely the study results are an accurate reflection of reality. Often researchers identify either the attrition rate or the retention rate but not both. It is better to provide a rate in addition to the number of subjects withdrawing or completing a study. In the example just presented with a sample size of 160, if 40 subjects withdrew from the study, then 120 subjects were retained or completed the study. The retention rate is calculated by dividing the number of subjects completing the study by the initial sample size and multiplying by 100%.

Sample retention rate formula = number subjects completing study ÷ sample size × 100%

Retention rate = 120 (number retained) ÷ 160 (sample size) = 0.75 × 100% = 75%

The study by Twiss et al. (2009) of the effects of ST exercises on muscle strength, balance, and falls of BCSs with bone loss was introduced earlier in this chapter with the discussion of sampling criteria; the following excerpt presents the acceptance rate and sample attrition for this study.

"A sample of 249 participants met the screening criteria and they were enrolled in the study.... Of the 249 women, 223 completed the 24-month testing and were included in the analysis (exercise [treatment group] = 110; comparison = 113). The remaining 26

women (exercise = 14; comparison = 12) withdrew from the study before 24 months. Reasons for withdrawal included the desire for a different exercise program (n = 7); insufficient time (n = 6); intolerance to meds (n = 5); cancer recurrence (n = 5); health problems (n = 2); and relocation (n = 1)." (Twiss et al., 2009, p. 22)

Twiss et al. (2009) identified that 249 participants or subjects met the sampling criteria and 249 were enrolled in the study indicating that the acceptance rate for the study was 100%. The sample retention was 223 women for a retention rate of 90% (223 ÷ 249 × 100% = 89.6% = 90%), and the sample attrition rate was 26 women for an attrition rate of 10% (100% − 90% = 10%). The treatment group retention was 110 women with a retention rate of 89% (110 ÷ 124 × 100% = 88.7% = 89%). The comparison group retention was 113 women with a retention rate of 90% (113 ÷ 125 = 90.4% = 90%). This study has an excellent acceptance rate (100%) and a very strong sample retention rate of 90% for a 24-month-long study. The retention rates for both groups were very strong and comparable (treatment group 89% and comparison group 90%). Twiss et al. (2009) also provided a rationale for the subjects' attrition, and the reasons were varied and seemed appropriate and typical for a study lasting 24 months. The acceptance rate, the sample and group retention rates, and the reasons for subjects' attrition indicate limited potential for systematic variation in the study sample. The likelihood is increased that the sample is representative of the target population and the results are an accurate reflection of reality. The study would have been strengthened if the researchers would have included not only the numbers but also the sample and group retention rates.

Randomization

From a sampling theory point of view, randomization means that each individual in the population should have a greater than zero opportunity to be selected for the sample. The method of achieving this opportunity is referred to as random sampling. In experimental studies that use a control group, subjects are randomly selected and randomly assigned to either the control group or the experimental group. The use of the term control group—the group not receiving the treatment—is usually limited to studies using random sampling and random assignment to the treatment and control groups. The control group usually receives no care. If nonrandom sampling methods are used for sample selection, the group not receiving a treatment receives usual or standard care and is generally referred to as a **comparison group**. With a comparison group, there is an increase in the possibility of preexisting differences between that group and the experimental group receiving the treatment.

Random sampling increases the extent to which the sample is representative of the target population. However, random sampling must take place in an accessible population that is representative of the target population. Exclusion criteria limit true randomness. Thus, a study that uses random sampling techniques may have such restrictive sampling criteria that the sample is not truly random. In any case, it is rarely possible to obtain a purely random sample for nursing studies because of informed consent requirements. Even if the original sample is random, persons who volunteer or consent to participate in a study may differ in important ways from persons who are unwilling to participate. All samples with human subjects must be **volunteer samples**, which includes individuals willing to participate in the study, to protect the rights of the individuals (Fawcett & Garity, 2009). Methods of achieving random sampling are described later in the chapter.

Sampling Frame

For each person in the target or accessible population to have an opportunity to be selected for the sample, each person in the population must be identified. To accomplish this goal, the researcher must acquire a list of every member of the population through the use of the sampling criteria to define membership. This listing of members of the population is referred to as the **sampling frame**. The researcher selects subjects from the sampling frame using a sampling plan. Djukic, Kovner, Budin, and Norman (2010) studied the effect of nurses' perceived physical work environment on their job satisfaction and described their sampling frame in the following excerpt.

"The study was conducted at a large urban hospital in the U.S. northeast region that is a nongovernment, not-for-profit, general medical and surgical major teaching hospital. About 1,300 staff RNs [population] were employed at the hospital at the time of the study.... A total of 746 RNs who met eligibility criteria were invited to participate in the study [sampling frame of target population]. The eligible RNs were those who had a functioning work e-mail account and who worked fulltime, on inpatient units, providing direct patient care." (Djukic et al., 2010, pp. 444-445)

The sampling frame in this study included the names of the 746 RNs who were asked to participate in the study.

Sampling Plan

A **sampling plan** describes the strategies that will be used to obtain a sample for a study. The plan is developed to enhance representativeness, reduce systematic bias, and decrease the sampling error. Sampling strategies have been devised to accomplish these three tasks and to optimize sample selection. The sampling plan may use probability (random) sampling methods or nonprobability (nonrandom) sampling methods.

A **sampling method** is the process of selecting a group of people, events, behaviors, or other elements that represent the population being studied. A sampling method is similar to a design; it is not specific to a study. The sampling plan provides detail about the application of a sampling method in a specific study. The sampling plan must be described in detail for purposes of critical appraisal, replication, and future meta-analyses. The sampling method implemented in a study varies with the type of research being conducted. Quantitative, outcomes, and intervention research apply a variety of probability and nonprobability sampling methods. Qualitative research usually includes nonprobability sampling methods. The sampling methods to be included in this text are identified in Table 15-1 and are linked to the types of research that most commonly incorporate them. The following sections describe the different types of probability and nonprobability sampling methods most commonly used in quantitative, qualitative, outcomes, and intervention research in nursing.

Probability (Random) Sampling Methods

Probability sampling methods have been developed to ensure some degree of precision in estimations of the population parameters. Probability samples reduce sampling error. The term **probability sampling method** refers to the fact that every member (element) of the population has a probability higher than zero of being selected for the sample. Inferential statistical analyses are based on the assumption that the sample from which data were derived has been obtained randomly. Thus, probability sampling methods are often referred to as **random sampling methods**. These samples are more likely to represent the population than samples obtained with nonprobability sampling methods. All subsets of the population, which may differ from one another but contribute to the

TABLE 15-1 Probability and Nonprobability Sampling Methods Commonly Applied in Nursing Research

Sampling Method	Common Applications
Probability Sampling Methods	
Simple random sampling	Quantitative, outcomes, and intervention research
Stratified random sampling	Quantitative, outcomes, and intervention research
Cluster sampling	Quantitative, outcomes, and intervention research
Systematic sampling	Quantitative, outcomes, and intervention research
Nonprobability Sampling Methods	
Convenience sampling	Quantitative, qualitative, outcomes, and intervention research
Quota sampling	Quantitative, outcomes, and intervention research
Purpose or purposeful sampling	Qualitative and sometimes quantitative research
Network or snowball sampling	Qualitative and sometimes quantitative research
Theoretical sampling	Qualitative research

parameters of the population, have a chance to be represented in the sample. Probability sampling methods are most commonly applied in quantitative, outcomes, and intervention research.

There is less opportunity for systematic bias if subjects are selected randomly, although it is possible for a systematic bias to occur by chance. Using random sampling, the researcher cannot decide that person *X* would be a better subject for the study than person *Y*. In addition, a researcher cannot exclude a subset of people from selection as subjects because he or she does not agree with them, does not like them, or finds them hard to deal with. Potential subjects cannot be excluded just because they are too sick, not sick enough, coping too well, or not coping adequately. The researcher, who has a vested interest in the study, could (consciously or unconsciously) select subjects whose conditions or behaviors are consistent with the study hypothesis. It is tempting to exclude uncooperative or assertive individuals. Random sampling leaves the selection to chance and decreases sampling error and increases the validity of the study (Thompson, 2002).

Theoretically, to obtain a probability sample, the researcher must develop a sampling frame that includes every element in the population. The sample must be randomly selected from the sampling frame. According to sampling theory, it is impossible to select a sample randomly from a population that cannot be clearly defined. Four sampling designs have been developed to achieve probability sampling: simple random sampling, stratified random sampling, cluster sampling, and systematic sampling.

Simple Random Sampling

Simple random sampling is the most basic of the probability sampling methods. To achieve simple random sampling, elements are selected at random from the sampling frame. This goal can be accomplished in various ways, limited only by the imagination of the researcher. If the sampling frame is small, the researcher can write names on slips of paper, place the names in a container, mix well, and draw out one at a time until the desired sample size has been reached. Another technique is to assign a number to each name in the sampling frame. In large population sets, elements may already have assigned numbers. For example, numbers are assigned to medical records, organizational memberships, and professional licenses. The researcher can use a computer to select these numbers randomly to obtain a sample.

There can be some differences in the probability for the selection of each element, depending on whether the name or number of the selected element is replaced before the next name or number is selected. Selection with replacement, the most conservative random sampling approach, provides exactly equal opportunities for each element to be selected (Thompson, 2002). For example, if the researcher draws names out of a hat to obtain a sample, each name must be replaced before the next name is drawn to ensure equal opportunity for each subject.

Selection without replacement gives each element different levels of probability for selection. For example, if the researcher is selecting 10 subjects from a population of 50, the first name has a 1 in 5 chance (10 draws, 50 names), or a 0.2 probability, of being selected. If the first name is not replaced, the remaining 49 names have a 9 in 49 chance, or a 0.18 probability, of being selected. As further names are drawn, the probability of being selected decreases.

There are many ways to achieve random selection, such as with the use of a computer, a random numbers table, drawing names out of a hat, or a roulette wheel. The most common method of random selection is the computer, which can be programmed to select a sample randomly from the sampling frame with replacement. However, some researchers still use a table of random numbers to select a random sample.

TABLE 15-2		Section from a Random Numbers Table							
06	84	10	22	56	72	25	70	69	43
07	63	10	34	66	39	54	02	33	85
03	19	63	93	72	52	13	30	44	40
77	32	69	58	25	15	55	38	19	62
20	01	94	54	66	88	43	91	34	28

Table 15-2 shows a section from a random numbers table. To use a table of random numbers, the researcher places a pencil or a finger on the table with the eyes closed. The number touched is the starting place. Moving the pencil or finger up, down, right, or left, the researcher uses the numbers in order until the desired sample size is obtained. For example, the researcher places a pencil on 58 in Table 15-2, which is in the fourth column from the left and fourth row down. If five subjects are to be selected from a population of 100 and the researcher decides to go across the column to the right, the subject numbers chosen are 58, 25, 15, 55, and 38. Table 15-2 is useful only if the population number is less than 100. However, tables are available for larger populations, such as the random numbers table provided in the online resources for this textbook or the Thompson (2002, pp. 14-15) sampling text.

Degirmen, Ozerdogan, Sayiner, Kosgeroglu, and Ayranci (2010, p. 153) conducted a pretest-posttest randomized controlled experimental study to determine the effect of hand and foot massage and foot massage only interventions on the postoperative pain of women who had a cesarean operation. These researchers obtained their sample using a simple random sampling method that is described in the following excerpt from their study.

"The study was conducted in obstetric intensive care units and services of all the public and university hospitals in the province of Eskisehir, Turkey.... During the 4 month study, 281 patients attended for the cesarean operations to the obstetric intensive care units and services of all hospitals concerned [target population and settings]. The total 75 study patients [sample] out of the 281 were selected by random sampling method from the patients' presenting orders [sampling frame] and evenly divided into three groups; a control group, a foot and hand massage group, and a foot massage group, each of which included 25

patients.... Because some patients accepted the intervention before the operation, but changed their mind after the operation (3 patients in total), not all patients participated in the study." (Degirmen et al., 2010, p. 154)

Degirmen et al. (2010) clearly identified their target population as women needing cesarean operations, and the 281 women with presenting orders provided the sampling frame for the study. The sample of 75 women was randomly selected, but the researchers did not indicate the process for the random selection. The use of a computer to select a sample randomly is usually the most efficient and unbiased process. The subjects were evenly divided with 25 in each group, but the researchers do not indicate if the assignment to groups was random or based on the convenience of the subjects or researchers. Application of simple random sampling and the attrition of only three (4%) subjects from the study seem to provide a sample representative of the target population. However, the study would have been strengthened by a discussion of the process for random sampling and a clarification of how the subjects were assigned to groups. The outcomes of the study were that foot and hand massage interventions significantly reduced postoperative pain experienced by the women and that foot and hand massage was significantly more effective than foot massage only.

Stratified Random Sampling

Stratified random sampling is used when the researcher knows some of the variables in the population that are critical to achieving representativeness. Variables commonly used for stratification are age, gender, ethnicity, socioeconomic status, diagnosis, geographical region, type of institution, type of care, care provider, and site of care. The variable or variables chosen for stratification need to be correlated with the dependent variables being examined in the study. Subjects within each stratum are expected to be more similar (homogeneous) in relation to the study variables than they are to be similar to subjects in other strata or the total sample. In stratified random sampling, the subjects are randomly selected on the basis of their classification into the selected strata.

For example, if in conducting your research you selected a stratified random sample of 100 adult subjects using age as the variable for stratification, the sample might include 25 subjects in the age range 18 to 39 years, 25 subjects in the age range 40 to 59 years, 25 subjects in the age range 60 to 79 years, and 25 subjects 80 years or older. Stratification ensures that all levels of the identified variable, in this example age, are adequately represented in the sample. With a stratified random sample, you could use a smaller sample size to achieve the same degree of representativeness as a large sample acquired through simple random sampling. Sampling error decreases, power increases, data collection time is reduced, and the cost of the study is lower if stratification is used (Fawcett & Garity, 2009; Thompson, 2002).

One question that arises in relation to stratification is whether each stratum should have equivalent numbers of subjects in the sample (termed **disproportionate sampling**) or whether the numbers of subjects should be selected in proportion to their occurrence in the population (termed **proportionate sampling**). For example, if stratification is being achieved by ethnicity and the population is 45% white non-Hispanic, 25% Hispanic nonwhite, 25% African American, and 5% Asian, your research team would have to decide whether to select equal numbers of each ethnic group or to calculate a proportion of the sample. Good arguments exist for both approaches. Stratification is not as useful if one stratum contains only a small number of subjects. In the aforementioned situation, if proportions are used and the sample size is 100, the study would include only five Asians, hardly enough to be representative. If equal numbers of each group are used, each group would contain at least 25 subjects; however, the white non-Hispanic group would be underrepresented. In this case, mathematically weighting the findings from each stratum can equalize the representation to ensure proportional contributions of each stratum to the total score of the sample. Most textbooks on sampling describe this procedure (Levy & Lemsbow, 1980; Thompson, 2002; Yates, 1981).

Ulrich et al. (2006) used a stratified random sampling method to obtain their sample of nurse practitioners (NPs) and physician assistants (PAs) for the purpose of studying the ethical conflict of these healthcare providers associated with managed care. The following excerpt from this study describes the sampling method used to obtain the final sample of 1536 providers (833 NPs and 689 PAs).

"A self-administered questionnaire was mailed to an initial stratified random sample [sampling method] of 3,900 NPs and PAs practicing in the United States. The sample was selected from the national lists provided by Medical Marketing Services, an independently owned organization that manages medical industry lists (www.mmslists.com/main.asp). The list for PAs was derived from the American Academy of Physicians Assistants (AAPA), and a comprehensive list of NPs was derived from the medical and nursing boards of the 50 states and the District of Columbia [sampling frames for NPs and PAs].... After undeliverable (1.9%) and other disqualified respondents (13.2%, i.e., no longer practicing, non-primary-care practitioner) were removed, the overall adjusted response rate was 50.6%." (Ulrich et al., 2006, p. 393)

The study sampling frames for the NPs and PAs are representative of all 50 states and the District of Columbia, and the lists for the sampling frames were from quality sources. The study has a strong response rate of 50.6% for a mailed questionnaire, and the researchers identified why certain respondents were disqualified. The final sample was large (1536 subjects) with strong representation for both NPs (833 subjects) and PAs (689 subjects). The study sample might have been stronger with a more equal number of NP and PA subjects. The 833 NPs and 689 PAs add to 1522 subjects and it is unclear why the sample size is identified as 1536 unless there are missing data from subjects. However, the sample was a great strength of this study and appeared to represent the target population of NPs and PAs currently practicing in primary care in the United States.

Cluster Sampling

Cluster sampling is a probability sampling method applied when the population is heterogeneous; it is similar to stratified random sampling but takes advantage of the natural clusters or groups of population units that have similar characteristics (Fawcett & Garity, 2009). Cluster sampling is used in two situations. The first situation is when a simple random sample would be prohibitive in terms of travel time and cost. Imagine trying to arrange personal meetings with 100 people, each in a different part of the United States. The second situation is in cases in which the individual elements making up the population are unknown, preventing the development of a sampling frame. For example, there is no list of all the heart surgery patients who complete rehabilitation programs in the United States. In these cases, it is often possible to obtain lists of institutions or organizations with which the elements of interest are associated.

In cluster sampling, the researcher develops a sampling frame that includes a list of all the states, cities, institutions, or organizations with which elements of the identified population would be linked. States, cities, institutions, or organizations are selected randomly as units from which to obtain elements for the sample. In some cases, this random selection continues through several stages and is referred to as **multistage cluster sampling**. For example, the researcher might first randomly select states and next randomly select cities within the sampled states. Hospitals within the randomly selected cities might then be randomly selected. Within the hospitals, nursing units might be randomly selected. At this level, either all the patients on the nursing unit who fit the criteria for the study might be included, or patients could be randomly selected.

Cluster sampling provides a means for obtaining a larger sample at a lower cost. However, it has some disadvantages. Data from subjects associated with the same institution are likely to be correlated and not completely independent. This correlation can cause a decrease in precision and an increase in sampling error. However, such disadvantages can be offset to some extent by the use of a larger sample.

Fouladbakhsh and Stommel (2010, p. E8) used multistage cluster sampling in their study of the "complex relationships among gender, physical and psychological symptoms, and use of specific CAM [complementary and alternative medicine] health practices among individuals living in the United States who have been diagnosed with cancer." These researchers described their sampling method in the following excerpt from their study.

"The NHIS [National Health Interview Survey] methodology employs a multistage probability cluster sampling design [sampling method] that is representative of the NHIS target universe, defined as 'the civilian noninstitutionalized population' (Botman, Moore, Moriarty, & Parsons, 2000, p. 14; National Center for Health Statistics). In the first stage, 339 primary sampling units were selected from about 1,900 area sampling units representing counties, groups of adjacent counties, or metropolitan areas covering the 50 states and the District of Columbia [1st stage cluster sampling]. The selection included all of the most populous primary sampling units in the United States and stratified probability samples (by state, area poverty level, and population size) of the less populous ones. In a second step, primary sampling units were partitioned into substrata (up to 21) based on concentrations of African American and Hispanic populations [2nd stage

cluster sampling]. In a third step, clusters of dwelling units form the secondary sampling units selected from each substratum [3rd stage cluster sampling]. Finally, within each secondary sampling unit, all African American and Hispanic households were selected for interviews, whereas other households were sampled at differing rates within the substrata. Therefore, the sampling design of the NHIS includes oversampling of minorities." (Fouladbakhsh & Stommel, 2010, pp. E8-E9)

These researchers detailed their use of multistage cluster sampling and clearly identified the three stages implemented and the rationale for each stage. The study had a large, national sample that seemed representative of all 50 states and the District of Columbia with an oversampling of minorities to accomplish the purpose of the study. The complex cluster sampling method used in this study provided a representative sample, which decreases the likelihood of sampling error and increases the validity of the study findings. The findings reported by Fouladbakhsh and Stommel (2010, p. E7) indicated that "CAM practice use was more prevalent among female, middle-aged, Caucasian, and well-educated subjects. Pain, depression, and insomnia were strong predictors of practice use, with differences noted by gender and practice type."

Systematic Sampling

Systematic sampling can be conducted when an ordered list of all members of the population is available. The process involves selecting every kth individual on the list, using a starting point selected randomly. If the initial starting point is not random, the sample is not a probability sample. To use this design in your research, you must know the number of elements in the population and the size of the sample desired. Divide the population size by the desired sample size, giving k, the size of the gap between elements selected from the list. For example, if the population size is $N = 1200$ and the desired sample size is $n = 100$, then you could calculate the value of k:

$$k = \textbf{population size} \div \textbf{sample size desired}$$

Example: $k = 1200$ (population size) $\div$ 100 (sample size desired) $= 12$

Thus, $k = 12$, which means that every 12th person on the list would be included in the sample. Some authors argue that this procedure does not truly give each element an opportunity to be included in the sample; it provides a random but unequal chance for inclusion (Thompson, 2002).

Researchers must be careful to determine that the original list has not been set up with any ordering that could be meaningful in relation to the study. The process is based on the assumption that the order of the list is random in relation to the variables being studied. If the order of the list is related to the study, systematic bias is introduced. In addition to this risk, it is difficult to compute sampling error with the use of this design (Floyd, 1993).

Li and Mukamel (2010, p. S256) conducted a secondary data analysis of National Nursing Home Survey (NNHS) data to identify any "racial disparities in the receipt and documentation of influenza and pneumococcus vaccinations among nursing-home residents." The NNHS data were obtained using stratified random sampling and systematic sampling for selection of the nursing homes and random sampling of the residents for interviews. The researchers described the sampling plan for the NNHS and the participants for their study in the following study excerpt.

"We obtained the public-use resident file of the Centers for Disease Control and Prevention's 2004 NNHS, which includes a nationally representative sample of nursing homes, their residents, and the services the residents received.... The 2004 NNHS involved a stratified 2-stage probability design. The first stage was the selection of nursing homes stratified by geographical location (state, county, and zip code), bed-size category (number of beds), and ownership status (profit vs. nonprofit). Nursing homes were finally selected by systematic sampling, with the probability proportional to bed-size category. The second stage, sampling of current residents, was carried out by interviewers at the time of their visits to the facilities. Individuals were randomly selected from patient rosters, and a sample of up to 12 current residents per facility was selected for the final interview. The final NNHS comprised 13,507 residents in 1174 nursing homes, with an overall response rate of 78%.... Our analyses were limited to 11,448 nonHispanic Whites and 1384 Blacks, excluding 765 residents (5.7%) of other races/ethnicities.... The final sample comprised 10,562 residents for analysis of influenza and 12,134 residents for the analysis of pneumococcus vaccinations." (Li & Mukamel, 2010, p. S256)

Li and Mukamel (2010) used a national database developed with strong probability sampling methods (stratified random sampling and systematic sampling). The database included a nationally representative sample of nursing homes and their residents, which decreases the potential for sampling error and supports the validity of the findings. The study design was limited to an examination of data from white and black subjects, who were the largest groups represented in the nursing homes surveyed. The sample size was extremely large, which increases the potential to generalize the findings to these two ethnic groups. The study would have been strengthened by a more detailed discussion of the systematic sampling of the nursing homes and the random sampling of the residents. The researchers found that disparities existed in vaccination coverage of white and black nursing home residents and recommended interventions to improve coverage.

Nonprobability (Nonrandom) Sampling Methods Commonly Applied in Quantitative Research

In nonprobability sampling, not every element of the population has an opportunity to be included in the sample. Nonprobability sampling methods increase the likelihood of obtaining samples that are not representative of their target populations. However, most nursing studies use nonprobability sampling, especially convenience sampling, to select study samples. In conducting studies in nursing and other health disciplines, limited subjects are available, and it is often impossible to obtain a random sample. Researchers often include any subjects willing to participate who meet the eligibility criteria.

There are several types of nonprobability (nonrandom) sampling designs. Each addresses a different research need. The five nonprobability sampling designs described in this textbook are (1) convenience sampling, (2) quota sampling, (3) purposive or purposeful sampling, (4) network or snowball sampling, and (5) theoretical sampling. These sampling methods are applied in both quantitative and qualitative research. However, convenience sampling and quota sampling are applied more often in quantitative, outcomes, and intervention research than in qualitative studies and are discussed in this section (see Table 15-1). Purposive sampling, network sampling, and theoretical sampling are more commonly applied in qualitative studies than in quantitative studies and are discussed later in this chapter.

Convenience Sampling

In convenience sampling, subjects are included in the study because they happened to be in the right place at the right time. Researchers simply enter available subjects into the study until they have reached the desired sample size. Convenience sampling, also called accidental sampling, is considered a weak approach to sampling because it provides little opportunity to control for biases. Multiple biases may exist in convenience sampling; these biases range from minimal to serious. Researchers need to identify and describe known biases in their samples. You can identify biases by carefully thinking through the sample criteria used to determine the target population and taking steps to improve the representativeness of the sample. For example, in a study of home care management of patients with complex healthcare needs, educational level would be an important extraneous variable. One solution for controlling this extraneous variable would be to redefine the sampling criteria to include only patients with a high school education. Doing so would limit the extent of generalization but decrease the bias created by educational level. Another option would be to select a population known to include individuals with a wide variety of educational levels. Data could be collected on educational level so that the description of the sample would include information on educational level. With this information, one could judge the extent to which the sample was representative with respect to educational level (Thompson, 2002).

Decisions related to sample selection must be carefully described to enable others to evaluate the possibility of biases. In addition, data need be gathered to allow a thorough description of the sample that can also be used to evaluate for possible biases. Data on the sample can be used to compare the sample with other samples and to estimate the parameters of populations through meta-analyses.

Many strategies are available for selecting a convenience sample. A classroom of students might be used. Patients who attend a clinic on a specific day, subjects who attend a support group, patients currently admitted to a hospital with a specific diagnosis, and every fifth person who enters the emergency department are examples of types of commonly selected convenience samples.

Convenience samples are inexpensive and accessible, and they usually require less time to acquire than other types of samples. Convenience samples provide means to conduct studies on topics that could not be examined through the use of probability sampling. Convenience sampling enables researchers to acquire information in unexplored areas. According to Kerlinger and Lee (2000), a convenience sample is probably not that bad when it is used with reasonable knowledge and care in implementing a study. Healthcare studies are usually conducted with particular types of patients experiencing varying numbers of health problems; these patients often are reluctant to participate in research. Thus, researchers often find it very difficult to recruit subjects for their studies and frequently must use a sample of convenience versus random sampling to obtain their sample.

O'Shea, Wallace, Griffin, and Fitzpatrick (2011, p. 35) used convenience sampling to determine the "effectiveness of a spiritual educational session on pediatric nurses' perspectives concerning the provision of pediatric spiritual care." The following excerpt describes their sampling method.

> "The setting for the data collection was a large university-affiliated children's hospital located in the northeast. Participants represented a convenience sample [sampling method] from a potential 355 registered neonatal and pediatric staff nurses employed at the hospital [target population]. Forty-one nurses voluntarily consented to participate. Number of participants per session varied from approximately two to five, depending on the day and time of the session." (O'Shea et al., 2011, p. 37)

O'Shea et al. (2011) clearly identified their sampling method, target population, and sample size. The acceptance rate for the study was 41 neonatal and pediatric nurses, which is only 12% of the 355 nurses in the target population. The nurses volunteering to participate in the study might be different in some way from the nurses refusing to participate. The small sample size ($N = 41$) and low acceptance rate increase the chance for sampling error and decrease the representativeness of the sample. However, all 41 participants completed this quasi-experimental study (0% attrition rate), which decreases the potential for bias. The sample was homogeneous for registered nurse status, employed on pediatric units, and gender (female $n = 40$). The sample was heterogeneous for education ranging from associate's degree to master's in nursing and for years of experience ranging from less than 2 years to more than 20 years. In a quasi-experimental study, a homogeneous sample decreases the extraneous variables that might influence the findings. Based on the sampling method (nonprobability convenience sample), small sample size, high refusal rate, and differences in the education and years of experience of the nurses, the findings from this study are best generalized to the sample and not the accessible or target populations. The researchers found that the educational sessions had a positive effect on the nurses' perspectives toward providing spiritual care, but additional research is needed to confirm the effect of this intervention. Additional studies with large convenience samples that have similar results would indicate the effectiveness of this intervention for practice.

Quota Sampling

Quota sampling uses a convenience sampling technique with an added feature, a strategy to ensure the inclusion of subject types or strata in a population that are likely to be underrepresented in the convenience sample, such as women, minority groups, elderly adults, poor people, rich people, and undereducated adults. This method may also be used to mimic the known characteristics of the target population or to ensure adequate numbers of subjects in each stratum for the planned statistical analyses. The technique is similar to the technique used in stratified random sampling, but the initial sample is not random. If necessary, mathematical weighting can be used to adjust sample values so that they are consistent with the proportion of subgroups found in the population. Quota sampling offers an improvement over convenience sampling and tends to decrease potential biases. In most studies in which convenience samples are used, quota sampling could be used and should be considered (Thompson, 2002).

Pieper, Templin, Kirsner, and Birk (2010) used quota sampling to examine the impact of vascular leg disorders, such as chronic venous disorders and peripheral arterial disease, on the physical activity levels of opioid-addicted adults in a methadone-maintained program. The following excerpt describes their sampling process.

"The sample (N = 713) was obtained from September 2005 to December 2007 from 12 methadone treatment clinics located in a large urban area [convenience sampling]. The sample was stratified on four variables: age (25-39 years, 40-49 years, 50-65 years); gender (male, female); ethnicity (African American, White); and drug use (nonIDU [injection drug use], arm/upper body injection only, or legs ± upper body injection; Pieper, Templin, Kirsner, & Birk, 2009) [quota sampling]. The purpose of the stratification was to allow comparisons of type of drug use with minimal confounding by age, gender, or ethnicity. Additional inclusion criteria included presence of both legs, able to walk, and able to speak and understand English. The analyses reported here are on the 569 participants who completed the revised LDUQ [Legs in Daily Use Questionnaire], which were edited after examining the test-retest data from 104 participants, not included in the 569, who were tested first." (Pieper et al., 2010, p. 429)

Pieper et al. (2010) clearly identified that the original sample was one of convenience because it included people attending 12 methadone treatment clinics who were willing to participate in the study. The quota sampling involved stratification of the sample on four variables with a clear rationale for the variables selected for stratification. The study was completed by 569 participants, but 104 participants were used for examining the test-retest reliability of the LDUQ and not included in the final data collection. The study had an attrition of 40 participants (attrition rate = 40 ÷ 569 × 100% = 7%).

The study by Pieper et al. (2010) has several strengths in the sampling process. The use of quota sampling ensured that the study sample was more representative of the target population than using convenience sampling only. In addition, the participants were obtained from 12 different clinics and the sample size was large (N = 713 − 104 [used only for instrument reliability testing] = 569) with a small attrition rate (7%). The sample appeared to be representative of the target population with limited potential for sampling error. The findings indicated that motivation was the strongest predictor of physical activity and that healthcare professionals need to evaluate the vascular health of legs of drug injection users before encouraging exercise.

Nonprobability Sampling Methods Commonly Applied in Qualitative Research

Qualitative research is conducted to gain insights and discover meaning about a particular experience, situation, cultural element, or historical event. The intent is an in-depth understanding of a purposefully selected sample and not the generalization of the findings from a randomly selected sample to a target population, as in quantitative, outcomes, and intervention research. In qualitative research, experiences, events, and incidents are more the focus of sampling than people (Marshall & Rossman, 2011; Munhall, 2012; Patton, 2002). The researcher attempts to select participants or informants who can provide extensive information about the experience or event being studied. For example, if the goal of your study was to describe the phenomenon of living with chronic pain, you would purposefully select participants who were articulate and reflective, had a history of chronic pain, and were willing to share their chronic pain experience (Coyne, 1997).

The three common sampling methods applied in qualitative research are purposive or purposeful sampling, network or snowball sampling, and theoretical sampling (see Table 15-1). These sampling methods enable the researcher to select the specific participants who would provide the most extensive information about the phenomenon, event, or situation being studied (Marshall & Rossman, 2011). The sample selection process can have a profound effect on the quality of the research and should be described in enough depth to promote the interpretation of the findings and the replication of the study (Munhall, 2012; Patton, 2002).

Purposive Sampling

In **purposive sampling**, sometimes referred to as *purposeful, judgmental,* or *selective sampling,* the researcher consciously selects certain participants, elements, events, or incidents to include in the study. In purposive sampling, qualitative researchers select **information-rich cases**, or cases that can teach them a great deal about the central focus or purpose of the study (Green & Thorogood, 2004; Patton, 2002). Efforts might be made to include typical and atypical participants or situations. Researchers also seek **critical cases**, or cases that make a point clearly or are extremely important in understanding the purpose of the study (Munhall, 2012). The researcher might select participants or informants of various ages, participants with differing diagnoses or illness severity, or participants who received an ineffective treatment versus an effective treatment for their illness.

This sampling plan has been criticized because it is difficult to evaluate the precision of the researcher's judgment. How does one determine that the patient or element was typical or atypical, good or bad, effective or ineffective? Researchers need to indicate the characteristics that they desire in participants and provide a rationale for selecting these types of participants to obtain essential data for their study. Purposive sampling method is used in qualitative research to gain insight into a new area of study or to obtain in-depth

understanding of a complex experience or event (Munhall, 2012).

Sternberg and Barry (2011, p. 64) applied purposive and snowball sampling methods in conducting their phenomenological study of "the experiences of transnational Latina mothers who immigrated to the United States without legal documentation or their children." Snowball sampling, discussed in the next section, involves current study participants identifying additional potential study participants who are similar to them. Sternberg and Barry describe their sampling methods in the following study excerpt.

"A purposive sample of Latina mothers who immigrated to the United States without their children was selected. Interviews were conducted and analyzed until saturation and redundancy was achieved (Munhall, 2007). Eight women in total participated in the study. Three women visiting a free community clinic in southeast Florida were invited to participate in the study by the nurse researcher; the other five were recruited using snowball sampling. Snowball sampling was chosen over random sampling because of the difficulty in gaining access to a population with so many undocumented members (Munhall, 2007). Further, it enabled the researcher to establish a trusting relationship with the participants and obtain a more heterogeneous sample group. To be included in this study, participants had to be mothers who were 18 years of age or older, Spanish or English speaking, and immigrants to the United States from Latin America who had left their child or children in their country of origin." (Sternberg & Barry, 2011, pp. 65-66)

Sternberg and Barry (2011) clearly identified their sampling methods that were appropriate for the qualitative study they conducted. The initial three participants were identified through purposive sampling so that they could achieve a group reflective of their sampling criteria. Individuals without legal documentation are hard to locate, so use of snowball sampling was appropriate to identify five additional participants. The eight participants provided an adequate-sized sample because the researchers were able to reach saturation and redundancy of themes during their data analysis. The findings from the study included seven essential themes: "living in extreme poverty, having hope, choosing to walk from poverty, suffering through the trip to and across the U.S.-Mexican border, mothering from afar, valuing family, and changing personally" (Sternberg & Barry, 2011, p. 67).

Network (Snowball) Sampling

Network sampling, sometimes referred to as *snowball* or *chain sampling,* holds promise for locating samples difficult or impossible to obtain in other ways or that had not been previously identified for study. Network sampling takes advantage of social networks and the fact that friends tend to have characteristics in common. When you have found a few participants with the necessary criteria, you can ask for their assistance in getting in touch with others with similar characteristics. The first few participants are often obtained through convenience or purposive sampling methods, and the sample size is expanded using network or snowball sampling. This sampling method is occasionally used in quantitative studies, but it is more commonly used in qualitative studies. In qualitative research, network sampling is an effective strategy for identifying participants who know other potential participants who can provide the greatest insight and essential information about an experience or event that is identified for study (Marshall & Rossman, 2011; Munhall, 2012; Patton, 2002).

This strategy is also particularly useful for finding participants in socially devalued populations, such as alcoholics, child abusers, sex offenders, drug addicts, and criminals. These individuals are seldom willing to make themselves known. Other groups, such as widows, grieving siblings, or individuals successful at lifestyle changes, can be located using this strategy. These individuals are outside the existing healthcare system and are difficult to find. Biases are built into the sampling process because the participants are not independent of one another. However, the participants selected have the expertise to provide the essential information needed to address the study purpose. The study by Sternberg and Barry (2011) presented in the previous section applied snowball or network sampling to identify additional study participants who had immigrated to the United States without legal documentation. These researchers clearly identified their use of snowball sampling and their rationale for using this method in their study.

Theoretical Sampling

Theoretical sampling is usually applied in grounded theory research to advance the development of a selected theory throughout the research process (Munhall, 2012). The researcher gathers data from any individual or group that can provide relevant data for theory generation. The data are considered relevant if they include information that generates, delimits, and saturates the theoretical codes in the study needed for theory generation. A code is saturated if it is complete and the researcher can see how it fits in the theory. The researcher continues to seek sources and gather data until the codes are saturated and the theory evolves from the codes and the data. Diversity in the sample is encouraged so that the theory developed covers a wide range of behavior in varied situations (Marshall & Rossman, 2011; Patton, 2002).

Beaulieu, Kools, Kennedy, and Humphreys (2011, p. 41) conducted a qualitative study using grounded theory methods to "explore and better understand the reasons for the apparent underuse of emergency contraceptive pills (ECPs) in young people in coupled relationships." These researchers applied three sampling methods: (1) convenience sampling, (2) snowball sampling, and (3) theoretical sampling. They described their sampling methods in the following study excerpt.

"A convenience sample was recruited via public notices and snowball sampling (Fain, 2004). Inclusion criteria were women 18 to 25 years of age, English speaking, with basic knowledge of ECPs, and currently involved in a sexual relationship with a partner who was also willing to participate in the study.... Analysis began simultaneously with data collection as dictated by the tenets of grounded theory.... The initial analysis of interviews and field notes consisted of strategies of open coding and memoing (Glaser & Strauss, 1967).... As new categories emerged, the original interview guide was revised and additional couples were recruited to allow for theoretical sampling, that is, sampling specifically to fill in theoretical gaps, strengthen categories and their relationships, and verify or challenge emerging conceptualizations (Strauss & Corbin, 1998) and forced coding (Charmaz, 2006)." (Beaulieu et al., 2011, p. 43)

Beaulieu et al. (2011) clearly identified their sampling methods that were appropriate for a qualitative study conducted with grounded theory methodology. Both convenience and snowball sampling methods were applied because the researchers wanted an adequate number of couples to participate in their study and discuss their decision making regarding ECPs use. Beaulieu et al. also provided a detailed rationale for their use of theoretical sampling to develop a theory about decision making of young couples related to ECPs use. The sampling methods provided a strong sample of 22 couples, who provided the essential information for grounded theory development (Glaser & Strauss, 1967; Strauss & Corbin, 1998). More details on this study are presented later in this chapter in the discussion of sample size in qualitative studies.

Sample Size in Quantitative Research

One of the questions beginning researchers commonly ask is, "What size sample should I use?" Historically, the response to this question has been that a sample should contain at least 30 subjects for each study variable measured. Statisticians consider 30 subjects as the minimum number for data on a single variable to approach a normal distribution. So if a study includes 4 variables, researchers need at least 120 subjects in their final sample. Researchers are encouraged to determine the possible attrition rate for their study to ensure an adequate sample size at the completion of their study. For example, researchers might anticipate a 10-15% attrition rate in their study and need to obtain a sample of 130 to 140 subjects to ensure the final sample size after attrition is 120. The best method of determining sample size is a power analysis but if information is not available to conduct a power analysis, this recommendation of 30 subjects per study variable might be used.

The deciding factor in determining an adequate sample size for correlational, quasi-experimental, and experimental studies is power. Power is the capacity of the study to detect differences or relationships that actually exist in the population. Expressed another way, power is the capacity to reject a null hypothesis correctly. The minimum acceptable power for a study is commonly recommended to be 0.80 (80%) (Aberson, 2010; Cohen, 1988; Kraemer & Thiemann, 1987). If you do not have sufficient power to detect differences or relationships that exist in the population, you might question the advisability of conducting the study. You determine the sample size needed to obtain sufficient power by performing a power analysis. Power analysis includes the standard power (usually 80%), level of significance (usually set at 0.05 in nursing studies), effect size (discussed in the next section), and sample size.

An increasing number of nurse researchers are using power analysis to determine sample size, but it is essential that the results of the power analyses be included in the published studies. Not conducting a power analysis for a study and omitting the power analysis results in a published study are significant problems if the study failed to detect significant differences or relationships, which might be due to an inadequate sample size. The calculation of the power analysis varies with the types of statistical analyses used to analyze study data. Statistical programs are available to conduct a power analysis for a study (see Chapter 21). However, you can get a general idea about sample size using the power tables in Appendix F in this textbook.

The adequacy of sample sizes must be evaluated more carefully in future nursing studies before data collection. Studies with inadequate sample sizes should not be approved for data collection unless they are preliminary pilot studies conducted before a planned larger study. If it is impossible for you to obtain a larger sample because of time or numbers of available subjects, you should redesign your study so that the available sample is adequate for the planned analyses. If you cannot obtain a sufficient sample size, you should not conduct the study.

Large sample sizes are difficult to obtain in nursing studies, require long data collection periods, and are costly. In developing the methodology for a study, you must evaluate the elements of the methodology that affect the required sample size. Kraemer and Thiemann (1987) identified the following factors that must be taken into consideration in determining sample size:

1. The more stringent the significance level (e.g., 0.001 versus 0.05), the greater the necessary sample size. Most nursing studies include a level of significance or alpha $(\alpha) = 0.05$.
2. Two-tailed statistical tests require larger sample sizes than one-tailed tests. (Tailedness of statistical tests is explained in Chapters 21 and 25.)
3. The smaller the effect size, the larger the necessary sample size. The effect size is a determination of the effectiveness of a treatment on the outcome (dependent) variable or the strength of the relationship between two variables.
4. The larger the power required, the larger the necessary sample size. Thus, a study requiring a power of 90% requires a much larger sample than a study with power set at 80%.
5. The smaller the sample size, the smaller the power of the study (Aberson, 2010; Cohen, 1988; Kraemer & Thiemann, 1987).

The factors that must be considered in decisions about sample size (because they affect power) are effect size, type of study, number of variables, sensitivity of the measurement methods, and data analysis techniques. These factors are discussed in the following sections.

Effect Size

Effect is the presence of a phenomenon. If a phenomenon exists, it is not absent, and the null hypothesis is in error. However, effect is best understood when not considered in a dichotomous way—that is, as either present or absent. If a phenomenon exists, it exists to some degree. **Effect size** (*ES*) is the extent to which a phenomenon is present in a population. In this case, the term *effect* is used in a broader sense than the term *cause and effect*. For example, you might examine the impact of distraction on the experience of pain during an injection. To examine this question, you might obtain a sample of subjects receiving injections and measure the perception of pain in a group of subjects who were distracted during injection and a group of subjects who were not distracted. The null hypothesis would be: "There is no difference in the level of pain perceived by the treatment group receiving distraction than the comparison group receiving no distraction." If this were so, you would say that the effect of distraction on the perception of pain was zero, and the null hypothesis would be accepted. In another study, you might be interested in using the Pearson product moment correlation *r* to examine the relationship between coping and anxiety. Your null hypothesis is that the population *r* would be zero, or coping is not related to anxiety (Cohen, 1988).

In a study, it is easier to detect large differences between groups than to detect small differences. Strong relationships between variables in a study are easier to detect than weak relationships. Thus, smaller samples can detect large *ESs*; smaller *ESs* require larger samples. *ESs* can be positive or negative because variables are positively and negatively correlated. A negative *ES* is calculated if a treatment causes a decrease in the study mean, such as an exercise program that decreases the weight of subjects. Broadly speaking, the definitions for *ES* strengths might be as follows:

Small *ES* would be <0.3 or <−0.3

Medium *ES* would be about 0.3 to 0.5 or −0.3 to −0.5

Large *ES* would be >0.5 or >−0.5

These broad ranges are provided because the *ES* definitions of small, medium, and large vary based on the analysis being conducted. For example, the *ESs* for comparing two means, such as the treatment group mean with the comparison group mean (expressed as *d*), are small = 0.2 or −0.2, medium = 0.5 or −0.5, and large = 0.8 or −0.8. The *ESs* for relationships (expressed as *r*) might be defined as small = 0.1 or −0.1, medium = 0.3 or −0.3, and large = 0.5 or −0.5 (Aberson, 2010; Cohen, 1988).

Extremely small *ESs* (e.g., <0.1) may not be clinically important because the relationships between the variables are small or the differences between the treatment and comparison groups are limited. Knowing the *ES* that would be regarded as clinically important allows us to limit the sample to the size needed to detect that level of *ES* (Kraemer & Thiemann, 1987). A result is clinically important if the effect is large enough to alter clinical decisions. For example, in comparing glass thermometers with electronic thermometers, an effect size of $0.1° F$ in oral temperature is probably not important enough to influence selection of a particular type of thermometer in clinical practice. The clinical importance of an *ES* varies on the basis of the variables being studied and the population.

ESs vary according to the population being studied. Researchers must determine the *ES* for the particular relationship or effect being studied in a selected population. The most desirable source of this information is evidence from previous studies (Aberson, 2010; Melnyk & Fineout-Overholt, 2011). The correlation value (*r*) is equal to the *ES* for the relationship between two variables. For example, if depression is correlated with anxiety at $r = 0.45$, then the $ES = r = 0.45$, a medium *ES*.

$$ES \text{ formula for relationships} = r$$

Example: $ES = r = 0.45$

In published studies with treatments, means and standard deviations can be used to calculate the *ES* (Grove, 2007). For example, if the mean weight loss for the treatment or intervention group is 5 pounds per month with a standard deviation $(SD) = 4.5$, and the mean weight loss of the control or comparison group is 1 pound per month with $SD = 6.5$, you can calculate the *ES*, which is usually expressed as *d*.

$$ES \text{ formula for group differences} = d = \text{mean of}$$
$$\text{the treatment group} - \text{mean of the control group}$$
$$\div \text{ standard deviation of control group}$$

Example: $ES = d = 5 - 1 \div 6.5 = 4 \div 6.5 = 0.615 = 0.62$

This calculation can be used only as an estimate of *ES* for the study. If the researcher changes the measurement method used, the design of the study, or the population being studied, the *ES* will be altered. When estimating *ES* based on previous studies, you might note the *ESs* vary from 0.33 to 0.45; it is best to choose the lower *ES* of 0.33 to calculate a sample size for a study. The best estimate of a population parameter of

ES is obtained from a meta-analysis in which an estimated population *ES* is calculated through the use of statistical values from all studies included in the analysis (Aberson, 2010; Cohen, 1988).

If few relevant studies have been conducted in the area of interest, a small pilot study can be performed, and data analysis results can be used to calculate the *ES*. If pilot studies are not feasible, dummy power table analysis can be used to calculate the smallest *ES* with clinical or theoretical value. Yarandi (1991) described the process of calculating a dummy power table. If all else fails, *ES* can be estimated as small, medium, or large. Numerical values would be assigned to these estimates and the power analysis performed. Cohen (1988) and Aberson (2010) indicated the numerical values for small, medium, and large effects on the basis of specific statistical procedures. In new areas of research, *ESs* for studies are usually set as small (<0.3) (Aberson, 2010).

Jones, Duffy, and Flanagan (2011) conducted a randomized clinical trial to test the efficacy of a nurse-coached telephone intervention on the distress symptoms and functional health status of ambulatory arthroscopic surgery patients. These researchers conducted a power analysis to identify the sample size for their study, and it is described in the following excerpt.

"The inclusion criteria were as follows: adults (18 years or older) who were able to read and write English, would undergo ambulatory arthroscopic surgery under general anesthesia, had telephone access at home, and were discharged home on the day of surgery [target population]. According to power calculations, a sample size of 102 participants would assure a power >.80, given a significance level [alpha] of .05, three measurement times, a minimum correlation of repeated measure of .30, and a low to moderate effect size (*d* = .75)." (Jones et al., 2011, p. 94)

Jones et al. (2011) clearly identified their target population and the process for determining their sample size using power analysis. The standard power of 0.80 or 80% was used, and alpha was set at 0.05, which is common in nursing studies. The focus of the study was determining differences between the treatment and comparison groups, so the *ES* was expressed as $d = 0.75$, which is a moderate ES for examining differences between groups (see previous discussion of *ESs*). Jones et al. (2011, p. 92) found the "intervention participants had significantly less

symptom distress at 72 hours and 1 week postsurgery and significantly better overall physical and mental health at 1 week postsurgery than those who received usual practice." The significant results indicate the study had an adequate sample size to determine differences between the intervention or experimental group and usual practice or comparison group. If the study findings had been nonsignificant, the researchers would have needed to conduct a power analysis to determine the power achieved in the study.

Type of Study

Descriptive case studies tend to use small samples. Groups are not compared, and problems related to sampling error and generalization have little relevance for such studies. A small sample size may better serve the researcher who is interested in examining a situation in depth from various perspectives. Other descriptive studies, particularly studies using survey questionnaires, and correlational studies often require large samples. In these studies, multiple variables may be examined, and extraneous variables are likely to affect subject responses to the variables under study. Statistical comparisons are often made among multiple subgroups in the sample, requiring that an adequate sample be available for each subgroup being analyzed. In addition, subjects are likely to be heterogeneous in terms of demographic variables, and measurement tools are sometimes not adequately refined. Although target populations may have been identified, sampling frames may be unavailable, and parameters have not usually been well defined by previous studies. All of these factors decrease the power of the study and require increases in sample size (Aberson, 2010; Kraemer & Thiemann, 1987).

In the past, quasi-experimental and experimental studies often used smaller samples than descriptive and correlational studies. As control in the study increases, the sample size can decrease and still approximate the population. Instruments in these studies tend to be refined, improving precision. However, sample size must be sufficient to achieve an acceptable level of power (0.8) and reduce the risk of a type II error (indicating the study findings are nonsignificant, when they are really significant) (Aberson, 2010; Kraemer & Thiemann, 1987).

The study design influences power, but the design with the greatest power may not always be the most valid design to use. The experimental design with the greatest power is the pretest-posttest design with a historical control or comparison group. However, this design may have questionable validity because of the historical control group. Can the researcher demonstrate that the historical control group is comparable to the experimental group? The repeated measures design increases power if the trait being assessed is relatively stable over time. Designs that use blocking or stratification usually require an increase in the total sample size. The sample size increases in proportion to the number of cells included in the data analysis. Designs that use matched pairs of subjects have greater power and require a smaller sample (see Chapter 11 for a discussion of these designs). The higher the degree of correlation between subjects on the variable on which the subjects are matched, the greater the power (Kraemer & Thiemann, 1987).

Kraemer and Thiemann (1987) classified studies as *exploratory* or *confirmatory*. According to their approach, confirmatory studies should be conducted only after a large body of knowledge has been gathered through exploratory studies. Confirmatory studies are expected to have large samples and to use random sampling techniques. These expectations are lessened for exploratory studies. Exploratory studies are not intended for generalization to large populations. They are designed to increase the knowledge of the field of study. For example, pilot or preliminary studies to test a methodology or provide estimates of an *ES* are often conducted before a larger study. In other studies, the variables, not the subjects, are the primary area of concern. Several studies may examine the same variables using different populations. In these types of studies, the specific population used may be incidental. Data from these studies may be used to define population parameters. This information can be used to conduct confirmatory studies using large, randomly selected samples.

Confirmatory studies, such as studies testing the effects of nursing interventions on patient outcomes or studies testing the fit of a theoretical model, require large sample sizes. Clinical trials are being conducted in nursing for these purposes. The power of these large, complex studies must be carefully analyzed (Leidy & Weissfeld, 1991). For the large sample sizes to be obtained, subjects are acquired in numerous clinical settings, sometimes in different parts of the United States. Kraemer and Thiemann (1987) believed that these studies should not be performed until extensive information is available from exploratory studies. This information should include meta-analysis and the definition of a population *ES*.

Number of Variables

As the number of variables under study grows, the needed sample size may also increase. Adding variables such as age, gender, ethnicity, and education to the analysis plan (just to be on the safe side) can increase the sample size by a factor of 5 to 10 if the selected variables are uncorrelated with the dependent variable. In this case, instead of a sample of 50, you may need a sample of 250 to 500 if you plan to use the variables in the statistical analyses. (Using them only to describe the sample does not cause a problem in terms of power.) If the variables are highly correlated with the dependent variable, however, the effect size will increase, and the sample size can be reduced.

Variables included in the data analysis must be carefully selected. They should be essential to the research purpose or should have a documented strong relationship with the dependent variable (Kraemer & Thiemann, 1987). Sometimes researchers have obtained sufficient sample size for the primary analyses but failed to plan for analyses involving subgroups, such as analyzing the data by age categories or by ethnic groups, which require a larger sample size. A larger sample size is also needed if multiple dependent variables have been included.

Measurement Sensitivity

Well-developed instruments measure phenomena with precision. For example, a thermometer measures body temperature precisely. Instruments measuring psychosocial variables tend to be less precise. However, a scale with strong reliability and validity tends to measure more precisely than an instrument that is less well developed. Variance tends to be higher in a less well-developed tool than in one that is well developed. An instrument with a smaller variance is preferred because the power of a test always decreases when within-group variance increases (Kraemer & Thiemann, 1987). If you were measuring anxiety and the actual anxiety score for several subjects was 80, the subjects' scores on a less well-developed scale might range from 70 to 90, whereas a well-developed scale would tend to show a score closer to the actual score of 80 for each subject. As variance in instrument scores increases, the sample size needed to gain an accurate understanding of the phenomenon under study increases.

The range of measured values influences power. For example, a variable might be measured in 10 equally spaced values, ranging from 0 to 9. *ESs* vary according to how near the value is to the population mean. If the mean value is 5, *ESs* are much larger in the extreme values and lower for values near the mean. If you decided to use only subjects with values of 0 and 9, the *ES* would be large, and the sample could be small. The credibility of the study might be questionable, however, because the values of most individuals would not be 0 or 9 but rather would tend to be in the middle range of values. If you decided to include subjects who have values in the range of 3 to 6, excluding the extreme scores, the *ES* would be small, and you would require a much larger sample. The wider the range of values sampled, the larger the *ES* (Kraemer & Thiemann, 1987). If you had a heterogeneous group of study participants, you would expect them to have a wide range of scores on a depression scale, which would increase the *ES*. A strong measurement method has validity and reliability and measures variables at the interval or ratio level. The stronger the measurement methods used in a study, the smaller the sample that is needed to identify significant relationships among variables and differences between groups.

Data Analysis Techniques

Data analysis techniques vary in their ability to detect differences in the data. Statisticians refer to this as the power of the statistical analysis. For your data analysis, choose the most powerful statistical test appropriate to the data. Overall, parametric statistical analyses are more powerful than nonparametric techniques in detecting differences and should be used if the data meet criteria for parametric analysis. However, in many cases, nonparametric techniques are more powerful if your data do not meet the assumptions of parametric techniques. Parametric techniques vary widely in their capacity to distinguish fine differences and relationships in the data. Parametric and nonparametric analyses are discussed in Chapter 21.

There is also an interaction between the measurement sensitivity and the power of the data analysis technique. The power of the analysis technique increases as precision in measurement increases. Larger samples must be used when the power of the planned statistical analysis is low.

For some statistical procedures, such as the *t*-test and analysis of variance (ANOVA), having equal group sizes increases power because the effect size is maximized. The more unequal the group sizes are, the smaller the effect size. In unequal groups, the total sample size must be larger (Kraemer & Thiemann, 1987).

The chi-square (χ^2) test is the weakest of the statistical tests and requires very large sample sizes to achieve acceptable levels of power. As the number of categories (cells in the chi-square analysis) in a study grows, the sample size needed increases. Also, if there are small numbers in some of the categories, you must increase the sample size. Kraemer and Thiemann (1987) recommended that the chi-square test be used only when no other options are available. In addition, the categories should be limited to those essential to the study.

Sample Size in Qualitative Research

In quantitative research, the sample size must be large enough to describe variables, identify relationships among variables, or determine differences between groups. However, in qualitative research, the focus is on the quality of information obtained from the person, situation, event, or documents sampled versus the size of the sample (Marshall & Rossman, 2011; Munhall, 2012; Patton, 2002; Sandelowski, 1995). The sample size and sampling plan are determined by the purpose and philosophical basis of the study. The sample size required is determined by the depth of information needed to gain insight into a phenomenon, explore and describe a concept, describe a cultural element, develop a theory, or describe a historical event. The sample size can be too small when the data collected lack adequate depth or richness. An inadequate sample size can reduce the quality and credibility of the research findings. Many qualitative researchers use purposive or purposeful sampling methods to select the specific participants, events, or situations that they believe would provide them the rich data needed to gain insights and discover new meaning in an area of study (Sandelowski, 2000).

The adequacy of the sample size in a study should be justified by the researchers. Often the number of participants in a qualitative study is adequate when saturation of information is achieved in the study area (Fawcett & Garity, 2009). **Saturation of data** occurs when additional sampling provides no new information, only redundancy of previously collected data. Important factors that must be considered in determining sample size to achieve saturation of data are (1) scope of the study, (2) nature of the topic, (3) quality of the data, and (4) study design (Marshall & Rossman, 2011; Morse, 2000; Munhall, 2012; Patton, 2002).

Scope of the Study

If the scope of a study is broad, researchers need extensive data to address the study purpose, and it takes longer to reach data saturation. A study with a purpose that has a broad scope requires more sampling of participants, events, or documents than a study with a narrow scope (Morse, 2000). A study that has a clear focus and provides focused data collection usually has richer, more credible findings. The depth of a study's scope and its clarity of focus influence the number of participants needed for the study sample. For example, fewer participants would be needed to describe the phenomenon of chronic pain in adults with rheumatoid arthritis than would be needed to describe the phenomenon of chronic pain in elderly adults. A study of chronic pain experienced by elderly adults has a much broader focus, with less clarity, than a study of chronic pain experienced by adults with a specific medical diagnosis of rheumatoid arthritis.

Nature of the Topic

If the topic of your study is clear and the participants can easily discuss it, fewer individuals are needed to obtain the essential data. If the topic is difficult to define and awkward for people to discuss, you will probably need a larger number of participants or informants to saturate the data (Morse, 2000; Patton, 2002). For example, a phenomenological study of the experience of an adult living with a history of child sexual abuse is a sensitive, complex topic to investigate. This type of topic would probably require a greater number of participants and increased interview time to collect the essential data.

Quality of the Data

The quality of information obtained from an interview, observation, or document review influences the sample size. The higher the quality and richness of the data, the fewer the research participants needed to saturate data in the area of study. Quality data are best obtained from articulate, well-informed, and communicative participants. These participants are able to share more rich data in a clear and concise manner. In addition, participants who have more time to be interviewed usually provide data with greater depth and breadth. Qualitative studies require that you critically appraise the quality of the richness of communication elicited from the participants, the degree of access provided to events in a culture, or the number and quality of documents studied. These characteristics directly affect the richness of the data collected and influence the sample size needed to achieve quality study findings (Fawcett & Garity, 2009; Munhall, 2012).

Study Design

Some studies are designed to increase the number of interviews with participants. The more interviews conducted with a participant, the greater the quality of the data collected. For example, a study design that includes an interview both before and after an event would produce more data than a single interview. Designs that involve interviewing a family or a group of individuals produce more data than an interview

with a single study participant. In critically appraising a qualitative study, determine if the sample size is adequate for the design of the study.

Beaulieu et al. (2011) provided a detailed discussion of how they determined their final sample size. This qualitative study conducted with grounded theory methodology was introduced earlier in the discussion of theoretical sampling. The study focused on developing a theory about decision making of young adult couples regarding their use of ECPs. The sample was obtained with convenience, snowball, and theoretical sampling and resulted in a sample size of 22 couples. The following study excerpt provides the researchers' rationale for the final sample size of their study.

"A convenience sample was recruited via public notices and snowball sampling.... All interested young women initiated the first contact with the researcher by e-mail or telephone.... At the first meeting, which also included partners, study procedures were reviewed with participants, after which written consent and demographic information were obtained....

Analysis began simultaneously with data collection as dictated by the tenets of grounded theory.... As these processes progressed, axial coding was performed to identify core categories and their relationships. As new categories emerged, the original interview guide was revised and additional couples were recruited to allow for theoretical sampling, that is sampling specifically to fill in theoretical gaps, strengthen categories and their relationships, and verify or challenge emerging conceptualizations (Strauss & Corbin, 1998) and focused coding (Charmaz, 2006). Member checking occurred throughout the analysis by sharing the preliminary findings with subsequent couples to meet the requirements of confirmability of developing conceptualizations (Denzin & Lincoln, 2000). Saturation—when no new categories emerge (Strauss & Corbin, 1998)— was reached after interviewing 18 couples, but five more couples were included to ensure comprehensive analysis as well as theoretical verification. As the analysis continued through the processes of grounded theorizing, salient categories consistent with contemporary grounded theory principles (Clarke, 2005) were constructed to characterize the experience of young couples regarding ECPs. A theoretical model was developed to describe and explain the process of emergency contraceptive decision making in young couples." (Beaulieu et al., 2011, p. 43)

The study by Beaulieu et al. (2011) has many strengths in the area of sampling, including quality sampling methods (convenience, snowball, and theoretical), strong sample size ($N = 22$ couples), and conscientious participants. The investigators provide extensive details of the theoretical sampling conducted to ensure saturation was achieved with no new categories emerging. The saturation occurred after 18 couples, but the researchers interviewed 5 more couples to ensure depth and breadth in the data for theoretical verification. Beaulieu et al. (2011) described how they were able to develop successfully a theoretical model of experiences of young couples regarding use of ECPs. The study would have been strengthened by knowing how many study participants were obtained by each of the sampling methods (convenience, snowball, and theoretical). Also the researchers mentioned saturation was obtained with 18 couples but 5 more couples were included or $N = 23$ but the sample size identified was $N = 22$. A rationale is needed for the attrition of one of the couples from the study.

Research Settings

The setting is the location where a study is conducted. There are three common settings for conducting nursing research: natural, partially controlled, and highly controlled. A natural setting, or *field setting,* is an uncontrolled, real-life situation or environment (Kerlinger & Lee, 2000). Conducting a study in a natural setting means that the researcher does not manipulate or change the environment for the study. Descriptive and correlational quantitative studies and qualitative studies are often conducted in natural settings. For example, in the study by Beaulieu et al. (2011) discussed previously, the investigators made no attempt to manipulate the settings when they conducted the interviews for their qualitative study. All the data were conducted in natural settings as the interviews of the couples took place in various public settings or in their homes. The intent of the study was to develop a theory of the decision making of young adult couples regarding ECP use in a natural environment.

A partially controlled setting is an environment that the researcher manipulates or modifies in some way. An increasing number of nursing studies, usually correlational, quasi-experimental, and experimental studies, are being conducted in partially controlled settings. In a study that was introduced earlier in the discussion of sampling criteria, Twiss et al. (2009) conducted a quasi-experimental study to determine the effects of a strength training (ST) intervention on

muscle strength, balance, and falls of breast cancer survivors (BCSs) with bone loss. These researchers used both partially controlled and natural settings in their studies, which are described in the following excerpt.

> "This was a multisite, randomized controlled trial of a 24-month multi-component intervention with follow-up data collection at 36 months....
>
> **"Setting**
>
> "Exercise activities were performed in participants' homes [natural setting] or at investigator-approved fitness centers [partially controlled setting], and Biodex and balance testing were performed by physical therapists at hospitals or rehabilitation centers [partially controlled settings] at each of the four sites." (Twiss et al., 2009, p. 22)

Twiss et al. (2009) partially controlled the fitness centers by approving them but did not try to control the specific activities of each center. The researchers also ensured that the measurements were taken in a precise and accurate way by an expert (physical therapist) in partially controlled settings of hospitals and rehabilitation centers. The natural and partially controlled settings seemed appropriate in this study for the implementation of the ST intervention and for the precise and accurate measurement of the outcome variables.

A highly controlled setting is an artificially constructed environment developed for the sole purpose of conducting research. Laboratories, research or experimental centers, and test units in hospitals or other healthcare agencies are highly controlled settings where experimental studies are often conducted. This type of setting reduces the influence of extraneous variables, which enables the researcher to examine accurately the effect of one variable on another. Highly controlled settings are commonly used to conduct experimental research. Sharma, Ryals, Gajewski, and Wright (2010) conducted an experimental study to examine the effects of a moderate-intensity aerobic exercise program on painlike behavior and neurotrophin-3 (NT-3) in female mice. The rationale for conducting this study was that the literature and clinical practice supported the use of aerobic exercise in reducing pain and improving function in people with chronic pain, but the molecular basis for these positive actions was poorly understood. This study was conducted in a laboratory using a selected type of mouse, and the setting is described in the following excerpt.

"All experiments were approved by the Institutional Animal Care and Use Committee of the University of Kansas Medical Center and adhered to the university's animal care guidelines. Forty CF-1 female mice (weight = 25 g) were used to examine the effects of moderately intense exercise on primary (muscular) and secondary (cutaneous) hyperalgesia and NT-3 synthesis. Because women develop wide-spread pain syndromes at a greater rate than age-matched men, hyperalgesia was induced in female mice. The mice were exposed to 12-hour light/dark cycle and had access to food and water *ad libitum*....

Initially, the mice were randomly assigned to either the acidic saline injection (experimental) group or the normal saline injection (placebo) group. Five days after inducing hyperalgesia with acidic saline injection into the right limb, the animals were further assigned to either exercise or no-exercise group.... Two 6-lane, motorized treadmills were used for the exercise training." (Sharma et al., 2010, pp. 715-716)

Sharma et al. (2010) conducted their study in a highly controlled laboratory setting in terms of the housing and feeding of the mice, the light and temperature of the environment, implementation of the treatments, and the measurements of the dependent variables. Only with animals could this type of setting control be achieved in conducting this study. This type of highly controlled setting removes the effect of numerous extraneous variables, so the effects of the independent variables on the dependent variables can be clearly determined. However, because this research was conducted on animals, the findings cannot be generalized to humans, and additional research is needed to determine the molecular basis of the influence of aerobic exercise on pain and functioning in humans.

Recruiting and Retaining Research Participants

After a research team makes a decision about the size of the sample, the next step is to develop a plan for recruiting research participants, which involves identifying, accessing, and communicating with potential study participants who are representative of the target population. Recruitment strategies differ, depending on the type of study, population, and setting. Special attention must focus on recruiting subjects who tend to be underrepresented in studies, such as minorities, women, children, and elderly adults (Fulmer, 2001; Gul & Ali, 2010; Hendrickson, 2007; Hines-Martin, Speck, Stetson, & Looney, 2009). The sampling plan, initiated at the beginning of data collection, is almost always more difficult than expected. In addition to subject recruitment, retaining acquired subjects is critical to achieve an acceptable sample size and requires researchers to consider the effects of the data collection strategies on subject attrition. Retaining research participants involves the participants or subjects completing the required behaviors of a study to its conclusion. The problems with retaining participants increase as the data collection period lengthens. Some researchers never obtain their planned sample size because of the problems they encounter as they try to recruit and retain subjects. These researchers often are forced to complete their study with a smaller sample size, which could decrease the power of the study and potentially produce nonsignificant results (Aberson, 2010). With an increasing number of studies being conducted in health care, recruiting and retaining subjects have become more complex issues for researchers to manage (Gul & Ali, 2010; McGregor, Parker, LeBlanc, & King, 2010).

Recruiting Research Participants

The effective recruitment of subjects is crucial to the success of a study. A few studies examining the effectiveness of various strategies of participant recruitment and retention have appeared in the literature (Davidson, Cronk, Harrar, Catley, & Good, 2010; Hines-Martin et al., 2009; Whitebird, Bliss, Savik, Lowry, & Jung, 2010). However, most of the information available to guide researchers comes from the personal experiences of skilled researchers, some of whom have published their ideas (Gul & Ali, 2010; McGregor et al., 2010). Some of the positive and negative factors that influence a subject's decision to participate in a study are (1) the attitudes and ethics of the researchers, (2) the subject's need for a treatment, (3) the subject's interest in the study topic, (4) financial compensation, (5) fear of the unknown, (6) time and travel constraints, (7) language barriers, and (8) the nature of the informed consent (Gul & Ali, 2010; Hine-Martin et al., 2009; Madsen et al., 2002; Papadopoulos & Lees, 2002; Sullivan-Bolyai et al., 2007).

The researcher's initial communication with a potential subject usually strongly affects the subject's decision about participating in the study. Therefore, the approach must be pleasant, positive, informative, culturally sensitive, and nonaggressive. The researcher needs to explain the importance of the study and clarify exactly what the subject will be asked to do, how much of the subject's time will be involved, and what the duration of the study will be. Research participants are valuable resources, and the researcher must communicate this value to the potential subject. High-pressure techniques, such as insisting that the subject make an instant decision to participate in a study, usually lead to resistance and a higher rate of refusals. If the study involves minorities, researchers must be culturally competent or knowledgeable and skilled in relating to the particular ethnic group being studied (Hines-Martin et al., 2009; Papadopoulos & Lees, 2002). If the researcher is not of the same culture as the potential subjects, he or she may employ a data collector who is of the same culture. Hendrickson (2007) used a video for recruiting Hispanic women for her study, and she provided all the details related to the study in the subjects' own language in the video. This approach greatly improved the subjects' understanding of the study and their desire to participate.

If a potential subject refuses to participate in a study, you must accept the refusal gracefully—in terms of body language as well as words. Your actions can influence the decision of other potential subjects who observe or hear about the encounter. Studies in which a high proportion of individuals refuse to participate have a serious validity problem. The sample is likely to be biased because often only a certain type of individual has agreed to participate. You should keep records of the numbers of persons who refuse and, if possible, their reasons for refusal. With this information, you can include the refusal rate in the published research report with the reasons for refusal. It would also be helpful if you could determine if the potential subjects who refused to participate differed from the individuals who agreed to participate in the study. This information will help you to determine the representativeness of your sample (Thompson, 2002).

Recruiting minority subjects for a study can be particularly problematic. Minority individuals may be difficult to locate and are often reluctant to participate in studies because of feelings of being "used" while receiving no personal benefit from their involvement or because of their distrust of the medical community. Effective strategies for recruiting minorities include developing partnerships with target groups, community leaders, and potential participants in the community; using active face-to-face recruitment in nonthreatening settings; and using appropriate language to communicate clearly the purpose, benefits, and risks of the study (Alvarez, Vasquez, Mayorga, Feaster, & Mitrani, 2006). Hines-Martin et al. (2009)

studied the recruitment and retention process for intervention research conducted with a sample of primarily low-income African American women. Their complex, multistage recruitment strategies are introduced in the following excerpt.

> "Phase I involved the development of a recruitment team, composed of a co-investigator, in addition to an African American nurse familiar with the target population, and two women who were long-standing community members.
>
> Phase I activities began with periods of observation in the community setting and discussions with community center personnel to improve the investigators' understanding of who used the community center services and when. It became increasingly clear that only two of the three communities felt a connection with or used the community center routinely.... Therefore, the recruitment team, with the assistance from nursing graduate students, walked every block of the two relevant communities at different times of the day and different days of the week to better understand when and where community women could be found in their daily lives.... Community women were informed of new initiatives at the center and were provided with recruitment flyers including pictures of the research team. The recruitment team then undertook usual recruitment activities, such as meeting with women's groups in the communities and recruitment at community fairs." (Hines-Martin et al., 2009, pp. 665-666)

If researchers use data collectors in their studies, they need to verify the data collectors are following the sampling plan, especially in random samples. When the data collectors encounter difficult subjects or are unable to make contact easily, they may simply shift to the next person without informing the principal investigator. This behavior could violate the rules of random sampling and bias the sample. If data collectors do not understand, or do not believe in, the importance of randomization, their decisions and actions can undermine the intent of the sampling plan. Thus, data collectors must be carefully selected and thoroughly trained. A plan for the supervision and follow-up of data collectors to increase their accountability should be developed (Thompson, 2002).

If you conduct a survey study, you may never have personal contact with the subjects. To recruit such subjects, you must rely on the use of attention-getting techniques, persuasively written material, and strategies for following up on individuals who do not respond to the initial written or email communication. The strategies need to be appropriate to the potential subjects; mailed surveys are probably still the best way to obtain information from elderly adults. Because of the serious problems of low response rates in survey studies, using strategies to increase the response rate is critical. For instance, we have received a teabag or packet of instant coffee with a questionnaire, accompanied by a recommendation in the letter to have a cup of tea or coffee "on" the researcher while we complete the questionnaire. Creativity is required in the use of such strategies because they tend to lose their effect on groups who receive questionnaires frequently. In some cases, small amounts of money ($1.00 to $5.00) are enclosed with the letter, which may suggest that the recipient buy a soft drink or that the money is a small offering for completing the questionnaire. This strategy imposes some sense of obligation on the recipient to complete the questionnaire, but it is not thought to be coercive. Also, you should plan emailing or mailings to avoid holidays or times of the year when activities are high for potential subjects, possibly reducing the return rate.

Researchers frequently use the Internet to recruit subjects and to collect survey data. This method makes it easier for you to contact potential subjects and for the subjects to provide the requested data. However, an increased number of surveys are being sent by the Internet, which can decrease the response rate of potential subjects who are frequently surveyed. In studies with surveys, the letter emailed to potential subjects must be carefully composed. It may be your only chance to persuade the subject to invest the time needed to complete the questionnaire. You must sell the reader on the importance of both your study and his or her response. The tone of your letter will be the potential subject's only image of you as a person; yet, for many subjects, their response to the perception of you as a person most influences their decision about completing the questionnaire. Seek examples of letters sent by researchers who have had high response rates, and save letters you received to which you responded positively. You also might pilot-test your letter on potential research participants who can give you feedback about their reactions to the letter's tone.

The use of follow-up emails, letters, or cards has been repeatedly shown to raise response rates to surveys. The timing is important. If too long a period has lapsed, the potential subject may have deleted the questionnaire from his or her email box or discarded the mailed copy. However, sending the follow-up too soon could be offensive. Before the questionnaires are emailed or mailed, precise plans need to be made for monitoring the return of each questionnaire. A bar graph could be developed to record the return of each questionnaire as a means of suggesting when the follow-up mailing or emailing should occur. The cumulative number and percentage of responses would be logged on the graph to reflect the overall data collection process. The data from emailed questionnaires can be immediately analyzed so that researchers can easily keep track of the numbers of participants responding. When the daily or weekly responses decline, a follow-up email or first-class letter could be sent encouraging individuals to complete the questionnaire. Study participants and questionnaires are assigned the same code numbers, and nonrespondents are identified by checking the list of code numbers of unreturned questionnaires. A third follow-up questionnaire with a further modified cover letter could be emailed or mailed to increase the return rate for the questionnaires.

The factors involved in the decision of whether to respond to a questionnaire are not well understood. One factor is the time required to respond; this includes the time needed to orient to the directions and the emotional energy necessary to deal with the threats and anxieties generated by the questions. There is also a cognitive demand for thinking. Subjects seem to make a judgment about the relevance of the research topic and the potential for personal application of findings. Previous experience with questionnaires is also a deciding factor.

Traditionally, subjects for physiological nursing studies have been sought in the hospital setting. However, access to these subjects is becoming more difficult—in part because of the larger numbers of nurses and other healthcare professionals now conducting research. The largest involvement of research subjects within a healthcare agency usually occurs with medical research and mainly with clinical trials that include large samples (Gul & Ali, 2010). Nurse researchers are recruiting subjects from a variety of clinical settings. Whitebird et al. (2010) identified three successful recruitment methods to use in healthcare agencies: (1) identifying potential participants using administrative databases, (2) obtaining referrals of potential participants through healthcare providers and other sources, and (3) approaching directly a known potential subject. An initial phase of recruitment may involve obtaining community and institutional support for the study. Support from other healthcare professionals, such as nurses and physicians, and clinical agency staff is usually crucial to the successful recruitment of research participants.

Recruitment of subjects for clinical trials requires a different set of strategies because the recruitment may be occurring simultaneously in several sites (perhaps in different cities). Many of these studies never achieve their planned sample size. The number of subjects meeting the sampling criteria who are available in the selected clinical sites may not be as large as anticipated. Researchers must often screen twice as many patients as are required for the study to obtain a sufficient sample size. Screening logs must be kept during the recruiting period to record data on patients who met the criteria but were not entered into the study. Researchers commonly underestimate the amount of time required to recruit subjects for a clinical trial. In addition to defining the number of subjects and the time set aside for recruitment, it may be helpful to develop short-term or interim recruitment goals designed to maintain a constant rate of patient entry (Gul & Ali, 2010). Hellard, Sinclair, Forbes, and Fairley (2001) studied methods to improve the recruitment and retention of subjects in clinical trials and found that the four most important strategies were to (1) use nonaggressive recruitment methods, (2) maintain regular contact with the participants, (3) ensure that the participants are kept well informed of the progress of the study, and (4) provide constant encouragement to subjects to continue participation. Sullivan-Bolyai et al. (2007) identified the barriers and strategies to improve the recruitment of study participants from clinical settings. Table 15-3 identifies these common barriers to research participant recruitment and provides possible strategies to manage them.

Studies may also benefit from the endorsement of community leaders, such as city officials; key civic leaders; and leaders of social, educational, religious, or labor groups. In some cases, these groups may be involved in planning the study, leading to a sense of community ownership of the project. Community groups may also help researchers to recruit subjects for the study. Subjects who meet the sampling criteria sometimes are found in the groups assisting with the study. Endorsement may involve letters of support and, in some cases, funding. These activities can add legitimacy to the study and make involvement in the study more attractive to potential subjects (Alvarez et al., 2006; Davidson et al., 2010; Hines-Martin et al., 2009).

Media support can be helpful in recruiting subjects. Researchers can place advertisements in local newspapers and church and neighborhood bulletins. Radio stations can make public service announcements. Members of the research team can speak to groups relevant to the study population. Your team can place posters in public places, such as supermarkets, drugstores, and public laundries. With permission, you can set up tables in shopping malls with a member of the research team present to recruit subjects. Plan for possible challenges in recruitment and include multiple methods and locations in your application for human subject approval for your study. Otherwise, you would need to submit a modified protocol to the institutional review board when you add a method or site for recruitment.

Davidson et al. (2010) used multiple strategies to recruit and retain college smokers in a cessation clinical trial. Their four-phase recruitment process is presented in the following study excerpt.

> "Participants in this study were members of Greek fraternities and sororities enrolled at a large Midwestern university, and data were collected from 2006 to 2009.... The clinical trial involved testing a four-session, MI [motivational interviewing] counseling intervention on smoking cessation. Participants were recruited from college fraternity and sorority chapters regardless of their interest in quitting smoking. Recruitment involved four phases. First, out of 41 fraternity and sorority chapters from a large Midwestern university, the 30 chapters with the larger memberships were invited to participate. Second, within these invited chapters, individuals were recruited to participate in an initial, 5-minute, 8-item screening survey (i.e., Screener).
>
> Third, individual members of these 30 chapters who met the inclusion criteria based on the Screener and who were interested in participating in the study were recruited to participate in a more extensive (30-45 minute) computerized baseline assessment approximately 1-4 days following the Screener.... Fourthly, eligible individuals who completed the baseline assessment were recruited for enrollment in the clinical trial." (Davidson et al., 2010, pp. 146-147)

The recruitment for this smoking cessation clinical trial was accomplished by using the Greek chapters. Davidson et al. (2010) developed relationships with these Greek organizations by meeting with leaders and members and attending special events. To accomplish phases two and three, the researchers met with the participants at convenient times and in accessible locations. The participants were also provided incentives of food (cookies and pizza), small cash gifts, and raffles for iPods. These creative strategies increased the recruitment and retention of the study participants.

TABLE 15-3 **Barriers to Recruitment with Actions and Strategies for Engaging Health Care Providers in the Referral Process**

Barriers and Actions	Strategies
HIPAA* Create alternative recruitment methods	Ask Clinicians to distribute letters to potential study participants Obtain institutional review board waiver of authorization requirement for the use or disclosure of personal health information Work with clinics to secure a consent that meets HIPAA* regulations and allows the staff to provide names and contact information of patients with specific conditions that may be of interest to researchers Recognize and acknowledge the burden that recruitment places on healthcare providers
Work burden Create compensations	Provide Salary support Provide educational incentives (e.g., purchase laptop, journals, books, pay for conference attendance in the field under study) for healthcare providers who do not normally have access to such opportunities as part of their job Assess administrative or managerial perceptions of healthcare providers' recruitment-related responsibilities, and if salary support is given, how that money will be used Discuss the designated recruitment tasks and responsibilities with the assigned staff to determine their perceptions and expectations
Financial disincentives Recognize that patient numbers or productivity may be linked to the clinic's livelihood	Assess the clinic's financial situation and determine if it is realistic, pragmatic, or feasible to use that site, especially if its funding depends on patient numbers Help keep participants linked to the clinical site while they are participating in the study
Provider competition Create a partnership with healthcare providers involved in recruitment so that they are rewarded and acknowledged for their participation in the research process	Develop a research proposal that reflects the clinical site's philosophical and policy perspectives and priorities Include healthcare providers in the development of a study Hire and pay a clinical staff member to be responsible for introducing the study to potential participants Link recruitment activities to nursing clinical ladder or organization values Maintain open communication between the clinical and research teams regarding the workings of the study
Provider concerns Demystify research process Develop a team atmosphere and a spirit of "we're all in this together"	Assess healthcare providers' perceptions of research Encourage healthcare providers to participate in developing the research proposal Include healthcare providers in developing study-related manuscripts Include healthcare providers in research team meetings at a mutually convenient time Express appreciation in an ongoing basis for healthcare providers' involvement in recruitment process Share recruitment status information on a monthly basis with healthcare providers Share pilot or feasibility data with healthcare providers to support the study rationale and choice of specific methods
Desire to protect patients Work with healthcare providers to acknowledge and respect patient decision-making abilities Encourage healthy partnerships between patients and healthcare providers	Acknowledge responsibility of healthcare providers to protect patients from harm Address concerns of healthcare providers by emphasizing the pilot data that supports the protocol Model respectful partnerships with study participants

From Sullivan-Bolyai, S., Bova, C., Deatrick, J. A., Knafl, K., Grey, M., Leung, K., et al. (2007). Barriers and strategies for recruiting study participants in clinical settings. *Western Journal of Nursing Research, 29*(4), 498–499.

*HIPAA, Health Insurance Portability and Accountability Act.

Retaining Subjects

A serious problem in many studies is subject retention, and sometimes participant attrition cannot be avoided. Subjects move, die, or withdraw from a treatment. If you must collect data at several points over time, subject attrition can become a problem. Subjects who move frequently and subjects without phones pose a particular problem. Numerous strategies have been found to be effective in maintaining the sample. It is a good idea to obtain the names, email addresses, and phone numbers (cell and home numbers if possible) of at least two family members or friends when you enroll the participant in the study. Ask if the participant would agree to give you access to unlisted phone numbers in the event of changes in his or her number.

In some studies, subjects are reimbursed for time and expenses related to participation. A bonus payment may be included for completing a certain phase of the study. Gifts can be used in place of money. Sending greeting cards for birthdays and holidays helps maintain contact. Researchers found that money was more effective than gifts in retaining subjects in longitudinal studies. However, some people pointed out the moral issues related to providing monetary payment to subjects. This strategy can compromise the voluntariness of participation in a study and particularly has the potential of exploiting low-income persons.

Collecting data takes time. The participant's time is valuable and should be used frugally. During data collection, it is easy to begin taking the participant for granted. Taking time for social amenities with participants may also pay off. However, take care that these interactions do not influence the data being collected. Beyond that, nurturing subjects participating in the study is critical. In some situations, providing refreshments and pleasant surroundings is helpful. During the data collection phase, you also may need to nurture others who interact with the participants; these may be volunteers, family, staff, students, or other professionals. It is important to maintain a pleasant climate for the data collection process, which pays off in the quality of data collected and the retention of subjects (Davidson et al., 2010; Gul & Ali, 2010; Hines-Martin et al., 2009; McGregor et al., 2010).

Qualitative studies and longitudinal studies require extensive time commitment from subjects. They are asked to participate in detailed interviews or to complete numerous forms at various intervals during a study (Marshall & Rossman, 2011; Munhall, 2012; Patton, 2002). Sometimes data are collected with diaries that require daily entries over a set period of time. These studies face the greatest risk of participant mortality. Chapters 4 and 12 provide more details on the recruitment and retention of research participants for qualitative studies.

Clinical trials can also require extensive time commitments from subjects. Gul and Ali (2010) mentioned the importance of overcoming participant barriers to continuing in a study, such as time to complete data collection forms, transportation problems, and conflicts with work and family commitments. There is no formula for compensating study participants, but many studies mention small monetary payments, gifts, or free health or child care. It is important that the incentives used to recruit and retain research participants be documented in the published study. Communication is one of the most important facets to retaining study participants. Davidson et al. (2010), whose recruitment strategies were introduced earlier, describe their success with retention in their smoking cessation clinical trial in the following excerpt.

> "A very high proportion of participants (89%) completed at least one session (90% treatment; 87% comparison). The majority (73%) were retained, completing three or more sessions (75% treatment; 70% comparison), and over half completed the maximum of four sessions (63% treatment; 61% comparison). At the follow-up assessment occurring 6 months after the baseline assessment, 79% of the participants ($n = 357$) were retained (80% treatment; 78% comparison)." (Davidson et al., 2010, p. 150)

Research participants who have a personal investment in the study are more likely to complete the study. This investment occurs through interactions with and nurturing by the researcher. A combination of the participant's personal belief in the significance of the study, the perceived altruistic motives of the researcher in conducting the study, the ethical actions of the researcher, and the nurturing support provided by the researcher during data collection can greatly diminish subject attrition (Hines-Martin et al., 2009; Madsen et al., 2002; McGregor et al., 2010). The recruitment and retention of subjects will continue to be significant challenges for researchers, and creative strategies are needed to manage these challenges.

KEY POINTS

- Sampling involves selecting a group of people, events, behaviors, or other elements with which to conduct a study. Sampling denotes the process of making the selections; sample denotes the selected group of elements.

- A sampling plan is developed to increase representativeness, decrease systematic bias, and decrease the sampling error; there are two main types of sampling plans—probability and nonprobability.

- Sampling error includes random variation and systematic variation. Refusal and attrition rates are important to calculate in a study to determine potential systematic variation or bias.

- Four sampling designs have been developed to achieve probability or random sampling: simple random sampling, stratified random sampling, cluster sampling, and systematic sampling.

- In nonprobability (nonrandom) sampling, not every element of the population has an opportunity for selection in the sample. The five nonprobability sampling designs described in this textbook are (1) convenience sampling, (2) quota sampling, (3) purposive or purposeful sampling, (4) network or snowball sampling, and (5) theoretical sampling.

- In quantitative studies, sample size is best determined by a power analysis, which is calculated using the level of significance (usually $\alpha = 0.05$), standard power of 0.80 (80%), and effect size. Factors important to sample size in quantitative research include (1) type of study, (2) number of variables studied, (3) measurement sensitivity, and (4) data analysis techniques.

- The number of participants in a qualitative study is adequate when saturation of information is achieved in the study area, which occurs when additional sampling provides no new information, only redundancy of previously collected data. Important factors that must be considered in determining sample size to achieve saturation of data are (1) scope of the study, (2) nature of the topic, (3) quality of the data, and (4) study design.

- The three common settings for conducting nursing research are natural, partially controlled, and highly controlled. A natural setting, or field setting, is an uncontrolled, real-life situation or environment. A partially controlled setting is an environment that the researcher has manipulated or modified in some way. A highly controlled setting is an artificially constructed environment, such as a laboratory or research unit in a hospital, developed for the sole purpose of conducting research.

- Recruiting and retaining research participants have become significant challenges in research; some strategies to assist researchers with these challenges are provided so that their samples might be more representative of their target population.

REFERENCES

Aberson, C. L. (2010). *Applied power analysis for the behavioral sciences*. New York, NY: Routledge Taylor & Francis Group.

Alvarez, R. A., Vasquez, E., Mayorga, C. C., Feaster, D. J., & Mitrani, V. B. (2006). Increasing minority research participation through community organization outreach. *Western Journal of Nursing Research*, 28(5), 541–560.

Barhyte, D. Y., Redman, B. K., & Neill, K. M. (1990). Population or sample: Design decision. *Nursing Research*, 39(5), 309–310.

Beaulieu, R., Kools, S. M., Kennedy, H. P., & Humphreys, J. (2011). Young adult couples' decision making regarding emergency contraceptive pills. *Journal of Nursing Scholarship*, 43(1), 41–48.

Botman, S. L., Moore, T. F., Moriarty, C. L. & Parsons, V. L. (2000). Design and estimation for the National Health Interview Survey, 1995-2004. *National Center for Health Statistics, Vital Health Statistics, Series 2, No. 130*, 1–32.

Charmaz, K. (2006). *Constructing grounded theory: A practical guide through qualitative analysis*. Thousand Oaks, CA: Sage.

Clarke, A. (2005). *Situational analysis grounded theory after the postmodern turn*. Thousand Oaks, CA: Sage.

Cohen, J. (1988). *Statistical power analysis for the behavioral sciences* (2nd ed.). New York, NY: Academic Press.

Coyne, I. T. (1997). Sampling in qualitative research. Purposeful and theoretical sampling; merging or clear boundaries. *Journal of Advanced Nursing*, 26(3), 623–630.

Davidson, M. M., Cronk, N. J., Harrar, S., Catley, D., & Good, G. E. (2010). Strategies to recruit and retain college smokers in cessation trials. *Research in Nursing & Health*, 33(2), 144–155.

Degirmen, N., Ozerdogan, N., Sayiner, D., Kosgeroglu, N., & Ayranci, U. (2010). Effectiveness of foot and hand massage in post-cesarean pain control in a group of Turkish pregnant women. *Applied Nursing Research*, 23(3), 153–158.

Denzin, N., & Lincoln, Y. (2000). *Handbook of qualitative research* (2nd ed.). Thousand Oaks, CA: Sage.

Djukic, M., Kovner, C., Budin, W. C., & Norman, R. (2010). Physical work environment: Testing an expanded model of job satisfaction in a sample of registered nurses. *Nursing Research*, 59(6), 441–451.

Fain, J. (2004). *Reading, understanding, and applying nursing research* (2nd ed.). Philadelphia, PA: F. A. Davis Company.

Fawcett, J., & Garity, J. (2009). *Evaluating research for evidence-based nursing practice*. Philadelphia, PA: F. A. Davis.

Floyd, J.A. (1993). Systematic sampling: Theory and clinical methods. *Nursing Research*, 42(5), 290–293.

Foulabakhsh, J. M., & Stommel, M. (2010). Gender, symptom experience, and use of complementary and alternative medicine practices among cancer survivors in the U.S. cancer population. *Oncology Nursing Forum*, 37(1), E7–E15. Retrieved from *Oncology Nursing Forum* online.

Fulmer, T. (2001). Editorial: Recruiting older adults in our studies. *Applied Nursing Research*, 14(2), 63.

Glaser, B. G., & Strauss, A. L. (1967). *The discovery of grounded theory: Strategies for qualitative research*. Chicago: IL. Aldine.

Green, J., & Thorogood, N. (2004). *Qualitative methods for health research*. Thousand Oaks, CA: Sage Publications.

Grove, S. K. (2007). *Statistics for health care research: A practical workbook*. St. Louis, MO: Saunders.

Gul, R. B., & Ali, P. A. (2010). Clinical trials: The challenge of recruitment and retention of participants. *Journal of Clinical Nursing*, *19*(1-2), 227–233.

Hellard, M.E., Sinclair, M.I., Forbes, A.B., & Fairley, C.K. (2001). Methods used to maintain a high level of participant involvement in a clinical trial. *Journal of Epidemiology & Community Health*, *55*(5), 348–351.

Hendrickson, S. G. (2007). Video recruitment of non-English-speaking participants. *Western Journal of Nursing Research*, *29*(2), 232–242.

Hines-Martin, V., Speck, B. J., Stetson, B., & Looney, S. W. (2009). Understanding systems and rhythms for minority recruitment in intervention research. *Research in Nursing & Health*, *32*(6), 657–670.

Jones, D., Duffy, M. E., & Flanagan, J. (2011). Randomized clinical trial testing efficacy of a nurse-coached intervention in arthroscopy patients. *Nursing Research*, *60*(2), 92–99.

Kerlinger, F. N., & Lee, H. B. (2000). *Foundations of behavioral research* (4th ed.). Fort Worth, TX: Harcourt College Publishers.

Kraemer, H. C., & Thiemann, S. (1987). *How many subjects? Statistical power analysis in research*. Newbury Park, CA: Sage.

Larson, E. (1994). Exclusion of certain groups from clinical research. *Image: Journal of Nursing Scholarship*, *26*(3), 185–190.

Leidy, N. K., & Weissfeld, L. A. (1991). Sample sizes and power computation for clinical intervention trials. *Western Journal of Nursing Research*, *13*(1), 138–144.

Levy, P. S., & Lemsbow, S. (1980). *Sampling for health professionals*. Belmont, CA: Lifetime Learning.

Li, Y., & Mukamel, D. B. (2010). Racial disparities in receipt of influenza and pneumococcus vaccinations among US nursing-home residents. *American Journal of Public Health*, *100*(S1), S256–S262.

Madsen, S. M., Mirza, M. R., Holm, S., Hilsted, K. L., Kampmann, K., & Riis, P. (2002). Attitudes towards clinical research amongst participants and nonparticipants. *Journal of Internal Medicine*, *251*(2), 156–168.

Marshall, C., & Rossman, G. B. (2011). *Designing qualitative research* (5th ed.). Thousand Oaks, CA: Sage Publications.

McGregor, L., Parker, K., LeBlanc, P., & King, K. M. (2010). Using social exchange theory to guide successful study recruitment and retention. *Nurse Researcher*, *17*(2), 74–82.

Melnyk, B. M., & Fineout-Overholt, E. (2011). *Evidence-based practice in nursing & healthcare: A guide to best practice* (2nd ed.). Philadelphia: PA: Lippincott Williams & Wilkins.

Morse, J. M. (2000). Determining sample size. *Qualitative Health Research*, *10*(1), 3–5.

Munhall, P. L. (2007). *Nursing research: A qualitative perspective* (4th ed.). Sudbury, MA: Jones & Bartlett.

Munhall, P. L. (2012). *Nursing research: A qualitative perspective* (5th ed.). Sudbury, MA: Jones & Bartlett.

Neumark, D. E., Stommel, M., Given, C. W., & Given, B. A. (2001). Brief report: Research design and subject characteristics predicting nonparticipation in panel survey of older families with cancer. *Nursing Research*, *50*(6), 363–368.

O'Shea, E. R., Wallace, M., Griffin, M. Q., & Fitzpatrick, J. J. (2011). The effect of an educational session on pediatric nurses' perspectives toward providing spiritual care. *Journal of Pediatric Nursing*, *26*(1), 34–43.

Papadopoulos, I., & Lees, S. (2002). Developing culturally competent researchers. *Journal of Advanced Nursing*, *37*(3), 258–264.

Patton, M. Q. (2002). *Qualitative evaluation and research methods* (3rd ed.). Thousand Oaks, CA: Sage.

Pieper, B., Templin, T. N., Kirsner, R. S., & Birk, T. J. (2009). Impact of injection drug use on distribution and severity of chronic venous disorders. *Wound Repair & Regeneration*, *17*(4), 485–491.

Pieper, B., Templin, T. N., Kirsner, R. S., & Birk, T. J. (2010). The impact of vascular leg disorders on physical activity in methadone-maintained adults. *Research in Nursing & Health*, *33*(5), 426–440.

Sandelowski, M. (1995). Sample size in qualitative research. *Research in Nursing & Health*, *18*(2), 179–183.

Sandelowski, M. (2000). Combining qualitative and quantitative sampling, data collection, and analysis techniques in mixed-method studies. *Research in Nursing & Health*, *23*(3), 246–255.

Sharma, N. K., Ryals, J. M., Gajewski, B. J., & Wrights, D. E. (2010). Aerobic exercise alters analgesia and neurotrophin-3 synthesis in an animal model of chronic widespread pain. *Physical Therapy*, *90*(5), 714–725.

Strauss, A., & Corbin, J. (1998). *Basics of qualitative research, techniques, and procedures for developing grounded theory* (2nd ed.). Thousand Oaks, CA: Sage.

Sternberg, R. M., & Barry, C. (2011). Transnational mothers crossing the border and bringing their health care needs. *Journal of Nursing Scholarship*, *43*(1), 64–71.

Sullivan-Bolyai, S., Bova, C., Deatrick, J. A., Knafl, K., Grey, M., Leung, K., et al. (2007). Barriers and strategies for recruiting study participants in clinical settings. *Western Journal of Nursing Research*, *29*(4), 486–500.

Thompson, S. K. (2002). *Sampling* (2nd ed.). New York, NY: John Wiley & Sons.

Twiss, J. J., Waltman, N. L., Berg, K., Ott, C. D., Gross, G. J., & Lindsey, A. M. (2009). An exercise intervention for breast cancer survivors with bone loss. *Journal of Nursing Scholarship*, *41*(1), 20–27.

Ulrich, C. M., Danis, M., Ratcliffe, S. J., Garrett-Mayer, E., Koziol, D., Soeken, K. L., et al. (2006). Ethical conflict in nurse practitioners and physician assistants in managed care. *Nursing Research*, *55*(6), 391–401.

Whitebird, R. R., Bliss, D. Z., Savik, K., Lowry, A., & Jung, H. G. (2010). Comparing community and specialty provider-based recruitment in a randomized clinical trial: Clinical trial in fecal incontinence. *Research in Nursing & Health*, *33*(6), 500–511.

Yarandi, H. N. (1991). Planning sample sizes: Comparison of factor level means. *Nursing Research*, *40*(1), 57–58.

Yates, F. (1981). *Sampling methods for censuses and surveys*. New York, NY: Macmillan.

16
CHAPTER

Measurement Concepts

Measurement is the process of assigning numbers to objects, events, or situations in accord with some rule (Kaplan, 1963). The numbers assigned can indicate numerical values or categories for the objects being measured for research or practice. **Instrumentation**, a component of measurement, is the application of specific rules to develop a measurement device such as a scale or questionnaire. Quality instruments are essential for obtaining trustworthy data when measuring outcomes for research and practice (Doran, 2011; Melnyk & Fineout-Overhold, 2011; Waltz, Strickland, & Lenz, 2010).

The rules of measurement were developed so that the assigning of values or categories might be done consistently from one subject (or event) to another and eventually, if the measurement method is found to be meaningful, from one study to another. The rules of measurement established for research are similar to the rules of measurement implemented in nursing practice. For example, when nurses measure the urine output from patients, they use an accurate measurement device, observe the amount of urine in the device or container in a consistent way, and precisely record the urine output in the medical record. This practice promotes accuracy and precision and reduces the amount of error in measuring physiological variables such as urine output.

When measuring a subjective concept such as pain experienced by a child, researchers and nurses in practice need to use an instrument that captures the pain the child is experiencing. A commonly used scale to measure a child's pain is the Wong-Baker FACES Pain Rating Scale (Hockenberry & Wilson, 2009). By using this valid and reliable rating scale to measure the child's pain, any change in the measured value can be attributed to a change in the child's pain rather than measurement error. A copy of the Wong-Baker FACES Pain Rating Scale is provided in Chapter 17. Selecting accurate and precise physiological measurement

methods and valid and reliable scales and questionnaires is essential in measuring study variables and outcomes in practice (Bannigan & Watson, 2009; Bialocerkowski, Klupp, & Bragge, 2010; DeVon, et al., 2007).

Researchers need to understand the logic within measurement theory so that they can select and use existing instruments or develop new quality measurement methods for their studies. Measurement theory, as with most theories, uses terms with meanings that can be best understood within the context of the theory. The following explanation of the logic of measurement theory includes definitions of directness of measurement, measurement error, levels of measurement, and reference of measurement. The reliability and validity of measurement methods, such as scales and questionnaires, are detailed. The accuracy, precision, and error of physiological measures are described. The chapter concludes with a discussion of sensitivity; specificity; and likelihood ratios examined to determine the quality of diagnostic tests and instruments used in healthcare research and practice.

Directness of Measurement

Measurement begins by clarifying the object, characteristic, or element to be measured. Only then can one identify or develop strategies or methods to measure it. In some cases, identification of the measurement object and measurement strategies can be objective, specific, and straightforward, as when we are measuring concrete factors, such as a person's weight or waist circumference; this is referred to as **direct measurement**. Healthcare technology has made direct measures of objective elements—such as height, weight, temperature, time, space, movement, heart rate, and respiration—familiar to us. Technology is also available to measure many biological and chemical characteristics, such as laboratory values, pulmonary functions, and sleep patterns. Nurses are also experienced in gathering direct measures of demographic variables, such as age, gender, ethnicity, diagnosis, marital status, income, and education.

However, in nursing, the characteristic we want to measure often is an abstract idea or concept, such as pain, stress, depression, anxiety, caring, or coping. If the element to be measured is abstract, it is best clarified through a conceptual definition (see Chapter 8). The conceptual definition can be used to select or develop appropriate means of measuring the concept. The instrument or measurement strategy used in the study must match the conceptual definition. An abstract concept is not measured directly; instead, indicators or attributes of the concept are used to represent the abstraction. This is referred to as **indirect measurement**. For example, the complex concept of coping might be defined by the frequency or accuracy of identifying problems, the creativity in selecting solutions, and the speed or effectiveness in resolving the problem. A single measurement strategy rarely, if ever, can completely measure all aspects of an abstract concept. Multi-item scales have been developed to measure abstract concepts, such as the Spielberger State-Trait Anxiety Inventory developed to measure individuals' innate anxiety trait and their anxiety in a specific situation (Spielberger, Gorsuch, & Lushene, 1970).

Measurement Error

There is no perfect measure. Error is inherent in any measurement strategy. **Measurement error** is the difference between what exists in reality and what is measured by an instrument. Measurement error exists in both direct and indirect measures and can be random or systematic. Direct measures, which are considered to be highly accurate, are subject to error. For example, the weight scale may not be accurate, laboratory equipment may be precisely calibrated but may change with use, or the tape measure may not be placed in the same location or held at the same tension for each measurement.

There is also error in indirect measures. Efforts to measure concepts usually result in measuring only part of the concept or measures that identify an aspect of the concept but also contain other elements that are not part of the concept. Figure 16-1 shows a Venn diagram of the concept *A* measured by instrument *A-1*. In this figure, *A-1* does not measure all of concept *A*. In addition, some of what *A-1* measures is outside the concept of *A*. Both of these situations are examples of errors in measurement and are shaded in Figure 16-1.

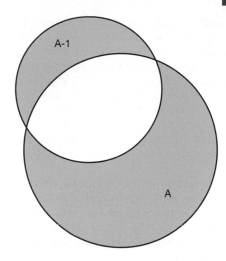

Figure 16-1 Measurement error when measuring a concept.

Types of Measurement Errors

Two types of errors are of concern in measurement: random error and systematic error. To understand these types of errors, we must first understand the elements of a score on an instrument or an observation. According to measurement theory, there are three components to a measurement score: true score, observed score, and error score. The **true score** (T) is what we would obtain if there was no error in measurement. Because there is always some measurement error, the true score is never known. The **observed score** (O) is the measure obtained for a subject using a selected instrument during a study. The **error score** (E) is the amount of random error in the measurement process. The theoretical equation of these three measures is as follows:

$$\text{Observed score} = \text{true score} + \text{random error}$$

This equation is a means of conceptualizing random error and not a basis for calculating it. Because the true score is never known, the random error is never known but only estimated. Theoretically, the smaller the error score, the more closely the observed score reflects the true score. Therefore, using instruments that reduce error improves the accuracy of measurement (Waltz et al., 2010).

Several factors can occur during the measurement process that can increase random error. These factors include (1) transient personal factors, such as fatigue, hunger, attention span, health, mood, mental status, and motivation; (2) situational factors, such as a hot stuffy room, distractions, the presence of significant others, rapport with the researcher, and the playfulness or seriousness of the situation; (3) variations in the administration of the measurement procedure, such as interviews in which wording or sequence of questions is varied, questions are added or deleted, or researchers code responses differently; and (4) processing of data, such as errors in coding, accidentally marking the wrong column, punching the wrong key when entering data into the computer, or incorrectly totaling instrument scores (Devon et al., 2007; Waltz et al., 2010).

Random error causes individuals' observed scores to vary in no particular direction around their true score. For example, with random error, one subject's observed score may be higher than his or her true score, whereas another subject's observed score may be lower than his or her true score. According to measurement theory, the sum of random errors is expected to be zero, and the random error score (E) is not expected to correlate with the true score (T). Random error does not influence the mean to be higher or lower but rather increases the amount of unexplained variance around the mean. When this occurs, estimation of the true score is less precise.

If you were to measure a variable for three subjects and diagram the random error, it might appear as shown in Figure 16-2. The difference between the true score of subject 1 (T_1) and the observed score (O_1) is two positive measurement intervals. The difference between the true score (T_2) and observed score (O_2) for subject 2 is two negative measurement intervals. The difference between the true score (T_3) and observed score (O_3) for subject 3 is zero. The random error for these three subjects is zero ($+2 - 2 + 0 = 0$). In viewing this example, one must remember that this is only a means of conceptualizing random error.

Measurement error that is not random is referred to as **systematic error**. A scale that weighs subjects 3 pounds more than their true weights is an example of systematic error. All of the body weights would be higher, and, as a result, the mean would be higher than it should be. Systematic error occurs because something else is being measured in addition to the concept. A conceptualization of systematic error is presented in Figure 16-3. Systematic error (represented by the shaded area in the figure) is due to the part of A-1 that is outside of A. This part of A-1 measures factors other than A and biases scores in a particular direction.

Systematic error is considered part of T (true score) and reflects the true measure of A-1, not A. Adding the true score (with systematic error) to the random error

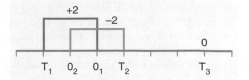

Figure 16-2 Conceptualization of random error.

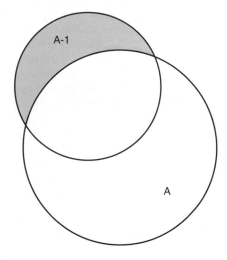

Figure 16-3 Conceptualization of systematic error.

(which is 0) yields the observed score, as shown by the following equations:

$$T \text{ (true score with systematic error)} + E \text{ (random error of 0)} = O \text{ (observed score)}$$

or

$$T + E = O$$

Some systematic error is incurred in almost any measure; however, a close link between the abstract theoretical concept and the development of the instrument can greatly decrease systematic error. Because of the importance of this factor in a study, researchers spend considerable time and effort in selecting and developing quality measurement methods to decrease systematic error.

Another effective means of diminishing systematic error is to use more than one measure of an attribute or a concept and to compare the measures. To make this comparison, researchers use various data collection methods, such as scale, interview, and observation. Campbell and Fiske (1959) developed a technique

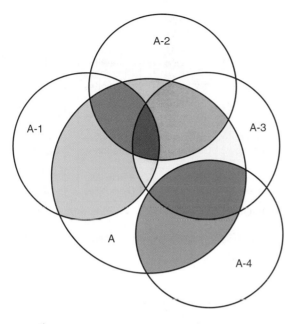

Figure 16-4 Multiple measures of an abstract concept.

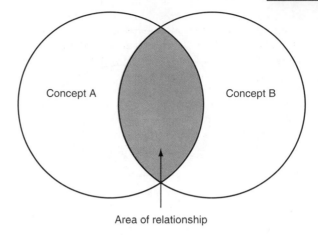

Area of relationship

Figure 16-5 True relationship of concepts *A* and *B*.

of using more than one method to measure a concept, referred to as the **multimethod-multitrait technique**. More recently, the technique has been described as a version of mixed methodology, as discussed in Chapter 10. These techniques allow researchers to measure more dimensions of abstract concepts, and the effect of the systematic error on the composite observed score decreases. Figure 16-4 illustrates how more dimensions of concept *A* are measured through the use of four instruments, designated *A-1, A-2, A-3,* and *A-4.*

For example, a researcher could decrease systematic error in measures of anxiety by (1) administering the Spielberger State-Trait Anxiety Inventory, (2) recording blood pressure readings, (3) asking the subject about anxious feelings, and (4) observing the subject's behavior. Multimethod measurement strategies decrease systematic error by combining the values in some way to give a single observed score of anxiety for each subject. However, sometimes it may be difficult logically to justify combining scores from various measures, and a mixed-methods approach might be the most appropriate to use in the study. Mixed-methods study uses a combination of quantitative and qualitative approaches in their implementation (Creswell, 2009).

In some studies, researchers use instruments to examine relationships. Consider a hypothesis that tests the relationship between concept *A* and concept *B.* In Figure 16-5, the shaded area enclosed in the dark lines represents the true relationship between concepts *A* and *B,* such as the relationship between anxiety and depression. For example, two instruments, *A-1* (Spielberger State Anxiety Scale) and *B-1* (Center for Epidemiological Studies Depression Scale, Radloff, 1977), are used to examine the relationship between concepts *A* and *B.* The part of the true relationship actually reflected by *A-1* and *B-1* measurement methods is represented by the colored area in Figure 16-6. Because two instruments provide a more accurate measure of concepts *A* and *B,* more of the true relationship between concepts *A* and *B* can be measured.

If additional instruments (*A-2* and *B-2*) are used to measure concepts *A* and *B,* more of the true relationship might be reflected. Figure 16-7 demonstrates with different colors the parts of the true relationship between concepts *A* and *B* that is measured when concept *A* is measured with two instruments (*A-1* and *A-2*) and concept *B* is measured with two instruments (*B-1* and *B-2*).

Levels of Measurement

The traditional levels of measurement have been used for so long that the categorization system has been considered absolute and inviolate. In 1946, Stevens organized the rules for assigning numbers to objects so that a hierarchy in measurement was established called the **levels of measurement**. The levels of measurement, from lower to higher, are nominal, ordinal, interval, and ratio.

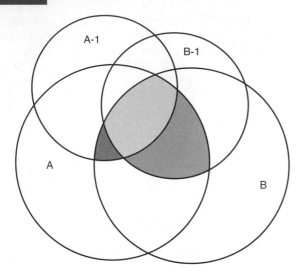

Figure 16-6 Examining a relationship using one measure of each concept.

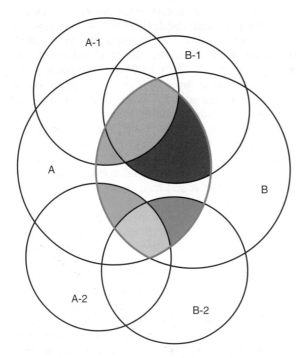

Figure 16-7 Examining a relationship using two measures of each concept.

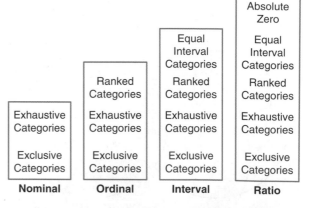

Figure 16-8 Summary of the rules for levels of measurement.

Nominal Level of Measurement

Nominal level of measurement is the lowest of the four measurement levels or categories. It is used when data can be organized into categories of a defined property but the categories cannot be ordered. For example, diagnoses of chronic diseases are nominal data with categories such as hypertension, type 2 diabetes, and dyslipidemia. One cannot say that one category is higher than another or that category A (hypertension) is closer to category B (diabetes) than to category C (dyslipidemia). The categories differ in quality but not quantity. One cannot say that subject A possesses more of the property being categorized than does subject B. (*Rule:* **The categories must be unorderable.**) Categories must be established so that each datum fits into only one of the categories. (*Rule:* **The categories must be exclusive.**) All the data must fit into the established categories. (*Rule:* **The categories must be exhaustive.**)

Figure 16-8 provides a summary for the rules for the four levels of measurement—nominal, ordinal, interval, and ratio. Data such as ethnicity, gender, marital status, religion, and diagnoses are examples of nominal data. When data are coded for entry into the computer, the categories are assigned numbers. For example, gender may be classified as 1 = male and 2 = female. The numbers assigned to categories in nominal measurement are used only as labels and cannot be used for mathematical calculations.

Ordinal Level of Measurement

Data that can be measured at the **ordinal level** can be assigned to categories of an attribute that can be ranked. There are rules for how one ranks data. As with nominal-scale data, the categories must be exclusive and exhaustive. With ordinal level data, the quantity of the attribute possessed can be identified. However, it cannot be shown that the intervals between the ranked categories are equal (see Figure 16-8). Ordinal data are considered to have unequal intervals. Scales with unequal intervals are sometimes referred to as ordered metric scales.

Many scales used in nursing research are ordinal levels of measure. For example, one could rank intensity of pain, degrees of coping, levels of mobility, ability to provide self-care, or daily amount of exercise on an ordinal scale. For daily exercise, the scale could be 0 = no exercise; 1 = moderate exercise, no sweating; 2 = exercise to the point of sweating; 3 = strenuous exercise with sweating for at least 30 minutes per day; 4 = strenuous exercise with sweating for at least 1 hour per day. This type of scale may be referred to as a metric ordinal scale.

Interval Level of Measurement

In interval level of measurement, distances between intervals of the scale are numerically equal. Such measurements also follow the previously mentioned rules: mutually exclusive categories, exhaustive categories, and rank ordering. Interval scales are assumed to be a continuum of values (see Figure 16-8). The researcher can identify the magnitude of the attribute much more precisely. However, it is impossible to provide the absolute amount of the attribute because of the absence of a zero point on the interval scale.

Fahrenheit and Celsius temperatures are commonly used as examples of interval scales. A difference between a temperature of 70° F and one of 80° F is the same as the difference between a temperature of 30° F and one of 40° F. We can measure changes in temperature precisely. However, it is impossible to say that a temperature of 0° C or 0° F means the absence of temperature because these indicate very cold temperatures.

Ratio Level of Measurement

Ratio level of measurement is the highest form of measure and meets all the rules of the lower forms of measures: mutually exclusive categories, exhaustive categories, rank ordering, equal spacing between intervals, and a continuum of values. In addition, ratio level measures have absolute zero points (see Figure 16-8). Weight, length, and volume are common examples of ratio scales. Each has an absolute zero point, at which a value of zero indicates the absence of the property being measured: Zero weight means the absence of weight. In addition, because of the

absolute zero point, one can justifiably say that object A weighs twice as much as object B, or that container A holds three times as much as container B. Laboratory values are also an example of ratio level of measurement where the individual with a fasting blood sugar (FBS) of 180 has an FBS twice that of an individual with a normal FBS of 90. To help expand understanding of levels of measurement (nominal, ordinal, interval, and ratio) and to apply this knowledge, Grove (2007) developed a statistical workbook focused on examining the levels of measurement, sampling methods, and statistical results in published studies.

Importance of Level of Measurement for Statistical Analyses

An important rule of measurement is that one should use the highest level of measurement possible. For example, you can collect data on age (measured) in a variety of ways: (1) you can obtain the actual age of each subject (ratio level of measurement); (2) you can ask subjects to indicate their age by selecting from a group of categories, such as 20 to 29, 30 to 39, and so on (ordinal level of measurement); or (3) you can sort subjects into two categories of younger than 65 years of age and 65 years of age and older (nominal level of measurement). The highest level of measurement in this case is the actual age of each subject, which is the preferred way to collect these data. If you need age categories for specific analyses in your research, the computer can be instructed to create age categories from the initial age data (Waltz et al., 2010).

The level of measurement is associated with the types of statistical analyses that can be performed on the data. Mathematical operations are limited in the lower levels of measurement. With nominal levels of measurement, only summary statistics, such as frequencies, percentages, and contingency correlation procedures, can be used. However, if a variable such as age is measured at the ratio level (actual age of the subject), the data can be analyzed with more sophisticated analysis techniques. Variables measured at the interval or ratio level can be analyzed with the strongest statistical techniques available, which are more effective in identifying relationships among variables or determining differences between groups (Corty, 2007; Grove, 2007).

Controversy over Measurement Levels

There is controversy over the system that is used to categorize measurement levels, dividing researchers into two factions: fundamentalists and pragmatists.

Pragmatists regard measurement as occurring on a continuum rather than by discrete categories, whereas *fundamentalists* adhere rigidly to the original system of categorization (Nunnally & Bernstein, 1994; Stevens, 1946).

The primary focus of the controversy relates to the practice of classifying data into the categories ordinal and interval. This controversy developed because, according to the fundamentalists, many of the current statistical analysis techniques can be used only with interval and ratio data. Many pragmatists believe that if researchers rigidly adhered to rules developed by Stevens (1946), few if any measures in the social sciences would meet the criteria to be considered interval-level data. They also believe that violating Stevens' criteria does not lead to serious consequences for the outcomes of data analysis. Pragmatists often treat ordinal data from multi-item scales as interval data, using statistical methods (parametric analysis techniques) to analyze them, such as Pearson's product-moment correlation coefficient, *t*-test, and analysis of variance (ANOVA), which are traditionally reserved for interval or ratio level data (Armstrong, 1981; Knapp, 1990). Fundamentalists insist that the analysis of ordinal data be limited to statistical procedures designed for ordinal data, such as nonparametric procedures. Parametric statistical analysis techniques were developed to analyze interval and ratio level data, and nonparametric techniques were developed to analyze nominal and ordinal data (see Chapter 21).

The Likert scale uses scale points such as "strongly disagree," "disagree," "uncertain," "agree," and "strongly agree." Numerical values (e.g., 1, 2, 3, 4, and 5) are assigned to these categories. Fundamentalists claim that equal intervals do not exist between these categories. It is impossible to prove that there is the same magnitude of feeling between "uncertain" and "agree" as there is between "agree" and "strongly agree." Therefore, they hold this is ordinal level data, and parametric analyses cannot be used. Pragmatists believe that with many measures taken at the ordinal level, such as scaling procedures, an underlying interval continuum is present that justifies the use of parametric statistics (Knapp, 1990; Nunnally & Bernstein, 1994).

Our position agrees more with the pragmatists than with the fundamentalists. Many nurse researchers analyze data from Likert scales and other rating scales as though the data were interval level (Waltz et al., 2010). However, some of the data in nursing research are obtained through the use of crude measurement methods that can be classified only into the lower levels of measurement (ordinal or nominal).

Therefore, we have included the nonparametric statistical procedures needed for their analysis in Chapters 22 to 25 on statistics.

Reference Testing of Measurement

Referencing involves comparing a subject's score against a standard. Two types of testing involve referencing: norm-referenced testing and criterion-referenced testing. Norm-referenced testing addresses the question, "How does the average person score on this test or instrument?" This testing involves standardization of scores for an instrument that is accomplished by data collection over several years, with extensive reliability and validity information available on the instrument. Standardization involves collecting data from thousands of subjects expected to have a broad range of scores on the instrument. From these scores, population parameters such as the mean and standard deviation (described in Chapter 22) can be developed. Evidence of the reliability and validity of the instrument can also be evaluated through the use of the methods described later in this chapter. The best-known norm-referenced test is the Minnesota Multiphasic Personality Inventory (MMPI), which is used commonly in psychology and occasionally in nursing research and practice to diagnosis personality disorders. The Graduate Record Examination (GRE) is another norm-referenced test commonly used as one of the admission criteria for graduate study.

Criterion-referenced testing asks the question, "What is desirable in the perfect subject?" It involves comparing a subject's score with a criterion of achievement that includes the definition of target behaviors. When the subject has mastered these behaviors, he or she is considered proficient in the behavior (DeVon et al., 2007; Sax, 1997). The criterion might be a level of knowledge or desirable patient outcomes. Criterion measures have been used for years to evaluate outcomes in healthcare agencies and to determine clinical expertise of students. For example, a clinical evaluation form would include the critical behaviors the nurse practitioner (NP) student is expected to master in a pediatric course to be clinically competent to care for pediatric patients at the end of the course. Criterion-reference testing is also used in nursing research. Criterion-referenced testing might be used to measure the clinical expertise of a nurse or the self-care of a cardiac patient after cardiac rehabilitation.

Reliability

The reliability of an instrument denotes the consistency of the measures obtained of an attribute, item, or situation in a study or clinical practice. The greater the reliability or consistency of the measures of a particular instrument, the less random error in the measurement method (Bannigan & Watson, 2009; Bialocerkowski et al., 2010; DeVon et al., 2007). If the same measurement scale is administered to the same individuals at two different occasions, the measurement is reliable if the individuals' responses to the items remain the same (assuming that nothing has occurred to change their responses). For example, if you use a scale to measure the anxiety levels of 10 individuals at two points in time 30 minutes apart, you would expect the individuals' anxiety levels to be relatively unchanged from one measurement to the next if the scale is reliable. If two data collectors observe the same event and record their observations on a carefully designed data collection instrument, the measurement would be reliable if the recordings from the two data collectors are comparable. The equivalence of their results would indicate the reliability of the measurement technique. If responses vary each time a measure is performed, there is a chance that the instrument is unreliable, meaning that it yields data with a large random error.

Reliability plays an important role in the selection of measurement methods for use in a study. Researchers need instruments that are reliable and provide values with only a small amount of error. Reliable instruments enhance the power of a study to detect significant differences or relationships actually occurring in the population under study. It is important to examine the reliability of an instrument from previous research before using it in a study. Estimates of instrument reliability are specific to the population and sample being studied. High reported reliability values on an established instrument do not guarantee that its reliability would be satisfactory in another sample from a different population (Waltz et al., 2010). Researchers need to perform reliability testing on each instrument used in their study before performing other statistical analyses. The reliability values must be included in the published report of a study to document that the instruments used were reliable for the study sample (Bialocerkowski et al., 2010; DeVon et al., 2007).

Reliability testing examines the amount of measurement error in the instrument being used in a study. Reliability is concerned with the dependability, consistency, stability, precision, reproducibility, and comparability of a measurement method (Bartlett & Frost, 2008). The strongest measure of reliability is obtained from heterogeneous samples versus homogeneous samples. Heterogeneous samples have more between-participant variability, and this is a stronger evaluation of reliability than homogeneous samples with little between-participant variation. When critically appraising the reliability of an instrument in a study, you need to examine the sample for heterogeneity by determining the variability of the scores among study participants (Bartlett & Frost, 2008; Bialocerkowski et al., 2010).

All measurement techniques contain some random error, and the errors might be due to the measurement method used, the study participants, or the researchers gathering the data. Reliability exists in degrees and is usually expressed as a form of correlation coefficient, with 1.00 indicating perfect reliability and 0.00 indicating no reliability (Bialocerkowski et al., 2010). For example, reliability coefficients of 0.80 or higher are considered strong values for an established psychosocial scale such as the State-Trait Anxiety Inventory by Spielberger et al. (1970). With test-retest, the closer that reliability coefficient is to 1.00, the more stable the measurement method. The reliability coefficient varies based on the type of reliability being examined. The three most common types of reliability discussed in healthcare studies are (1) stability reliability, (2) equivalence reliability, and (3) internal consistency (Bannigan & Watson, 2009; Bialocerkowski et al., 2010; DeVon et al., 2007; Waltz et al., 2010).

Stability Reliability

Stability reliability is concerned with the consistency of repeated measures of the same attribute with the use of the same scale or instrument over time. It is usually referred to as test-retest reliability. This measure of reliability is generally used with physical measures, technological measures, and paper-and-pencil scales. The technique requires an assumption that the factor to be measured remains the same at the two testing times and that any change in the value or score is a consequence of random error.

The optimal time period between test-retest measurements depends on the variability of the variable being measured, complexity of the measurement process, and characteristics of the participants (Bialocerkowski et al., 2010). Physical measures and equipment can be tested and then immediately retested, or the equipment can be used for a time and then retested to determine the necessary frequency of recalibration. For example, in measuring blood pressure (BP), researchers often take two to three BP readings 5 minutes apart and average the readings to obtain a reliable or precise measure of BP. Researchers can follow the standards for recalibration of equipment or be more conservative. The standard requirements might be to recalibrate the BP equipment every 6 months, but researchers might choose to recalibrate the equipment every month or even every week if multiple BP readings are being taken each day for a study. The test-retest of a measurement method might have a longer period of time if the variable being measured changes slowly. For example, the diagnosis of osteoporosis is made by bone mineral density (BMD) study of the hip, spine, and wrist. The BMD score is determined with a dual-energy x-ray absorptiometry (DEXA) scan. Because the BMD does not change rapidly in people even with treatment, test-retest over a 1- to 2-month time period could be used to show reliable or consistent DEXA scan scores for patients.

With paper-and-pencil educational tests, a period of 2 to 4 weeks is recommended between the two testing times, but the time period for retesting does depend on what is measured and the instrument used (Sax, 1997). After the same participants have been retested with the same instrument, the investigators perform a correlational analysis on the scores from the two measurement times. This correlation is called the coefficient of stability, and the closer the coefficient is to 1.00, the more stable the instrument (Waltz et al., 2010). For some scales, test-retest reliability has not been as effective as originally anticipated. The procedure presents numerous problems. Subjects may remember their responses from the first testing time, leading to overestimation of the reliability. Subjects may be changed by the first testing and may respond to the second test differently, leading to underestimation of the reliability (Bialocerkowski et al., 2010).

Test-retest reliability requires the assumption that the factor being measured has not changed between the measurement points. Many of the phenomena studied in nursing, such as hope, coping, pain, and anxiety, do change over short intervals. Thus, the assumption that if the instrument is reliable, values will not change between the two measurement periods may not be justifiable. If the factor being measured does change, the test is not a measure of reliability. If the measures stay the same even though the factor being measured has changed, the instrument may lack reliability. If researchers are going to examine the reliability of an instrument with test-retest, they need to determine the optimum time between administrations of the instrument based on the variable being measured and the study participants (Devon et al., 2007).

Stability of a measurement method is important and needs to be examined as part of instrument development and discussed when the instrument is used in a study. When describing test-retest results, researchers need to discuss the process and the time period between administering an instrument and the rationale for this time frame. If a scale was administered twice 30 minutes apart or there was 1 month between test and retesting, the consistency of the subjects' scores need to be discussed in terms of the timing for retesting (Bannigan & Watson, 2009; Bialocerkowski et al., 2010; DeVon et al., 2007).

Equivalence Reliability

Equivalence reliability compares two versions of the same paper-and-pencil instrument or two observers measuring the same event. Comparison of two observers is referred to as interrater reliability. Comparison of two paper-and-pencil instruments is referred to as alternate-forms reliability or parallel-forms reliability. Alternative forms of instruments are of more concern in the development of normative knowledge testing. However, when repeated measures are part of the design, alternative forms of measurement, although not commonly used, would improve the design. Demonstrating that one is actually testing the same content in both tests is extremely complex, and the procedure is rarely used in clinical research (Bialocerkowski et al., 2010).

The procedure for developing parallel forms involves using the same objectives and procedures to develop two like instruments. These two instruments when completed by the same group of study participants on the same occasion or two different occasions should have approximately equal means and standard deviations. In addition, these two instruments should correlate equally with another variable. For example, if two instruments were developed to measure pain, the scores from these two scales should correlate equally with perceived anxiety score. If both forms of the instrument are administered during the same occasion, a reliability coefficient can be calculated to determine equivalence. A coefficient of 0.80 or higher indicates equivalence (Waltz et al., 2010).

Determining interrater reliability is a concern when studies include observational measurement, which is common in qualitative research. Interrater reliability values need to be reported in any study in which observational data are collected or judgments are made by two or more data gatherers. Two techniques determine interrater reliability. Both techniques require that two or more raters independently observe and record the same event using the protocol developed for the study or that the same rater observes and records an event on two occasions. To judge interrater reliability adequately, the raters need to observe at least 10 subjects or events (DeVon et al., 2007; Waltz et al., 2010). A digital recorder can be used to record the raters to determine their consistency in recording essential study information. Every data collector used in the study must be tested for interrater reliability and trained to a consistency in data collection.

One procedure for calculating interrater reliability requires a simple computation involving a comparison of the agreements obtained between raters on the coding form with the number of possible agreements. This calculation is performed through the use of the following equation:

Number of agreements ÷ number of possible agreements = interrater reliability

This formula tends to overestimate reliability, a particularly serious problem if the rating requires only a dichotomous judgment, such as present or absent. In this case, there is a 50% probability that the raters will agree on a particular item through chance alone. If more than two raters are involved, a statistical procedure to calculate coefficient alpha (discussed later in this chapter) may be used. ANOVA may also be used to test for differences among raters. There is no absolute value below which interrater reliability is unacceptable. However, any value less than 0.80 (80%) should generate serious concern about the reliability of the data because there is 20% chance of error. The more ideal interrater reliability value is 0.90, which means 90% reliability and 10% error. The process for determining interrater reliability and the value achieved need to be included in the research report (DeVon et al., 2007).

When raters know they are being watched, their accuracy and consistency are considerably better than when they believe they are not being watched. Interrater reliability declines (sometimes dramatically) when the raters are assessed covertly (Topf, 1988). You can develop strategies to monitor and reduce the decline in interrater reliability, but they may entail considerable time and expense.

Internal Consistency

Tests of instrument internal consistency or homogeneity, used primarily with paper-and-pencil tests or scales, address the correlation of various items within the instrument. The original approach to determining internal consistency was split-half reliability. This strategy was a way of obtaining test-retest reliability without administering the test twice. The instrument items were split in odd-even or first-last halves, and a correlational procedure was performed between the two halves. In the past, researchers generally reported the Spearman-Brown correlation coefficient in their studies (Nunnally & Bernstein, 1994; Sax, 1997). One of the problems with the procedure was that although items were usually split into odd-even items, it was possible to split them in a variety of ways. Each approach to splitting the items would yield a different reliability coefficient. The researcher could continue to split the items in various ways until a satisfactorily high coefficient was obtained.

More recently, testing the internal consistency of all the items in the instrument has been seen as a better approach to determining reliability. Although the mathematics of the procedure are complex, the logic is simple. One way to view it is as though one conducted split-half reliabilities in all the ways possible and then averaged the scores to obtain one reliability score. Internal consistency testing examines the extent to which all the items in the instrument consistently measure a concept. Cronbach's alpha coefficient is the statistical procedure used for calculating internal consistency for interval and ratio level data. This reliability coefficient is essentially the mean of the inter-item correlations and can be calculated using most data analysis programs such as the Statistical Program for the Social Sciences (SPSS). If the data are dichotomous, such as a symptom list that has responses of present or absent, the Kuder-Richardson formulas (*KR 20* or *KR 21*) can be used to calculate the internal consistency of the instrument (DeVon et al., 2007). The *KR 21* assumes that all the items on a scale or test are equally difficult; the *KR 20* is not based on this assumption. Waltz et al. (2010) provided the formulas for calculating both *KR 20* and *KR 21*.

Cronbach's alpha coefficients can range from 0.00, indicating no internal consistency or reliability, to 1.00, indicating perfect internal reliability with no measurement error. Alpha coefficients of 1.00 are not obtained in study results because all instruments have some measurement error. However, many respected psychosocial scales used for 15 to 30 years to measure study variables in a variety of populations have strong 0.8 or greater internal reliability coefficients. The coefficient of 0.80 (or 80%) indicates the instrument is 80% reliable with 20% random error (DeVon et al., 2007; Fawcett & Garity, 2009; Grove, 2007). Scales with 20 or more items usually have stronger internal consistency coefficients than scales with 10 to 15 items or less. Often scales that measure complex constructs such as quality of life (QOL) have subscales that measure different aspects of QOL, such as health, physical functioning, and spirituality. Some of these complex scales with distinct subscales, such as the QOL scale, might have lower Cronbach's alpha coefficients since the scale is measuring different aspects of QOL. The subscales have fewer items than the total scale and usually lower Cronbach's alpha coefficients but do need to show internal consistency in measuring a concept (Bialocerkowski et al., 2010; Waltz et al., 2010).

Newer instruments, developed in the last 5 years, might show moderate internal reliability (0.70 to 0.79) when used in measuring variables in a variety of samples. The subscales of these new instruments might have internal reliability from 0.60 to 0.69. The authors of these scales might continue to refine them based on additional reliability and validity information to improve the reliability of the total scale and subscales. Reliability coefficients less than 0.60 are considered low and indicate limited instrument reliability or consistency in measurement with high random error. Higher levels of reliability or precision (0.90 to 0.99) are important for physiological measures that are used to determine critical physiological functions such as arterial pressure and oxygen saturation (Bialocerkowski et al., 2010; DeVon et al., 2007).

The quality of the instrument reliability needs to be examined in terms of the type of study, measurement method, and population (DeVon et al., 2007; Kerlinger & Lee, 2000). In published studies, researchers need to identify the reliability coefficients of an instrument from previous research and for their particular study. Because the reliability of an instrument can vary from one population or sample to another, it is important that the reliability of the scale and subscales be determined and reported for the sample in each study (Bialocerkowski, et al., 2010).

Dickerson, Kennedy, Wu, Underhill, and Othman (2010) conducted a study of QOL and anxiety levels of patients with implantable defibrillators. They provided the following discussion of the reliability of the scales they used in their study.

"**Anxiety.** Anxiety was measured by the Spielberger State-Trait Anxiety Inventory (STAI), which determines a subject's current state of anxiety. This instrument differentiates between the temporary condition of 'state anxiety' and the longstanding quality of 'trait anxiety.' The STAI is a 40-item instrument that gages emotional reactions to the environment (e.g., 'I am tense,' 'I feel upset,' or 'I am worried'). Subjects rate themselves on a 4-point scale of 1 (not at all) to 4 (very much so). The median α [alpha] reliability of the inventory was reported to be 0.93 [from previous studies].... Cronbach's α scores for the present study ranged from 0.90 to 0.96 for the 3 time periods. Only the state anxiety score was used in this analysis.

"**Quality-of-life measure.** Quality-of-life was measured using the Ferrans and Powers Quality of Life Index, Cardiac Version (QLI: CV) (Bliley & Ferrans, 1993). The QLI: CV measures the subject's perception of QOL, according to a 72-item scale consisting of 2 parts. The first part measures satisfaction with various aspects of life and the second part measures the importance of these aspects to a subject. In part 1, subjects respond to a 6-point scale, ranging from 'very important' (6 points) to 'very unimportant' (1 point). Scores are calculated by weighing the satisfaction responses with the importance responses. They reflect how satisfied subjects are with the aspects of life that are important to them. The 4 subscales of QOL scored include health and functioning, social and economic, psychological/spiritual, and family. The reliability of the total scale's internal consistency was supported by α coefficients ranging from 0.90 to 0.95. Stability and reliability were supported by a test-retest correlation of 0.87 at a 2-week interval, and 0.81 at a 1-month interval.... Cronbach's α scores for the present study ranged from 0.95 to 0.96 for total QLI: CV, and for the subscales, Cronbach's α scores ranged from 0.88 to 0.94." (Dickerson et al., 2010, p. 468)

Dickerson et al. (2010) used two very reliable scales to measure their study variables and documented this in their article. They measured anxiety with the Spielberger STAI, which was developed more than 40 years ago (Spielberger et al., 1970), has shown strong internal consistency in previous research (median alpha = 0.93), and was reliable in this study (Cronbach's alpha = 0.90 to 0.96). In previous studies, the QLI: CV had strong internal consistency for the total scale (alpha = 0.90-0.95) and stability reliability with test-retest over 2 weeks and 1 month. In addition to the strong stability reliability coefficients, the researchers also provided the time frames for the test-retests that were run on the scale. Another strength is that the QLI: CV showed strong internal consistency for the total scale (alpha = 0.95 to 0.96) and the four subscales (alpha = 0.88 to 0.94) with the population in this study.

Other approaches to testing internal consistency are (1) Cohen's kappa statistic, which determines the percentage of agreement with the probability of chance being taken out; (2) correlating each item with the total score for the instrument; and (3) correlating each item with each other item in the instrument. This procedure, often used in instrument development, allows researchers to identify items that are not highly correlated and delete them from the instrument. Factor analysis may also be used to develop instrument reliability. The number of factors being measured influences the reliability of the instrument, and total instrument scores may be more reliable than the scores of the subscales. After performing the factor analysis, the researcher can delete instrument items with low factor weights. After these items have been deleted, reliability scores on the instrument are higher. For instruments with more than one factor, correlations can be performed between items and factor scores (see Chapter 23 for a discussion of factor analysis).

It is essential that an instrument be both reliable and valid for measuring a study variable in a population. If the instrument has low reliability values, it cannot be valid because its measurement is inconsistent and has high measurement error (DeVon et al., 2007; Waltz et al., 2010). An instrument that is reliable cannot be assumed to be valid for a particular study or population. You need to determine the validity of the instrument you are using for your study, which you can accomplish in a variety of ways.

Validity

The **validity** of an instrument determines the extent to which it actually reflects or is able to measure the construct being examined. Several types of validity are discussed in the literature, such as content validity, predictive validity, criterion validity, and construct validity. Within each of these types, subtypes have been identified. These multiple types of validity are very confusing, especially because the types are not discrete but are interrelated (Bannigan & Watson, 2009; DeVon et al., 2007; Fawcett & Garity, 2009).

In this text, validity is considered a single broad measurement evaluation that is referred to as **construct validity** and includes various types, such as content validity, validity from factor analysis, convergent and divergent validity, validity from contrasting groups, and validity from prediction of future and current events (DeVon et al., 2007). All of the previously identified types of validity are now considered evidence of construct validity. In 1999, in its *Standards for Educational and Psychological Testing,* the American Psychological Association's Committee to Develop Standards published standards used to judge the evidence of validity. This important work greatly extends our understanding of what validity is and how to achieve it. According to the American Psychological Association's Committee to Develop Standards (1999), validity addresses the appropriateness, meaningfulness, and usefulness of the specific inferences made from instrument scores. It is the inferences made from the scores, not the scores themselves, that are important to validate (Devon et al., 2007; Goodwin & Goodwin, 1991).

Validity, similar to reliability, is not an all-or-nothing phenomenon but rather a matter of degree. No instrument is completely valid. One determines the degree of validity of a measure rather than whether or not it has validity. Determining the validity of an instrument often requires years of work. Many authors equate the validity of the instrument with the rigorousness of the researcher. The assumption is that because the researcher develops the instrument, the researcher also establishes the validity. However, this is an erroneous assumption because validity is not a commodity that researchers can purchase with techniques. Validity is an ideal state—to be pursued, but not to be attained. As the roots of the word imply, *validity* includes truth, strength, and value. Some authors might believe that validity is a tangible "resource," which can be acquired by applying enough appropriate techniques. However, we reject this view and believe measurement validity is similar to integrity, character, or quality, to be assessed relative to purposes and circumstances and built over time by researchers conducting a variety of studies (Brinberg & McGrath, 1985).

Figure 16-9 illustrates validity (the shaded area) by the extent to which the instrument *A-1* reflects concept

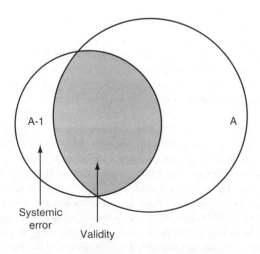

Figure 16-9 Representation of instrument validity.

A. As measurement of the concept improves, validity improves. The extent to which the instrument *A-1* measures items other than the concept is referred to as systematic error (identified as the unshaded area of *A-1* in Figure 16-9). As systematic error decreases, validity increases.

Validity varies from one sample to another and from one situation to another; therefore, validity testing affirms the appropriateness of an instrument for a specific group or purpose rather than the instrument itself (DeVon et al., 2007; Waltz et al., 2010). An instrument may be valid in one situation but not valid in another. Instruments used in nursing studies that were developed for use in other disciplines need to be examined for validity in terms of nursing knowledge. An instrument developed to measure cognitive function in educational studies might not capture the cognitive function level of elderly adults measured in a nursing study. Researchers are encouraged to reexamine validity in each of their study situations. The types of validity covered in this section include face and content validity, readability of an instrument, validity from factor analysis, validity from structural analysis, validity from contrasting (or known) groups, convergent and divergent validity, validity from discriminant analysis, validity from prediction of future and concurrent events, and successive verification validity.

Face and Content Validity

In the 1960s and 1970s, the only type of validity that most studies addressed was referred to as **face validity**, which verified basically that the instrument looked like it was valid or gave the appearance of measuring the construct it was supposed to measure. Face validity is a subjective assessment that might be made by the researchers or potential subjects. Because this is a subjective judgment with no clear guidelines for making the judgment, this is considered the weakest form of validity (DeVon et al., 2007). However, it is still an important aspect of the usefulness of the instrument because the willingness of subjects to complete the instrument relates to their perception that the instrument measures the construct they agreed to provide (Thomas, 1992). Face validity is often considered a step before or an aspect of content validity.

Content validity examines the extent to which the measurement method includes all the major elements relevant to the construct being measured. This evidence is obtained from the following three sources: the literature, representatives of the relevant populations, and content experts (DeVon et al., 2007; Fawcett & Garity, 2009; Waltz et al., 2010).

Documentation of content validity begins with development of the instrument. The first step of instrument development is to identify *what* is to be measured; this is referred to as the *universe* or *domain* of the construct. You can determine your domain through a concept analysis or an extensive literature search. Qualitative methods can also be used for this purpose. Johnson and Rogers (2006) developed the Medication-Taking Questionnaire (MTQ) based on purposeful action dimensions to determine the decision-making process of individuals for adherence to medication treatment for hypertension. They described their initial instrument development process as follows.

"A total of 20 items (need, $n = 8$; effectiveness, $n = 6$; and safety, $n = 6$) were initially developed to tap the three underlying dimensions of purposeful action based on the statements given by participants in a qualitative study (Johnson, 2002; Johnson, Williams, & Marshall, 1999). The method for item construction was guided by the principles outlined in DeVellis (1991) and Streiner and Norman (1995).... The MTQ: Purposeful Action items were arranged in a 7-point, Likert-type format describing responses based on agreement (7 = *always agree*, 6 = *very frequently agree*, 5 = *usually agree*, and 4 = *occasionally agree*, 3 = *rarely agree*, 2 = *almost never agree*, 1 = *never agree*). The 7-response option was used in an attempt to obtain optimal variance while discouraging a ceiling effect (Steiner & Norman, 1995). Higher scores for the MTQ: Purposeful Action indicated greater intent to take medications based on perceived need, effectiveness, and safety." (Johnson & Rogers, 2006, p. 339)

Researchers need to describe the procedures used to develop or select items for the instrument that represent the domain of the construct. One helpful strategy commonly used is to develop a blueprint or matrix, such as was used in developing test items for an examination that was done by Johnson (2002) in her dissertation focused on development of the MTQ. However, before developing such items, the blueprint specifications must be submitted to an expert panel to validate that they are appropriate, accurate, and representative. At least five experts are recommended, although a minimum of three experts is acceptable if you cannot locate additional individuals with expertise in the area. Researchers might seek out individuals with expertise in various fields—for example, one individual with knowledge of instrument development, a second with clinical expertise in an appropriate field of practice, and a third with expertise in another discipline relevant to the content area.

The experts need specific guidelines for judging the appropriateness, accuracy, and representativeness of the specifications. Berk (1990) recommended that the experts first make independent assessments and then meet for a group discussion of the specifications. The instrument specifications then can be revised and resubmitted to the experts for a final independent assessment. Davis (1992) recommended that the researcher provide expert reviewers with theoretical definitions of concepts and a list of which instrument items are expected to measure each of the concepts. The researcher asks the reviewers to judge how well each of the concepts has been represented in the instrument.

Researchers need to determine how to measure the domain. The item format, item content, and procedures for generating items must be carefully described. Items are then constructed for each cell in the matrix, or observational methods are designated to gather data related to a specific cell. Researchers are expected to describe the specifications used in constructing items or selecting observations. Sources of content for items must be documented. Then researchers can assemble, refine, and arrange the items in a suitable order before submitting them to the content experts for evaluation. Specific instructions for evaluating each item and the total instrument must be given to the experts.

In developing content validity for an instrument, researchers can calculate a **content validity ratio** (CVR) for each item on a scale by rating it 0 (not necessary), 1 (useful), or 3 (essential). A method for calculating the CVR was developed by Lawshe (1975) and is presented in Table 16-1 (DeVon et al., 2007). Minimum CVR scores for including items in an instrument can be based on a one-tailed test with a 0.05 level of significance.

The content validity score calculated for the complete instrument is called the **content validity index** (CVI). The CVI was developed to obtain a numerical value that reflects the level of content-related validity evidence for a measurement method (Waltz & Bausell, 1981). In calculating CVI, experts rate the content relevance of each item in an instrument using a 4-point rating scale. Lynn (1986, p. 384) recommended standardizing the options on this scale to read as follows: "1 = not relevant; 2 = unable to assess relevance without item revision or item is in need of such revision that it would no longer be relevant; 3 = relevant but needs minor alteration; 4 = very relevant and

succinct." In addition to evaluating existing items, the experts were asked to identify important areas not included in the instrument. The calculation for the CVI is presented in Table 16-1 using the format developed by Lynn (1986). Complete agreement needs to exist among the expert reviewers to retain an item with seven or fewer reviewers. If few reviewers are used and many of the experts support most of the items on an instrument, this often results in an inflated CVI and an inflation in the content validity of the instrument (DeVon et al., 2007).

As presented earlier, Johnson and Rogers (2006) developed the MTQ: Purposeful Action and described their content validity testing process and outcomes as follows.

"Content validity testing was undertaken to determine clarity and relevance of content. Participants and experts were given verbal instructions and a packet consisting of a consent form, written instructions, clarity instrument, content validity instrument, and demographic questionnaire. The clarity instrument asked participants to rate items as clear or unclear (Imle & Atwood, 1988). Participants were given a definition of each subscale and asked to rate each item's relevancy using a 4-point scale from 1 (irrelevant) to 4 (extremely relevant; Lynn, 1986). Space was provided to make comments after each rating procedure. (p. 339)

Items met clarity criterion if 70% of participants rated the item as clear and the content validity criterion if 80% of participants rated the item as 3 or 4 (Imle & Atwood, 1988; Lynn, 1986). The comments from the clarity and content validity criterion were used to revise the MTQ: Purposeful Action items and subscales....

Of the 20 MTQ: Purpose Action items, 19 achieved clarity and content validity agreement. The 1 item that had an unacceptable clarity agreement was eventually eliminated from the questionnaire. Professionals expressed a concern about the lack of specificity in the questions, but that was not an issue for the hypertensive participants. For example, one professional indicated that the item, 'Blood pressure pills keep me from having problems,' lacked specificity. Because the purpose of this questionnaire was to establish a general screening tool for individuals who potentially may choose not to take their medications rather than to create a diagnostic tool, the participants' scores were given priority. Of the 20 items [see

TABLE 16-1 Two Methods of Calculating the Content Validity Ratio (CVR) and the Content Validity Index (CVI)

	Lawshe (1975)	Lynn (1986)
Rating scale	Scale used for rating items 0 1 3 Not necessary Useful Essential	Scale used for rating items 1 2 3 4 Irrelevant Extremely Relevant
Calculations	To calculate CVR (a score for individual scale items) $$CVR = (n_e - N/2)/(N/2)$$ *Note:* n_e = The number of experts who rated an item as "essential" N = the total number of experts. *Example:* If 8 of 10 experts rated an item as essential, CVR would be $(8 - 5/5) = 0.60$	CVI for each scale item is the proportion of experts who rate the item as a 3 or 4 on a 4-point scale. *Example:* If 4 of 6 content experts rated an item as relevant (3 or 4), CVI would be: 4/6 = 0.67 This item would not meet the 0.83 level of endorsement required to establish content validity using a panel of 6 experts at the 0.05 level of significance. Therefore, it would be dropped CVI for the entire scale is the proportion of the total number of items deemed content valid. *Example:* If 77 of 80 items were deemed content valid, CVI would be: 77/80 = 0.96
Acceptable range	Depends on number of reviewers	Depends on number of reviewers

From DeVon, H. A., Block, M. E., Moyle-Wright, P., Ernst, D. M., Hayden, S. J., Lazzara, D. J., Savoy, S. M., & Kostas-Polston, E. (2007). A psychometric toolbox for testing validity and reliability. *Journal of Nursing Scholarship, 39*(2), 158.

Table 16-2 for the 20 items in the original questionnaire], 12 underwent minor grammatical revisions guided by the comments of both the participants and professionals. For example, items were made specific to blood pressure and the term medication was changed to pills. Several items were reworded, or the tense of the verb was changed." (Johnson & Rogers, 2006, pp. 341-342)

Before sending the instrument to experts for evaluation, researchers need to decide how many experts must agree on each item and on the total instrument for the content to be considered valid. Items that do not achieve minimum agreement by the expert panel must be either eliminated from the instrument or revised (DeVon et al., 2007; Lynn, 1986). Johnson and Rogers (2006) described their panel of reviewers, who were health professionals and patients prescribed antihypertensive medications, for the MTQ in the following excerpt.

"Content validity testing was conducted in a sample of five hypertensive patients and five health care professionals who examined the MTQ for clarity and content relevance (Imle & Atwood, 1988; Lynn, 1986). Professionals were invited to participate in the study based on their known experience with antihypertensive treatment and included two family physicians, a cardiology nurse practitioner, a nurse working with a statewide cardiovascular disease program, and a nurse researcher who had published articles on adherence. All professionals were Anglo American and were nearly equally divided with regard to gender.

Participants for the content validity phase who had been prescribed antihypertensive medications and lived in a situation in which they managed their own medications were recruited through healthy aging clinics, worksite wellness programs, hospital outpatient clinics, and hospital emergency departments in the intermountain west. The five hypertensive participants were Anglo American, had at least a high school education and ranged in age from 48 to 90 years (M = 62.0 ± 16.4)." (Johnson & Rogers, 2006, p. 338)

Johnson and Rogers (2006) provided excellent detail about the development of their instrument and

TABLE 16-2   Medication-Taking Questionnaire: Purposeful Action—Initial 20 Items Statistics

	M	SD	Item-Total Correlation	Mann-Whitney Adherence p Values*
Perceived Need				
My blood pressure pills keep me from having a stroke.	5.8	1.5	0.58	0.08
I need to take my blood pressure pills.	6.4	1.4	0.77	0.01
I take my blood pressure pills for my health.	6.5	1.3	0.75	0.01
Blood pressure pills keep me from having health-related problems.	5.7	1.5	0.63	0.17
I could have health problems if I do not take my blood pressure pills.	6.1	1.3	0.74	0.13
It's not a problem if I miss my blood pressure pills.†	5.1	2.0	0.30	0.02
I would rather treat my blood pressure without pills.†	4.1	2.3	0.37	0.26
I am OK if I do not take my blood pressure pills.†	5.6	1.8	0.64	0.012
Perceived Effectiveness				
My blood pressure will come down enough without pills.†	5.4	1.8	0.40	0.10
I will have problems if I don't take my blood pressure pills.	6.1	1.4	0.63	0.001
My blood pressure pills control my blood pressure.	6.0	1.4	0.66	0.46
Blood pressure pills benefit my health.	6.1	1.4	0.74	0.01
I feel better when I take my blood pressure pills.	5.4	1.8	0.56	0.01
I have problems finding pills that will control my blood pressure.†	5.7	1.8	0.09	0.059
Perceived as Safe				
The side effects from my blood pressure pills are a problem.†	5.2	1.9	0.40	0.10
The side effects from my blood pressure pills are harmful.†	5.6	1.8	0.63	0.27
My blood pressure pills are safe.	5.8	1.4	0.66	0.47
Taking my blood pressure pills is not a problem because they benefit my health.	6.0	1.4	0.74	0.02
My blood pressure pills cause other health problems.†	5.4	1.8	0.56	0.35
I will become dependent on my blood pressure pills.†	3.9	2.3	−0.5	0.20

From Johnson, M. J., & Rogers, S. (2006). Development of the Purposeful Action Medication-Taking Questionnaire. *Western Journal of Nursing Research,* *28*(3), 344.

*Difference between low (scored 1-3) versus high (scored 7-10) adherence.

†Reverse coded.

M, Mean; *SD,* standard deviation.

the process for determining content validity. They also provided extensive information about the expert review panel for conducting the content validity testing. The strength of the review panel is that it included both health professionals and patients taking medications for hypertension. However, since all the reviewers were Anglo American, there was no ethnic diversity in the review process. The MTQ was a Likert scale with 7-point response options (described earlier), so it would be clearer if the researchers had called the MTQ a Likert scale versus a questionnaire (Waltz et al., 2010).

With some modifications, the content validity procedure previously described can be used with existing instruments, many of which have never been evaluated for content-related validity. With the permission of the author or researcher who developed the instrument, you could revise the instrument to improve its content-related validity (Lynn, 1986). In addition, the panel of experts or reviewers evaluating the items of the instrument for content validity might also examine it for readability and language acceptability to possible subjects or data gatherers (Berk, 1990; DeVon et al., 2007).

Readability of an Instrument

Readability is an essential element of the validity and reliability of an instrument. Assessing the level of readability of an instrument is simple and takes seconds with the use of a computer. There are more than 30 readability formulas. These formulas count language elements in the document and use this information to estimate the degree of difficulty a reader may have in comprehending the text. Readability formulas are now a standard part of word-processing software. Box 16-1 provides instructions for using the Fog formula to determine the readability of a measurement method.

Although readability has never been formally identified as a component of content validity, it is essential that the items of an instrument be comprehended by subjects. Miller and Bodie (1994) suggested that the researcher should directly assess the reading comprehension level of the study population before using a formula to calculate an instrument's readability. They indicated that it is a mistake to assume that someone's literacy is equivalent to the last grade level the individual completed. Miller and Bodie (1994) recommended that researchers use the Classroom Reading

Inventory (CRI), which is based on the Flesch, Space, Dale, and Fry reading comprehension scales (Flesch 1984; Silvaroli, 1986). This instrument determines the level at which an individual can comprehend written material without assistance. Johnson and Rogers (2006) described the readability of their MTQ: Purposeful Action as follows.

"Items were worded at approximately a sixth-grade reading level, evaluated by using the Flesch-Kincaid grade-level assessment program in Microsoft Word (2000) (Rasin, 1997). Items ranged from a 1.0 to 6.2 grade level, with a 3.5 grade level readability score for the overall questionnaire." (Johnson & Rogers, 2006, p. 339)

Validity from Factor Analysis

Factor analysis is a valuable approach for determining evidence of an instrument's construct validity. This analysis technique is used to determine the various dimensions or subcomponents of a phenomenon of interest. To employ factor analysis, the instrument must be administered to a large, representative sample of participants at one time. Usually the data are initially analyzed with exploratory factor analysis (EFA) to examine relationships among the various items of the instrument. Items that are closely related are clustered into a factor. The researcher needs to preset the minimum loading for an item to be included in a factor. The minimum loading is usually set at 0.30 but might be as high as 0.50 (Waltz et al., 2010). The factors identified are the subcomponents of the construct the instrument was developed to measure. Determining and naming the factors identified through EFA require detailed work on the part of the researcher. The researcher can validate the number of factors or subcomponents in the instrument and measurement equivalence among comparison groups through the use of confirmatory factor analysis (CFA). Items that do not fall into a factor (because they do not correlate with other items) may be deleted (DeVon et al., 2007; Munro, 2005; Stommel, Wang, Given, & Given, 1992; Waltz et al., 2010). A more extensive discussion of EFA and CFA is presented in Chapter 23.

Johnson and Rogers (2006) conducted an EFA to determine the factor structure for their MTQ: Purposeful Action scale. The EFA identifies the specific factors or subscales for the scale and the items that fit each of these subscales. The original scale had 20 items sorted into three subscales (labeled perceived need, perceived effectiveness, and perceived as safe) that are identified in Table 16-2. The EFA and the results are presented in Table 16-3 and described as follows.

Box 16-1	**How to Find the Fog Index (Fog Formula)**

1. Pick a sample of writing 100 to 125 words long. Count the average number of words per sentence. In counting, treat independent clauses as separate sentences. "In school we studied; we learned; we improved" is three sentences.

2. Count the words of three syllables or more. Do not count: (a) capitalized words, (b) combinations of short words such as butterfly or manpower, or (c) verbs made into three syllables by adding "-es" or "-ed" such as trespasses or created. Divide the count of long words by the number of words in the passage to get the percentage.

3. Add the results from no. 1 (average sentence length) and no. 2 (percentage of long words). Multiply the sum by 0.4. Ignore the numbers after the decimal point.

4. The result is the years of schooling needed to understand the passage tested easily. Few readers have more than 17 years of schooling, so give any passage higher than 17 a Fog Index of 17-plus.

Adapted from Gunning, R., & Kallan, R. A. (1994). *How to take the fog out of business writing.* Chicago, IL: Dartnell. The Fog Index is a service mark licensed exclusively to RK Communication Consultants by D. and M. Mueller.

"Factor analysis is a grouping technique that allows for evaluation of the dimensionality of scales (Munro, 2001; Nunnally & Bernstein, 1994). A principal axis factoring solution with an oblimen rotation, considered the best analysis for achieving a theoretical solution uncontaminated by unique and random error variability was undertaken....

The EFA yielded two interpretable factors [see Table 16-3], which eliminated six additional items because of factor loadings < 0.40. The first factor merged the need and effectiveness items along with one item from the Safe subscale. This factor was renamed treatment benefits (benefits). The second factor, renamed medication safety (safety), was reduced to three of the original safe subscales items.

The Benefits subscale retained nine items that focused on the actual perceived benefits of treatment, such as preventing a stroke, controlling blood pressure, preventing further health problems, and feeling better when taking medications, which indicated a desire to control blood pressure to maintain and promote health and well-being. The subscale had an eigenvalue of 5.5 and a total item variance explained by the factor of 46%....

The Safety subscale (three items) focused on side effects of medications. This subscale had an eigenvalue of 1.9 and a total item variance explained by the factor of 16%.... Together, the two factor solution had a coefficient alpha [Cronbach alpha] of 0.87 and an explained variance of 62%." (Johnson & Rogers, 2006, pp. 343-346)

TABLE 16-3 Principal Axis Factor Analysis with Oblimen Rotation Pattern (and Structure in Parentheses) Coefficients for the Medication-Taking Questionnaire: Purposeful Action Two-Factor Solution

	Factor Loadings				Eigen-value	% Variance Explained	Coefficient Alpha
	1	2	h^2				
Treatment benefits					5.5	45.9	0.90
I need to take my blood pressure pills.	0.84	(0.85)	(0.34)	0.73			
Taking my blood pressure pills is not a problem because they benefit my health.	0.82	(0.84)	(0.35)	0.72			
I could have problems if I do not take my blood pressure pills.	0.81	(0.84)	(0.21)	0.70			
Blood pressure pills keep me from having health-related problems.	0.81	(0.79)	(0.16)	0.63			
My blood pressure pills keep me from having a stroke.	0.75	(0.75)	(0.23)	0.55			
I feel better when I take my blood pressure pills.	0.74	(0.74)	(0.21)	0.55			
My blood pressure pills control my blood pressure.	0.74	(0.74)	(0.26)	0.55			
I am OK if I do not take my blood pressure pills.*	0.72	(0.71)		0.52			
My blood pressure will come down enough without pills.*	0.54	(0.48)		0.30			
Medication safety					1.9	15.6	0.80
The side effects from my blood pressure pills are harmful.*	(0.19)	0.87	(0.86)	0.74			
The side effects from my blood pressure pills are a problem.*	(0.27)	0.84	(0.86)	0.71			
My blood pressure pills cause other health problems.*	(0.29)	0.82	(0.83)	0.70			
Total					7.4	61.5	0.88

From Johnson, M. J., & Rogers, S. (2006). Development of the Purposeful Action Medication-Taking Questionnaire. *Western Journal of Nursing Research,* 28(3), 345.
Note: *n* = 229.
*Item required reverse coding. Factor loadings in parentheses represent structure coefficients. If patterned or structure coefficient is not listed, the value was <0.15.

Johnson and Rogers (2006) provided a clear, concise rationale for the revisions that they made in their MTQ: Purposeful Action scale. In this study, the revised scale showed internal consistency (Cronbach alpha = 0.87) and construct validity obtained through content analysis and EFA. Johnson and Rogers (2006, p. 348) also conducted CFA that "supported the hypothesis that benefits and safety [factors or subscales] underlie the cognitive component of medication taking in hypertensive medications."

Validity from Structural Analysis

Structural analysis is used to examine the structure of relationships among the various items of an instrument. This approach provides insights beyond that provided by factor analysis. Factor analysis determines what items group together. Structural analysis determines how each item is related to other items. Structural analysis goes a step beyond factor analysis. The exact relationship of each item in a factor is examined through correlational analyses.

Convergent Validity

In some cases, instruments are available to measure a construct, such as depression. However, for many possible reasons, the existing instruments may be unsatisfactory for a particular purpose or a particular population, such as measuring major depression in young children, and the researcher may choose to develop a new instrument for a study. In examining the validity of the new instrument, it is important to determine how closely the existing instruments measure the same construct as the newly developed instrument (**convergent validity**). One can administer all of the instruments (the new one and the existing ones) to a sample concurrently and evaluate the results using correlational analyses. If the measures are highly positively correlated, the validity of each instrument is strengthened.

Johnson and Rogers (2006) strengthened the validity of their 12-item MTQ: Purposeful Action scale and its subscales (benefit and safety) by correlating them with a variety of other instruments (Hamilton Health Belief Model Hypertension [HBM] Scale with the HBM subscales of Susceptibility, Severity, Benefits, and Barriers; Lifestyle Busyness Questionnaire with Busyness and Routine subscales; and Blood Pressure Feedback Log). The results of these correlations are presented in Table 16-4. The significant positive correlations of 0.3 to 0.63 between the existing scales (Hamilton HBM Scale with Susceptibility and Benefits subscales and the Blood Pressure Feedback Log for adherent group) and the MTQ and the benefits subscale add to the construct validity of these instruments. This is an example of examining convergent validity for this scale, which was strong for the

---

TABLE 16-4 Validity Correlation Coefficients for the Medication-Taking Questionnaire: Purposeful Action and Subscales

	MTQ: Purposeful Action	MTQ Benefit Subscale	MTQ Safe Subscale
Hamilton HBM Scale[a]	0.30**	0.43**	−0.12
HBM: Susceptibility subscale	0.36**	0.41**	0.01
HBM: Severity subscale	0.00	0.12	−0.27**
HBM: Benefits subscale	0.58**	0.63**	0.19
HBM: Barriers subscale	−0.49**	−0.42**	−0.41**
Lifestyle Busyness Questionnaire[b]	0.08	0.11	−0.02
Busyness subscale	0.10	0.13	0.01
Routine subscale	−0.07	−0.06	−0.06
Blood Pressure Feedback Log[c]			
Adherent	0.53**	0.54**	0.25*
Nonadherent	−0.60**	−0.50**	−0.53**

From Johnson, M. J., & Rogers, S. (2006). Development of the Purposeful Action Medication-Taking Questionnaire. *Western Journal of Nursing Research,* 28(3), 347.

HBM, Health Belief Model Hypertension Scale.

[a]$n = 107$.

[b]$n = 104$.

[c]$n = 102$.

*$p < 0.05$, two-tailed.

**$p < 0.01$, two-tailed.

MTQ and the benefit subscale but not the safety subscale.

Divergent Validity

Sometimes, instruments can be located that measure a construct opposite to the construct measured by the newly developed instrument (divergent validity). For example, if the newly developed instrument measures hope, you could search for an instrument that measures hopelessness or despair. If possible, you could administer this instrument and the instruments used to test convergent validity at the same time. This approach of combining convergent and divergent validity testing of instruments is called multitrait-multimethod (MT-MM).

The MT-MM approach can be used when researchers are examining two or more constructs being measured by two or more measurement methods (DeVon et al., 2007). Correlational procedures are conducted with the different scales and subscales. If the convergent measures positively correlate and the divergent measures negatively correlate with other measures, validity for each of the instruments is strengthened. Johnson and Rogers (2006) used an MT-MM approach in examining convergent and divergent validity related to their MTQ: Purposeful Action. The convergent validity findings were discussed in the previous section. Table 16-4 shows that the MTQ and the subscales benefits and safety were significantly, negatively correlated with HBM Barriers subscale and the Blood Pressure Feedback Log for nonadherent hypertensive patients. These scales measure the opposite construct from the MTQ and its subscales, so these significant negative correlations indicated that the construct validity was strengthened for these instruments. The correlations with the Lifestyle Busyness Questionnaire were too low (−0.07 to 0.13) to add to the convergent or divergent validity of the MTQ: Purposeful Action scale and subscales (see Table 16-4).

Validity from Contrasting (or Known) Groups

To test the validity of an instrument, identify groups that are expected (or known) to have contrasting scores on the instrument. Generate hypotheses about the expected response of each of these known groups to the construct. Next, select samples from at least two groups that are expected to have opposing responses to the items in the instrument. Hagerty and Patusky (1995) developed a measure called the Sense of Belonging Instrument (SOBI). They tested the instrument on the following three groups: community college students, clients diagnosed with major

depression, and retired Roman Catholic nuns, as described in the following excerpt.

> "The community college sample was chosen for its heterogeneous mix of students and ease of access. Depressed clients were included based on the literature and the researcher's clinical experience that interpersonal relationships and feeling 'connected' are difficult when one is depressed. It was hypothesized that the depressed group would score significantly lower on the SOBI than the student group. The nuns were selected to examine the performance of the SOBI with a group that, in accordance with the theoretical basis of the instrument, should score significantly higher than the depressed and student groups." (Hagerty & Patusky, 1995, p. 10)

The nuns had the highest sense of belonging, the student groups followed, and the depressed group had the lowest sense of belonging. This test increased the validity of the instrument in that the scores of groups were as anticipated.

Evidence of Validity from Discriminant Analysis

Instruments sometimes have been developed to measure constructs closely related to the construct measured by a newly developed instrument. For example, an instrument might exist to measure medication management in patients with diabetes that is similar to the MTQ: Purposeful Action developed by Johnson and Rogers (2006) for patients with hypertension. If such instruments can be located, you can strengthen the validity of the MTQ instrument and the other medication management instrument by testing the extent to which the two instruments can finely discriminate between these related concepts. Testing of this discrimination involves administering the two instruments simultaneously to a sample and performing a discriminant analysis (see Kerlinger & Lee, 2000, for a discussion of discriminant analysis).

Validity from Prediction of Future Events and Concurrent Events

The ability to predict future performance or attitudes on the basis of instrument scores adds to the validity of an instrument. Nurse researchers often want to determine the ability of scales developed to measure selected health behaviors to predict the future health status of individuals. One approach might be to examine reported stress levels of selected individuals in highly stressful careers such as nursing and see if stress is linked to the nurses' future incidence of hypertension. If study analysis links stress to future hypertension, measuring a nurse's stress could be used to predict his or her future likelihood of becoming hypertensive. For example, the validity of the Nursing Stress Scale (NSS) could be tested in this manner. French, Lenton, Walters, and Eyles (2000) did an expanded evaluation of the reliability and validity of the NSS with a random sample of 2280 nurses working in a wide range of healthcare settings. They noted that the NSS included nine subscales: death and dying, conflict with physicians, inadequate preparation, problems with supervisors, workload, problems with peers, uncertainty concerning treatment, patients and their families, and discrimination. Confirmatory factor analyses supported the factor structure. Cronbach alpha coefficients of eight of the subscales were 0.70 or higher. The NNS showed reliability and validity in measuring stress in nurses and could be used in a study to determine the link to hypertension. The accuracy of **predictive validity** is determined through regression analysis.

Validity can be tested by examining the ability to predict the current value of one measure on the basis of the value obtained on the measure of another concept. For example, you might be able to predict the self-esteem score of an individual who had a high score on an instrument to measure coping. A person who received a high score on coping might be expected also to have a high self-esteem score. If these results held true in a study in which both measures were obtained concurrently, the two instruments would have evidence of **concurrent validity**.

Successive Verification of Validity

After the initial development of an instrument, it is hoped that other researchers would begin using the instrument in additional studies. Each of these studies could add to the validity and reliability information on the instrument. There is a successive verification of the validity of the instrument over time when used in a variety of studies with different populations and settings. For example, additional researchers are using the MTQ: Purposeful Action in their studies, which has the potential to add to the validity of this questionnaire (Lehane & McCarthy, 2007).

Accuracy, Precision, and Error of Physiological Measures

Accuracy and precision of physiological and biochemical measures tend not to be reported in published studies. These routine **physiological measures** are assumed to be accurate and precise, an assumption that is not always correct. The most common physiological measures used in nursing studies are blood pressure, heart rate, weight, and temperature. These measures are often obtained from the patient's record with no consideration given to their accuracy. It is important to consider the possibility of differences between the obtained value and the true value of physiological measures. Thus, researchers using physiological measures need to provide evidence of the accuracy and precision of their measures (Ryan-Wenger, 2010).

The evaluation of physiological measures may require a slightly different perspective from that applied to behavioral measures, in that standards for most biophysical measures are defined by national and international organizations such as the International Organization of Standardization (IOS) (2011a) and the Clinical Laboratory Standards Institute (CLSI) (2011). CLSI develops standards for laboratory and other healthcare-related biophysical measures. The IOS is the world's largest developer and publisher of international standards and includes a network of 160 countries (see IOS website for details at http://www.iso.org/iso/home.htm). The ISO standards were developed to accomplish the following:

- Make the development, manufacturing, and supply of products and services more efficient, safer, and cleaner
- Facilitate trade between countries and make it fairer
- Provide governments with a technical base for health, safety, and environmental legislation and conformity assessment
- Share technological advances and good management practice
- Disseminate innovations
- Safeguard consumers and users in general of products and services
- Make life simpler by providing solutions to common problems (ISO, 2011b)

You can locate the standards for different biophysical equipment, products, or services that you might use in a study or in clinical practice. Within IOS, the Joint Committee for Guides in Metrology (JCGM) has two major areas of focus: (1) Guide to the Expression of Uncertainty in Measurement (GUM) and (2) International Vocabulary of Basic and General Terms in Metrology (VIM) (JCGM, 2011). VIM is a document that standardizes terminology related to biophysical measurements, such as accuracy, precision, error, sensitivity, specificity, and likelihood ratio that are described in this section.

Accuracy

Accuracy involves determining the closeness of the agreement between the measured value and the true value of the quantity being measured (JCGM, 2011). Accuracy is similar to validity, in which evidence of content-related validity addresses the extent to which the instrument measured the construct or domain defined in the study. New measurement devices are compared with existing standardized methods of measuring a biophysical property or concept. For example, measures of oxygen saturation with a pulse oximeter were correlated with arterial blood gas measures of oxygen saturation to determine the accuracy of the pulse oximeter. Thus, there should be a very strong, positive correlation (≥ 0.95) between pulse oximeter and blood gas measures of oxygen saturation to support the accuracy of the pulse oximeter (CLSI, 2011).

Accuracy of physiological measures depends on the (1) quality of the measurement equipment or device, (2) detail of the data collection plan, and (3) expertise of the data collector (Ryan-Wenger, 2010). The data collector or person conducting the biophysical measures must do the measurements in a standardized way that is usually directed by a measurement protocol. For example, BP readings in a study need to be taken using a protocol: (1) place the subject in a chair and allow 5 minutes of rest; (2) remove restrictive clothing from the subject's arm; (3) measure the subject's upper arm and select the appropriate cuff size; (4) instruct the subject to place his or her feet flat on the floor; (5) support the subject's arm when taking the BP reading; and (6) take three BP readings each 5 minutes apart, average the readings, and enter the averaged BP reading into a computer. Some measurements, such as arterial pressure, can be obtained by the biomedical device producing the reading and automatically recorded in a computerized database. This type of data collection greatly reduces the potential for error and increases accuracy and precision.

The biomedical device or equipment used to measure a study variable must be examined for accuracy. Researchers need to document the extent to which the biophysical measure is an accurate measurement of a study variable and the level of error expected. Reviewing the ISO (2011b) and CLSI (2011) standards could provide essential accuracy information and information about the company that developed the device or equipment.

Selectivity, an element of accuracy, is "the ability to identify correctly the signal under study and to distinguish it from other signals" (Gift & Soeken, 1988, p. 129). Because body systems interact, the researcher must choose instruments that have selectivity for the dimension being studied. For example, electrocardiographic readings allow one to differentiate electrical signals coming from the myocardium from similar signals coming from skeletal muscles.

To determine the accuracy of biochemical measures, review the standards set by CLSI (2011) and determine if the laboratory where the measures are going to be obtained is certified. Most laboratories are certified, so researchers could contact experts in the agency on the laboratory procedure and ask them to describe the process for collection, analysis, and values obtained for specimens. You might also ask these experts to judge the appropriateness of the biophysical device for the construct being measured in the study. Use contrasted groups' techniques by selecting a group of subjects known to have high values on the biochemical measures and comparing them with a group of subjects known to have low values on the same measure. In addition, to obtain concurrent validity, compare the results of the test with results from the use of a known standard (CLSI, 2011), such as the example of the comparison of pulse oximeter values with blood gas values for oxygen saturation.

Precision

Precision is the degree of consistency or reproducibility of measurements made with physiological instruments or devices. There should be close agreement in the replicated measures of the same variable or object under specified conditions (Ryan-Wenger, 2010). Precision is similar to reliability. The precision of most physiological devices or equipment is determined by the manufacturer and is part of quality control testing done in the agency using the device. Similar to accuracy, precision depends on the collector of the biophysical measures and the consistency of the measurement equipment or device. The protocol for collecting the biophysical measures improves precision and accuracy (see the previous example of protocol to measure BP).

The data collectors need to be trained to ensure consistency, which is documented with intrarater (within a single data collector) and interrater (among data collectors) percentages of agreements. The kappa coefficient of agreement is one of the most common and simplest statistics to determine intrarater and interrater accuracy and precision for nominal level data (Cohen, 1960; Ryan-Wenger, 2010). The equipment and devices used to measure physiological variables need to be maintained according to the standards set by IOS and the manufacturers of the devices. Many devices need to be recalibrated according to set criteria to ensure consistency in measurements. Because of fluctuations in some physiological measures, test-retest reliability might be inappropriate.

Two procedures are commonly used to determine the precision of biochemical measures. One is the Levy-Jennings chart. For each analysis method, a control sample is analyzed daily for 20 to 30 days. The control sample contains a known amount of the substance being tested. The mean, the standard deviation, and the known value of the sample are used to prepare a graph of the daily test results. Only 1 value of 22 is expected to be greater than or less than 2 standard deviations from the mean. If two or more values are more than 2 standard deviations from the mean, the method is unreliable in that laboratory. Another method of determining the precision of biochemical measures is the duplicate measurement method. The same technician performs duplicate measures on randomly selected specimens for a specific number of days. The results are essentially the same each day if there is high precision. Results are plotted on a graph, and the standard deviation is calculated on the basis of difference scores. The use of correlation coefficients is not recommended (DeKeyser & Pugh, 1990).

Sensitivity

Sensitivity of physiological measures relates to "the amount of change of a parameter that can be measured precisely" (Gift & Soeken, 1988, p. 130). If changes are expected to be small, the instrument must be very sensitive to detect the changes. Thus, sensitivity is associated with effect size (see Chapter 15). With some instruments, sensitivity may vary at the ends of the spectrum. This is referred to as the *frequency response*. The stability of the instrument is also related to sensitivity. This feature may be judged in terms of the ability of the system to resume a steady state after a disturbance in input. For electrical systems, this feature is referred to as *freedom from drift* (Gift & Soeken, 1988).

Error

Sources of error in physiological measures can be grouped into the following five categories: environment, user, subject, machine, and interpretation. The environment affects both the machine and the subject. Environmental factors include temperature, barometric pressure, and static electricity. User errors are caused by the person using the instrument and may be associated with variations by the same user, different users, changes in supplies, or procedures used to operate the equipment. Subject errors occur when the subject alters the machine or the machine alters the

subject. In some cases, the machine may not be used to its full capacity. Machine error may be related to calibration or to the stability of the machine. Signals transmitted from the machine are also a source of error and can cause misinterpretation (Ryan-Wenger, 2010).

Sources of error in biochemical measures are biological, preanalytical, analytical, and postanalytical. Biological variability in biochemical measures is due to factors such as age, gender, and body size. Variability in the same individual is due to factors such as diurnal rhythms, seasonal cycles, and aging. Preanalytical variability is due to errors in collecting and handling of specimens. These errors include sampling the wrong patients; using an incorrect container, preservative, or label; lysis of cells; and evaporation. Preanalytical variability may also be due to patient intake of food or drugs, exercise, or emotional stress. Analytical variability is associated with the method used for analysis and may be due to materials, equipment, procedures, and personnel used. The major source of postanalytical variability is transcription error. This source of error can be greatly reduced by entering data into the computer directly (DeKeyser & Pugh, 1990).

When the scores obtained in a study are at the interval or ratio level, a commonly used method of evaluating precision and accuracy errors is the Bland-Altman chart (Bland & Altman, 1986). This chart is a scatter plot of the differences between observed scores on the Y-axis and the combined mean of the two methods on the X-axis. The distribution of the difference scores is examined in context of the limits of agreement that are drawn as a horizontal line across the chart or scatter plot (see Chapter 23). The limits are set by the researchers and might include 1 or 2 standard deviations from the mean or might be the clinical standards of the maximum amount of error that is safe. The data points are examined for level of agreement (congruence) and for level of bias (systematic error). Outliers are readily visible from the chart, and each outlier case should be examined to identify the cause of such a large discrepancy. Clinical laboratory standards indicate that "more than 3 outliers per 100 observations suggest there are major flaws in the measurement system" (Ryan-Wenger, 2010, p. 381).

Schell et al. (2011) conducted a study to compare upper arm and calf automatic noninvasive BPs in children in a pediatric intensive care unit (PICU). The researchers documented the accuracy of their BP monitoring equipment, training of their data collectors, and the procedures for taking the BPs in their study. The errors in precision and accuracy are documented with Bland-Altman charts for systolic BP, diastolic BP, and mean arterial pressure readings. The chart of the systolic BP is included as an example in Figure 16-10. This study was conducted to determine an alternative method of obtaining BP when the injuries of the child prevent BP readings using the upper arm.

"BP Monitor

"BP was obtained using a Spacelabs Ultraview SL monitoring system (Spacelabs Healthcare, Issaquah, WA), which consists of hemodynamic parameter modules that can be inserted into stationary bedside and portable monitor housings. All monitoring functions were controlled through the modules. During data collection, each set of arm and calf BP measurements was obtained simultaneously using two identical parameter modules: one inserted into the subject's stationary bedside housing and the other inserted into a portable monitor housing brought to the subject's bedside. Modules and housings are inspected and tested annually by Biomedical Support Services to ensure accurate functioning. The accuracy of these monitors for arm BPs meets or exceeds SP10-1992 Association for the Advancement of Medical Instrumentation standards (mean error = ±4.5 mm Hg, *SD* = ±7.3 mm Hg) for arm measurements (White et al., 1993). Spacelabs Healthcare did not report data regarding accuracy of calf BPs.

"Training of Data Collectors

"Data were collected by five pediatric intensive care nurses who attended a data training session that addressed location of arm and calf sites, measurement of limb circumference, and use of the RASS [Richmond Agitation Sedation Scale]. The nurses also attended a BP monitor in-service offered by the Spacelab representative when the monitors were adopted in the PICU in January 2006....

"Procedure

"Subjects were placed in a supine position with the head of bed elevated 30° as determined by a handheld protractor or the degree indicator incorporated into the bed frame. Subjects remained in this position for at least 5 minutes prior to data collection. Cuff sizes were selected based on limb circumferences measured to the nearest 0.5 cm. Spacelabs cuff sizes were as follows: neonate, 6-11 cm; infant, 8-11 cm; child, 12-19 cm; small adult, 17-26 cm; and adult, 24-32 cm. Per manufacturer's recommendations, if circumference overlapped two categories of cuff size, the

---

larger cuff was selected. Using a paper tape measure, arm circumference was obtained at the point halfway between the elbow and the shoulder. Calf circumference was measured at the point midway between the ankle and the knee. The BP cuffs were applied to the arm and calf on the same side. Subjects' extremities were positioned at the side of their bodies, resting on the bed, for all measurements.... Systolic, diastolic, and mean BP values for the arm and calf as well as a simultaneous heart rate were documented. Data collectors notified the child's nurse or physician if an abnormal arm reading was obtained." (Schell et al., 2011, pp. 6-7)

"To promote best practice, clinicians should base treatment choices on individual patient data, not group data. Therefore, Bland-Altman analyses were used to determine agreement between arm and calf oscillometric BPs for individual subjects. Perfect agreement occurs when all data points lie on the line of equality of the *X*-axis. The bias (mean difference between arm and calf pressures) systolic BP was 8.0 mm Hg with the limits of agreement −18.9 and 34.9 mm Hg. Limits of agreement indicated that 95% of the sample falls between these values [see Figure 16-10]. The limits of agreement for diastolic BP were −22.7 and 25.0 mm Hg with a bias of 1.1 mm Hg." (Schell et al., 2011, p. 9)

Schell et al. (2011) provided evidence of the accuracy, precision, and error of the BP monitoring equipment used in their study. They also provided a detailed discussion of the procedures for data collection that followed a rigorous protocol to ensure accurate and precise BP readings were obtained for all ages of children based on their measured arm and calf sizes. The data collectors were trained in BP monitoring by the Spacelab representative, which would increase their expertise in the use of the equipment. However, the study would have been strengthened by a discussion of the intrarater and interrater percentage of agreement for the data collectors. The use of the Bland-Altman plot to identify the error in precision and accuracy for systolic BPs, diastolic BPs, and mean arterial pressures added to the credibility of the findings. The researchers found that the arm and calf BPs were not interchangeable for many of the children 1 to 8 years old. "Clinical BP differences were the greatest in children between ages 2 and less than 5 years. Calf BPs are not recommended for this population. If the calf is unavoidable due to medical reasons, trending of BP from this site should remain consistent during the child's stay" (Schell et al., 2011, p. 10).

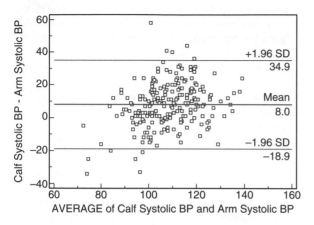

Figure 16-10 Bland-Altman plot of systolic BP. (From Schell, K., Briening, E., Lebet, R., Pruden, K., Rawheiser, S., & Jackson, B. [2011]. Comparison of arm and calf automatic noninvasive blood pressures in pediatric intensive care patients. *Journal of Pediatric Nursing, 26*[1], 9.)

Sensitivity, Specificity, and Likelihood Ratios

An important part of building evidence-based practice (EBP) is the development, refinement, and use of quality diagnostic tests and measures in research and practice. Researchers want to use the most accurate and precise measure or test in their study to promote quality outcomes. If a quality diagnostic test does not exist, some nurses have participated in the development and refinement of new biophysical tests. Clinicians want to know what diagnostic test, such as laboratory or imaging study, to order to help screen for and accurately determine the absence or presence of an illness (Sackett, Straus, Richardson, Rosenberg,

& Haynes, 2000). When you order a diagnostic test, how can you be sure that the results are valid or accurate? This question is best answered by current, quality research to determine the sensitivity and specificity of the test.

Sensitivity and Specificity

The accuracy of a screening test or a test used to confirm a diagnosis is evaluated in terms of its ability to assess correctly the presence or absence of a disease or condition as compared with a gold standard. The gold standard is the most accurate means of currently diagnosing a particular disease and serves as a basis for comparison with newly developed diagnostic or screening tests (Campo, Shiyko, & Lichtman, 2010). If the test is positive, what is the probability that the disease is present? If the test is negative, what is the probability that the disease is not present? When you talk to the patient about the results of their tests, how sure are you that they do or do not have the disease? Sensitivity and specificity are the terms used to describe the accuracy of a screening or diagnostic test (Table 16-5). There are four possible outcomes of a screening test for a disease: (1) true positive, which accurately identifies the presence of a disease; (2) false positive, which indicates a disease is present when it is not; (3) true negative, which indicates accurately that a disease is not present; or (4) false negative, which indicates that a disease is not present when it is (Campo et al., 2010; Grove, 2007). The 2 × 2 contingency table shown in Table 16-5 should help you to visualize sensitivity and specificity and these four outcomes (Craig & Smyth, 2012; Sackett et al., 2000).

Sensitivity and specificity can be calculated based on research findings and clinical practice outcomes to determine the most accurate diagnostic or screening tool to use in identifying the presence or absence of a disease for a population of patients. The calculations for sensitivity and specificity are provided as follows:

TABLE 16-5 Results of Sensitivity and Specificity of Screening Tests			
Diagnostic Test Result	**Disease Present**	**Disease Not Present or Absent**	**Total**
Positive test	a (true positive)	b (false positive)	a + b
Negative test	c (false negative)	d (true negative)	c + d
Total	a + c	b + d	a + b + c + d

From Grove, S. K. (2007). *Statistics for health care research: A practical workbook*. Philadelphia, PA: Saunders, p. 335.

a = The number of people who have the disease and the test is positive (true positive).

b = The number of people who do not have the disease and the test is positive (false positive).

c = The number of people who have the disease and the test is negative (false negative).

d = The number of people who do not have the disease and the test is negative (true negative).

Sensitivity calculation = probability of disease
$$= a/(a + c)$$
$$= \text{true positive rate}$$

Specificity calculation = probability of disease
$$= d/(b + d)$$
$$= \text{true negative rate}$$

Sensitivity is the proportion of patients with the disease who have a positive test result or true positive. The ways the researcher or clinician might refer to the test sensitivity include the following:

- *Highly sensitive test* is very good at identifying the patient with a disease.
- If a test is highly sensitive, it has a low percentage of false negatives.
- *Low sensitivity test* is limited in identifying the patient with a disease.
- If a test has low sensitivity, it has a high percentage of false negatives.
- If a sensitive test has negative results, the patient is less likely to have the disease.
- Use the acronym *SnNout:* High sensitivity (*Sn*), test is negative (*N*), rules the disease out (*out*) (Campo et al., 2010; Grove, 2007).

Specificity of a screening or diagnostic test is the proportion of patients without the disease who have a negative test result or true negative. The ways the researcher or clinician might refer to the test specificity include the following:

- *Highly specific test* is very good at identifying patients without a disease.
- If a test is very specific, it has a low percentage of false positives.
- *Low specificity test* is limited in identifying patients without a disease.
- If a test has low specificity, it has a high percentage of false positives.
- If a specific test has positive results, the patient is more likely to have the disease.

- Use the acronym *SpPin:* High specificity (*Sp*), test is positive (*P*), rules the disease in (*in*).

Sarikaya, Aktas, Ay, Cetin, and Celikmen (2010) conducted a study to determine the sensitivity and specificity of rapid antigen diagnostic testing (RADT) for diagnosing pharyngitis in patients in the emergency department. Acute pharyngitis is primarily a viral infection, but in 10% of the cases it is caused by bacteria. Most cases of bacterial pharyngitis are caused by group A beta-hemolytic streptococci (GABHS). One laboratory method for diagnosing GABHS is RADT, which has become more popular than a throat culture because it can be processed rapidly during an emergency department and primary care visit.

> "We conducted a study to define the sensitivity and specificity of RADT, using throat culture results as the gold standard, in 100 emergency department patients who presented with symptoms consistent with streptococal pharyngitis. We found that RADT had a sensitivity of 68.2% (15 of 22), a specificity of 89.7% (70 of 78), a positive predictive value of 65.2% (15 of 23), and a negative predictive value of 90.9% (70 of 77). We conclude that RADT is useful in the emergency department when the clinical suspicion is GABHS, but results should be confirmed with a throat culture in patients whose RADT results are negative." (Sarikaya et al., 2010, p. 180)

The results of the study by Sarikaya et al. (2010) were put into Table 16-6 so that you might see how the sensitivity and specificity were calculated in this study.

Sensitivity calculation = probability of disease
$$= a/(a + c) = \text{true positive rate}$$

Sensitivity = probability of GABHS pharyngitis
$$= 15/(15 + 7) = 15/22 = 68.18\% = 68.2\%$$

TABLE 16-6 Results of Sensitivity and Specificity of Rapid Antigen Diagnostic Testing (RADT)

RADT Result	GABHS Disease Present	GABHS Disease Absent	Total
Positive test	a (true positive) = 15	b (false positive) = 8	a + b = 15 + 8 = 23
Negative test	c (false negative) = 7	d (true negative) = 70	c + d = 7 + 70 = 77
Total	a + c = 15 + 7 = 22	b + d = 8 + 70 = 78	a + b + c + d = 100

GABHS, Group A beta-hemolytic streptococci.

a = The number of people who have GABHS pharyngitis disease and the test is positive (true positive).

b = The number of people who do not have GABHS pharyngitis disease and the test is positive (false positive).

c = The number of people who have GABHS pharyngitis disease and the test is negative (false negative).

d = The number of people who do not have GABHS pharyngitis disease and the test is negative (true negative).

Specificity calculation = probability of disease
$$= d/(b+d) = \text{true negative rate}$$

Specificity = probability no GABHS pharyngitis
$$= 70/(8+70) = 70/78 = 89.74\% = 89.7\%$$

The sensitivity of 68.2% indicates the percentage of patients with a positive RADT who had GABHS pharyngitis (true positive rate). The specificity of 89.7% indicates the percentage of patients with a negative RADT who did not have GABHS pharyngitis (true negative rate). In developing a diagnostic or screening test, researchers need to achieve the highest sensitivity and specificity possible. In selecting screening tests to diagnose illnesses, clinicians need to determine the most sensitive and specific screening test but also need to examine cost and ease of access to these tests in making their final decision (Craig & Smyth, 2012; Grove, 2007; Sackett et al., 2000).

Likelihood Ratios

Likelihood ratios (LRs) are additional calculations that can help researchers to determine the accuracy of diagnostic or screening tests, which are based on the sensitivity and specificity results. LRs are calculated to determine the likelihood that a positive test result is a true positive and a negative test result is a true negative. The ratio of the true positive results to false positive results is known as the positive LR (Campo et al., 2010). The positive LR is calculated as follows using the data from the study by Sarikaya et al. (2010):

Positive LR = sensitivity ÷ 100% − specificity

Positive LR for GABHS pharyngitis
$$= 68.2\% \div 100\% - 89.7\% = 68.2\% \div 10.3\% = 6.62$$

The negative LR is the ratio of true negative results to false negative results, and it is calculated as follows:

Negative LR = 100% − sensitivity ÷ specificity

Negative LR for GABHS pharyngitis
$$= 100\% - 68.2\% \div 89.7\% = 31.8\% \div 89.7\% = 0.35$$

The very high LRs (or LRs that are >10) rule in the disease or indicate that the patient has the disease. The very low LRs (or LRs that are <0.1) virtually rule out the chance that the patient has the disease (Campo et al., 2010; Craig & Smyth, 2012; Melnyk & Fineout-Overholt, 2011; Sackett et al., 2000). Understanding sensitivity, specificity, and LR increases your ability to read clinical studies and to determine the most accurate diagnostic test to use in research and clinical practice.

KEY POINTS

- Measurement is the process of assigning numbers to objects, events, or situations in accord with some rule.
- Instrumentation is the application of specific rules to develop a measurement device or instrument.
- Measurement theory and the rules within this theory have been developed to direct the measurement of abstract and concrete concepts.
- There is direct measurement and indirect measurement.
- Healthcare technology has made researchers familiar with direct measures of concrete elements, such as height, weight, heart rate, temperature, and blood pressure.
- Indirect measurement is used with abstract concepts, when the concepts are not measured directly, but when the indicators or attributes of the concepts are used to represent the abstraction. Common abstract concepts measured in nursing include anxiety, stress, coping, quality of life, and pain.
- Measurement error is the difference between what exists in reality and what is measured by a research instrument.
- The levels of measurement, from lower to higher, are nominal, ordinal, interval, and ratio.
- Reliability refers to how consistently the measurement technique measures the concept of interest and includes stability reliability, equivalence reliability, and internal consistency.
- The validity of an instrument is determined by the extent to which the instrument actually reflects the abstract construct being examined and includes such types as face and content validity, validity from factor analysis, validity from structural analysis, convergent validity, divergent validity, validity from contrasting groups, validity from discriminant analysis, validity from prediction of future and concurrent events, and successive verification validity.
- Evaluation of physiological measures requires a different perspective from that of behavioral measures and requires evaluation for accuracy, precision, and error.
- The accuracy of screening or diagnostic tests is determined by calculating the sensitivity, specificity, and likelihood ratios for the test.

REFERENCES

American Psychological Association's Committee to Develop Standards. (1999). *Standards for educational and psychological testing*. Washington, DC: American Psychological Association.

Armstrong, G. D. (1981). Parametric statistics and ordinal data: A pervasive misconception. *Nursing Research*, *30*(1), 60–62.

Bannigan, K., & Watson, R. (2009). Reliability and validity in a nutshell. *Journal of Clinical Nursing*, *18*(23), 3237–3243.

Bartlett, J. W., & Frost, C. (2008). Reliability, repeatability and reproducibility: Analysis of measurement errors in continuous variables. *Ultrasound Obstetric Gynecology*, *31*(4), 466–475.

Berk, R. A. (1990). Importance of expert judgment in content-related validity evidence. *Western Journal of Nursing Research*, *12*(5), 659–671.

Bialocerkowski, A., Klupp, N., & Bragge, P. (2010). Research methodology series: How to read and critically appraise a reliability article. *International Journal of Therapy & Rehabilitation*, *17*(3), 114–120.

Bland, J. M., & Altman, D. G. (1986). Statistical methods for assessing agreement between two methods of clinical measurement. *Lancet*, *1*(8476), 307–310.

Bliley, A. V., & Ferrans, C. E. (1993). Quality of life after coronary angioplasty. *Heart & Lung*, *22*(3), 193–199.

Brinberg, D., & McGrath, J. E. (1985). *Validity and the research process*. Beverly Hills, CA: Sage.

Campbell, D. T., & Fiske, D. W. (1959). Convergent and discriminant validation by the multitrait-multimethod matrix. *Psychological Bulletin*, *56*(2), 81–105.

Campo, M., Shiyko, M. P., & Lichtman, S. W. (2010). Sensitivity and specificity: A review of related statistics and controversies in the context of physical therapist education. *Journal of Physical Therapy Education*, *24*(3), 69–78.

Clinical and Laboratory Standards Institute (CLSI). (2011). *Harmonized terminology database*. Retrieved from http://www.clsi.org/Content/NavigationMenu/Resources/HarmonizedTerminologyDatabase/Harmonized_Terminolo.htm.

Cohen, J. A. (1960). A coefficient of agreement for nominal scales. *Education & Psychological Measurement*, *20*(1), 37–46.

Corty, E. W. (2007). *Using and interpreting statistics: A practical text for the health, behavioral, and social sciences*. St. Louis, MO: Mosby.

Craig, J. V., & Smyth, R. L. (2012). *The evidence-base practice manual for nurses* (3rd ed.). Edinburgh, Scotland: Churchill Livingstone.

Creswell, J. W. (2009). *Research design: Qualitative, quantitative, and mixed methods approaches* (3rd ed.). Los Angeles, CA: Sage.

Davis, L. L. (1992). Instrument review: Getting the most from a panel of experts. *Applied Nursing Research*, *5*(4), 194–197.

DeKeyser, F. G., & Pugh, L. C. (1990). Assessment of the reliability and validity of biochemical measures. *Nursing Research*, *39*(5), 314–317.

DeVellis, R. F. (1991). *Scale development: Theory and applications*. Newbury Park, CA: Sage.

DeVon, H. A., Block, M. E., Moyle-Wright, P., Ernst, D. M., Hayden, S. J., Lazzara, D. J., et al. (2007). A psychometric toolbox for testing validity and reliability. *Journal of Nursing Scholarship*, *39*(2), 155–164.

Dickerson, S. S., Kennedy, M., Wu, Y. B., Underhill, M., & Othman, A. (2010). Factors related to quality-of-life pattern changes in recipients of implantable defibrillators. *Heart & Lung*, *39*(6), 466–476.

Doran, D. M. (2011). *Nursing outcomes: The state of the science* (2nd ed.). Sudbury, MA: Jones & Bartlett Learning.

Fawcett, J., & Garity, J. (2009). *Evaluating research for evidence-based nursing practice*. Philadelphia: F.A. Davis.

Flesch, R. (1984). A new readability yardstick. *Journal of Applied Psychology*, *32*, 221–233.

French, S. E., Lenton, R., Walters, V., & Eyles, J. (2000). An empirical evaluation of an expanded nursing stress scale. *Journal of Nursing Measurement*, *8*(2), 161–178.

Gift, A. G., & Soeken, K. L. (1988). Assessment of physiologic instruments. *Heart & Lung*, *17*(2), 128–133.

Goodwin, L. D., & Goodwin, W. L. (1991). Estimating construct validity. *Research in Nursing & Health*, *14*(3), 235–243.

Grove, S. K. (2007). *Statistics for health care research: A practical workbook*. Philadelphia, PA: Saunders.

Gunning, R., & Kallan, R. A. (1994). *How to take the fog out of business writing*. Chicago, IL: Dartnell.

Hagerty, B. M. K., & Patusky, K. (1995). Developing a measure of sense of belonging. *Nursing Research*, *44*(1), 9–13.

Hockenberry, M. J., & Wilson, D. (2009). *Wong's essentials of pediatric nursing* (8th ed.). St. Louis, MO: Mosby.

Imle, M. A., & Atwood, J. R. (1988). Retaining qualitative validity while gaining reliability and validity: Development of the Transition to Parenthood Concerns Scale. *Advanced Nursing Science*, *11*(1), 61–75.

International Organization for Standardization (ISO). (2011a). *Standards development*. Retrieved from http://www.iso.org/iso/standards_development.htm.

International Organization for Standardization (ISO). (2011b). *Discover IOS: What standards do*. Retrieved from http://www.iso.org/iso/about/discover-iso_what-standards-do.htm.

Johnson, M. J. (2002). *The development and testing of three medication-taking questionnaires for the medication adherence model constructs for hypertensive patients*. Unpublished doctoral dissertation. University of Utah, Salt Lake City, UT.

Johnson, M. J., & Rogers, S. (2006). Development of the Purposeful Action Medication-Taking Questionnaire. *Western Journal of Nursing Research*, *28*(3), 335–351.

Johnson, M. J., Williams, M., & Marshall, E. S. (1999). Adherent and nonadherent medication-taking elderly hypertensive patients. *Clinical Nursing Research*, *8*(4), 318–335.

Joint Committee for Guides in Metrology. (2011). *JCGM: Joint Committee for Guides in Metrology*. Retrieved from http://www.iso.org/sites/JCGM/GUM-introduction.htm.

Kaplan, A. (1963). *The conduct of inquiry: Methodology for behavioral science*. New York, NY: Harper & Row.

Kerlinger, F. N., & Lee, H. B. (2000). *Foundations of behavioral research* (4th ed.) Fort Worth, TX: Harcourt College Publishers.

Knapp, T. R. (1990). Treating ordinal scales as interval scales: An attempt to resolve the controversy. *Nursing Research*, *39*(2), 121–123.

Lawshe, C. H. (1975). A quantitative approach to content validity. *Personnel Psychology*, *28*, 563–575.

Lehane, E., & McCarthy, G. (2007). An examination of intentional and unintentional aspects of medication non-adherence in patients diagnosed with hypertension. *Journal of Clinical Nursing, 16*(4), 698–706.

Lynn, M. R. (1986). Determination and quantification of content validity. *Nursing Research, 35*(6), 382–385.

Melnyk, B. M., & Fineout-Overholt, E. (2011). *Evidence-based practice in nursing & healthcare: A guide to best practice* (2nd ed.). Philadelphia, PA: Lippincott Williams & Wilkins.

Miller, B., & Bodie, M. (1994). Determination of reading comprehension level for effective patient health-education materials. *Nursing Research, 43*(2), 118–119.

Munro, B. H. (2001). *Statistical methods for health care research* (4th ed.). Philadelphia, PA: Lippincott Williams & Wilkins.

Munro, B. H. (2005). *Statistical methods for health care research* (5th ed.). Philadelphia, PA: Lippincott Williams & Wilkins.

Nunnally, J. C., & Bernstein, I. H. (1994). *Psychometric theory* (3rd ed.). New York, NY: McGraw-Hill.

Radloff, L. S. (1977). The CES-D scale: A self-report depression scale for research in the general population. *Applied Psychological Measures, 1*, 385–394.

Rasin, J. H. (1997). Measurement issues with the elderly. In M. Frank-Stromberg & S. J. Olsen (Eds.), *Instruments for clinical health-care research* (2nd ed., pp. 44–53). Boston, MA: Jones & Bartlett.

Ryan-Wenger, N. A. (2010). Evaluation of measurement precision, accuracy, and error in biophysical data for clinical research and practice. In C. F. Waltz, O. L. Strickland, & E. R. Lenz (Eds.), *Measurement in nursing and health research* (4th ed.) (pp. 371–383). New York, NY: Springer Publishing Company.

Sackett, D. L., Straus, S. E., Richardson, W. S., Rosenberg, W., & Haynes, R. B. (2000). *Evidence-based medicine: How to practice and teach EBM* (2nd ed.). Edinburgh: Churchill Livingstone.

Sarikaya, S., Aktas, C., Ay, D., Cetin, A., & Celikmen, F. (2010). Sensitivity and specificity of rapid antigen detection testing for diagnosing pharyngitis in emergency department. *Ear Nose & Throat Journal, 89*(4), 180–182.

Sax, G. (1997). *Principles of educational and psychological measurement and evaluation* (4th ed.). Belmont, CA: Wadsworth Publishing Company.

Schell, K., Briening, E., Lebet, R., Pruden, K., Rawheiser, S., & Jackson, B. (2011). Comparison of arm and calf automatic non-invasive blood pressures in pediatric intensive care patients. *Journal of Pediatric Nursing, 26*(1), 3–12.

Silvaroli, N. J. (1986). *Classroom reading inventory* (5th ed.). Dubuque, IA: William C. Brown.

Spielberger, C. D., Gorsuch, R. L., & Lushene, P. R. (1970). *Manual for the State-Trait Anxiety Inventory (Form Y)*. Palo Alto, CA: Consulting Psychologists Press.

Stevens, S. S. (1946). On the theory of scales of measurement. *Science, 103*, 677–680.

Stommel, M., Wang, S., Given, C. W., & Given, B. (1992). Confirmatory factor analysis (CFA) as a method to assess measurement equivalence. *Research in Nursing & Health, 15*(5), 399–405.

Streiner, D. L., & Norman, G. R. (1995). *Health measurement scales: A practical guide to their development and use* (2nd ed.). Oxford, UK: Oxford University Press.

Thomas, S. (1992). Face validity. *Western Journal of Nursing Research, 14*(1), 109–112.

Topf, M. (1988). Interrater reliability decline under covert assessment. *Nursing Research, 37*(1), 47–49.

Waltz, C. W., & Bausell, R. B. (1981). *Nursing research: Design, statistics and computer analysis*. Philadelphia: F. A. Davis.

Waltz, C. F., Strickland, O. L., & Lenz, E. R. (2010). *Measurement in nursing and health research* (4th ed.). New York, NY: Springer Publishing Company.

White, W. B., Berson, A. S., Robbins, C., Jamieson, M. J., Prisant, L. M., Roccella, E., et al. (1993). National standard for measurement of resting and ambulatory blood pressures with automated sphygmomanometers. *Hypertension, 21*(4), 504–509.

17

CHAPTER

Measurement Methods Used in Developing Evidence-Based Practice

Nursing research examines a wide variety of phenomena, requiring an extensive array of measurement methods. However, nurse researchers have sometimes found limited instruments available to measure phenomena central to the studies essential for generating evidence-based practice (EBP). Thus, for the last 30 years, nurse researchers have made it a priority to develop valid and reliable instruments to measure phenomena of concern to nursing. As a result, the number and quality of measurement methods have greatly increased (DeVon et al., 2007; Waltz, Strickland, & Lenz, 2010).

Knowledge of measurement methods is important to all aspects of nursing. To perform a critical appraisal of a study, nurses need knowledge of measurement theory and an understanding of the state of the art for developing instruments to examine the phenomena under study. For example, when evaluating someone else's research, you might want to know whether the researcher was using an older tool that has been surpassed by more precise and accurate physiological measures. It might help you to know that measuring a particular phenomenon has been a problem with which nurse researchers have struggled for many years. Your understanding of the successes and struggles in measuring nursing phenomena may stimulate your creative thinking and lead you to contribute your own research to the development of measurement approaches. Some nursing phenomena have not been adequately examined because reliable and valid instruments are not available to measure them, which makes it difficult for nurse researchers to generate the essential evidence needed for practice (Brown, 2009; Craig & Smyth, 2012; Melnyk & Fineout-Overholt, 2011).

This chapter describes the common measurement approaches used in nursing research, including physiological measures, observations, interviews, questionnaires, and scales. Other methods of measurement discussed include Q-sort methodology, the Delphi technique, diaries, and use of existing databases. The chapter also describes the process for locating existing instruments, determining their reliability and validity, and assessing their readability. Directions are provided for describing an instrument in a written report. The chapter concludes with a description of the process of scale construction and issues related to translating an instrument into another language.

Physiological Measurement

Much of nursing practice is oriented toward physiological dimensions of health. Therefore, many of our questions require us to be able to measure these dimensions. Of particular importance are studies linking physiological, psychological, and social variables. The need for physiological research reached national attention in 1993 when the National Institute of Nursing Research (NINR) recommended an increase in physiologically-based nursing studies because 85% of NINR-funded studies involved nonphysiological variables. According to NINR staff, a review of physiological studies funded by the NINR found that "the biological measurements used in the funded grants often were not state-of-the-science, and the biological theory underlying the measurements often was underutilized" (Cowan, Heinrich, Lucas, Sigmon, & Hinshaw, 1993, p. 4). Cowan et al. proposed a 10-year plan to enhance the education of nurse researchers in physiological measurement, expand the number and quality of physiological studies conducted, and increase the funding for physiological research. Rudy and Grady (2005) noted in their small study of funded researchers ($N = 31$) that nursing is building a group of nurse scientists who are committing their research careers to studying various biological and pathological phenomena. Over the last 15 years, nurse researchers have expanded their use and development of precise and accurate physiological measures. An example is the current research taking place in genetics, which was encouraged by Grady, Director of the NINR, with the implementation of the Summer Genetics Institute (SGI) to expand the conduct of genomic research (NINR, 2012).

The 2011 Strategic Plan for NINR emphasized the conduct of biological research to provide a foundation for understanding and managing diseases and to test preventive care and self-management strategies. NINR (2011) proposed to invest in research to "[i]mprove quality of life by managing symptoms of chronic illness," which will require expansion in the number of biologically based studies and the quality of physiological measurements used in these studies (see the NINR most current Mission and Strategic Plan document at http://www.ninr.nih.gov/AboutNINR/NINRMission andStrategicPlan/). The increased number of biological researchers and the expanded funding for biological research have increased the quality and quantity of physiological measures used in nursing studies.

Physiological measures include two categories, biophysical and biochemical. Biophysical measures might include the use of the stethoscope and sphygmomanometer to measure blood pressure, and a biochemical measure might include the laboratory value for total cholesterol. Physiological measures can be acquired in a variety of ways from instruments within the body (in vivo), such as a reading from an arterial line, or from application of an instrument on the outside of a subject (in vitro), such as a blood pressure cuff (Stone & Frazier, 2010). The following sections describe how to obtain physiological measures by self-report, observation, direct or indirect measurement, laboratory tests, electronic monitoring, and the creative development of new instruments. The measurement of physiological variables across time is also addressed. This section concludes with a discussion of how to select physiological measures for a particular study.

Obtaining Physiological Measures by Self-Report

Self-report has been used effectively to obtain physiological information and may be particularly useful when the subjects are not in closely monitored settings such as hospitals, clinics, or research facilities. Phenomena that have been or could be measured by self-report include hours of sleep, patterns of daily activities, eating patterns, dieting patterns, stool frequency and consistency, patterns of joint stiffness, variations in degree of mobility, and exercise patterns. For some variables, self-report may be the only means of obtaining the information. Such may be the case

when study participants experience a physiological phenomenon that cannot be observed or measured by others. Nonobservable physiological phenomena include pain, nausea, dizziness, indigestion, patterns of hunger or thirst, hot flashes, tinnitus, pruritus, fatigue, malaise, and dyspnea (DeVon et al., 2007; Waltz et al., 2010).

Bhengu et al. (2011) studied the physiological symptoms experienced by individuals infected with human immunodeficiency virus (HIV) and receiving antiretroviral therapy. These physiological symptoms were measured using a self-report checklist completed by the HIV-infected patients. The measurement method was the revised Sign and Symptom Checklist for HIV patients (SSC-HIVrev) developed by Holzemer et al. (1999) and revised by Holzemer, Hudson, Kirksey, Hamilton, and Bakken (2001). The SSC-HIVrev instrument is described in the following excerpt.

"[The SSC-HIVrev has been widely used and] found to be valid and reliable for measuring HIV-related symptoms.... Respondents report the presence and intensity of the symptoms based on the following:

'Below is a list of potential problems related to HIV that you may be experiencing today. If you have the problems, please rate the degree of intensity of the problem. If you do not have the problem, do not check a box.'

Items are scored using the following scale: 0 = not checked, 1 = mild, 2 = moderate, and 3 = severe. Total symptom score is a count of the number of symptoms checked as present on the day of completing the questionnaire, ranging from 0 to 72. A total symptom intensity score is a weighting of symptoms based on the 1-to-3 scale of mild, moderate, or severe. Prior studies indicate that the six factors have strong reliability estimates and stable factor structure that supports the construct validity of the 26-item instrument. Additional evidence supports the concurrent validity of the scale as well as its sensitivity to change over time. The final version of the SSC-HIVrev (Parts I and II; Holzemer et al., 2001) used in this study is a 26-item scale available for use by clinicians and researchers to measure the patient's self-report of HIV-related signs and symptoms. In this study, alpha reliabilities ranged from .77 to .91 (malaise/fatigue = .91, confusion/distress/pain = .89, fever/chills = .83, gastrointestinal discomfort = .85, shortness of breath = .80, and nausea/vomiting = .77)." (Bhengu et al., 2011, pp. 4-5)

The self-report SSC-HIVrev scale was refined by Holzemer et al. (1999, 2001) over the years and has documented reliability and validity. The SSC-HIVrev has demonstrated construct validity through factor analysis, with six factors being identified, and concurrent validity. The scale has strong reliability in previous studies and in this study for the total scale and the six subscales (alpha reliabilities ranging from 0.77 to 0.91). Using self-report measures may enable nurses to study research questions that were not previously considered, which could be an important means to build knowledge in areas not yet explored. The insight gained could alter the way nurses manage patient situations that are now considered problematic and improve patient outcomes (Doran, 2011). However, self-report is a subjective way to measure physiological variables, and studies are strengthened by having both subjective and objective measurements of physiological variables.

Obtaining Physiological Measures by Observation

Researchers sometimes obtain data on physiological parameters by using observational data collection measures. These measures provide criteria for quantifying various levels or states of physiological functioning. In addition to collecting clinical data, this method provides a means to gather data from the observations of caregivers. This source of data has been particularly useful in studies involving critically ill patients in intensive care units (ICUs) and patients with Alzheimer's disease, advanced cancer, and severe mental illness. Observation is also an effective way to gather data on frail elderly adults, infants, and young children. Studies involving home health agencies and hospices often use observation tools to record physiological dimensions of patient status. These data are sometimes stored electronically and are available to researchers for large database analysis. Measuring physiological variables using observation requires a quality tool for data collection and consistent use of this tool by data collectors. If the observations in a study are being conducted using multiple data collectors, it is essential that the consistency or interrater reliability of the data collectors be determined (see Chapter 16) (Bialocerkowski, Klupp, & Bragge, 2010; DeVon et al., 2007; Waltz et al., 2010).

Klein, Dumpe, Katz, and Bena (2010) developed a Nonverbal Pain Assessment Tool (NPAT) to measure the pain experience by nonverbal adult patients in the ICU. Testing of the tool occurred in three phases that focused on the internal reliability, content validity, and criterion validity of the tool and the interrater reliability of the data collectors. The following excerpt describes development of the NPAT and its demonstrated reliability and validity.

> "Content validity examines the extent of the tool's ability to measure the construct under consideration (in this study, pain). Construction of the scale began with an in-depth review of the literature to determine commonly accepted signs and behaviors of pain. Three nurse experts, including 2 clinical nurse specialists and a nurse from the Pain Management Service, reviewed the tool and selected behaviors.
>
> Criterion-related validity compares the new tool to a 'gold standard.'… We hypothesized that a significant correlation would be found between the NPAT score and the patient's self-report of pain, the 'gold standard' for pain assessment." (Klein et al., 2010, p. 523)
>
> "The internal reliability for the entire scale was .82 (Cronbach's alpha).… Subscale internal reliability scores comprised: emotion, .77; movement, .78; verbal, .79; facial, .77; and position, .78.… To determine the interrater reliability of the revised NPAT, a convenience sampling included all patients more than 16 years old and admitted to any of the 4 ICUs during the data collection period. The same teams of nurses were used. Data were collected for 50 patients, although data from only 39 patients were useable. The concordance correlation coefficient was .72 (95% confidence interval), demonstrating strong interrater reliability.… The criterion validity of the revised NPAT was again tested.… The concordance correlation coefficient was .66 (95% confidence interval), indicating moderate to strong validity." (Klein et al., 2010, pp. 525-526)

Klein et al. (2010) found the NPAT had strong internal reliability for both the total scale (Cronbach's alpha = 0.82) and the subscales (Cronbach's alpha ranging from 0.77 to 0.79). Because the NPAT is a new tool, these researchers described the content and criterion validity of the tool and recognized the need for additional research to determine the reliability and validity of the tool with different samples. The final copy of this tool is presented later in this chapter.

Obtaining Physiological Measures Directly or Indirectly

Physiological variables can be measured either directly or indirectly. **Direct measures** are more accurate because there is an objective measurement of the study variable. For example, patients might be asked to report any irregular heartbeats during waking hours over a 24-hour period, which is an indirect measurement of heart rhythm, and each patient's heart could be monitored with a Holter monitor over the same 24-hour time frame (direct measure of heart rhythm). Whenever possible, researchers usually select direct measures of study variables because of the accuracy and precision of these measurement methods. However, if a direct measurement method does not exist, an indirect measurement method could be used in the initial investigation of a physiological variable. Sometimes researchers use both direct and indirect measurement methods to expand the understanding of a physiological variable. Dubbert, White, Grothe, O'Jile, and Kirchner (2006) studied the physical activity of patients who are severely mentally ill. These researchers measured the variable physical activity with indirect and direct measurement methods that are described in the following excerpt.

"Self-Reported Physical Activity [Indirect Measurement]

"The 42-item Community Health Activities Model Program for Seniors (CHAMPS) … was used to assess frequency and duration of a variety of physical activities for the previous 4 weeks. The CHAMPS yields estimates of kilocalorie (kcal) energy expenditure per unit time and physical activity frequency. In nonclinical samples, CHAMPS scores have test-retest reliability intraclass correlations (ICCS) $R = 0.76$ for moderate and $R = 0.66$ for total estimated kcal expenditure over 6 months and validity correlations in the $R = 0.20$ to 0.30 range with performance on a 6-minute walk test….

"Objectively Measured Physical Activity [Direct Measurement]

"Participants wore RT3 (Stayhealthy, Inc., Monrovia, CA) accelerometers to obtain objective estimates of daily physical activity. The RT3 instrument, about the size of a pager, measures acceleration of movement along three axes, which was averaged into a composite score (i.e., vector movement [VM]), representing the overall magnitude of activity for each minute. RT3 software transformed VM into an estimate of energy expenditure (i.e., kcal per day and per hour), using participant's height, weight, age, and gender." (Dubbert et al., 2006, p. 206)

Obtaining Physiological Measures from Laboratory Tests

Laboratory tests are usually very precise and accurate and provide direct measures of many physiological variables. Biochemical measures, such as total cholesterol, triglycerides, hemoglobin, and hematocrit, must be obtained through invasive procedures. Sometimes these invasive procedures are part of routine patient care, and researchers, with institutional review board (IRB) approval, can obtain the results from the patient's record. Although nurses are now performing some biochemical measures in the nursing unit, these measures often require laboratory analysis. When invasive procedures are not part of routine care but are instead performed specifically for a study, great care must be taken to protect the subjects and to follow guidelines for informed consent and IRB approval. Neither the patients nor their insurers can be billed for invasive procedures that are not part of routine care; thus, the researcher must seek external funding or the institution in which the patient is receiving care must agree to forego billing for the procedure.

Researchers need to ensure the accuracy and precision of laboratory measures and the methods of collecting specimens for their studies. The laboratory performing the analyses needs to be certified and in compliance with national standards developed by the Clinical and Laboratory Standards Institute (CLSI, 2011). The data collectors need to be trained to ensure that intrarater reliability and interrater reliability are maintained during the data collection process (see Chapter 16) (Bialocerkowski et al., 2010; Waltz et al., 2010). Smith, Annesi, Walsh, Lennon, and Bell (2010) examined the effects of a behavioral treatment on voluntary physical activity, self-efficacy, and risk factors for type 2 diabetes in obese preadolescents 10 to 14 years old. The risk factors for diabetes measured in this study included lipid values and glucose/insulin ratio that were determined before and after the 12-week behavioral treatment. The following excerpt describes the blood analyses that were conducted in this study.

"Blood Analyses

"Total cholesterol, low-density lipoprotein (LDL) cholesterol, and high-density lipoprotein (HDL) cholesterol are measures of lipids in the blood. Each is expressed as milligram per deciliter. For ages less than 18 years, normal ranges are 125 to 170 mg/dl, less than 110 mg/dl, and 38 to 76 mg/dl, respectively. Generally, lower values on total cholesterol and LDL cholesterol and a higher value on HDL cholesterol are preferable. Glucose/insulin ratio is a measure of metabolic functioning and expressed as a ratio of glucose (mg/dl) to insulin (mcIU/ml). The target value is 7.0 or above (Silfen et al., 2001). Generally, a higher score is preferable. Blood was drawn while participants were in a fasting state and analyzed by Quest Diagnostics (Madison, NJ) at no cost to participants' families." (Smith et al., 2010, p. 395)

These researchers clearly described the blood analyses performed in their study and the normal values for preadolescents. To promote precision and accuracy in the lipid values and the glucose/insulin ratios obtained, the participants were instructed to fast and the blood was analyzed in a certified laboratory (Quest Diagnostics). The blood was drawn in a physician's office and transferred to the laboratory for analysis. The study report would have been strengthened by a discussion of the data collection process in the physician's office to ensure that the blood specimens were consistently collected and managed in the delivery to the laboratory.

Obtaining Physiological Measures through Electronic Monitoring

The availability of electronic monitoring equipment has greatly increased the possibilities of physiological measurement in nursing studies, particularly in critical care environments. Understanding the processes of electronic monitoring can make the procedure less formidable to individuals critically appraising published studies and individuals considering using the method for measurement.

To use electronic monitoring, usually sensors are placed on or within study participants. The sensors measure changes in body functions such as electrical energy. Figure 17-1 shows the process of electronic measurement. Many sensors need an external stimulus to trigger the measurement process. Transducers convert the electrical signal to numerical data. Electrical signals often include interference signals as well as the desired signal, so you may choose to use an amplifier to decrease interference and amplify the desired signal. The electrical signal is digitized (converted to numerical digits or values) and stored in a computer. In addition, it is immediately displayed on a monitor. The display equipment may be visual or auditory or both. One type of display equipment is an oscilloscope that displays the data as a waveform; it may provide information such as time, phase, voltage, or frequency of the target event or behavior. The final phase is the recording, data processing, and transmission that might be done through computer, camera, graphic recorder, or magnetic tape recorder (Stone & Frazier, 2010). A graphic recorder provides a printed version of the data. Some electronic equipment simultaneously records multiple physiological measures that are displayed on a monitor. The equipment is often linked to a computer or might be wireless, which allows the researcher to review the data. The computer often contains complex software for detailed analysis of the data and provides a printed report of the analysis results (Pugh & DeKeyser, 1995; Stone & Frazier, 2010).

The advantages of using electronic monitoring equipment are the collection of accurate and precise data, recording of data accurately within a computerized system, potential for collection of large amounts of data frequently over time, and transmission of data electronically for analysis. One disadvantage of using certain sensors to measure physiological variables is that the presence of a transducer within the body can alter the reading. For example, the presence of a flow

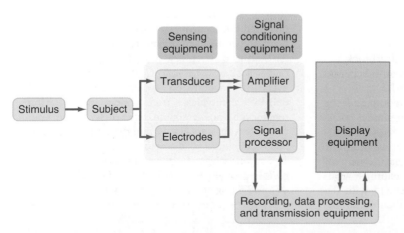

Figure 17-1 **Process of electronic measurement.**

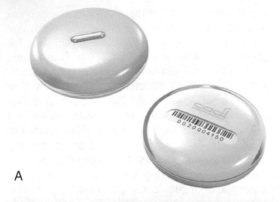

A

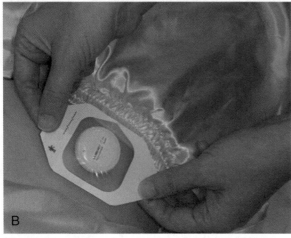

B

Figure 17-2 **A,** OR wireless thermometer. The disc has an elliptical cross section, and the sensing element consists of a metal strip located at the center of the skin-contact side. **B,** ThermoSENSOR. The device has been placed over the first piece of hypoallergenic adhesive film dressing on the lower abdomen and is about to be secured to the lower abdomen by a second piece of the same dressing. (From Ng, K., Wong, S., Lim, S., & Goh, Z. [2010]. Evaluation of the Cadi ThermoSENSOR wireless skin-contact thermometer against ear and axillary temperatures in children. *Journal of Pediatric Nursing, 25*[3], 177.)

transducer in a blood vessel can partially block the vessel and alter blood flow resulting in an inaccurate reflection of the flow (Ryan-Wenger, 2010).

Ng, Wong, Lim, and Goh (2010) compared the Cadi ThermoSENSOR wireless skin-contact thermometer (Figure 17-2) readings with the ear and axillary temperatures in children. The ThermoSENSOR thermometer provides a continuous measurement of body temperature and transmits the readings wirelessly to a central server. The measurement with the ThermoSENSOR thermometer is described in the following excerpt.

"Developed by Cadi Scientific in Singapore as part of an integrated wireless system for temperature monitoring and location tracking, this system uses a reusable skin-contact thermometer or sensor called the ThermoSENSOR. This thermometer takes the form of a small disc that can be easily adhered to the patient's skin, and each disc is assigned a unique radio frequency identification (RFID) number [see Figure 17-2]. The thermometer measures body temperature continuously and transmits a temperature reading and the RFID number approximately every 30 seconds to a computer or server through one or more signal receivers (nodes) installed in the vicinity of the patient [Figure 17-3]." (Ng et al., 2010, pp. 176-177)

"Before the study, a ThermoSENSOR wireless temperature monitoring system was installed in the ward. A wireless signal receiver (node) was installed in the ceiling of each of the five-bedded rooms.... These receivers were connected to the hospital's local area network (LAN). The system worked in such a way that temperature readings and RFID numbers transmitted by a sensor were received by one or more wireless receivers in the vicinity of the sensor and transferred through the LAN to a personal computer.... Web-based application software designed for use with the wireless system and installed on the computer was used to configure the computer to receive, store, and display the temperature and RFID data. A total of 32 sensors were used for the study.

The ThermoSENSOR uses a thermistor as the sensing element. When in use, the sensor is attached to the patient using a two-layer dressing system that prevents the sensor from coming in direct contact with the skin [see Figure 17-2]. The sensor is water resistant and can be cleaned by immersing it in a cleaning and disinfectant solution. The manufacturer provided the following specifications for the sensor: operating ambient temperature range, 10° C to 50° C; thermistor accuracy, ± 0.2° C for temperature range of 32.0° C to 42.0° C; data transmission rate, every 30 seconds on average; radio frequency, 868.4 MHz; typical transmission range, 10 m (unblocked); power source, internal 3-V lithium coin-cell battery; battery life, 12 months (continuous operation); dimensions, diameter of 36 mm, height of 11.6 mm; weight, 10 g without battery; applicable radio equipment standards, ETSI 300 220, ETSI EN 301 489." (Ng et al., 2010, pp 177-178)

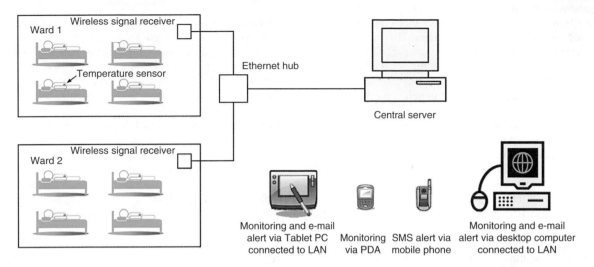

Figure 17-3 Setup of the ThermoSENSOR wireless temperature monitoring system. Each sensor transmits data wirelessly to a signal receiver (node) that is within the prescribed transmission range. The signal receiver uploads the data to a central server through the local area network (LAN), through which the data can be accessed from computers and other devices that are connected, wirelessly or by wired means, to the LAN. The server can be configured to send out e-mail and short message service (SMS) alerts. (From Ng, K., Wong, S., Lim, S., & Goh, Z. [2010]. Evaluation of the Cadi ThermoSENSOR wireless skin-contact thermometer against ear and axillary temperatures in children. *Journal of Pediatric Nursing, 25*[3], 177.)

Ng et al. (2010) provided detailed descriptions and pictures of both the ThermoSENSOR thermometer and the wireless setup. The thermometer was consistently applied to the abdomen of each child and was cleaned in a precise way. The manufacturer specifications of the thermometer documented that it was an accurate device to measure temperature. The wireless system was described in detail with documentation of its precision and accuracy in obtaining and transferring the children's temperatures to a computer for recording, display, and analysis of the data. The findings of the study indicated that the ThermoSENSOR wireless skin-contact thermometer readings were comparable to the ear and axillary temperature readings.

Genetic Advancements in Measuring Nucleic Acids

The Human Genome Project has greatly expanded the understanding of deoxyribonucleic acid (DNA) that contains the code for controlling human development. The U.S. Human Genome Project was begun in 1990 by the Department of Energy and the National Institutes of Health and was completed in 2003. The genome is the entire DNA sequence in an organism, including its genes. The genes carry information for making all the proteins required by the organism that are used to determine how the body looks, functions,

and behaves. The DNA is a double-stranded helix and serves as the code for the production of the single-stranded messenger ribonucleic acid (RNA) (Stone & Frazier, 2010).

"The project goals were to:
- Identify all the approximately 20,000-25,000 genes in human DNA,
- Determine the sequences of the 3 billion chemical base pairs that make up human DNA,
- Store this information in databases,
- Improve tools for data analysis,
- Transfer related technologies to the private sector, and
- Address the ethical, legal, and social issues (ELSI) that may arise from the project" (Department of Education Genomic Science, 2011)

The advancements in genetics have facilitated the development of new technologies that have permitted the analysis of normal and abnormal genes for the detection and diagnosis of genetic diseases. Through the use of molecular cloning, sufficient quantities of DNA and RNA have been produced to permit analysis in research. The Southern blotting technique is the standard way for analyzing the structure of DNA. The Northern blotting technique is used for RNA analysis. Analyses of both normal and mutant genes are of interest, and the Western blotting technique is used to examine the mutant proteins in cells obtained from patients with diseases. In addition, polymerase chain reaction can selectively amplify DNA and RNA molecules for study (Stone & Frazier, 2010).

It is important that nurses be aware of the advances in technologies to measure nucleic acids and use them in their programs of research. Nurses are becoming more aware of the conduct of genetic research through doctoral and postdoctoral programs specialized in this area. In addition, the NINR provides the SGI to expand researchers' expertise in conducting genetic research. You can access information on the SGI at the following NINR (2012) website: http://www.ninr.nih.gov/Training/TrainingOpportunitiesIntramural/Summer GeneticsInstitute/. These educational opportunities have expanded genetic research in nursing and increased the number of studies focused on the measurement of nucleic acids by nurses.

Jones, Munro, Grap, Kitten, and Edmond (2010) conducted a study to determine the impact of oral care on the bacteremia risk in mechanically ventilated adults. The researchers wanted to determine if tooth brushing induced transient bacteremia in this group of patients. They used DNA typing to identify organisms for the blood and oral cultures collected before and 1 minute and 30 minutes after tooth brushing. Their measurement of oral microbial organisms is presented in the following excerpt.

> "**Oral microbial culture.** A swab of the oral cavity for microbial culture was performed immediately preceding the first tooth brushing intervention. The oral cavity was swabbed in the following order using a single swab: upper and lower buccal and lingual gingival margin (obtaining organisms from the gum line and tooth surface), and palate. The oral microbial cultures were performed using BBL Culture Swab Plus collection and transport media (Becton, Dickinson and Co, Sparks, MD) and were analyzed using standard operations for the clinical microbiology laboratory. Cultures were analyzed and quantified for the following potentially pathogenic organisms: viridians group Streptococci, *Staphylococcus aureus, Pseudomonas aeruginosa, Enterococcus* spp., *Klebsiella pneumoniae,* and *Candida* spp. These organisms are most commonly cited as causes of bloodstream infections in mechanically ventilated patients. Positive cultures were frozen and stored for comparison with blood culture organisms by DNA typing. We prospectively planned the microbial analysis using multi-locus sequence typing to identify species at the strain level. Multi-locus sequence typing is a relatively new and powerful technique that

> involves molecular comparison of collections of essential genes also referred to as the 'housekeeping' genes.... Comparison of DNA sequences from isolates found in blood cultures and oral cultures would enhance the determination of whether the isolates were identical or different, and differentiate transient bacteremia from intravenous line or sample contamination from bacteremia of oral origin. DNA typing would reduce the likelihood that confounding variables in the ICU (e.g., the presence of invasive lines, frequent and invasive procedures, intubation, comorbidities, and immunosuppression) would adversely affect the analysis." (Jones et al., 2010, p. S59)

Through the use of DNA typing, Jones et al. (2010) were able to measure very precisely bacteremia risk associated with oral care in mechanically ventilated patients. By comparison of DNA sequences in the blood and oral cultures, other confounding potential causes of bacteremia could be eliminated. The researchers found that tooth brushing did not induce transient bacteremia in the patient population. This research provides a basis for future research focused on standardizing effective and safe oral care in this population.

Developing New Physiological Measures

Some studies require imaginative approaches to measuring phenomena that are traditionally observed in clinical practice but are not measured. The first step in this process is to recognize that the phenomenon being observed by the nurse can be measured. Once that idea has emerged, one can begin envisioning various means of measuring the phenomenon. As new physiological measurements are developed, they must be compared with previous methods to determine the best strategy for measuring each physiological outcome based on the patient's condition. Gelinas et al. (2010) developed a new approach for detecting pain in adults by measuring the cerebral regional oxygen saturation (rSO_2) using near-infrared spectroscopy (NIRS). The NIRS technique (IN-VOS-4100 system; Somanetics, Troy, MI) was used to measure pain during the nociceptive procedures, such as intravenous and arterial line insertions, sternal bone incision, and thorax opening, during cardiac surgery. The rSO_2 measurements were compared with the scores from the Critical-Care Pain Observation Tool (CPOT) and the faces pain thermometer (FPT) to determine discriminant and criterion validity. These physiological measures used in this study are presented in the following excerpt.

"Measurement Instruments

"**Near-infrared spectroscopy.** Near-infrared spectroscopy technology is based on the property of near-infrared light to diffuse throughout biological tissue. At near-infrared wavelengths, hemoglobin and cytochrome c-oxydase, also known as the enzyme cytochrome aa3, are the main chromophores (i.e., substances absorbing light at a given wave-length). The light source of the oximeter provides two continuous wavelengths of near-infrared light (730 and 810 nm) in the frontal region.... The ratio of oxygenated hemoglobin and total hemoglobin is measured, and a subtraction of the superficial signal from the deeper signal is performed by the monitor to obtain the regional hemoglobin oxygen saturation (rSO_2) in the frontal cortex, i.e., the main variable in this study.... Brain-activity imaging was associated with changes in cerebral oxygenation indicators as measured with the NIRS, supporting the validity of this noninvasive technique. The NIRS system used in the present study was the INVOS-4100. It continuously monitors rSO_2, and was used according to the manufacturer's instructions.

"**Critical-Care Pain Observation Tool.** The CPOT was a key pain measure in this study, because it was used to examine criterion validity of rSO_2. This behavioral pain scale includes 4 behaviors (facial expression, body movements, muscle tension, and vocalization), with a possible total score ranging from 0 to 8. It was developed and validated in different ICU groups.... The CPOT showed good interrater reliability (ICC = .80 to .93), discriminant validity (significantly higher CPOT scores during procedural pain), and criterion validity. During procedural pain (turning), correlation coefficients of .59 and .71 ($p \leq .05$) were obtained between patients' self-reports of pain intensity and their CPOT scores, whereas correlation coefficients of .49 and .40 ($p \leq .05$) were evident when patients were at rest before and after turning. Finally, a sensitivity of 86% and a specificity of 78% were obtained for a cutoff score >2 in the presence of pain on the CPOT during nociceptive exposure of postoperative ICU adults.

"**Faces pain thermometer.** The faces pain thermometer (FPT) consists of a thermometer graded from 0 to 10, including 6 faces.... The FPT was another key pain measure in this study, because it provided a standardized indicator of the patient's self-report of pain intensity, which was also used to determine the criterion validity of rSO_2. This scale demonstrated good convergent (r = .80 to .86, $p \leq$

.001, using the 5-point descriptive pain scale) and discriminant ($t = -5.10$, $p \leq .001$, comparing patients' pain intensity at rest and during turning) validity in cardiac-surgery patients, showing an association with a higher pain intensity score during turning." (Gelinas et al., 2010, p. 488)

These researchers detailed the use of the NIRS technique to measure rSO_2, and this measurement of pain was comparable to the CPOT and the FPT. Comparison of the rSO_2 with the CPOT and FPT added to the criterion, convergent, and discriminant validity of the measurement methods. Gelinas et al. (2010, p. 485) concluded, "Although further research is needed in critically ill adult patients undergoing more painful procedures, the NIRS may become a promising technique for assessing pain."

Obtaining Physiological Measures across Time

Many nursing studies using physiological measurement methods focused on a single point in time. Thus, there is insufficient information on normal variations in physiological measures across time and much less information on changes in physiological measures across time in individuals with abnormal physiological states. In some cases, physiological states exhibit cyclic activity and are associated with circadian rhythms and day-night patterns. An important question to ask is "How labile is the measure?" Some measures vary within the individual from time to time, even when conditions are similar. Circadian rhythms, activities, emotions, dietary intake, or posture can also affect physiological measures. Researchers need to determine to what extent these factors would affect the ability to interpret measurement outcomes. When a clinician observes variation in a physiological value, it is important to know whether the variation is within the normal range or signals a change in the patient's condition. Thus, additional studies need to be conducted to describe patterns of physiological function over time.

In the previously discussed study using NIRS, Gelinas et al. (2010) conducted a repeated-measures design that involved obtaining measurements from 40 subjects at two test periods. The first test period occurred while patients were awake, and the rSO_2, CPOT, and FPT measurements were recorded for each subject. The second test period took place after the induction of anesthesia, and it was possible to record only the rSO_2. These simultaneous measurements of pain using various instruments as well as the repeated measures of the rSO_2 when patients were anesthetized allowed the examination of reliability and validity of the NIRS technique to measure rSO_2 as a pain indicator over time.

Selecting a Physiological Measure

Researchers designing a physiological study have less assistance in selecting methods of measurement than researchers conducting studies using psychosocial variables. Multiple books and electronic sources are available that discuss various methods for measuring psychosocial variables. In addition, numerous articles in nursing journals describe the development of psychosocial variables or discuss various means of measuring a particular psychosocial variable. However, literature guiding the selection of physiological variables is still sparse. You might consider the following factors when selecting a physiological measure for a study:

1. What physiological variables are relevant to the study?
2. Do the variables need to be measured continuously or at a particular point in time?
3. Are repeated measures needed?
4. Do certain characteristics of the population under study place limits on the measurement approaches that can be used?
5. How has the variable been measured in previous research?
6. Is more than one measurement method available to measure the physiological variable being studied (Stone & Frazier, 2010)?
7. Which measurement method is the most accurate and precise for the population you are studying (Fawcett & Garity, 2009; Ryan-Wenger, 2010)?
8. Could the study be designed to include more than one measurement method for the variable being studied (DeVon et al., 2007; Fawcett & Garity, 2009)?
9. Where can the measurement device or devices be obtained to measure the physiological variable being studied?
10. Can the measurement device be obtained from the manufacturer for use in the study, or must it be purchased?
11. What are the standards for the measurement device or equipment that has been designated nationally and internationally (International Organization for Standardization [IOS], 2011)?

It is more difficult to identify previous research on physiological measures than it is to find research on psychosocial measures. The sources most commonly used to identify physiological measurement methods are previous studies that have measured a particular physiological variable. Literature reviews or meta-analyses can provide reference lists of relevant studies. Because the measure might have been used in studies unrelated to the current research topic, it is usually important to examine the research literature broadly.

Physiological measures must be linked conceptually with the framework of the study. The logic of operationalizing the concept in a particular way must be well thought out and expressed clearly (see Chapter 7). It is often a good idea to use diverse physiological measures of a single concept, which reduces the impact of extraneous variables that might affect measurement. The operationalization of a physiological variable in a study should clearly indicate the physiological measure to be used. The link of the physiological variable to the concept in the framework must be made explicit in the published report of your study.

You also need to evaluate the accuracy and precision of physiological measures. Until more recently, researchers commonly used information from the equipment manufacturer to describe the accuracy of measurement. This information is useful, but it is insufficient to evaluate accuracy and precision. The accuracy and precision of physiological measures are discussed in Chapter 16 (CLSI, 2011; IOS, 2011; Ryan-Wenger, 2010).

You need to consider problems you might encounter when using various approaches to physiological measurement. One factor of concern is the sensitivity of the measure. Will the measure detect differences finely enough to avoid a type II error—known as a false negative—that occurs when the investigator claims there is no difference between groups or relationships among variables when one really exists (see Chapter 21)? Physiological measures are usually norm referenced. Data obtained from a study participant are compared with a norm as well as with other participants. You need to determine whether the norm used for comparison is relevant for the population you are studying. Laboratories are certified by ensuring that the analyses conducted in the laboratory meet a national standard (CLSI, 2011). New physiological measures are compared with the "gold standard" or the current best measurement method for a physiological variable. For example, Klein et al. (2010) compared their NPAT with the "gold standard" of the patients' self-reports of pain using the CPOT.

Many measurement strategies require the use of specialized equipment. In many cases, the equipment is available in the patient care area and is part of routine patient care in that unit. Otherwise, the researcher may need to purchase, rent, or borrow the equipment specifically for the study. You need to be skilled in operating the equipment or obtain the assistance of someone who has these skills. You need to ensure that the equipment is operated in an optimal fashion and is used in a consistent manner. Sometimes equipment must be recalibrated, or reset, regularly to ensure consistent readings. For example, weight scales are recalibrated periodically to ensure that the weight indicated is accurate and precise. According to federal guidelines, recalibration must be performed as follows:

- In accordance with the manufacturers' instructions
- In accordance with national and international standards (IOS, 2011)
- In accordance with criteria set up by the laboratory (CLSI, 2011)
- At least every 6 months
- After major preventive maintenance or replacement of a critical part
- When quality control indicates a need for recalibration

Reporting Physiological Measures in Studies

When publishing the results of a physiological study, researchers must describe the measurement technique in considerable detail to allow an adequate critical appraisal of the study, enable others to replicate the study, and promote clinical application of the results. At the present time, only a few physiological replication studies have been reported in the nursing literature. A detailed description of physiological measures in a research report includes the following:

1. Description of the equipment or device used in performing the measurement
2. Identification of the name of the equipment manufacturer
3. Account of the accuracy and precision of the equipment or device based on previous research, the manufacturers' specifications, and national and international standards
4. Explanation of the exact procedure followed to measure the physiological variable
5. Overview of the process the device used to record, retrieve, and store data

The examples discussed in this section can be used as models for describing the methods for obtaining and implementing physiological measures to obtain accurate and precise measures of physiological variables to ensure quality study outcomes.

Observational Measurement

Observational measurement is the use of unstructured and structured inspection to gauge a study variable. This section focuses on structured observational measurement; unstructured observational measurement is described in Chapter 12. Although data collection by observation is most common in qualitative research, it is used to some extent in all types of studies (Marshall & Rossman, 2011; Munhall, 2012). First, you must decide what you want to observe, and then you need to determine how to ensure that every variable is observed in a similar manner in each instance. Much attention must be given to training data collectors, especially when the observations are complex and examined over time (Waltz et al., 2010). You must create opportunities for the observational technique to be pilot-tested and to generate data on interrater reliability. Observational measurement tends to be more subjective than other types of measurement and is often seen as less credible. However, in many cases, observation is the only possible way to obtain important evidence for practice.

Structured Observations

The first step in a **structured observation** is to define carefully what specific behaviors or events are to be inspected or observed in a study. From that point, researchers determine how the observations are to be made, recorded, and coded. In most cases, the research team develops an observational checklist or category system to direct collecting, organizing, and sorting of the specific behaviors or events being observed. The extent to which these categories are exhaustive varies with the study.

Category Systems

The observational categories should be mutually exclusive. If the categories overlap, the observer will be faced with making judgments regarding which category should contain each observed behavior, and data collection and recording may be inconsistent. In some category systems, only the behavior that is of interest is recorded. Most category systems require the observer to make some inference from the observed event to the category. The greater the degree of inference required, the more difficult the category system is to use. Some systems are applicable in a wide variety of studies, whereas others are specific to the study for which they were designed. The number of categories used varies considerably with the study. An optimal number for ease of use and therefore effectiveness of observation is 15 to 20 categories.

Klein et al. (2010) developed the NPAT that was introduced earlier in this chapter. The NPAT included categories of behaviors that were to be observed to determine the pain level for nonverbal adults in the ICU (see Figure 17-4). The interrater reliability of the tool in this study was ensured when "Two RNs, trained in the use and scoring of the NPAT, simultaneously observed a patient unable to verbalize his or her pain" (Klein et al., 2010, p. 523).

Another type of category system used to direct the collection of observational data is a checklist. Observational checklists are techniques used to establish whether a behavior occurred. The observer places a tally mark on a data collection form each time he or she witnesses the behavior. Behavior other than that on the checklist is ignored. In some studies, the observer may place multiple tally marks in various categories while witnessing a particular event. However, in other studies, the observer is required to select a single category in which to place the tally mark.

Rating Scales

Rating scales (discussed in detail later in this chapter) can be used for observation and for self-reporting. A rating scale allows the observer to rate the behavior or event on a scale. This method provides more information for analysis than the use of dichotomous data, which indicate only that the behavior either occurred or did not occur. The NPAT also included a rating scale in which each observational category was scored on a scale or 0 to 2 or 0 to 3 (see Figure 17-4). The tool resulted in a total score between 0 and 10, with 0 indicating no pain and 10 indicating the worst pain ever experienced by the patient (Klein et al., 2010).

Interviews

Interviews involve verbal communication during which the subject provides information to the researcher. Although this measurement strategy is most common in qualitative and descriptive studies, it also can be used in other types of studies. The various approaches to conducting interviews range from very unstructured interviews in which study participants control content (see Chapter 12) to interviews in which the participants respond to a questionnaire that the researcher has carefully designed (Waltz et al., 2010). Although most interviews are conducted face to face, telephone interviews are also commonly used.

Using the interview method for measurement requires careful detailed work with a scientific approach. Excellent books are available on the techniques of developing interview questions (Briggs, 1986; Dillman, Smyth, & Christian, 2009; Dillon, 1990; Foddy, 1993; Fowler, 1990; Gorden, 1987, 1998; McLaughlin, 1990; Mishler, 1986). If you plan to use this strategy, consult a text on interview methodology before designing your instrument. Because nurses frequently use interview techniques in nursing assessment, the dynamics of interviewing are familiar; however, using this technique for measurement in research requires greater sophistication.

Structured Interviews

Structured interviews are verbal interactions with subjects that allow the researcher to exercise increasing amounts of control over the content of the interview to obtain essential data for a study. The researcher designs the questions before data collection begins, and the order of the questions is specified. In some cases, the interviewer is allowed to explain the meaning of the question further or modify the way in which the question is asked so that the subject can understand it better. In more structured interviews, the interviewer is required to ask the question precisely as it has been designed. If the subject does not understand the question, the interviewer can repeat it only. The subject may be limited to a range of responses previously developed by the researcher, similar to those in a questionnaire. If the possible responses are lengthy or complex, they may be printed on a card so that study participants can review them visually before selecting a response.

Designing Interview Questions

The process for developing and sequencing interview questions is similar to the process used to design questionnaires and is explained in the section on questionnaires. Briefly, questions progress from broad and general to narrow and specific. Questions are grouped by topic, with fairly "safe" topics being addressed first and sensitive topics reserved until late in the interview process. Other data such as age, educational level, income, and other demographic information are usually collected last. These data are best obtained from other sources, such as patient records, to allow more time for the primary interview questions. The wording of questions in an interview depends on the educational level of the study participants. Different participants may interpret the wording of certain questions in a variety of ways, and researchers need to anticipate this possibility. After the interview protocol has been developed, it is wise to seek feedback from an expert on interview technique and from a content expert.

Is patient able to make vocalizations or sound cues?
Score under the yes **or** no column; add scores for total score (range 0-10)

YES   **NO**

SCORE	EMOTION	An affective response to a situation	EMOTION		SCORE
	0	Smiling; calm; relaxed or none due to coma state or analgesia		0	
	1	Anxious; irritable; withdrawn; closes eyes; does not engage with physical environment		1	
	2	Tearful/crying **or** uncooperative		2	
	MOVEMENT	Change in placement and positioning of the body and extremities when not engaged in any care activities	**MOVEMENT**		
	0	None; sleeping comfortable; no unusual movements; **or** none due to coma state or analgesia		0	
	1	Restless **or** slow, decreased movement; reluctant to move; muscle tenseness		2	
	2	Rigidity; increasing motion; stiffening; tossing; turning; flapping of arms; stiffening		3	
	VERBAL CUES	Sound cues or vocalizations other than speech			
	0	No vocalization			
	1	Whimpering; moaning; sighing		n/a	
	2	Screaming; crying out			
	FACIAL CUES	Expressions on face	**FACIAL CUES**		
	0	Relaxed, calm expression **or** none due to coma state or analgesia		0	
	1	Drawn around the mouth and eyes; narrowed eyes		1	
	2	Wincing; grimacing; clenched teeth; furrowed brows; tightened lips		2	
	POSITIONING/GUARDING	Body responses that imply a protection of the body from contact with external touch	**POSITIONING/GUARDING**		
	0	Relaxed body **or** none due to coma state or analgesia		0	
	1	Guarding/tense		2	
	2	Jumpy when touched; clutching of siderails; withdraws when touched		3	
		TOTAL			

Choose only one behavior per category

Figure 17-4 Nonverbal Pain Assessment Tool–Final. (From Klein, D. G., Dumpe, M., Katz, E., & Bena, J. [2010]. Pain assessment in the intensive care unit: Development and psychometric testing of the nonverbal pain assessment tool. *Heart & Lung, 39*[6], 527.)

Pilot-Testing the Interview Protocol

After the research team has satisfactorily developed the interview protocol, team members need to pretest or pilot-test it on subjects similar to the individuals who will be included in their study. Pilot-testing allows the research team to identify problems in the design of questions, sequencing of questions, or procedure for recording responses. It also provides an opportunity to assess the reliability and validity of the interview instrument (Waltz et al., 2010).

Training Interviewers

Skilled interviewing requires practice, and interviewers must be familiar with the content of the interview. They need to anticipate situations that might occur during the interview and develop strategies for dealing with them. One of the most effective methods of developing a polished approach is role-playing. Playing the role of the subject can give the interviewer insight into the experience and facilitate an effective response to unscripted situations.

The interviewer must establish a permissive atmosphere in which the subject is encouraged to respond to sensitive topics. He or she also needs to develop an unbiased verbal and nonverbal manner. The wording of a question, the tone of voice, a raised eyebrow, and a shifting body position all can communicate a positive or negative reaction to the subject's responses—either of which can alter the data.

Preparing for an Interview

If you are serving as the interviewer and expect the meeting to be lengthy, you need to make an appointment. Dress nicely for the meeting, but do not overdress, and be prompt. Choose a site for the interview that is quiet and private and provides a pleasant environment. Before the appointment, carefully plan the instructions you will give to the subject. For example, you might say, "I am going to ask you a series of questions about …. Before you answer each question you need to …. Select your answer from the following …, and then you may elaborate on your response. I will record your answer and then, if it is not clear, I may ask you to explain some aspect further."

Probing

Interviewers use **probing** to obtain more information in a specific area of the interview. In some cases, you may have to repeat a question. If your subject answers, "I don't know," you may have to press for a response. In other situations, you may have to explain the question further or ask the subject to explain statements that he or she has made. At a deeper level, you may pick up on a comment the participant made and begin asking questions to understand better what the subject meant. Probes should be neutral to avoid biasing participants' responses. Probing for additional information needs to be done within reasonable guidelines so that participants do not feel they are being cross-examined.

Recording Interview Data

Data obtained from interviews are recorded, either during the interview or immediately afterward. The recording may be in the form of handwritten notes, video recordings, or audio recordings. If you hand-record your notes, you must have the skill to identify key ideas (or capture essential data) in an interview and concisely record this information. Data must be recorded without distracting the interviewee. Some interviewees have difficulty responding if it is obvious that the interviewer is taking notes or recording the conversation. In such a case, the interviewer may need to record data *after* completing the interview. If you wish to record the interview, you first must obtain IRB approval and then obtain the participant's permission. Plan to prepare verbatim transcriptions of the recordings before data analysis. In some studies, researchers use content analysis to capture the meaning within the data (see Chapter 12).

Advantages and Disadvantages of Interviews

Interviewing is a flexible technique that can allow researchers to explore greater depth of meaning than they can obtain with other techniques. Use your interpersonal skills to encourage your subject's cooperation and elicit more information. The response rate to interviews is higher than the response rate to questionnaires; thus interviews can offer a more representative sample. Interviews allow researchers to collect data from participants who are unable or unlikely to complete questionnaires, such as very ill subjects or subjects whose reading, writing, and ability to express themselves are marginal. Interviews are a form of self-report, and the researcher must assume that the information provided is accurate. Interviewing requires much more time than questionnaires and scales and is more costly. Because of time and cost, sample size is usually limited. Subject bias is always a threat to the validity of the findings, as is inconsistency in data collection from one subject to another (Dillman et al., 2009).

Interviewing children requires a special understanding of the art of asking children questions. The interviewer must use words that children tend to use to define situations and events. Interviewers also must be familiar with the language skills that exist at different stages of development. Children view topics differently than adults do. Their perception of time, past and present, is also different. Holaday and Turner-Henson (1989) provided detailed suggestions for developing an interview guide or questionnaire appropriate for children.

Some researchers use a combination of structured interview questions and open-ended or unstructured interview questions to gather the data needed for a study. Harralson (2007, p. 96) used structured and unstructured questions to examine the "factors associated with delay in seeking emergency medical attention for acute ischemic symptoms in a sample of predominantly African American women." Harralson interviewed female patients who presented with symptoms of acute myocardial infarction in a large, urban teaching hospital in the United States. The following excerpt describes the interview process used in this study.

"Structured Interview

"The study used a structured interview to explore the variables of interest. The 45-minute interview included questions pertaining to sociodemographics, social support, general physical health, medical comorbidities, perceived and practical barriers to seeking health care, and CHD [coronary heart disease] symptoms and severity. Open-ended questions addressed the patients' experiences from symptom onset until a decision was made to seek medical attention. Open-ended questions included questions about patients' physical and emotional feelings during the experience, decision-making processes (i.e., who they told and who they sought advice from), and beliefs about what was happening to them at the onset of the symptoms of AMI [acute myocardial infarction].

The structured interview was developed specifically for this study on the basis of a systematic review of the literature that examined concepts and factors associated with delay in seeking medical treatment. In addition, several nurses, cardiologists, and social scientists reviewed the interview.

To reduce recall bias in this study, interviews were conducted within 5 days of the acute ischemic event. This recall time frame is similar to time periods used in other studies reviewed in the background section." (Harralson, 2007, p. 98)

Questionnaires

A questionnaire is a printed self-report form designed to elicit information that can be obtained from a subject's written responses. The information derived through questionnaires is similar to information obtained by interview, but the questions tend to have less depth. The subject is unable to elaborate on responses or ask for questions to be clarified, and the data collector cannot use probe strategies. However, questions are presented in a consistent manner, and there is less opportunity for bias than in an interview.

Questionnaires can be designed to determine facts about the study participants or persons known by the participants; facts about events or situations known by the participants; or beliefs, attitudes, opinions, levels of knowledge, or intentions of the participants. Questionnaires can be distributed to large samples directly or indirectly through email or mail. The design, development, and administration of questionnaires have been addressed in many excellent books that focus on survey techniques (Berdie, Anderson, & Niebuhr, 1992; Converse & Presser, 1986; Saris & Gallhofer, 2007; Thomas, 2004). Two nursing methodology texts (Shelley, 1984; Waltz et al., 2010) provide detailed explanations of the procedure for questionnaire development.

Although questions on a questionnaire appear easy to design, a well-designed item requires considerable effort. Similar to interviews, questionnaires can have varying degrees of structure. Some questionnaires ask open-ended questions that require written responses. Others ask closed-ended questions with options that the researcher has selected. Data from open-ended questions are often difficult to interpret, and content analysis may be used to extract meaning. Open-ended questionnaire items are not advised if your data are being obtained from large samples.

Researchers frequently use computers to gather questionnaire data (Saris, 1991; Thomas, 2004). Computers are sometimes set up at the data collection site, such as a clinic or hospital; the questionnaire is presented on screen; and subjects respond by using the keyboard or mouse. Data are stored in a computer file and are immediately available for analysis. Data entry errors are greatly reduced. Most researchers email subjects and direct them to a website where they can complete the questionnaire online, allowing the data to be stored and analyzed immediately. Thus, researchers can keep track of the number of subjects completing their questionnaire and the evolving results.

Development of Questionnaires

The first step in either selecting or developing a questionnaire is to identify the information desired. For this purpose, the research team develops a blueprint or table of specifications. The blueprint identifies the essential content to be covered by the questionnaire; the content must be at the educational level of the potential subjects. It is difficult to stick to the blueprint when designing the questionnaire because it is tempting to add "just one more question" that seems to be a "neat idea" or a question that someone insists "really should be included." However, as a questionnaire lengthens, fewer subjects are willing to respond, and more questions are left blank.

The second step is to search the literature for questionnaires or items in questionnaires that match the blueprint criteria. Sometimes published studies include questionnaires, but frequently you must contact the authors of a study to request a copy of their questionnaire. Researchers are encouraged to use questions in exactly the same form as questionnaires in previous studies to determine the validity of the questionnaire for new samples. However, questions that are poorly written need to be modified, even if rewriting makes it more difficult to compare the validity results of the questionnaire directly with questionnaires from previous studies.

In some cases, you may find a questionnaire in the literature that matches the questionnaire blueprint that you have developed for your study. However, you may have to add items to or delete items from an existing questionnaire to accommodate your blueprint. In some situations, items from several questionnaires are combined to develop an appropriate questionnaire.

An item on a questionnaire has two parts: a question (or stem) and a response set. Each question must be carefully designed and clearly expressed. Problems include ambiguous or vague language, leading questions that influence the response, questions that assume a preexisting state of affairs, and double questions.

In some cases, respondents interpret terms used in the question in one way when the researcher intended a different meaning. For example, the researcher might ask how heavy the traffic is in the neighborhood in which the family lives. The researcher might be asking about automobile traffic, but the respondent interprets the question in relation to drug traffic. The researcher might define *neighborhood* as a region composed of a three-block area, whereas the respondent considers a neighborhood to be a much larger area. *Family* could be defined as people living in one house or as all close blood relations. If a question includes a term that is unfamiliar to the respondent or

for which several meanings are possible, the term must be defined (Saris & Gallhofer, 2007; Waltz et al., 2010).

Leading questions suggest to the respondent the answer the researcher desires. These types of questions often include value-laden words and indicate the researcher's bias. For example, a researcher might ask, "Do you believe physicians should be coddled on the nursing unit?" or "All hospitals are stressful places to work, aren't they?" These examples are extreme, and leading questions are usually constructed more subtly. The degree of formality with which the question is expressed and the permissive tone of the questions are, in many cases, important for obtaining a true measure. A permissive tone suggests that any of the possible responses would be acceptable.

Questions implying a preexisting state of affairs often lead respondents to admit to a previous behavior regardless of how they answer. Examples are "How long has it been since you used drugs?" or, to an adolescent, "Do you use a condom when you have sex?"

Double questions ask for more than one bit of information: "Do you like critical care nursing and working closely with physicians?" It would be possible for the respondent to like working in critical care settings but dislike working closely with physicians. In this case, the question would be impossible to answer accurately. A similar question is, "Was the in-service program educational and interesting?"

Questions with double negatives are often difficult for study participants to interpret. For example, one might ask, "Do you believe nurses should not question doctors' orders? Yes or No." In this case, the wording of this question can be easily misinterpreted and the word "not" possibly overlooked. This situation can lead participants to respond in a way contrary to how they actually think or feel.

Each item in a questionnaire has a **response set** that provides the parameters within which the respondent can answer. This response set can be open and flexible, as it is with open-ended questions, or it can be narrow and directive, as it is with closed-ended questions. For example, an open-ended question might have a response set of three blank lines. With closed-ended questions, the response set includes a specific list of alternatives from which to select.

Response sets can be constructed in various ways. The cardinal rule is that every possible answer must have a response category. If the sample includes respondents who might not have an answer, a response category of "don't know" or "uncertain" should be included. If the information sought is factual, include "other" as one of the possible responses. However, recognize that the item "other" is essentially lost data. Even if the response is followed by a statement such as "Please explain," it is rarely possible to analyze the data meaningfully. If a large number of study participants (>10%) select the alternative "other," the alternatives included in the response set might not be appropriate for the population studied (Saris & Gallhofer, 2007).

The simplest response set is the dichotomous yes/no option. Arranging responses vertically preceded by a blank reduces errors. For example,

_____ Yes
_____ No

is better than

_____ Yes _____ No

because in the latter example, the respondent might not be sure whether to indicate yes by placing a response before or after the "Yes."

Response sets must be mutually exclusive, which might not be the case in the following response set because a respondent might legitimately need to select two responses:

_____ Working full-time
_____ Full-time graduate student
_____ Working part-time
_____ Part-time graduate student

Cazzell (2010) developed the Self-Report College Student Risk Behavior Questionnaire, an eight-item questionnaire with response set of yes and no possible answers. This questionnaire was developed and refined as part of her dissertation at The University of Texas at Arlington. Cazzell's questionnaire was developed based on the 87 risk behaviors identified in a national survey conducted by the U.S. Centers for Disease Control and Prevention on the *Youth Risk Behavior Surveillance System* (Brener et al., 2004). Cazzell's (2010) Self-Report College Student Risk Behavior Questionnaire was developed based on the eight most commonly identified adolescent risk behaviors from the Centers for Disease Control and Prevention survey. Content validity of this eight-item questionnaire was developed by having two addiction experts, a doctorally prepared social worker and a pediatric clinical nurse specialist evaluate the items. The content validity index calculated for the questionnaire was 0.88, supporting the inclusion of these eight items in the questionnaire. Cazzell (2011) continued her development and refinement of this questionnaire and expanded question #2 on use of alcohol to target binge drinking (see Figure 17-5).

The questionnaire instructions should be pilot-tested on naive subjects who are willing and able to express their reactions to the instructions. Each question should clearly instruct the subject how to respond (i.e., choose one, mark all that apply), or instructions should be included at the beginning of the questionnaire. The subject must know whether to circle, underline, or fill in a circle as he or she responds to items. Clear instructions are difficult to construct and usually require several attempts. Cazzell (2011) provided clear directions and an example of how to complete her questionnaire and directed the students to report their participation in these risk behaviors over the past 30 days (see Figure 17-5).

After the questionnaire items have been developed, you need to plan carefully how they will be ordered. Questions related to a specific topic must be grouped together. General items are included first with progression to more specific items. More important items might be included first, with subsequent progression to items of lesser importance. Questions of a sensitive nature or questions that might be threatening should appear last on the questionnaire. In some cases, the response to one item may influence the response to another. If so, the order of such items must be carefully considered. Open-ended questions should be presented last because their responses require more time than needed for closed-ended questions. The general trend is to ask for demographic data about the subject at the end of the questionnaire.

An introductory page in the computer or a cover letter for a mailed questionnaire is needed to explain the purpose of the study and identify the researchers, the approximate amount of time required to complete the form, and organizations or institutions supporting the study. Often researchers indicate that completion of the questionnaire implies informed consent. A questionnaire on the computer when completed can be easily submitted, and the data can be analyzed immediately. Returning mailed questionnaires is much more complex. The instructions need to include an address to which the questionnaire can be returned. This address must be at the end of the questionnaire and on the cover letter and envelope. Respondents often discard both the envelope and the cover letter and do not know where to send the questionnaire after completing it. It is also wise to provide a stamped, addressed envelope for the subject to return the questionnaire. If possible, the best way to provide questionnaires to potential subjects is by emailing a web address so participants can easily complete the questionnaire in their own time, and their responses are automatically submitted at the end of the questionnaire. Sending questionnaires by email has many advantages, but one disadvantage is being able to access only individuals with email. Researchers need

Unique ID:

Self-Report College Student Risk Behavior Measure

Shade Circles Like This --> ●
Not Like This --> ⊠ ✓

Answer YES or NO based on your participation in these behaviors over the past 30 days.

1. I smoked a cigarette (even a puff). ○ Yes ○ No

2. I drank alcohol (even one drink). ○ Yes ○ No
   If you answered YES to Question #2:

   a. If you are a female, did you have 4 or ○ Yes ○ No
   more drinks on one occasion?

   b. If you are a male, did you have 5 or ○ Yes ○ No
   more drinks on one occasion?

3. I used an illegal drug (even once). ○ Yes ○ No

4. I had sexual intercourse without a condom. ○ Yes ○ No

5. I rode in a car without wearing my seatbelt ○ Yes ○ No
   (even once).

6. I drove a car without wearing my seatbelt ○ Yes ○ No
   (even once).

7. I rode in a car with a person driving under ○ Yes ○ No
   the influence (even once).

8. I drove a car while under the influence ○ Yes ○ No
   (even once).

Figure 17-5 Self-Report College Student Risk Behavior Questionnaire. (From Cazzell, M. [personal communication, March 20, 2011]. Self-report college student risk behavior questionnaire. The University of Texas at Arlington, Arlington, TX.)

to determine if the population they are studying has email access (Thomas, 2004).

Your questionnaire must be pilot-tested to determine the clarity of questions, effectiveness of instructions, completeness of response sets, time required to complete the questionnaire, and success of data collection techniques. As with any pilot test, the subjects and techniques must be as similar as possible to those planned for the main study. In some cases, the open-ended questions are included in a pilot test to obtain information for the development of closed-ended response sets for the main study.

Questionnaire Validity

One of the greatest risks in developing response sets is leaving out an important alternative or response. For example, if the questionnaire item addressed the job position of nurses working in a hospital and the sample included nursing students, a category must be added to represent the student role. When seeking opinions, there is a risk of obtaining a response from an individual who actually has no opinion on the research topic. When an item requests knowledge that the respondent does not possess, the subject's guessing interferes with obtaining a true measure of the study variables.

The response rate to questionnaires is generally lower than that with other forms of self-reporting, particularly if the questionnaires are mailed out. If the response rate is less than 50%, the representativeness of the sample is seriously in question. The response rate for mailed questionnaires is usually small (25% to 35%), so researchers are frequently unable to obtain a representative sample, even with randomization. There seems to be a stronger response rate for questionnaires that are sent by email, but the response is still usually less than 50%. Strategies that can increase the response rate for an emailed or mailed questionnaire are discussed in Chapter 20.

Study participants commonly fail to respond to all the questions on a questionnaire. This problem, especially with long questionnaires, can threaten the validity of the instrument. In some cases, study participants may write in an answer if they do not agree with the available choices, or they might write comments in the margin. Generally, these responses cannot be included in the analysis; however, you should keep a record of such responses. These responses might be used later to refine the questionnaire questions and responses.

Consistency in the way the questionnaire is administered is important to validity. Variability that could confound the interpretation of the data reported by the study participants is introduced by administering some questionnaires in a group setting, mailing some questionnaires, and emailing some questionnaires. There should not be a mix of mailing or emailing to business addresses and to home addresses. If questionnaires are administered in person, the administration needs to be consistent. Several problems in consistency can occur: (1) Some subjects may ask to take the form home to complete it and return it later, whereas others will complete it in the presence of the data collector; (2) some subjects may complete the form themselves, whereas others may ask a family member to write the responses that the respondent dictates; and (3) in some cases, a secretary or colleague may complete the form, rather than the individual whose response you are seeking. These situations may lead to biases in responses that are unknown to the researcher and can alter the true measure of the variables.

Analysis of Questionnaire Data

Data from questionnaires are often at the nominal or ordinal level of measurement, which limit analyses for the most part to descriptive statistics, such as frequencies and percentages, and nonparametric inferential statistics, such as chi square, Spearman rank-order correlation, and Mann-Whitney U (see Chapters 22 through 25). However, in certain cases, ordinal data from questionnaires are treated as interval data, and t-tests and analysis of variance are used to test for differences between responses of various subsets of the sample (Grove, 2007). Discriminant analysis may be used to determine the ability to predict membership in various groups from responses to particular questions.

Scales

Scales, a form of self-report, are a more precise means of measuring phenomena than questionnaires. Most scales have been developed to measure psychosocial variables. However, self-reports can be obtained on physiological variables such as pain, nausea, or functional capacity by using scaling techniques as discussed earlier in this chapter. Scaling is based on mathematical theory, and there is a branch of science whose primary concern is the development of measurement scales. From the point of view of scaling theory, considerable measurement error, both random and systematic error, is expected in a single item. Therefore, in most scales, the various items on the scale are summed to obtain a single score, and these scales are referred to as summated scales. Less random and systematic error exists when using the total score of a scale in conducting data analyses, although subscale comparisons are usually of interest and are conducted. Using several items in a scale to measure a concept is comparable to using several instruments to measure a concept (see Figure 16-4 in Chapter 16). The various items in a scale increase the dimensions of the concept that are reflected in the instrument. The types of scales commonly used in nursing studies include rating scale, Likert scale, semantic differential scale, and visual analogue scale (VAS).

Rating Scale

A rating scale lists an ordered series of categories of a variable that are assumed to be based on an underlying continuum. A numerical value is assigned to each category, and the fineness of the distinctions between categories varies with the scale, making this one of the crudest forms of scaling technique. The general public commonly uses rating scales. In conversations, one can hear statements such as "On a scale of 1 to 10, I would rank that …." Rating scales are easy to develop; however, one must be careful to avoid end statements that are so extreme that no subject would select them.

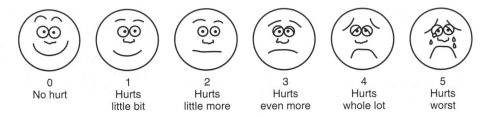

Figure 17-6 Wong-Baker FACES Pain Rating Scale. (From Hockenberry, M. J., & Wilson, D. [2009]. *Wong's essentials of pediatric nursing* [8th ed., p. 1203]. St. Louis, MO: Mosby.).

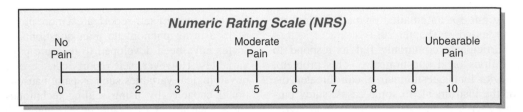

Figure 17-7 Numeric Rating Scale (NRS).

A rating scale could be used to rate the degree of cooperativeness of the patient or the value placed by the subject on nurse-patient interactions. This type of scale is often used in observational measurement to guide data collection. The Wong-Baker FACES Pain Rating Scale is commonly used to assess the pain of children in clinical practice and has been shown to be valid and reliable over the years (Figure 17-6) (Hockenberry & Wilson, 2009). Pain in adults is often assessed with a numeric rating scale such as the one presented in Figure 17-7. Klein et al. (2010) developed the NPAT rating scale, which was introduced earlier in this chapter to determine the pain level for nonverbal adults in the ICU (see Figure 17-4).

Likert Scale

The Likert scale determines the opinion or attitude of a subject and contains a number of declarative statements with a scale after each statement. The Likert scale is the most commonly used of the scaling techniques in nursing and healthcare studies. The original version of the scale included five response categories. Each response category was assigned a value, with a value of 1 given to the most negative response and a value of 5 given to the most positive response (Nunnally & Bernstein, 1994).

Response choices in a Likert scale most commonly address agreement, evaluation, or frequency. Agreement options may include statements such as *strongly agree, agree, uncertain, disagree,* and *strongly disagree*. Evaluation responses ask the respondent for an evaluative rating along a good/bad continuum, such as positive to negative or excellent to poor. Frequency responses may include statements such as *never, rarely, sometimes, frequently,* and *all the time*. The terms used are versatile and must be selected for their appropriateness to the stem (Spector, 1992). Sometimes seven options are given, and sometimes only four options are given.

Use of the uncertain or neutral category is controversial because it allows the subject to avoid making a clear choice of positive or negative statements. Thus, sometimes only four or six options are offered, with the uncertain category omitted. This type of scale is referred to as a forced choice version. Sometimes respondents become annoyed at forced choice items and refuse to complete them. Researchers who use the forced choice version consider an item that is left blank as a response of "uncertain." However, responses of "uncertain" are difficult to interpret, and if a large number of respondents select that option or leave the question blank, the data may be of little value.

How the researcher phrases item stems depends on the type of judgment that the respondent is being asked to make. Agreement items are declarative statements such as "Nurses should be held accountable for managing a patient's pain." Frequency items can be behaviors, events, or circumstances to which the respondent can indicate how often they occur. A frequency stem might be "You read research articles in nursing journals." An evaluation stem could be "The effectiveness of 'X' drug for relief of nausea after chemotherapy." Items must be clear, concise, and concrete (Spector, 1992).

An instrument using a Likert scale usually consists of 15 to 30 items, each addressing an element of the concept being measured. Half the statements should be expressed positively and half should be expressed negatively, termed *counterbalancing,* to avoid inserting response-set bias into the participants' responses. Response-set bias tends to occur when participants anticipate that either the positive or the negative (agree or disagree) response is consistently provided either in the right or left hand columns of the scale. Participants might note a pattern that agreeing with scale items consistently falls to the right and disagreeing to the left. Thus, they might fail to read all questions carefully and just mark the right or left column based on whether they agree or disagree with scale items. Response-set bias can be avoided by wording some scale items positively and other items negatively. Participants would need to mark some items in the right column (agree) and others in the left column (disagree) of the scale based on their sentiments.

Scale values of negatively worded items must be reversed before analysis so that the participants' agreement with certain positively worded items and, accordingly, their disagreement with negatively worded items on the same scale have higher scale values or scores reflecting their agreement. Usually, the values obtained from each item in the instrument are summed to obtain a single score for each subject. Although the values of each item are technically ordinal-level data, the summed score is often treated as interval-level data, allowing more sophisticated parametric statistical analyses (Nunnally & Bernstein, 1994).

The Center for Epidemiological Studies Depression Scale (CES-D) is an example of a 4-point Likert scale that is commonly used to measure depression in nursing studies (Figure 17-8). The CES-D was developed by Radloff in 1977 and has shown to be a reliable and valid measure of depression. Beckie, Beckstead, Schocken, Evans, and Fletcher (2011) implemented a tailored cardiac rehabilitation program to determine its effect on the depressive symptoms of women with coronary heart disease. In this randomized clinical trial, the CES-D was used to measure depressive symptoms in the women and is described in the following excerpt.

Psychological Outcome

"The 20-item Center for Epidemiological Studies Depression Scale (CES-D) (Radloff, 1977) measured depressive symptoms [see Figure 17-8]. Participants reported the frequency of occurrence of depressive symptoms during the past week ranging from 0 ([Rarely or none of the time or] < a day) to 3 (Most of the time [5-7 days]). Scores range from 0 to 60 with higher scores reflecting greater depressive symptoms. Used extensively in CHD [coronary heart disease] populations (Beckie, Fletcher, Beckstead, Schocken, & Evans, 2008; Dunn, Corser, Stommel, & Holmes-Rovner, 2006; Scholz, Knoll, Sniehotta, & Schwarzer, 2006; Swardfager et al., 2008), a score of 16 is typically the cut-off score for an elevated level of depressive symptoms. Evidence of concurrent validity, construct validity, and reliability of the CES-D has also been provided for community samples (Radloff, 1977). Cronbach's alpha in the current study at all three time-points was over .90." (Beckie et al., 2011, p. 6)

Beckie et al. (2011) clearly described the CES-D used to measure depression in their study. The scoring of the scale was discussed with a score of 16 indicating elevated depressive symptoms in women with coronary heart disease. The reliability of the scale for this study was strong ($r = .90$). The discussion of the scale would have been strengthened by expanding the validity and reliability information from previous research. Beckie et al. (2011) found that the gender-tailored cardiac rehabilitation program significantly reduced the depressive symptoms of the women compared with the traditional cardiac rehabilitation program.

Semantic Differential Scale

The semantic differential scale was developed by Osgood, Suci, and Tannenbaum (1957) to measure attitudes or beliefs. It is now used more broadly to measure variations in views of a concept. A semantic differential scale consists of two opposite adjectives with a 7-point scale between them. The subject is to select 1 point on the scale that best describes his or her view of the concept being examined. The scale is designed to measure the connotative meaning of the concept to the subject. Although the adjectives may not seem to be particularly related to the concept being examined, the technique can be used to distinguish varying degrees of positive and negative attitudes

Center for Epidemiologic Studies Depression Scale
DEPA

THESE QUESTIONS ARE ABOUT HOW YOU HAVE BEEN FEELING LATELY.
AS I READ THE FOLLOWING STATEMENTS, PLEASE TELL ME HOW OFTEN YOU FELT OR
BEHAVED THIS WAY IN THE <u>LAST WEEK</u>. [*Hand card*]. **FOR EACH STATEMENT, DID YOU FEEL
THIS WAY:** [Interviewer: You may help respondent focus on the whichever "style" answer is easier]

    0 = **R**arely or none of the time (or less than 1 day)?
    1 = **S**ome or a little of the time (or 1-2 days)?
    2 = **O**ccasionally or a moderate amount of time (or 3-4 days)?
    3 = **M**ost or all of the time (or 5-7 days)?

		R	S	O	M	NR
1.	I WAS BOTHERED BY THINGS THAT USUALLY DON'T BOTHER ME.	0	1	2	3	--
2.	I DID NOT FEEL LIKE EATING; MY APPETITE WAS POOR.	0	1	2	3	--
3.	I FELT THAT I COULD NOT SHAKE OFF THE BLUES EVEN WITH HELP FROM MY FAMILY AND FRIENDS.	0	1	2	3	--
4.	I FELT THAT I WAS JUST AS GOOD AS OTHER PEOPLE.	0	1	2	3	--
5.	I HAD TROUBLE KEEPING MY MIND ON WHAT I WAS DOING.	0	1	2	3	--
6.	I FELT DEPRESSED.	0	1	2	3	--
7.	I FELT THAT EVERYTHING I DID WAS AN EFFORT.	0	1	2	3	--
8.	I FELT HOPEFUL ABOUT THE FUTURE.	0	1	2	3	--
9.	I THOUGHT MY LIFE HAD BEEN A FAILURE.	0	1	2	3	--
10.	I FELT FEARFUL.	0	1	2	3	--
11.	MY SLEEP WAS RESTLESS.	0	1	2	3	--
12.	I WAS HAPPY.	0	1	2	3	--
13.	I TALKED LESS THAN USUAL.	0	1	2	3	--
14.	I FELT LONELY.	0	1	2	3	--
15.	PEOPLE WERE UNFRIENDLY.	0	1	2	3	--
16.	I ENJOYED LIFE.	0	1	2	3	--
17.	I HAD CRYING SPELLS.	0	1	2	3	--
18.	I FELT SAD.	0	1	2	3	--
19.	I FELT PEOPLE DISLIKED ME.	0	1	2	3	--
20.	I COULD NOT GET GOING.	0	1	2	3	--

Figure 17-8 Center for Epidemiologic Studies Depression Scale (CES-D). (From Radloff, L. S. [1977]. The CES-D scale: A self-report depression scale for research in the general population. *Applied Psychological Measures, 1,* 385–394.)

toward a concept. Figure 17-9 illustrates the form used for this type of scale.

In a semantic differential scale, values from 1 to 7 are assigned to each of the spaces, with 1 being the most negative response and 7 the most positive. Placement of negative responses to the left or right of the scale should be randomly varied to avoid global responses (in which the subject places checks in the same column of each scale). Each line is considered one scale, and the values for the scales are summed to obtain one score for each subject. Factor analysis is used to determine the factor structure, which is expected to reflect three factors or dimensions: (1) evaluation, (2) potency, and (3) activity (Osgood et al., 1957). Researchers need to explain theoretically why particular items on the scale cluster together in the factor analysis. Thus, development of the instrument contributes to theory development. Factor analysis is also used to evaluate the construct validity of the instrument. With some of these instruments, three

Nursing Research

| Logical | |____|____|____|____|____|____|____| | Illogical |

| Insignificant | |____|____|____|____|____|____|____| | Significant |

| Structured | |____|____|____|____|____|____|____| | Unstructured |

| Active | |____|____|____|____|____|____|____| | Passive |

| Organized | |____|____|____|____|____|____|____| | Disorganized |

Figure 17-9 Example items from a semantic differential scale to measure nursing research.

| Scientific | |____|____|____|____|____|____|____| | Unscientific |

| Important to Practice | |____|____|____|____|____|____|____| | Unimportant to Practice |

| Lacking Rigor | |____|____|____|____|____|____|____| | Rigorous |

| Detailed | |____|____|____|____|____|____|____| | Vague |

| Boring | |____|____|____|____|____|____|____| | Exciting |

factor scores, each representing one of the dimensions, are used to describe the subject's responses and provide for further analysis (Nunnally & Bernstein, 1994).

Chase (2011) conducted a quasi-experimental study to examine the effect of an intergenerational email project on the attitudes of college students toward older adults. The college students were paired with older adults with whom they exchanged emails for 6 weeks. The students' attitudes toward the older adults were measured with the Aging Semantic Differential (ASD). The ASD includes 32 bipolar adjectives with a 7-point linear scale between them. The college students indicated their degree of agreement with each pair of the adjectives on a scale from 1 to 7. Chase found that the emailing intervention significantly improved the college students' attitudes toward older adults in the experimental group versus the students in the comparison group.

Visual Analogue Scale

One of the problems with scaling procedures is the difficulty of obtaining a fine discrimination of values. In an effort to resolve this problem, the visual analogue scale was developed to measure magnitude, strength, and intensity of an individual's sensations or

feelings (Wewers & Lowe, 1990). The VAS is referred to as *magnitude scaling* (Gift, 1989). This technique seems to provide interval-level data, and some researchers argue that it provides ratio-level data (Sennott-Miller, Murdaugh, & Hinshaw, 1988). It is particularly useful in scaling stimuli. This scaling technique has been used to measure pain, mood, anxiety, alertness, craving for cigarettes, quality of sleep, attitudes toward environmental conditions, functional abilities, and severity of clinical symptoms (Waltz et al., 2010; Wewers & Lowe, 1990).

The stimuli must be defined in a way that the subject clearly understands. Only one major cue should appear for each scale. The scale is a line 100 mm in length with right-angle stops at each end. The line may be horizontal or vertical as shown in Figure 17-10. Bipolar anchors are placed beyond each end of the line. The anchors should *not* be placed underneath or above the line before the stop. These end anchors should include the entire range of sensations possible in the phenomenon being measured. Examples include "all" and "none," "best" and "worst," and "no pain" and "worst pain imaginable" (see Figure 17-10).

The VAS is frequently used in healthcare research because it is easy to construct, administer, and score.

Figure 17-10 Example of a visual analogue scale to measure pain.

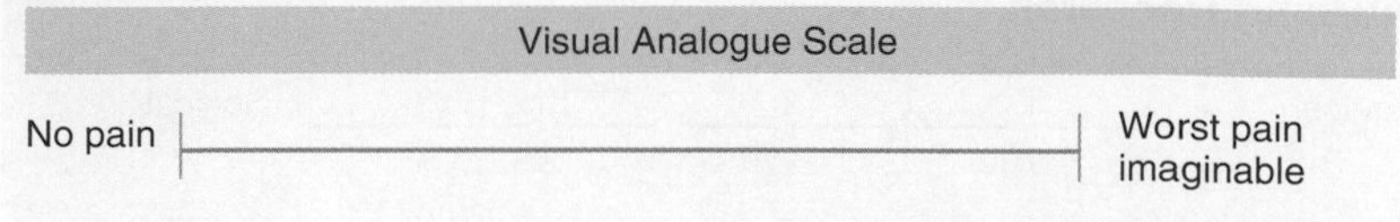

Visual Analogue Scale

No pain |——————————————————————————————| Worst pain imaginable

A VAS can be administered using a drawn, printed, or computer-generated 100-mm line (Raven et al., 2008; Waltz et al., 2010). The research participant is asked to place a mark through the line to indicate the intensity of the sensation or stimulus. A ruler is used to measure the distance between the left end of the line and the mark placed by the subject. This measure is the value of the subject's sensation. With a computer-generated VAS, research participants can touch the VAS line on the computer screen to indicate the degree of their sensations, such as pain. The computer can determine the value of the sensation for each subject and store it in a database (Raven et al., 2008). The scale is designed to be used while the subject is seated. Whether use of the scale from the supine position influences the results by altering perception of the length of the line has yet to be determined (Gift, 1989). A VAS can be developed for children by using pictorial anchors at each end of the line rather than words (Lee & Kieckhefer, 1989).

Wewers and Lowe (1990) published an extensive evaluation of the reliability and validity of VAS, although reliability is difficult to determine. Reliability of the VAS is most often determined with the test-retest method, which is effective if the variable being measured is fairly stable, such as chronic pain. Because most of the variables measured with the VAS are labile, test-retest consistency is not applicable, and because a single measure is obtained, internal consistency cannot be examined. The VAS is more sensitive to small changes than numerical and rating scales and can discriminate between two dimensions of pain.

Validity of the VAS has most commonly been determined by comparing VAS scores with other measures of a concept. Winkelman, Norman, Maloni, and Kless (2008) compared VAS scores with dermatome assessment in measuring pain during labor. The following study excerpt describes the agreement between these two measures of pain in laboring women who received an epidural analgesia.

"The Visual Analogue Sensation of Pain Scale was used to measure patient reports of labor pain. The solid line was vertical in this study, with *no pain* anchoring the bottom of the line and *worst pain*

imaginable at the top of the line (Gagliese, Weizblit, Ellis, & Chan, 2005). A mark at the bottom (i.e., zero) indicated no pain; 100 was the greatest value of pain. Each subject placed a mark on the vertical line to represent the level of pain or discomfort. A superimposed transparency marked in 1-mm increments was used to record the distance of each subject's mark from the bottom of the line. Intrarater reliability for VAS values was set at 2 mm; 90% agreement was maintained.... A standard dermatome chart was also used in data collection.... Dermatomes represent sensory input from spinal nerves to specific areas of the skin." (Winkelman et al., 2008, pp. 105-106)

"VAS and dermatome levels were moderately correlated at each time point with Pearson's r ranging from .331 to .546 ($p > .05$).... Overall, there was insufficient agreement on the intensity of pain sensation between dermatome level and VAS scores.... The lack of agreement between dermatome levels and VAS scores indicates that one value cannot be substituted for another. Specifically, the assessment of dermatome level provided an equivalent substitute for the VAS as a measure of pain in laboring women only at 20 minutes following epidural analgesia administration." (Winkelman et al., 2008, pp. 107-108)

Winkelman et al. (2008) clearly described the VAS used in their study and how the scale was administered and scored. These researchers found that both the VAS and the dermatome assessment were easy to use during labor and were good measures of pain shortly after epidural anesthesia. However, one measure could not be substituted for the other, and the best measure of pain in laboring women is currently dermatome assessment. Other studies comparing the VAS with other instruments measuring the same construct have had varying positive and negative results. Additional research is needed with the VAS to ensure it is a reliable and valid measure of certain patients' sensations (Waltz et al., 2010).

Q-Sort Methodology

Q-sort methodology is a technique of comparative rating that preserves the subjective point of view of the individual (McKeown & Thomas, 1988). Cards are used to categorize the importance placed on various words or phrases in relation to the other words or phrases in the list. Each phrase is placed on a separate card. The number of cards should range from 40 to 100 (Tetting, 1988). The subject is instructed to sort the cards into a designated number of piles, usually 7 to 10 piles ranging from the most to the least important. However, the subject is limited in the number of cards that may be placed in each pile. If the subject must sort 60 cards, category 1 (of greatest importance) may allow only 2 cards; category 2, 5 cards; category 3, 10 cards; category 4, 26 cards; category 5, 10 cards; category 6, 5 cards; and category 7 (the least important), 2 cards. Placement of the cards fits the pattern of a normal curve. The subject is usually advised to select first the cards that he or she wishes to place in the two extreme categories and then work toward the middle category (which contains the largest number of cards), rearranging cards until he or she is satisfied with the results. When sorting the cards, subjects might be encouraged to make comments about the statements on the cards and provide a rationale for the categories where they placed the cards (Akhtar-Danesh, Baumann, & Cordingley, 2008; Dariel, Wharrad, & Windle, 2010).

The Q-sort method can also be used to determine the priority of items or the most important items to include in the development of a scale. In the previously mentioned example, the behaviors sorted into categories 1, 2, and 3 might be organized into a 17-item scale. Correlational or factor analysis is used to analyze the data (Dariel et al., 2010; Dennis, 1986; Tetting, 1988). Simpson (1989) suggested using the Q-sort method for cross-cultural research, with pictures rather than words used for nonliterate groups.

Dariel et al. (2010) used the Q-sort methodology to examine faculty views toward the use of technology in nursing education. They described the Q-sort methodology in-depth in their article, and the following excerpt includes the Q-sort methodology they used in their study.

"The Q-sort [methodology] typically consists of a number of statements printed on small cards, which participants rank according to a 'condition of instruction.' This act of ranking each statement in relation to others, rather than evaluating them individually, is designed to capture the way people think about ideas in relation to other ideas rather than in isolation (Akhtar-Danesh et al., 2008)." (Dariel et al., 2010, p. 60)

"Statements with which participants most agree are placed on the far right of the grid, whereas those with which they most disagree are placed on the far left. Cards are then placed in each subsequent column based on their views towards the previous cards. While participants read the statements, they are asked to make comments about their interpretation of the statements and their placement on the grid.

"During the pilot study, participants were asked to read the statements using a specific 'condition of instruction' to guide the sort and provide a lens through which to read each statement. The guiding statement was 'Think about the issues which might be influencing your approach to using technology in your teaching practice as you read and sort the statements according to how you most agree or most disagree with how they each impact your use (or decision not to use) e-learning.' Participants then placed each statement into a quasi-normal distribution grid with 11 categories ranging from −5 to +5." (Dariel et al., 2010, pp. 67-68)

Delphi Technique

The Delphi technique measures the judgments of a group of experts for the purpose of making decisions, assessing priorities, or making forecasts (Vernon, 2009). Using this technique allows a wide variety of experts to express opinions and provide feedback, nationally and internationally, without meeting together. When the Delphi technique is used, the opinions of individuals cannot be altered by the persuasive behavior of a few people at a meeting. Three types of Delphi techniques have been identified: classic or consensus Delphi, dialectic Delphi, and decision Delphi. In classic Delphi, the focus is on reaching consensus. Dialectic Delphi is sometimes called policy Delphi, and the aim is not consensus but rather to identify and understand a variety of viewpoints and resolve disagreements. In decision Delphi, the panel consists of individuals in decision-making positions. The purpose is to come to a decision (Vernon, 2009; Waltz et al., 2010). Mitchell (1998) assessed the validity of the Delphi technique in nursing education planning and found that 98.1% of the predicted events had either occurred or were still expected to occur.

To implement the Delphi technique, researchers identify a panel of experts, who have a variety of

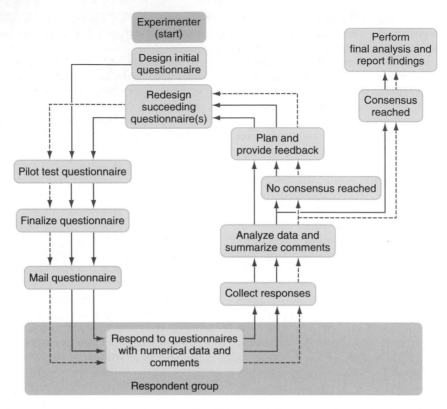

Figure 17-11 **Delphi technique sequence model. Multiple arrows indicate repeated cycles of review by experts.**

perceptions, personalities, interests, and demographics to reduce biases in the process. Members of the panel usually remain anonymous to each other. A questionnaire is developed that addresses the topics of concern. Although most questions call for closed-ended responses, the questionnaire usually contains opportunities for open-ended responses by the expert. Once they have completed the questionnaires, the respondents return them to the researcher, who then analyzes and summarizes the results. The statistical analyses usually include measures of central tendency and measures of dispersion. The role of the researcher is to maintain objectivity. The outcome of the statistical analysis is returned to the panel of experts, along with a second questionnaire. Respondents with extreme responses to the first round of questions may be asked to justify their responses. The respondents return the second round of questionnaires to the researcher for analysis. This procedure is repeated until the data reflect a consensus among the panel. Limiting the process to two or three rounds is not a good idea if consensus is the goal. In some studies, true consensus is reached, whereas in others, "majority rules." Some authors question whether the agreement reached is genuine (Vernon, 2009; Waltz et al., 2010). Couper (1984) developed a model of the Delphi technique, which is presented in Figure 17-11. This model might assist you in implementing a Delphi technique in a study.

Vernon (2009) identified benefits and limitations of the Delphi technique. The benefits include increased access to experts and usually good response rates. The Delphi design has simplicity and flexibility in its use; it is easily understood and implemented by researchers. Because the participants are anonymous, views can be expressed freely without direct persuasion from others.

There are also several potential problems that researchers could encounter when using the Delphi technique. There has been no documentation that the responses of "experts" are different from responses one would receive from a random sample of subjects. Because the panelists are anonymous, they have no accountability for their responses. Respondents could make hasty, ill-considered judgments because they know that no negative feedback would result. Feedback on the consensus of the group tends to centralize opinion, and traditional analysis with the use of means and medians may mask the responses of individuals who are resistant to the consensus sentiment. Conclusions could be misleading (Vernon, 2009).

Some nursing specialty organizations have established their research priorities by using Delphi techniques. Lindeman (1975) conducted one of the initial studies using the Delphi technique to determine research priorities in clinical nursing. She used a panel of 433 experts, nurses and nonnurses, with a wide range of interests. The panel was sent four rounds of a 150-item questionnaire. The report, published in *Nursing Research,* had an important influence on the research conducted in nursing for clinical practice.

Wilkes, Mohan, Luck, and Jackson (2010) used the Delphi technique to develop a violence assessment tool for a hospital emergency department. The following excerpt from their study describes the methodology they used.

"The aim of this study was to develop a violence assessment tool by refining a list of predictive cues identified from both a previous study and existing literature. Using the Delphi technique, a panel of 11 expert nurse academics and clinicians developed a 37-item questionnaire and used three rounds of Delphi to refine the violence assessment questionnaire. The resulting tool comprises 17 cues of potential violence that can be easily observed and requires no prior knowledge of the perpetrators' medical history." (Wilkes et al., 2010, p. 70)

Diaries

A **diary** is a recording of events over time by an individual to document experiences, feelings, or behavior patterns. Diaries are also called logs or journals and have been used since the 1950s to collect data for research from various populations including children, patients with acute and chronic illness, pregnant women, and elderly adults (Aroian & Wal, 2007; Nicholl, 2010). A diary, which allows recording shortly after an event, is thought to be more accurate than obtaining the information through recall during an interview. In addition, the reporting level of incidents is higher, and one tends to capture the participant's immediate perception of situations.

The diary technique gives nurse researchers a means to obtain data on topics of particular interest within nursing that have not been accessible by other means. Some potential topics for diary collection include expenses related to a healthcare event (particularly out-of-pocket expenses), self-care activities

(frequency and time required), symptoms of disease, eating behavior, exercise behavior, sexual activities, the child development process, and care provided by family members in a home-care situation. Although diaries have been used primarily with adults, they are also an effective means of collecting data from school-age children.

Health diaries have been used to document health problems, responses to symptoms, and efficacy of responses. Diaries may also be used to determine how people spend their days; this information could be particularly useful in managing the care needs of individuals with chronic illnesses. In experimental studies, diaries may be used to determine responses of subjects to experimental treatments. Diaries can take a variety of forms and might include filling in blanks, selecting the best response from a list of options, or checking a column. Figure 17-12 shows a page from a diary for patients to record their symptoms and how they were managed. This diary includes blanks to identify the symptoms and an option to check how the symptoms were managed. This type of diary is used to collect numerical data for a quantitative study. Validity and reliability have been examined by comparing the results with data obtained through interviews and have been found to be acceptable. Participation in studies using health diaries has been good, and attrition rates are reported as low. Some diaries include the collection of narrative data and are more common in qualitative studies (Alaszewski, 2006).

Nicholl (2010) and Burman (1995) provide some key points to consider when selecting a diary for collecting data in a study:

1. Analyze the phenomenon of interest to determine if it can be adequately captured using a diary. Also, determine if a diary is the best data collection approach when compared with interviews, questionnaires, and scales.
2. Decide if the diary will be used alone or with other measurement methods.
3. Determine which format of the diary to use so that the most valid information can be obtained to address the study purpose without burdening the study participants. Diaries can be paper, online, or phone text-messaging formats. Some researchers are using blogs as a way to collect diary data (Lim, Sacks-Davis, Aitken, Hocking, & Hellard, 2010). The format of the questions in diaries can also vary based on the purpose of the study. Diaries with closed-ended questions are usually used in quantitative research, and participants are provided specific direction on the data to be recorded. Diaries with open-ended questions are more common in

Date	What symptom did you have?	Did you talk with a family member or friend about the symptom?		Did you talk with a health professional about it?		Did you take any pills or treatments for the symptom?	
		No	Yes	No	Yes	No	Yes, Specify

Figure 17-12 **Sample diary page.**

qualitative research with the narrative data requiring content analysis (Alaszewski, 2006; Nicholl, 2010).

4. Pilot-test any new or refined diary with the target population of interest to identify possible problems, determine if the instructions and terminology are clear, ensure that the data can be recorded with this approach, and examine the ability of participants to complete diaries.

5. Determine the period of time that the diary will be completed to accomplish the purpose of the study, taking into consideration the burden on the participants. Typical diary periods are 2 to 8 weeks.

6. Provide clear instructions to all participants on the use of a diary before the study begins to enhance the quality of data collected. Participants need to know how to use the diaries, what types of events are to be reported, and how to contact the researcher or clinician with questions.

7. Use follow-up procedures, such as phone calls or emails, during data collection to enhance completion rates. Diaries might be emailed, mailed, or picked up by the researchers. Picking up the diary in person promotes a higher completion rate than mailing.

8. Plan data analysis procedures during diary development and refine these plans to ensure the most appropriate analyses are used. Diary data are very dense and rich, and carefully prepared analysis plans can minimize problems (Burman, 1995; Nicholl, 2010).

The use of diaries has some disadvantages. In some cases, keeping the diary may alter the behavior or events under study. For example, if a person were keeping a diary of the nursing care that he or she was providing to patients, the insight that the person gained from recording the information in the diary might lead to changes in care. In addition, patients can become more sensitive to items (e.g., symptoms or problems) reported in the diary, which could result in overreporting. Subjects may also become bored with keeping the diary and become less thorough in recording items, which could result in underreporting (Aroian & Wal, 2007; Nicholl, 2010).

Lim et al. (2010) conducted a randomized controlled trial to determine the best diary format for collecting sexual behavior information from adolescents. The three formats for the diaries were paper, online, and phone text messaging (short message service); these were compared for response rate, timeliness, completeness of data, and acceptability. The following excerpt describes the use of the diaries for data collection and the outcomes.

"Participants were recruited by telephone and randomized into one of three groups. They completed weekly sexual behavior diaries for 3 months by SMS [short message service], online, or paper (by post). An online survey was conducted at the end of 3 months to compare retrospective reports with the diaries and assess opinions on the diary collection method.... Conclusions were that the SMS is a convenient and timely method of collecting brief behavioral data, but online data collection was

> preferable to most participants and more likely to be completed. Data collected in retrospective sexual behavior questionnaires were found to agree substantially with data collected through weekly self-report diaries." (Lim et al., 2010, p. 885)

Lim et al. (2010) provided some valuable information about the formats for collecting data with diaries. Researchers might want to consider using online or phone text messaging to collect diary data from younger populations. These formats could significantly increase the response rate and the completeness of the data collected. The paper format for collecting diary data also provides quality information and might be better for populations with limited access to technology.

Measurement Using Existing Databases

Nurse researchers are increasing their use of existing databases to address the research problems they have identified as essential in generating evidence for practice. The reasons for using these databases in studies are varied. With the computerization of healthcare information, more large data sets have been developed internationally, nationally, regionally, at the state level, and within clinical agencies. These databases include large amounts of information that have relevance in developing research evidence needed for practice (Brown, 2009; Melnyk & Fineout-Overholt, 2011). The costs and technology for storage of data have improved over the last 10 years making these large data sets more reliable and accessible. Using existing databases makes it possible to conduct complex analyses to expand understanding of healthcare outcomes (Doran, 2011). Another reason is that the primary collection of data in a study is limited by the availability of participants and the expense of the data collection process. By using existing databases, researchers are able to have larger samples, conduct more longitudinal studies, experience less costs during the data collection process, and limit the burdens placed on study participants (Johantgen, 2010).

There are also problems with using data from existing databases. The data in the database might not clearly address the researchers' study purpose. Most researchers identify a study problem and purpose and then develop a methodology to address these. The data collected are specific to the study and clearly focused on answering the research questions or testing the study hypotheses. However, with existing databases, researchers need to ensure that the data they require for their study is in the database they are planning to use. Sometimes researchers must revise their study questions and variables based on what data exist in the database. The level of measurement of the study variables might limit the analysis techniques that can be used. There is also the question of the validity and reliability of the data in existing databases; unless these are specifically reported, researchers using these data files need to be cautious in their interpretation of findings.

Existing Healthcare Data

Existing healthcare data consist of two types: secondary and administrative. Data that are collected for a particular study are considered primary data. Data that are collected from previous research and stored in a database are considered secondary data when used by other researchers to address their study purposes. Because these data were collected as part of research, details can be obtained about the data collection and storage process. Researchers usually clearly indicate in their article in the methodology section when secondary data analyses were conducted as part of their research (Johantgen, 2010).

Data that are collected for reasons other than research are considered administrative data. Administrative data are collected within clinical agencies; obtained by national, state, and local professional organizations; and collected by federal, state, and local agencies. The processes for collection and storage of administrative data are more complex and often more unclear than the data collection process for research (Johantgen, 2010). The data in administrative databases are collected by different people in different sites using different methods. However, the data elements collected for most administrative databases include demographics, organizational characteristics, clinical diagnosis and treatment, and geographical information. These database elements were standardized by the Health Insurance Portability and Accountability Act (HIPAA) of 1996, which improved the quality of the databases. The HIPAA regulations can be viewed online at http://www.hhs.gov/ocr/privacy/ (U.S. Department of Health & Human Services, 2011).

When using secondary data and administrative data in a study, researchers need to determine the reliability and validity of the data in the database they plan to access. They also need to ensure that the data in the data set address the research questions or hypotheses of their study Lake, Shang, Klaus, and Dunton (2010) used an existing database entitled the National Database of Nursing Quality Indicators (NDNQI) for the conduct of their study. The NDNQI was designed to measure nursing quality and patient safety. Lake et al. examined the relationships between patient falls, nursing unit staffing, and hospital Magnet status. The following excerpt describes the database they used.

"NDNQI Database Overview

The NDNQI, a unique database that was well-suited to our study aims, is part of the American Nurses Association's (ANA) Safety and Quality Initiative. This initiative started in 1994 with information gathering from an expert panel and focus groups to specify a set of 10 nurse-sensitive indicators to be used in the database.... The database was pilot tested in 1996 and 1997 and was established in 1998 with 35 hospitals. Use of the NDNQI has grown rapidly.... In 2009, 1,450 hospitals—one out of every four general hospitals in the U.S.—participated in it.

The NDNQI has served as a unit-level benchmarking resource, but research from this data repository has been limited. NDNQI researchers have published two studies on the association between characteristics of nursing workforce and fall rates.... The scope of work on this topic was extended in the current study by: (a) specifying nurse staffing separately for RNs [registered nurses], LPNs [licensed practical nurses], and NAs [nursing assistants], (b) using the entire NDNQI database, (c) selecting the most detailed level of observation (month), and (d) applying more extensive patient risk adjustment than had been evaluated previously." (Lake et al., 2010, p. 415)

Lake et al. (2010) provide a detailed description of the national database that they used in their study. This database was selected because it was "well-suited" to the study's aims and because the focus of the study was to expand on previous research that had been done using this database information. The development of the database was very structured, which increases the reliability and validity of the field data.

Selection of an Existing Instrument

Selecting an instrument to measure the variables in a study is a critical process in research. The method of measurement selected must fit closely the conceptual definition of the variable. Researchers need to conduct an extensive search of the literature to identify appropriate methods of measurement. In many cases, they find instruments that measure some of the needed elements but not all, or the content may be related to but somehow different from what is needed for a study. Instruments found in the literature may have little or no documentation of their validity and reliability.

Beginning researchers often conclude that no appropriate method of measurement exists and that they must develop a tool. At the time, this solution seems to be the most simple because the researcher has a clear idea of what needs to be measured. This solution is not recommended unless all else fails. Tool development is a lengthy process and requires sophisticated research. Using a new instrument in a study without first evaluating its validity and reliability can be problematic and lead to questionable findings.

For novice researchers developing their first study, it is essential to identify existing instruments to measure study variables. Jones (2004) developed a flow chart that might help you to select an existing instrument for your study (Figure 17-13). The major steps include (1) identifying an instrument from the literature, (2) determining if the instrument is appropriate for measuring a study variable, and (3) examining the performance of the instrument by evaluating its reliability and validity. These steps are detailed in the following sections.

Locating Existing Instruments

Locating existing measurement methods has become easier in recent years. A computer database, the Health and Psychological Instruments Online (HAPI), is available in many libraries and can be used to search for instruments that measure a particular concept or for information on a particular instrument. Sometimes a search on Medline or CINAHL might uncover an instrument that is useful. Many reference books have compiled published measurement tools, some that are specific to instruments used in nursing research. Dissertations often contain measurement tools that have never been published, so a review of *Dissertation Abstracts* online might be helpful.

Another important source of recently developed measurement tools is word-of-mouth communication among researchers. Information on tools is often presented at research conferences years before publication. There are usually networks of researchers conducting studies on similar nursing phenomena. These researchers are frequently associated with nursing organizations and keep in touch through

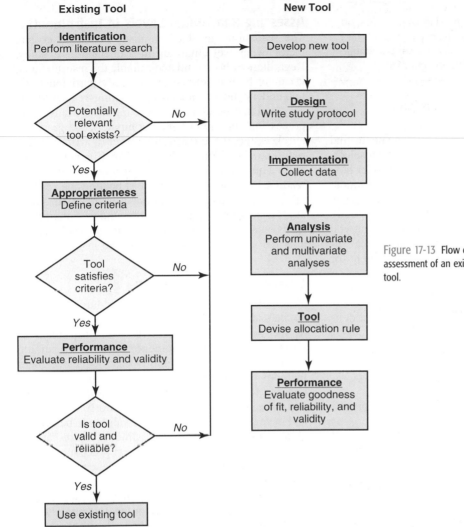

Figure 17-13 Flow chart depicting the identification and assessment of an existing tool and development of a new tool.

newsletters, correspondence, telephone, email, computer discussion boards, and web pages. Questioning available nurse investigators can lead to a previously unknown tool. These researchers can often be reached by telephone, letter, or email and are usually willing to share their tools in return for access to the data to facilitate work on developing validity and reliability information. The Sigma Theta Tau *Directory of Nurse Researchers* provides email address and phone information on nurse researchers. In addition, it lists nurse researchers by category according to their area of research.

Waltz and colleagues (2010) made the following suggestions to facilitate locating existing instruments for studies:

"(1) [S]earch computerized databases by using the name of the instrument or keywords or phrases; (2) generalize the search to the specific area of interest and related topics (research reports are particularly valuable); (3) search for summary articles describing, comparing, contrasting, and evaluating the instruments used to measure a given concept; (4) search journals, such as *Journal of Nursing Measurement*, that are devoted specifically to measurement; (5) after identifying a publication in which relevant instruments are used, use citation indices to locate other publications that used them; (6) examine computer-based and print indices, and compendia of instruments developed by nursing, medicine, and other disciplines; and (7) examine copies of published proceedings and abstracts from relevant scientific meetings." (Waltz et al., 2010, pp. 393-394)

Evaluating Existing Instruments for Appropriateness and Performance

You may need to examine several instruments to find the one most appropriate for your study. When selecting an instrument for research, carefully consider how the instrument was developed, what the instrument measures, and how to administer it. Before you review existing instruments, be sure you have conceptually defined your study variable and are clear on what you desire to measure. You then need to address the following questions to determine the best instrument for measuring your study variable:

1. Does this instrument measure what you want to measure?
2. Does the instrument reflect your conceptual definition of the variable?
3. Is the instrument well constructed?
4. Does your population resemble populations previously studied with the instrument? (Waltz et al., 2010)
5. Is the readability level of the instrument appropriate for your population?
6. How sensitive is the instrument in detecting small differences in the phenomenon you want to measure (what is the effect size)?
7. What is the process for obtaining, administering, and scoring the instrument? Are there costs associated with the instrument?
8. What skills are required to administer the instrument? Do you need training or a particular credential to administer the instrument?
9. How are the scores interpreted?
10. What is the time commitment of the study participants and researcher for administration of the instrument?
11. What evidence is available related to the reliability and validity of the instrument? Have multiple types of validity been examined (content validity, validity from factor analysis, validity from examining measures assessing for convergence and divergence, or evidence of validity from prediction of concurrent and future events)? Chapter 16 provided a detailed discussion of reliability and validity (Bartlett & Frost, 2008; Bialocerkowski et al., 2010; DeVon et al., 2007; Fawcett & Garity, 2009).

Assessing Readability Levels of Instruments

The readability level of an instrument is a critical factor when selecting an instrument for a study. Regardless of how valid and reliable the instrument is, it cannot be used effectively if study participants do not understand the items. Calculating readability is easy and can be done in a few minutes. Many word processing programs and computerized grammar checkers report the readability level of written material. The Fog formula described in Chapter 16 provides a quick and easy way to assess readability. If the reading level of an instrument is beyond the reading level of the study population, you need to select another instrument for use in your study. Changing the items on an instrument to reduce the reading level can alter the validity and reliability of the instrument.

Constructing Scales

Scale construction is a complex procedure that should not be undertaken lightly. There must be firm evidence of the need for developing another instrument to measure a particular phenomenon important to nursing practice. However, in many cases, measurement methods have not been developed for phenomena of concern to nurse researchers, or measurement tools that have been developed may be poorly constructed and have insufficient evidence of validity to be acceptable for use in studies. It is possible for the researcher to carry out instrument development procedures on an existing scale with inadequate evidence of validity before using it in a study. Neophyte nurse researchers could assist experienced researchers in carrying out some of the field studies required to complete the development of scale validity and reliability.

The procedures for developing a scale have been well defined. The following discussion describes this theory-based process and the mathematical logic underlying it. The theories on which scale construction is most frequently based include classic test theory (Nunnally & Bernstein, 1994), item response theory (Hulin, Drasgow, & Parsons, 1983), multidimensional scaling (Borg & Groenen, 2010; Kruskal & Wish, 1990), and unfolding theory (Coombs, 1950). Most existing instruments used in nursing research have been developed with classic test theory, which assumes a normal distribution of scores.

Constructing a Scale by Using Classic Test Theory

In classic test theory, the following process is used to construct a scale:

1. *Define the concept.* A scale cannot be constructed to measure a concept until the nature of the concept has been delineated. The more clearly the concept is defined, the easier it is to write items to measure it (Spector, 1992). Concepts are defined through the process of concept analysis, a procedure discussed in Chapter 7.

2. *Design the scale.* Items should be constructed to reflect the concept as fully as possible. The process of construction differs depending on whether the scale is a rating scale, Likert scale, or semantic differential scale. Items previously included in other scales can be used if they have been shown empirically to be good indicators of the concept (Hulin et al., 1983). A blueprint may ensure that all elements of the concept are covered. Each item must be stated clearly and concisely and express only one idea. The reading level of items must be identified and considered in terms of potential respondents. The number of items constructed must be considerably larger than planned for the completed instrument because items are discarded during the item analysis step of scale construction. Nunnally and Bernstein (1994) suggested developing an item pool at least twice the size of that desired for the final scale.

3. *Review the items.* As items are constructed, it is advisable to ask qualified individuals to review them. Crocker and Algina (1986) recommended asking for feedback in relation to accuracy, appropriateness, or relevance to test specifications; technical flaws in item construction; grammar; offensiveness or appearance of bias; and level of readability. The items should be revised according to the critical appraisal.

4. *Conduct preliminary item tryouts.* While items are still in draft form, it is helpful to test them on a limited number of subjects (15 to 30) who represent the target population. The reactions of respondents should be observed during testing to note behaviors such as long pauses, answer changing, or other indications of confusion about specific items. After testing, a debriefing session needs to be held during which respondents are invited to comment on items and offer suggestions for improvement. Descriptive and exploratory statistical analyses are performed on data from these tryouts while noting means, response distributions, items left blank, and outliers. Items need to be revised based on this analysis and comments from respondents.

5. *Perform a field test.* All the items in their final draft form are administered to a large sample of subjects who represent the target population. Spector (1992) recommended a sample size of 100 to 200 subjects. However, the sample size needed for the statistical analyses to follow depends on the number of items in the instrument. Some experts recommend including 10 subjects for each item being tested. If the final instrument was expected to have 20 items, and 40 items were constructed for the field test, 400 subjects could be required.

6. *Conduct item analyses.* The purpose of item analysis is to identify items that form an internally consistent or reliable scale and to eliminate items that do not meet this criterion. Internal reliability implies that all the items are consistently measuring a concept. Before these analyses are conducted, negatively worded items must be reverse-scored or given a score as though the item was stated positively. For example, the item might read "I do not believe exercise is important to health," with the responses of 1 = strongly disagree, 2 = disagree, 3 = uncertain, 4 = agree, and 5 = strongly agree. If the subject marked a 1 for strongly disagree, this item would be reverse-scored and given a 5, indicating the subject thinks exercise is very important to health. The analyses examine the extent of intercorrelation among the items. The statistical computer programs currently providing the set of statistical procedures needed to perform item analyses (as a package) are SPSS, SPSS/PC, and SYSTAT. These packages perform item-item correlations and item-total correlations. In some cases, the value of the item being examined is subtracted from the total score, and an item-remainder coefficient is calculated. This latter coefficient is most useful in evaluating items for retention in the scale.

7. *Select items to retain.* Depending on the number of items desired in the final scale, items with the highest coefficients are retained. Alternatively, a criterion value for the coefficient (e.g., 0.40) can be set, and all items greater than this value are retained. The greater the number of items retained, the smaller the item-remainder coefficients can be and still have an internally consistent scale. After this selection process, a coefficient alpha is calculated for the scale. This value is a direct function of the number of items and the magnitude of intercorrelation. Thus, one can increase the value of a coefficient alpha by increasing the number of items or raising the intercorrelations through inclusion of more highly intercorrelated items. Values of coefficient alphas range from 0 to 1. The

alpha value should be at least 0.70 to indicate sufficient internal consistency in a new tool (Nunnally & Bernstein, 1994). An iterative process of removing or replacing items or both, recalculating item-remainder coefficients, and recalculating the alpha coefficient are repeated until a satisfactory alpha coefficient is obtained. Deleting poorly correlated items raises the alpha coefficient, but decreasing the number of items lowers it (Spector, 1992). The initial attempt at scale development may not achieve a sufficiently high coefficient alpha. In this case, additional items need to be written, more data collected, and the item analysis redone. This scenario is most likely to occur when too few items were developed initially or when many of the initial items were poorly written. It may also be a consequence of attempts to operationalize an inadequately defined concept (Spector, 1992).

8. *Conduct validity studies.* When scale development is judged to be satisfactory, studies must be performed to evaluate the validity of the scale. (See the discussion of validity in Chapter 16.) These studies require the researcher to collect additional data from large samples. As part of this process, scale scores must be correlated with scores on other variables proposed to be related to the concept being put into operation. Hypotheses must be generated regarding variations in mean values of the scale in different groups. Exploratory and confirmatory factor analysis (discussed in Chapters 16 and 23) is usually performed as part of establishing the validity of the instrument. As many different types of evidence of validity as possible should be collected (Spector, 1992).

9. *Evaluate the reliability of the scale.* Various statistical procedures are performed to determine the reliability of the scale. These analyses can be performed on the data collected to evaluate validity for this scale. (See Chapter 16 for a discussion of the procedures performed to examine reliability.)

10. *Compile norms on the scale.* To determine norms, the scale must be administered to a large sample that is representative of the groups to which the scale is likely to be administered. Norms should be acquired for as many diverse groups as possible. Data acquired during validity and reliability studies can be included for this analysis. To obtain the large samples needed for this purpose, many researchers permit others to use their scale with the condition that data from these studies be provided for compiling norms.

11. *Publish the results of development of the scale.* Scales are often not published for many years after the initial development because of the length of time required to validate the instrument. Some researchers never publish the results of this work. Studies using the scale are published, but the instrument development process may not be available except by writing to the author. This information needs to be added to the body of knowledge, and colleagues should encourage instrument developers to complete the work and submit it for publication (Lynn, 1989; Norbeck, 1985). Klein et al. (2010) provided a detailed discussion of their development of the NPAT that was presented earlier in this chapter. The validity and reliability of the tool were addressed and a copy of the tool was included in the article (see Figure 17-4).

Constructing a Scale by Using Item Response Theory

Using item response theory to construct a scale proceeds initially in a fashion similar to that of classic test theory. There is an expectation of a well-defined concept to operationalize. Items are initially written in a manner similar to that previously described, and item tryouts and field testing are also similar. However, the process changes with the initiation of item analysis. The statistical procedures used are more sophisticated and complex than the procedures used in classic test theory. Using data from field testing, item characteristic curves are calculated by using logistic regression models (Hulin et al., 1983; Nunnally & Bernstein, 1994). After selecting an appropriate model based on information obtained from the analysis, item parameters are estimated. These parameters are used to select items for the scale. This strategy is used to avoid problems encountered with classic test theory measures.

Scales developed by using classic test theory effectively measure the characteristics of subjects near the mean. The statistical procedures used assume a linear distribution of scale values. Items reflecting responses of respondents closer to the extremes tend to be discarded because of the assumption that scale values should approximate the normal curve. Scales developed in this manner often do not provide a clear understanding of study participants at the high or low end of values.

One purpose of item response theory is to choose items in such a way that estimates of characteristics at each level of the concept being measured are accurate. To accomplish this goal, researchers use maximal likelihood estimates. A curvilinear distribution of scale values is assumed. Rather than choosing items on the basis of the item remainder coefficient, the researcher specifies a test information curve. The scale can be tailored to have the desired measurement accuracy. By comparing a scale developed by classic test theory with one developed from the same items with item response theory, one would find differences in some of the items retained. Biserial correlations would be lower in the scale developed from item response theory than in the scale developed from classic test theory. Item bias is lower in scales developed by using item response theory and occurs when respondents from different subpopulations having the same amount of an underlying trait have different probabilities of responding to an item positively (Hambleton & Swaminathan, 2010; Hulin et al., 1983).

Constructing a Scale by Using Multidimensional Scaling

Multidimensional scaling is used when the concept being operationalized is actually an abstract construct believed to be represented most accurately by multiple dimensions. The scaling techniques used allow the researcher to uncover the hidden structure in the construct. The analysis techniques use proximities among the measures as input. The outcome of the analysis is a spatial representation, or a geometrical configuration of data points, that reveals the hidden structure. The procedure tends to be used to examine differences in stimuli rather than differences in people. A researcher might use this method to measure differences in perception of light or pain. Scales developed by using this procedure reveal patterns among items. The procedure is used in the development of rating scales and semantic differentials (Borg & Groenen, 2010; Kruskal & Wish, 1990).

Constructing a Scale by Using Unfolding Theory

When a scale is being constructed with the use of unfolding theory, researchers ask study participants to respond to the items in the rating scale. Next, participants are asked to rank the various response options in relation to the response option that they selected for that item. This procedure is followed for each item in the scale. By using this procedure, the underlying continuum for each scale item is "unfolded." As an example, suppose researchers developed the following item:

My preference for a diet to lose weight is
1. A low-fat diet
2. A low-calorie diet
3. A low-carbohydrate diet
4. A vegetarian diet

Study participants would be asked to select their response to the item and then rank the other options according to the proximity to their choice. The participant might choose a low-calorie diet as number 1, a low-carbohydrate diet as number 2, a low-fat diet as number 3, and a vegetarian diet as number 4. Although the preferences of other study participants would differ, the results can be plotted to reveal patterns of an underlying continuum. Items selected for the scale would be the items with evidence of a pattern of responses.

Translating a Scale to Another Language

Contrary to expectations, translating an instrument from the original language to a target language is a complex process. By translating a scale, researchers can compare concepts among respondents of different cultures. The comparison requires that they first infer and then validate that the conceptual meaning in which the scale was developed is the same in both cultures. This process is highly speculative, and conclusions about the similarities of meanings in a measure must be considered tentative (Hulin et al., 1983).

Four types of translations can be performed: pragmatic translations, aesthetic-poetic translations, ethnographic translations, and linguistic translations. Pragmatic translations communicate the content from the source language accurately in the target language. The primary concern is the information conveyed. An example of this type of translation is the use of translated instructions for assembling a computer. Aesthetic-poetic translations evoke moods, feelings, and affect in the target language that are identical to those evoked by the original material. In ethnographic translations, the purpose is to maintain meaning and cultural content. In this case, translators must be familiar with both languages and cultures. Linguistic translations strive to present grammatical forms with equivalent meanings. Translating a scale is generally done in the ethnographic mode (Hulin et al., 1983).

One strategy for translating scales is to translate from the original language to the target language and then back-translate from the target language to the original language by using translators not involved in the original translation (Fawcett & Garity, 2009). Discrepancies are identified, and the procedure is repeated until troublesome problems are resolved. After this procedure, the two versions are administered to bilingual subjects and scored by standard procedures. The resulting sets of scores are examined to determine the extent to which the two versions yield similar information from the subjects. This procedure assumes that the subjects are equally skilled in both languages. One problem with this strategy is that bilingual subjects may interpret meanings of words differently from monolingual subjects. This difference in interpretation is a serious concern because the target subjects for most cross-cultural research are monolingual (Hulin et al., 1983).

Yu, Lee, and Woo (2004) provided an excellent description of their process of translating the Medical Outcomes Study Social Support Survey (MOS-SSS) from English to Chinese. These researchers used the forward and backward translation process previously discussed, and the steps they took are outlined in the following excerpt.

"This translation model includes a cycle of four steps as follows.

Forward translation of the MOS-SSS by a bilingual health professional. The translation process began with forward translation of the original source language (SL) version (English) of the MOS-SSS into the target language (TL) of Chinese by a bilingual native Chinese registered nurse....

Review of the Chinese MOS-SSS by a monolingual reviewer. The Chinese version of the MOS-SSS was then reviewed by a Chinese monolingual reviewer for incomprehensible or ambiguous wordings....

Backward translation of the Chinese MOS-SSS by a bilingual health professional. In this step, the reviewed Chinese version of the MOS-SSS (as discussed in Step 2) was back translated by another bilingual nurse, who was 'blinded' to the original English version....

Comparison of the SL version and back-translated version. The researcher, at this stage, compared the back-translated version of the MOS-SSS with its original version for linguistic congruence and cultural relevancy. Items with apparent discrepancies were examined to ascertain whether the problems originated in the forward translation or the backward translation. The error in items resulting from the forward translation had to go through the whole-cycle again from Steps 1 to 4, whereas the latter type of error was subjected to further back translation. This process was repeated until a maximum equivalence between the SL and back-translated versions was achieved." (Yu et al., 2004, pp. 309-310)

In 1997, the Medical Outcomes Trust introduced new translation criteria that are much more comprehensive. The discussion of these criteria is available at www.outcomes-trust.org/bulletin/0797blltn.htm. Hulin et al. (1983) suggested the use of item response theory procedures to address some of the problems of translation. These procedures can provide direct evidence about the meanings of items in the two languages. Item characteristic curves for an item in the two languages can be compared, as can scale scores in the two languages. This procedure eliminates the need for bilingual samples. It also eliminates the need for the two populations to be equivalent in terms of the distributions of their scores on the trait being measured.

Rather than translating an instrument into each language, Turner, Rogers, Hendershot, Miller, and Thornberry (1996) tested the use of electronic technology involving multilingual audio computer-assisted self-interviewing (Audio-CASI) to enable researchers to include multiple linguistic minorities in nationally representative studies and clinical studies. The Audio-CASI system uses electronic translation from one language to another. In the funded project to develop and test Audio-CASI, a backup phone bank was available to provide multilingual assistance if needed. Whether this strategy will provide equivalent validity of a translated tool is unclear.

KEY POINTS

- Measurement approaches used in nursing research include physiological measures; observations; interviews; questionnaires; scales; and specialized instruments such as Q-sort method, Delphi technique, diaries, and analyses using existing databases.
- Measurements of physiological variables can be either direct or indirect and sometimes require the use of specialized equipment or laboratory analysis.
- The Human Genome Project has increased the opportunities for nurses to be involved in genetic research and to include the measurement of nucleic acids in their studies.
- To measure observations, every variable is observed in a similar manner in each instance, with careful attention given to training data collectors.
- In structured observational studies, category systems must be developed; checklists or rating scales are developed from the category systems and used to guide data collection.

- Interviews involve verbal communication between the researcher and the study participant, during which the researcher acquires information. Interviewers must be trained in the skills of interviewing, and the interview protocol must be pretested.
- A questionnaire is a printed or electronic self-report form designed to elicit information through the responses of a study participant. The information obtained through questionnaires is similar to information obtained by interview, but the questions tend to have less depth. An item on a questionnaire usually has two parts: a lead-in question and a response set.
- Scales, another form of self-reporting, are more precise in measuring phenomena than questionnaires and have been developed to measure psychosocial and physiological variables. The types of scales included in this text are rating scale, Likert scale, semantic differential scale, and visual analogue scale.
- A rating scale is a crude form of measurement that includes a list of an ordered series of categories of a variable, which are assumed to be based on an underlying continuum. A numerical value is assigned to each category.
- The Likert scale contains declarative statements with a scale after each statement to determine the opinion or attitude of a study participant.
- A semantic differential scale consists of two opposite adjectives with a 7-point scale between them and measures the connotative meaning of a concept to a subject.
- The visual analogue scale, sometimes referred to as magnitude scaling, is a 100-mm line with right-angle stops at each end with bipolar anchors placed beyond each end of the line. These end anchors must cover the entire range of sensations possible in the phenomenon being measured.
- The Delphi technique measures the judgments of a group of experts to assess priorities or make forecasts. It provides a means for researchers to obtain the opinions of a wide variety of experts across the United States without the need for the experts to meet.
- A diary, which allows one to record an experience shortly after an event, is more accurate than obtaining the information through recall at an interview. In addition, the reporting level of incidents is higher, and one tends to capture the participant's immediate perception of situations.
- Nurse researchers are expanding their use of data from existing databases to answer their research questions and test their research hypotheses. Health data are usually categorized into secondary data and administrative data.
- The choice of tools for use in a particular study is a critical decision that can have a major impact on the significance of the study.
- The researcher first must conduct an extensive search for existing tools. Once found, the tools must be carefully evaluated. Tools that are selected for a study need to be described in great detail in the proposal and in the final research report for publication.
- Scale construction is a complex procedure that should not be undertaken lightly. Theories on which scale construction is most frequently based include classic test theory, item response theory, multidimensional scaling, and unfolding theory. Most existing instruments used in nursing research have been developed through the use of classic test theory.
- Translating a scale to another language is a complex process that allows concepts among respondents of different cultures to be compared if care is taken to ensure that concepts have the same or similar meanings across cultures.

REFERENCES

Akhtar-Danesh, N., Baumann, A., & Cordingley, L. (2008). Q-methodology in nursing research: A promising method for the study of subjectivity. *Western Journal of Nursing Research*, 30(6), 759–773.

Alaszewski, A. (2006). *Using diaries for social research*. London, UK: Sage.

Aroian, K. J. & Wal, J. S. V. (2007). Measuring elders' symptoms with daily diaries and retrospective reports. *Western Journal of Nursing Research*, 29(3), 322–337.

Bartlett, J. W. & Frost, C. (2008). Reliability, repeatability and reproducibility: Analysis of measurement errors in continuous variables. *Ultrasound Obstetric Gynecology*, 31(4), 466–475.

Beckie, T. M., Beckstead, J. W., Schocken, D. D., Evans, M. E., & Fletcher, G. F. (2011). The effects of a tailored cardiac rehabilitation program on depressive symptoms in women: A randomized clinical trial. *International Journal of Nursing Studies*, 48(1), 3–12.

Beckie, T. M., Fletcher, G. F., Beckstead, J. W., Schocken, D. D., & Evans, M. E. (2008). Adverse baseline physiological and psychosocial profiles of women enrolled in a cardiac rehabilitation clinical trial. *Journal of Cardiopulmonary Rehabilitation & Prevention*, 28(1), 52–60.

Berdie, D. R., Anderson, J. F., & Niebuhr, M. A. (1992). *Questionnaires: Design and use* (2nd ed.). Metuchen, NJ: Scarecrow Press.

Bhengu, B. R., Ncama, B. P., McInerney, P. A., Wantland, D. J., Nicholas, P. D., Corless, I. B., et al. (2011). Symptoms experienced by HIV-infected individuals on antirctroviral therapy in KwaZulu-Natal, South Africa. *Applied Nursing Research*, 24(1), 1–9.

Bialocerkowski, A., Klupp, N., & Bragge, P. (2010). Research methodology series: How to read and critically appraise a reliability article. *International Journal of Therapy & Rehabilitation, 17*(3), 114–120.

Borg, J. & Groenen, P. J. (2010). *Modern multidimensional scaling: Theory and application* (2nd ed.). New York, NY: Springer.

Brener, N. D., Kann, L., Kinchen, S. A., Grunbaum, J. A., Whalen, L., Eaton, D.; Department of Health and Human Services, Centers for Disease Control and Prevention. (2004). Methodology of the Youth Risk Surveillance System. *Morbidity & Mortality Weekly Report, 53*(Sept. 24), 1–13.

Briggs, C. L. (1986). *Learning how to ask: A sociolinguistic appraisal of the role of the interview in social science research.* Cambridge, MA: Cambridge University Press.

Brown, S. J. (2009). *Evidence-based nursing: The research-practice connection.* Boston, MA: Jones & Bartlett.

Burman, M.E. (1995). Health diaries in nursing research and practice. *Image Journal of Nursing Scholarship, 27*(2), 147–152.

Cazzell, M. (2010). *College student risk behavior: The implications of religiosity and impulsivity.* Ph.D. dissertation, The University of Texas at Arlington, United States: Texas. Proquest Dissertations & Theses. (Publication No. AAT 3391108).

Cazzell, M. (personal communication, March 20, 2011). Self-report college student risk behavior questionnaire. The University of Texas at Arlington, Arlington, TX.

Chase, C. A. (2011). An intergenerational e-mail pal project on attitudes of college students toward older adults. *Educational Gerontology, 37*(1), 27–37.

Clinical and Laboratory Standards Institute (CLSI). (2011). *Harmonized terminology database.* Retrieved from http://www.clsi.org/Content/NavigationMenu/Resources/HarmonizedTerminologyDatabase/Harmonized_Terminolo.htm.

Converse, J. M., & Presser, S. (1986). *Survey questions: Handcrafting the standardized questionnaire.* Newbury Park, CA: Sage.

Coombs, C. H. (1950). Psychological scaling without a unit of measurement. *Psychological Review, 57*(3), 145–158.

Couper, M. R. (1984). The Delphi technique: Characteristics and sequence model. *Advances in Nursing Science, 7*(1), 72–77.

Cowan, M. J., Heinrich, J., Lucas, M., Sigmon, H., & Hinshaw, A. S. (1993). Integration of biological and nursing sciences: A 10-year plan to enhance research and training. *Research in Nursing & Health, 16*(1), 3–9.

Craig, J. V., & Smyth, R. L. (2012). *The evidence-base practice manual for nurses* (3rd ed.). Edinburgh, UK: Churchill Livingstone.

Crocker, L., & Algina, J. (1986). *Introduction to classical modern test theory.* New York, NY: Holt, Rinehart & Winston.

Dariel, O. P., Wharrad, H., & Windle, R. (2010). Developing Q-methodology to explore staff views toward the use of technology in nurse education. *Nurse Researcher, 18*(1), 58–71.

Dennis, K. E. (1986). Q methodology: Relevance and application to nursing research. *Advances in Nursing Science, 8*(3), 6–17.

Department of Education Genomic Science. (2011). *Human Genome Project information.* Retrieved from http://www.ornl.gov/sci/techresources/Human_Genome/home.shtml.

DeVon, H. A., Block, M. E., Moyle-Wright, P., Ernst, D. M., Hayden, S. J., Lazzara, D. J., et al. (2007). A psychometric toolbox for testing validity and reliability. *Journal of Nursing Scholarship, 39*(2), 155–164.

Dillman, D. A., Smyth, J. D., & Christian, L. M. (2009). *Internet, mail, and mixed-mode surveys: The tailored design method.* Hoboken, NJ: John Wiley & Sons.

Dillon, J. T. (1990). *The practice of questioning.* New York, NY: Routledge.

Doran, D. M. (2011). *Nursing outcomes: The state of the science* (2nd ed.). Sudbury, MA: Jones & Bartlett Learning.

Dubbert, P. M., White, J. D., Grothe, K. B., O'Jile, J., & Kirchner, K. A. (2006). Physical activity in patients who are severely mentally ill: Feasibility of assessment for clinical and research applications. *Archives of Psychiatric Nursing, 20*(5), 205–209.

Dunn, S. L., Corser, W., Stommel, M., & Holmes-Rovner, M. (2006). Hopelessness and depression in the early recovery period after hospitalization for acute coronary syndrome. *Journal of Cardiopulmonary Rehabilitation, 26*(3), 152–159.

Fawcett, J., & Garity, J. (2009). *Evaluating research for evidence-based nursing practice.* Philadelphia: F.A. Davis.

Foddy, W. H. (1993). *Constructing questions for interviews and questionnaires: Theory and practice in social research.* Cambridge, UK: Cambridge University Press.

Fowler, F. J. (1990). *Standardized survey interviewing: Minimizing interviewer-related error.* Newbury Park, CA: Sage.

Gagliese, L., Weizblit, N., Ellis, W., & Chan, V. W. (2005). The measurement of postoperative pain: A comparison in younger and older surgical patients. *Pain, 117*(3), 412–420.

Gelinas, C., Choiniere, M., Ranger, M., Denault, A., Deschamps, A., & Johnston, C. (2010). Toward a new approach for the detection of pain in adult patients undergoing cardiac surgery: Near-infrared spectroscopy—a pilot study. *Heart & Lung, 39*(6), 485–943.

Gift, A. G. (1989). Visual analogue scales: Measurement of subjective phenomena. *Nursing Research, 38*(5), 286–288.

Gorden, R. L. (1987). *Interviewing: Strategy, techniques, and tactics.* Chicago, IL: Dorsey Press.

Gorden, R. L. (1998). *Basic interviewing skills.* Chicago, IL: Dorsey Press.

Grove, S. K. (2007). *Statistics for health care research: A practical workbook.* Philadelphia, PA: Saunders.

Hambleton, R. K., & Swaminathan, H. (2010). *Item response theory: Principles and applications.* Boston, MA: Kluwer Academic Publishers Group.

Harralson, T. L. (2007). Factors influencing delay in seeking treatment for acute ischemic symptoms among lower income, urban women. *Heart & Lung, 36*(2), 96–104.

Hockenberry, M. J., & Wilson, D. (2009). *Wong's essentials of pediatric nursing* (8th ed.). St. Louis, MO: Mosby.

Holaday, B., & Turner-Henson, A. (1989). Response effects in surveys with school-age children. *Nursing Research, 38*(4), 248–250.

Holzemer, W. L., Henry, S. B., Nokes, K. M., Corless, I. B., Brown, M. A., Powell-Cope, G. M., et al. (1999) Validation of the Sign and Symptom Checklist for persons with HIV disease (SSC-HIV). *Journal of Advanced Nursing, 30*(5), 1041–1049.

Holzemer, W. L., Hudson, A., Kirksey, K. M., Hamilton, M. J., & Bakken, S. (2001). The revised Sign and Symptom Checklist for

HIV (SSC-HIVrev). *Journal of the Association of Nurses in AIDS Care*, *12*(1), 60–70.

Hulin, C. L., Drasgow, F., & Parsons, C. K. (1983). *Item response theory: Application to psychological measurement*. Homewood, IL: Dow Jones-Irwin.

International Organization for Standardization. (ISO). (2011). *Standards development*. Retrieved from http://www.iso.org/iso/standards_development.htm.

Johantgen, M. (2010). Using existing administrative and national databases. In C. F. Waltz, O. L. Strickland, & E. R. Lenz (Eds.), *Measurement in nursing and health research* (4th ed., pp. 241–250). New York, NY: Springer Publishing Company.

Jones, D. J., Munro, C. L., Grap, M. J., Kitten, T., & Edmond, M. (2010). Oral care and bacteremia risk in mechanically ventilated adults. *Heart & Lung*, *39*(6S), S57–S65.

Jones, J. M. (2004). Nutritional methodology: Development of a nutritional screening or assessment tool using a multivariate technique. *Nutrition*, *20*(3), 298–306.

Klein, D. G., Dumpe, M., Katz, E., & Bena, J. (2010). Pain assessment in the intensive care unit: Development and psychometric testing of the nonverbal pain assessment tool. *Heart & Lung*, *39*(6), 521–528.

Kruskal, J. B., & Wish, M. (1990). *Multidimensional scaling*. Newbury Park, CA: Sage.

Lake, E. T., Shang, J., Klaus, S., & Dunton, N. E. (2010). Patient falls: Association with hospital Magnet status and nursing unit staffing. *Research in Nursing & Health*, *33*(5), 413–425.

Lee, K. A., & Kieckhefer, G. M. (1989). Measuring human responses using visual analogue scales. *Western Journal of Nursing Research*, *11*(1), 128–132.

Lim, M., Sacks-Davis, R., Aitken, C. K., Hocking, J. S., & Hellard, M. E. (2010). Randomized controlled trial of paper, online, and SMS diaries for collecting sexual behavior information from young people. *Journal of Epidemiology & Community Health*, *64*(10), 885–889.

Lindeman, C. A. (1975). Delphi survey of priorities in clinical nursing research. *Nursing Research*, *24*(6), 434–441.

Lynn, M. R. (1989). Instrument reliability: How much needs to be published? *Heart & Lung*, *18*(4), 421–423.

Marshall, C., & Rossman, G. B. (2011). *Designing qualitative research* (5th ed.). Thousand Oaks, CA: Sage.

McKeown, B., & Thomas, D. (1988). *Q methodology*. Newbury Park, CA: Sage.

McLaughlin, P. (1990). *How to interview: The art of asking questions* (2nd ed.). North Vancouver, BC: International Self-Counsel Press.

Melnyk, B. M., & Fineout-Overholt, E. (2011). *Evidence-based practice in nursing and healthcare: A guide to best practice* (2nd ed.). Philadelphia, PA: Lippincott Williams & Wilkins.

Mishler, E. G. (1986). *Research interviewing: Context and narrative*. Cambridge, MA: Harvard University Press.

Mitchell, M. P. (1998). Nursing education planning: A Delphi study. *Journal of Nursing Education*, *37*(7), 305–307.

Munhall, P. L. (2012). *Nursing research: A qualitative perspective* (5th ed.). Miami, FL: Jones & Bartlett.

National Institute of Nursing Research (NINR). (2012). *Summer Genetics Institute (SGI)*. Retrieved from http://www.ninr.nih.gov/Training/TrainingOpportunitiesIntramural/Summer GeneticsInstitute.

National Institute of Nursing Research (NINR). (2011). *Strategic plan National Institute of Nursing Research: Areas of research emphasis*. Retrieved from http://www.ninr.nih.gov/AboutNINR/NINRMissionandStrategicPlan/.

Ng, K., Wong, S., Lim, S., & Goh, Z. (2010). Evaluation of the Cadi ThermoSENSOR wireless skin-contact thermometer against ear and axillary temperatures in children. *Journal of Pediatric Nursing*, *25*(3), 176–186.

Nicholl, H. (2010). Diaries as a method of data collection in research. *Paediatric Nursing*, *22*(7), 16–20.

Norbeck, J. S. (1985). What constitutes a publishable report of instrument development? *Nursing Research*, *34*(6), 380–381.

Nunnally, J. C., & Bernstein, I. H. (1994). *Psychometric theory* (3rd ed.). New York, NY: McGraw-Hill.

Osgood, C. E., Suci, G. J., & Tannenbaum, P. H. (1957). *The measurement of meaning*. Urbana, IL: University of Illinois Press.

Pugh, L. C., & DeKeyser, F. G. (1995). Use of physiologic variables in nursing research. *Image Journal of Nursing Scholarship*, *27*(4), 273–276.

Radloff, L. S. (1977). The CES-D scale: A self-report depression scale for research in the general population. *Applied Psychological Measures*, *1*, 385–394.

Raven, E. E., Haverkamp, D., Sierevelt, I. N., Van Montfoort, D. O., Poll, R. G., Blankevoort, L., et al. (2008). Construct validity and reliability of the disability of arm, shoulder, and hand questionnaire for upper extremity complaints in rheumatoid arthritis. *Journal of Rheumatology*, *35*(12), 2334–2338.

Rudy, E., & Grady, P. (2005). Biological researchers: Building nursing science. *Nursing Outlook*, *53*(2), 88–94.

Ryan-Wenger, N. A. (2010). Evaluation of measurement precision, accuracy, and error in biophysical data for clinical research and practice. In C. F. Waltz, O. L. Strickland, & E. R. Lenz (Eds.), *Measurement in nursing and health research* (4th ed., pp. 371–383). New York, NY: Springer Publishing Company.

Saris, W. E. (1991). *Computer-assisted interviewing*. Newbury Park, CA: Sage.

Saris, W. E., & Gallhofer, I. N. (2007). *Design, evaluation, and analysis of questionnaires for survey research*. Hoboken, NJ: John Wiley & Son.

Scholz, J., Knoll, N., Sniehotta, F. F., & Schwarzer, R. (2006). Physical activity and depressive symptoms in cardiac rehabilitation: Long-term effects of a self-management intervention. *Social Science & Medicine*, *62*(12), 3109–3120.

Sennott-Miller, L., Murdaugh, C., & Hinshaw, A. S. (1988). Magnitude estimation: Issues and practical applications. *Western Journal of Nursing Research*, *10*(4), 414–424.

Shelley, S. I. (1984). *Research methods in nursing and health*. Boston, MA: Little, Brown.

Silfen, M. E., Manibo, A. M., McMahon, D. J., Levine, L. S., Murphy, A. R., & Oberfield, S. E. (2001). Comparison of simple measures of insulin sensitivity in young girls with premature adrenarche: The fasting glucose to insulin ratio may be a simple and useful measure. *Journal of Clinical Endocrinology & Metabolism*, *86*(6), 2863–2868.

Simpson, S. H. (1989). Use of Q-sort methodology in cross-cultural nutrition and health research. *Nursing Research*, *38*(5), 289–290.

Smith, A. E., Annesi, J. J., Walsh, A. M., Lennon, V., & Bell, R. A. (2010). Association of changes in self-efficacy, voluntary physical activity, and risk factors for type 2 diabetes in a behavioral treatment for obese preadolescents: A pilot study. *Journal of Pediatric Nursing*, *25*(5), 393–399.

Spector, P. E. (1992). *Summated rating scale construction: An introduction*. Newbury Park, CA: Sage.

Stone, K. S., & Frazier, S. K. (2010). Measurement of physiological variables using biomedical instrumentation. In C. F. Waltz, O. L. Strickland, & E. R. Lenz (Eds.), *Measurement in nursing and health research* (4th ed., pp. 335–370). New York, NY: Springer Publishing Company.

Swardfager, W., Herrmann, N., Dowlati, Y., Oh, P., Kiss, A., & Lanctot, K. L. (2008). Relationship between cardiopulmonary fitness and depressive symptoms in cardiac rehabilitation patients with coronary artery disease. *Journal of Rehabilitation Medicine*, *40*(3), 213–218.

Tetting, D. W. (1988). Q-sort update. *Western Journal of Nursing Research*, *10*(6), 757–765.

Thomas, S. J. (2004). *Using web and paper questionnaires for database-based decision making: From design to interpretation of the results*. Thousand Oaks, CA: Corwin Press.

Turner, C. F., Rogers, S. M., Hendershot, T. P., Miller, H. G., & Thornberry, J. P. (1996). Improving representation of linguistic minorities in health surveys. *Public Health Reports*, *111*(3), 276–279.

U.S. Department of Health and Human Services. (2011). *Health information privacy*. Retrieved from http://www.hhs.gov/ocr/privacy/.

Vernon, W. (2009). The Delphi technique: A review. *International Journal of Therapy & Rehabilitation*, *16*(2), 69–76.

Waltz, C. F., Strickland, O. L., & Lenz, E. R. (2010). *Measurement in nursing and health research* (4th ed.). New York, NY: Springer Publishing Company.

Wewers, M. E., & Lowe, N. K. (1990). A critical review of visual analogue scales in the measurement of clinical phenomena. *Research in Nursing & Health*, *13*(4), 227–236.

Wilkes, L., Mohan, S., Luck, L., & Jackson, D. (2010). Development of a violence tool in the emergency hospital setting. *Nurse Researcher*, *17*(4), 70–82.

Winkelman, C., Norman, D., Maloni, J. A., & Kless, J. R. (2008). Pain measurement during labor: Comparing the visual analog scale with dermatome assessment. *Applied Nursing Research*, *21*(2), 104–109.

Yu, D. S. F., Lee, D. T. F., & Woo, J. (2004). Issues and challenges of instrument translation. *Western Journal of Nursing Research*, *26*(3), 307–320.

18
CHAPTER

Critical Appraisal of Nursing Studies

ℯvolve http://evolve.elsevier.com/Grove/practice/

The nursing profession continues to strive for evidence-based practice, which includes critically appraising studies, synthesizing research findings, and applying sound scientific evidence in practice. Researchers also critically appraise studies in a selected area, develop a summary of current knowledge, and identify areas for future studies. Critically appraising research is essential for evidence-based nursing practice and the conduct of future research. The **critical appraisal of research** involves a systematic, unbiased, careful examination of all aspects of studies to judge their strengths, weaknesses, meaning, and significance. The ability of a nurse to appraise studies critically is based on the nurse's previous research experience and knowledge of a topic. To conduct a critical appraisal of research, one must possess analysis and logical reasoning skills to examine the credibility and integrity of a study. This chapter provides a background for critically appraising studies in nursing and other healthcare disciplines. The expanding roles of nurses in conducting critical appraisals of research are addressed. Detailed guidelines are provided to direct you in critically appraising both quantitative and qualitative studies.

Evolution of Critical Appraisal of Research in Nursing

The process for critically appraising research has evolved gradually in nursing from a few to now many nurses who are prepared to conduct comprehensive, scholarly critiques. During the 1940s and 1950s, presentations of nursing research were followed by critiques of the studies. These critiques often focused on the weaknesses or limitations of the studies and tended

to be harsh and traumatic for the researcher (Meleis, 2007). As a consequence of these early unpleasant experiences, nurse researchers began to protect and shelter their nurse scientists from the threat of criticism. Public critiques, written or verbal, were rare in the 1960s and 1970s. Nurses responding to research presentations focused on the strengths of studies, and the limitations were either critically not mentioned or were minimized. Thus, the effects of the limitations on the meaning, validity, and significance of studies were often lost.

Incomplete critiques or the absence of critiques may have served a purpose as nurses gained basic research skills. However, the nursing discipline has moved past this point, and it is recognized that comprehensive critical appraisals of research are essential to strengthen the scientific investigations needed for evidence-based practice (EBP; Brown, 2009; Craig & Smyth, 2012; Fawcett & Garity, 2009). As a result of advances in the nursing profession over the last 30 years, many nurses now have the educational preparation and expertise to conduct critical appraisals of research. Nursing research textbooks provide detailed information on the critical appraisal process. Skills in critical appraisal are introduced at the baccalaureate level of nursing education and are expanded at the master's and doctoral levels. Specialty organizations provide workshops on the critical appraisal process to promote the use of scientific evidence in practice.

The critical appraisal of studies is essential for the development and refinement of nursing knowledge. Nurses need these skills to examine the meaning and credibility of study findings and to ask searching questions. Was the methodology of a study sound to produce credible findings? Are the findings an accurate reflection of reality? Do they increase our understanding of the nature of phenomena that are important in nursing? Are the findings from the present study consistent with findings from previous studies? The answers to these questions require careful examination of the research problem and purpose, the theoretical or philosophical basis of the study, and the study's methodology. Not only must the mechanics of conducting the study be evaluated, but also the abstract and logical reasoning the researchers used to plan and implement the study (Fawcett & Garity, 2009; Munhall, 2012). If the reasoning process used to develop a study has flaws, there are probably flaws in interpreting the meaning of the findings, decreasing the credibility of the study.

All studies have flaws, but if all flawed studies were discarded, there would be no scientific knowledge base for practice. In fact, science itself is flawed. Science does not completely or perfectly describe, explain, predict, or control reality. However, improved understanding and an increased ability to predict and control phenomena depend on recognizing the flaws in studies and in science. New studies can then be planned to minimize the flaws or limitations of earlier studies. A researcher must critically analyze previous studies to determine their limitations and then interpret the study findings in light of those limitations. The limitations can lead to inaccurate data, inaccurate outcomes of analysis, and decreased ability to generalize the findings. You must decide if a study is too flawed to be used in a systematic review of knowledge in an area. Although we recognize that knowledge is not absolute, we need to have confidence in the research evidence synthesized for practice.

All studies have strengths as well as limitations. Recognition of these strengths is also essential to the generation of sound research evidence for practice. If only weaknesses are identified, nurses might discount the value of studies and refuse to invest time in reading and examining research. The continued work of the researcher also depends on recognizing the strengths of the study. If no study is good enough, why invest time conducting research? The strong points of a study, added to the strong points from multiple other studies, slowly build solid research evidence for practice.

When Are Critical Appraisals of Research Implemented in Nursing?

In general, research is critically appraised to broaden understanding, summarize knowledge for practice, and provide a knowledge base for future studies. In addition, critical appraisals are often conducted after verbal presentations of studies, after a published research report, for an abstract section for a conference, for article selection for publication, and for evaluation of research proposals for implementation or funding. Nursing students, practicing nurses, nurse educators, and nurse researchers all are involved in the critical appraisal of research.

Critical Appraisal of Studies by Students

In nursing education, conducting a critical appraisal of a study is often seen as a first step in learning the research process. Part of learning this process is being able to read and comprehend published research reports. However, conducting a critical appraisal of a study is not a basic skill, and the content presented in previous chapters is essential for implementing this process. Nurses usually acquire basic knowledge of the research process and critical appraisal skills early in their nursing education. Advanced analysis skills are usually taught at the master's and doctoral levels. Performing a critical appraisal of a study involves (1) identifying the elements or steps of the study, (2) determining the study strengths and limitations, and (3) evaluating the credibility and meaning of study findings for nursing knowledge and practice. By critically appraising studies, students expand their analysis skills, strengthen their knowledge base, and increase their use of research evidence in practice.

Critical Appraisal of Research by Practicing Nurses

Practicing nurses need to appraise studies critically so that their practice is based on current research evidence and not tradition and trial and error (Brown, 2009; Melnyk & Fineout-Overholt, 2011). Nursing actions must be updated in response to the current evidence that is generated through research and theory development. Practicing nurses need to design methods for remaining current in their practice areas. Reading research journals and posting or emailing current studies at work can increase nurses' awareness of study findings but are insufficient for the purposes of critical appraisal. Nurses need to question the quality of the studies and the credibility of the findings and share their concerns with other nurses. For example, nurses may form a research journal club in which studies are presented and critically appraised by members of the group (Gloeckner & Robinson, 2010). Skills in critical appraisal of research enable practicing nurses to synthesize the most credible, significant, and appropriate evidence for use in their practice. EBP is essential in agencies either seeking or maintaining Magnet status. The Magnet Recognition Program®

was developed by the American Nurses Credentialing Center (ANCC, 2012) to recognize healthcare organizations that provide nursing excellence with care based on the most current research evidence (see http://www.nursecredentialing.org/Magnet/Program Overview.aspx).

Critical Appraisal of Research by Nurse Educators

Educators critically appraise research to expand their knowledge base and to develop and refine the educational process. The careful analysis of current nursing studies provides a basis for updating curriculum content for use in clinical and classroom settings. Educators act as role models for their students by examining new studies, evaluating the information obtained from research, and indicating what research evidence to use in practice. In addition, educators collaborate in the conduct of studies, which requires a critical appraisal of previous relevant research.

Critical Appraisal of Studies by Nurse Researchers

Nurse researchers critically appraise previous research to plan and implement their next study. Many researchers have a program of research in a selected area, and they update their knowledge base by critiquing new studies in this area. The outcomes of these appraisals influence the selection of research problems and purposes, the implementation of research methodologies, and the interpretations of findings in future studies. The critical appraisal and synthesis of previous studies for the literature review section in a research proposal or report were described in Chapter 6.

Critical Appraisal of Research Presentations and Publications

Critical appraisals following research presentations can assist researchers in identifying the strengths and weaknesses of their studies and generating ideas for further research. Participants listening to study critiques might gain insight into the conduct of research. Experiencing the critical appraisal process can increase the ability of participants to evaluate studies and judge the usefulness of the research evidence for practice.

At the present time, at least two nursing research journals, *Scholarly Inquiry for Nursing Practice: An International Journal* and *Western Journal of Nursing Research,* include commentaries after the research articles. In these journals, other researchers critically appraise the authors' studies, and the authors have a chance to respond to these comments. Published research critical appraisals often increase the

reader's understanding of the study and the quality of the study findings (American Psychological Association [APA], 2010; Pyrczak, 2008). Another, more informal critique of a published study might appear in a letter to the editor, in which readers have the opportunity to comment on the strengths and weaknesses of published studies by writing to the journal editor.

Critical Appraisal of Abstracts for Conference Presentations

One of the most difficult types of critical appraisal is examining abstracts. The amount of information available is usually limited because many abstracts are restricted to 100 to 250 words. Nevertheless, reviewers must select the best-designed studies with the most significant outcomes for presentation at nursing conferences. This process requires an experienced researcher who needs few cues to determine the quality of a study. Critical appraisal of an abstract usually addresses the following criteria: (1) appropriateness of the study for the program; (2) completeness of the research project; (3) overall quality of the study problem, purpose, methodology, and results; (4) contribution of the study to the knowledge base of nursing; (5) contribution of the study to nursing theory; (6) originality of the work (not previously published); (7) implication of the study findings for practice; and (8) clarity, conciseness, and completeness of the abstract (APA, 2010).

Critical Appraisal of Research Articles for Publication

Nurse researchers who serve as peer reviewers for professional journals evaluate the quality of research articles submitted for publication. The role of these scientists is to ensure that the studies accepted for publication are well designed and contribute to the body of knowledge. Most of these reviews are conducted anonymously so that friendships or reputations do not interfere with the selection process (Pyrczak, 2008; Tilden, 2002). In most refereed journals, the experts who examine the research report have been selected from an established group of peer reviewers. Their comments or summaries of their comments are sent to the researcher. The editor also uses these comments to make selections for publication. The process for publishing a study is described in Chapter 27.

Critical Appraisal of Research Proposals

Critical appraisals of research proposals are conducted to approve student research projects; to permit data collection in an institution; and to select the best studies for funding by local, state, national, and international organizations and agencies. The process researchers use to seek the approval to conduct a study is presented in Chapter 28. The peer review process in federal funding agencies involves an extremely complex critical appraisal. Nurses are involved in this level of research review through the national funding agencies, such as the National Institute of Nursing Research (NINR, 2012), National Institutes of Health, and the Agency for Healthcare Research and Quality. Some of the criteria used to evaluate the quality of a proposal for possible funding include the (1) significance of the research problem and purpose for nursing, (2) appropriate use of methodology for the types of questions that the research is designed to answer, (3) appropriate use and interpretation of analysis procedures, (4) evaluation of clinical practice and forecasting of the need for nursing or other appropriate interventions, and (5) construction of models to direct the research and interpret the findings. The NINR (2012) website (http://www.ninr.nih.gov/ResearchAnd Funding/) provides details on grant development and research funding, and Chapter 29 focuses on seeking funding for research.

TABLE 18-1	Educational Level and Expected Level of Expertise in Critical Appraisal of Research
Educational Level	**Expected Level of Expertise in Critical Appraisal of Research**
Baccalaureate	Identify the steps of the quantitative research process in a study
	Identify the elements of a qualitative study
Master's	Determine study strengths and weaknesses in quantitative and qualitative studies
	Evaluate the credibility and meaning of a study and its contribution to nursing knowledge and practice
Doctorate or postdoctorate	Synthesize multiple studies in systematic reviews, meta-analyses, meta-syntheses, and mixed-methods systematic reviews

Nurses' Expertise in Critical Appraisal of Research

Conducting a critical appraisal of a study is a complex mental process that is stimulated by raising questions. The level of critique conducted is influenced by the sophistication of the individual appraising the study (Table 18-1). The initial critical appraisal of research by an undergraduate student often involves the identification of the steps of the research process in a quantitative study. Some baccalaureate programs include more in-depth research courses that include critical appraisals of the steps of quantitative studies and identification of the aspects of qualitative studies. A critical appraisal of research conducted by a student at the master's level usually involves description of study strengths and weaknesses and evaluation of the credibility and meaning of the study findings for nursing knowledge and practice. Critical appraisals might focus on quantitative, qualitative, and outcomes studies.

At the doctoral level, students often critically appraise several studies in an area of interest and perform a complex synthesis of the research findings to determine the current empirical knowledge base for the phenomenon. These complex syntheses of quantitative, qualitative, outcomes, and intervention research include (1) systematic review of research, (2) meta-analysis, (3) meta-synthesis, and (4) mixed methods systematic review (see Table 18-1). These summaries of current research evidence are essential for providing EBP and directing future research (Craig & Smyth, 2012; Higgins & Green, 2008; Sandelowski & Barroso, 2007; Whittemore, 2005). Definitions of these types of complex syntheses are presented in Chapter 2, and Chapter 19 provides guidelines for critically appraising and conducting these syntheses.

The major focus of this chapter is conducting critical appraisals of quantitative and qualitative studies. These critical appraisals involve implementing some initial guidelines that are outlined in Box 18-1. These guidelines stress the importance of examining the expertise of the authors, reviewing the entire study, addressing the strengths and weaknesses of the study, and evaluating the credibility of the study findings (Fawcett & Garity, 2009; Marshall & Rossman, 2011; Munhall, 2012; Shadish, Cook, & Campbell, 2002). These guidelines provide a basis for the critical appraisal process for quantitative research that is discussed in the next section and the critical appraisal process for qualitative research discussed later.

Critical Appraisal Process for Quantitative Research

The **critical appraisal process for quantitative research** includes three steps: (1) identifying the steps of the research process, (2) determining study strengths

Box 18-1	Guidelines for Conducting Critical Appraisals of Quantitative and Qualitative Research

1. *Read and evaluate the entire study.* A research appraisal requires comprehension of a study that includes the identification and examination of all steps of the research process.
2. *Examine the research, clinical, and educational background of the authors.* The authors need a clinical and scientific background that is appropriate for the study conducted.
3. *Examine the organization and presentation of the research report.* The title of the research report needs to indicate clearly the focus of the study. The report usually includes an abstract, introduction, methods, results, discussion, and references. The abstract of the study needs to present the purpose of the study clearly and to highlight the methodology and major results. The body of the report needs to be complete, concise, clearly presented, and logically organized. The references need to be complete and presented in a consistent format.
4. *Identify the strengths and weaknesses of a study.* All studies have strengths and

weaknesses, and you can use the questions in this chapter to facilitate identification of them. Address the quality of the problem, purpose, methodology, results, and findings of quantitative and qualitative studies.
5. *Provide specific examples of the strengths and weaknesses of a study.* These examples provide a rationale and documentation for your critical appraisal of the study.
6. *Be objective and realistic in identifying a study's strengths and weaknesses.* Do not be overly critical when identifying the weaknesses of a study or overly flattering when identifying the strengths.
7. *Suggest modifications for future studies.* Modifications should increase the strengths and decrease the weaknesses in the study.
8. *Evaluate the study.* Indicate the overall quality of the study and its contribution to nursing knowledge. Discuss the consistency of the findings of this study with the findings of previous studies. Discuss the need for further research and the potential implications of the findings for practice.

and weaknesses, and (3) evaluating the credibility and meaning of a study to nursing knowledge and practice. These steps occur in sequence, vary in depth, and presume accomplishment of the preceding steps. However, an individual with critical appraisal experience frequently performs several steps of this process simultaneously.

This section includes the three steps of the quantitative research critical appraisal process and provides relevant questions for each step. These questions are not comprehensive but have been selected as a means for stimulating the logical reasoning and analysis necessary for conducting a study review. Persons experienced in the critical appraisal process formulate additional questions as part of their reasoning processes. We cover the identification of the steps of the research process separately because persons who are new to critical appraisal start with this step. The questions for determining the study strengths and weaknesses are covered together because this process occurs simultaneously in the mind of the person conducting the critical appraisal. Evaluation is covered separately because of the increased expertise needed to perform this step.

Step I: Identifying the Steps of the Research Process in Studies

Initial attempts to comprehend research articles are often frustrating because the terminology and stylized manner of the report are unfamiliar. Identification of the steps of the research process in a quantitative study is the first step in critical appraisal. It involves understanding the terms and concepts in the report; identifying study elements; and grasping the nature, significance, and meaning of the study elements. The following guidelines are presented to direct you in identifying the elements or steps of a study.

Guidelines for Identifying the Steps of the Research Process

The first step involves reviewing the abstract and reading the study from beginning to end (see the guidelines in Box 18-1). As you read, address the following questions about the presentation of the study: Does the title clearly identify the focus of the study by including the major study variables and the population? Does the title indicate the type of study conducted—descriptive, correlational, quasi-experimental, or experimental (Kerlinger & Lee,

2000; Shadish et al., 2002)? Was the abstract clear? Was the writing style of the report clear and concise? Were the different parts of the research report plainly identified (APA, 2010)? Were relevant terms defined? You might underline the terms you do not understand and determine their meaning from the glossary at the end of this textbook. Read the article a second time and highlight or underline each step of the quantitative research process. An overview of these steps is presented in Chapter 3. To write a critical appraisal identifying the study steps, you need to identify each step of the research process concisely and respond briefly to the following guidelines and questions:

I. Introduction
   A. Describe the qualifications of the authors to conduct the study, such as research expertise, clinical experience, and educational preparation. Doctoral education, such as a PhD, provides experience in conducting research. Have the researchers conducted previous studies, especially studies in this area? Are the authors involved in clinical practice or certified in their area of clinical expertise?
   B. Discuss the clarity of the article title (type of study, variables, and population identified).
   C. Discuss the quality of the abstract (includes purpose; highlights design, sample, and intervention [if applicable]; and presents key results).
II. State the problem.
   A. Significance of the problem
   B. Background of the problem
   C. Problem statement
III. State the purpose.
IV. Examine the literature review.
   A. Are relevant previous studies and theories described?
   B. Are the references current? (Number and percentage of sources in the last 10 years and in the last 5 years?)
   C. Are the studies described, critically appraised, and synthesized (Fawcett & Garity, 2009)?
   D. Is a summary provided of the current knowledge (what is known and not known) about the research problem?
V. Examine the study framework or theoretical perspective.
   A. Is the framework explicitly expressed, or must the reviewer extract the framework from implicit statements in the introduction or literature review?
   B. Is the framework based on tentative, substantive, or scientific theory? Provide a rationale for your answer.
   C. Does the framework identify, define, and describe the relationships among the concepts of interest? Provide examples of this.
   D. Is a model of the framework provided for clarity? If a model is not presented, develop one that represents the framework of the study and describe it.
   E. Link the study variables to the relevant concepts in the model.
   F. How is the framework related to the body of knowledge of nursing (Alligood, 2010; Smith & Liehr, 2008)?
VI. List any research objectives, questions, or hypotheses.
VII. Identify and define (conceptually and operationally) the study variables or concepts that were identified in the objectives, questions, or hypotheses. If objectives, questions, or hypotheses are not stated, identify and define the variables in the study purpose and the results section of the study. If conceptual definitions are not found, identify possible definitions for each major study variable. Indicate which of the following types of variables were included in the study. A study usually includes independent and dependent variables or research variables but not all three types of variables.
   A. Independent variables: Identify and define conceptually and operationally.
   B. Dependent variables: Identify and define conceptually and operationally.
   C. Research variables or concepts: Identify and define conceptually and operationally.
VIII. Identify demographic variables and other relevant terms.
IX. Identify the research design.
   A. Identify the specific design of the study. Draw a model of the design by using the sample design models presented in Chapter 11.
   B. Does the study include a treatment or intervention? If so, is the treatment clearly described with a protocol and consistently implemented, which indicates intervention fidelity (Forbes, 2009; Mittlbock, 2008)?

C. If the study has more than one group, how were subjects assigned to groups (Mittlbock, 2008; Shadish et al., 2002)?

D. Are extraneous variables identified and controlled? Extraneous variables are usually discussed as a part of quasi-experimental and experimental studies (Shadish et al., 2002).

E. Were pilot study findings used to design this study? If yes, briefly discuss the pilot and the changes made in this study based on the pilot.

X. Describe the sample and setting.

A. Identify inclusion or exclusion sample or eligibility criteria.

B. Identify the specific type of probability or nonprobability sampling method that was used to obtain the sample. Did the researchers identify the sampling frame for the study (Thompson, 2002)?

C. Identify the sample size. Discuss the refusal rate and include the rationale for refusal if presented in the article. Discuss the power analysis if this process was used to determine sample size (Aberson, 2010).

D. Identify the sample attrition (number and percentage) and rationale for the study.

E. Identify the characteristics of the sample.

F. Discuss the institutional review board approval. Describe the informed consent process used in the study.

G. Identify the study setting, and indicate if it is appropriate for the study purpose.

XI. Identify and describe each measurement strategy used in the study. The following table includes the critical information about two measurement methods, the Beck Likert scale to measure depression and the physiological instrument to measure blood pressure. Completing this table allows you to cover essential measurement content for a study (Waltz, Strickland, & Lenz, 2010).

A. Identify each study variable that was measured.

B. Identify the name and author of each measurement strategy.

C. Identify the type of each measurement strategy (e.g., Likert scale, visual analogue scale, physiological measure, and existing database).

D. Identify the level of measurement (nominal, ordinal, interval, or ratio) achieved by each measurement method used in the study (Grove, 2007).

E. Describe the reliability of each scale for previous studies and this study. Identify the precision of each physiological measure (Bialocerkowski, Klupp, & Bragge, 2010; DeVon et al., 2007).

F. Identify the validity of each scale and the accuracy of physiological measures (DeVon et al., 2007; Ryan-Wenger, 2010).

Variable Measured	Name of Measurement Method/ Author	Type of Measurement Method	Level of Measurement	Reliability or Precision	Validity or Accuracy
Depression	Beck Depression Inventory/Beck	Likert scale	Interval	Cronbach alpha of 0.82-0.92 from previous studies and 0.84 for this study. Reading level at 6th grade.	Construct validity: Content validity from concept analysis, literature review, and reviews of experts. Convergent validity with Zung Depression Scale. Prediction validity of patients' future depression episodes. Successive use validity with previous studies and this study.
Blood pressure (BP)	Omron BP equipment/ Health Care Equipment Agency	Physiological measurement method	Ratio	Test-retest values of BP measurements in previous studies. BP equipment new and recalibrated every 50 BP readings in this study. Average 3 BP readings to determine BP.	Documented accuracy of systolic and diastolic BPs to 1 mm Hg by company developing Omron BP cuff. Designated protocol for taking BP. Average 3 BP readings to determine BP.

XII. Describe the procedures for data collection.
XIII. Describe the statistical techniques performed to analyze study data.
   A. List the statistical procedures conducted to describe the sample.
   B. Was the level of significance or alpha identified? If so, indicate what it was (0.05, 0.01, or 0.001).
   C. Complete the following table with the analysis techniques conducted in the study: (1) identify the focus (description, relationships, or differences) for each analysis technique; (2) list the statistical analysis technique performed; (3) list the statistic; (4) provide the specific results; and (5) identify the probability (*p*) of the statistical significance achieved by the result (Corty, 2007; Grove, 2007).

Purpose of Analysis	Analysis Technique	Statistic	Results	Probability (*p*)
Description of subjects' pulse rate	Mean	*M*	71.52	
	Standard deviation	*SD*	5.62	
	Range	Range	58-97	
Difference between men and women in systolic and diastolic blood pressures respectively	*t*-test	*t*	3.75	0.001
	t-test	*t*	2.16	0.042
Differences of diet group, exercise group, and comparison group for pounds lost by adolescents	Analysis of variance	*F*	4.27	0.04
Relationship of depression and anxiety in elderly adults	Pearson correlation	*r*	0.46	0.03

XIV. Describe the researcher's interpretation of findings.
   A. Are the findings related back to the study framework? If so, do the findings support the study framework?
   B. Which findings are consistent with the expected findings?
   C. Which findings were not expected?
   D. Are the findings consistent with previous research findings (Fawcett & Garity, 2009)?
XV. What study limitations did the researcher identify?
XVI. How did the researcher generalize the findings?
XVII. What were the implications of the findings for nursing practice?
XVIII. What suggestions for further study were identified?
XIX. Is the description of the study sufficiently clear for replication?

Step II: Determining Study Strengths and Weaknesses

The next step in critically appraising a quantitative study requires determining the strengths and weaknesses of the study. To do this, you must have knowledge of what each step of the research process should be like from expert sources such as this textbook and other research sources (Aberson, 2010; Bartlett & Frost, 2008; Bialocerkowski et al., 2010; Borglin &

Richards, 2010; Burns & Grove, 2011; DeVon et al., 2007; Doran, 2011; Fawcett & Garity, 2009; Grove, 2007; Houser, 2008; Morrison et al., 2009; Ryan-Wenger, 2010; Santacroce, Maccarelli, & Grey, 2004; Shadish et al., 2002; Thompson, 2002; Waltz et al., 2010). The ideal ways to conduct the steps of the research process are compared with the actual study steps. During this comparison, you examine the extent to which the researcher followed the rules for an ideal study and identify the study elements that are strengths or weaknesses.

You also need to examine the logical links connecting one study element with another. For example, the problem needs to provide background and direction for the statement of the purpose. In addition, you need to examine the overall flow of logic in the study. The variables identified in the study purpose need to be consistent with the variables identified in the research objectives, questions, or hypotheses. The variables identified in the research objectives, questions, or hypotheses need to be conceptually defined in light of the study framework. The conceptual definitions provide the basis for the development of operational definitions. The study design and analyses need to be appropriate for the investigation of the study purpose and for the specific objectives, questions, or hypotheses (Fawcett & Garity, 2009). Most of the limitations or weaknesses in a study result from breaks in logical reasoning. For example, biases caused by sampling and design impair the logical flow from design to interpretation of findings (Borglin & Richards, 2010).

The previous level of critical appraisal addressed concrete aspects of the study. During analysis, the process moves to examining abstract dimensions of the study, which requires greater familiarity with the logic behind the research process and increased skill in abstract reasoning.

You also need to gain a sense of how clearly the researcher grasped the study situation and expressed it. The clarity of the researchers' explanation of study elements demonstrates their skill in using and expressing ideas that require abstract reasoning. With this examination of the study, you can determine which aspects of the study are strengths and which are weaknesses and provide rationale and documentation for your decisions.

Guidelines for Determining Study Strengths and Weaknesses

The following questions were developed to assist you in examining the different aspects of a study and determining if it is a strength or weakness. The intent is not to answer each of these questions but to read the questions and make judgments about the elements or steps in the study. You need to provide a rationale for your decisions and document from relevant research sources such as those listed in the previous section and in the references at the end of this chapter. For example, you might decide the study purpose is a strength because it addresses the study problem, clarifies the focus of the study, and is feasible to investigate (Burns & Grove, 2011; Fawcett & Garity, 2009; Pyrczak, 2008).

I. Research problem and purpose
  A. Is the problem sufficiently delimited in scope so that it is researchable but not trivial?
  B. Is the problem significant to nursing and clinical practice (Brown, 2009)?
  C. Does the purpose narrow and clarify the aim of the study?
  D. Was this study feasible to conduct in terms of money commitment; the researchers' expertise; availability of subjects, facilities, and equipment; and ethical considerations?

II. Review of literature
  A. Is the literature review organized to show the progressive development of evidence from previous research?
  B. Is a theoretical knowledge base developed for the problem and purpose?
  C. Is a clear, concise summary presented of the current empirical and theoretical knowledge in the area of the study

(Craig & Smyth, 2012; Fawcett & Garity, 2009)?
  D. Does the literature review summary identify what is known and not known about the research problem and provide direction for the formation of the research purpose?

III. Study framework
  A. Is the framework presented with clarity? If a model or conceptual map of the framework is present, is it adequate to explain the phenomenon of concern?
  B. Is the framework linked to the research purpose? If not, would another framework fit more logically with the study?
  C. Is the framework related to the body of knowledge in nursing and clinical practice?
  D. If a proposition or relationship from a theory is to be tested, is the proposition clearly identified and linked to the study hypotheses (Alligood, 2010; Fawcett & Garity, 2009; Smith & Liehr, 2008)?

IV. Research objectives, questions, or hypotheses
  A. Are the objectives, questions, or hypotheses expressed clearly?
  B. Are the objectives, questions, or hypotheses logically linked to the research purpose?
  C. Are hypotheses stated to direct the conduct of quasi-experimental and experimental research (Kerlinger & Lee, 2000; Shadish et al., 2002)?
  D. Are the objectives, questions, or hypotheses logically linked to the concepts and relationships (propositions) in the framework (Fawcett & Garity, 2009; Smith & Liehr, 2008)?

V. Variables
  A. Are the variables reflective of the concepts identified in the framework?
  B. Are the variables clearly defined (conceptually and operationally) and based on previous research or theories (Smith & Liehr, 2008)?
  C. Is the conceptual definition of a variable consistent with the operational definition?

VI. Design
  A. Is the design used in the study the most appropriate design to obtain the needed data?
  B. Does the design provide a means to examine all the objectives, questions, or hypotheses?

C. Is the treatment clearly described (Forbes, 2009)? Is the treatment appropriate for examining the study purpose and hypotheses? Does the study framework explain the links between the treatment (independent variable) and the proposed outcomes (dependent variables) (Sidani & Braden, 1998)? Was a protocol developed to promote consistent implementation of the treatment to ensure intervention fidelity (Morrison et al., 2009)? Did the researcher monitor implementation of the treatment to ensure consistency (Santacroce et al., 2004)? If the treatment was not consistently implemented, what might be the impact on the findings?

D. Did the researcher identify the threats to design validity (statistical conclusion validity, internal validity, construct validity, and external validity) and minimize them as much as possible (Shadish et al., 2002)?

E. Is the design logically linked to the sampling method and statistical analyses?

F. If more than one group is used, do the groups appear equivalent (Borglin & Richards, 2010)?

G. If a treatment was implemented, were the subjects randomly assigned to the treatment group, or were the treatment and comparison groups matched? Were the treatment and comparison group assignments appropriate for the purpose of the study (Borglin & Richards, 2010)?

VII. Sample, population, and setting

A. Is the sampling method adequate to produce a representative sample?

B. What are the potential biases in the sampling method? Are any subjects excluded from the study because of age, socioeconomic status, or ethnicity without a sound rationale (Borglin & Richards, 2010; Thompson, 2002)?

C. Did the sample include an understudied population, such as young, elderly, or minority subjects?

D. Were the sampling criteria (inclusion and exclusion) appropriate for the type of study conducted?

E. Is the sample size sufficient to avoid a type II error? Was a power analysis conducted to determine sample size? If a power analysis was conducted, were the results of the analysis clearly described and used to determine the final sample size? Was the attrition rate projected in determining the final sample size (Aberson, 2010)?

F. Are the rights of human subjects protected?

G. Is the setting used in the study typical of clinical settings (Borglin & Richards, 2010)?

H. Was the refusal to participate rate a problem? If so, how might this weakness influence the findings?

I. Was sample attrition a problem? Did the researchers provide a rationale for the attrition of study participants? How did attrition influence the final sample and the study results and findings (Aberson, 2010; Fawcett & Garity, 2009)?

VIII. Measurements

A. Do the measurement methods selected for the study adequately measure the study variables?

B. Are the measurement methods sufficiently sensitive to detect small differences between subjects? Should additional measurement methods have been used to improve the quality of the study outcomes (Waltz et al., 2010)?

C. Do the measurement methods used in the study have adequate validity and reliability? What additional reliability or validity testing is needed to improve the quality of the measurement methods (Bartlett & Frost, 2008; Bialocerkowski et al., 2010; DeVon et al., 2007; Roberts & Stone, 2004)?

D. Respond to the following questions, which are relevant to the measurement approaches used in the study:

1. Scales and questionnaires

   (a) Are the instruments clearly described?

   (b) Are techniques to complete and score the instruments provided?

   (c) Are validity and reliability of the instruments described (DeVon et al., 2007)?

   (d) Did the researcher reexamine the validity and reliability of instruments for the present sample?

   (e) If the instrument was developed for the study, is the instrument development process described (Waltz et al., 2010)?

2. Observation
   (a) Is what is to be observed clearly identified and defined?
   (b) Is interrater reliability described?
   (c) Are the techniques for recording observations described (Waltz et al., 2010)?
3. Interviews
   (a) Do the interview questions address concerns expressed in the research problem?
   (b) Are the interview questions relevant for the research purpose and objectives, questions, or hypotheses?
   (c) Does the design of the questions tend to bias subjects' responses?
   (d) Does the sequence of questions tend to bias subjects' responses (Waltz et al., 2010)?
4. Physiological measures
   (a) Are the physiological measures or instruments clearly described (Ryan-Wenger, 2010)? If appropriate, are the brand names, such as Space Labs or Hewlett-Packard, of the instruments identified?
   (b) Are the accuracy, precision, and error of the physiological instruments discussed (Ryan-Wenger, 2010)?
   (c) Are the physiological measures appropriate for the research purpose and objectives, questions, or hypotheses?
   (d) Are the methods for recording data from the physiological measures clearly described? Is the recording of data consistent?

IX. Data collection
   A. Is the data collection process clearly described (Fawcett & Garity, 2009; Kerlinger & Lee, 2000)?
   B. Are the forms used to collect data organized to facilitate computerizing the data?
   C. Is the training of data collectors clearly described and adequate?
   D. Is the data collection process conducted in a consistent manner (Borglin & Richards, 2010)?
   E. Are the data collection methods ethical?

F. Do the data collected address the research objectives, questions, or hypotheses?
G. Did any adverse events occur during data collection, and were these appropriately managed?

IX. Data analysis
   A. Are data analysis procedures appropriate for the type of data collected (Corty, 2007; Grove, 2007)?
   B. Are data analysis procedures clearly described? Did the researcher address any problems with missing data and how this problem was managed?
   C. Do the data analysis techniques address the study purpose and the research objectives, questions, or hypotheses (Fawcett & Garity, 2009)?
   D. Are the results presented in an understandable way by narrative, tables, or figures, or a combination of methods (APA, 2010)?
   E. Are the statistical analyses logically linked to the design (Borglin & Richards, 2010)?
   F. Is the sample size sufficient to detect significant differences if they are present?
   G. Was a power analysis conducted for nonsignificant results (Aberson, 2010)?
   H. Are the results interpreted appropriately?

X. Interpretation of findings
   A. Are findings discussed in relation to each objective, question, or hypothesis?
   B. Are various explanations for significant and nonsignificant findings examined?
   C. Are the findings clinically significant (Gatchel & Mayer, 2010; LeFort, 1993; Melnyk & Fineout-Overholt, 2011)?
   D. Are the findings linked to the study framework (Smith & Liehr, 2008)?
   E. Are the study findings an accurate reflection of reality and valid for use in clinical practice (Houser, 2008)?
   F. Do the conclusions fit the results from the data analyses? Are the conclusions based on statistically significant and clinically important results (Gatchel & Mayer, 2010)?
   G. Does the study have limitations not identified by the researcher?
   H. Did the researcher generalize the findings appropriately?
   I. Were the identified implications for practice appropriate based on the study findings and the findings from previous

research (Brown, 2009; Fawcett & Garity, 2009)?

J. Were quality suggestions made for further research?

Step III: Evaluating a Study

Evaluation involves determining the validity, credibility, significance, and meaning of the study by examining the links between the study process, study findings, and previous studies. The steps of the study are evaluated in light of previous studies, such as an evaluation of present hypotheses based on previous hypotheses, present design based on previous designs, and present methods of measuring variables based on previous methods of measurement. The findings of the present study are also examined in light of the findings of previous studies. Evaluation builds on conclusions reached during the first two stages of the critical appraisal so that the credibility, validity, and meaning of the study findings can be determined for nursing knowledge and practice.

Guidelines for Evaluating a Study

You need to reexamine the findings, conclusions, and implications sections of the study and the researchers' suggestions for further study. Using the following questions as a guide, summarize your evaluation of the study, and document your responses.

I. What rival hypotheses can be suggested for the findings?

II. Do you believe the study findings are valid? How much confidence can be placed in the study findings (Borglin & Richards, 2010; Fawcett & Garity, 2009)?

III. To what populations can the findings be generalized (Thompson, 2002)?

IV. What questions emerge from the findings, and does the researcher identify them?

V. What future research can be envisioned?

VI. Could the limitations of the study have been corrected?

VII. When the findings are examined in light of previous studies, what is now known and not known about the phenomenon under study?

You need to read previous studies conducted in the area of the research being examined and summarize your responses to the following questions:

I. Are the findings of previous studies used to generate the research problem and purpose?

II. Is the design an advancement over previous designs (Borglin & Richards, 2010; Shadish et al., 2002)?

III. Do sampling strategies show an improvement over previous studies? Does the sample selection have the potential for adding diversity to samples previously studied (Aberson, 2010; Thompson, 2002)?

IV. Does the current research build on previous measurement strategies so that measurement is more precise or more reflective of the variables (DeVon et al., 2007; Waltz et al., 2010)?

V. How do statistical analyses compare with analyses used in previous studies (Corty, 2007)?

VI. Do the findings build on the findings of previous studies?

VII. Is current knowledge in this area identified?

VIII. Does the author indicate the implication of the findings for practice?

The evaluation of a research report should also include a final discussion of the quality of the report. This discussion should include an expert opinion of the contribution of the study to nursing knowledge and the need for additional research in selected areas. You also need to determine if the empirical evidence generated by this study and previous research is ready for use in practice (Brown, 2009; Craig & Smyth, 2012; Fawcett & Garity, 2009; Melnyk & Fineout-Overholt, 2011; Whittemore, 2005).

Critical Appraisal Process for Qualitative Studies

Critical appraisal of qualitative studies requires a different approach than the steps and processes used when appraising a quantitative study (Sandelowski, 2008). However, appraisal of quantitative and qualitative studies has a common purpose—determining the rigor with which the methods were applied. The integrity of the design and methods affects the credibility and meaningfulness of the findings and their usefulness in clinical practice (Pickler & Butz, 2007). Burns (1989) first described the standards for rigorous qualitative research 20 years ago. Since that time, other criteria have been published (Cesario, Morin, & Santa-Donato, 2002; Clissett, 2008; Fossey, Harvey, McDermott, & Davidson, 2002; Morse, 1991; Pickler & Butz, 2007) and have been the source of considerable debate (Cohen & Crabtree, 2008; Mackey, 2012; Nelson, 2008; Stige, Malterud, & Midtgarden, 2009; Whittemore, Chase, & Mandle, 2001). Nurses critically appraising qualitative studies need three prerequisite characteristics in applying rigorous appraisal standards. Without these prerequisites, nurses may miss potential valuable contributions qualitative studies might make to the knowledge base of nursing for practice. These required prerequisite characteristics are addressed in the following section.

Prerequisites for Critical Appraisal of Qualitative Studies

The first prerequisite for appraising qualitative studies is an appreciation for the philosophical foundation of qualitative research. Qualitative researchers design their studies to be congruent with one of a wide range of philosophies, such as phenomenology, symbolic interactionism, and hermeneutics, each of which espouses slightly different approaches to gaining new knowledge (Liamputtong & Ezzy, 2005). Although unique, the qualitative philosophies are similar in their view of the uniqueness of the individual and the value of the individual's perspective. Without an appreciation for the philosophical perspective supporting the study being critically appraised, the appraiser may not appropriately apply the standards of rigor consistent with that perspective (Sale, 2008). Chapter 4 contains more information on the different philosophies that are foundational to qualitative research.

Guided by an appreciation of qualitative philosophical perspectives, nurses appraising a qualitative study can evaluate the approach used to gather, analyze, and interpret the data. A basic knowledge of different qualitative approaches is as essential for appraisal of qualitative studies as knowledge of quantitative research designs is for appraising quantitative studies. Spending time in the culture, organization, or setting that is the focus of the study is an expectation for ethnography studies but would not be expected for a phenomenological study. A researcher using a grounded theory approach is expected to analyze data to extract social processes and construct connections among emerging concepts. Phenomenological researchers are expected to produce a rich, detailed description of a lived experience. Knowing these distinctions is a prerequisite to fair and objective critical appraisal of qualitative studies. What one expects to find in a qualitative research report may be the most important influence on one's appraisal of the study (Sandelowski & Barroso, 2007).

Appreciating philosophical perspectives and knowing qualitative approaches are superficial, however, without empathy for the participant's perspective. Empathy creates an openness to knowing a participant within a naturalistic holistic framework. This openness allows qualitative researchers and nurses applying the findings to acknowledge the depth, richness, and complexity inherent in the lives of the patients we serve. These prerequisites of philosophical foundation, type of qualitative study, and openness to study participants direct the implementation of the following guidelines for critically appraising qualitative studies.

Critical Appraisal Guidelines for Qualitative Studies

Problem Statement

1. Identify the clinical problem and research problem that led to the study. Were the clinical problem and research problem explicitly stated?
2. How did the author establish the significance of the study? In other words, why should the reader care about this study? Look for statements about human suffering, costs of treatment, or the number of people affected by the clinical problem.
3. Did the researcher identify a personal connection or motivation for selecting this topic to study? For example, the researcher may choose to study the lived experience of men undergoing radiation for prostate cancer after the researcher's father underwent the same treatment. Acknowledging motives and potential biases is an expectation for qualitative researchers (Munhall, 2012).

Purpose and Research Questions

1. Identify the purpose of the study. Is the purpose a logical approach to addressing the research problem of the study (Fawcett & Garity, 2009; Munhall, 2012)? Does the purpose have an intuitive fit with the problem?
2. List research questions that the study was designed to answer. If the author does not explicitly provide the questions, attempt to infer the questions from the answers. What information did the author include as findings?
3. Were the research questions related to the problem and purpose?
4. Were qualitative methods appropriate to answer the research questions?

Literature Review

1. Did the author cite quantitative and qualitative studies relevant to the focus of the study? What other types of literature did the author include?
2. Are the references current? For qualitative studies, the author may have included studies older than the 5-year limit typically used for quantitative studies. Findings of older qualitative studies may be relevant to a qualitative study.

3. Identify the disciplines of the authors of studies cited in the article. Does it appear that the author searched databases outside of the Cumulative Index to Nursing and Allied Health Literature for relevant studies? Research publications in other disciplines as well as literary works in the humanities may have relevance for some qualitative studies.

4. Did the author evaluate or indicate the weaknesses of the available studies?

5. Did the literature review include adequate synthesized information to build a logical argument? Another way to ask the question: Did the author provide enough evidence to support the verdict that the study was needed?

Philosophical Foundation

The methods used by qualitative researchers are determined by the philosophical foundation of their work. The researcher may not have stated explicitly the philosophical stance on which the study is based. Despite this omission, a knowledgeable reader can recognize the philosophy through the description of the problem, formulation of the research questions, and selection of the methods to address the research questions. A well-designed qualitative study is congruent at each stage with the underlying philosophical perspective, and it is clearest if the researcher identifies this perspective in his or her research report (Fawcett & Garity, 2009; Marshall & Rossman, 2011; Munhall, 2012).

1. Did the author identify a specific perspective from which the study was developed? If so, what was it?

2. If a broad philosophy, such as phenomenology, was identified, did the researcher identify the specific philosopher, such as Husserl or Heidegger?

3. Did the researcher cite a primary source for the philosophical foundation?

Qualitative Approach

1. Identify the stated or implied research approach used for the study.

2. Provide a paraphrased description of the research approach used. See Chapter 4 for descriptions of the different qualitative research perspectives or traditions.

3. Were the methods of the study consistent with the research tradition?

Sampling and Sample

1. Identify how study participants were selected.

2. At what sites were participants recruited for the study? Did the sites for recruitment fit the sampling needs of the study?

3. What were the inclusion and exclusion criteria for the sample?

4. Were the selected participants able to provide data relevant to the study purpose and research questions?

5. How many people participated in the study? Did any potential study participants refuse to participate? Did any of the participants start but not finish the study, which determines the study attrition rate?

Data Collection

1. How were data collected in this study? What rationale did the author provide for using this data collection method?

2. Identify the period of time during which data collection occurred.

3. Describe the sequence of data collection events for a participant. For example, were data collected from one interview or a series of interviews? Were focus group participants given an opportunity to provide additional data or review the preliminary conclusions of the researcher?

4. Did the researcher describe changes that were made in the methods in response to the context and early data collection? Were data collection procedures proscriptively applied or allowed to emerge with some flexibility? Flexibility within parameters of the method is considered appropriate for qualitative studies (Fossey et al., 2002).

Protection of Human Study Participants

Qualitative studies tend to address areas of human life that are "sensitive" and require care in the way they are addressed by researchers (Cowles, 1988). For example, many of the topics studied by qualitative researchers are social or moral issues not talked about in common society. Other qualitative studies explore emotional topics that may cause the participant discomfort, anxiety, or grief. A qualitative report should provide clues that the researcher was aware of these concerns and addressed them appropriately.

1. Identify the benefits and risks of participation addressed by the authors. Were there benefits or risks the authors do not identify?

2. How were recruitment and consent techniques adjusted to accommodate the sensitivity of the subject matter and psychological distress of potential participants?

3. How were data collection and management techniques adapted in acknowledgment of participant sensitivity and vulnerability? For example, did the authors have a counselor or other resources

available for participants who might become upset or disturbed by the interview?

Data Management and Analysis

1. Describe the data management and analysis methods used in the study (Marshall & Rossman, 2011; Munhall, 2012).
2. Did the author discuss how the rigor of the process was ensured? For example, does the author describe maintaining a paper trail of critical decisions that were made during the analysis of the data?
3. Analysis of qualitative data is influenced by the experiences and perspectives of the individuals doing the analysis. What measures were used to minimize or allow for the effects of researcher bias? For example, did two researchers independently analyze the data and compare their analyses? Some qualitative researchers believe that comparability of interpretation across researchers is more consistent with a positivist philosophy (Fossey et al., 2002) and would not include this as a criterion for appraisal.
4. Did the data management and analysis methods fit the research purposes and data?

Findings

1. Did the findings address the purpose of the study (Marshall & Rossman, 2011; Munhall, 2012)?
2. Were the data analyzed sufficiently? Findings in a qualitative study are expected to be more than the words that participants said. The researcher is expected to identify themes or abstract concepts that emerged from the data (Fawcett & Garity, 2009).
3. Were the interpretations of data congruent with data collected?
4. Did the researcher address variations in the findings by relevant sample characteristics?

Discussion

1. Did the results offer new information about the target phenomenon?
2. Were the findings linked to findings in other studies or other relevant literatures (Fawcett & Garity, 2009; Munhall, 2012)?
3. Describe the clinical, policy, theoretical, and other significance of the findings. Does the author explore these applications?

Logic and Form of Findings

The study report is the means of communicating the findings. Producing knowledge can occur only through communication (Sandelowski & Barroso, 2007); the logic and form of the findings are critical to the appraisal of the study.

1. Were readers able to hear the voice of the participants and gain an understanding of the phenomenon studied?
2. Were readers able to identify easily the elements of the research report?
3. Did the overall presentation of the study fit its purpose, method, and findings (Fawcett & Garity, 2009; Marshall & Rossman, 2011; Munhall, 2012)?
4. Was there a coherent logic to the presentation of findings?

Evaluation Summary

"The sense of rightness and feeling of comfort readers experience reading the report of a study constitute the very judgments they make about the validity or trustworthiness of the study itself" (Sandelowski & Barroso, 2007, p. xix). Critical appraisal is not complete without making judgments about the validity of the study. Synthesis of the evaluative criteria for qualitative studies can be reframed as philosophical congruence, methodological coherence, intuitive comprehension, and intellectual contribution (Cesario et al., 2002; Clissett, 2008; Fossey et al, 2002; Morse, 1991; Nelson, 2008; Pickler & Butz, 2007; Stige et al., 2009).

1. *Philosophical congruence:* Were the development and implementation of the study congruent with the philosophical foundation of the study?
2. *Methodological coherence:* Did the data collection, analysis, and interpretation processes fit together to form a coherent approach to address the research problem?
3. *Intuitive comprehension:* Do the findings provide a credible reflection of reality and expand the reader's comprehension of the study topic? If so, how can the findings be used in nursing practice?
4. *Intellectual contribution:* What do the findings contribute to the current body of knowledge?
5. State the conclusion of the critical appraisal of the study.

KEY POINTS

- Critical appraisal of research involves carefully examining all aspects of a study to judge its merits, limitations, meaning, validity, and significance in light of previous research experience, knowledge of the topic, and clinical expertise.
- Critical appraisals of research are conducted (1) to summarize evidence for practice, (2) to provide a

basis for future research, (3) to evaluate presentations and publications of studies, (4) for abstract selection for a conference, (5) to select an article for publication, and (6) to evaluate research proposals for funding and implementation in clinical agencies.

- Nurses' levels of expertise in conducting critical appraisals depend on their educational preparation; nurses with baccalaureate, master's, doctorate, and postdoctorate preparation all have a role in examining the quality of research.

- The critical appraisal process for quantitative research includes the following steps: identifying the steps of the research process in a study; determining the study strengths and weaknesses; and evaluating the credibility, validity, and meaning of a study to nursing knowledge and practice.

- The identification step involves understanding the terms and concepts in the report and identifying study elements.

- The second step of determining study strengths and weaknesses involves comparing what each step of the research process should be like with how the steps of the study were conducted. The logical development and implementation of the study steps also need to be examined for strengths and weaknesses.

- Study strengths and weaknesses need to be clearly identified, supported with a rationale, and documented with current research sources.

- The evaluation step involves examining the meaning, validity, and significance of the study according to set criteria.

- To perform fair critical appraisals of qualitative studies, nurses need the prerequisites of an appreciation for the philosophical foundations of qualitative research, knowledge of different qualitative approaches, and empathy for the study participant's perspective.

- Each aspect of a qualitative study, such as problem, purpose, research questions, sample, data collection and analysis, and findings, needs to be examined for strengths and weaknesses.

- Philosophical congruence, methodological coherence, intuitive comprehension, and intellectual contribution are evaluative standards for qualitative studies.

- Philosophical congruence is the extent to which the development and implementation of the study reflected the philosophical underpinnings of the qualitative approach used for the study.

- Methodological coherence is the extent to which the data collection, implementation, and analysis

formed a coherent whole to address the research problem.

- Intuitive comprehension is the enhanced understanding gained by readers of the participant perspective on the study topic.

- Intellectual contribution is the degree to which the findings add to the knowledge of the discipline.

REFERENCES

Aberson, C. L. (2010). *Applied power analysis for the behavioral sciences.* New York, NY: Routledge Taylor & Francis Group.

Alligood, M. R. (2010). *Nursing theory: Utilization & application.* St Louis, MO: Mosby.

American Nurses Credentialing Center (ANCC). (2012). Magnet program overview. Retrieved from http://www.nursecredentialing.org/Magnet/ProgramOverview.aspx.

American Psychological Association (APA). (2010). *Publication manual of the American Psychological Association* (6th ed.). Washington, DC: Author.

Bartlett, J. W., & Frost, C. (2008). Reliability, repeatability and reproducibility: Analysis of measurement errors in continuous variables. *Ultrasound in Obstetrics & Gynecology, 31*(4), 466–475.

Bialocerkowski, A., Klupp, N., & Bragge, P. (2010). Research methodology series: How to read and critically appraise a reliability article. *International Journal of Therapy and Rehabilitation, 17*(3), 114–120.

Borglin, G., & Richards, D. A. (2010). Bias in experimental nursing research: Strategies to improve the quality and explanatory power of nursing science. *International Journal of Nursing Studies, 47*(1), 123–128.

Brown, S. J. (2009). *Evidence-based nursing: The research-practice connection.* Sudbury, MA: Jones & Bartlett Publishers.

Burns, N. (1989). Standards for qualitative research. *Nursing Science Quarterly, 2*(1), 44–52.

Burns, N., & Grove, S. K. (2011). *Understanding nursing research* (5th ed.). Philadelphia, PA: Saunders.

Cesario, S., Morin, K., & Santa-Donato, A. (2002). Evaluating the level of evidence of qualitative research. *Journal of Obstetric, Gynecologic, and Neonatal Nursing, 31*(6), 708–714.

Clissett, P. (2008). Evaluating qualitative research. *Journal of Orthopedic Nursing, 12*(2), 99–105.

Cohen, D. J., & Crabtree, B. F. (2008). Evaluative criteria for qualitative research in health care: Controversies and recommendations. *Annals of Family Medicine, 6*(4), 331–339.

Corty, E. W. (2007). *Using and interpreting statistics: A practical text for the health, behavioral, and social sciences.* St. Louis, MO: Mosby.

Cowles, K. V. (1988). Issues in qualitative research on sensitive topics. *Western Journal of Nursing Research, 10*(2), 163–179.

Craig, J. V., & Smyth, R. L. (2012). *The evidence-based practice manual for nurses* (3rd ed.). Edinburgh, UK: Churchill Livingstone.

DeVon, H. A., Block, M. E., Moyle-Wright, P., Ernst, D. M., Hayden, S. J., Lazzara, D. J., et al. (2007). A psychometric toolbox for testing validity and reliability. *Journal of Nursing Scholarship*, *39*(2), 155–164.

Doran, D. M. (2011). *Nursing-sensitive outcomes: State of the science*. Sudbury, MA: Jones & Bartlett.

Fawcett, J., & Garity, J. (2009). *Evaluating research for evidence-based nursing practice*. Philadelphia, PA: F.A. Davis.

Forbes, A. (2009). Clinical intervention research in nursing. *International Journal of Nursing Studies, 46*(4), 557–568.

Fossey, E., Harvey, C., McDermott, F., & Davidson, L. (2002). Understanding and evaluating qualitative research. *Australian and New Zealand Journal of Psychiatry, 36*(6), 717–732.

Gatchel, R. J., & Mayer, T. G. (2010). Testing minimal clinically important difference: Consensus or conundrum? *The Spine Journal, 35*(19), 1739–1743.

Gloeckner, M. B., & Robinson, C. B. (2010). A nursing journal club thrives through shared governance. *Journal for Nurses in Staff Development, 26*(6), 267–270.

Grove, S. K. (2007). *Statistics for health care research: A practical workbook*. St. Louis, MO: Saunders.

Higgins, J. P. T., & Green, S. (2008). *Cochrane handbook for systematic reviews of interventions*. West Sussex, UK: Wiley-Blackwell & The Cochrane Collaboration.

Houser, J. (2008). *Nursing research: Reading, using, and creating evidence*. Sudbury, MA: Jones & Bartlett.

Kerlinger, F. N., & Lee, H. B. (2000). *Foundations of behavioral research* (4th ed.). Fort Worth, TX: Harcourt College.

LeFort, S. M. (1993). The statistical versus clinical significance debate. *Image Journal of Nursing Scholarship, 25*(1), 57–62.

Liamputtong, P., & Ezzy, D. (2005). *Qualitative research methods* (2nd ed.). Melbourne, VIC, Australia: Oxford University Press.

Mackey, M. C. (2012). Evaluation of qualitative research. In P. L. Munhall (Ed.). *Nursing research: A qualitative perspective* (5th ed., pp. 517–532). Sudbury, MA: Jones & Bartlett.

Marshall, C., & Rossman, G. B. (2011). *Designing qualitative research* (5th ed.). Los Angeles, CA: Sage.

Meleis, A. I. (2007). *Theoretical nursing: Development and progress* (4th ed.). Philadelphia, PA: Lippincott.

Melnyk, B. M., & Fineout-Overholt, E. (2011). *Evidence-based practice in nursing & healthcare: A guide to best practice* (2nd ed.). Philadelphia, PA: Lippincott Williams & Wilkins.

Mittlbock, M. (2008). Critical appraisal of randomized clinical trials: Can we have faith in the conclusions? *Breast Care, 3*(5), 341–346.

Morrison, D. M., Hoppe, M. J., Gillmore, M. R., Kluver, C., Higa, D., & Wells, E. A. (2009). Replicating an intervention: The tension between fidelity and adaptation. *AIDS Education and Prevention, 21*(2), 128–140.

Morse, J. M. (1991). Evaluating qualitative research. *Qualitative Health Research, 1*(3), 283–286.

Munhall, P. L. (2012). *Nursing research: A qualitative perspective* (5th ed.). Sudbury, MA: Jones & Bartlett Learning.

National Institute of Nursing Research (NINR, 2011). Research and funding. Retrieved from http://www.ninr.nih.gov/ResearchAndFunding/.

Nelson, A. M. (2008). Addressing the threat of evidence-based practice to qualitative inquiry through increasing attention to quality: A discussion paper. *International Journal of Nursing Studies, 45*(2), 316–322.

Pickler, R. H., & Butz, A. (2007). Evaluating qualitative research studies. *Journal of Pediatric Health Care, 21*(3), 195–197.

Pyrczak, F. (2008). *Evaluating research in academic journals: A practical guide to realistic evaluation* (4th ed.). Los Angeles, CA: Pyrczak.

Roberts, W. D., & Stone, P. W. (2004). Ask an expert: How to choose and evaluate a research instrument. *Applied Nursing Research, 16*(10), 70–72.

Ryan-Wenger, N. A. (2010). Evaluation of measurement precision, accuracy, and error in biophysical data for clinical research and practice. In C. F. Waltz, O. L. Strickland, & E. R. Lenz (Eds.). *Measurement in nursing and health research* (4th ed., pp. 371–383). New York, NY: Springer Publishing Company.

Sale, J. E. M. (2008). How to assess rigor … or not in qualitative research. *Journal of Evaluation in Clinical Practice, 14*(5), 912–913.

Sandelowski, M. (2008). Justifying qualitative research. *Research in Nursing & Health, 31*(3), 193–195.

Sandelowski, M., & Barroso, J. (2007). *Handbook for synthesizing qualitative research*. New York, NY: Springer Publishing Company.

Santacroce, S. J., Maccarelli, L. M., & Grey, M. (2004). Methods: Intervention fidelity. *Nursing Research, 53*(1), 63–66.

Shadish, W. R., Cook, T. D., & Campbell, D. T. (2002). *Experimental and quasi-experimental designs for generalized causal inference*. Chicago, IL: Rand McNally.

Sidani, S., & Braden, C. J. (1998). *Evaluation of nursing interventions: A theory-driven approach*. Thousand Oaks, CA: Sage.

Smith, M. J., & Liehr, P. R. (2008). *Middle range theory for nursing* (2nd ed.). New York, NY: Springer Publishing Company.

Stige, B., Malterud, K., & Midtgarden, T. (2009). Toward an agenda for evaluation of qualitative research. *Qualitative Health Research, 19*(10), 1504–1516.

Thompson, S. K. (2002). *Sampling* (2nd ed.). New York, NY: John Wiley & Sons.

Tilden, V. (2002). Editorial. Peer review: Evidence-based or sacred cow? *Nursing Research, 51*(5), 275.

Waltz, C. F., Strickland, O. L., & Lenz, E. R. (2010). *Measurement in nursing and health research* (4th ed.). New York, NY: Springer Publishing Company.

Whittemore, R. (2005). Methods. Combining evidence in nursing research: Methods and implications. *Nursing Research, 54*(1), 56–62.

Whittemore, R., Chase, S. K., & Mandle, C. L. (2001). Validity in qualitative research. *Qualitative Health Research, 11*(4), 522–537.

19
CHAPTER

Evidence Synthesis and Strategies for Evidence-Based Practice

esearch evidence has greatly expanded since the 1990s as numerous quality studies in nursing, medicine, and other healthcare disciplines have been conducted and disseminated. These studies are commonly communicated via journal publications, the Internet, books, conferences, and television. The expectations of society and the goals of healthcare systems are the delivery of high-quality, cost-effective health care to patients, families, and communities nationally and internationally. To ensure the delivery of quality health care, the care must be based on the current, best research evidence available. Healthcare agencies are emphasizing the delivery of evidence-based health care, and nurses and physicians are focused on evidence-based practice (EBP). With the emphasis on EBP over the last 2 decades, outcomes have improved for patients, healthcare providers, and healthcare agencies (Brown, 2009; Craig & Smyth, 2012; Doran, 2011; Gerrish et al., 2011; Higgins & Green, 2008; Melnyk & Fineout-Overholt, 2011; Sackett, Straus, Richardson, Rosenberg, & Haynes, 2000).

Evidence-based practice (EBP) is an important theme in this textbook and was defined earlier as the conscientious integration of best research evidence with clinical expertise and patient values and needs in the delivery of quality, cost-effective health care (see Chapter 1) (Craig & Smyth, 2012; Institute of Medicine, 2001; Sackett et al., 2000). **Best research evidence** is produced by the conduct and synthesis of numerous high-quality studies in a selected health-related area. The concept of best research evidence was described in Chapter 2, and the processes for synthesizing research evidence (systematic review, meta-analysis, meta-synthesis, and mixed-methods systematic review) are defined.

This chapter builds on previous EBP discussions to provide you with strategies for implementing the best research evidence in your practice and moving the profession of nursing toward EBP. This chapter examines the benefits and barriers related to implementing evidence-based care in nursing. Guidelines are provided for synthesizing research to determine the best research evidence. Two nursing models developed to facilitate evidence-based practice in healthcare agencies are introduced. Expert researchers, clinicians, and consumers—through government agencies, professional organizations, and healthcare agencies—have developed an extensive number of evidence-based guidelines. This chapter offers a framework for reviewing the quality of these evidence-based guidelines and for using them in practice. The chapter concludes with a discussion of the nationally designated EBP centers and Institutional Clinical Translational Science Awards. These centers and awards are supported by the U.S. government to expand the research evidence generated, synthesized, and developed into evidence-based guidelines for practice.

Benefits and Barriers Related to Evidence-Based Nursing Practice

EBP is a goal for the profession of nursing and each practicing nurse. At the present time, some nursing interventions are evidence-based, or supported by the best research knowledge available from systematic reviews, meta-analyses, meta-syntheses, and mixed-methods systematic reviews. However, many nursing interventions require additional research to generate essential knowledge for making changes in practice. Some nurses readily use research-based interventions, and others are slower to make changes in their practice based on research. Some clinical agencies are supportive of EBP and provide resources to facilitate this process, but other agencies have limited support for the EBP process. This section identifies some of the benefits and barriers related to EBP to assist you in promoting EBP in your agency and delivering evidence-based care to your patients.

Benefits of Evidence-Based Practice in Nursing

The greatest benefits of EBP are improved outcomes for patients, providers, and healthcare agencies. Organizations and agencies nationally and internationally have promoted the synthesis of the best research evidence in thousands of healthcare areas by teams of expert researchers and clinicians. These research syntheses, such as systematic reviews and meta-analyses, have provided the basis for developing strong evidence-based guidelines for practice. These guidelines identify the best treatment plan or gold standard for patient care in a selected area to promote quality health outcomes. Healthcare providers have easy access to numerous evidence-based guidelines to assist them in making the best clinical decisions for their patients. These evidence based syntheses and guidelines are communicated by presentations and publications and can be easily accessed online through the National Guideline Clearinghouse (NGC, 2012b) in the United States (http://www.guidelines.gov/), Cochrane Collaboration (2012) in England (http://www.cochrane.org/), and Joanna Briggs Institute (2012) in Australia (http://www.joannabriggs.edu.au/).

Individual studies, research syntheses, and evidence-based guidelines assist students, educators, registered nurses (RNs), and advanced practice nurses (APNs) to provide the best possible care. Expert APNs, such as nurse practitioners, clinical nurse specialists, nurse anesthetists, and nurse midwives, are resources to other nurses and facilitate access to evidence-based guidelines to ensure patient care is based on the best research evidence available (Gerrish et al., 2011). Nurse researchers and APNs are involved in the development of systematic reviews, meta-analyses, meta-syntheses, and evidence-based guidelines to manage patient health problems, prevent illnesses, and promote health.

Healthcare agencies are highly supportive of EBP because it promotes quality, cost-effective care for patients and families and meets accreditation requirements. The Joint Commission revised their accreditation criteria to emphasize patient care quality achieved through EBP. Approximately 25% of chief nursing officers (CNOs) identified the movement toward evidence-based nursing practice as their number one priority (Nurse Executive Center, 2005; The Joint Commission, 2012).

Many CNOs and healthcare agencies are trying either to obtain or to maintain Magnet status, which documents the excellence of nursing care in an agency. Approval for Magnet status is obtained through the American Nurses Credentialing Center (ANCC). The national and international healthcare agencies that currently have Magnet status can be viewed online at the ANCC (2012) website (http://www.nursecredentialing.org/FindaMagnetHospital.aspx). The Magnet Recognition Program® recognizes EBP as a way to improve the quality of patient care and to revitalize the nursing environment. Selection criteria for Magnet status that require healthcare agencies to promote the conduct of research and the use of research evidence in practice follow.

"FORCE 6: Quality Care

"Research and Evidence-Based Practice

"22. Describe how current literature, appropriate to the practice setting, is available, disseminated, and used to change administrative and clinical practices.

"23. Discuss the institution's policies and procedures that protect the rights of participants in research protocols. Include evidence of consistent nursing involvement in the governing body responsible for protection of human subjects in research.

"24. Provide evidence that research consultants are actively involved in shaping nursing research infrastructure, capacity, and mentorship.

"25. Provide a copy of the nursing budget or other sources of funding for the past year, the current year-to-date, and the future projection, highlighting the allocation and utilization of resources for nursing research.

"26. Supply documentation of all nursing research activities that are ongoing, including internal validation studies, internal and external research, and participation in surveys completed within the past twelve (12) month period.

"27. Provide evidence of education and mentoring activities that have effectively engaged staff nurses in research- and/or evidence-based practice activities.

"28. Describe resources available to nursing staff to support participating in nursing research and nursing research utilization activities." (Nurse Executive Center, 2005, p. 15)

These selection criteria include critical elements for EBP, especially financial support for and outcomes related to research activities. Important research-related outcomes to be documented by agencies for Magnet status include nursing studies conducted and professional publications and presentations by nurses. For each study, the following needs to be documented: title of the study, principal investigator or investigators, role of nurses in the study, and study status (Horstman & Fanning, 2010). In working toward EBP, nurses are encouraged to embrace the benefits of EBP, use the evidence-based guidelines available, synthesize current research evidence, and support or participate in the research needed to determine the effectiveness of selected nursing interventions.

Barriers of Evidence-Based Practice in Nursing

Barriers to the EBP movement have been both practical and conceptual. One of the most serious barriers is the lack of research evidence available regarding the effectiveness of many nursing interventions. EBP requires synthesizing research evidence from randomized controlled trials (RCTs) and other types of intervention studies, and these types of studies are still limited in nursing. Mantzoukas (2009) reviewed the research evidence in 10 high-impact nursing journals, including *Nursing Research, Research in Nursing & Health, Western Journal of Nursing Research, Journal of Nursing Scholarship,* and *Advances in Nursing Science,* between 2000 and 2006 and found that the studies were 7% experimental, 6% quasi-experimental, and 39% nonexperimental. However, RCTs and quasi-experimental studies conducted to determine the effectiveness of nursing interventions continue to increase.

Systematic reviews and meta-analyses conducted in nursing have been limited compared with other disciples. In addition, nurse authors of these research syntheses have sometimes indicated there is inadequate research evidence to support using certain nursing interventions in practice (Craig & Smyth, 2012; Mantzoukas, 2009). Bolton, Donaldson, Rutledge, Bennett, and Brown (2007, p. 123S) conducted a review of "systematic/integrative reviews and meta-analyses on nursing interventions and patient outcomes in acute care settings." Their literature search covered 1999-2005 and identified 4000 systematic/ integrative reviews and 500 meta-analyses covering the following seven topics selected by the authors: staffing, caregivers, incontinence, elder care, symptom management, pressure ulcer prevention and treatment, and developmental care of neonates and infants. The authors found a limited association between nursing interventions and processes and patient outcomes in acute care settings. Their findings included the following.

"The strongest evidence was for the use of patient risk-assessment tools and interventions implemented by nurses to prevent patient harm. We observed significant variation in the methods to measure the effect of independent variables (nursing interventions) on patient outcomes. Results indicate the need for more research measuring the effect of specific nursing interventions that may impact acute care patient outcomes." (Bolton et al., 2007, p. 123S)

Extensive evidence has been generated through nursing research, but additional studies are needed that focus on determining the effectiveness of nursing interventions on patient outcomes (Bolton et al., 2007; Craig & Smyth, 2012; Doran, 2011; Mantzoukas, 2009). Identifying the areas where research evidence is lacking is an important first step in developing the evidence needed for practice. Well-designed experimental and quasi-experimental studies are needed to test selected nursing interventions and to use that understanding to generate sound evidence for practice (see Chapter 14). Nurses also need to be more active in conducting quality syntheses (systematic reviews, meta-analyses, and meta-syntheses) of research evidence in selected areas (Finfgeld-Connett, 2010; Higgins & Green, 2008; Rew, 2011; Sandelowski & Barroso, 2007). The next section of this chapter provides guidelines to direct different types of research syntheses.

Another concern is that the research evidence is generated based on population data and then is applied in practice to individual patients. Sometimes it is difficult to transfer research knowledge to individual patients, who respond in unique ways or have unique needs (Biswas et al., 2007). More work is needed to promote the use of evidence-based guidelines with individual patients. The National Institutes of Health (NIH) is supporting translational research to improve the use of research evidence with different patient populations in various settings. Patients who have poor outcomes when managed according to an evidence-based guideline need to be reported, and, if possible, their circumstances should be published as a case study. Electronic patient records now make it possible to determine patient outcomes of care delivered using EBP guidelines.

Best research evidence is generated mainly from RCTs and other intervention studies with limited focus on the contributions of descriptive-correlational studies, qualitative research, mixed-methods studies, and theories. These types of studies do make contributions to the research evidence in many areas and need to be synthesized for use in practice (Mantzoukas, 2009) (see Chapter 10 for mixed-methods studies). Qualitative researchers have developed several synthesis processes for qualitative studies, and these are discussed later in this chapter.

Another concern of the EBP movement is that the development of evidence-based guidelines has led to a "cookbook" approach to health care. Health professionals are expected to follow these guidelines in their practice as developed. However, the definition of EBP describes it as the conscientious *integration* of best research evidence with clinical expertise and patient values and needs. Nurse clinicians have a major role in determining how the best research evidence will be implemented to achieve quality care and outcomes. For example, a nurse practitioner uses the national evidence-based guidelines for the treatment of patients with hypertension (Joint National Committee on Prevention, Detection, Evaluation, and Treatment of High Blood Pressure [JNC 7]) (Chobanian et al., 2003) but also makes clinical decisions based on the needs and values of individual patients. If a patient has a dry, persistent, irritating cough when taking angiotensin-converting enzyme inhibitor medications, this type of medication would not be used to manage the patient's high blood pressure if possible. If a patient refuses a treatment based on cultural or religious reasons, these reasons would be taken into consideration in developing the patient's treatment plan. Evidence-based guidelines provide the gold standard for managing a particular health condition, but the healthcare provider and patient individualize the treatment plan.

Another serious barrier is that some healthcare agencies and administrators do not provide the resources necessary for nurses to implement EBP. Their lack of support might include the following: (1) inadequate access to research journals and other sources of synthesized research findings and evidence-based guidelines, (2) inadequate knowledge on how to implement evidence-based changes in practice, (3) heavy workload with limited time to make research-based changes in practice, (4) limited authority to change patient care based on research findings, (5) limited support from nursing administrators or medical staff to make evidence-based changes in practice, (6) limited funds to support research projects and research-based changes in practice, and (7) minimal rewards for providing evidence-based care to patients and families (Butler, 2011; Eizenberg, 2010; Gerrish et al., 2011). The success of EBP is determined by all involved including healthcare agencies, administrators, nurses, physicians, and other healthcare professionals. We all need to take an active role in ensuring that the health care provided to patients and families is based on the best research available.

Guidelines for Synthesizing Research Evidence

Many nurses lack the expertise and confidence to synthesize research evidence in a selected area of nursing. They need additional knowledge and skills in critically appraising studies and synthesizing research evidence. Synthesizing research evidence can focus on a specific area or intervention for practice or on complex clinical problems. Master's and doctoral students often focus on clearly defined interventions when conducting research syntheses. Synthesis of research in complex clinical areas is best done with a team of expert researchers and clinicians. However, novice researchers need to be included in these teams to increase their understanding of the synthesis processes for determining the best research evidence in an area.

In this section, guidelines are provided for conducting systematic reviews, meta-analyses, meta-syntheses, and mixed-methods systematic reviews to guide you in synthesizing research evidence for nursing practice. Numerous research syntheses have been conducted in nursing and medicine, so be sure to search for an existing synthesis or review of research in an area before undertaking such a project. More recent data suggest that at least 2500 new systematic reviews are reported in English and indexed in MEDLINE each year (Liberati et al., 2009). Table 19-1 identifies some common databases and EBP organizational websites for nurses to search for nursing syntheses of research. The Cochrane Collaboration library of systematic reviews is an excellent resource with more than 11,000 entries relevant to nursing and health care (http://www.cochrane.org/cochrane-reviews). In 2009, the Cochrane Nursing Care Field was developed to support the conduct, dissemination, and use of systematic reviews in nursing. The Joanna Briggs Institute also provides resources for locating and conducting research syntheses in nursing (see Table 19-1). If you can find no synthesis of research for a selected nursing intervention or the review you find is outdated, you

TABLE 19-1   Evidence-Based Practice Resources

Resource	Description
Electronic Databases	
CINAHL (Cumulative Index to Nursing and Allied Health Literature)	CINAHL is an authoritative resource covering the English-language journal literature for nursing and allied health. Database was developed in the U.S. and includes sources published from 1982 forward
MEDLINE (PubMed—National Library of Medicine)	Database was developed by the National Library of Medicine in the U.S. and provides access to >11 million MEDLINE citations back to the mid-1960s and additional life science journals
MEDLINE with MeSH	Database provides authoritative medical information on medicine, nursing, dentistry, veterinary medicine, the healthcare system, preclinical services, and more
PsychINFO	Database was developed by the American Psychological Association and includes professional and academic literature for psychology and related disciplines from 1887 forward
CANCERLIT	Database of information on cancer was developed by the U.S. National Cancer Institute
National Library Sites	
Cochrane Library	Cochrane Library provides high-quality evidence to inform people providing and receiving health care and people responsible for research, teaching, funding, and administration of health care at all levels. Included in the Cochrane Library is the Cochrane Collaboration (2012), which has many systematic reviews of research. Cochrane Reviews are available at http://www.cochrane.org/reviews/
National Library of Health (NLH)	NLH is located in the United Kingdom. You can search for evidence-based sources at http://www.evidence.nhs.uk/
Evidence-Based Practice Organizations	
Cochrane Nursing Care Network	Cochrane Collaboration includes 11 different fields, one of which is the Cochrane Nursing Care Field (CNCF), which supports the conduct, dissemination, and use of systematic reviews in nursing; see http://cncf.cochrane.org/
National Guideline Clearinghouse (NGC)	Agency for Healthcare Research and Quality (AHRQ) developed NGC to house the thousands of evidence-based guidelines that have been developed for use in clinical practice. The guidelines can be accessed online at http://www.guidelines.gov
National Institute for Health and Clinical Excellence (NICE)	NICE was organized in the United Kingdom to provide access to the evidence-based guidelines that have been developed. These guidelines can be accessed at http://nice.org.uk
Joanna Briggs Institute	This international evidence-based organization, originating in Australia, has a search website that includes evidence summaries, systematic reviews, systematic review protocols, evidence-based recommendations for practice, best practice information sheets, consumer information sheets, and technical reports; see *Search the Joanna Briggs Institute* (2012) at http://www.joannabriggs.edu.au/Search.aspx

might use the following guidelines to conduct a systematic review of relevant research.

Guidelines for Implementing and Evaluating Systematic Reviews

A systematic review is a structured, comprehensive synthesis of the research literature to determine the best research evidence available to address a healthcare question. A systematic review involves identifying, locating, appraising, and synthesizing quality research evidence for expert clinicians to use to promote an EBP (Bettany-Saltikov, 2010a; Craig & Smyth, 2012; Higgins & Green, 2008; Liberati et al., 2009; Rew, 2011). Systematic reviews are often conducted by two or more researchers or clinicians (or researchers and clinicians) in a selected area of interest to determine the best research knowledge in that area. Systematic reviews need to be conducted with rigorous research methodology to promote the accuracy of the findings and minimize the reviewers' bias.

Table 19-2 is a checklist for critically appraising the steps of a systematic review, and these steps are discussed in the following section. These steps are based on the Preferred Reporting Items for Systematic

TABLE 19-2 Checklist for Critically Appraising Published Systematic Reviews

Systematic Review Steps	Step Complete (Yes or No)	Comments: Quality and Rationale
1. Was the clinical question clearly expressed and significant? Was the PICOS (participants, intervention, comparative interventions, outcomes, and study design) format used to develop the question and focus the review?		
2. Were the purpose and objectives or aims of the review clearly expressed and used to direct the review?		
3. Were the search criteria clearly identified? Was the PICOS format used to identify the search criteria and were the years covered, language, and publication status of sources identified in the search criteria?		
4. Was a comprehensive, systematic search of the literature conducted using explicit criteria identified in Step 3? Were the search strategies clearly reported with examples? Did the search include published studies, grey literature, and unpublished studies?		
5. Was the process for the selection of studies for the review clearly identified and consistently implemented? Was the selection process expressed in a flow diagram such as Figure 19-1?		
6. Were key elements (population, sampling process, design, intervention, outcomes, and results) of each study clearly identified and presented in a table?		
7. Was a quality critical appraisal of the studies conducted? Were the results related to participants, types of intervention, outcomes, outcome measurement methods, and risks of bias clearly discussed related to each study (i.e., in table and narrative format)?		
8. Was a meta-analysis conducted as part of the systematic review? Was a rationale provided for conducting the meta-analysis? Were the details of the meta-analysis process and results clearly described?		
9. Were the results of the review clearly described (i.e., in narrative and table)? Were details of the study interventions compared and contrasted in a table? Were the outcome variables clearly identified and the quality of the measurement methods addressed?		
10. Did the report conclude with a clear discussion section? a. Were the review findings summarized to identify the current best research evidence? b. Were the limitations of the review and how they might have affected the findings addressed? c. Were the recommendations for further research, practice, and policy development addressed?		
11. Did the authors of the review develop a clear, concise, quality report for publication? Was the report inclusive of the items identified in the PRISMA Statement (Liberati et al., 2009)?		

Reviews and Meta-Analyses (PRISMA) Statement and other relevant sources to guide nurses in conducting systematic reviews (Bettany-Saltikov, 2010a, 2010b; Higgins & Green, 2008; Rew, 2011). The PRISMA Statement was developed in 2009 by an international group of expert researchers and clinicians to improve the quality of reporting for systematic reviews and meta-analyses. The PRISMA Statement includes 27 items, which can be found at http://prisma-statement.org/ and are detailed in the article by Liberati et al. (2009). If the review process is clearly detailed in the report, others can replicate the process and verify the findings (Rew, 2011). A systematic review conducted by Goulding, Furze, and Birks (2010) is presented as an example with the discussion of the review steps outlined in Table 19-2. Goulding et al. conducted a systematic review of only RCTs to determine the best interventions to use in changing maladaptive illness beliefs of people with coronary heart disease (CHD).

Step 1: Formulate a Relevant Clinical Question to Direct the Review

A systemic review or meta-analysis is best directed by a relevant clinical question that focuses the review process and promotes the development of a quality synthesis of research evidence. Formulating the question involves identifying a relevant topic, developing a question of interest that is worth investigating, deciding if the question will generate significant information for practice, and determining if the question will clearly direct the review process and synthesis of findings. A well-stated question will define the nature and scope of the literature search, identify keywords for the search, determine the best search strategy, provide guidance in selecting articles for the review, and guide the synthesis of results (Bettany-Saltikov, 2010a, 2010b; Higgins & Green, 2008; Liberati et al., 2009).

The question developed might focus on an intervention or therapy, health promotion action, illness prevention strategy, diagnostic process, prognosis, causation, or experiences (Bettany-Saltikov, 2010a). One of the most common formats used to develop a relevant clinical question to guide a systematic review is the PICO or PICOS format described in the *Cochrane Handbook for Systematic Reviews of Interventions* (Higgins & Green, 2008). **PICOS format** includes the following elements:

P—Population or participants of interest (see Chapter 15 on sampling)

I—Intervention needed for practice (see Chapter 14 on intervention research)

C—Comparisons of the intervention with control, placebo, standard care, variations of the same intervention, or different therapies (see Chapter 14)

O—Outcomes needed for practice (see Chapter 13 on outcomes research and Chapter 17 on measurement methods)

S—Study design (see Chapter 11 on types of study designs)

Goulding et al. (2010) noted that interventions to change maladaptive illness beliefs were beneficial to people with CHD because positive illness representations may lead to improved lifestyle behaviors of exercise, smoking cessation, and balanced diet. What was not known was "[w]hich types of intervention to change illness cognitions (e.g. counseling, education, or cognitive behavioural) are most effective" (Goulding et al., 2010, p. 948) for people with CHD. The *population* was people with CHD, and the *intervention* was focused on changing maladaptive illness beliefs of these individuals. The different types of this intervention, including counseling, education, and

cognitive behavioral therapy, were compared. The intervention group was *compared* with groups receiving standard care, no treatment, or a variation of the treatment. The primary *outcome* measured was the change in beliefs about CHD at follow-up. The *study design* included synthesis of only RCTs using guidelines from the Cochrane Collaboration handbook (Higgins & Green, 2008) (see Chapters 11 and 14 about conducting RCTs). The study design (RCTs) clearly focused the literature review but might have eliminated some important studies that could have expanded the knowledge related to the intervention of changing illness beliefs.

Step 2: State the Purpose and Objectives or Aims of the Review

Most systematic reviews of research include a purpose and specific aims or objects to guide the synthesis process (Bettany-Saltikov, 2010a; Rew, 2011). The purpose identifies the major goal or focus of the review. Goulding et al. (2010, p. 948) identified their purpose as follows: "This systematic review was therefore necessary to collate and present evidence of the effectiveness of maladaptive belief change interventions for people with CHD." The specific aims direct the remaining steps of the research synthesis and become the focus of the discussion of the findings. Goulding et al. (2010) identified the following.

"Aims

"The aims of the systematic review were to establish whether interventions can significantly change maladaptive illness cognitions in people with CHD and to demonstrate which types of intervention are most effective. We also aimed to assess whether change in cognition was accompanied by changes in behavioural, functional, and psychological outcomes." (Goulding et al., 2010, p. 948)

Step 3: Identify the Literature Search Criteria and Strategies

Researchers conducting a systematic review or meta-analysis need to identify the inclusion and exclusion criteria to be used to direct their literature search. The PICOS format might be used to develop the search criteria with more detail being developed for each of the elements. These search criteria might focus on the following: (1) type of research methods, such as quantitative, qualitative, or outcomes research; (2) the population or type of study participants; (3) study designs, such as description, correlational, quasi-experimental, experimental, qualitative, or mixed methods; (4) sampling processes, such as probability or nonprobability sampling methods; (5) intervention and comparison interventions; and (6) specific outcomes to be measured. The PICOS format is effective in identifying the key terms to be included in the search process. The search criteria also need to indicate the years for the review, language, and publication status. The focus of the review might be narrowed by limiting the years reviewed, the language to English, and only studies in print (Bettany-Saltikov, 2010b; Higgins & Green, 2008; Rew, 2011).

Often searches have been limited to *published sources* in common databases, which excludes the grey literature from the research synthesis. Grey literature refers to studies that have limited distributions, such as theses and dissertations, unpublished research reports, articles in obscure journals, articles in some online journals, conference papers and abstracts, conference proceedings, research reports to funding agencies, and technical reports (Benzies, Premji, Hayden, & Serrett, 2006; Conn, Valentine, Cooper, & Rantz, 2003). Most grey literature is difficult to access through database searches and is often not peer-reviewed with limited referencing information. These are some of the main reasons for not including grey literature in searches for systematic reviews and meta-analyses. However, excluding grey literature from these searches might result in misleading, biased results. Studies with significant findings are more likely to be published than studies with non-significant findings and are usually published in more high-impact, widely distributed journals that are indexed in computerized databases (Conn et al., 2003). Studies with significant findings are more likely to have duplicate publications that need to be excluded when selecting studies to include in a research synthesis. Benzies et al. made the following recommendations related to including grey literature in a systematic review or meta-analysis.

- "Intervention and outcome are complex with multiple components.
- Lack of consensus is present concerning measurement of outcome.
- Context is important to implementing the intervention.
- Availability of research-based evidence is low volume and quality." (Benzies et al., 2006, p. 60)

Authors of systematic reviews also need to identify the search strategies that they will use. Many sources are identified through searches of electronic databases using the criteria previously discussed. However, publication bias might best be reduced with more rigorous searches of the following areas for grey literature and other unpublished studies:

1. Review the references of identified studies for additional studies. These are ancestry searches to use citations in relevant studies to identify additional studies.
2. Hand search certain journals for selected years, especially for older studies that were not identified in the electronic search.
3. Identify expert researchers in an area and search their names in the databases.
4. Contact the expert researchers regarding studies they have conducted that have not been published yet.
5. Search thesis and dissertation databases for relevant studies.
6. Review abstracts and conference reports of relevant professional organizations.
7. Search the websites of funding agencies for relevant research reports (Bettany-Saltikov, 2010b; Conn et al., 2003; Liberati et al., 2009).

Often it is best to construct a table that includes the search criteria so that they can be applied consistently throughout the search process (Liberati et al., 2009) (see Chapter 6). Goulding et al. (2010) used the PICOS format to determine inclusion criteria for the studies in the search. The *participants* had to be adults with at least one of the following: angina, CHD, myocardial infarction, or eligible for or recently received revascularization by percutaneous coronary intervention or coronary artery bypass graft surgery. The studies needed to focus on an *intervention* to change knowledge, attitudes, perceptions, and misconceptions about CHD. The interventions to change maladaptive beliefs were *compared* with different interventions, usual care, or no intervention. The primary *outcome* was change in beliefs about CDH, and the secondary outcomes were focused on quality of life, behavior change, anxiety level, depression, psychological well-being, and modifiable risk factors. The *study design* was limited to only RCTs that included a comparison of the intervention group with a control group or another intervention.

Goulding et al. (2010) designed their literature search strategies and their protocol for conducting their systematic review using sources such as the Cochrane Collaboration handbook (Higgins & Green, 2008) and the Quality of Reporting of Meta-analyses

(QUOROM) Statement (Moher et al., 1999). No date restriction was applied to the search for studies, but because of the lack of funds, only studies reported in English were identified. The databases searched are discussed in Step 4. The researchers did not include grey literature in their review and recognized this as a limitation in their discussion section.

Step 4: Conduct a Comprehensive Search of the Research Literature

The next step for conducting a systematic review or meta-analysis requires an extensive search of the literature focused by the criteria and strategies identified in Step 3. The different databases searched, date of the search, and search results need to be recorded for each database (see Chapter 6 for details on conducting and storing searches of databases). Table 19-1 identifies common databases that are searched by nurses in conducting syntheses of research and in searching for evidence-based guidelines. Usually the key search terms are identified in the report. Sometimes authors of systematic reviews provide a table that identifies the search terms and criteria. The PRISMA Statement recommends presenting the full electronic search strategy used for at least one major database such as CINAHL or MEDLINE (Liberati et al., 2009). The search strategies used to identify grey literature and other unpublished studies need to be identified.

Goulding et al. (2010) searched the following electronic databases: MEDLINE, EMBASE, CINAHL, BNI, PsychINFO, The Cochrane Library (including the Cochrane Database of Systematic Reviews, CENTRAL, and DARE), and Web of Knowledge. They provided an extensive table that detailed their electronic search of the five databases identified. The search criteria included the participants with different types of CHD; interventions of education and cognitive and behavioral therapies; comparisons with control, standard care, and placebo groups; outcomes of health knowledge, attitudes, and illness perceptions; and study design of RCT. The authors noted that the electronic search identified 3526 citations and that they obtained one source from an expert researcher and seven by reviewing the references of other studies.

Step 5: Selection of Studies for Review

The selection of studies for inclusion in the systematic review or meta-analysis is a complex process that initially involves review and removal of duplicate sources. The abstracts of the remaining studies are reviewed by two or more authors and sometimes an external reviewer to ensure they meet the criteria

identified in Step 3. The abstracts might be excluded based on the study participants, interventions, outcomes, or design not meeting the search criteria. Sometimes the abstracts are not in English, are incomplete, or are of studies not attainable. If contacting the authors of the abstracts cannot produce essential information, often the abstracts are excluded from the review (Bettany-Saltikov, 2010b; Higgins & Green, 2008; Liberati et al., 2009).

After the abstracts meeting the designated criteria are identified, the next step is to retrieve the full-text citation for each study. It is best to enter these studies into a table and document how each study meets the eligibility criteria. If studies do not meet criteria, they need to be removed with a rationale provided. Two or more authors of the review need to examine the studies to ensure that the eligibility or inclusion criteria are consistently implemented. Often the study selection process includes all members of the review team. This selection process is best demonstrated by a flow diagram that was developed by the PRISMA Group (Liberati et al., 2009). Figure 19-1 shows this diagram, which has four phases: (1) identification of the sources, (2) screening of the sources based on set criteria, (3) determining if the sources meet eligibility requirements, and (4) identifying the studies included in the review.

Goulding et al. (2010) provided the following description of their section of sources and a flow diagram (see Figure 19-2) that documented the final results of the 13 RCTs included in their systematic review.

"Search Outcome

"The electronic search produced 3526 citations, which were reduced to 115 on citation review. A check of 10% of these citations was undertaken by an independent researcher from another university, with 100% concordance on abstracts to be retrieved. A review of abstracts identified 74 papers to retrieve in full. A further seven papers were identified from reference checks, and an additional relevant study was uncovered via contact with an expert in the field. After a consensus meeting between all authors of the review, 13 studies were included. Each of these was a published journal article. The study selection flow-chart shown in [Figure 19-2] documents this process." (Goulding et al., 2010, p. 950)

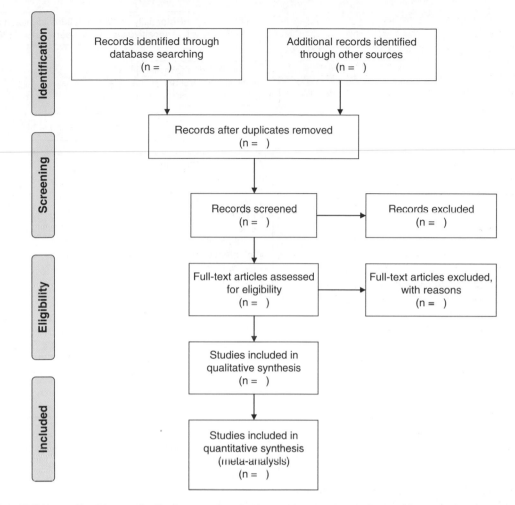

Figure 19-1 PRISMA 2009 Flow Diagram. Identification, screening, eligibility, and inclusion of research sources in systematic reviews and meta-analyses. (From Moher, D., Liberati, A., Tetzlaff, J., Altman, D. G., & PRISMA Group. [2009]. *Preferred Reporting Items for Systematic Reviews and Meta-Analyses: The PRISMA Statement.* Retrieved from http://www.prisma-statement.org.)

Step 6: Critical Appraisal of the Studies Included in Review

An initial critical appraisal of the methodological quality of the studies occurs during the selection of the studies to be included in the systematic review. Once the studies are selected, a more thorough critical appraisal takes place. This critical appraisal is best done by constructing a table describing the characteristics of the included studies, such as the purpose of the studies, population, sampling method, sample size, sample acceptance and attrition rates, design, intervention (independent variable), dependent variables, measurement methods for each dependent variable,

and major results (Bettany-Saltikov, 2010b; Higgins & Green, 2008; Liberati et al., 2009).

It is best if two or more experts independently review the studies and make judgments about their quality. The authors of the review usually contact the study investigators if needed to obtain important information about the study design or results not included in the publication. Chapter 18 provides guidelines for critically appraising quantitative and qualitative studies. The critical appraisal of the studies is often difficult because of the differences in types of participants, designs, sampling methods, intervention protocols, outcome variables and measurement methods,

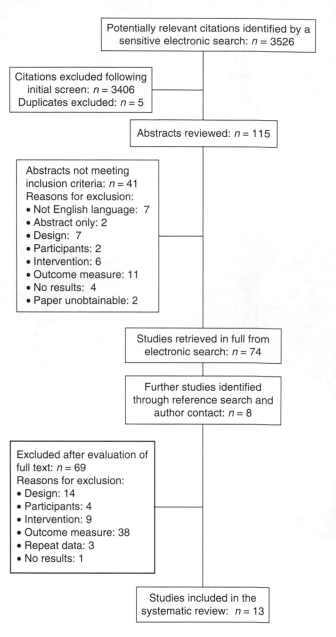

Figure 19-2 Study selection flow chart. (From Goulding, L., Furze, G., & Birks, Y. [2010]. Randomized controlled trials of interventions to change maladaptive illness beliefs in people with coronary heart disease: Systematic review. *Journal of Advanced Nursing, 66*[5], 950.)

and presentation of results. The studies are often rank-ordered based on their quality and contribution to the development of the review (Bettany-Saltikov 2010b; Liberati et al., 2009).

Goulding et al. (2010) developed a detailed table of essential content from the 13 studies included in the systematic review and labeled the headings of the columns in the table as (1) authors, year, and country of the study; (2) participants and setting; (3) design, sample size per group, and follow-up; (4) intervention; (5) control or comparison group; (6) study outcomes; and (7) results with statistical significance set at alpha = 0.05. Two reviewers independently assessed the quality of each study. They provided a detailed description of the appraisal process and their findings for each study. You may want to access this systematic review to view their table of studies and examine their critical appraisal process.

Step 7: Conduct a Meta-Analysis If Appropriate

Some systematic reviews include published meta-analyses as sources in the review. Because a meta-analysis involves the use of statistics to summarize results of different studies, it usually provides strong, objective information about the effectiveness of an intervention or solid knowledge about a clinical problem. Other authors conduct a meta-analysis in the synthesis of sources for their systematic review (Liberati et al., 2009). The authors of the review need to provide a rationale for conducting the meta-analysis and detail the process they used to conduct this analysis. For example, a meta-analysis might be conducted on a small group of similar studies to determine the effect of an intervention. The next section provides more details on conducting a meta-analysis.

The systematic review conducted by Goulding et al. (2010) did not include a meta-analysis as a source, and a meta-analysis was not conducted during the review process. A meta-analysis was probably not appropriate because of the limited number of studies that had been conducted to examine the effectiveness of the intervention to change maladaptive illness beliefs in people with CHD.

Step 8: Results of the Review

The results of the authors' reviews need to include a description of the study participants, types of interventions, and outcomes. The results of the different types of interventions might be best summarized in a table that includes the following: (1) study source; (2) structure of the intervention (stand-alone or multi-faceted); (3) specific type of intervention such as physiological treatment, education, counseling, or behavioral therapy; (4) delivery method such as demonstration and return demonstration, verbal, video, or self-administered; and (5) statistical difference between the intervention and the control, standard care, placebo, or alternative intervention groups (Liberati et al., 2009).

The specific outcomes, including primary and secondary outcomes, of the studies might also be best summarized in a table. This table might include (1) the study source; (2) outcome variable, with an indication as to whether it was a primary or secondary outcome in the study; (3) measurement method used for each study outcome variable; and (4) the quality of the measurement methods, such as the reliability and validity of a scale or the precision and accuracy of a physiological measure (see Chapter 16).

Goulding et al. (2010, p. 955) described their participants for their 13 studies as "male and female adults of all ages with a diagnosis of CHD (including people diagnosed with MI [myocardial infarction] or angina or those receiving revascularization). There was no clear link between patient group and effectiveness of interventions to change beliefs." These authors also provided two detailed tables: one addressing the types of interventions and the other identifying the measurement methods of the study outcomes and quality of these methods. Numerous outcome measures were used in the 13 studies, and some had poor reliability and validity, which limit the results of this systematic review. Goulding et al. also summarized key findings related to the effectiveness of the interventions and reached the following conclusion.

> "Overall, the majority of interventions designed to elicit positive and correct illness cognitions regarding CHD were effective. Such interventions can be effective either as part of a multifaceted intervention or as a stand-alone intervention. However, because of the numerous differences in the structure of each intervention, method of belief change, and method of delivery, it is difficult to ascertain whether there is a relationship between type of intervention and effect on belief change." (Goulding et al., 2010, p. 956)

Step 9: Discussion Section of the Review

In a systematic review or meta-analysis, the discussion of the findings needs to include an overall evaluation of the types of interventions implemented and the outcomes measured. The methodological issues or limitations of the review also need to be addressed. The discussion section needs to include a theoretical link back to the studies' frameworks to indicate the theoretical implications of the findings. Lastly, the discussion section needs to provide recommendations for further research, practice, and policy development (Bettany-Saltikov, 2010b; Higgins & Green, 2008; Liberati et al., 2009). Goulding et al. (2010) provided the following discussion of their findings; review limitations; and recommendations for research, practice, and policy development.

> "We found that interventions to change beliefs can be successful, with cognitive behavioral interventions being the most consistently effective. The evidence on whether interventions to change maladaptive beliefs can improve psychological, functional, and behavioural outcomes was unclear. It is therefore not

possible to determine which types of intervention are most effective in creating improvements in these important outcomes.

Methodological Issues

The major weakness of the review methodology was the lack of a search for non-English language literature, unpublished trials, and grey literature because of time and resource constraints.... It is therefore possible that the review has a publication bias. However, as one of the authors (GF) is internationally collaborative in the review area, it is unlikely that a large number of studies of good quality was missed....

The purpose of including only RCTs was to synthesize the results of the best quality research available, yet some of the included studies did not meet the anticipated quality standard. This said, the overall review methodology was good....

Leventhal's CSM [Common Sense Model] can be used to explain the relationships between illness beliefs, coping, and medical, psychological, and social outcomes. Four of the reports included in the review explicitly mentioned the theoretical framework of the CSM as informing the design of the intervention or interpretation of results....

Implications for Future Research

The review demonstrates the need for methodologically sound and adequately powered trials of interventions to change maladaptive illness cognitions.... The follow-up time of such interventions should be long enough to determine whether any positive effects remain stable over time.... Cognitive behavioral interventions appear promising, and could perhaps be used in conjunction with education and counseling. It is important that researchers choose a valid and reliable measure to assess change in the cognition(s) of interest." (Goulding et al., pp. 957-959)

Goulding et al. stressed the importance of interventions to change maladaptive illness beliefs of people with CHD. However, the impact of changing those beliefs on behavior, functional, and psychological outcomes is unclear. Additional research is needed on the use of cognitive behavioral interventions to change maladaptive illness beliefs and how this affects people with CHD health outcomes.

Step 10: Development of the Final Report for Publication

The final step is the development of the systematic review report for publication and presentation. The report should include a title that identifies it as either a systematic review or a meta-analysis for ease of location in database searches. An abstract also needs to be included that identifies background, purpose, data sources, review methods, results, and conclusions. The body of the report needs to include the content discussed in the previous nine steps: (1) clinical question to be addressed by the review; (2) purpose and aims or objectives to be accomplished by the review; (3) search criteria and strategies used to identify essential studies; (4) comprehensive search of the literature and results; (5) selection of studies to be included in the review; (6) critical appraisal process and findings; (7) description of the meta-analysis conducted and results if appropriate; (8) presentation of the review results in table and narrative format; and (9) discussion of the systematic review findings, limitations, and implications for further research, practice, and policy development.

The PRISMA Group developed a 27-item checklist to use in developing the final reports for systematic reviews and meta-analyses. This PRISMA Group checklist is presented in Table 19-3 and discussed on PRISMA Group website (http://www.prisma-statement.org) and in the articles by Liberati et al. (2009) and Moher, Liberati, Tetzlaff, Altman, and PRISMA Group (2009). This checklist is an excellent guide to use in developing the final report of a systematic review or meta-analysis for publication. This checklist was developed to improve the quality, completeness, and consistency of the syntheses developed and published in nursing, medicine, and other healthcare professions.

Critical Appraisal of a Published Systematic Review

Your critical appraisal of a systematic review might be guided by the checklist provided in Table 19-2. This table includes the steps of a systematic review, and you need to assess if each step was completed or not in the review. You also need to provide comments and rationale for the appraised strengths and limitations of the review. Using this checklist, you could develop a formal critical appraisal paper for a systematic review. In developing and critically appraising systematic reviews, you might also use the articles by Bettany-Saltikov (2010a, 2010b), the Cochrane Collaboration handbook (Higgins & Green, 2008), the EBP manual for nurses by Craig and Smyth (2012), and other sources identified by your faculty or experts in this area.

The critical appraisal of a systematic review or meta-analysis also needs to include an assessment of how current the literature synthesis is. This leads to the following question: How quickly do systematic reviews become out of date? Shojania et al. (2007,

TABLE 19-3 Checklist of Items to Include When Reporting a Systematic Review or Meta-Analysis

Section/Topic	No.	Checklist Item	Reported on Page No.
Title			
Title	1	Identify the report as a systematic review, meta-analysis, or both	
Abstract			
Structured summary	2	Provide a structured summary including, as applicable, background; objectives; data sources; study eligibility criteria, participants, and interventions; study appraisal and synthesis methods; results; limitations; conclusions and implications of key findings; systematic review registration number	
Introduction			
Rationale	3	Describe the rationale for the review in the context of what is already known	
Objectives	4	Provide an explicit statement of questions being addressed with reference to PICOS (participants, interventions, comparisons, outcomes, and study design)	
Methods			
Protocol and registration	5	Indicate if a review protocol exists; if and where it can be accessed (e.g., Web address); and, if available, provide registration information including registration number	
Eligibility criteria	6	Specify study characteristics (e.g., PICOS, length of follow-up) and report characteristics (e.g., years considered, language, publication status) used as criteria for eligibility, giving rationale	
Information sources	7	Describe all information sources (e.g., databases with dates of coverage, contact with study authors to identify additional studies) in the search and date last searched	
Search	8	Present full electronic search strategy for at least one database, including any limits used, such that it could be repeated	
Study selection	9	State the process for selecting studies (i.e., screening, eligibility, included in systematic review, and, if applicable, included in the meta-analysis)	
Data collection process	10	Describe method of data extraction from reports (e.g., piloted forms, independently, in duplicate) and any processes for obtaining and confirming data from investigators	
Data items	11	List and define all variables for which data were sought (e.g., PICOS, funding sources) and any assumptions and simplifications made	
Risk of bias in individual studies	12	Describe methods used for assessing risk of bias of individual studies (including specification of whether this was done at the study or outcome level), and how this information is to be used in any data synthesis	
Summary measures	13	State the principal summary measures (e.g., risk ratio, difference in means)	
Synthesis of results	14	Describe the methods of handling data and combining results of studies, if done, including measures of consistency (e.g., I^2) for each meta-analysis	

From Moher, D., Liberati, A., Tetzlaff, J., Altman, D. G., & PRISMA Group. (2009). *Preferred Reporting Items for Systematic Reviews and Meta-Analyses: The PRISMA Statement*. Retrieved from http://www.prisma-statement.org.

p. 224) conducted a survival analysis on 100 quantitative systematic reviews published from 1995-2005 "to estimate the average time to changes in evidence that is sufficiently important to warrant updating systematic reviews." They found the average time before a systematic review should be updated was 5.5 years. However, 23% of the reviews signaled a need for updating within 2 years, and 15% needed updating within 1 year. Shojania et al. (2007) stressed that high-quality systematic reviews that were directly relevant to clinical practice require frequent updating to stay current. There are numerous nursing and medical sources of systematic reviews, but it is important for you to know the steps of the systematic review process and to be able to appraise critically the quality of these reviews.

Conducting Meta-Analyses to Synthesize Research Evidence

A meta-analysis is conducted to pool statistically the results from previous studies into a single quantitative analysis that provides one of the highest levels of evidence about the effectiveness of an intervention (Andrel, Keith, & Leiby, 2009; Craig & Smyth, 2012; Higgins & Green, 2008; Liberati et al., 2009). This approach has objectivity because it includes analysis techniques to determine the effect of an intervention while examining the influences of variations in the studies selected for the meta-analysis. The studies to be included in the analysis need to be examined for variations or heterogeneity in such areas as sample characteristics, sample size, design, types of intervention, and outcomes variables and measurement methods (Higgins & Green, 2008). Heterogeneity in the studies to be included in a meta-analysis can lead to different types of biases, which are detailed in the next section.

Statistically combining data from several studies results in a large sample size with increased power to determine the true effect of a specific intervention on a particular outcome (see Chapter 15 for discussion of power). The ultimate goal of a meta-analysis is to determine if an intervention (1) significantly improves outcomes, (2) has minimal or no effect on outcomes, or (3) increases the risk of adverse events. Meta-analysis is also an effective way to resolve conflicting study findings and controversies that have arisen related to a selected intervention. When conducting a systematic review, authors might conduct a meta-analysis on a group of similar studies to determine the effectiveness of an intervention (Higgins & Green, 2008).

Strong evidence for using an intervention in practice can be generated from a meta-analysis of multiple, quality studies such as RCTs and quasi-experimental studies. However, the conduct of a meta-analysis depends on the accuracy, clarity, and completeness of information presented in studies. Box 19-1 provides a list of information that needs to be included in a research report to facilitate the conduct of a meta-analysis.

The steps for conducting a meta-analysis are similar to the steps for conducting a systematic review that were detailed in the previous section. The PRISMA Statement introduced earlier provides clear directions

Box 19-1	Recommended Reporting for Authors to Facilitate Meta-Analysis

Demographic Variables Relevant to Population Studied

Age
Gender
Marital status
Ethnicity
Education
Socioeconomic status

Methodological Characteristics

Sample size (experimental and control groups)
Type of sampling method
Sampling refusal rate and attrition rate
Sample characteristics
Research design
Groups included in study—experimental, control, comparison, placebo groups
Intervention protocol and fidelity discussion
Data collection techniques
Outcome measurements
    Reliability and validity of instruments
    Precision and accuracy of physiological measures

Data Analysis

Name of statistical tests
Sample size for each statistical test
Degrees of freedom for each statistical test
Exact value of each statistical test
Exact p value for each test statistic
One-tailed or two-tailed statistical test
Measures of central tendency (mean, median, and mode)
Measures of dispersion (range, standard deviation)
Post hoc test values for ANOVA (Analysis of variance) test of three or more groups

for developing a report for either a systematic review or a meta-analysis (see Table 19-3) (Liberati et al., 2009). The following information is provided to increase your ability to appraise critically meta-analysis studies and to conduct a meta-analysis for a selected intervention. The PRISMA Statement, Cochrane Collaboration guidelines for meta-analysis (Higgins & Green, 2008), and other resources (Andrel et al., 2009; Conn & Rantz, 2003; Noordzij, Hooft,

Dekker, Zoccali, & Jager, 2009; Turlik, 2010) were used to provide detail for conducting a meta-analysis. Conn's (2010) meta-analysis to determine the effect of physical activity interventions on depressive symptom outcomes in healthy adults is presented as an example.

Clinical Question for Meta-Analysis

The clinical question developed for a meta-analysis is usually clearly focused as: "What is the effectiveness of a selected intervention?" The PICOS (participants, intervention, comparative interventions, outcomes, and study design) format discussed earlier might be used to generate the clinical question (Higgins & Green, 2008; Liberati et al., 2009; Moher et al., 2009). Conn (2010) indicated that only one previous meta-analysis had examined the effect of physical activities (PA) on depressive symptoms among subjects without clinical depression. Thus, she wanted to address the following clinical question: "What is the effect of PA on depressive symptoms in healthy adults?"

Purpose and Questions to Direct Meta-Analysis

Researchers need to identify clearly the purpose of their meta-analysis and the questions or objectives that guide the analysis. The Cochrane Collaboration identified the following four basic questions to guide a meta-analysis to determine the effect of an intervention:

"1. What is the direction of effect?
"2. What is the size of effect?
"3. Is the effect consistent across studies?
"4. What is the strength of evidence for the effect?" (Higgins & Green, 2008, p. 244)

Conn clearly identified the following purpose:

"This meta-analysis synthesized depressive symptom outcomes of supervised and unsupervised PA interventions among healthy adults.... This meta-analysis addressed the following research questions:
"(1) What are the overall effects of supervised PA and unsupervised PA interventions on depressive symptoms in healthy adults without clinical depression?
"(2) Do interventions' effects on depressive symptom outcomes vary depending on

intervention, sample, and research design characteristics?
"(3) What are the effects of interventions on depressive symptoms among studies comparing treatment subjects with before versus after interventions?" (Conn, 2010, pp. 128, 129)

Search Criteria and Strategies for Meta-Analyses

The methods for identifying search criteria and selecting search strategies are similar for meta-analyses and systematic reviews. The search criteria are usually narrowly focused for meta-analysis to identify selective studies examining the effect of a particular intervention. The search needs to be rigorous and include published sources identified through varied databases and unpublished studies and grey literature identified through other types of searches (see previous section). Conn (2010) clearly identified her search strategies in the following excerpt.

"Primary Study Search Strategies

"Multiple search strategies were used to ensure a comprehensive search and thus limit bias while moving beyond previous reviews. An expert reference librarian searched 11 computerized databases (e.g., MEDLINE, PsychINFO, EMBASE) using broad search terms.... Search terms for depressive symptoms were not used to narrow the search because many PA interventions studies report depressive symptom outcomes but do not consider these the main outcomes of the study and thus papers are not indexed by these terms. Several research registers were examined including Computer Retrieval of Information on Scientific Projects and mRCT, which contains 14 active registers and 16 archived registers. Computerized author searches were completed for project principal investigators located from research registers and for the first three authors on eligible studies. Author searches were completed for dissertation authors to locate published papers. Ancestry searches were conducted on eligible and review papers. Hand searches were completed for 114 journals which frequently report PA intervention research." (Conn, 2010, p. 129)

Possible Biases for Meta-Analyses and Systematic Reviews

Even with rigorous literature searches, authors of meta-analyses and systematic reviews are often limited to mainly published studies. The nature of the sources can lead to biases and flawed or inaccurate conclusions in the research syntheses. The common biases that can occur in conducting and reporting research syntheses include publication bias such as time lag bias, location bias, duplicate publication bias, citation bias, and language bias; bias from poor study methodology; and outcome reporting bias. Publication bias occurs because studies with positive results are more likely to be published than studies with negative or inconclusive results. Higgins and Green (2008) found that the odds were four times greater that positive study results would be published versus negative results. Time-lag bias, a type of publication bias, occurs because studies with negative results are usually published later, sometimes 2 to 3 years later, than studies with positive results. Sometimes studies with negative results are not published at all, whereas studies with positive results might be published more than once (duplicate publication bias). Location bias can occur if studies are published in lower impact journals and indexed in less-searched databases. A citation bias occurs when certain studies are cited more often than others and are more likely to be identified in database searchers. Language bias can occur if searches focus just on studies in English and important studies exist in other languages.

Biases in studies' methodologies are often related to design and data analysis problems. The strengths and threats to design validity need to be examined during critical appraisal of the studies for inclusion in a meta-analysis or systematic review (see Chapter 10 for discussion of design validity). The analyses conducted in studies need to be appropriate and complete (see Chapters 20 through 25 on data analysis). Outcome reporting bias occurs when study results are not reported clearly and with complete accuracy. For example, reporting bias occurs when researchers selectively report positive results and not negative results; or positive results might be addressed in detail with limited discussion of negative results. Higgins and Green (2008) provided a much more detailed discussion of potential biases in systematic reviews and meta-analyses.

An analysis method called the funnel plot can be used to assess for biases in a group of studies. Funnel plots provide graphic representations of possible effect sizes (ESs) or odds ratios (ORs) for interventions in selected studies. The ES or strength of an intervention

in a study can be calculated by determining the difference between the experimental and control groups for the outcome variable. The mean difference between the experimental and control groups for several studies is easily determined if the outcome variable is measured by the same scale or instrument in each study (see Chapter 15 for calculation of ES). However, the standardized mean difference (SMD) must be calculated in a meta-analysis when the same outcome, such as depression, is measured by different scales or methods. More details are provided on SMD later in this section. Figure 19-3 shows a funnel plot of the SMDs from 13 individual studies. The SMDs from the studies are fairly symmetrical or equally divided by the line through the middle of the funnel in the graph. A symmetrical funnel plot indicates limited or no publication bias. Asymmetry of the funnel plot is due to publication bias, but Egger, Smith, Schneider, and Minder (1997) also believed it reflects methodological bias, reporting bias, heterogeneity in the studies' sample size and interventions, and chance. In Figure 19-3, the studies with small sample sizes are toward the bottom of the graph, and the studies with larger samples are toward the top.

Figure 19-4 includes two example funnel plots with the plot in Figure 19-4A showing no apparent publication bias. An unbiased sample of studies should appear basically symmetrical in the funnel with the ORs of the studies fairly equally divided on either side of the line (see Chapter 24 for calculating OR). The funnel plot shown in Figure 19-4B demonstrates publication bias in favor of larger studies with positive results when the studies having smaller effect and sample sizes are removed. This collection of studies in a meta-analysis could lead to the conclusion that a treatment was effective when it might not be when looking at a larger collection of studies with negative and positive

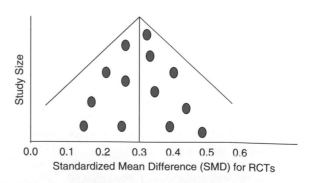

Figure 19-3 Funnel plot of standardized mean differences (SMDs) for randomized controlled trials (RCTs) with limited bias.

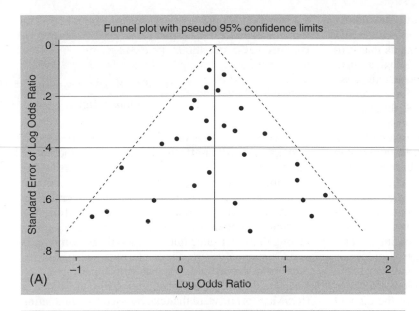

(A)

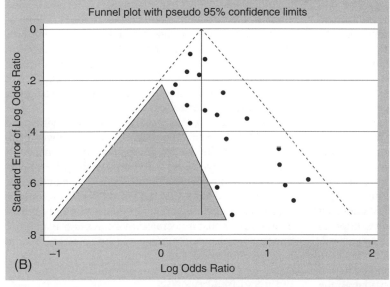

(B)

Figure 19-4 **A** and **B,** Funnel plots examining publication bias. (From Andrel, J. A., Keith, S. W., & Leiby, B. E. [2009]. Meta-analysis: A brief introduction. *Clinical & Translational Science, 2*[5], 376.)

results as in the plot in Figure 19-4A. Conn (2010) discussed her search results and risk of publication bias in the following excerpt.

"Comprehensive searchers yielded 70 reports.... The supervised PA two-group comparison included 1,598 subjects. The unsupervised PA two-group comparison included 1,081 subjects. The treatment single-group comparisons included 1,639 supervised PA and 3,420 unsupervised PA subjects.... Most primary studies were published articles (s=54), and the remainder were dissertations (s=14), book chapter (s=1), and conference presentation materials (s=1; s indicates the number of reports). Publication bias was evident in the funnel plots for supervised and unsupervised PA two-group outcome comparisons and for treatment group, pre- vs. post-intervention supervised PA and unsupervised PA comparisons. The control group pre- and post-comparison distributions on the funnel plots suggested less publication bias than plots of treatment groups. Unless otherwise specified, all results are from the treatment vs. control comparisons." (Conn, 2010, p. 131)

Results of Meta-Analysis for Continuous Outcomes

Many nursing studies examine continuous outcomes or outcomes that are measured by methods that produced interval or ratio level data. Physiological measures to examine blood pressure produce ratio level data. Likert scales such as the Center for Epidemiologic Studies Depression (CES-D) Scale produce interval level data (see Figure 17-8 for a copy of CES-D Scale). Blood pressure and depression are continuous outcomes. Meta-analysis includes a two-step process: Step 1 is the calculation of a summary statistic for each study to describe the intervention effect, and step 2 is the summary (pooled) intervention effect that is the weighted average of the interventions effects estimated from the different studies. In step 1, to determine the effect of an intervention on continuous outcomes, the mean difference between two groups is calculated. The mean difference is a standard statistic that is calculated to determine the absolute difference between two groups. It is an estimate of the amount of change caused by the intervention (e.g., physical activity) on the outcome (e.g., depression) on average compared with the control group. The mean difference can be calculated to determine the effect of an intervention only if the outcome is measured by the same scale in all the studies (Higgins & Green, 2008).

A standardized mean difference (SMD), or *d,* is used in studies as a summary statistic that is calculated in a meta-analysis when the same outcome is measured by different scales or methods. The SMD is also sometime referred to as the standardized mean effect size. For example, in the meta-analysis by Conn (2010), depression was commonly measured with three different scales: Profile of Mood States, Beck Depression Inventory, and CES-D Scale. Studies that have differences in means in the same proportion to the standard deviations have the same SMD (*d*) regardless of the scales used to measure the outcome variable. The differences in the means and standard deviations in the studies are assumed to be due to the measurement scales and not variability in the outcome (Higgins & Green, 2008). The SMD is calculated by meta-analysis software, and the formula is provided as follows:

$$\text{SMD}\,(d) = \frac{\text{difference in mean outcome between groups}}{\text{standard deviation of outcome among participants}}$$

In step 2 of meta-analysis of summarizing the effects of an intervention across studies, the pooled intervention effect estimate is "calculated as a weighted average of the intervention effects estimated in the individual studies. A weighted average" is defined by Higgins and Green (2008, p. 263) as:

$$\text{Weighted average} = \frac{\text{sum of (estimate} \times \text{weight)}}{\text{sum of weights}}$$

In combining intervention effect estimates across studies, a random-effects meta-analysis model or fixed-effect meta-analysis model can be used. The assumption of using the random-effects model is that all the studies are not estimating the same intervention effect but related effects over studies that follow a distribution across studies. When each study is estimating the exact same quality, a fixed-effect model is used. Meta-analysis results can be obtained using software from SPSS and SAS statistical packages (see Chapter 21). Cochrane Collaboration Review Manager (RevMan) is software that can be used for conducting meta-analyses. This chapter provides a very basic discussion of key ideas related to conducting meta-analyses, and you are encouraged to review Higgins and Green (2008) and other meta-analysis sources to increase your understanding of this process (Andrel et al., 2009; Fernandez & Tran, 2009; Turlik, 2010). We also recommend the assistance of a statistician in conducting these analyses.

Conn's (2010) meta-analysis result identified a standardized mean effect size of 0.372 between the treatment and the control groups for the 38 supervised PA studies and SMD of 0.522 among the 22 unsupervised PA studies. This meta-analysis documented that supervised and unsupervised PA reduced symptoms of depression in healthy adults or adults without clinical depression. Thus, a decrease in depression is another important reason for encouraging patients to be involved in physical activities.

Results of Meta-Analysis for Dichotomous Outcomes

If the outcome data to be examined in a meta-analysis are dichotomous, risk ratios, odds ratios, and risk differences are usually calculated to determine the effect of the intervention on the measured outcome. These terms are introduced in this chapter but more information is available in Craig and Smyth (2012), Higgins and Green (2008), and Sackett et al. (2000). With dichotomous data, every participant fits into one of two categories, such as clinically improved or no clinical improvement, effective screening device or ineffective screening device, or alive or dead. Risk ratio (*RR*), also called relative risk, is the ratio of the risk of subjects in the intervention group to the risk of subjects in the control group for having a particular health outcome. The health outcome is usually adverse, such as the risk of a disease (e.g., cancer) or the risk of complications or death (Higgins & Green, 2008). The calculation for *RR* follows and is:.

$$\text{Relative risk } (RR) = \frac{\text{risk of event in experimental group}}{\text{risk of event in control group}}$$

The odds ratio (*OR*) is defined as the ratio of the odds of an event occurring in one group, such as the treatment group, to the odds of it occurring in another group, such as the standard care group. The *OR* is a way of comparing whether the odds of a certain event is the same for two groups (see Chapter 24). An example is the odds of medication adherence or non-adherence for an experimental group receiving an intervention of education and specialized medication packaging intervention versus a group receiving standard care. The calculation for *OR* is:

$$\text{Odds ratio } (OR) = \frac{\text{odds of event in experimental group}}{\text{odds of event in control or comparison group}}$$

The risk difference (*RD*), also called the *absolute risk reduction,* is the risk of an event in the experimental group minus the risk of the event in the control or standard care group.

$$\text{Risk difference } (RD) = \text{risk of experimental group} - \text{risk of control group}$$

Meta-analysis results from studies with dichotomous data are often presented using a forest plot. Fernandez and Tran (2009) provided a format for presenting a forest plot in a meta-analysis study (Figure 19-5). A forest plot usually includes the following information: (1) author, year, and name of the study; (2) raw data from the intervention and control groups and total number in each group; (3) point estimate (*OR* or *RR*) and confidence internal (*CI*) for each study shown as a line and block on the graph; (4) numerical values for point estimate (*OR* or *RR*) and *CI* for each study; and (5) percent weights given to each study (Fernandez & Tran, 2009; Higgins & Green, 2008). In Figure 19-5, column 1 identifies each of the studies using the clearest format for the studies being analyzed. Column 2 includes the number of participants with the outcome (*n*) and total number of participants in the intervention or experimental group, expressed as *n/N*. Column 3 includes the number of participants with the outcome and total number in the control group. Column 4 graphically presents the *OR* with a block and the 95% *CI* with a line. Column 5 provides the percent weights given to each of the three studies in this example. Column 6 provides the numerical values for the *OR* and 95% *CI*.

The bottom of the forest plot in Figure 19-5 provides a summary of results and significance including total events for intervention and control groups, test for heterogeneity, and test for overall effect. The large diamond in the plot is the summary of the effect of the studies included in the analysis. If the diamond is left of the line that is positioned at 1, the results favor the intervention or treatment, and the *CI* does not include 1 if the results are statistically significant (Fernandez & Tran, 2009). If the point estimates are consistently more on one side of the vertical line, this shows homogeneity of the studies. If the point estimates are fairly equally distributed on both the left and the right side of the veridical line, this shows heterogeneity of the studies included in the meta-analysis. The term *heterogeneity* was introduced earlier; heterogeneity can exist in the sample size and characteristics, types of intervention, designs, and outcomes of the studies. Heterogeneity statistics for random-effects meta-analyses include chi-square tests (see Chapter 25), the I^2, and a test for differences across subgroups if they are appropriate (Higgins & Green, 2008).

Magnus, Ping, Shen, Bourgeois, and Magnus (2011) conducted a meta-analysis of the effectiveness of mammography screening in reducing breast cancer mortality in women 39 to 49 years old. Because mammography screening is significant in reducing breast cancer mortality of women older than 50 years and early detection of breast cancer increases survival, annual routine mammography screening has been recommended for all women 40 to 47 years old in the United States. Thus, "the primary aim of the current study was, after a quality assessment of identified randomized controlled trials (RCTs), to conduct a meta-analysis of the effectiveness of mammography screening [*intervention*] in women aged 39-49 [*population*] in reducing breast cancer mortality [*dichotomous outcome*]. The second aim was to compare and discuss the results of previously published meta-analyses" (Magnus et al., 2011, p. 845). The following excerpts describe the methods, results, and conclusions of this meta-analysis.

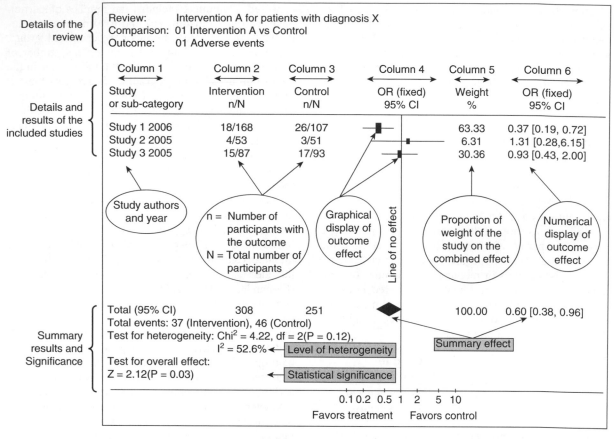

Figure 19-5 Meta-analysis graph for dichotomous data. CI, confidence interval; OR, odds ratio. (From Fernandez, R. S., & Tran, D. T. [2009]. The meta-analysis graph: Clearing the haze. *Clinical Nurse Specialist, 23*[2], 58.)

"**Methods:** PubMed/MEDLINE, OVID, COCHRANE, and Educational Resources Information Center (ERIC) databases were searched, and extracted references were reviewed. Dissertation abstracts and clinical trials databases available online were assessed to identify unpublished works. All assessments were independently done by two reviewers. All trials included were RCTs, published in English, included data on women aged 39-49, and reported relative risk (*RR*)/odds ratio (*OR*) or frequency data.

Results: Nine studies were identified.... The individual trials were quality assessed, and the data were extracted using predefined forms. Using the DerSimonian and Laird random effects model, the results from the seven RCTs with the highest quality score were combined, and a significant pooled *RR* estimate of 0.83 (95% confidence interval [CI] 0.72-0.97) was calculated." (Magnus et al., 2011, p. 845)

The results of the study were graphically represented using a forest plot (Figure 19-6). The plot clearly identifies the names of the seven studies included in the meta-analysis on the left side of the figure. The *RR* and *CI* for each study are identified with a block and horizontal line. The numerical *RR* and *95% CI* values are identified on the right side of the plot with the percent of weight given to each study. Most of the studies show homogeneity with odds ratios left of the vertical line except for the Stockholm study. The forest plot would have been strengthened by including the results from the test for heterogeneity and test for overall effect. Magnus et al. (2011, p. 845) concluded, "Mammography screenings were effective and generate a 17% reduction in breast cancer mortality in women 39-49 years of age. The quality of the trials varies, and providers should inform women in this age group about the positive and negative aspects of mammography screenings."

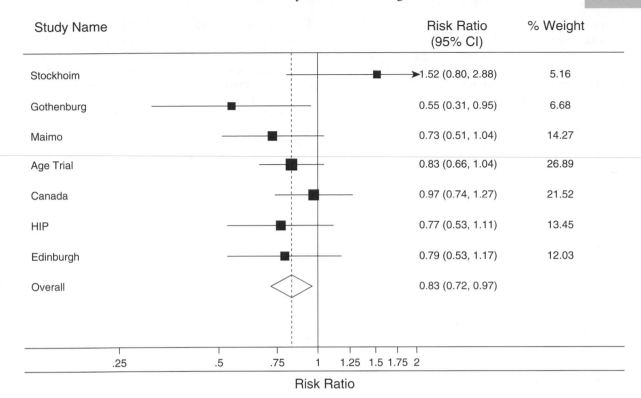

Study Name		Risk Ratio (95% CI)	% Weight
Stockhoim		1.52 (0.80, 2.88)	5.16
Gothenburg		0.55 (0.31, 0.95)	6.68
Maimo		0.73 (0.51, 1.04)	14.27
Age Trial		0.83 (0.66, 1.04)	26.89
Canada		0.97 (0.74, 1.27)	21.52
HIP		0.77 (0.53, 1.11)	13.45
Edinburgh		0.79 (0.53, 1.17)	12.03
Overall		0.83 (0.72, 0.97)	

Risk Ratio

Figure 19-6 Forest plot showing the individual randomized controlled trials and the overall pooled estimate from the seven original randomized controlled trials with a high-quality score addressing the impact of mammography screening on breast cancer mortality in women 39 to 49 years old. *CI*, Confidence interval. (From Magnus, M. C., Ping, M., Shen, M. M., Bourgeois, J., & Magnus, J. H. [2011]. Effectiveness of mammography screening in reducing breast cancer mortality in women aged 39-49 years: A meta-analysis. *Journal of Women's Health, 20*[6], 848.)

Conducting Meta-Synthesis of Qualitative Research

Qualitative research synthesis is the process and product of systematically reviewing and formally integrating the findings from qualitative studies (Sandelowski & Barroso, 2007). The process for conducting a synthesis of qualitative research is still in the developmental phase. Various synthesis methods have appeared in the literature, such as meta-synthesis, meta-ethnography, meta-study, meta-narrative, qualitative metasummary, qualitative meta-analysis, and aggregated analysis (Barnett-Page & Thomas, 2009; Kent & Fineout-Overholt, 2008; Sandelowski & Barroso, 2007; Walsh & Downe, 2005). Qualitative researchers are not in agreement at the present time about the method to use for synthesizing qualitative research or if one method is possible to accomplish this process. Although the methodology is not clearly developed for qualitative research synthesis, researchers recognize the importance of summarizing qualitative findings to determine knowledge that might

be used in practice and for policy development (Barnett-Page & Thomas, 2009; Finfgeld-Connett, 2010; Sandelowski & Barroso, 2007). The Cochrane Collaboration recognizes the importance of synthesizing qualitative research, and the Cochrane Qualitative Methods Group was developed as a forum for discussion and development of methodology in this area (Higgins & Green, 2008).

The qualitative research synthesis method that seems to be gaining momentum in the nursing literature is meta-synthesis. Methodological articles have been published to describe meta-synthesis, but this method is still in early phases of development (Finfgeld-Connett, 2010; Kent & Fineout-Overholt, 2008; Walsh & Downe, 2005). Meta-synthesis is defined as the systematic compiling and integration of qualitative study results to expand understanding and develop a unique interpretation of study findings in a selected area. The focus is on interpretation rather than the combining of study results as with quantitative research synthesis. Meta-synthesis involves the breaking down of findings from different studies to discover essential features and then the combining of these ideas into a unique, transformed whole. Sandelowski and Barroso (2007) identified metasummary as a step in conducting meta-synthesis. Metasummary is the summarizing of findings across qualitative reports to identify knowledge in a selected area. A process for conducting a meta-synthesis is described in the following section. A meta-synthesis conducted by Denieffe and Gooney (2011) of the symptom experience of women with breast cancer is presented as an example.

Framing a Meta-Synthesis Exercise

Initially, researchers need to provide a frame for the meta-synthesis to be conducted (Kent & Fineout-Overholt, 2008; Walsh & Downe, 2005). Framing involves identifying the focus and scope of the meta-synthesis to be conducted. The focus of the meta-synthesis is usually an important area of interest for the individuals conducting it and a topic with an adequate body of qualitative studies. The scope of a meta-synthesis is an area of debate, with some qualitative researchers recommending a narrow, precise approach and others recommending a broader, more inclusive approach. However, researchers recognize framing is essential for making the synthesis process manageable and the findings meaningful and potentially transferable to practice. Framing the meta-synthesis is facilitated by the authors' research and clinical expertise, initial review of the relevant qualitative literature, and discussion with expert qualitative researchers. Usually a research question is developed to direct the meta-synthesis process.

Denieffe and Gooney (2011) conducted their meta-synthesis based on the stages developed by Sandelowski and Barroso (2007). These stages included "identifying a research question, collecting relevant data (qualitative studies), appraising the studies, performing a metasummary and meta-synthesis" (Denieffe and Gooney, 2011, p. 425). Denieffe and Gooney developed the following question to direct their meta-synthesis and provided a rationale for their scope and focus.

"In this study the question was set as 'What is the symptom experience of women with breast cancer from time of diagnosis to completion of treatment?' The time frame selected from time of diagnosis to completion of treatment, has been conceptualized ... as the 'acute stage,' encompassing initial diagnosis and treatment in the first of a three-stage process of survivorship." (Denieffe & Gooney, 2011, p. 425)

Searching the Literature and Selecting Sources

Most authors agree that a rigorous search of the literature needs to be conducted. The search needs to include databases, books and book chapters, and full reports of theses and dissertations. Special search strategies that were identified earlier need to be engaged to identify grey literature because qualitative studies might be published in more obscure journals. The search criteria need to identify the years of the search, keywords to be searched, and language of sources. Meta-syntheses are usually limited to qualitative studies only and do not included mix-method studies (Walsh & Downe, 2005). Also, qualitative findings that have not been interpreted but are unanalyzed quotes, field notes, case histories, stories, or poems are usually excluded (Finfgeld-Connett, 2010). The search process is usually very fluid with the conduct of additional computerized and hand searches to identify more studies. Sandelowski and Barroso (2007) identified a berry-picking process to search for sources, which includes a dynamic process of modifying search terms and methods to identify relevant sources. However, it is important for researchers to document systematically the strategies that they used to search the literature and the sources found through these different search strategies.

The final selection of studies to include in the meta-synthesis depends on the focus and scope of the synthesis. Some authors focus on one type of qualitative research, such as ethnography, or one investigator in a particular area. Others include studies with different qualitative methodologies and investigators in a field or related fields. The search criteria need to be consistently implemented in determining the studies to be included and excluded in the synthesis. A flow diagram might be developed to identify the process for selecting the studies similar to the one identified for systematic reviews and meta-analyses (see Figure 19-1) (Sandelowski & Barroso, 2007). Denieffe and Gooney (2011) provided the following description of their literature search, search criteria, and selection of studies for their meta-synthesis.

"Relevant qualitative research studies were located and retrieved using computer searches in CINAHL, PsychLIT, Academic Search Premier, Embase, and MEDLINE. The research reports selected for this synthesis met the following inclusion criteria: (1) the study focused on women with breast cancer; (2) there were explicit references to the use of qualitative research methods; and (3) the study focused on women's perspectives and experiences of symptoms with breast cancer. There were no restrictions related to the date the research was published. Keywords used were breast cancer, experience, symptom, and symptom experience.... The search using electronic databases was supplemented by ... footnote chasing using reference lists, citation searching, in addition to hand searching of journals, and consultation with clinical colleagues and researchers in the area. A total of 253 studies were identified as being possibly relevant.... Only 31 studies were found to be relevant to the research question and included in the meta-synthesis. Reasons for this reduction included papers that provided limited qualitative data, ... did not address the research question, ... addressed post-treatment/survivor concerns, ... or data given may not have related to patients with breast cancer." (Denieffe & Gooney, 2011, pp. 425-426)

Appraisal of Studies and Analysis of Data

The critical appraisal process for qualitative research varies among sources. We recommend that you use the critical appraisal guidelines for qualitative research presented in Chapter 18. These guidelines might be used for examining the quality of individual studies and a group of studies for a meta-synthesis. Usually a table is developed as part of the appraisal process, but this is also an area of debate. The table headings might include (1) author and year of source, (2) aim or goal of the study, (3) theoretical orientation, (4), methodological orientation, (5) type of findings, (6) sampling plan, (7) sample size, and (8) other key content relevant for comparison. This table provides a display of relevant study elements so that a comparative appraisal might be conducted (Sandelowski & Barroso, 2007; Walsh & Downe, 2005). The comparative analysis of studies involves examining methodology and findings across studies for similarities and differences. The frequency of similar findings might be recorded. The differences or contradictions in studies need to be resolved or explained (or both). Varied analysis techniques often are used by the researchers to translate the findings of the different studies into a new or unique description.

Denieffe and Gooney (2011) developed a detailed comparative analysis table of the 31 studies they included in their meta-synthesis. Their table included the headings mentioned in the previous paragraph and

the following: time frame from diagnosis, treatment, age range, and ethnic origin. They indicated that the "final stage of data analysis was the qualitative meta-synthesis, interpreting the findings. Constant targeted comparison within and between study findings was undertaken, utilizing external literature to facilitate interpretation of the emerging findings" (Denieffe & Gooney, 2011, p. 426).

Discussion of Meta-Synthesis Findings

A meta-synthesis report might include findings presented in different formats based on the knowledge developed and the perspective of the authors. A synthesis of qualitative studies in an area might result in the discovery of unique or more refined themes explaining the area of synthesis. The findings from a meta-synthesis might be presented in narrative format or graphically presented in a model. The discussion of findings also needs to include identification of the limitations of the meta-synthesis. The report often concludes with recommendations for further research and possibly implications for practice or policy development or both.

The synthesis by Denieffe and Gooney (2011) of 31 qualitative studies in the area of symptoms experienced by women with breast cancer resulted in the identification of four emerging themes: (1) breast cancer and the impact on self, (2) self-image and stigma, (3) self and self-control, and (4) more than just a symptom. The researchers linked each of these themes with the appropriate studies and presented this information clearly in a table. Denieffe and Gooney (2011) also developed a detailed model that linked the themes about self to the diagnosis and treatment of the women and the symptoms they experienced (Figure 19-7). The following excerpt provides the conclusions from this meta-synthesis.

"The overarching idea emerging from this meta-synthesis is that the symptoms experience for women with breast cancer has effects on the very 'self' of the individual. Emerging is women's need to consider the existential issues that they face while simultaneously dealing with a multitude of physical and psychological symptoms. This meta-synthesis develops a new, integrated, and more complete interpretation of findings on the symptom experience of women with breast cancer. The results offer the clinician a greater understanding in depth and breadth than the findings from individual studies on symptom experiences." (Denieffe & Gooney, 2011, p. 424)

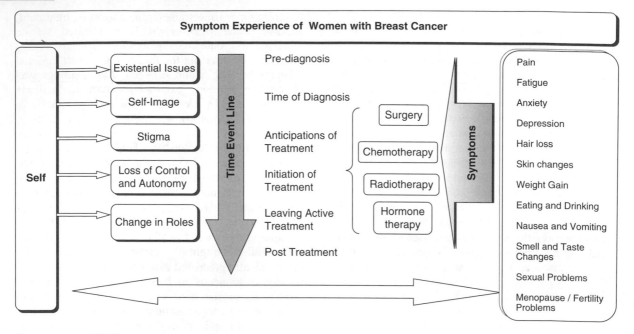

Figure 19-7 Overall findings of meta-synthesis. (From Denieffe, S., & Gooney, M. [2011]. A meta-synthesis of women's symptoms experience and breast cancer. *European Journal of Cancer Care, 20*[4], 430.)

Mixed-Methods Systematic Reviews

In recent years, nurse researchers have been conducting mixed-methods studies that include both quantitative and qualitative research methods (Creswell, 2009) (see Chapter 10 for different types of mixed-methods designs). Researchers recognize the importance of synthesizing the findings of these studies to determine important knowledge for practice and policy development. For some synthesis areas, researchers need to combine the findings from both quantitative and qualitative studies to determine the current knowledge in that area. Harden and Thomas (2005) identified this process of combining findings from quantitative and qualitative studies as mixed-methods synthesis. Higgins and Green (2008) referred to this synthesis of quantitative, qualitative, and mixed-methods studies as a *mixed-method systematic review*.

The systematic reviews discussed earlier in this chapter included only studies of a quantitative methodology, such as meta-analyses, RCTs, and quasi-experimental studies, to determine the effectiveness of an intervention. Mixed-methods systematic reviews might include various study designs, such as qualitative research and quasi-experimental, correlational, and descriptive studies (Bettany-Saltikov, 2010b; Higgins & Green, 2008; Liberati et al., 2009). Reviews that include syntheses of various quantitative and qualitative study designs are referred to as **mixed-methods systematic reviews** in this text. Mixed-methods systematic reviews have the potential to contribute to Cochrane Interventions reviews for practice and health policy in the following ways:

> "1. **In forming** reviews by using evidence from qualitative research to help define and refine a question... .
>
> "2. **Enhancing** reviews by synthesizing evidence from qualitative research identified whilst looking for evidence ... .
>
> "3. **Extending** reviews by undertaking a search and synthesis specially of evidence from qualitative studies to address questions directly related to the effectiveness review.
>
> "4. **Supplementing** reviews by synthesizing qualitative evidence to address questions on aspects other than effectiveness." (Higgins & Green, 2008, p. 574)

Conducting mixed-methods systematic reviews involves implementing a complex synthesis process that includes expertise in synthesizing knowledge from quantitative, qualitative, and mixed-methods studies. Higgins and Green (2008) recommended two types of approaches to integrate the findings from quantitative, qualitative, and mixed-methods studies: (1) multilevel syntheses and (2) parallel syntheses. Multilevel synthesis involves synthesizing the findings from quantitative studies separate from qualitative studies and integrating the findings from these two syntheses in the final report. Parallel synthesis involves the separate synthesis of quantitative and qualitative studies, but the findings from the qualitative synthesis are used in interpreting the synthesized quantitative studies.

Further work is needed to develop the methodology for conducting a mixed-methods systematic review. The steps overlap with the systematic review and meta-synthesis processes that have been previously described. The process might best be implemented with a team of researchers with expertise in conducting different types of studies and research syntheses. The basic structure for the mixed-methods systematic review might include the following: (1) identify purpose and questions or aims of review; (2) develop the review protocol that includes search strategies for quantitative, qualitative, and mixed-methods studies; (3) identify search criteria for quantitative studies; (4) identify search criteria for qualitative and mixed-methods studies; (5) conduct a rigorous search of the literature; (6) select relevant quantitative, qualitative, and mixed-method studies for synthesis; (7) construct a table of information of studies to allow comparative appraisal of the studies; (8) conduct critical appraisals of the quality of quantitative and qualitative studies; (9) synthesize study findings; and (10) develop a report that integrates the results of syntheses for both quantitative, qualitative, and mixed-method studies. The reader is encouraged to refer to the steps in systematic review and meta-analysis for conducting quantitative research syntheses and to the meta-synthesis discussion for synthesizing qualitative studies.

Wulff, Cummings, Marck, and Yurtseven (2011) conducted a mixed-methods systematic review to examine the association of medication administration technologies and patient safety. This review included 12 studies with the following designs: five preintervention and postintervention studies, five correlational studies, and two qualitative studies. The major focus of this review was the synthesis of the 10 quantitative studies that identified the benefits of implementing medication administration technologies to improve patient safety. However, the problem identified by both the quantitative and the qualitative studies was that nurses develop workarounds in implementing different types of medication administration technologies that could compromise patient safety.

Models to Promote Evidence-Based Practice in Nursing

Two models commonly used to facilitate EBP in nursing are the Stetler Model of Research Utilization to Facilitate EBP (Stetler, 2001) and the Iowa Model of Evidence-Based Practice to Promote Quality of Care (Titler et al., 2001). This section introduces these two models that might be used to implement evidence-based protocols, algorithms, and guidelines in clinical agencies.

Stetler Model of Research Utilization to Facilitate Evidence-Based Practice

An initial model for research utilization in nursing was developed by Stetler and Marram in 1976 and expanded and refined by Stetler in 1994 and 2001 to promote EBP for nursing. The Stetler model (2001) (see Figure 19-8) provides a comprehensive framework to enhance the use of research evidence by nurses to facilitate EBP. The research evidence can be used at the institutional or individual level. At the institutional level, synthesized research knowledge is used to develop or update protocols, algorithms, policies, procedures, or other formal programs implemented in the institution. Individual nurses, including practitioners, educators, and policy makers, summarize research and use the knowledge to influence educational programs, make practice decisions, and impact political decision making. Stetler's model is included in this text to guide individual nurses and healthcare institutions in using research evidence in practice. The following sections briefly describe the five phases of the Stetler model: (I) preparation, (II) validation, (III) comparative evaluation and decision making, (IV) translation and application, and (V) evaluation (see Figure 19-8).

Phase I: Preparation

The intent of the Stetler model (2001) is to make using research evidence in practice a conscious, critical thinking process that is initiated by the user. The first phase (preparation) involves determining the purpose, focus, and potential outcomes of making an evidence-based change in a clinical agency. The agency's priorities and other external and internal factors that could be influenced by or could influence the proposed practice change need to be examined. After the purpose of the evidence-based project has been identified and

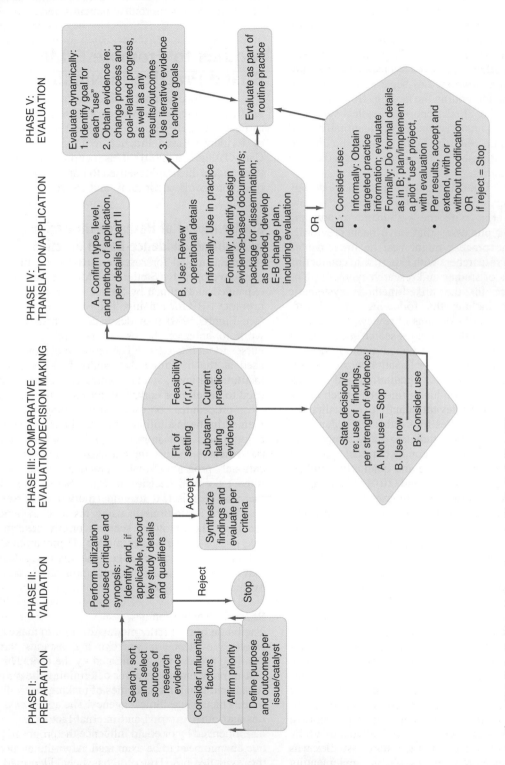

Figure 19-8 Stetler Model, part I: Steps of research utilization to facilitate EBP.
Stetler, C. B. (2001). Updating the Stetler Model of Research Utilization to facilitate evidence-based practice. *Nursing Outlook, 42*(6), 276.

approved by the agency, a detailed search of the literature is conducted to determine the strength of the evidence available for use in practice. The research literature might be reviewed to solve a difficult clinical, managerial, or educational problem; to provide the basis for a policy, standard, algorithm, or protocol; or to prepare for an in-service program or other type of professional presentation.

Phase II: Validation

In the validation phase, research reports are critically appraised to determine their scientific soundness. If the studies are limited in number or are weak or both, the findings and conclusions are considered inadequate for use in practice, and the process stops. The quality of the research evidence is greatly strengthened if a systematic review or meta-analysis has been conducted in the area where you want to make an evidence-based change. If the research knowledge base is strong in the selected area, a decision must be made regarding the priority of using the evidence in practice by the clinical agency.

Phase III: Comparative Evaluation and Decision Making

Comparative evaluation includes four parts: (1) substantiation of the evidence, (2) fit of the evidence with the healthcare setting, (3) feasibility of using research findings, and (4) concerns with current practice (Figure 19-8). Substantiating evidence is produced by replication, in which consistent, credible findings are obtained from several studies in similar practice settings. The studies generating the strongest research evidence are RCTs and meta-analyses of RCTs and quasi-experimental studies, which provide extremely strong evidence about the effectiveness of nursing interventions. To determine the fit of the evidence in the clinical agency, the characteristics of the setting are examined to determine the forces that would facilitate or inhibit the evidence-based change. Stetler (2001) believed the feasibility of using research evidence in practice involved examining the three R's related to making changes in practice: (1) potential risks, (2) resources needed, and (3) readiness of the people involved. The final comparison involves determining whether the research information provides credible, empirical evidence for making changes in the current practice. The research evidence needs to document that an intervention increased the quality in current practice by solving practice problems and improving patient outcomes. By conducting phase III, the overall benefits and risks of using the research evidence in a practice setting can be assessed. If the benefits

(improved patient, provider, or agency outcomes) are much greater than the risks (complications, morbidity, mortality, or increased costs) for the organization, the individual nurse, or both, using the research-based intervention in practice is feasible.

Three types of decisions (decision making) are possible during this phase: (1) to use the research evidence, (2) to consider using the evidence, and (3) not to use the research evidence. The decision to use research knowledge in practice is determined mainly by the strength of the evidence. Depending on the research knowledge to be used in practice, the individual practitioner, hospital unit, or agency might make this decision. Another decision might be to consider using the available research evidence in practice. When a change is complex and involves multiple disciplines, the individuals involved often need additional time to determine how the evidence might be used and what measures will be taken to coordinate the involvement of different health professionals in the change. A final option might be not to make a change in practice because of the poor quality of the research evidence, costs, and other potential problems.

Phase IV: Translation and Application

The translation and application phase involves planning for and using the research evidence in practice. The translation phase involves determining exactly what knowledge will be used and how that knowledge will be applied to practice. The use of the research evidence can be cognitive, instrumental, or symbolic. Cognitive application is a more informal use of the research knowledge to modify one's way of thinking or appreciation of an issue (Stetler, 2001). Cognitive application may improve the nurse's understanding of a situation, allow analysis of practice dynamics, or improve problem-solving skills for clinical problems. Instrumental and symbolic applications are formal ways to make changes in practice. Instrument application involves using research evidence to support the need for change in nursing interventions or practice protocols, algorithms, and guidelines. Symbolic or political use occurs when information is used to support or change an agency policy. The application phase includes the following steps for planned change: (1) assess the situation to be changed, (2) develop a plan for change, and (3) implement the plan. During the application phase, the protocols, policies, procedures, or algorithms developed with research knowledge are implemented in practice (Stetler, 2001). A pilot project on a single hospital unit might be conducted to implement the change in practice, and the results of this project could be evaluated to determine if the change should be extended throughout the healthcare agency or corporation.

Phase V: Evaluation

The final stage is to evaluate the effect of the evidence-based change on selected agency, personnel, or patient outcomes. The evaluation process can include both formal and informal activities that are conducted by administrators, nurse clinicians, and other health professionals (see Figure 19-8). Informal evaluations might include self-monitoring or discussions with patients, families, peers, and other professionals. Formal evaluations can include case studies, audits, quality assurance, and outcomes research projects. The goal of the Stetler model (2001) is to increase the use of research evidence in nursing to facilitate EBP. This model provides detailed steps to encourage nurses to become change agents and make the necessary improvements in practice based on the best current research evidence.

Iowa Model of Evidence-Based Practice

Nurses are actively involved in conducting research, synthesizing research evidence, and developing evidence-based guidelines for practice. Nurses have a strong commitment to EBP and can benefit from the direction provided by the Iowa model to expand their research-based practice. The Iowa Model of Evidence-Based Practice provides direction for the development of EBP in a clinical agency. Titler et al. initially developed this EBP model in 1994 and revised it in 2001. In a healthcare agency, triggers initiate the need for change, and the focus should always be to make changes based on best research evidence. These triggers can be problem-focused and evolve from risk management data, process improvement data, benchmarking data, financial data, and clinical problems (see Figure 19-9). The triggers can also be knowledge-focused, such as new research findings, changes in national agencies or organizational standards and guidelines, an expanded philosophy of care, or questions from the institutional standards committee. The triggers are evaluated and prioritized based on the needs of the clinical agency. If a trigger is considered an agency priority, a group is formed to search for the best evidence to manage the clinical concern (Titler et al., 2001).

In some situations, the research evidence is inadequate to make changes in practice, and additional studies are needed to strengthen the knowledge base. Sometimes the research evidence can be combined with other sources of knowledge (theories, scientific principles, expert opinion, and case reports) to provide fairly strong evidence for developing research-based protocols for practice. The strongest evidence is generated from meta-analyses of several RCTs, systematic reviews that usually include meta-analyses, and individual studies. Systematic reviews provide the best research evidence for developing evidence-based guidelines. The research-based protocols or evidence-based guidelines are pilot-tested on a particular unit and then evaluated to determine the impact on patient care (see Figure 19-9). If the outcomes are favorable from the pilot test, the change is made in practice and monitored over time to determine its impact on the agency environment, staff, costs, and the patient and family (Titler et al., 2001). An agency can promote EBP by using the Iowa model to identify triggers for change, implement patient care based on the best research evidence, and monitor changes in practice to ensure quality care.

Implementing Evidence-Based Guidelines in Practice

EBP of nursing and medicine has expanded extensively since the 1990s. Research knowledge is generated every day that needs to be critically appraised and synthesized to determine the best evidence for use in practice (Craig & Smyth, 2012; Higgins & Green, 2008; Melnyk & Fineout-Overholt, 2011). This section discusses the development of EBP guidelines and provides a model for using these guidelines in practice. Chobanian et al. (2003) conducted an excellent systematic review to determine the best research evidence available for assessing, diagnosing, and managing hypertension. This systematic review, which included several meta-analyses and integrative reviews, was used to develop the JNC 7 evidence-based guideline for hypertension (U.S. Department of Health and Human Services, National Institutes of Health, National Heart, Lung, and Blood Institute, 2003). The JNC 7 evidence-based guideline is presented later in this chapter. JNC-8 is being developed by a national panel of expert researchers and clinicians with an expected availability to the public for review and comment by 2012 and publication to follow (see the status of the guideline at http://www.nhlbi.nih.gov/guidelines/hypertension/jnc8/index.htm). This section focuses on the development and use of evidence-based guidelines in practice.

Development of Evidence-Based Guidelines

Once a significant health topic or condition has been selected, guidelines are developed to promote

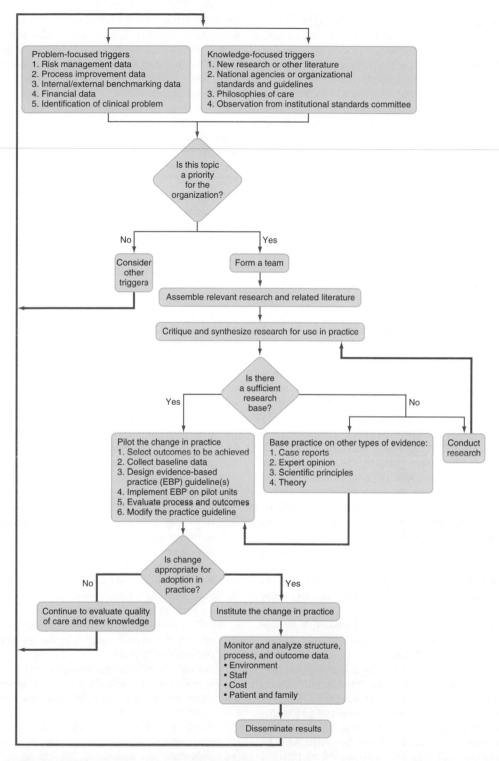

Figure 19-9 Iowa Model of Evidence-Based Practice to Promote Quality Care.
Titler, M. G., Kleiber, C., Steelman, V. J., Rakel, B. A., Budreau, G., Everett, L. Q., et al. (2001). The Iowa Model of Evidence-Based Practice to promote quality care. *Critical Care Nursing Clinics of North America, 13*(4), 500.

effective management of this health condition. Since the 1980s, the Agency for Healthcare Research and Quality (AHRQ) has had a major role in identifying health topics and developing evidence-based guidelines for these topics (http://www.ahrq.gov). In the late 1980s and early 1990s, a panel or team of experts was often charged with developing guidelines for the AHRQ. The AHRQ solicited the members of the panel, who usually included nationally recognized researchers in the topic area; expert clinicians, such as physicians, nurses, pharmacists, and social workers; healthcare administrators; policy developers; economists; government representatives; and consumers. The group designated the scope of the guidelines and conducted extensive reviews of the literature including relevant systematic reviews, meta-analyses, qualitative research syntheses, mixed-methods systematic reviews, individual studies, and theories.

The best research evidence available was synthesized to develop recommendations for practice. Most of the evidence-based guidelines included systematic reviews, meta-analyses, and multiple individual studies. The guidelines were examined for their usefulness in clinical practice, their impact on health policy, and their cost-effectiveness. Consultants, other researchers, and additional expert clinicians often were asked to review the guidelines and provide input. Based on the experts' critique, the AHRQ revised and packaged the guidelines for distribution to healthcare professionals. Some of the first guidelines focused on the following healthcare problems: (1) acute pain management in infants, children, and adolescents; (2) prediction and prevention of pressure ulcers in adults; (3) urinary incontinence in adults; (4) management of functional impairments with cataracts; (5) detection, diagnosis, and treatment of depression; (6) screening, diagnosis, management, and counseling about sickle cell disease; (7) management of cancer pain; (8) diagnosis and treatment of heart failure; (9) low back problems; and (10) otitis media diagnosis and management in children.

At the present time, standardized guideline development ranges from a structured process such as the one just discussed to a less structured process in which a guideline might be developed by a healthcare organization, healthcare plan, or professional organization. The AHRQ initiated the National Guideline Clearinghouse (NGC, 2012b) in 1998 to store the evidence-based practice guidelines. Initially, the NGC had 200 guidelines, but now the collection has expanded to thousands of clinical practice guidelines. The NGC is a publicly available database of evidence-based clinical practice guidelines and related documents. Free Internet access to guidelines is available at http://www.guideline.gov. The NGC is updated weekly with new content that the AHRQ produces in partnership with the American Medical Association and the American Association of Health Plans (now America's Health Insurance Plans). The key components of the NGC and its user-friendly resources can be found on the AHRQ website at http://www.guideline.gov/index.aspx. Some of the critical information on the NGC is provided here to show you what is available and how to access the NGC resources:

* "Structured abstracts (summaries) about the guideline and its development.
* Links to full-text guidelines, where available, and/or ordering information for print copies.
* Downloads of the Complete NGC Summary for all guidelines represented in the database.
* A Guideline Comparison utility that gives users the ability to generate side-by-side comparisons for any combination of two or more guidelines.
* Unique guideline comparisons called Guideline Syntheses prepared by NGC staff, compare guidelines covering similar topics, highlighting areas of similarity and difference. NGC Guideline Syntheses often provide a comparison of guidelines developed in different countries, providing insight into commonalities and differences in international health practices.
* An electronic forum, NGC-L for exchanging information on clinical practice guidelines, their development, implementation, and use.
* An Annotated Bibliography database where users can search for citations for publications and resources about guidelines, including guideline development and methodology, structure, evaluation, and implementation.

Other features include the following:

* What's New enables users to see what guidelines have been added each week and includes an index of all guidelines in NGC.
* NGC Update Service is a weekly electronic mailing of new and updated guidelines posted to the NGC Web site.
* Detailed Search enables users to create very specific search queries based on the various attributes found in the NGC Classification Scheme.
* NGC Browse permits users to scan for guidelines available on the NGC site by disease/condition, treatment/intervention, or developing organization.

- Full-text guidelines and/or companion documents available through the guideline developer that can be downloaded.
- Glossary provides definitions of terms used in the standardized abstracts (summaries)." (NGC, 2012a, http://www.guideline.gov/browse/by-topic.aspx)

Criteria for submitting clinical practice guidelines and the application process are provided online. Following are the criteria that an evidence-based guideline must meet to be submitted to the NGC:

- "The guideline must contain systematically developed recommendations, strategies, or other information to assist healthcare decision-making in specific clinical circumstances.
- The guideline must have been produced under the auspices of a relevant professional organization (e.g., medical specialty society, government agency, healthcare organization, or health plan).
- The guideline development process must have included a verifiable, systematic literature search and review of existing evidence published in peer-reviewed journals.
- The guideline must be current and the most recent version (i.e., developed, reviewed, or revised within the last 5 years)." (NGC, 2012b, http://www.guideline.gov/)

The NGC provides varied audiences with an easy-to-use mechanism for obtaining objective, detailed information on clinical practice guidelines. In addition, the NGC (2012a) provides a list of the guidelines that are in the process of being developed (http://www.guideline.gov/browse/by-topic.aspx).

In addition to the evidence-based guidelines, the AHRQ has developed many tools to assess the quality of care that is provided by the evidence-based guidelines. You can search the AHRQ (2012a, 2012c) website (http://www.qualitymeasures.ahrq.gov/) for an appropriate tool to measure a variable in a research project or to evaluate outcomes of care in a clinical agency.

Numerous professional organizations, healthcare agencies, universities, and other groups provide evidence-based guidelines for practice. Websites are as follows:

- Academic Center for Evidence-Based Nursing: http://www.acestar.uthscsa.edu
- Association of Women's Health, Obstetric, and Neonatal Nurses: http://awhonn.org
- Centers for Health Evidence.net: http://www.cche.net
- CMA InfoBase: http://mdm.ca/cpgsnew/cpgs/index.asp
- Guidelines Advisory Committee: http://www.gacguidelines.ca
- Guidelines International Network: http://www.g-i-n.net/
- HerbMed: Evidence-Based Herbal Database, 1998, Alternative Medicine Foundation: http://www.herbmed.org/
- MD Consult: http://www.mdconsult.com/php/286943359-1063/homepage
- National Association of Neonatal Nurses: http://www.nann.org/
- National Institute for Clinical Excellence (NICE): http://www.nice.org.uk/catcg2.asp?c=20034
- Oncology Nursing Society: http://www.ons.org/
- PIER—the Physicians' Information and Education Resource (authoritative, evidence-based guidance to improve clinical care; ACP-ASIM members only): http://pier.acponline.org/index.html
- Primary Care Clinical Practice Guidelines: http://www.medscape.com/pages/editorial/public/pguidelines/index-primarycare
- U.S. Preventive Services Task Force: http://www.uspreventiveservicestaskforce.org/about.htm

Implementing the Joint National Committee on Prevention, Detection, Evaluation, and Treatment of High Blood Pressure Evidence-Based Guideline in Practice

Evidence-based guidelines have become the standards for providing care to patients in the United States and other nations. A few nurses have participated in committees that have developed these evidence-based guidelines, and many APNs are using these guidelines in their practices. An evidence-based guideline for the assessment, diagnosis, and management of high blood pressure is provided as an example. This guideline was developed from JNC 7 and was published in the *Journal of the American Medical Association* (Chobanian et al., 2003). The NIH Department of Health and Human Services National Heart, Lung, and Blood Institute developed educational materials to communicate the specifics of this guideline to promote its use by healthcare providers. This guideline is presented in

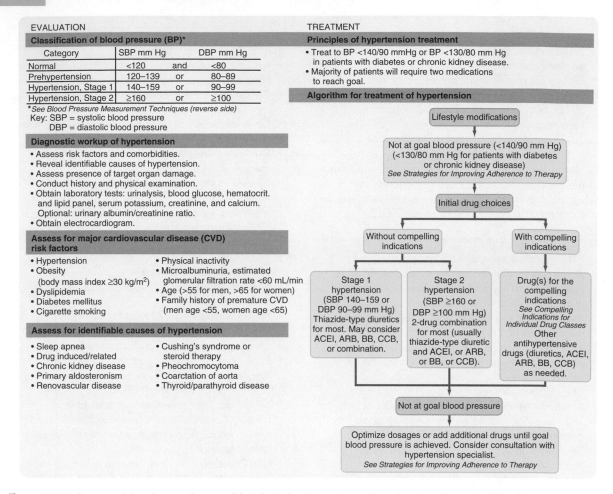

EVALUATION

Classification of blood pressure (BP)*

Category	SBP mm Hg		DBP mm Hg
Normal	<120	and	<80
Prehypertension	120–139	or	80–89
Hypertension, Stage 1	140–159	or	90–99
Hypertension, Stage 2	≥160	or	≥100

**See Blood Pressure Measurement Techniques (reverse side)*
Key: SBP = systolic blood pressure
       DBP = diastolic blood pressure

Diagnostic workup of hypertension

- Assess risk factors and comorbidities.
- Reveal identifiable causes of hypertension.
- Assess presence of target organ damage.
- Conduct history and physical examination.
- Obtain laboratory tests: urinalysis, blood glucose, hematocrit. and lipid panel, serum potassium, creatinine, and calcium. Optional: urinary albumin/creatinine ratio.
- Obtain electrocardiogram.

Assess for major cardiovascular disease (CVD) risk factors

- Hypertension
- Obesity (body mass index ≥30 kg/m²)
- Dyslipidemia
- Diabetes mellitus
- Cigarette smoking
- Physical inactivity
- Microalbuminuria, estimated glomerular filtration rate <60 mL/min
- Age (>55 for men, >65 for women)
- Family history of premature CVD (men age <55, women age <65)

Assess for identifiable causes of hypertension

- Sleep apnea
- Drug induced/related
- Chronic kidney disease
- Primary aldosteronism
- Renovascular disease
- Cushing's syndrome or steroid therapy
- Pheochromocytoma
- Coarctation of aorta
- Thyroid/parathyroid disease

TREATMENT

Principles of hypertension treatment

- Treat to BP <140/90 mmHg or BP <130/80 mm Hg in patients with diabetes or chronic kidney disease.
- Majority of patients will require two medications to reach goal.

Algorithm for treatment of hypertension

Lifestyle modifications

Not at goal blood pressure (<140/90 mm Hg) (<130/80 mm Hg for patients with diabetes or chronic kidney disease) *See Strategies for Improving Adherence to Therapy*

Initial drug choices

Without compelling indications

With compelling indications

Stage 1 hypertension (SBP 140–159 or DBP 90–99 mm Hg) Thiazide-type diuretics for most. May consider ACEI, ARB, BB, CCB, or combination.

Stage 2 hypertension (SBP ≥160 or DBP ≥100 mm Hg) 2-drug combination for most (usually thiazide-type diuretic and ACEI, or ARB, or BB, or CCB).

Drug(s) for the compelling indications *See Compelling Indications for Individual Drug Classes* Other antihypertensive drugs (diuretics, ACEI, ARB, BB, CCB) as needed.

Not at goal blood pressure

Optimize dosages or add additional drugs until goal blood pressure is achieved. Consider consultation with hypertension specialist. *See Strategies for Improving Adherence to Therapy*

Figure 19-10 Reference card from the seventh report of the Joint National Committee on Prevention, Detection, Evaluation, and Treatment of High Blood Pressure (JNC 7). U.S. Department of Health and Human Services, National Institutes of Health, National Heart, Lung, and Blood Institute. (2003). *Reference card from the Seventh report of the Joint National Committee on Prevention, Detection, Evaluation, and Treatment of High Blood Pressure (JNC 7).* Bethesda, MD: NIH Publication No. 03-5231. Retrieved from www.nhlbi.nih.gov/guidelines/hypertension/jnc7card.htm.

Figure 19-10 and provides clinicians with direction for the following: (1) classification of blood pressure as normal, prehypertension, hypertension stage 1, and hypertension stage 2; (2) conduct a diagnostic workup of hypertension; (3) assessment of the major cardiovascular disease risk factors; (4) assessment of the identification of causes of hypertension; and (5) treatment of hypertension. An algorithm provides direction for the selection of the most appropriate treatment methods for each patient diagnosed with hypertension (U.S. Department of Health and Human Services, National Institutes of Health, National Heart, Lung, and Blood Institute, 2003).

APNs and RNs need to assess the usefulness and quality of each evidence-based guideline before they

implement it in their practice. Figure 19-11 presents the **Grove Model for Implementing Evidence-Based Guidelines in Practice**. In this model, nurses identify a practice problem, search for the best research evidence to manage the problem in their practice, and note that an evidence-based guideline has been developed. The quality and usefulness of the guideline must be assessed by the healthcare provider before it is used in practice, and that involves examining the following: (1) the authors of the guideline, (2) the significance of the healthcare problem, (3) the strength of the research evidence, (4) the link to national standards, and (5) the cost-effectiveness of using the guideline in practice. The quality of the JNC 7 guideline is examined as an example using the four criteria identified in the Grove

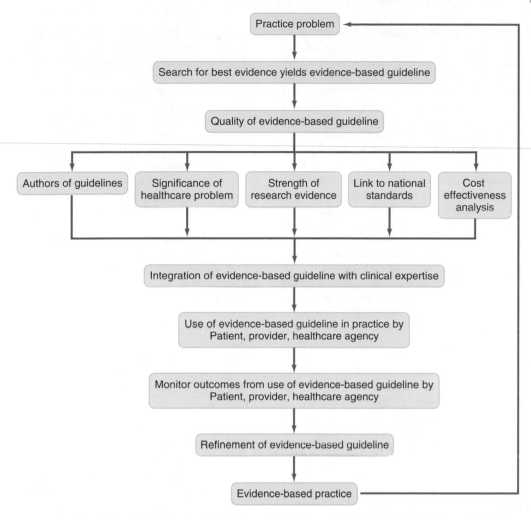

Figure 19-11   Grove Model for Implementing Evidence-Based Guidelines in Practice.

model (see Figure 19-11). The authors of the JNC 7 guideline were expert researchers, clinicians (physicians), policy developers, healthcare administrators, and the National High Blood Pressure Education Program Coordinating Committee. These authors have the expertise to develop an evidence-based guideline for the significant health problem of hypertension.

"Hypertension is a significant healthcare problem because it affects approximately 50 million individuals in the United States and approximately 1 billion individuals worldwide.... Hypertension is the most common primary diagnosis in the United States with

35 million office visits as the primary diagnosis.... Recent clinical trials have demonstrated that effective BP [blood pressure] control can be achieved in most patients with hypertension, but the majority will require 2 or more antihypertensive drugs." (Chobanian et al., 2003, p. 2562)

The research evidence for the development of the JNC 7 guideline was extremely strong. The JNC 7 report included 81 references; 9 (11%) of the references were meta-analyses, and 35 (43%) were RCTs (experimental studies); 44 (54%) sources are considered extremely strong research evidence. The other references were strong and included retrospective analyses or case-controlled studies, prospective or cohort studies, cross-sectional surveys or prevalence studies, and clinical intervention studies (nonrandom) (Chobanian et al., 2003). The JNC 7 provides the national standard for the assessment, diagnosis, and treatment of hypertension. The recommendations from the JNC 7 are supported by the Department of Health and Human Services and disseminated through NIH publication no. 03-5231. Use of the JNC 7 guideline in practice is cost-effective because the clinical trials have shown that "antihypertensive therapy has been associated with 35% to 40% mean reductions in stroke incidence; 20% to 25% in myocardial infarction [MI]; and more than 50% in HF [heart failure]" (Chobanian et al., 2003, p. 2562).

The next step is for APNs and physicians to use the JNC 7 guideline in their practice (see Figure 19-11). Healthcare providers can assess the adequacy of the guideline for their practice and modify the hypertension treatments based on the individual health needs and values of their patients. The outcomes for the patient, provider, and healthcare agency need to be examined. The outcomes would be recorded in the patients' charts and possibly in a database owing to the electronic medical records and would include the following: (1) blood pressure readings for patients; (2) incidence of diagnosis of hypertension based on the JNC 7 guidelines; (3) appropriateness of the treatments implemented to manage hypertension; and (4) incidence of stroke, MI, and HF over 5, 10, 15, and 20 years. The healthcare agency outcomes include the access to care by patients with hypertension, patient satisfaction with care, and the cost related to diagnosis and treatment of hypertension and the complications of stroke, MI, and HF. This EBP guideline will be refined in the future based on clinical outcomes, outcome studies, and new controlled clinical trials (see previous discussion of JNC 8). The use of this evidence-based guideline and additional guidelines promote an EBP for APNs (see Figure 19-10).

Evidence-Based Practice Centers

In 1997, the AHRQ launched its initiative to promote EBP by establishing 12 evidence-based practice centers (EPCs) in the United States and Canada.

"[The EPCs develop evidence reports and technology assessments on] topics relevant to clinical, social science/behavioral, economic, and other health care

organization and delivery issues—specifically those that are common, expensive, and/or significant for the Medicare and Medicaid populations. With this program, AHRQ became a 'science partner' with private and public organizations in their efforts to improve the quality, effectiveness, and appropriateness of health care by synthesizing the evidence and facilitating the translation of evidence-based research findings. Topics are nominated by non-federal partners such as professional societies, health plans, insurers, employers, and patient groups." (AHRQ, 2012b, http://www.ahrq.gov/clinic/epc/)

Under the EPC Program, the AHRQ awards 5-year contracts to institutions to serve as EPCs. EPCs review all relevant scientific literature on clinical, behavioral, organizational, and financial topics to produce evidence reports and technology assessments. These reports are used to inform and develop coverage decisions, quality measures, educational materials, tools, guidelines, and research agendas. The EPCs also conduct research on methodology of systematic reviews. The AHRQ developed the following criteria as the basis for selecting a topic to be managed by an EPC:

- "High incidence or prevalence in the general population and in special populations, including women, racial and ethnic minorities, pediatric and elderly populations, and those of low socioeconomic status.
- Significance for the needs of the Medicare, Medicaid, and other Federal health programs.
- High costs associated with a condition, procedure, treatment, or technology, whether due to the number of people needing care, high unit cost of care, or high indirect costs.
- Controversy or uncertainty about the effectiveness or relative effectiveness of available clinical strategies or technologies.
- Impact potential for informing and improving patient or provider decision making.
- Impact potential for reducing clinically significant variations in the prevention, diagnosis, treatment, or management of a disease or condition; in the use of a procedure or technology; or in the health outcomes achieved.
- Availability of scientific data to support the systematic review and analysis of the topic.

• Submission of the nominating organization's plan to incorporate the report into its managerial or policy decision making, as defined above.
• Submission of the nominating organization's plan to disseminate derivative products to its members and plan to measure members' use of these products, and the resultant impact of such use on clinical practice." (AHRQ, 2012b)

The AHRQ (2012b) website (http://www.ahrq.gov/clinic/epc) provides the names of the EPCs and the focus of each center. This site also provides a link to the evidence-based reports produced by these centers. These EPCs have had an important role in the development of evidence-based guidelines since the 1990s and will continue to make significant contributions to EBP in the future. They are also involved in the development of measurement tools to examine the outcomes from EBP.

Introduction to Translational Research

Some of the barriers to EBP have resulted in the development of a new type of research to improve the translation of research knowledge to practice. This new research methodology is called transitional research and is being supported by the NIH (2012). Translational research is an evolving concept that is defined by the NIH as the translation of basic scientific discoveries into practical applications. Basic research discoveries from the laboratory setting need to be tested in studies with humans. In addition, the outcomes from human clinical trials need to be adopted and maintained in clinical practice. Translational research is being encouraged by both medicine and nursing to increase the implementation of evidence-based interventions in practice and to determine if these interventions are effective in producing the outcomes desired in clinical practice (Chesla, 2008; NIH, 2012). Translational research was originally part of the National Center for Research Resources. However, in December 2011, the National Center for Advancing Translation Sciences (NCATS) was developed as part of the NIH Institutes and Centers (NIH, 2012).

The NIH wanted to encourage researchers to conduct translational research and developed the Clinical and Translational Science Awards (CTSA) Consortium in October 2006. The consortium started with 12 centers located throughout the United States and expanded to 39 centers in April 2009. The program is projected to be fully implemented in 2012 with about 60 institutions involved in clinical and translational science. A website has been developed to enhance communication and encourage sharing of information related to translational research projects at http://www.ctsaweb.org/.

The CTSA Consortium is mainly focused on expanding the translation of medical research to practice. Titler (2004, p. S1) defined transitional research for the nursing profession as the: "Scientific investigation of methods, interventions, and variables that influence adoption of evidence-based practices (EBPs) by individuals and organizations to improve clinical and operational decision making in health care. This includes testing the effect of interventions on promoting and sustaining the adoption of EBPs." Baumbusch et al. (2008) developed a collaborative model for knowledge translation between research and practice in clinical settings. As you search the literature for relevant research syntheses and studies, you will note that translation studies are being published in nursing. Whittemore, Melkus, Wagner, Dziura, Northrup, and Grey (2009) conducted a translation study to promote the transfer of a Diabetic Prevention Program to primary care. These types of studies will assist you in translating research findings to your practice and determining the impact of EBP on patients' health. However, national funding is needed to expand the conduct of transitional research in nursing.

We hope that the content in this chapter increases your understanding of EBP, the conduct of research syntheses, the application of EBP models, and the implementation of EBP guidelines. We encourage you to take an active role in moving nursing toward EBP that improves outcomes for patients, healthcare professionals, and healthcare agencies.

KEY POINTS

• Evidence-based practice (EBP) is the conscientious integration of best research evidence with clinical expertise and patient values and needs in the delivery of quality, cost-effective health care. Best research evidence is produced by the conduct and synthesis of numerous, high-quality studies in a health-related area.
• There are benefits and barriers associated with EBP. The benefits of EBP are that the standards for hospital accreditation by the Joint Commission

support EBP as does the Magnet Hospital Program® managed by the American Nurses' Credentialing Center.

- Guidelines are provided for conducting the research synthesis processes of systematic review, meta-analysis, meta-synthesis, and mixed-methods systematic review. These synthesis processes are used to determine the best research evidence in a selected area and the quality of the research evidence available for practice.
- A systematic review is a structured, comprehensive synthesis of the research literature to determine the best research evidence available to address a healthcare question. A systematic review involves identifying, locating, appraising, and synthesizing quality research evidence for expert clinicians to use to promote EBP.
- A meta-analysis is conducted to pool statistically the results from previous studies into a single quantitative analysis that provides one of the highest levels of evidence about the effectiveness of an intervention.
- Meta-synthesis is defined as the systematic compiling and integration of qualitative study results to expand understanding and develop a unique interpretation of study findings in a selected area. The focus is on interpretation rather than the combining of study results as with quantitative research synthesis.
- Reviews that include syntheses of various quantitative, qualitative, and mixed-methods studies are referred to as mixed-methods systematic reviews in this text.
- Two models have been developed to promote EBP in nursing: the Stetler Model of Research Utilization to Facilitate EBP (Stetler, 2001) and the Iowa Model of Evidence-Based Practice to Promote Quality of Care (Titler et al., 2001).
- The phases of the revised Stetler model are (I) preparation, (II) validation, (III) comparative evaluation and decision making, (IV) translation and application, and (V) evaluation.
- The Iowa model provides guidelines for implementing patient care based on the best research evidence and monitoring changes in practice to ensure quality care.
- The process for developing evidence-based guidelines is described, and an example of the guideline for assessment, diagnosis, and treatment of hypertension is provided.
- The Grove Model for Implementing Evidence-Based Guidelines in Practice is provided to assist nurses in determining the quality of evidence-based guidelines and the steps for using these guidelines in practice.
- An excellent source for evidence-based guidelines is the National Guideline Clearinghouse (NGC) that was initiated by the AHRQ in 1998.
- Evidence-based practice centers (EPCs), created by the AHRQ in 1997, have had an important role in the conduct of research, development of systematic reviews, and formulation of evidence-based guidelines in selected practice areas.
- Translational research is an evolving concept that is defined by the NIH as the translation of basic scientific discoveries into practical applications.

REFERENCES

Agency for Healthcare Research and Quality (AHRQ). (2012a). *AHRQ tools and resources for better health care*. Retrieved from http://www.ahrq.gov/qual/tools/toolsria.htm.

Agency for Healthcare Research and Quality (AHRQ). (2012b). *Evidence-based practice centers: Synthesizing scientific evidence to improve quality and effectiveness in health care*. Retrieved from http://www.ahrq.gov/clinic/epc/.

Agency for Healthcare Research and Quality (AHRQ). (2012c). *National Quality Measures Clearinghouse (NQMC)*. Retrieved October 7, 2011, from http://qualitymeasures.ahrq.gov/.

American Nurses Credentialing Center (ANCC). (2012). *Magnet program overview*. Retrieved from http://www.nursecredentialing.org/Magnet/ProgramOverview.aspx.

Andrel, J. A., Keith, S. W., & Leiby, B. E. (2009). Meta-analysis: A brief introduction. *Clinical & Translational Science, 2*(5), 374–378.

Barnett-Page, E., & Thomas, J. (2009). Methods for the synthesis of qualitative research: A critical review. *BMC Medical Research Methodology, 9*, 59. DOI: 10.1186/147-2288-9-59.

Baumbusch, J. L., Kirkham, S. R., Khan, K. B., McDonald, H., Semeniuk, P., Tan, E., et al. (2008). Pursuing common agendas: A collaborative model for knowledge translation between research and practice in clinical settings. *Research in Nursing & Health, 31*(2), 130–140.

Benzies, K. M., Premji, S., Hayden, K. A., & Serrett, K. (2006). State-of-the-evidence reviews: Advantages and challenges of including grey literature. *Worldviews on Evidence-Based Nursing, 3*(2), 55–61.

Bettany-Saltikov, J. (2010a). Learning how to undertake a systematic review: Part 1. *Nursing Standard, 24*(50), 47–56.

Bettany-Saltikov, J. (2010b). Learning how to undertake a systematic review: Part 2. *Nursing Standard, 24*(51), 47–58.

Biswas, R., Umakanth, S., Strumberg, J., Martin, C. M., Hande, M., & Nagra, J. S. (2007). The process of evidence-based medicine and the search for meaning. *Journal of Evaluation in Clinical Practice, 13*(4), 529–532.

Bolton, L. B., Donaldson, N. E., Rutledge, D. N., Bennett, C., & Brown, D. S. (2007). The impact of nursing interventions: Overview of effective interventions, outcomes, measures, and priorities for future research. *Medical Care Research & Review, 64*(Suppl 2), 123S–143S.

Brown, S. J. (2009). *Evidence-based nursing: The research-practice connection*. Sudbury, MA: Jones & Bartlett Publishers.

Butler, K. D. (2011). Nurse practitioners and evidence-based nursing practice. *Clinical Scholars Review, 4*(1), 53–57.

Chesla, C. A. (2008). Translational research: Essential contributions from interpretive nursing science. *Research in Nursing & Health, 31*(4), 381–390.

Chobanian, A. V., Bakris, G. L., Black, H. R., Cushman, W. C., Green, L. A., Izzo, J. L., et al. (2003). The seventh report of the Joint National Committee on Prevention, Detection, Evaluation, and Treatment of high blood pressure: The JNC 7 report. *Journal of the American Medical Association, 289*(19), 2560–2572.

Cochrane Collaboration. (2012). *Cochrane reviews*. Retrieved from http://www.cochrane.org/cochrane-reviews.

Conn, V. S. (2010). Depressive symptom outcomes of physical activity interventions: Meta-analysis findings. *Annals of Behavioral Medicine, 39*(2), 128–138.

Conn, V. S., & Rantz, M. J. (2003). Research methods: Managing primary study quality in meta-analyses. *Research in Nursing & Health, 26*(4), 322–333.

Conn, V. S., Valentine, J. C., Cooper, H. M., & Rantz, M. J. (2003). Methods: Grey literature in meta-analyses. *Nursing Research, 52*(4), 256–261.

Craig, J. V., & Smyth, R. L. (2012). *The evidence-based practice manual for nurses* (3rd ed.). Edinburgh, UK: Churchill Livingstone.

Creswell, J. W. (2009). *Research design: Qualitative, quantitative, and mixed-methods approaches*. Los Angeles, CA: Sage.

Denieffe, S., & Gooney, M. (2011). A meta-synthesis of women's symptoms experience and breast cancer. *European Journal of Cancer Care, 20*(4), 424–435.

Doran, D. (2011). *Nursing sensitive outcomes: The state of the science* (2nd ed.). Sudbury, MA: Jones & Bartlett Learning.

Egger, M., Smith, G. D., Schneider, M., & Minder, C. (1997). Bias in meta-analysis detected by a simple graphical test. *British Medical Journal, 315*, 629–634.

Eizenberg, M. M. (2010). Implementation of evidence-based nursing practice: Nurses' personal and professional factors? *Journal of Advanced Nursing, 67*(1), 33–42.

Fernandez, R. S., & Tran, D. T. (2009). The meta-analysis graph: Clearing the haze. *Clinical Nurse Specialist, 23*(2), 57–60.

Finfgeld-Connett, D. (2010). Generalizability and transferability of meta-synthesis research findings. *Journal of Advanced Nursing, 66*(2), 246–254.

Gerrish, K., Guillaume, L., Kirshbaum, M., McDonnell, A., Tod, A., & Nolan, M. (2011). Factors influencing the contribution of advanced practice nurses to promoting evidence-based practice among front-line nurses: Findings from a cross-sectional survey. *Journal of Advanced Nursing, 67*(5), 1079–1090.

Goulding, L., Furze, G., & Birks, Y. (2010). Randomized controlled trials of interventions to change maladaptive illness beliefs in people with coronary heart disease: Systematic review. *Journal of Advanced Nursing, 66*(5), 946–961.

Harden, A., & Thomas, J. (2005). Methodological issues in combining diverse study types in systematic reviews. *International Journal of Social Research Methodology, 8*(3), 257–271.

Higgins, J. P. T., & Green, S. (2008). *Cochrane handbook for systematic reviews of interventions*. West Sussex, UK: Wiley-Blackwell & The Cochrane Collaboration.

Horstman, P., & Fanning, M. (2010). Tips for writing magnet evidence. *Journal of Nursing Administration, 40*(1), 4–6.

Institute of Medicine. (2001). *Crossing the quality chasm: A new health system for the 21st century*. Washington, DC: National Academy Press.

Joanna Briggs Institute. (2012). *Search the Joanna Briggs Institute*. Retrieved from http://www.joannabriggs.edu.au/Search.aspx.

Kent, B., & Fineout-Overholt, E. (2008). Using meta-synthesis to facilitate evidence-based practice. *Worldviews on Evidence-Based Nursing, 5*(3), 160–162.

Liberati, A., Altman, D. G., Tetzlaff, J., Mulrow, C., Gotzsche, P. C., Ioannidis, J. P., et al. (2009). The PRISMA Statement for reporting systematic reviews and meta-analyses of studies that evaluate healthcare interventions: Explanation and elaboration. *Annals of Internal Medicine, 151*(4), W-65-W-94.

Magnus, M. C., Ping, M., Shen, M. M., Bourgeois, J., & Magnus, J. H. (2011). Effectiveness of mammography screening in reducing breast cancer mortality in women aged 39-49 years: A meta-analysis. *Journal of Women's Health, 20*(6), 845–852.

Mantzoukas, S. (2009). The research evidence published in high impact nursing journals between 2000 and 2006: A quantitative content analysis. *International Journal of Nursing, 46*(4), 479–489.

Melnyk, B. M., & Fineout-Overholt, E. (2011). *Evidence-based practice in nursing & healthcare: A guide to best practice* (2nd ed.). Philadelphia, PA: Lippincott Williams & Wilkins.

Moher, D., Cook, D. J., Eastwook, S., Olkin, I., Rennie, D., & Stroup, E. F. (1999). Improving the quality of reports of meta-analyses of randomized controlled trials: The QUOROM statement. *The Lancet, 354*, 1896–1900.

Moher, D., Liberati, A., Tetzlaff, J., Altman, D. G., & PRISMA Group. (2009). *Preferred Reporting Items for Systematic Reviews and Meta-Analyses: The PRISMA Statement*. Retrieved from http://www.prisma-statement.org.

National Guideline Clearinghouse (NGC). (2012a). *National Guideline Clearinghouse: Guidelines by topics. Agency for Healthcare Research and Quality*. Retrieved from http://www.guideline.gov/browse/by-topic.aspx.

National Guideline Clearinghouse (NGC). (2012b). *National Guideline Clearinghouse: Home. Agency for Healthcare Research and Quality*. Retrieved from http://www.guideline.gov/.

National Institutes of Health (NIH). (2012). *NIH: National Center for Translational Science*. Bethesda, MD: Author. Retrieved from http://www.ncrr.nih.gov/clinical_research_resources/clinical_and_translational_science_awards/index.asp.

Noordzij, M., Hooft, L., Dekker, F. W., Zoccali, C., & Jager, K. J. (2009). Systematic reviews and meta-analyses: When they are useful and when to be careful. *Kidney International, 76*(11), 1130–1136.

Nurse Executive Center. (2005). *Evidence-based nursing practice: Instilling rigor into clinical practice*. Washington, DC: The Advisory Board Company.

Rew, L. (2011). The systematic review of literature: Synthesizing evidence for practice. *Journal for Specialists in Pediatric Nursing, 16*(1), 64–69.

Sackett, D. L., Straus, S. E., Richardson, W. S., Rosenberg, W., & Haynes, R. B. (2000). *Evidence-based medicine: How to practice & teach EBM* (2nd ed.). London, UK: Churchill Livingstone.

Sandelowski, M., & Barroso, J. (2007). *Handbook for synthesizing qualitative research*. New York, NY: Springer.

Shojania, K. G., Sampson, M., Ansari, M. T., Ji, J., Doucette, S., & Moher, D. (2007). How quickly do systematic reviews go out of date? Survival analysis. *Annals of Internal Medicine*, *147*(4), 224–234.

Stetler, C. B. (1994). Refinement of the Stetler/Marram model for application of research findings to practice. *Nursing Outlook*, *42*(1), 15–25.

Stetler, C. B. (2001). Updating the Stetler Model of Research Utilization to facilitate evidence-based practice. *Nursing Outlook*, *49*(6), 272–279.

Stetler, C. B., & Marram, G. (1976). Evaluating research findings for applicability in practice. *Nursing Outlook*, *24*(9), 559–563.

The Joint Commission. (2012). *About our standards*. Retrieved from http://www.jointcommission.org/standards_information/standards.aspx.

Titler, M. G. (2004). Overview of the U.S. invitational conference "Advancing Quality Care Through Translation Research." *Worldviews on Evidence-Based Nursing*, *1*(1), S1–S5.

Titler, M. G., Kleiber, C., Steelman, V. J., Rakel, B. A., Budreau, G., Everett, L. Q., et al. (1994). Research-based practice to promote the quality of care. *Nursing Research*, *43*(5), 307–313.

Titler, M. G., Kleiber, C., Steelman, V. J., Rakel, B. A., Budreau, G., Everett, L. Q., et al. (2001). The Iowa Model of Evidence-Based Practice to promote quality care. *Critical Care Nursing Clinics of North America*, *13*(4), 497–509.

Turlik, M. (2010). Evaluating the results of a systematic review/meta-analysis. *Podiatry Management*. Retrieved from www.podiatrym.com.

U.S. Department of Health and Human Services, National Institutes of Health, National Heart, Lung, and Blood Institute. (2003). *Reference card from the Seventh report of the Joint National Committee on Prevention, Detection, Evaluation, and Treatment of High Blood Pressure (JNC 7)*. Bethesda, MD: NIH Publication No. 03-5231. Retrieved from www.nhlbi.nih.gov/guidelines/hypertension/jnc7card.htm.

Walsh, D., & Downe, S. (2005). Meta-synthesis method for qualitative research: A literature review. *Journal of Advanced Nursing*, *50*(2), 204–211.

Whittemore, R., Melkus, G., Wagner, J., Dziura, J., Northrup, V., & Grey, M. (2009). Translating the diabetes prevention program to primary care: A pilot study. *Nursing Research*, *58*(1), 2–12.

Wulff, K., Cummings, G. G., Marck, P., & Yurtseven, O. (2011). Medication administration technologies and patient safety: A mixed-method systematic review. *Journal of Advanced Nursing*, *67*(10), 2080–2085.

20

Collecting and Managing Data

*e*volve http://evolve.elsevier.com/Grove/practice/

ata collection is one of the most exciting parts of research. After all the planning, writing, and negotiating, you should be eager and well prepared for this active part of research. The passion that comes from wanting to know the answer to your research question brings a sense of excitement and eagerness to start collecting your data. However, before you leap into data collection, you need to spend some time carefully planning this adventure and pilot test each step. Planning data collection begins with identifying all the data to be collected. The data to be collected are determined by the research questions, objectives, or hypotheses of the proposed study. As you develop the data collection plan, be sure that you gather all the data needed to answer the research questions, achieve the study objectives, or test the hypotheses. Chapter 16 includes detailed information about measurement, so the focus in this chapter is on the logistical and pragmatic aspects of quantitative data collection. Data collection strategies for qualitative studies are described in Chapter 12.

To start planning the data collection process, you need to determine the best mode by which the data can be collected. Factors that influence the plan to collect and enter data into a database for analysis include cost, time, the availability of assistance, and the need for consistency. The development of the data collection plan is followed by developing data collection forms and a codebook for data entry. Conducting a pilot test with a small group of subjects is the next recommended step. The pilot test may result in modifications of the plan, and then the actual data collection can begin. During data collection, various problems may arise. Potential situations are described in this chapter along with problem-solving strategies. The chapter concludes with the discussion of data entry and management.

Data Collection Modes

Data can be collected by interview (face-to-face or telephone); observations; focus groups; self-administered questionnaires (online or hard copy); or extraction from existing documents such as patient medical records, motor vehicle department accident records, or state birth records (Figure 20-1). Many factors need to be considered when a researcher is deciding on the mode for collecting data. Harwood and Hutchinson (2009) describe four factors that need to be part of your decision-making process: (1) purpose and complexity of the study, (2) availability of financial and physical resources, (3) characteristics of study participants and how best to gain access to them from the population, and (4) your skills and preferences as a researcher.

Researcher-Administered or Participant-Administered Instruments

If you need a subject's accurate blood pressure or height and weight, a self-report measure may be neither valid nor reliable for the purpose of your study. However, if the purpose of your study can be accomplished with a self-report survey method, you must decide whether the format will be researcher-administered or self-administered. It may be best for the researcher to administer self-report paper-and-pencil instruments if the potential subjects have minimal language or literacy ability, whereas it may be best to consider electronic data collection or medical record extraction if the subjects are likely to have hearing impairments, transportation problems, or physical difficulties.

If the researcher is administering the survey, will it be in person or by telephone? If self-administered, will

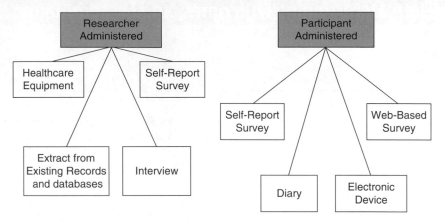

Figure 20-1 Data collection modes.

the participant complete a pencil-and-paper copy or an online electronic copy? Internet survey centers specialize in this mode of data collection and have expert help or tutorials for assessing the best mode for your study purpose. For example, in deciding on a telephone survey, how many times will you try to reach a potential subject before you give up, what days of the week or hours of the day will you call and how might that bias your sample or their responses, and how will you accurately determine the response rate (Harwood, 2009)? If you decide on a mailed paper-and-pencil survey, what will you do with undelivered or incomplete returns? Will you search for correct mailing addresses and try again? Will you send a reminder if the survey is not received within a particular time frame, and, if so, what time frame will you give a respondent, and how many reminders will you send (Harwood, 2009)?

Electronic Data Collection

When you are using an existing instrument, you may need permission to convert the questions into an online format, a special type of form that allows the data to be scanned into a database, or into an application for a phone or other electronic device. Each of these modes of data collection may require special hardware and software. Universities, schools of nursing, and funded researchers are purchasing these sometimes expensive products because the costs of acquiring the hardware and software are considerably less than the costs of entering data manually.

Scannable Forms

Other software allows the preparation of special data collection forms that rely on optical character recognition (OCR), which requires exact placement on the page for each potential response. To maintain the precise location of each response on print copies of these instruments, careful attention must be given to printing or copying these forms. The complete form is scanned, and the answers (data) are automatically recorded in a database. Additional features include data accuracy verification, selective data extraction and analysis, auditing and tracking, and flexible export interfaces. Figure 20-2 shows the scannable version of the Parents and Newborn Screening Survey developed by Patricia Newcomb, PhD, RN, CPNP, and Barbara True, MSN, CNS. Subjects completing the survey fill in the circle that corresponds to the appropriate option for each question.

Online Data Collection

Computer software packages developed by a variety of companies (e.g., Zoomerang and SurveyMonkey) enable researchers to provide an online copy of instruments and other data collection forms. These types of software programs have unique features that allow the researcher to develop point-and-click automated forms that can be distributed electronically. The following questions need to be considered with use of these programs. For an online survey, is it a secure site for the purposes of confidentiality and anonymity? How will you ensure that only eligible participants complete the survey? Will potential subjects receive a personalized email from you with a link to a website? How will you obtain the email addresses? Can you offer help if the subjects have any questions about your study?

Online services can be easy to use for both the researcher and study participants but may be costly and require specific assurances about confidentiality

Text continued on p. 513

ID | 1 | 0 | 6 | 1

Parents and Newborn Screening Survey
The University of Texas at Arlington College of Nursing
Andrews Women's Hospital

Instructions: Please use a BLACK PEN for completing the survey. Do not use pencil.

Please shade circles like this: ●
Not like this: ✗ ✓

---

1. My age is:

○ Less than 18   ○ 18-24   ○ 25-30   ○ 31-35   ○ 36+

2. My race/ethnic group is:

○ African-American   ○ Asian   ○ Caucasian   ○ Hispanic   ○ Other

3. My highest level of education is:

○ Less than high school   ○ High school diploma   ○ Some college   ○ Bachelor's degree   ○ Master's degree or more

4. I work in the healthcare field:

○ Yes   ○ No

5. I started pregnancy care:
○ In the first 3 months of my pregnancy
○ In the second 3 months of my pregnancy
○ In the last 3 months of my pregnancy
○ I did not get medical care during my pregnancy

6. My care for this pregnancy and birth was paid for by:
○ Medicaid
○ Private insurance
○ I paid for it by myself
○ I don't know how it will be paid for

7. I learned about newborn screening from (may circle more than one):
○ I never heard of newborn screening before this
○ My doctor or midwife
○ My child's doctor or nurse practitioner
○ A book, video, or brochure
○ My hospital nurse
○ My doctor's nurse
○ Internet
○ Friend or family member
○ Other

109
Parents and Newborn Screening Survey
08/22/2011

Please Turn Over
Page 1

0534001092

Figure 20-2 Scannable form: Parents and Newborn Screening Survey. (Developed by Patricia Newcomb, PhD, RN, CPNPN, and Barbara True, MSN, CNS; Teleform designed by Denise Cauble and Whitney Mildren, Graduate Research Assistants and PhD students, College of Nursing, The University of Texas at Arlington.) *Continued*

ID [ ][ ][ ][ ]

8. I have other children.

○ Yes   ○ No

9. I learned about newborn screening before this baby was born.

○ Yes   ○ No

10. The language I speak most of the time is:

○ English   ○ Spanish   ○ Other_____

Please put a check in the box that shows how much you agree or disagree with the statement.

	Strongly Agree	Agree	Not sure	Disagree	Strongly Disagree
11. I understand what I need to know about newborn screening.	○	○	○	○	○
12. I know when my baby should have another newborn screening.	○	○	○	○	○
13. If my baby has a disease that shows up on newborn screening, serious problems can be prevented if my baby gets treatment right away.	○	○	○	○	○
14. I will get the results of the newborn screening tests by mail.	○	○	○	○	○
15. My baby's doctor will get the results of the newborn screening tests by mail.	○	○	○	○	○
16. Doing the newborn screening is worth the discomfort the baby feels.	○	○	○	○	○
17. I know what genetic testing is.	○	○	○	○	○
18. I know where to take my baby for the second newborn screening test.	○	○	○	○	○
19. Newborn screening can identify babies with certain serious inherited diseases.	○	○	○	○	○
20. I understand what DNA does.	○	○	○	○	○
21. If my baby's newborn test is abnormal, my baby's father might have something wrong with his DNA.	○	○	○	○	○

109
Parents and Newborn Screening Survey
08/22/2011

Please Go To Next Page
Page 2

8572001092

Figure 20-2, cont'd

ID

Instructions: Please use a BLACK PEN for completing the survey. Do not use pencil.

	Strongly Agree	Agree	Not sure	Disagree	Strongly Disagree
22. All babies should have genetic testing when they are born.	O	O	O	O	O
23. If my baby's newborn test is abnormal, I might have something wrong in my DNA.	O	O	O	O	O
24. Newborn screening will test for some, but not all, serious diseases that run in families.	O	O	O	O	O
25. Babies with serious disorders may look healthy when they are born.	O	O	O	O	O
26. I am scared that the newborn test might find something wrong with my baby.	O	O	O	O	O
27. I know what newborn screening bloodspots are.	O	O	O	O	O
28. The state of Texas will keep my baby's bloodspots unless I mail them a form telling them not to.	O	O	O	O	O
29. I wish I had more information about newborn screening.	O	O	O	O	O
30. Some of the tests in the newborn screening are genetic tests.	O	O	O	O	O
31. There is DNA in my baby's blood spots.	O	O	O	O	O
32. It would be OK to use my baby's bloodspots for research to find treatments for serious diseases.	O	O	O	O	O
33. It is OK for the state to keep my baby's bloodspots for research without getting special permission from me.	O	O	O	O	O
34. It would be OK to keep my baby's DNA for future study if my baby's name or other private information is not connected to the DNA sample.	O	O	O	O	O

109
Parents and Newborn Screening Survey
08/22/2011

Please Turnover
Page 3

6735001091

Figure 20-2, cont'd

Continued

ID

Instructions: Please use a BLACK PEN for completing the survey. Do not use pencil.

Please shade circles like this: ●
Not like this: ✗ ✓

35. It would be OK with me for the state to share my baby's bloodspots with researchers all over the nation.	○	○	○	○	○
36. It would be OK to let the state share my baby's bloodspots with researchers if an ethics committee reviews the research first.	○	○	○	○	○
37. If future research is done on my baby's bloodspots I want to know.	○	○	○	○	○
38. I do not want the state or any other group to keep the bloodspots from my baby's testing for any reason.	○	○	○	○	○
39. I want my baby to have newborn screening.	○	○	○	○	○
40. My baby will have another newborn screening, but I do not really want it.	○	○	○	○	○

This is the End. Thank you!

Please share any comments that would help us improve the newborn screening process:

If you would like to learn more about newborn screening, please pick up some of our information about newborn screening at the desk or from your nurse when you leave today.

109
Parents and Newborn Screening Survey
08/22/2011

5991001094

Figure 20-2, cont'd

of data and anonymity of subjects. The National Institutes of Health (NIH) supports a secure Internet environment for building online data surveys and data management packages (Harris et al., 2009). This service, developed by experts at Vanderbilt University, is called REDCap (Research Electronic Data Capture) and may be available at your university research site (http://project-redcap.org/).

Im et al. (2007) conducted a survey in the United States of gender and ethnic differences in the experience of cancer pain. These researchers administered their questionnaire over the Internet and through a paper-and-pencil format based on subject preference. The following excerpt describes the data collection procedure for their study:

"To administer the Internet questionnaire, a Web site conforming to the Health Insurance Portability and Accountability Act standards, the System Administration, Networking, and Security Institute Federal Bureaus of Investigation recommendations, and the Institutional Review Board [IRB] policy of the institution where the researchers were affiliated was developed and published on an independent, dedicated Web site server. When potential participants visited the project Web site, informed consent was obtained by asking them to click a button labeled *I agree to participate*. After this, questions on specific diagnoses, cancer therapies, and medications were asked, and the appropriateness of answers was checked automatically through a server-side program; participants were connected automatically to the Internet survey web page if the answers were appropriate.

"Upon request, pen-and-pencil questionnaires were provided by mail to the community consultants, who distributed the questionnaires in person only to those who were identified as cancer patients. These questionnaires accompanied hard copies of the same informed consent form included in the Internet format of the questionnaire, and the pen-and-pencil questionnaire included a sentence 'Filling out this questionnaire means that you are aged over 18 years old and giving your consent to participate in this survey.' After the self-administered questionnaires were completed, community consultants retrieved all except five (these were mailed directly to the research team by the participants) in person at the community settings and mailed them to the research team. Supplementing pen-and-pencil questionnaires was essential to recruit the target number of ethnic minority cancer patients across the nation who did not have access to the Internet but were interested in participating in the study. Among the 276 participants who were recruited through community settings, 246 ... used the pen-and-pencil questionnaires. ... There were no statistically significant differences in psychometric properties between the Internet format and the pen-and-pencil format of the questionnaire. ... It took an average of 30-40 minutes for the participants to complete either the Internet format or the pen-and-pencil format of the questionnaire." (Im et al., 2007, pp. 299-300)

Im et al. (2007) maximized their sample size and obtained a more representative sample by giving participants an option to complete their questionnaire on the Internet or using paper-and-pencil format. The researchers took steps to ensure that the data collected by the two formats were comparable by testing for significant differences and finding none. The time to complete the Internet and paper-and-pencil questionnaires did not vary. Im et al. (2007) also ensured that an ethical study was conducted and subjects' rights were protected.

The additional advantage of Internet data collection is that responses can be time/date stamped. For example, if subjects are instructed to complete the questionnaire before bedtime, the time can be verified. If subjects are instructed to complete a daily diary, date of entry would be documented, and subjects would be discouraged from entering all diary days on the last day just before returning the diary to the researcher (Fukuoka, Kamitani, Dracup, & Jong, 2011).

Computer-Based Data Collection

With the advent of laptop and tablet computers, data collectors can code data directly into an electronic file at the data collection site. If a computer is used for data collection, a program must be written for entering, cleaning, and storing data. A computer enables users to collect large amounts of data with few errors that can be readily analyzed with a variety of statistical software packages. In addition to researchers using technology at the point of data collection to record data, technology has made it possible to interface physiological monitoring systems with computers for data collection. An advantage of using computers for the acquisition and storage of physiological data is the increased accuracy and precision that can be achieved by reducing errors associated with manually recording or transcribing physiological data from a monitor. Another advantage is that more data points can be recorded electronically than could be recorded manually. Computers linked to physiological monitoring systems can store multiple data for multiple indicators, such as blood pressures, oxygen saturation levels, and sleep stages. Because data can be electronically recorded, data collection is less labor intensive, and the data are ready to analyze more quickly. The initial cost of equipment may be high, but it is reasonable when the cost of hiring and training human data collectors is considered.

There are some concerns with the use of computerized data acquisition systems, but physiological data are usually best gathered and stored directly into a computer database to ensure accurate, complete data collection. Physiological data typically require large computer storage space. The computer-equipment interface may require more space in an already crowded clinical setting; when possible, existing equipment should be used to collect data. Purchasing the equipment, setting it up, and installing the software can be time-consuming and expensive at the start of your project. Thus, initial studies usually require substantial funding. Another concern is that the nurse researcher may focus on the machine and technology and neglect observing and interacting with the subject.

The most serious disadvantage of computerized data collection is the possibility of measurement error that can occur with equipment malfunctions and software errors. Regular maintenance and calibrations, or reliability checks of the equipment and software, reduce this problem. The benefits of collecting repeated measures over time may outweigh the risk of missing data because of poor compliance. For example, collecting continuous rectal temperature data from a subject is easier and less burdensome than asking the subject to measure an oral temperature every 1 to 2 hours.

Savian, Paratz, and Davies (2006) conducted a single-blind randomized, crossover study with 14 mechanically ventilated intensive care unit patients.

"[The purpose of the study was to determine the effectiveness of] manual hyperinflation (MHI) and ventilator hyperinflation (VHI) on respiratory mechanics (static compliance [C_{st}]), oxygenation (arterial oxygen tension [PaO_2]/fraction of inspired oxygen [FIO_2] ratio), and secretion removal (wet weight of sputum and peak expiratory flow rate [PEFR]) at different levels of PEEP [positive end-expiratory pressure] ... a secondary aim was to investigate the hemodynamics heart rate [HR], mean arterial pressure [MAP] and metabolic response (carbon dioxide output [VCO_2]) during MHI and VHI." (Savian et al., 2006, p. 335)

The computerized systems used to collect and record data in the study by Savian et al. (2006) are detailed in the following excerpt:

"PEFR and CO_2 [carbon dioxide] production were measured using a flow and CO_2 sensor connected to the patient's airways and to the CO_2SMO [carbon dioxide] respiratory mechanics monitor (CO_2SMO Plus Model 8000, Novametrix Medical Systems Inc., Wallingford, CT). All information from the CO_2SMO monitor was simultaneously recorded in the Analysis Plus computer program.

"Static lung compliance was recorded by the static measures function device on the Bennett 7200 ventilator where a plateau pressure was obtained by including an inspiratory pause of 2 seconds into the mandatory breath. ...

"PaO_2/FIO_2 ratio was calculated from arterial blood samples taken immediately before and immediately after MHI and VHI. Four milliliters of arterial blood were drawn into a syringe containing heparin and analyzed by a blood gas machine (Bayer Australian Limited 865, Pymble, NSW, CAN 000128714). This procedure was standardized across subjects.

"HR and MAP were read directly from the monitoring system (Merlin pressure module M1006A Hewlett Packard, Palo Alto, CA) and recorded every minute before, during, and for 5 minutes after MHI and VHI." (Savian et al., 2006, p. 336)

The use of computerized data collection by Savian et al. (2006) enabled them to collect repeated measures on several physiological variables in an accurate and precise way. The data were collected by sensors and stored in the computer to reduce error and facilitate data analysis.

Phones and Other Electronic Devices

Software applications for mobile phones have evolved from personal digital assistants (PDAs) that allow the researcher to collect and download data directly into the computer from observations as they occur. Healthcare providers load applications that facilitate accurate assessment, diagnosis, and pharmacological and nonpharmacological management of patients. PDAs are also used to store deidentified data from office computers in a form that is easily transportable. PDA software is currently available that may help nurse practitioners collect data for research. Multiple nurse practitioners involved in a research project could forward data electronically from PDAs to a central research site for analysis. Encrypted electronic devices are needed to protect the confidentiality of data during transmission. These electronic devices can be misplaced or stolen, threatening confidentiality. Researchers need to protect the data with a security code to ensure that no one but themselves can access data in these formats.

Mobile phones and computers are becoming more similar with the increased sophistication of applications for mobile phones. Some of these applications can be used to collect various data. Other electronic devices include pill containers that record when pills are accessed and watches with timers to remind participants to take certain health-related actions. However, the use of these devices for research may require considerable preparation. You may need to hire programmers with the needed expertise, and you may need to purchase, rent, or borrow the needed number of devices or monitors.

Factors Influencing Data Collection

When planning data collection, cost, time, the availability of assistance, and the need for consistency are critical factors to consider. The researcher balances these factors with the need to maintain the reliability and validity of the study in the development of the data collection plan.

Cost Factors

Cost is a major consideration when planning a study. Measurement tools, such as continuous electrocardiogram monitors (Holter monitor), wrist activity monitors (accelerometers), spirometers, pulse oximeters, or glucometers, used in physiological studies may need to be rented, purchased, or loaned from the manufacturer or other company. You may need to pay a fee to use instruments or questionnaires. Some instruments and questionnaires are available only if a copy is purchased for each participant. Data collection forms may need to be formatted or developed for electronic use. In some cases, printing costs for materials such as teaching materials or questionnaires that will be used during the study must be considered. Providing the required copy of the signed consent form doubles the expense of consent forms. Small payments to participants in the form of cash or gift cards should be considered as compensation for a subject's time and effort in providing the data. Sometimes childcare may need to be provided for parents and other caregivers who

would not otherwise be able to participate in your study. In some studies, postage is an additional expense. There may be costs involved in coding the data for entry into the computer and for conducting data analyses. Consultation with a statistician early in the development of a research project and during data analysis must also be budgeted. You may need to hire someone who can remain blinded for data entry or analysis or someone who can type the final report, develop graphics or presentations, or type and edit manuscripts for publication.

In addition to the above-described direct costs of a research project, there are costs associated with the researcher's time and travel to and from the study site. You also must estimate the expense of presenting the research findings at conferences and include those expenses in the budget. To prevent unexpected expenses from delaying the study, examine all costs in an organized manner. A budget is best developed early in the planning process and revised as plans are modified. Seeking funding for at least part of the study costs can facilitate the conduct of a study.

Time Factors

Researchers often underestimate the time required for participants to complete data collection forms and for the research team to recruit and enroll subjects for a study. The first aspect of time—the participant's time commitment—must be determined early in the process because the time needed for participant involvement must be included in the informed consent process and document. While conducting your pilot study, make note of the time required to collect data from a subject. You may need to revise your timeline and consent form to reflect the expected time commitment accurately.

The second aspect of time—the time needed to complete data collection—is especially challenging to predict because events during the data collection period sometimes are not under the researcher's control. For example, a sudden heavy staff workload may make data collection temporarily difficult or impossible, or the number of potential subjects might be reduced for a period. In some situations, researchers must obtain permission from each subject's physician before they are permitted to collect data on that subject. Activities required for this stipulation, such as contacting physicians, explaining the study, and obtaining permission, require extensive time. In some cases, potential subjects are lost before the researcher can obtain the mandatory permission, extending the time required to obtain the necessary number of subjects.

How long will it take to identify potential subjects, explain the study, and obtain consent? How much time will be needed for activities such as completing questionnaires or obtaining physiological measures? Novice researchers have difficulty making reasonable estimates of time and costs related to a study. Validating the time and cost estimates with an experienced researcher can be very informative. Experienced researchers know the challenges of data collection and have learned that data collection may take two to three times longer than predicted. If the cost and time factors are prohibitive, you may need to simplify your study so that fewer variables are measured, fewer instruments are used, or fewer subjects are needed. Make the design less complex, and use fewer data collectors. A blinded intervention study involves more research staff and is generally not feasible for a novice researcher. These are serious modifications, however, with implications for the validity of the findings, so you and your team should thoroughly examine the consequences before making such revisions. If preliminary time or cost estimates go beyond expectations, you can revise the time schedules and budget with new projections for completing the study.

Consistency

Consistency in data collection across subjects is critical. What time of year will data be collected? For example, if you collect data during holiday seasons, data about sleeping, eating, or exercising may vary. Pediatric patients with asthma may experience more symptoms during the winter months than during summer. Planning data collection for a study of symptom management with this population would need to take this possibility into consideration.

The specific days and hours of data collection may influence the consistency of the data collected and must be carefully considered. For example, the energy level and state of mind of subjects from whom data are gathered in the morning may differ from that of subjects from whom data are gathered in the evening. With hospitalized study participants, visitors are more likely to be present at certain times of day and may interfere with data collection or influence participant responses. Patient care routines vary with the time of day. In some studies, the care recently received or the care currently being provided may alter the data you gather. The subjects you approach on Saturday to participate in the study may differ from the subjects you approach on weekday mornings. Subjects seeking care on Saturday may have a full-time job, whereas subjects seeking care on weekday mornings may be either unemployed or too ill to work.

Who will collect the data? If you decide to use data collectors, they must be trained in responsible conduct of research and issues of informed consent, ethics, and confidentiality and anonymity (see Chapter 9). They must be informed about the research project, familiar with the instruments to be used, and have equivalent training in the data collection process. In addition to training, data collectors need written guidelines or protocols that indicate which instruments to use, the order in which to introduce the instruments, how to administer the instruments, and a time frame for the data collection process (Harwood, 2009; Kang, Davis, Habermann, Rice, & Broome, 2005).

If more than one person is collecting the data, consistency among data collectors (interrater reliability) must be ensured through testing (see Chapter 16). The training needs to continue until interrater reliability estimates are at least 85% to 90% agreement between the expert and the trainee or trainees. Waltz, Strickland, and Lenz (2010) suggest that a minimum of 10% of the data needs to be compared across raters before interrater reliability can be adequately reported. The trained data collector's interrater reliability with the expert trainer should be assessed intermittently throughout data collection to ensure consistency from the first to the last participant in the study. Data collectors also must be encouraged to identify and record any problems or variations in the environment that affect the data collection process. The description of the training of the data collectors is usually reported in the methods section of an article so that others can assess the data collection process (Harwood & Hutchinson, 2009).

Availability of Assistance

Who is going to help you with the study? If you are a student, will your mentor or supervising faculty member participate? Does your mentor or supervising faculty member have research assistants who could assist in your study? Will nurses, physicians, and other health professionals assist with recruitment? Do they have time to do this? Are they willing to help?

Will the researcher collect all the data, or will data collectors be employed for this purpose? Can data collectors be nurses working in the area? Data collection may be delayed when nurses providing patient care are also expected to be data collectors. Even when a nurse agrees to help you with subject recruitment or data collection, patient care takes priority over data collection and increases the risk for missing data or missing the opportunity to enroll eligible subjects.

If clinicians are going to recruit subjects or collect data, the clinicians need to complete training for protection of human subjects during research. An IRB requires documentation of this training for each person involved in recruitment and data collection. If you are going to be doing all the data collection yourself, will you be available every day of the week? What hours will you be available? If others will be involved in collecting data, allow time for training on data collection procedures. You need to be available by telephone or other means for questions and emergencies when others are collecting data for your study. Keeping these factors in mind, you are now ready to plan the data collection process for your study.

Data Collection and Coding Plan

The factors of cost, time, availability of assistance, and need for consistency shape the data collection plan that you develop. A data collection plan details how you will implement your study. The plan for collecting data is specific to the study being conducted and requires that you consider some common elements of research. You need to map out procedures you will use to collect data, anticipate the time and cost of data collection, develop data collection forms that ease data entry, and prepare a codebook that will help you to code the variables to be entered in a database. This extensive planning increases the accuracy of the data collected and the validity of the study findings. The validity and strength of the findings from several carefully planned studies increase the quality of the research evidence that is then available for implementing into clinical practice (Melnyk & Fineout-Overholt, 2010).

Identifying data include variables such as patient record number, home address, and date of birth (see Chapter 9). Avoid collecting these data unless they are essential to answer the research question. For example, collect a patient's age instead of date of birth. Review regulations by the Health Insurance Portability and Accountability Act about the participant's private health information (www.hhs.gov/ocr/hipaa).

The methodology of a study may include contacting subjects later for additional data collection. In this case, you will need to obtain the subject's address and telephone number and protect the information appropriately. Names and phone numbers of family members or friends may also be useful if subjects are likely to move or may be difficult to contact. This information can be obtained only with subjects' permission as part of their informed consent. Consider the importance of each piece of data and the subject's time required to collect it. If the data can be obtained from patient records or any other written sources, you do not need to ask the subject to provide this information. To collect data from a patient's records, make sure to include permission to do this in the consent form, and ensure that the IRB has authorized your team to do this.

Data Collection Forms

Before data collection begins, you may need to develop or modify forms on which to record data. These forms can be used to record demographic data, information from the patient record, observations, or values from physiological measures. The demographic variables commonly collected in nursing studies include age, gender, race, education, income, employment status, diagnosis, and marital status. You may want to collect additional demographic data if researchers have identified participant characteristics that affect the study variables. You also might need to collect other data that may be extraneous or confounding variables, such as the subject's physician, stage of illness, length of illness or hospitalization, complications, date of data collection, time of day and day of week of data collection, and any untoward events that occur during the data collection period. If there are only women in your sample, the subject's age and reproductive status, parity, and number of children in the home may be confounding variables. In a study of patients with ventilator-associated pneumonia, the researcher needs to record the length of time between when the patient was intubated and when ventilator-associated pneumonia was diagnosed. The researcher for this study also needs to record whether the patient had a preexisting pulmonary disease.

Data collection forms must be designed so that the data are easily recorded, coded, and entered into the computer. You need to decide whether data will be collected in raw form or coded at the time of collection. Coding in quantitative studies is the process of transforming data into numerical symbols that can be entered easily into the computer. For example, variables such as race, gender, ethnicity, and diagnoses can be categorized and given numerical labels. For gender, the male category could be identified by a "1" and the female category by a "2." You may also want to include an "other" category (coded "3") for participants who are transgendered or transsexual. To be able to compare your sample with samples in federally funded studies, you may need to separate the questions about ethnicity and race. In 2003, the Office of Management and Budget of the U.S. government directed researchers and others collecting data for federal purposes or at federal expense to separate the questions of race and ethnicity (Office of Minority Health,

2010). At the same time, the Office of Management and Budget specified the categories for each. The following questions are correct according to these federal guidelines. How would a subject who is biracial or multiracial complete the form? You may want to word the question to ask the participant's primary race or allow multiple responses.

Ethnicity
(1) Hispanic or Latino
(2) Non-Hispanic or Latino

Race
(1) American Indian or Alaskan Native
(2) Asian
(3) Black or African American
(4) Native Hawaiian or Other Pacific Islander
(5) White

The coding categories developed for a study not only must be mutually exclusive but also exhaustive, which means that the value for a specific variable fits into only one category, and each observation must fit into a category. For example, a subject is highly unlikely to want to reveal his or her exact income but would be more willing to indicate that the income is in a particular range. The income ranges would not be mutually exclusive or exhaustive if they were categorized in the following way on a demographic questionnaire:

Income range (please check the range that most accurately reflects your income)
____ (1) $30,000 to $40,000
____ (2) $40,000 to $50,000
____ (3) $50,000 to $59,000
____ (4) $60,000 to $70,000
____ (5) $70,000 or more

These categories are not exclusive because they overlap, and a subject with a $40,000 income could mark category 1 or category 2 or both. The categories are not exhaustive because a subject may have an income of either $25,000 or $59,500, yet the questionnaire does not contain categories that include each of these incomes. How much detail do you need on income? Do you want to know if the participant's household income is below poverty level? To determine poverty level, you must know not only the household income but also how many people live in the household and compare this information with federal poverty guidelines (http://aspe.hhs.gov/poverty/09poverty.shtml).

The following income ranges are both exclusive and exhaustive and would be appropriate for collecting demographic data from subjects:

Income range (please check the range that most accurately reflects your family's income for a year, before taxes)

____ (1) Less than $30,000
____ (2) $30,000 to $49,999
____ (3) $50,000 to $69,999
____ (4) $70,000 or greater

Data collection forms offer many response styles. The person completing the form (subject or data collector) might be asked to check a blank space before or after the words "male," "female," or "other" or to circle one of the words. If code numbers or variable name codes are used, the meaning of the codes should be clearly indicated on the collection forms so that the individual completing the form understands them and is not confused or misled by the code. Developing a codebook for your data collection forms and data entry is discussed later.

Placement of the data on the forms is important because careful placement makes it easier for subjects to complete the form without missing an item and for data entry staff to locate responses for computer entry. Placement of blanks on the left side of the page seems to be most efficient for data entry, but this layout may prove problematic when subjects are completing the forms. The least effective arrangement is when the data are positioned irregularly on the form because the risk of data being missed during data entry is high. Subjects' names should not be on the data collection forms; only the subject's identification number should appear. The researcher may keep a master list of subjects and their code numbers, which is stored in a separate location and either encrypted in an electronic file or data repository or locked in a file drawer to ensure the subjects' privacy. Often this master list of subjects and codes is kept with the subjects' consent forms in a locked file drawer. This master list is required if collecting data later or recontacting the subject is a necessary component of your study.

You should always organize your data collection forms and instruments to begin with less personal types of questions about age and education before delving into more personal questions about contraceptives or feelings and attitudes. Also, you would not want to save your most important items for the last page of the questionnaire and risk missing data if a participant becomes too fatigued or bored to finish the questions. Different types of questions require more or less time to complete, a factor that needs to be considered. Also, questions may ask for a response related to different time frames. For example, if one questionnaire asks about the past week and two other questionnaires ask about the past month, these should be organized so that the subject is not confused by going back and forth between time frames. If you have several instruments or forms, you may want to put them together in a booklet to minimize the likelihood that a questionnaire or form will be missed.

Figure 20-3 provides a sample data collection form. It includes four items that could be problematic for coding, data analysis, or both. The blank used to enter "Surgical Procedure Performed" would lead to problems when it is time to enter the data into a computerized data set. Because multiple surgical procedures could have been performed, developing codes for the various surgical procedures would be difficult and time-consuming. In addition, different words might be used to record the same surgical procedure. It may be necessary to tally the surgical procedures manually. Unless this degree of specification of procedures is important to the study, an alternative would be to develop larger categories of procedures before data collection and place the categories on the data collection form. A category of "Other" might be useful for less commonly performed surgical procedures. This method would require the data collector to make a judgment regarding which category was appropriate for a particular surgical procedure. Another option would be to write in the category code number for a particular surgical procedure after the data collection form is completed but before data entry. If the specific surgical procedure is important to your study, you may want to record the code the facility uses to bill for the procedure. Similar problems occur with the items "Narcotics Ordered after Surgery" and "Narcotic Administration." Unless these data are to be used in statistical analyses, it might be better to categorize this information manually for descriptive purposes. If these items are needed for planned statistical procedures, use care to develop appropriate coding. You may need detailed information if you want to know the appropriateness of the narcotic doses given. The researcher might be interested in determining differences in the amount of narcotics administered in a given period in relation to weight and height. For blinded studies, you do not want to record the treatment group assignments on the data collection form. Placing the treatment group code on the data collection form would be problematic because the information is no longer blinded and could influence the data recorded by the data collectors.

Data Collection Detailed Plan

To ensure consistency in the data collection process, you need to develop a detailed plan. Envision the overall activities that will be occurring during data collection. Write each step and develop the forms, training, and equipment needed for that step. Focus on who, what, when, where, why, and how. How will you

---

DATA COLLECTION FORM

Demographics
____Subject Identification Number
____Age
____Gender
  1. Male
  2. Female
____Weight (in pounds)
____Height (in inches)
_____Surgical Procedure Performed
__/__/__Surgery Date (Month/Day/Year)
__/__/__Surgery Time (Hour/Minute/AM or PM)
Narcotics Ordered After Surgery_____

_____

Narcotic Administration
  Date   Time   Narcotic   Dose
1.
2.
3.
4.
5.
Instruction on Use of Pain Scale
__/__/__Date (Month/Day/Year)
__/__/__Time (Hour/Minute/AM or PM)
Comments:

    __Treatment Group
    1. TENS
    2. Placebo-TENS
    3. No-Treatment Control

Treatment Implemented
__/__/__Date (Month/Day/Year)
__/__/__Time (Hour/Minute/AM or PM)
Comments:

Dressing Change
__/__/__Date (Month/Day/Year)
__/__/__Time (Hour/Minute/AM or PM)
_____Hours since surgery
Comments:

Measurement of Pain
_____Score on Visual Analogue Pain Scale
__/__/__Date Pain Measured
    (Month/Day/Year)
__/__/__Time Pain Measured
    (Hour/Minute/AM or PM)
_____Hours since surgery
Comments:

    _____Data Collector Code
Comments:

Figure 20-3 **Data collection form.**

recruit subjects? At what point is a subject assigned to a group? It is optimal to assign subjects randomly to an intervention group or control group after baseline data are collected but before introducing the intervention. In this way, all subjects demonstrate the ability to complete the questions and measures and have the opportunity to decline further participation before group assignment. When and how will you implement the intervention? Will data be collected from more than one subject at a time, or is it necessary to focus attention on one subject at a time? How much time is needed to collect data from each subject? The length of time per subject is determined by study design, setting, and available space. In addition, if you plan for three subjects in the morning and three in the afternoon, what are the contingencies for subjects who arrive late or need additional time? Some subjects may be available only during their lunch break or in the evening.

You might develop a data collection flow diagram to illustrate the process for collecting data in your study. An example is shown in Figure 20-4. The Consolidated Standards of Reporting Trials (CONSORT) guidelines for reporting randomized trials in publications (Bennett, 2006) would also be very useful for depicting the design and flow of your data collection process and expected enrollment numbers, expected attrition rates, and final sample sizes for each group (see Chapter 19).

Decision Points

Decision points that occur during data collection must be identified, and all options must be considered. One decision may pertain to whether too few potential subjects are meeting the sampling inclusion criteria. Will you review study progress every week or every month? If too few subjects from your potential pool are eligible, at what point will you consider changing exclusion criteria? For example, if you are recruiting only first-time mothers older than 30 years of age, and you are turning away willing participants because they are too young, you and your research team need to reconsider the rationale for that criterion and perhaps decide either to lower the age range or to seek different recruitment sites.

Other decisions include whether the subject understands the information needed to give informed consent, whether the subject comprehends instructions related to providing data, and whether the subject has provided all the data needed. As you look through the completed data forms, are all responses completed? If the subject skips a page, you will need to return that page to the subject for completion. If the question about income is not completed, how will you handle

that missing response? Your data collection flow chart should indicate how much missing data will be allowed per subject. At what point will you decide to exclude a participant from your study?

Developing a Codebook for Data Definitions

We advise that you develop your codebook before initiating data collection or during the pilot study. A codebook identifies and defines each variable in your study and includes an abbreviated variable name (*income*), a descriptive variable label (*gross household annual income*), and the range of possible numerical values for every variable entered in a computer file (*0 = none; 1 = <$30,000; 6 = >$100,000*). Some codebooks also identify the source of each datum, linking your codebook with your data collection forms and scales. The codebook keeps you in control and provides a safety net for when you access the data later. Some computer programs, such as SPSS for Windows, allow you to print out your data definitions after setting up a database. Figure 20-5 is an example of data definitions from SPSS for Windows. Another example of coding is presented in Figure 20-6.

Developing a logical method of abbreviating variable names can be challenging. For example, you might use a quality-of-life (QOL) questionnaire in your study. It will be necessary for you to develop an abbreviated variable name for each item in the questionnaire. For example, the fourth item on a QOL questionnaire might be given the abbreviated variable name *QOL4*. A question asking the last time a home health nurse visited might be abbreviated *HHN Lstvisit*. Although abbreviated variable names usually seem logical at the time the name is created, it is easy to confuse or forget these names unless they are clearly documented with a variable label.

During the piloting phase of your research with the first few pilot subjects, you can easily refine your variable names and labels and request your research team or a statistician to review the variables. This practice encourages you to identify places in your forms that might prove to be a problem during data entry because of lack of clarity. Also, you may find that a single question contains not one but five variables. For example, an item might ask whether the subject received support from her or his mother, father, sister, brother, or other relatives and ask the subject to circle the number that represents those who provided support. You might think that you could code mother as "1," father as "2," sister as "3," brother as "4," and other as "5." However, because the individual can circle more than one, each relative must be coded separately. Thus, mother is one variable and would be a

ENROLLMENT AND SURVEY ADMINISTRATION PROCEDURES

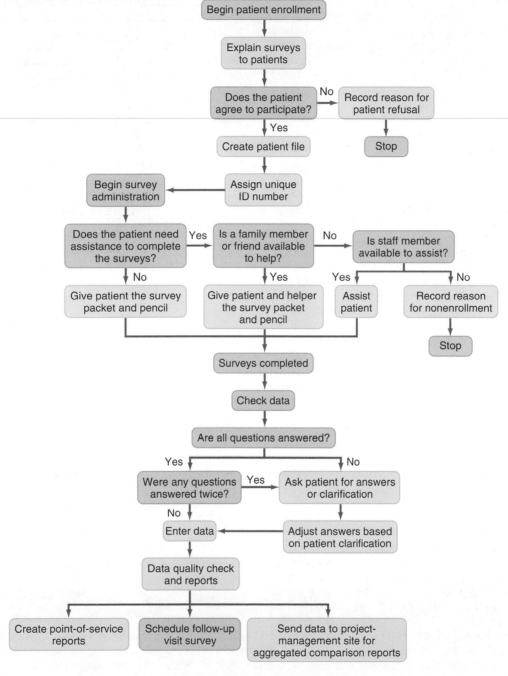

Figure 20-4 Data collection flow chart.

Q1		Value
Standard Attributes	Position	2
	Label	I was motivated to migrate from my country because my pay was too low.
	Type	Numeric
	Format	F8
	Measurement	Ordinal
	Role	Input
Valid Values	1	Strongly Disagree
	2	Disagree
	3	Neutral
	4	Agree
	5	Strongly Agree
Missing Values	System	

Q 39		Value
Standard Attributes	Position	40
	Label	What is your gender?
	Type	Numeric
	Format	F8
	Measurement	Nominal
	Role	Input
Valid Values	1	Male
	2	Female
Missing Values	System	

Q50		Value
Standard Attributes	Position	54
	Label	Which of the following best describes your current employment situation?
	Type	Numeric
	Format	F8
	Measurement	Nominal
	Role	Input
Valid Values	1	Employed and working full time
	2	Employed and working part time
	3	Employed, currently on leave
	4	Self-Employed
	5	Unemployed
	6	Other
Missing Values	System	

Figure 20-5 Example of data definitions from SPSS for Windows. (Source: Nurse International Relocation Questionnaire 2 [Gray & Johnson, 2009].)

Variable Name	Variable Label	Source	Value Levels	Valid Range	Missing Data	Comments
A1 to A5	Family Apgar	Q2Family Apgar	1=never 2=hardly ever 3=some of the time 4=almost always 5=always	1 – 5	9	Code as is (CAI)
MF3	Mother's feeling, Day 3	Tuesday diary, mother	1=poor 6=good	1 – 6	9	Code 1 to 6 left to right

Figure 20-6 Example of coding.

dichotomized value, coded "1" if circled and "0" if not circled. The father would be coded similarly as a second dichotomous variable, and so on. Identifying these items before data collection may allow you to restructure the item on the questionnaire or data collection form to simplify computer entry.

Give the codebook with its data definitions to the individual or individuals who will enter your data into the computer *before initiating data collection*. Decision rules for data entry should also be finalized. For example, if a subject selects two responses for a single item, will the variable be coded as missing, or does convention dictate that the lowest or highest value should be entered? Individuals who are entering data need to have clarity on the distinctions between coding a missing value or nonapplicable value as blank rather than entering a "0" value.

In addition, provide the following information to the person entering the data:

- Dates for data collection initiation and completion
- Estimated number of subjects to be included in the study and how often batches of subjects' data will be entered
- Plan for documenting refusal rate, sample size, and attrition during the study
- Copies of all scales, questionnaires, and data collection forms to be used in the study
- Location of every variable on scales, questionnaires, or data collection forms
- Statistical package to be used for analysis of the data
- Statistical analyses to be conducted to describe the sample and to address the research purpose and the objectives, questions, or hypotheses
- Contact information for the statistician or project director who is available to consult about data entry questions or data analysis
- Computer directory location of the database in which the data will be entered and copied for backup
- Timeline for receiving the data—for example, whether you will deliver the data in batches or wait until all the data have been gathered before delivering it

With this information, the assistant can develop the database in preparation for receiving the data. The time needed to prepare the database varies depending on the number of variables and the complexity of the response categories. Approximate dates for completion of the data entry, analyses, or both must be negotiated before beginning data collection. If you have a deadline for completing the study or presenting your results, you should share this information with the people performing data entry and analysis.

Pilot Study

Completing a pilot study may save you difficulty later when you implement the final steps of the research process. Pilot testing helps you to identify problems you might encounter while collecting data and helps you develop strategies for addressing potential problems. Chapter 3 provides reasons to conduct a pilot study. Following approval of the study by your IRB, use your research plan to recruit three to five subjects who meet your eligibility criteria. Use the data collection methods that you have selected and prepared. Pay attention to how long it takes to recruit a subject, obtain informed consent, and collect the data. Ask the participant to identify questions or aspects of the process that were unclear or confusing. Based on the pilot study and feedback of the first subjects, modify your data collection forms and methods of data collection to ensure the feasibility, validity, and reliability of the study.

Collecting Data

Data collection is the process of selecting subjects and gathering data from these subjects. The actual steps of collecting the data are specific to each study and depend on the research design and measurement methods. Data may be collected on subjects by observing, testing, measuring, questioning, recording, or any combination of these methods. The researcher is actively involved in this process either by collecting data or by supervising data collectors. You will apply ethical principles, people-management strategies, and problem-solving skills constantly as data collection tasks are implemented. Even after pilot testing, snags in the research plan can occur, and support systems are needed for data collectors who encounter situations in the home or clinic that require reporting to legal authorities. For example, during a home visit, a data collector may find that family members are neglecting a subject in the study who cannot get out of bed. Frequent interactions with data collectors on your team are also essential for assessing any minor or major risks and reporting adverse effects to your IRB.

Data Collection Tasks

In both quantitative and qualitative research, the investigator performs four tasks during the process of data collection. These tasks are interrelated and occur concurrently rather than in sequence. The tasks are (1) selecting subjects, (2) collecting data in a consistent way, (3) maintaining research controls as indicated in the study design, and (4) solving problems that threaten to disrupt the study. Selecting subjects is discussed in Chapter 15. Collecting data may involve administering Internet or paper-and-pencil scales; asking subjects to complete data collection forms in person or online; or recording data from observations, patient medical records, or monitoring equipment (Chapters 16 and 17 provide information on measurement strategies). Data collection tasks for qualitative studies are discussed in more detail in Chapter 12.

Maintaining Control

Maintaining control and consistency of the design and methods during subject selection and data collection protects the integrity or validity of the study. Researchers build controls into the design to minimize the influence of intervening forces on the study findings. Maintenance of these controls is essential. For example, a study to describe the changes in sleep stages during puberty may require controlling the environment of the bedroom to such an extent that a sleep laboratory is the only setting in which integrity can be maintained. Control is not always realistic in a natural field setting, and, in some cases, these controls can fail without the researcher realizing it. Often the researcher must opt for a randomized controlled study to address potential control failures so that they are equally likely to occur in either group.

In addition to maintaining controls identified in the research plan, you must continually watch for previously unidentified extraneous variables that might have an impact on the data being collected. These variables are often specific to a study and tend to become apparent during the data collection period. The extraneous variables identified during data collection must be considered during data analysis and interpretation. These variables also must be noted in the research report to allow future researchers to control them. For example, Lee and Gay (2011) studied sleep quality in new mothers and asked about the infant's sleep location, but the location at the beginning of the night was often not the same by morning and could not be controlled in the home setting.

Problem Solving

Little has been written about the problems encountered by nurse researchers. Research reports often read as though everything went smoothly. The implication is that if you are a good researcher, you will have no problems, which is not true. Research journals generally do not provide enough space for the researcher to describe the problems encountered, and inexperienced researchers may get a false impression. Some of the problems are hinted at in a published paper in either the limitations section or in a discussion of areas for future research. A more realistic sense of the problems encountered by a researcher can be obtained through personal discussions with the primary author about his or her process of data collection for a particular sample or using a particular method or instrument. Some common problems experienced by researchers are discussed in the following section.

A problem can be perceived either as a frustration or as a challenge. The fact that the problem occurred is not as important as successfully resolving it. The final and perhaps most important task during the data collection period may be debriefing with your research team in weekly meetings for problem resolution.

Data Collection Problems

Murphy's law (if anything can go wrong, it will, and at the worst possible time) seems to prevail in research, just as in other dimensions of life. For example, data collection frequently requires more time than was anticipated, and collecting the data is often more difficult than expected. Even following a pilot study, you may encounter challenges during the data collection process. Sometimes changes must be made in the way the data are collected, in the specific data collected, or in the timing of data collection. People react to the study in unpredictable ways. Institutional changes may force modifications in the research plan, or unusual or unexpected events may occur. You must be as consistent as possible during the data collection process, but you must also be flexible in dealing with unforeseen problems. Sometimes, sticking with the original plan at all costs is a mistake. Skills in finding ways to resolve problems that protect the integrity of the study can be critical.

In preparation for data collection, possible problems must be anticipated, and solutions for these problems must be explored. The following discussion describes some common problems and concerns and presents possible solutions. Problems that tend to occur with some regularity in studies have been categorized as people problems, researcher problems, institutional problems, and event problems.

People Problems

Nurses cannot place a subject in a laboratory test tube, instill one drop of the independent variable, and then measure the effect. Nursing studies are often conducted by examining subjects as they interact with their environments. Many aspects of the environment can be controlled by using a laboratory setting, but other studies require the natural setting to have external validity. When research involves people, nothing is completely predictable. People, in their complexity and wholeness, have an impact on all aspects of nursing studies. Researchers, potential subjects, family members of subjects, healthcare professionals, institutional staff members, and others ("innocent bystanders") interact within the study situation. You will need to observe closely and evaluate these interactions to determine their impact on your study.

Problems Selecting a Sample

The first step in initiating data collection—selecting a sample—may be the beginning of people problems. You may find that few people are available who fit your inclusion criteria or that many people you approach refuse to participate in the study even though the request seems reasonable. Appropriate subjects, who were numerous a month earlier, seem to have disappeared. Institutional procedures may change, which might make many potential subjects ineligible for participation in the study. You may have to evaluate the inclusion and exclusion criteria or seek additional sources for potential subjects. In research institutions that care for the indigent, patients tend to be reluctant to participate in research. This lack of participation might arise because these patients are frequently exposed to studies, feel manipulated, or misunderstand the research. Patients may feel that they are being used or fear that they will be harmed in some way. For example, recruiting Spanish-speaking women for a study of stress and acculturation may be met with high refusal rates if these women are worried about revealing their legal status in the United States. Recruiting women who are planning a pregnancy in the next 6 months may not yield participants because they are fearful that others (work colleagues or friends) will find out about their plan.

Subject Attrition

After you have selected a sample, certain problems might cause **subject attrition** (a loss of subjects from the study over time). For example, some subjects may agree to participate but then fail to follow through. Some may not complete needed forms and questionnaires or may fill them out incorrectly. To reduce these problems, a research team member can be available to subjects while they complete essential questions. Some subjects may not return for a second interview

or may not be home for a scheduled visit. Although you have invested time to collect data from these subjects, their data may have to be excluded from analysis because of incompleteness. Generally, the more data collection time points you require as part of your design, the higher the risk for attrition. Attrition can occur because of subject burden accumulating over time, because healthy adults relocate for employment or family reasons, or because of death in a more critically ill population.

Sometimes subjects must be dropped from the study by the research team because of changes in health status. For example, a patient may be transferred out of the intensive care unit where the study is being conducted. Another possibility might be that the patient's condition may worsen and the patient no longer meets the inclusion criteria. The limits of third-party reimbursement may force the healthcare provider to discontinue the services you are studying.

Subject attrition occurs to some extent in all longitudinal studies. One way for you to deal with this problem is to anticipate the attrition rate and increase the planned number of subjects to ensure that a minimally desired number will complete the full study. Review similar studies to anticipate the attrition rate. For example, Lim, Chiu, Dohrmann, and Tan (2010) reported a 31% attrition rate in their quasi-experimental study of the knowledge of registered nurses employed in long-term care. The investigators collected pretest data from 58 subjects and 4 weeks later collected post-test data from 40 subjects. If subject attrition is higher than expected, consider additional small incentives along the way or a bonus for completing the final assessment to achieve an adequate final sample size. Attrition is usually higher in the placebo or control group, but a well-designed, attention-control group should have an attrition rate that is similar to the attrition seen in your intervention group. Sometimes a study might end with a smaller than expected sample size. If so, the effect of a smaller sample on the power of planned statistical analyses must be considered because this smaller sample may be inadequate to test the hypotheses.

Researchers should report information about subjects' acceptance to participate in a study and attrition during the study to determine if the sample is representative of the study target population. Journal editors often require that manuscripts include a flow chart indicating the number of subjects meeting sample criteria, the numbers refusing to participate, and the reasons for refusal. If data are collected over time (repeated measures) or the study intervention is implemented over time, subjects often drop out of a

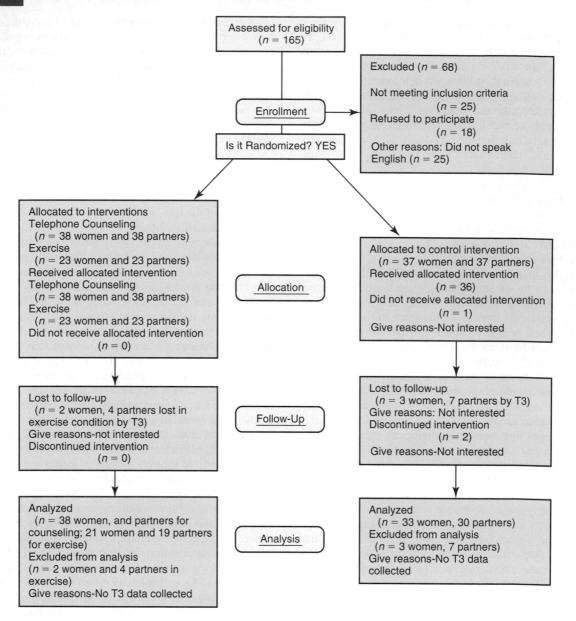

Figure 20-7 Sample selection and allocation.
T3 = Tumor more than 5cm across. (From Badger, T., Segrin, C., Dorros, S., Meek, P., & Lopez, A. M. [2007]. Depression and anxiety in women with breast cancer and their partners. *Nursing Research, 56*[1], 44–53.)

study, and it is important to document when and how much attrition occurred. Using the CONSORT guidelines published by Bennett (2006), Badger, Segrin, Dorros, Meek, and Lopez (2007) provided a flow chart to document participants' selection, refusal rate, assignment to group, and attrition over the weeks of data collection (see Figure 20-7). The flow chart clearly identifies important aspects of the sampling

process and reasons for attrition. This information enables researchers and clinicians to evaluate the representativeness of their sample for external validity and for any potential bias in interpreting the results.

Subject as an Object

The quality of interactions between the researcher and subjects during the study is a critical dimension for maintaining subject participation. When researchers are under pressure to complete a study, people can be treated as objects rather than as subjects, particularly if electronic data collection is used. In addition to being unethical, such impersonal treatment alters interactions, diminishes subject satisfaction, and increases likelihood for missing data and subject attrition. Subjects are scarce resources and must be treated with care. Treating the subject as an object can affect another researcher's ability to recruit from this population in the future. Treating the subject as an object can be minimized by building strategies into the consent process, such as offering them a personal copy of their results, recognizing their valuable participation with small gifts as tokens of appreciation, or providing monetary reimbursement for their time and effort.

External Influences on Subject Responses

People interacting with the subject, the researcher, or both can have an important impact on the data collection process. Family members may not agree to the subject's participation in the study or may not understand the study process. These individuals often influence the subject's decision to participate. Researchers benefit from taking the time to explain the study and seeking cooperation of family members. Family cooperation is essential when the potential subject is critically ill and unable to give informed consent.

Family members or other patients may also influence the subject's responses to scales or interview questions. In some cases, subjects may ask family members, friends, or other patients to complete study forms for them. The subject may discuss questions on the forms with other people who happen to be in the room, and therefore the data recorded do not reflect the subject's real feelings. If interviews are conducted while others are in the room, the subject's responses may depend on his or her need to meet the expectations of the other persons. Sometimes a family member may answer questions addressed verbally to the patient. The setting in which a questionnaire is completed or an interview is conducted may determine the extent to which the answers are a true reflection of a subject's feelings. If the privacy afforded by the setting varies from one subject to another, the subjects' responses may also vary and threaten both the internal and the external validity of the findings.

Usually, the most desirable setting for an interview is a private area away from distractions. If it is not possible to arrange for such a setting, the researcher can be present at the time the questionnaire is completed to decrease the influence of others. If the questionnaire is to be completed later or taken home and returned at a later time, the probability of influence by others increases, and return of the questionnaire packet becomes less likely, even if the subject is provided with a stamped return envelope. The impact of this problem on the integrity of the data depends on the nature of the questionnaire items. For example, a marital relationship questionnaire may have different responses if the subject is allowed to complete it alone and return it immediately to the researcher or have to complete it aloud with the spouse in attendance.

Passive Resistance

Healthcare professionals and institutional staff members working with the study participants in clinical settings may affect the data collection process. Some professionals verbalize strong support for the study and yet passively interfere with data collection. For example, nurses providing care may fail to follow the guidelines agreed on for providing the specific care activities being studied, or information needed for the study may be left off patient records. The researcher may not be informed when a potential subject has been admitted, and a physician who has agreed that his or her patients can be participants may decide as each patient is admitted that this one is not quite right for the study. In addition, when the permission of the physician or nurse practitioner is required, the provider might be unavailable to the researcher.

Nonprofessional staff members may not realize the impact of the data collection process on their work patterns until the process begins. The data collection process may violate their beliefs about how care should be provided (or has been provided). If ignored, their resistance can completely undo a carefully designed study. For example, research on skin care may disrupt a nursing aide's bathing routine, so he or she may continue the normal routine regardless of the study protocol and invalidate the study findings. When there is funding to support subject recruitment and data collection, funds can be used to reimburse the clinic or hospital staff members for their time, to create a raffle for one substantial gift, to offer a gift certificate to buy something needed for the clinic, or to send a nurse to a continuing education course. When funding is limited, staff members' enthusiasm for your study may be enhanced if they are able to participate in the research as authors or presenters in dissemination of the research findings.

Because of the potential impact of these problems, the researcher must maintain open communication and nurture positive relationships with other professionals and staff members during data collection. Problems that you and your team recognize early and deal with promptly have fewer serious consequences than problems you try to ignore. However, not all problems can be resolved. Sometimes you may need to seek creative ways to work around an individual or to counteract the harmful consequences of passive resistance.

Researcher Problems

Some problems are a consequence of the researcher's interaction with the study situation or lack of skill in data collection techniques. These problems are often difficult to identify because of the researcher's personal involvement. However, their effect on the study can be serious.

Researcher Interactions

Researcher interactions can interfere with data collection in interview situations. To gain the cooperation of the subject, the researcher needs to develop rapport with the subject. One way to do this is to select data collectors who resemble the types of subjects being recruited as much as possible. Rapport may suffer if a young man collects data from female caregivers of elderly adults about their experience with end-of-life care. Similarly, a white middle-aged woman collecting data from young African American men or Hispanic teens is likely to be more disadvantaged than a data collector who is more similar to the population of interest.

A balance is needed between rapport and over-involvement. The researcher can become so involved in interactions with a study participant that data collection on that particular subject is not completed. If you are collecting data from patient records while you are surrounded by professionals with whom you interact socially and professionally, it is sometimes difficult to focus completely on the study situation. This lack of attention usually leads to loss of data.

Lack of Skill in Data Collection Techniques

The researcher's skill in using a particular data collection technique can affect the quality of the data collected. A researcher who is unskilled at the beginning of data collection might practice the data collection techniques with the assistance of an experienced researcher. A pilot study to test data collection techniques is always helpful. If data collectors are being used, they also need opportunities to practice data collection techniques before the study is initiated. Sometimes a skill is developed during the course of a study; if this is the case, as one's skill increases, the data being collected may change and confound the study findings and threaten the validity of the study. If more than one data collector is used, the degree to which skills improve may vary across time and data collectors. The consistency of data collectors must be evaluated during the study to detect any changes in their data collection techniques.

Researcher Role Conflict

As a researcher, one is observing and recording events. Nurses who conduct clinical research often experience a conflict between their researcher role and their clinician role during data collection. In some cases, the researcher's involvement in the event, such as providing physical or emotional care to a patient during data collection, could alter the event and bias the results. It would be difficult to generalize the findings to other situations in which the researcher was not present to intervene. However, the needs of patients must take precedence over the needs of the study.

The dilemma is to determine when the needs of patients are great enough to warrant researcher intervention. Some patient questions or situations are life-threatening, such as respiratory distress and changes in cardiac function, and require immediate action by anyone present. Other patient needs are simple, can be addressed by any nurse available, and can be answered if the response is not likely to alter the results of your study. Examples of these interventions include giving the patient a bedpan, informing the nurse of the patient's need for pain medication, or helping the patient to open food containers. These situations seldom cause a dilemma.

Solutions to other situations are not as easy. For example, suppose that your study involves examining the emotional responses of patients' family members during and immediately after the patient's surgery. Your study includes an experimental group that receives one 30-minute family support session before and during the patient's surgery and a control group that receives no support session. Both sets of families are being monitored for 1 week after surgery to measure level of anxiety and coping strategies. You are currently collecting data on the control group. The data consist of demographic information and scales measuring anxiety and coping. One of the family members is in great distress. After completing the demographic information, she verbally expresses her fears and the lack of support she has received from the nursing staff. Two other subjects from different families hear the expressed distress and concur; they move closer to the conversation and look to you for information and support.

In this situation, a supportive response from you is likely to modify the results of the study because these responses are part of the treatment to be provided to the experimental group only. This interaction is likely to narrow the difference between the two groups and decrease the possibility that your results will show a significant difference between the two groups. How should you respond? Are you obligated to provide support? To some extent, almost any response would be supportive. One alternative is to provide the needed support and not include these family members in the control group. Another alternative is to recruit the help of a nonprofessional to collect the data from the control group. However, most people would provide some degree of support in the described situation, even though their skills in supportive techniques may vary.

Other dilemmas include witnessing unethical behavior that interferes with patient care or witnessing subjects' unethical or illegal behavior (Humphreys et al., 2011). Consent forms are often required to stipulate that any member of the research team is legally required to report illegal behaviors, such as neglect or abuse of children and elderly adults. Try to anticipate these dilemmas before data collection whenever possible and include this information in the consent form (Wong, Tiwari, Fong, Humphreys, & Bullock, 2011). Pilot studies can help you to identify dilemmas likely to occur in a study, and you can build strategies into the design to minimize or avoid them. However, some dilemmas cannot be anticipated, and you must respond to these problems spontaneously. There is no prescribed way to handle difficult dilemmas; each case must be dealt with individually. You should discuss any unethical and illegal behavior with members of your IRB or ethics committee or with legal advisors. These situations must be reported to the IRB, and experts there can advise you on the next step or course of action. After you have resolved the dilemma, it is wise to reexamine the situation for its effect on study results and consider options in case the situation arises again.

Another type of conflict arises when a subject makes inaccurate statements or asks a question about health practices or treatment. Rather than offering professional advice or responding to the question, the research nurse should acknowledge that it is a good question, but that the research protocol does not allow for a response during data collection. When data collection is complete, the research nurse can help formulate the question for the subject's healthcare provider or provide a readily available pamphlet or website for more information.

Maintaining Perspective
Data collection includes both joys and frustrations. Researchers must be able to maintain some degree of objectivity during the process and yet not take themselves too seriously. A sense of humor is invaluable. You must be able to experience the emotions and then become the rational problem solver. Management skills and mental health are as invaluable to a research career as being obsessive about data collection and data management.

Institutional Problems
Institutions are in a constant state of change. They will not stop changing for the period of a study, and these changes often affect data collection. A nurse who has been most helpful in your study may be promoted or transferred. The unit on which your study is conducted may be reorganized, moved, or closed during data collection. An area used for subject interviews may be transformed into an office or a storeroom. Patient record forms may be revised, omitting data that you and your team are collecting. The medical record personnel may be reorganizing files and temporarily unable to provide needed records.

These problems for the most part are completely outside of the researcher's control. Pay attention to the internal communication network of the institution for advanced warning of impending changes. Contacts within the institution's administrative decision makers could warn you about the impact of proposed changes on an ongoing study. In many cases, the IRB in the local hospital will have a nurse representative who can provide the needed consultation. However, in many cases, data collection strategies might have to be modified to meet the newly emerging situation. Balancing flexibility with maintaining the integrity of the study may be the key to successful data collection. As a data collection site, the subject's home setting may be more desirable and convenient for a subject than a complex facility or institution, and response rates may improve. The disadvantage is that home visits are time intensive for the researcher, and the subject may not be home at the agreed appointment time despite confirmed appointments and reminder calls.

Event Problems
Unpredictable events can be a source of frustration during a study. Research tools ordered from a testing company may be lost in the mail. The printer may break down just before 500 data collection forms are to be printed, or a machine to be used in data collection may break down and require 6 weeks for repair. A computer ordered for data collection may not arrive when promised or may malfunction. Data collection forms may be misplaced, misfiled, or lost.

Local, national, or world events can also influence a subject's response to a questionnaire or ability to enroll in a study. For example, a researcher conducting a study of the effects of fatigue on the health of air traffic controllers encounters a rash of national media reports about controllers falling asleep while on duty. This event could be expected to modify subjects' responses. In attempting to deal with the impact of the event on the study, the researcher could obtain IRB approval for a modification that would allow for continued data collection from the intended sample but to examine the impact of news such as this on subjects' responses rather than the original purpose. However, the emotional climate of the airports participating in the study may not be conducive to this option. The researcher may choose to wait 3 months before collecting additional data and examine the data before and after the event for statistically significant differences in responses. If no differences are found, the researcher could justify using all the data for analysis.

Other, less dramatic events can also have an impact on data collection. If data collection for the entire sample is planned for a single time, a snowstorm or a flood may require that the researcher cancel the session. Weather may decrease attendance far below that expected at a support group or series of teaching sessions. A bus strike can disrupt transportation systems to such an extent that subjects can no longer get to the data collection site. A new health agency may open in the city, which may decrease demand for the care activities being studied. Conversely, an external event can also increase attendance at clinics to such an extent that existing resources are stretched and data collection is no longer possible. These events are also outside the researcher's control and are impossible to anticipate. In most cases, however, restructuring the data collection period can salvage the study. To do so, it is necessary to examine all possible alternatives for collecting the study data. In some cases, data collection can simply be rescheduled; in other situations, the changes may need to be more complex. For example, recruiting women to participate in a study that requires an hour or longer of their time may necessitate that the researcher provide childcare. Providing childcare would be more costly and add complexity to the process, but it may be the best alternative for increasing participation.

Serendipity

Serendipity is the accidental discovery of something useful or valuable. During the data collection phase of studies, researchers often become aware of elements or relationships that they had not previously identified. These aspects may be closely related to the study being conducted or have little connection with it. They come from increased awareness and close observation of the study situation. Because the researcher is focused on close observation, other elements in the situation can come into clearer focus and take on new meaning. Serendipitous findings are important to the development of new insights in nursing theory. They can be important for understanding the totality of the phenomenon being examined. Additionally, they lead to areas of research that generate new knowledge. A relatively easy way to capture these insights as they occur is to keep a research journal. These events must be carefully recorded, even if their impact or meaning is not understood at the time.

Serendipitous findings can also lead the researcher astray. Sometimes researchers forget the original plan and redirect their attention to the newly discovered dimensions. Although modifying data collection to include data related to the new discovery may be valid, there has not been time to plan carefully a study related to the new findings. The study's approval by the IRB covers only information included in the submitted study proposal. Examination of the new data should be an offshoot only of the initial study and would require seeking additional IRB approval.

Having Access to Support Systems

The researcher must have access to individuals or groups who can provide mentorship, support, and consultation during the data collection period. Support can usually be obtained from academic committees, from IRB staff, and from colleagues on your research team.

Support of Academic Committees

Although thesis and dissertation committees are basically seen as stern keepers of the sanctity of the research process, they also serve as support systems for novice researchers. Committee members must be selected from faculty who are willing and able to provide the needed expertise and support. Experienced academic researchers are usually more knowledgeable about the types of support needed. Because they are directly involved in research, they tend to be sensitive to the needs of a novice researcher and more realistic about what can be accomplished in the designated time frame.

Institutional Support

A support system within the institution where the study is being conducted is also important. Support might come from people serving on the institutional research committee or from nurses working on the unit where the study is conducted. These people may have knowledge of how the institution functions, and their closeness to the study can increase their understanding of the problems experienced by the researcher and subjects. Do not overlook their ability to provide useful suggestions and assistance. Your ability to resolve some of the problems encountered during data collection may depend on having someone within the power structure of the institution who can intervene.

Colleague Support

In addition to professional support, having at least one peer in your research world with whom to share the joys, frustrations, and current problems of data collection is important. This colleague can often serve as a mirror to allow you to see the situation clearly and perhaps more objectively. With this type of support, the researcher can share and release feelings and gain some distance from the data collection situation. Alternatives for resolving the problem can be discussed in a less emotional context. Data collection is demanding but rewarding. With time, confidence and expertise of the novice researcher increase.

Data Safety and Monitoring Board as Source of Support

If you are conducting an intervention study that is deemed to be of low risk to the patient, such as a behavioral intervention to improve sleep quality, a data safety and monitoring plan will suffice. In these situations, less support for you as a researcher is needed. This plan is deemed adequate when it conforms to the IRB requirements for reporting any adverse event and includes annual progress reports. It requires that the researcher explicitly states the plan to review the data from each set number of subjects or from each 3-month or 6-month batch of recruited subjects, depending on the extent of the study.

If the study involves an intervention protocol that is higher risk to patient safety, a data safety and monitoring board is required. This board includes members who are not directly involved in the study and who can be objective about the findings to date. This board should meet at regular intervals and discuss whether the study should continue or be stopped based on the data collected to date. The board should consist of very experienced researchers and clinical experts. See Chapter 14 for more information on conducting intervention studies.

Managing Data

Once data collection begins, you have to be prepared to handle large quantities of data. To avoid a state of total confusion, make careful plans before data collection begins. Plans are needed to keep all data from a single subject together until analysis is initiated. Write the subject code number on each form, and check the forms for each subject to ensure that they all are present. Researchers have been known to sort their data by form, such as putting all the scales of one kind together, only to realize afterward that they had failed to code the forms with subject identification numbers first. They then had no idea which scale belonged to which subject, and valuable data were lost.

Allot space as needed for storing forms. Purchase file folders, and design a labeling method to allow easy access to data; color coding is often useful. If you are using multiple forms, the subject's demographic sheet could be one light color, with a different pastel color for the pain questionnaire and a contrasting light color for all the physiological data sheets used to record blood pressure, pulse, and respiration readings. Use envelopes to hold small pieces of paper or note cards that might fall out of a file folder. Plan to code data and enter them into the computer as soon as possible after data collection to reduce the loss or disorganization of data. If data are collected on a computer, make sure the data are backed up and stored in a separate space so that they are not lost if the computer fails.

Preparing Data for Computer Entry

Data must be carefully checked and problems corrected before you initiate the data entry phase. The data entry process should be essentially automatic and require no decisions regarding the data. Anything that alters the rhythm of data entry increases errors. For example, the subject's entry should be coded as it appears, and any reverse coding that may be needed should be done at a later time by computer manipulation in a consistent manner rather than trying to have the data entry person recode during data entry.

Such simplicity in data entry reduces the number of data entry errors and markedly decreases the time required for entry. It is not sufficient to establish general rules for individuals entering data such as "in this case always do X." This action still requires the person who is entering data to recognize a problem, refer to a general rule, and correct the data before entry. Correcting the data requires using a different color ink from the subject's mark, and the correction should be initialed by the researcher making the correction.

1. *Missing data.* Provide the data if possible or determine the impact of the missing data on your analysis. In some cases, the subject must be excluded from at least some of the analyses, so you must determine what data are essential.
2. *Items in which the subject provided two responses when only one was requested.* For example, if the question asked the subject to mark the most important item in a list of 10 items and the subject selected 2 items, you must decide how to resolve this problem; do not leave the decision to an assistant who is entering the data. In the codebook and on the form itself, indicate how that particular datum is to be coded and entered.
3. *Items in which the subject has marked a response between two options.* This problem commonly occurs with Likert-type scales, particularly scales using forced choice options. Given four options, the subject places a mark on the line between response 2 and response 3. In the codebook and on the form, indicate how the datum is to be coded. This is often best coded as a missing value, but coding rules should be consistent. A rationale can be made to take the highest value, the lowest value, or code toward the center value.
4. *Items that ask the subject to write in some information such as occupation or diagnosis.* Such items are a data enterer's nightmare. Develop a list of codes for entering such data. Rather than leaving it up to the assistant to determine which code matches the subject's written response, the researcher should enter this code in a different color and initial that change before turning the data over for entry. After the data have been checked and needed codes written in, it is prudent to make a copy rather than turning over the only set of your data to an assistant.

Data Entry Period

If you are entering your own data, develop a rhythm to your data entry process. Avoid distractions while entering data, and limit your data entry periods to 2-hour intervals to reduce fatigue, errors, and repetitive wrist strain or injury. Backup the database after each data entry period, and store it on an encrypted flash drive, on a secure website, or in a fireproof safe. It is possible for the computer to crash and lose all of your data. If an assistant is entering your data, make yourself as available as possible to respond to questions and address problems. After entry, the data

should be randomly checked for accuracy. Data checking is discussed in Chapter 21.

Storage and Retrieval of Data

In this time of flash drives and thumb drives, it is relatively easy to store data. The original data forms and database must be stored for a specified number of years dictated by the funding source or by the journal publisher. There are several reasons to store data. The data can be used for secondary analyses. For example, researchers participating in a project related to a particular research focus may pool data from various studies for access by all members of the group. Data should be available to document the validity of your analyses and the published results of your study. Because of nationally publicized incidents of scientific misconduct, where researchers fabricated data and published multiple manuscripts, you would be wise to preserve documentation that your data were obtained as you claim. Issues that have been raised include how long data should be stored, the need for institutional policy regarding data storage, and whether graduate students who conduct a study should leave a copy of their data at the university. Some researchers store their data for 5 years after publication, whereas others store their data until they retire from a research career. Researchers should check with their funding sponsors and publishers for guidelines on how long to keep the data. Most researchers store data in their office or laboratory; others archive their data in a central location with storage fees or retrieval fees. Graduate students do have a responsibility to keep and securely store data from their studies.

KEY POINTS

- Careful planning is needed before collecting and managing data.
- The researcher may need to develop data collection forms and format these forms to promote accuracy and ease of data entry.
- The researcher must determine exactly how and in what sequence data will be collected and the timing of the process. Information about the procedures to be used must be described in the subject's informed consent.
- The researcher must decide who will collect the data.
- If data collectors are used, they must be provided information about the research project, the instruments, and data collection protocol.

- Consistency in data collection across subjects is critical, and training is required to promote consistency among data collectors if more than one data collector is used.
- After training, data collectors must be evaluated periodically and randomly to determine their consistency.
- Decision points that occur during data collection must be identified, and all options must be considered.
- Data collection also involves maintaining research controls and solving problems that threaten to disrupt the study.
- Problems that arise during data collection involve recruitment and attrition issues, treatment of the subject as an object, external influences on subject responses, passive resistance from staff members or family, researcher interactions, lack of skill in data collection techniques, and researcher role conflicts.
- A successful study requires support that is often obtained from academic committees, healthcare agencies, and work colleagues.
- Data collected during a study must be accurately entered in an encrypted computer and safely stored in either a data repository or on an encrypted flash drive.

REFERENCES

Badger, T., Segrin, C., Dorros, S., Meek, P., & Lopez, A. M. (2007). Depression and anxiety in women with breast cancer and their partners. *Nursing Research*, 56(1), 44–53.

Bennett, J. M. (2006). The consolidated standards of reporting trials (CONSORT): Guidelines for reporting randomized trials. *Nursing Research*, 54(2), 128–132.

Fukuoka, Y., Kamitani, E., Dracup, K., & Jong, S. S. (2011). New insights into compliance with a mobile phone diary and pedometer use in sedentary women. *Journal of Physical Activity & Health*, 8(3), 398–403.

Gray, J. & Johnson, (2009). *Nurse International Relocation Questionnaire* 2. Unpublished research tool. Available from jgray@uta.edu.

Harris, P. A., Taylor, R., Thielke, R., Payne, J., Gonzalez, N., & Conde, J. G. (2009). Research electronic data capture (REDCap)——A metadata-driven methodology and workflow process for providing translational research informatics support. *Journal of Biomedical Informatics*, 42(2), 377–381.

Harwood, E. M. (2009). Data collection methods series: Part 3: Developing protocols for collecting data. *Journal of Wound Ostomy Continence Nursing*, 36(3), 246–250.

Harwood, E. M. & Hutchinson E. (2009). Data collection methods series: Part 2: Select the most feasible data collection mode. *Journal of Wound Ostomy Continence Nursing*, 36(2), 129–135.

Humphreys, J., Epel, E. S., Cooper, B. A., Lin, J., Blackburn, E. H., & Lee, K. A. (2011, March 8). Telomere shortening in formerly abused and never abused women. *Biological Research for Nursing*. Available from http://brn.sagepub.com/content/early/2011/03/07/1099800411398479.

Im, E., Chee, W., Guevara, E., Liu, Y., Lim, H., Tsai, H., et al. (2007). Gender and ethnic differences in cancer pain experience: A multiethnic survey in the United States. *Nursing Research*, 56(5), 296–306.

Kang, D. H., Davis, L., Habermann, B., Rice, M., & Broome, M. (2005). Hiring the right people and management of research staff. *Western Journal of Nursing Research*, 27(8), 1059–1066.

Lee, K. A. & Gay, C. L. (2011). Can modifications to the bedroom environment improve the sleep of new parents? Two randomized controlled trials. *Research in Nursing & Health*, 34(1), 7–19.

Lim, L. M., Chiu, L. H., Dohrmann, J., & Tan, K. (2010). Registered nurses' medication management of the elderly in aged care facilities. *International Nursing Review*, 57(1), 98–106.

Melnyk, B. M. & Fineout-Overholt, E. (2010). *Evidence-based practice in nursing and healthcare: A guide to best practice* (2nd ed.). Philadelphia, PA: Lippincott Williams & Wilkins.

Office of Minority Health. (2010). *OMB standards for data on race and ethnicity*. Retrieved from http://minorityhealth.hhs.gov/.

Savian, C., Paratz, J., & Davies, A. (2006). Comparison of the effectiveness of manual and ventilator hyperinflation at different levels of positive end-expiratory pressure in artificially ventilated and intubated intensive care patients. *Heart & Lung*, 35(5), 334–341.

Waltz, C. F., Strickland, O. L., & Lenz, E. R. (2010). *Measurement in nursing and health research* (4th ed.). New York, NY: Springer Publishing Company.

Wong, J. Y., Tiwari, A., Fong, D. Y., Humphreys, J., & Bullock, L. (2011). Depression among women experiencing intimate partner violence in a Chinese community. *Nursing Research*, 60(1), 58–65.

21
CHAPTER

Introduction to Statistical Analysis

Data analysis is often considered one of the most exciting steps of the research process. During this phase, you will finally obtain answers to the questions that led to the development of your study. Nevertheless, nurses probably experience greater anxiety about this phase of the research process than any other, as they question issues that range from their knowledge about critically appraising published studies to their ability to conduct research. Critical appraisal of the results section of a quantitative study requires you to be able to (1) identify the statistical procedures used; (2) judge whether these statistical procedures were appropriate for the hypotheses, questions, or objectives of the study and for the data available for analysis; (3) comprehend the discussion of data analysis results; (4) judge whether the author's interpretation of the results is appropriate; and (5) evaluate the clinical importance of the findings (see Chapter 18 for more details on critical appraisal).

As a neophyte researcher performing a quantitative study, you are confronted with many critical decisions related to data analysis that require statistical knowledge. To perform statistical analysis of data from a quantitative study, you need to be able to (1) determine the necessary sample size to power your study adequately; (2) prepare the data for analysis; (3) describe the sample; (4) test the reliability of measures used in the study; (5) perform exploratory analyses of the data; (6) perform analyses guided by the study objectives, questions, or hypotheses; and (7) interpret the results of statistical procedures. We recommend consulting with a statistician or expert researcher early in the research process to help you develop a plan for accomplishing these seven tasks. A statistician is also invaluable in conducting data analysis for a study and interpreting the results.

Critical appraisal of the results of studies and statistical analyses both require an understanding of the statistical theory underlying the process of analysis.

This chapter and the following four chapters provide you with the information needed for critical appraisal of the results sections of published studies and for performance of statistical procedures to analyze data in studies and in clinical practice. This chapter introduces the concepts of statistical theory and discusses some of the more pragmatic aspects of quantitative data analysis: the purposes of statistical analysis, the process of performing data analysis, the method for choosing appropriate statistical analysis techniques for a study, and resources for conducting statistical analysis procedures. Chapter 22 explains the use of statistics for descriptive purposes, such as describing the study sample or variables. Chapter 23 focuses on the use of statistics to examine proposed relationships among study variables, such as the relationships among the variables dyspnea, anxiety, and quality of life. Chapter 24 explores the use of statistics for prediction, such as using independent variables of age, gender, cholesterol values, and history of hypertension to predict the dependent variable of cardiac risk level. Chapter 25 guides you in using statistics to determine differences between groups, such as determining the difference in muscle strength and falls (dependent variables) between an experimental or intervention group receiving a strength training program (independent variable) and a comparison group receiving standard care.

Concepts of Statistical Theory

One reason nurses tend to avoid statistics is that many were taught the mathematical mechanics of calculating statistical formulas and were given little or no explanation of the logic behind the analysis procedure or the meaning of the results (Grove, 2007). This mathematical process is usually performed by computer, and information about it offers little assistance to the individuals making statistical decisions or explaining results. We approach data analysis from the perspective of enhancing your understanding of the meaning underlying statistical analysis. You can use this understanding either for critical appraisal of studies or for conducting data analyses.

The ensuing discussion explains some of the concepts commonly used in statistical theory. The logic of statistical theory is embedded within the explanations of these concepts. The concepts presented in this chapter include probability theory, classical hypothesis testing, Type I and Type II errors, statistical power, statistical significance versus clinical importance, inference, samples and populations, descriptive and inferential statistical techniques, measures of central tendency, the normal curve, sampling distributions, symmetry, skewness, modality, kurtosis, variation, confidence intervals, and parametric and nonparametric types of inferential statistical analyses.

Probability Theory

Probability theory addresses statistical analysis as the likelihood of accurately predicting an event or the extent of an effect. Nurse researchers might be interested in the probability of a particular nursing outcome in a particular patient care situation. For example, what is the probability of patients older than 75 years of age with cardiac conditions falling when hospitalized? With probability theory, you could determine how much of the variation in your data could be explained by using a particular statistical analysis. In probability theory, the researcher interprets the meaning of statistical results in light of his or her knowledge of the field of study. A finding that would have little meaning in one field of study might be important in another (Good, 1983; Kerlinger & Lee, 2000). Probability is expressed as a lowercase p, with values expressed as percentages or as a decimal value ranging from 0 to 1. For example, if the exact probability is known to be 0.23, it would be expressed as $p = 0.23$. The p in statistics is defined as the probability of rejecting the null hypothesis when the null is actually true. Nurse researchers typically consider a $p = 0.05$ value or less to indicate a real effect.

Classical Hypothesis Testing

Classical hypothesis testing refers to the process of testing a hypothesis to infer the reality of an effect. This process starts with the statement of a null hypothesis, which assumes no effect (e.g., no difference between groups, or no relationship between variables). The researcher sets the values of two theoretical probabilities: (1) the probability of rejecting the null hypothesis when it is in fact true (alpha [α], Type I error) and (2) the probability of retaining the null hypothesis when it is in fact false (beta [β], Type II error). In nursing research, alpha is usually set at 0.05, meaning that the researcher will allow a 5% or lower chance of making a Type I error. The beta is frequently set at 0.20, meaning that the researcher will allow for a 20% or lower chance of making a Type II error.

After conducting the study, the researcher culminates the hypothesis testing process by making a rational decision either to reject or to retain the null hypothesis, based on the statistical results. The following steps outline each of the components of statistical hypothesis testing.

1. State your primary null hypothesis. (Chapter 8 discusses the development of the null hypothesis.)
2. Set your study alpha (Type I error); this is usually $\alpha = 0.05$.
3. Set your study beta (Type II error); this is usually $\beta = 0.20$.
4. Conduct power analyses (Aberson, 2010; Cohen, 1988).
5. Design and conduct your study.
6. Compute the appropriate statistic on your obtained data.
7. Compare your obtained statistic with its corresponding theoretical distribution in the tables provided in the Appendices at the back of this book. For example, if you analyzed your data with a t-test, you would compare the t value from your study with the critical values of t in the table.
8. If your obtained statistic exceeds the critical value in the distribution table, you can reject your null hypothesis. If not, you must accept your null hypothesis. These ideas are discussed in more depth in Chapters 23 through 25 when the results of statistics are presented.

Cox (1958, p. 159) stated, "Significance tests, from this point of view, measure the adequacy of the data to support the qualitative conclusion that there is a true effect in the direction of the apparent difference." Thus, the decision is a judgment and can be in error. The level of statistical significance attained indicates the degree of uncertainty in taking the position that the difference between the two groups is real. Classical hypothesis testing has been largely criticized for such errors in judgments (Cohen, 1994; Loftus 1993). Much emphasis has been placed on researchers providing indicators of effect, rather than just relying on p values, specifically, providing the magnitude of the obtained effect (e.g., a difference or relationship) as well as confidence intervals associated with the statistical findings. These additional statistics give consumers of

TABLE 21-1 Type I and Type II Errors		Decision	
		Reject Null	**Accept Null**
True Population Status	**Null Is True**	Type I Error α	Correct Decision $1 - \alpha$
	Null Is False	Correct Decision $1 - \beta$	Type II Error β

research more information about the phenomenon being studied (Cohen 1994).

Type I and Type II Errors

We choose the probability of making a Type I error when we set alpha, and if we decrease the probability of making a Type I error, we increase the probability of making a Type II error. The relationships between Type I and Type II errors are defined in Table 21-1. Type II error occurs as a result of some degree of overlap between the values of different populations, so in some cases a value with a greater than 5% probability of being within one population may be within the dimensions of another population.

It is impossible to decrease both types of error simultaneously without a corresponding increase in sample size. The researcher needs to decide which risk poses the greatest threat within a specific study. In nursing research, many studies are conducted with small samples and instruments that lack precision and accuracy in the measurement of study variables. Many nursing situations include multiple variables that interact to lead to differences within populations. However, when one is examining only a few of the interacting variables, small differences can be overlooked and could lead to a false conclusion of no differences between the samples. In this case, the risk of a Type II error is a greater concern, and a more lenient level of significance is in order. Nurse researchers usually set the level of significance or $\alpha = 0.05$ for their studies versus a more stringent $\alpha = 0.01$ or 0.001. Setting $\alpha = 0.05$ reduces the risk of a Type II error of indicating study results are not significant when they are.

Statistical Power

Power is the probability that a statistical test will detect an effect when it actually exists. Power is the inverse of Type II error and is calculated as $1 - \beta$. Type II error is the probability of retaining the null hypothesis when it is in fact false. When the researcher sets Type II error at 0.20 before conducting a study, this means that the power of the planned statistic has been set to 0.80. In other words, the statistic will have an 80% chance of detecting an effect if it actually exists.

Reported studies failing to reject the null hypothesis (in which power is unlikely to have been examined) often have a low power level to detect an effect if one exists. Until more recently, the researcher's primary interest was in preventing a Type I error. Therefore, great emphasis was placed on the selection of a level of significance, but little emphasis was placed on power. This point of view is changing as we recognize the seriousness of a Type II error in nursing studies.

As stated in the steps of classical hypothesis testing previously, step 4 is "conducting a power analysis." Power analysis involves determining the required sample size needed to conduct your study after performing steps 1, 2, and 3. Cohen (1988) identified four parameters of power: (1) significance level, (2) sample size, (3) effect size, and (4) power (standard of 0.80). If three of the four are known, the fourth can be calculated by using power analysis formulas. Significance level and sample size are straightforward. Chapter 15 provides a detailed discussion of determining sample size in quantitative studies that includes power analysis. **Effect size** is "the degree to which the phenomenon is present in the population or the degree to which the null hypothesis is false" (Cohen, 1988, pp. 9-10). For example, suppose you were measuring changes in anxiety levels, measured first when the patient is at home and then just before surgery. The effect size would be large if you expected a great change in anxiety. If you expected only a small change in the level of anxiety, the effect size would be small.

Small effect sizes require larger samples to detect these small differences (see Chapter 15 for a detailed discussion of effect size). If the power is too low, it may not be worthwhile conducting the study unless a large sample can be obtained because statistical tests are unlikely to detect differences or relationships that exist. Deciding to conduct a study in these circumstances is costly in time and money, frequently does

TABLE 21-2	Software Applications for Statistical Analysis	
Software Application	**Website**
NCSS (Number Cruncher Statistical System)	www.ncss.com
SPSS (Statistical Packages for the Social Sciences)	www.spss.com
SAS (Statistical Analysis System)	www.sas.com
S+	spotfire.tibco.com
Stata	www.stat.com
JMP	www.jmp.com

not add to the body of nursing knowledge, and can lead to false conclusions. Power analysis can be conducted via hand calculations, computer software, or online calculators and should be performed to determine the sample size necessary for a particular study (Aberson, 2010). Power analysis can be calculated by using the free power analysis software G*Power (Faul, Erdfelder, Lang, & Buchner, 2007) or statistical software such as NCSS, SAS, and SPSS (Table 21-2). In addition, many free sample size calculators are available online that are easy to use and understand. If you have questions, you could consult a statistician.

The power achieved should be reported with the results of the studies, especially studies that fail to reject the null hypothesis (have nonsignificant results). If power is high, it strengthens the meaning of the findings. If power is low, researchers need to address this issue in the discussion of limitations and implications of the study findings. Modifications in the research methodology that resulted from the use of power analysis also need to be reported.

Statistical Significance versus Clinical Importance

The findings of a study can be statistically significant but may not be clinically important. For example, one group of patients might have a body temperature 0.1° F higher than that of another group. Data analysis might indicate that the two groups are statistically significantly different. However, the findings have little or no clinical importance because of the small difference in temperatures between groups. It is often important to know the magnitude of the difference between groups in studies. However, a statistical test that indicates significant differences between groups (e.g., a *t*-test) provides no information on the magnitude of the difference. The extent of the level of significance (0.01 or 0.0001) tells you nothing about the

magnitude of the difference between the groups or the relationship between two variables. The magnitude of group differences can best be determined through calculating effect sizes and confidence intervals (see Chapters 22 through 25).

Inference

Statisticians use the terms **inference** and **infer** in a similar way that a researcher uses the term *generalize*. Inference requires the use of inductive reasoning. One infers from a specific case to a general truth, from a part to the whole, from the concrete to the abstract, from the known to the unknown. When using inferential reasoning, you can never prove things; you can never be certain. However, one of the reasons for the rules that have been established with regard to statistical procedures is to increase the probability that inferences are accurate. Inferences are made cautiously and with great care. Researchers use inferences to infer from the sample in their study to the larger population.

Samples and Populations

Use of the terms *statistic* and *parameter* can be confusing because of the various populations referred to in statistical theory. A **statistic**, such as a mean ($\bar{X}$), is a numerical value obtained from a sample. A **parameter** is a true (but unknown) numerical characteristic of a population. For example, μ is the population mean or arithmetic average. The mean of the sampling distribution (mean of samples' means) can also be shown to be equal to μ. A numerical value that is the mean ($\bar{X}$) of the sample is a statistic; a numerical value that is the mean of the population (μ) is a parameter (Barnett, 1982).

Relating a statistic to a parameter requires an inference as one moves from the sample to the sampling distribution and then from the sampling distribution to the population. The population referred to is in one sense real (concrete) and in another sense abstract. These ideas are illustrated as follows:

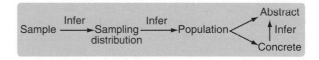

For example, perhaps you are interested in the cholesterol levels of women in the United States. Your population is women in the United States. You cannot measure the cholesterol level of every woman in the United States; therefore, you select a sample of women from this population. Because you wish your sample to be as representative of the population as possible, you obtain your sample by using random sampling techniques (see Chapter 15). To determine whether the cholesterol levels in your sample are similar to those in the population, you must compare the sample with the population. One strategy would be to compare the mean of your sample with the mean of the entire population. However, it is highly unlikely that you *know* the mean of the entire population; you must make an estimate of the mean of that population. You need to know how good your sample statistics are as estimators of the parameters of the population. First, you make some assumptions. You assume that the mean scores of cholesterol levels from multiple, randomly selected samples of this population would be normally distributed. This assumption implies another assumption: that the cholesterol levels of the population will be distributed according to the theoretical normal curve—that difference scores and standard deviations can be equated to those in the normal curve. The normal curve is discussed later in this chapter.

If you assume that the population in your study is normally distributed, you can also assume that this population can be represented by a normal sampling distribution. You infer from your sample to the sampling distribution, the mathematically developed theoretical population made up of parameters such as the mean of means and the standard error. The parameters of this theoretical population are the measures of the dimensions identified in the sampling distribution. You can infer from the sampling distribution to the population. You have both a concrete population and an abstract population. The concrete population consists of all the individuals who meet your study sample criteria, whereas the abstract population consists of individuals who will meet your sample criteria in the future or the groups addressed theoretically by your framework.

Types of Statistics

There are two major classes of statistics: descriptive statistics and inferential statistics. **Descriptive statistics** are computed to reveal characteristics of the sample and to describe study variables. **Inferential statistics** are computed to draw conclusions and make inferences about the greater population, based on the sample data set. The following sections define the concepts and rationale associated with descriptive and inferential statistics.

Descriptive Statistics

A basic yet important way to begin describing a sample is to create a frequency distribution of the variable or variables being studied. A frequency distribution is a plot of one variable, whereby the *x*-axis consists of the possible values of that variable, and the *y*-axis is the tally of each value. For example, if you assessed a sample for a variable such as pain using a visual analogue scale, and your subjects reported particular values for pain, you could create a frequency distribution as illustrated in Figure 21-1.

Measures of Central Tendency

The measures of central tendency are descriptive statistics. The statistics that represent *measures of central tendency* are the mean, median, and mode. All of these statistics are representations or descriptions of the center or middle of a frequency distribution. The **mean** is the arithmetic average of all of the values of a variable. The **median** is the exact middle value (or the average of the middle two values if there is an even number of observations). The **mode** is the most commonly occurring value in a data set (Grove, 2007; Munro, 2005). It is possible to have more than one mode in a sample, which is discussed later in this chapter. In a normal curve, the mean, median, and mode are equal or approximately equal (see Figure 21-2).

Normal Curve

The theoretical **normal curve** is an expression of statistical theory. It is a theoretical frequency distribution of all *possible* scores (see Figure 21-2). However, no real distribution fits the normal curve exactly. The idea of the normal curve was developed by an 18-year-old mathematician, Gauss, in 1795, who found that data measured repeatedly in many samples from the same population by using scales based on an underlying continuum can be combined into one large sample. From this large sample, one can develop a more accurate representation of the pattern of the curve in that population than is possible with only one sample. In most cases, the curve is similar, regardless of the specific data that have been examined or the population being studied. This theoretical normal curve is symmetrical and unimodal and has continuous values. The mean, median, and mode are equal. The distribution is completely defined by the mean and standard deviation, which are calculated and discussed further in Chapter 22.

Sampling Distributions

The shape of the distribution provides important information about the data. The outline of the distribution shape is obtained by using a histogram. Within this outline, the mean, median, mode, and standard

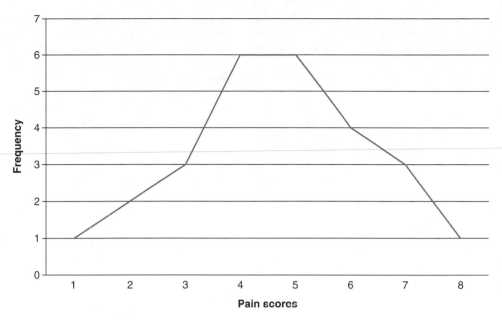

Figure 21-1 Frequency distribution of visual analogue scale pain scores.

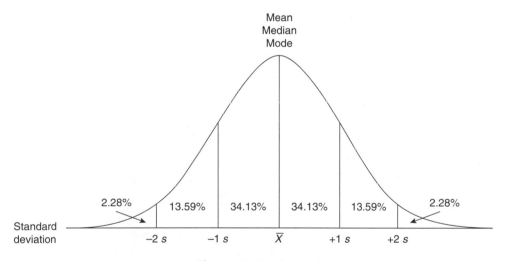

Figure 21-2 Normal curve.

deviation can be graphically illustrated (see Figure 21-2). This visual presentation of combined summary statistics provides insight into the nature of the distribution. As the sample size becomes larger, the shape of the distribution more accurately reflects the shape of the population from which the sample was taken. Even when statistics, such as means, come from a population with a skewed (asymmetrical) distribution, the sampling distribution developed from multiple means obtained from that skewed population tends to fit the pattern of the normal curve. This phenomenon is referred to as the **central limit theorem**.

Symmetry
Several terms are used to describe the shape of the curve (and the nature of a particular distribution). The shape of a curve is usually discussed in terms of symmetry, skewness, modality, and kurtosis. A

symmetrical curve is one in which the left side is a mirror image of the right side (see Figure 21-3). In these curves, the mean, median, and mode are equal and are the dividing point between the left and right sides of the curve.

Skewness

Any curve that is not symmetrical is referred to as **skewed** or **asymmetrical**. Skewness may be exhibited in the curve in various ways. A curve may be **positively skewed**, which means that the largest portion of data is below the mean. For example, data on length of enrollment in hospice are positively skewed. Most people die within the first 3 weeks of enrollment, whereas increasingly smaller numbers survive as time increases. A curve can also be **negatively skewed**, which means that the largest portion of data is above the mean. For example, data on the

occurrence of chronic illness by age in a population are negatively skewed, with most chronic illnesses occurring in older age groups. Figure 21-4 includes both a positively skewed distribution and a negatively skewed distribution.

In a *skewed distribution*, the mean, median, and mode are not equal. Skewness interferes with the validity of many statistical analyses; therefore, statistical procedures have been developed to measure the skewness of the distribution of the sample being studied. Few samples are perfectly symmetrical; however, as the deviation from symmetry increases, the seriousness of the impact on statistical analysis increases. In a positively skewed distribution, the mean is greater than the median, which is greater than the mode. In a negatively skewed distribution, the mean is less than the median, which is less than the mode (see Figure 21-4).

Modality

Another characteristic of distributions is their modality. Most curves found in practice are **unimodal**, which means that they have one mode, and frequencies progressively decline as they move away from the mode. Symmetrical distributions are usually unimodal. However, curves can also be **bimodal** (see Figure 21-5) or multimodal. When you find a bimodal

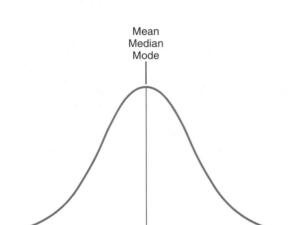

Figure 21-3 **Symmetrical curve.**

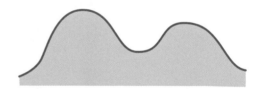

Figure 21-5 **Bimodal distribution.**

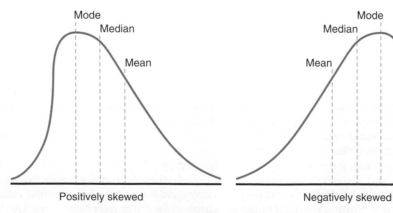

Figure 21-4 **Skewness.**

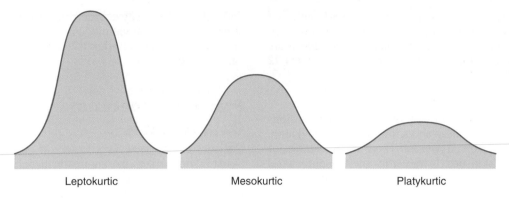

Leptokurtic   Mesokurtic   Platykurtic

Figure 21-6 Kurtosis.

sample, it usually means that you have not defined your population adequately.

Kurtosis

Another term used to describe the shape of the distribution curve is kurtosis. Kurtosis explains the degree of peakedness of the curve, which is related to the spread or variance of scores. An extremely peaked curve is referred to as leptokurtic, an intermediate degree of kurtosis is referred to as mesokurtic, and a relatively flat curve is referred to as platykurtic (see Figure 21-6). Extreme kurtosis can affect the validity of statistical analysis because the scores have little variation in a leptokurtic curve. Many computer programs analyze kurtosis before conducting statistical analyses. A kurtosis of zero indicates that the curve is mesokurtic. Kurtosis values above zero indicate that the curve is leptokurtic, and values below zero that are negative indicate a platykurtic curve (Box, Hunter, & Hunter, 1978).

Tests of Normality

Statistics are computed to obtain an indication of the skewness and kurtosis of a given frequency distribution. The Shapiro-Wilk's W test is a formal test of normality that assesses whether the distribution of a variable is skewed or kurtotic or both. This test has the ability to calculate both skewness and kurtosis for a study variable such as pain measured with a visual analog scale. For large samples ($n > 2000$), the Kolmogorov-Smirnov D test is an alternative test of normality for large samples.

Variation

The range, standard deviation, and variance are statistics that describe the extent to which the values in the sample vary from one another. The most common of these statistics to be reported in the literature is the standard deviation because of its direct association with the normal curve. If the frequency distribution of any given variable is approximately normal, knowing the standard deviation of that variable allows us to know what percentages of subjects' values on that variable fall between +1 and −1 standard deviation. Referring back to the hypothetical frequency distribution of pain in Figure 21-1, when we calculate a standard deviation, we know that 34.13% of the subjects' pain scores were between the mean pain score and 1 standard deviation above the mean pain score. We also know that 34.13% of the subjects' pain scores were between the mean pain score and 1 standard deviation below the mean. The middle 95.44% of the subjects' scores were between −2 standard deviations and +2 standard deviations.

Confidence Intervals

When the probability of including the value of the parameter within the interval estimate is known, this is referred to as a confidence interval. Calculating a confidence interval involves the use of two formulas to identify the upper and lower ends of the interval (see Chapter 22 for calculations). Confidence intervals are usually expressed as "(38.6, 41.4)," with 38.6 being the lower end and 41.4 being the upper end of the interval. Theoretically, we can produce a confidence interval for any parameter of a distribution. It is a generic statistical procedure. Confidence intervals can also be developed around correlation coefficients (Glass & Stanley, 1970). Estimation can be used for a single population or for multiple populations. In estimation, we are inferring the value of a parameter from sample data and have no preconceived notion of the value of the parameter. In contrast, in hypothesis testing, we have an a priori theory about the value of the parameter or parameters or some combination of parameters. A formula is provided for calculating conference intervals and example confidence intervals are provided for different analysis results in Chapters 22 through 25.

Inferential Statistics

Inferential statistics are computed to draw conclusions and make inferences about the greater population, based on the sample data set. There are two classes of inferential statistics: parametric and nonparametric statistics.

Parametric Statistics

The most commonly used type of statistical analysis is parametric statistics. The analysis is referred to as parametric statistical analysis because the findings are inferred to the parameters of a normally distributed population. These approaches to analysis emerged from the work of Fisher (1935) and require meeting the following three assumptions before they can justifiably be used.

1. The sample was drawn from a population for which the variance can be calculated. The distribution is usually expected to be normal or approximately normal (Conover, 1971, Munro, 2005).
2. Because most parametric techniques deal with continuous variables rather than discrete variables, the level of measurement should be at least interval level data or ordinal data with an approximately normal distribution.
3. The data can be treated as random samples (Box et al., 1978).

Nonparametric Statistics

Nonparametric statistical analysis, or distribution-free techniques, can be used in studies that do not meet the first two assumptions of normal distribution and at least interval level data. Most nonparametric techniques are not as powerful as their parametric counterparts (Tanizaki, 1997). In other words, nonparametric techniques are less able to detect differences and have a greater risk of a Type II error if the data meet the assumptions of parametric procedures; this is generally because nonparametric statistics are actually performed on ranks of the original data. When data have been converted into ranks, they inevitably lose accuracy. Because nonparametric statistics have lower statistical power, many researchers choose to submit ordinal data to parametric statistical procedures. If the instrument or measurement procedure yielding ordinal data has been rigorously evaluated, parametric statistics are justified (Fife-Schaw, 1995). For example,

researchers often analyze data from a Likert scale with strong reliability and validity as though they are interval level data (see Chapter 17 for a description of Likert scales).

Practical Aspects of Data Analysis

Statistics can be used for a variety of purposes, such as to (1) summarize, (2) explore the meaning of deviations in the data, (3) compare or contrast descriptively, (4) test the proposed relationships in a theoretical model, (5) infer that the findings from the sample are indicative of the entire population, (6) examine causality, (7) predict, or (8) infer from the sample to a theoretical model. These different purposes for data analysis are addressed in Chapters 22 through 25.

The process of quantitative data analysis consists of several stages: (1) preparation of the data for analysis; (2) description of the sample; (3) testing the reliability of measurement; (4) exploratory analysis of the data; (5) confirmatory analysis guided by the hypotheses, questions, or objectives; and (6) post hoc analysis. Statisticians such as Tukey (1977) divided the role of statistics into two parts: exploratory data analysis and confirmatory data analysis. You can perform exploratory data analysis to obtain a preliminary indication of the nature of the data and to search the data for hidden structure or models. Confirmatory data analysis involves traditional inferential statistics, which you can use to make an inference about a population or a process based on evidence from the study sample.

Although not all of these six stages are reflected in the final published report of the study, they all contribute to the insight you can gain from analyzing the data. Many novice researchers do not plan the details of data analysis until the data are collected and they are confronted with the analysis task. This research technique is poor and often leads to the collection of unusable data or the failure to collect the data needed to answer the research questions. Plans for data analysis need to be made during development of the study methodology. The following section covers the six stages of quantitative data analysis.

Preparing the Data for Analysis

Except in very small studies, computers are almost universally used for data analysis. Use of computers has increased over the last decade with easy-to-use data analysis packages becoming available for personal computers (PCs). When computers are used for analysis, the first step of the process is entering the data into the computer. Table 21-2 lists examples of common statistical packages used for nursing research.

Before entering data into the computer, the computer file that will contain the data needs to be carefully prepared with information from the codebook as described in Chapter 20. The location of each variable in the computer file needs to be identified. Each variable must be labeled in the computer so that the variables involved in a particular analysis are clearly designated on the computer printouts. Develop a systematic plan for data entry that is designed to reduce errors during the entry phase, and enter data during periods when you have few interruptions.

In some cases, data must be reverse-scored before initiating data analysis. Items in scales are often arranged so that sometimes a higher numbered response indicates more of the construct being studied, and sometimes a higher numbered response indicates less of the construct being studied. This arrangement prevents the subject from giving a global response to all items in the scale. To reduce errors, the values on these items need to be entered into the computer exactly as they appear on the data collection form. Values on the items are reversed by computer commands.

Cleaning the Data

Print the data file so that the data can be examined for errors. When the size of the data file allows, you need to cross-check every datum on the printout with the original datum for accuracy. Otherwise, randomly check the accuracy of data points. Correct all errors found in the computer file. Perform a computer analysis of the frequencies of each value of every variable as a second check of the accuracy of the data. Search for values outside the appropriate range of values for that variable. Data that have been scanned into a computer are less likely to have errors but should still be checked.

Identifying Missing Data

Identify all missing data points. Determine whether the information can be obtained and entered into the data file. If a large number of subjects have missing data on specific variables, you need to make a judgment regarding the availability of sufficient data to perform analysis with those variables. In some cases, subjects must be excluded from the analysis because of missing essential data. Missing data can also be imputed via missing data statistical procedures. The rules involving the appropriateness of missing data imputations are complex, and there are many choices

of statistical applications. The seminal publication on the subject of missing data imputation was written by Rubin (1976).

Data Transformations

Skewed or non–normally distributed data that do not meet the assumptions of parametric analysis can sometimes be transformed in such a way that the values are distributed closer to the normal curve. Various mathematical operations are used for this purpose. Examples of these operations include squaring each value, calculating the square root of each value, or calculating the logarithm of each value. These operations can allow the researcher to yield a frequency distribution that more closely approximates normality, freeing the researcher to compute parametric statistics.

Data Calculations and Scoring

Sometimes a variable used in the analysis is not collected but calculated from other variables and is referred to as a calculated variable. For example, if data are collected on the number of patients on a nursing unit and on the number of nurses on a shift, one might calculate a ratio of nurse to patient for a particular shift. The data are more accurate if this calculation is performed by computer rather than manually. The results can be stored in the data file as a variable rather than being recalculated each time the variable is used in an analysis (Shortliffe & Cimino, 2006).

Data Storage and Documentation

When the data-cleaning process is complete, backups need to be made again; labeled as the complete, cleaned data set; and carefully stored. Data cleaning is a time-consuming process that you will not wish to repeat unnecessarily. If your data are being stored on a PC hard disk drive, be sure to back up the information each time you enter more data. It is wise to keep a second copy of the data filed at a separate, carefully protected site. If your data are being stored on a network, ensure that the network drive is being backed up at least once a day. After data entry, you need to store the original data in secure files for safekeeping. The data files need to be secured as designated by institutional review board policies. This usually includes password protecting computer data files or storing data on encrypted flash drives to which only the research team has access.

Results of data analysis can easily become lost in the mountain of printer paper. Rather than keep paper printouts of statistical output, it is recommended that you make pdf (portable document format) files of each output file and store these files in the same folder as your data sets and reports. There are many free pdf converters available on the Internet for download. A pdf converter allows you to convert any file into a pdf file, which can be read by most computer operating systems. Converting output files into pdf files allows the researcher to transport those files and read them on any computer, even a computer that does not house the statistical software that created the original output file.

All files, including data sets and output files, need to be systematically named to allow easy access later when theses or dissertations are being written or research papers are being prepared for publication. We recommend naming files by time sequence. Name the file by its contents, and at the end of the file name, identify the date (month, day, and year) that the file was created or the analysis was performed. For example, the files named "Rehab Outcomes Data 03-29-12" and "Means and Standard Deviations of Pain Subscales 06-23-12" represent a data file saved on March 29, 2012, and a statistical output file containing means and standard deviations of subscale scores saved on June 23, 2012.

When you are preparing papers that describe your study, the results of each analysis reported in the paper need to be cross-indexed with the output file for reference as needed. As interpretation of the results proceeds and you attempt to link various findings, you may question some of the results. Selected results may not seem to fit with the rest of the results, or they may not seem logical. You may find that you have failed to include necessary statistical information. When rewriting a paper for publication, you may need to report additional results requested by reviewers. The search for a particular output can be time-consuming and frustrating if the printouts have not been carefully organized. It is easy to lose needed results and have to repeat the analysis.

Description of the Sample

After the data have been successfully entered in the computer and stored, researchers start conducting the essential analysis techniques for their studies. The first step is to obtain as complete a picture as possible of the sample. The demographic variables, such as age, gender, and economic status, are analyzed with the appropriate analysis techniques and used to develop the characteristics of the sample. The analysis techniques used in describing the sample are covered in Chapter 22.

Testing the Reliability of Measurement Methods

Examine the reliability of the methods of measurement used in the study. The reliability of observational measures or physiological measures may have been obtained during the data collection phase, but it needs to be noted at this point. Additional examination of the reliability of measurement methods, such as a Likert scale, is possible at this point. If you used a multiple-item Likert scale in data collection, alpha coefficients need to be calculated (Waltz, Strickland, & Lenz, 2010). The value of the coefficient needs to be compared with values obtained for the instrument in previous studies. If the alpha coefficient is unacceptably low (<0.6), you need to determine if you are justified in performing analysis on data from the instrument (see Chapter 16).

Exploratory Analysis of the Data

Examine all the data descriptively, with the intent of becoming as familiar as possible with the nature of the data. You might explore the data by conducting measures of central tendency and dispersion and examining outliers of the data. Neophyte researchers often omit this step and jump immediately into the analyses that were designed to test their hypotheses, questions, or objectives. However, they omit this step at the risk of missing important information in the data and performing analyses that are inappropriate for the data. The researcher needs to examine data on each variable by using measures of central tendency and dispersion. Are the data skewed or normally distributed? What is the nature of the variation in the data? Are there outliers with extreme values that appear different from the rest of the sample that cause the distribution to be skewed? The most valuable insights from a study sometimes come from careful examination of outliers (Tukey, 1977).

In many cases, as a part of exploratory analysis, inferential statistical procedures are used to examine differences and associations within the sample. From an exploratory perspective, these analyses are relevant only to the sample under study. There should be no intent to infer to a population. If group comparisons are made, effect sizes need to be determined for the variables involved in the analyses.

In some nursing studies, the purpose of the study is exploratory analysis. In such studies, it is often found that sample sizes are small, power is low, measurement methods have limited reliability and validity, and the field of study is relatively new. If treatments are tested, the procedure might be approached as a pilot study. The most immediate need is tentative exploration of the phenomena under study. Confirming the findings of these studies requires more rigorously designed studies with much larger samples. Many of these exploratory studies are reported in the literature as confirmatory studies, and attempts are made to infer to larger populations. Because of the unacceptably high risk of a Type II error in these studies, negative findings should be viewed with caution.

Using Tables and Graphs for Exploratory Analysis

Although tables and graphs are commonly thought of as a way of presenting the findings of a study, these tools may be even more useful in helping the researcher to become familiar with the data (see Figure 21-1 of the frequency distribution of visual analogue scale pain scores). Tables and graphs need to illustrate the descriptive analyses being performed, even though they will probably not be included in a research report. These tables and figures are prepared for the sole purpose of helping researchers to identify patterns in their data and interpret exploratory findings, but they are sometimes useful in reporting study results to selected groups (Munro, 2005). Visualizing the data in various ways can greatly increase insight regarding the nature of the data (see Chapter 22).

Confirmatory Analysis

As the name implies, confirmatory analysis is performed to confirm expectations regarding the data that are expressed as hypotheses, questions, or objectives. The findings are inferred from the sample to the population. Thus, inferential statistical procedures are used. The design of the study, the methods of measurement, and the sample size must be sufficient for this confirmatory process to be justified. A written analysis plan needs to describe clearly the confirmatory analyses that will be performed to examine each hypothesis, question, or objective.

1. Identify the level of measurement of the data available for analysis with regard to the research objective, question, or hypothesis (see Chapter 16).
2. Select a statistical procedure or procedures appropriate for the level of measurement that will respond to the objective, answer the question, or test the hypothesis.
3. Select the level of significance that you will use to interpret the results, which is usually $\alpha = 0.05$.
4. Choose a one-tailed or two-tailed test if appropriate to your analysis. The extremes of the normal curve are referred to as tails. In a one-tailed test of significance, the hypothesis is directional, and

the extreme statistical values that occur in a single tail of the curve are of interest. In a two-tailed test of significance, the hypothesis is nondirectional or null, and the extreme statistical values in both ends of the curve are of interest. Tailedness is discussed in more detail in Chapter 25.
5. Determine the sample size available for the analysis. If several groups will be used in the analysis, identify the size of each group.
6. Evaluate the representativeness of the sample (see Chapter 15).
7. Determine the risk of a Type II error in the analysis by performing a power analysis.
8. Develop dummy tables and graphics to illustrate the methods that you will use to display your results in relation to your hypotheses, questions, or objectives.
9. Determine the degrees of freedom for your analysis. Degrees of freedom (df) involve the freedom of a score's value to vary given the other existing scores' values. The calculation of df varies based on the analysis techniques conducted; Chapters 22 through 25 provide additional information and examples of df.
10. Perform the analyses with a computer and rarely manually.
11. Compare the statistical value obtained with the table value by using the level of significance, tailedness of the test, and df previously identified.
12. Most analyses are conducted by computer, and the computer printout includes the statistical value obtained by analyzing the data, p value, and df for each inferential analysis technique.
13. Reexamine the analysis to ensure that the procedure was performed with the appropriate variables and that the statistical procedure was correctly specified in the computer program.
14. Interpret the results of the analysis in terms of the hypothesis, question, or objective.
15. Interpret the results in terms of the framework.

Post Hoc Analysis

Post hoc analyses are commonly performed in studies with more than two groups when the analysis indicates that the groups are significantly different but does not indicate which groups are different. For example, an analysis of variance is conducted to examine the differences among three groups—experimental group, control group, and placebo group—and the groups are found to be significantly different. A post hoc analysis must be performed to determine which of the three groups are significantly different. Post hoc analysis is discussed in more detail in Chapter 25. In other studies, the insights obtained through the planned analyses generate further questions that can be examined with the available data.

Choosing Appropriate Statistical Procedures for a Study

Multiple factors are involved in determining the suitability of a statistical procedure for a particular study. These factors can be related to the nature of the study, the nature of the researcher, and the nature of statistical theory. Specific factors include (1) the purpose of the study; (2) hypotheses, questions, or objectives; (3) design; (4) level of measurement; (5) previous experience in statistical analysis; (6) statistical knowledge level; (7) availability of statistical consultation; (8) financial resources; and (9) access to computers. Use items 1 to 4 to identify statistical procedures that meet the requirements of the study, and narrow your options further through the process of elimination based on items 5 through 9.

The most important factor to examine when choosing a statistical procedure is the study hypothesis. The hypothesis that is clearly stated indicates the statistics needed to test it. An example of a clearly developed hypothesis is, "There is a difference in employment rates between veterans who receive vocational rehabilitation and veterans who are on a wait-list control." This statement tells the researcher that a statistic to determine differences between two groups is appropriate to address this hypothesis.

One approach to selecting an appropriate statistical procedure or judging the appropriateness of an analysis technique is to use a decision tree. A decision tree directs your choices by gradually narrowing your options through the decisions you make. A decision tree that can been helpful in selecting statistical procedures is presented in Figure 21-7.

One disadvantage of decision trees is that if you make an incorrect or uninformed decision (guess), you can be led down a path where you might select an inappropriate statistical procedure for your study. Decision trees are often constrained by space and do not include all the information needed to make an appropriate selection. A more extensive decision tree can be found in *A Guide for Selecting Statistical Techniques for Analyzing Social Science Data* by Andrews, Klem, Davidson, O'Malley, and Rodgers (1981). The following examples of questions designed to guide the selection or evaluation of statistical procedures were extracted from this book:

1. *How many variables does the problem involve?*
2. *How do you want to treat the variables with respect to the scale of measurement?*
3. *What do you want to know about the distribution of the variable?*
4. *Do you want to treat outlying cases differently from others?*
5. *What is the form of the distribution?*
6. *Is a distinction made between a dependent and an independent variable?*
7. *Do you want to test whether the means of the two variables are equal?*
8. *Do you want to treat the relationship between variables as linear?*
9. *How many of the variables are dichotomous?*
10. *Is the dichotomous variable a collapsing of a continuous variable?*
11. *Do you want to treat the ranks of ordered categories as interval scales?*
12. *Do the variables have the same distribution?*
13. *Do you want to treat the ordinal variable as though it were based on an underlying normally distributed interval variable?*
14. *Is the interval variable dependent?*
15. *Do you want a measure of the strength of the relationship between the variables or a test of the statistical significance of differences between groups (Kenny, 1979)?*
16. *Are you willing to assume that an interval-scaled variable is normally distributed in the population?*
17. *Is there more than one dependent variable?*
18. *Do you want to statistically remove the linear effects of one or more covariates from the dependent variable?*
19. *Do you want to treat the relationships among the variables as additive?*
20. *Do you want to analyze patterns existing among variables or among individual cases?*
21. *Do you want to find clusters of variables that are more strongly related to one another than to the remaining variables?*

Each question confronts you with a decision. The decision you make narrows the field of available statistical procedures (see Figure 21-7). Decisions must be made regarding the following:

1. Number of variables (one, two, or more than two)
2. Level of measurement (nominal, ordinal, or interval)
3. Type of variable (independent, dependent, or research)
4. Distribution of variable (normal or non-normal)
5. Type of relationship (linear or nonlinear)

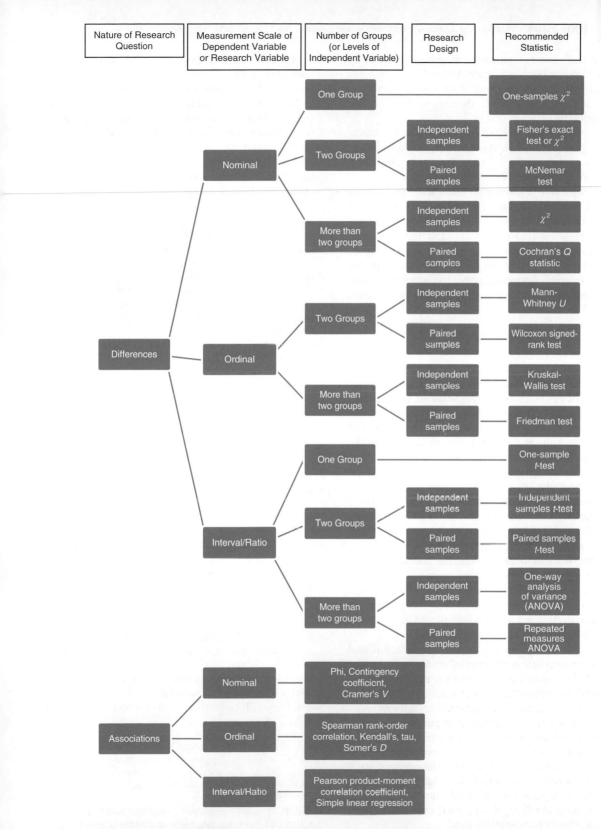

Figure 21-7 Statistical decision tree for selecting an appropriate analysis technique χ^2.

6. What you want to measure (strength of relationship or difference between groups)
7. Nature of the groups (equal or unequal in size, matched or unmatched, dependent [paired] or independent)
8. Type of analysis (descriptive, classification, methodological, relational, comparison, predicting outcomes, intervention testing, causal modeling, examining changes across time)

Selecting and evaluating statistical procedures requires that you make many judgments regarding the nature of the data and what you want to know. Knowledge of the statistical procedures and their assumptions is necessary for selecting appropriate procedures. You must weigh the advantages and disadvantages of various statistical options. Access to a statistician can be invaluable in selecting the appropriate procedures.

KEY POINTS

- This chapter introduces you to the concepts of statistical theory and discusses some of the more pragmatic aspects of quantitative data analysis, including the purposes of statistical analysis, the process of performing data analysis, the choice of the appropriate statistical procedures for a study, and resources for statistical analysis.
- Two types of errors can occur when making decisions about the meaning of a value obtained from a statistical test: Type I errors and Type II errors.
- A Type I error occurs when the researcher concludes a significant effect when no significant effect actually exists.
- A Type II error occurs when the researcher concludes no significant effect when an effect actually exists.
- The formal definition of the level of significance, or alpha (α), is the probability of making a Type I error when the null hypothesis is true.
- The p value is the exact value that can be calculated during a statistical computation to indicate the probability of making a Type I error.
- Power is the probability that a statistical test will detect a significant effect when it actually exists.
- Statistics can be used for various purposes, such as to (1) summarize, (2) explore the meaning of deviations in the data, (3) compare or contrast descriptively, (4) test the proposed relationships in a theoretical model, (5) infer that the findings from the sample are indicative of the entire population, (6) examine causality, (7) predict, or (8) infer from the sample to a theoretical model.

- The quantitative data analysis process consists of several stages: (1) preparation of the data for analysis; (2) description of the sample; (3) testing the reliability of measurement; (4) exploratory analysis of the data; (5) confirmatory analysis guided by hypotheses, questions, or objectives; and (6) post hoc analysis.
- A decision tree is provided to assist you in selecting appropriate analysis techniques to use in analyzing study or clinical data.

REFERENCES

Aberson, C. L. (2010). *Applied power analysis for the behavioral sciences.* New York, NY: Routledge Taylor & Francis Group.

Andrews, F. M., Klem, L., Davidson, T. N., O'Malley, P. M., & Rodgers, W. L. (1981). *A guide for selecting statistical techniques for analyzing social science data* (2nd ed.). Ann Arbor, MI: Survey Research Center, Institute for Social Research, University of Michigan.

Barnett, V. (1982). *Comparative statistical inference.* New York, NY: Wiley.

Box, G. E. P., Hunter, W. G., & Hunter, J. S. (1978). *Statistics for experimenters.* New York, NY: Wiley.

Cohen, J. (1988). *Statistical power analysis for the behavioral sciences* (2nd ed.). New York, NY: Academic Press.

Cohen, J. (1994). The earth is round ($p<.05$). *American Psychologist, 49*(12), 997–1003.

Conover, W. J. (1971). *Practical nonparametric statistics.* New York, NY: Wiley.

Cox, D. R. (1958). *Planning of experiments.* New York, NY: Wiley.

Faul, F., Erdfelder, E., Lang, A.-G., & Buchner, A. (2007). G*Power 3: A flexible statistical power analysis program for the social, behavioral, and biomedical sciences. *Behavior Research Methods, 39*(2), 175–191.

Fife-Schaw, C. (1995). Levels of measurement. In G. M. Breakwell, S. Hammond, & C. Fife-Schaw (Eds.), *Research methods in psychology.* Thousand Oaks, CA: Sage.

Fisher, R. A., Sir. (1935). *The designs of experiments.* New York, NY: Hafner.

Glass, G. V. & Stanley, J. C. (1970). *Statistical methods in education and psychology.* Englewood Cliffs, NJ: Prentice-Hall.

Good, I. J. (1983). *Good thinking: The foundations of probability and its applications.* Minneapolis, MN: University of Minnesota Press.

Grove, S. K. (2007). *Statistics for health care research: A practical workbook.* St. Louis, MO: Saunders.

Kenny, D. A. (1979). *Correlation and causality.* New York, NY: Wiley.

Kerlinger, F. N. & Lee, H. B. (2000). *Foundations of behavioral research* (4th ed.). New York, NY: Harcourt Brace.

Loftus, G. R. (1993). A picture is worth a thousand p values: On the irrelevance of hypothesis testing in the microcomputer age. *Behavior Research Methods, Instrumentation, & Computers, 25*(2), 250–256.

Munro, B. H. (2005). *Statistical methods for health care research* (5th ed.). Philadelphia, PA: Lippincott Williams & Wilkins.

Rubin, D. B. (1976). Inference and missing data. *Biometrika*, *63*(3), 581–592.

Shortliffe, E. H. & Cimino, J. J. (2006). *Biomedical informatics: Computer applications in health care and biomedicine*. New York, NY: Springer Science.

Tanizaki, H. (1997). Power comparison of non-parametric tests: Small-sample properties from Monte Carlo experiments. *Journal of Applied Statistics*, *24*(5), 603–632.

Tukey, J. W. (1977). *Exploratory data analysis*. Reading, MA: Addison-Wesley.

Waltz, C. F., Strickland, O. L., & Lenz, E. R. (2010). *Measurement in nursing and health research* (4th ed.). New York, NY: Springer Publishing Company.

22
CHAPTER

Using Statistics to Describe Variables

There are two major classes of statistics: descriptive statistics and inferential statistics. Descriptive statistics are computed to reveal characteristics of the sample data set. Inferential statistics are computed to gain information about effects in the population being studied. For some types of studies, descriptive statistics are the only approach to analysis of the data. For other studies, descriptive statistics are the first step in the data analysis process, to be followed by inferential statistics. For all studies that involve numerical data, descriptive statistics are crucial in understanding the fundamental properties of the variables being studied. This chapter focuses on descriptive statistics and includes the most common descriptive statistics conducted in nursing research with examples from clinical studies.

Using Statistics to Summarize Data

Frequency Distributions
A basic yet important way to begin describing a sample is to create a frequency distribution of the variable or variables being studied. A frequency distribution can be displayed in a table or figure. A line graph figure can be used to plot one variable, whereby the *x*-axis consists of the possible values of that variable, and the *y*-axis is the tally of each value. The frequency distributions presented in this chapter include values of continuous variables. With a continuous variable, the higher numbers represent more of that variable, and the lower numbers represent less of that variable. Common examples of continuous variables are age, income, blood pressure, weight, height, pain levels, and perception of quality of life.

The frequency distribution of a variable can be presented in a frequency table, which is a way of

organizing the data by listing every possible value in the first column of numbers and the frequency (tally) of each value in the second column of numbers. For example, consider the following hypothetical age data for patients from a primary care clinic. The ages of 20 patients were:

45, 26, 59, 51, 42, 28, 26, 32, 31, 55,
43, 47, 67, 39, 52, 48, 36, 42, 61, 57

First, we must sort the patients' ages from lowest to highest values:

26
26
28
31
32
36
39
42
42
43
45
47
48
51
52
55
57
59
61
67

Next, each age value is tallied to create the frequency. This is an example of an ungrouped frequency distribution. In an ungrouped frequency distribution, researchers list all categories of the variable on which they have data and tally each datum on the listing

TABLE 22-1	Grouped Frequency Distribution of Patient Ages with Percentages		
Adult Age Range	Frequency (*f*)	Percentage	Cumulative Percentage
20-29	3	15%	15%
30-39	4	20%	35%
40-49	6	30%	65%
50-59	5	25%	90%
60-69	2	10%	100%
Total	**20**	**100%**	

(Corty, 2007). In this example, all the different ages of the 20 patients are listed and then tallied for each age.

Age	Frequency
26	2
28	1
31	1
32	1
36	1
39	1
42	2
43	1
45	1
47	1
48	1
51	1
52	1
55	1
57	1
59	1
61	1
67	1

Because most of the ages in this data set have frequencies of "1," it is better to group the ages into ranges of values. These ranges must be mutually exclusive. A patient's age can be classified into only one of the ranges. In addition, the ranges must be exhaustive, meaning that each patient's age fits into at least one of the categories. For example, we may choose to have ranges of 10, so that the age ranges are 20 to 29, 30 to 39, 40 to 49, 50 to 59, and 60 to 69. We may choose to have ranges of 5, so that the age ranges are 20 to 24, 25 to 29, 30 to 34, and so on. The grouping should be devised to provide the greatest possible meaning to the purpose of the study. If the data are to be compared with data in other studies, groupings should be similar to groupings of other studies in this field of research. Classifying data into groups results in the development of a grouped frequency distribution (Munro, 2005).

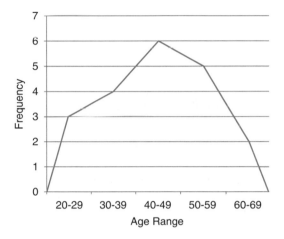

Figure 22-1 Frequency distribution of patient age ranges.

Table 22-1 presents a grouped frequency distribution of patient ages classified by ranges of 10 years. The range starts at "20" because there are no patient ages lower than 20; also, there are no ages higher than 69.

Table 22-1 also includes percentages of patients with an age in each range and the cumulative percentages for the sample, which should add to 100%. This table provides an example of a percentage distribution that indicates the percentage of the sample with scores falling in a specific group or range (Corty, 2007; Munro, 2005). Percentage distributions are particularly useful in comparing the data of the present study with results from other studies.

As discussed earlier, frequency distributions can be presented in figures. Frequencies are commonly presented in graphs, charts, histograms, and frequency polygons. Figure 22-1 is a line graph of the frequency distribution for age ranges, where the *x*-axis (horizontal line) represents the different age ranges, and the *y*-axis (vertical line) represents the frequencies of patients with ages in each of the ranges.

TABLE 22-2 Frequency Table of Smoking Status		
Smoking Status	Frequency	Percentage (%)
Current smoker	1	10%
Former smoker	6	60%
Never smoked	3	30%
Total	**10**	**100%**

TABLE 22-3 Data of Medication Use in Veterans with Rheumatoid Arthritis
Duration of Medication Use (years)
0.1
0.3
1.3
1.5
1.5
2.0
2.2
3.0
3.0
4.0

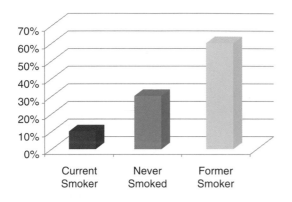

Figure 22-2 Histogram of smoking status.

A frequency table is also an important method to represent nominal data (Corty, 2007; Munro, 2005; Tukey, 1977). For example, a common nominal variable is smoking history. Many researchers assess subjects' history of smoking using nominal categories such as "never smoked," "former smoker," and "current smoker." Table 22-2 presents frequency and percentage distributions for data extracted from a sample of veterans with rheumatoid arthritis (Tran, Hooker, Cipher, & Reimold, 2009).

As shown in Table 22-2, the frequencies indicate that 6 of 10 (60%) veterans were former smokers, and 3 (30%) never smoked. For nominal variables such as smoking status, tables are a helpful method to inform researchers and others about the variable being studied. Graphically representing the values in a frequency table can yield visually important trends. Figure 22-2 is a histogram that was developed to represent the smoking status data visually.

Measures of Central Tendency

A **measure of central tendency** is a statistic that represents the center or middle of a frequency distribution (Corty, 2007; Glass & Stanley, 1970; Grove, 2007). The three measures of central tendency commonly reported in nursing studies include mode, median

(MD), and mean ($\bar{X}$) (Corty, 2007; Munro, 2005). The mode, median, and mean are defined and calculated in this section using data collected from veterans with rheumatoid arthritis (Tran et al., 2009). The data were extracted from a larger sample of veterans who had a history of biologic medication use. Examples of common biologic medications used to treat rheumatoid arthritis are adalimumab, etanercept, and infliximab (Deighton, O'Mahony, Tosh, Turner, & Rudolf, 2009). Table 22-3 contains the data collected from 10 veterans who had stopped taking biologic medications, and the variable represents the number of years that each veteran had taken the medication before the veteran stopped. Because the number of study subjects represented is 10, the correct statistical notation to reflect that number is:

$$n = 10$$

The letter "n" is lowercase because we are referring to a sample of veterans. If the data being presented represented the entire population of veterans, the correct notation would be uppercase "N" (Zar, 1999). Because most nursing research is conducted using samples, not populations, all formulas in Chapters 22 to 25 incorporate the sample notation, n.

Mode

The **mode** is the numerical value or score that occurs with the greatest frequency in a data set. It does not indicate the center of the data set. The data in Table 22-3 contain two modes: 1.5 years and 3.0 years of medication use. Each of these numbers occurred twice in the data set. When two modes exist, the data set is referred to as **bimodal** (see Chapter 21). A data set that contains more than two modes is referred to as **multimodal** (Zar, 1999).

Median

The median (*MD*) is the score at the exact center of the ungrouped frequency distribution. It is the 50th percentile. To obtain the *MD,* sort the values from lowest to highest. If the number of values is an uneven number, exactly 50% of the values are above the *MD* and 50% are below it. If the number of values is an even number, the *MD* is the average of the two middle values; thus, the *MD* may not be an actual value in the data set (Zar, 1999). For example, the data in Table 22-3 consist of 10 observations, and the *MD* is calculated as the average of the two middle values.

$$MD = \frac{(1.5 + 2.0)}{2} = 1.75$$

Mean

The mean is the arithmetic average of all the values of a variable in a study and is the most commonly reported measure of central tendency. The mean is the sum of the scores divided by the number of scores being summed. Similar to the *MD,* the mean may not be a member of the data set. The formula for calculating the mean is as follows:

$$\bar{X} = \frac{\Sigma X}{n}$$

where
$\bar{X}$ = mean
Σ = sigma, the statistical symbol for summation
X = a single value in the sample
n = total number of values in the sample

The mean number of years that the veterans used a biologic medication is calculated as follows:

$$\bar{X} = \frac{\begin{array}{c}(0.1 + 0.3 + 1.3 + 1.5 + 1.5 \\ + 2.0 + 2.2 + 3.0 + 3.0 + 4.0)\end{array}}{10}$$

$$\bar{X} = \frac{18.9}{10} = 1.89 \text{ years}$$

The mean is an appropriate measure of central tendency to calculate for approximately normally distributed populations with variables measured at the interval or ratio levels. It is also appropriate for ordinal level data such as Likert scale or rating scale values (as described in Chapter 17), where higher numbers represent more of the construct being measured, and lower numbers represent less of the construct, such as a 10-point pain rating scale, where 1 represents no noticeable pain and 10 represents dramatically intense pain (Clifford & Cipher, 2005).

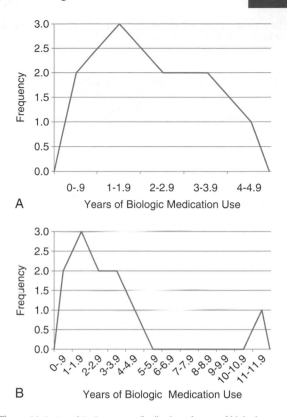

Figure 22-3 **A** and **B,** Frequency distribution of years of biologic medication use, without outlier and with outlier.

The mean is sensitive to extreme scores such as outliers. An outlier is a value in a sample data set that is unusually low or unusually high in the context of the rest of the sample data (Zar, 1999). An example of an outlier in the data presented in Table 22-3 might be a value such as medication use for 11 years. The existing values range from 0.1 to 4.0, indicating that no veteran used a biologic medication beyond 4 years. If an additional veteran was added to the sample, and that person used a biologic medication for 11 years, the mean would be much larger: 2.72 years (mean = 18.9 + 11 = 29.9 ÷ 11 = 2.718 rounded to 2.72). Simply adding this outlier to the sample nearly doubled the mean value. The outlier would also change the frequency distribution. Without the outlier, the frequency distribution is approximately normal, as shown in Figure 22-3. The inclusion of the outlier changes the shape from an approximately normal distribution to a positively skewed distribution (see Figure 22-3) (Zar, 1999). The median is a better measure of central tendency than the mean for these data that are positively skewed by the outlier (see Chapter 21 for discussion of skewness).

Using Statistics to Explore Deviations in the Data

Although the use of summary statistics has been the traditional approach to describing data or describing the characteristics of the sample before inferential statistical analysis, the ability of summary statistics to clarify the nature of data is limited. For example, using measures of central tendency, particularly the mean, to describe the nature of the data obscures the impact of extreme values or deviations in the data. Significant features in the data may be concealed or misrepresented. Often, anomalous, unexpected, problematic data and discrepant patterns are evident, but these are not regarded as meaningful. Measures of dispersion, such as the range, difference scores, variance, and standard deviation, provide important insight into the nature of the data.

Measures of Dispersion

Measures of dispersion or variability are measures of individual differences of the members of the population and sample (Munro, 2005). They indicate how values in a sample are dispersed around the mean. These measures provide information about the data that is not available from measures of central tendency. They indicate how different the scores are—the extent to which individual values deviate from one another. If the individual values are similar, measures of variability are small, and the sample is relatively homogeneous in terms of those values. When there are wide variations or differences in the scores, the sample is considered heterogeneous. The heterogeneity of sample scores or values is determined by measures of dispersion or variability (Zar, 1999). The measures of dispersion most commonly reported in nursing research are range, difference scores, variance, and standard deviation.

Range

The simplest measure of dispersion is the range (Corty, 2007; Munro, 2005). In published studies, range is presented in two ways: (1) the range is the lowest and highest scores, or (2) the range is calculated by subtracting the lowest score from the highest score. The range for the scores in Table 22-3 is 0.3 to 4.0 or can be calculated as follows: $4.0 - 0.3 = 3.7$. In this form, the range is a difference score that uses only the two extreme scores for the comparison. The range is generally reported in published studies but is not used in further analyses.

Difference Scores

Difference scores are obtained by subtracting the mean from each score. Sometimes a difference score is referred to as a deviation score because it indicates the extent to which a score deviates from the mean. Most variables in nursing research are not "scores"; however, the term *difference score* is used to represent the deviation of a value from the mean. The difference score is positive when the score is above the mean, and it is negative when the score is below the mean. The difference scores (both positive and negative) add to zero or approximately zero based on rounding. Difference scores are the basis for many statistical analyses and can be found within many statistical equations. The formula for difference scores is:

$$X - \bar{X}$$

The mean deviation is the average difference score, using the absolute values. The formula for the mean deviation is:

$$\bar{X}_{\text{deviation}} = \frac{\Sigma |X - \bar{X}|}{n}$$

$$\bar{X}_{\text{deviation}} = \frac{\begin{array}{c}1.8 + 1.6 + 0.6 + 0.4 + 0.4 \\ + 0.1 + 0.3 + 1.1 + 1.1 + 2.1\end{array}}{10}$$

$$\bar{X}_{\text{deviation}} = \frac{9.5}{10}$$

$$\bar{X}_{\text{deviation}} = 0.95$$

In this example using the data from Table 22-4, the mean deviation is 0.95. The result indicates that, on average, subjects' duration of biologic medication use deviated from the mean by 0.95 year.

Variance

Variance is another measure of dispersion commonly used in statistical analysis. The equation for a sample variance (s^2) is provided. The lowercase letter "s^2" is used to represent a sample variance. The lowercase Greek sigma "σ^2" is used to represent a population variance, in which the denominator is "N" instead of "$n - 1$." Because most nursing research is conducted using samples, not populations, all formulas in the next several chapters that contain a variance or standard deviation incorporate the sample notation and use

TABLE 22-4	Difference Scores of Duration of Biologic Medication Use	
X	**$-\bar{X}$**	**$X - \bar{X}$**
0.1	−1.9	−1.8
0.3	−1.9	−1.6
1.3	−1.9	−0.6
1.5	−1.9	−0.4
1.5	−1.9	−0.4
2.0	−1.9	0.1
2.2	−1.9	0.3
3.0	−1.9	1.1
3.0	−1.9	1.1
4.0	−1.9	2.1
	Σ of absolute values =	9.5

TABLE 22-5	Calculation of Variance for Duration of Medication Use		
X	**$\bar{X}$**	**$X - \bar{X}$**	**$(X - \bar{X})^2$**
0.1	−1.9	−1.8	3.24
0.3	−1.9	−1.6	2.56
1.3	−1.9	−0.6	0.36
1.5	−1.9	−0.4	0.16
1.5	−1.9	−0.4	0.16
2.0	−1.9	0.1	0.01
2.2	−1.9	0.3	0.09
3.0	−1.9	1.1	1.21
3.0	−1.9	1.1	1.21
4.0	−1.9	2.1	4.41
		Σ	13.41

"$n - 1$" as the denominator. Statistical software packages compute the variance and standard deviation using the sample formulas, not the population formulas.

$$s^2 = \frac{\Sigma(X - \bar{X})^2}{n-1}$$

The variance is always a positive value and has no upper limit. In general, the larger the calculated variance for a study variable is, the larger the dispersion or spread of scores is for the variable. The variance is most often computed to derive the standard deviation because in contrast to the variance, the standard deviation reflects important properties about the frequency distribution of the variable it represents. Table 22-4 displays how you might compute a variance by hand, using the medication use duration data. Table 22-5 shows calculation of variance for duration of medication use.

$$s^2 = \frac{13.41}{9}$$

$$s^2 = 1.49$$

Standard Deviation

Standard deviation (s) is a measure of dispersion that is the square root of the variance. The equation for obtaining a standard deviation is:

$$s = \sqrt{\frac{\Sigma(X - \bar{X})^2}{n-1}}$$

Table 22-5 displays the computations for the variance. To compute the standard deviation, simply take the square root of the variance. You know that the variance of biologic medication duration use is $s^2 = 1.49$. Therefore, the standard deviation of biologic duration is $s = 1.22$. In published studies, sometimes the statistic reported by researchers for standard deviation is *SD*. Either *SD* or *s* might be used in a research report to indicate the standard deviation for a study variable.

The standard deviation is an important statistic, both for understanding dispersion within a distribution and for interpreting the relationship of a particular value to the distribution. Grove's (2007) statistical workbook provides you with a resource for calculating and interpreting the measures of central tendency and measures of dispersion in published studies. The following section summarizes the properties of the standard deviation as it relates to a normal distribution.

Normal Curve

The standard deviation of a variable tells researchers much about the entire sample of values. A frequency distribution of a variable that is *perfectly normally distributed* is shown in Figure 22-4, otherwise known as the **normal curve.**

The normal curve is a perfectly symmetrical frequency distribution. The value at the exact center of a normal curve is the mean of the values. Note the lines to the left and to the right of the mean. Those lines are drawn at +1 standard deviation (which indicates 1 *s* above the mean) and −1 standard deviation (which indicates 1 *s* below the mean), +2 standard deviations above the mean, −2 standard deviations below the mean, and so forth. When a frequency distribution is shaped like the normal curve, we know that 34.13%

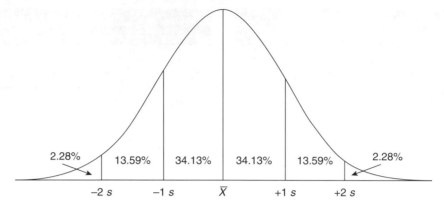

Figure 22-4 Normal curve. *s* = Standard deviation

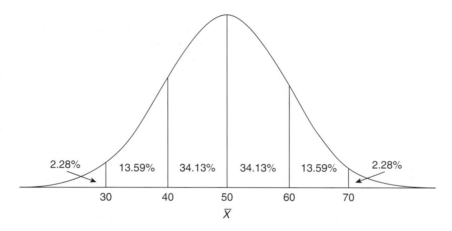

Figure 22-5 Frequency distribution of SF-36 Physical Functioning Scale values.

of the subjects scored between the mean and 1 standard deviation above the mean, and 34.13% of the subjects scored between the mean and 1 standard deviation below the mean. Because the normal curve is perfectly symmetrical, we also know that 50% of the subjects scored above the mean, and 50% of the subjects scored below the mean.

You can also say that 68.26% of the subjects scored between −1 and +1 standard deviation. This number is obtained by adding 34.13% and 34.13%. Furthermore, we can say that 95.44% of the subjects scored between −2 and +2 standard deviations. If we are given a mean and a standard deviation value for any variable that is normally distributed, we know certain facts about those data. For example, consider a score obtained on a subscale of the Short Form (36) Health survey (SF-36). The SF-36 is a widely used health survey that yields eight subscales that each represent a domain of subjective health status (Ware &

Sherbourne, 1992). The subscales have been normed on populations of respondents as having a mean of 50 and standard deviation of 10. The frequency distribution of responses for the subscale "Physical Functioning" can be drawn as seen in Figure 22-5.

The mean is marked as "50" in the middle, and the standard deviations are marked at the lines. Therefore, you know that 34.13% of the population scores between a 50 and a 60 on the Physical Functioning subscale. You also know that 95.44% of the population scores between 30 and 70 on the Physical Functioning subscale. Figure 22-5 shows that only 2.28% of the population scores above a value of 70 (this is computed by subtracting 34.13% and 13.59% from 50%). Likewise, only 2.28% of the population scores below a value of 30.

When using examples such as these, researchers often use the statistic "*z*" instead of the term "standard deviation." A *z* value is synonymous with a standard deviation unit. A z value of 1.0 represents 1 standard deviation unit above the mean. A z value of -1.0 represents 1 standard deviation unit below the mean. Although a standard deviation value cannot have a negative value, a z value can be negative or positive. A z of 0 represents exactly the mean value. Any value in a data set can be converted to a z by using the following formula:

$$z = \frac{(X - \bar{X})}{s}$$

For example, a person scoring a 61 on the SF-36 Physical Functioning scale would have a z value of 1.1:

$$z = \frac{(61 - 50)}{10}$$

$$z = 1.1$$

It is important to note how z values represent standard deviations on the normal curve because this knowledge becomes necessary when performing significance testing in inferential statistics. For example, observe how a z value of 1.0 or -1.0 is much more common than a z value of 3.0 or -3.0. The farther the z value is from the mean, the more uncommon, unusual, and unlikely that value is to occur. This principle is revisited in Chapters 23 through 25.

The distribution of the normal curve is drawn once more in Figure 22-6 but this time with the z statistic, where z represents 1 standard deviation unit. Common values of z are smaller values and closer to the mean. Uncommon and unusual z values are farther away from the mean (either lower than the mean or higher than the mean). When a variable is normally distributed, 95% of z values for that variable fall somewhere between a z of -1.96 and 1.96; 99% of z values for that variable fall somewhere between a z of -2.58 and 2.58 (see Figure 22-6). A table of z values can be found in Appendix A.

Sampling Error

A standard error describes the extent of **sampling error**. A **standard error of the mean** is calculated to determine the magnitude of the variability associated with the mean. A small standard error is an indication that the sample mean is close to the population mean. A large standard error yields less certainty that the sample mean approximates the population mean. The formula for the standard error of the mean ($s_{\bar{X}}$) is:

$$s_{\bar{X}} = \frac{s}{\sqrt{n}}$$

where
$s_{\bar{X}}$ = standard error of the mean
s = standard deviation
n = sample size

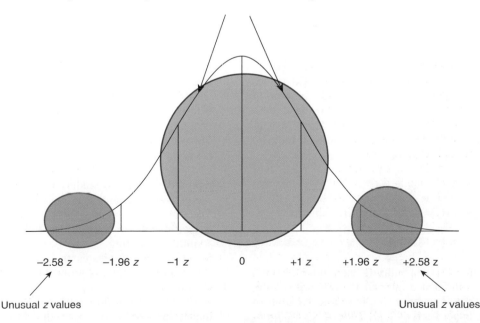

Figure 22-6 **Distribution of z values.**

Using the biologic medication duration data, we know that the standard deviation of biologic duration is $s = 1.22$. Therefore, the standard error of the mean for biologic duration is computed as follows:

$$s_{\bar{X}} = \frac{1.22}{\sqrt{10}}$$

$$s_{\bar{X}} = 0.39$$

The standard error of the mean for biologic duration is 0.39.

Confidence Intervals

To determine how closely the sample mean approximates the population mean, the standard error of the mean is used to build a **confidence interval**. A confidence interval can be created for many statistics, such as a mean, proportion, and odds ratio. To build a confidence interval around a statistic, you must have the standard error value and the t value to adjust the standard error. The t is a statistic for the t-test that is calculated to determine group differences and is discussed in more detail in Chapter 25. The degrees of freedom (df) to use to compute a confidence interval is:

$$df = n - 1$$

To compute the confidence interval for a mean, the lower and upper limits of that interval are created by multiplying the $s_{\bar{X}}$ by the t statistic, where $df = n - 1$. For a 95% confidence interval, the t value should be selected at alpha (α) = 0.05. For a 99% confidence interval, the t value should be selected at $\alpha = 0.01$.

Using the biologic medication duration data, we know that the standard error of the mean duration of biologic medication use is $s_{\bar{X}} = 0.39$. The mean duration of biologic medication use is 1.89. The 95% confidence interval for the mean duration of biologic medication use is computed as follows:

$$\bar{X} \pm s_{\bar{X}}t$$

$$1.89 \pm (0.39)(2.26)$$

$$1.89 \pm .88$$

As referenced in Appendix B, the t value required for the 95% confidence interval with $df = 9$ is 2.26. The previous computation results in a lower limit of 1.01 and an upper limit of 2.77. *Thus, it is 95% probable that the population mean is between 1.01 and*

2.77. If we were to compute a 99% confidence interval, we would require the t value that is referenced at $\alpha = 0.01$. The 99% confidence interval for the mean duration of biologic medication use is computed as follows:

$$1.89 \pm (0.39)(3.25)$$

$$1.89 \pm 1.27$$

As referenced in Appendix B, the t value required for the 99% confidence interval with $df = 9$ is 3.25. The previous computation results in a lower limit of 0.62 and an upper limit of 3.16. Thus, it is 99% probable that the population mean is between 0.62 and 3.16.

Degrees of Freedom

The concept of degrees of freedom was used in reference to computing a confidence interval. For any statistical computation, **degrees of freedom** is the number of independent pieces of information that are free to vary to estimate another piece of information (Zar, 1999). In the case of the confidence interval, the degrees of freedom (df) is $n - 1$. This means that there are $n - 1$ independent observations in the sample that are free to vary (to be any value) to estimate the lower and upper limits of the confidence interval.

--- **KEY POINTS** ---

- Data analysis begins with descriptive statistics in any study in which the data are numerical, including demographic variables for samples in quantitative and qualitative studies.
- Descriptive statistics allow the researcher to organize the data in ways that facilitate meaning and insight.
- Three measures of central tendency are the mode, median, and mean.
- The measures of dispersion most commonly reported in nursing studies are range, difference scores, variance, and standard deviation.
- The standard deviation and z represent certain properties of the normal curve that are used in significance testing.
- Standard error indicates the extent of sampling error, and a formula is provided for calculation of sampling error.
- To determine how closely the sample mean approximates the population mean, the standard error of the mean is used to build a confidence interval. The

formulas and calculations for the 95% and 99% confidence intervals are presented.

- For any statistical computation, degrees of freedom are the number of independent pieces of information that are free to vary to estimate another piece of information.

REFERENCES

Clifford, P. A. & Cipher, D. J. (2005). The Geriatric Multidimensional Pain and Illness Inventory: A new instrument measuring pain and illness in long-term care. *Clinical Gerontologist*, *28*(3), 45–61.

Corty, E. W. (2007). *Using and interpreting statistics: A practical text for the health, behavioral, and social sciences*. St. Louis, MO: Mosby Elsevier.

Deighton, C., O'Mahony, R., Tosh, J., Turner, C., & Rudolf, M. (2009). Guideline Development Group. Management of rheumatoid arthritis: Summary of NICE guidelines. *BMJ*, *338*, b702.

Glass, G. V. & Stanley, J. C. (1970). *Statistical methods in education and psychology*. Englewood Cliffs, NJ: Prentice-Hall.

Grove, S. K. (2007). *Statistics for health care research: A practical workbook*. St. Louis, MO: Saunders Elsevier.

Munro, B. H. (2005). *Statistical methods for health care research* (5th ed.). Philadelphia, PA: Lippincott Williams & Wilkins.

Tran, S., Hooker, R. S., Cipher, D. J., & Reimold, A. (2009). Patterns of biologic use in inflammatory diseases: Older males. *Drugs & Aging*, *26*(7), 607–615.

Tukey, J. W. (1977). *Exploratory data analysis*. Reading, MA: Addison-Wesley.

Ware, J. E. & Sherbourne, C. D. (1992). The MOS 36-Item Short-Form Health Survey (SF-36(r)): Conceptual framework and item selection. *Medical Care*, *30*(6), 473–483.

Zar, J. H. (1999). *Biostatistical analysis* (4th ed.). Upper Saddle River, NJ: Prentice-Hall.

23
CHAPTER

Using Statistics to Examine Relationships

Correlational analyses identify relationships or associations among variables. There are many different kinds of statistics that yield a measure of correlation. All of these statistics address a research question or hypothesis that involves an association or a relationship. Examples of research questions that are answered with correlation statistics are as follows: "Is there an association between weight loss and depression?" "Is there a relationship between patient satisfaction and health status?" A hypothesis is developed to identify the nature (positive or negative) of the relationship between the variables being studied. For example, a researcher may hypothesize that better self-reported health is associated with higher levels of patient satisfaction (Cipher & Hooker, 2006).

This chapter presents the common analysis techniques used to examine relationships in studies. The analysis techniques discussed include the use of scatter diagrams before correlational analysis, bivariate correlational analysis, testing the significance of a correlational coefficient, spurious correlations, correlations between two raters or measurements, the role of correlation in understanding causality, and multivariate correlational procedure–factor analysis.

Scatter Diagrams

Scatter plots or scatter diagrams provide useful preliminary information about the nature of the relationship between variables (Corty, 2007; Munro, 2005). The researcher should develop and examine scatter diagrams before performing a correlational analysis. Scatter plots may be useful for selecting appropriate correlational procedures, but most correlational procedures are useful for examining linear relationships only. A scatter plot can easily identify nonlinear relationships; if the data are nonlinear, the researcher should select statistical alternatives such as nonlinear regression analysis (Zar, 1999). A scatter plot is created by plotting the values of two variables on an *x*-axis and *y*-axis. As shown in Figure 23-1, pain levels from 14 long-term care residents were plotted against their number of behavioral disturbances (Cipher, Clifford, & Roper, 2006). Specifically, each resident's pair of values (pain score, behavior value) was plotted on the diagram. Pain was measured with the Geriatric Multidimensional Pain and Illness Inventory (GMPI), and behavioral disturbances were measured by the Geriatric Level of Dysfunction Scale (Clifford, Cipher, & Roper, 2005). The resulting scatter plot reveals a linear trend whereby higher levels of pain tend to correspond with higher behavioral disturbance values. The line drawn in Figure 23-1 is a regression line that represents the concept of **least-squares**. A **least-squares regression line** is a line drawn through a scatter plot that represents the smallest deviation of each value from the line (Cohen & Cohen, 1983). Regression analysis is discussed in detail in Chapter 24.

Bivariate Correlational Analysis

Bivariate correlational analysis measures the magnitude of linear relationship between two variables and is performed on data collected from a single sample (Munro, 2005). The particular correlation statistic that is computed depends on the scale of measurement of each variable. Correlational techniques are available for all levels of data: nominal (phi, contingency coefficient, Cramer's *V*, and lambda), ordinal (Spearman rank order correlation coefficient, gamma, Kendall's tau, and Somers' *D*), or interval and ratio (Pearson's product-moment correlation coefficient). Figure 21-7 in Chapter 21 illustrates the level of measurement for which each of these statistics is appropriate. Many of the correlational techniques (Kendall's tau, contingency coefficient, phi, and Cramer's *V*) are used in conjunction with contingency tables, which illustrate how values of one variable vary with values

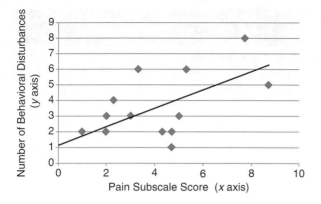

Figure 23-1 Scatter plot of pain and behavioral disturbances.

TABLE 23-1	Strength of Relationships	
Strength of Relationship	Positive Relationship	Negative Relationship
Weak relationship	0.00 to <0.30	0.00 to <−0.30
Moderate relationship	0.30 to 0.50	−0.30 to −0.50
Strong relationship	>0.50	>−0.50

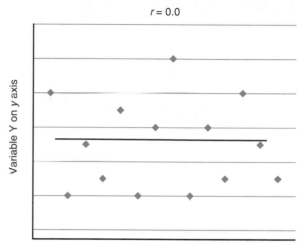

Figure 23-2 Scatter plot of r equal to approximately 0.00 representing no relationship between two variables.

for a second variable. Contingency tables are explained further in Chapter 25.

Correlational analysis provides two pieces of information about the data: the nature or direction of the linear relationship (positive or negative) between the two variables and the magnitude (or strength) of the linear relationship. *Correlation statistics are not an indication of causality,* no matter how strong the statistical result.

In a **positive linear relationship**, the values being correlated vary together (in the same direction). When one value is high, the other value tends to be high; when one value is low, the other value tends to be low. The relationship between weight and blood pressure is considered positive because the more a patient weighs, usually the higher his or her blood pressure. In a **negative linear relationship**, when one value is high, the other value tends to be low. There is a negative linear relationship between calories consumed and weight loss because the more calories a person consumes, the less his or her weight loss. A negative linear relationship is sometimes referred to as an **inverse linear relationship**—the terms *negative* and *inverse* are synonymous in correlation statistics.

Sometimes the relationship between two variables is **curvilinear**, which reflects a relationship between the variables that changes over the range of both variables. For example, one of the most famous curvilinear relationships is that of stress and test performance. Test performance tends to be better as test-takers have more stress but only up to a point. When students experience very high stress levels, test performance deteriorates (Lupien, Maheu, Tu, Fiocco, & Schramek, 2007; Yerkes & Dodson, 1908). Analyses designed to test for linear relationships or associations between two variables, such as Pearson's correlation, cannot detect a curvilinear relationship.

Pearson's Product-Moment Correlation Coefficient

Pearson's product-moment correlation was the first of the correlation measures developed and is the most commonly used (Corty, 2007; Munro, 2005). This coefficient (statistic) is represented by the letter r, and the value of r is always between −1.00 and +1.00. A value of zero indicates no relationship between the two variables. A positive correlation indicates that higher values of X are associated with higher values of Y, and lower values of X are associated with lower values of Y. A negative or inverse correlation indicates that higher values of X are associated with lower values of Y. The r value is indicative of the slope of the line (called a regression line) that can be drawn through a standard scatter plot of the values of two paired variables. The strengths of different relationships are identified in Table 23-1 (Aberson, 2010; Cohen, 1988). Figure 23-2 represents an r value approximately equal to zero, indicating no relationship or association between the two variables. An r value is rarely, if ever, equal to exactly zero. Figure 23-3 shows an r value equal to 0.50, which is a

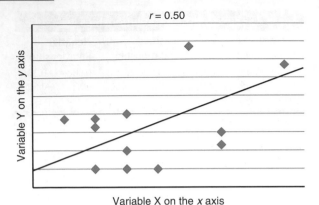

$r = 0.50$

Variable Y on the *y* axis

Variable X on the *x* axis

Figure 23-3 Scatter plot of variables where *r* is 0.50, representing a moderate positive correlation.

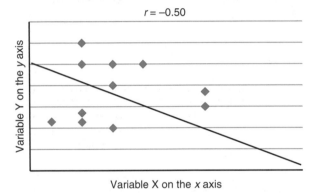

$r = -0.50$

Variable Y on the *y* axis

Variable X on the *x* axis

Figure 23-4 Scatter plot of variables where *r* is –0.50, representing a moderate inverse correlation.

moderate positive relationship. Figure 23-4 shows an *r* value equal to –0.50, which is a moderate negative or inverse relationship.

As discussed earlier, **Pearson's product-moment correlation coefficient** is used to determine the relationship between two variables measured at least at the interval level of measurement. The formula for Pearson's correlation coefficient is based on the following assumptions:

1. Interval or ratio measurement of both variables (e.g., age, income, blood pressure, cholesterol levels)
2. Normal distribution of at least one variable
3. Independence of observational pairs
4. Homoscedasticity

Data that are **homoscedastic** are evenly dispersed above and below the regression line, which indicates a linear relationship on a scatter plot. Homoscedasticity reflects equal variance of both variables. In other

TABLE 23-2	Computation of Pearson's Correlation				
Patient	X (Behaviors)	Y (Pain)	X^2	Y^2	XY
1	2	1.0	4	1.0	2.0
2	4	2.3	16	5.3	9.2
3	3	5.0	9	25.0	15.0
4	8	7.7	64	59.3	61.6
5	5	8.7	25	75.7	43.5
6	2	4.3	4	18.5	8.6
7	2	1.0	4	1.0	2.0
8	2	2.0	4	4.0	4.0
9	6	3.3	36	10.9	19.8
10	2	4.7	4	22.1	9.4
11	1	4.7	1	22.1	4.7
12	3	2.0	9	4.0	6.0
13	3	3.0	9	9.0	9.0
14	6	5.3	36	28.1	31.8
Total	**49**	**55**	**225**	**286**	**226.6**

words, for every value of *X*, the distribution of *Y* values should have equal variability. If the data for the two variables being correlated are not homoscedastic, inferences made during significance testing could be invalid (Cohen & Cohen, 1983).

Calculation

Pearson's product-moment correlation coefficient is computed using one of several formulas; the following formula is considered the "computational formula" because it makes computation by hand easier (Zar, 1999).

$$r = \frac{n\Sigma XY - \Sigma X\Sigma Y}{\sqrt{[n\Sigma X^2 - (\Sigma X)^2][n\Sigma Y^2 - (\Sigma Y)^2]}}$$

where

r = Pearson's correlation coefficient
n = total number of subjects
X = value of the first variable
Y = value of the second variable
XY = *X* multiplied by *Y*

Table 23-2 displays how one would set up data to compute a Pearson's correlation coefficient. This example includes a subset of data from a study introduced earlier in this chapter of long-term care residents (*n* = 14) with the most severe levels of dementia (Cipher et al., 2006). A subset of data was selected for this illustration so that the computation example would be small and manageable. In actuality, studies involving correlational analysis need to be adequately powered and involve a larger sample than is used here (Aberson, 2010; Cohen, 1988). However, all data presented in this chapter are actual, unmodified clinical data.

The first variable in Table 23-2 is the number of behavioral disturbances being exhibited by the residents. The second variable is the residents' scores on the Pain and Suffering subscale of the GMPI (Clifford & Cipher, 2005). The GMPI is a comprehensive pain assessment instrument that was designed to be used by nurses, social workers, and psychologists to assess pain experienced by a person residing in a long-term care facility. The GMPI Pain and Suffering subscale is scored on a scale of 1 to 10, with higher numbers indicating more severe pain. Higher numbers are also indicative of more behavioral disturbances. The null hypothesis being tested is: *There is no significant association between pain and behavioral disturbances among long-term care residents with severe dementia*. The data in Table 23-2 are arranged in columns, which correspond to the elements of the formula. The summed values in the last row of Table 23-2 are inserted into the appropriate place in the formula:

$$r = \frac{14(226.6) - (49)(55)}{\sqrt{[14(225) - 49^2][14(286) - 55^2]}}$$

$$r = \frac{14(226.6) - (49)(55)}{\sqrt{(749)(979)}}$$

$$r = \frac{477.4}{856.3} = 0.56$$

Interpretation of Results

The *r* value is 0.56, indicating a strong positive relationship between pain and behavioral disturbances among long-term care residents with severe dementia. To determine whether this relationship is improbable to have been caused by chance alone, we consult the *r* probability distribution table. The formula for **degrees of freedom** (*df*) for a Pearson's *r* is *n* − 2. Recall from Chapter 22 that every inferential statistic has its own formula for degrees of freedom (numbers of values that are free to vary). In our analysis, the *df*

is 14 − 2 = 12. With *r* of 0.56 and *df* = 12, you need to consult the table in Appendix C to identify the critical value of *r*. The critical *r* value at α = 0.05, *df* = 12 is 0.532. Our obtained *r* was 0.56, which exceeds the critical value in the table. Therefore, we can conclude that: *There was statistically significant positive correlation between pain and behavioral disturbances exhibited in long-term care residents with severe dementia, r (12) = 0.56,* p < 0.05. The null hypothesis is rejected.

Every inferential statistic can be reflected by a **probability distribution** of that statistic. The table we referred to in Appendix C to determine the significance of our obtained *r* was actually drawn from the probability distribution of *r*. Chapter 22 illustrated the probability distribution of *z*, which appears identical to the normal curve. The Pearson's *r* can be reflected by a theoretical distribution of *r* values. The shape of this distribution changes, depending on the size of the sample. When a Pearson's correlation is computed using a large number of values (*n* > 120), the corresponding distribution of *r* values appears similar to the normal curve. The smaller the sample size, the flatter the *r* distribution, and the larger the sample size, the more the *r* distribution approximates the normal curve reflecting the range of paired values obtained. Sample size matters because the shape of the probability distribution determines whether our obtained statistic is statistically significant (Zar, 1999).

For example, consider our obtained *r* of 0.56, previously calculated. At 12 *df*, the *r* probability distribution looks like that of Figure 23-5. With a sample size of 14 (and 12 *df*), the middle 95% of the *r* probability distribution is marked by −0.53 and 0.53. The mean *r*, theoretically, is *r* = 0. That is, most correlation coefficients computed between two variables equal zero, reflecting no relationships between the two variables. Therefore, an *r* value of 0 is the most common and probable *r* value. It is much more improbable to obtain a high *r* value. At 12 *df*, *r* values within the limits of −0.53 and 0.53 are considered common and likely, and

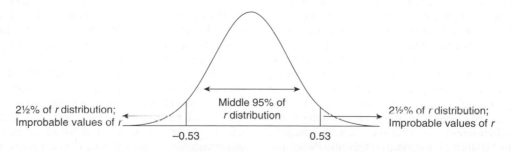

Figure 23-5 Probability distribution of *r* at *df* = 12.

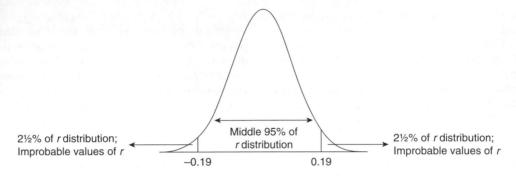

2½% of *r* distribution;
Improbable values of *r*

Middle 95% of
r distribution

2½% of *r* distribution;
Improbable values of *r*

−0.19   0.19

Figure 23-6 **Probability distribution of *r* at *df* = 100.**

values outside of these limits are uncommon, unlikely, and improbable to have occurred by chance. The values outside of these limits constitute 5% of the *r* distribution, which is where the concept of alpha (Type I error) originates. We obtained an *r* of 0.56 and rejected the null hypothesis. In rejecting the null hypothesis, there is less than a 5% chance that we are making a Type I error.

Compare Figure 23-5 with Figure 23-6, in which the probability distribution of *r* at *df* = 100 is displayed. Appendix C tells us that the critical *r* value at alpha (α) = 0.05, *df* = 100 (and a sample size of 102) is *r* = 0.19. This means that the middle 95% of the *r* probability distribution at *df* = 100 is marked by −0.19 and 0.19. Furthermore, *r* values within the limits of −0.19 and 0.19 are considered common and likely, and values outside of these limits are uncommon, unlikely, and improbable to have occurred by chance. Observe the difference that the larger sample size makes in the critical *r* value to achieve significance. The larger the sample size, the smaller the obtained *r* value can be to be considered still statistically significant.

Effect Size

After establishing the statistical significance of *r*, the relationship subsequently must be examined for clinical importance. There are ranges for strength of association suggested by Cohen (1988), as displayed in Table 23-1. One can also assess the magnitude of association by obtaining the **coefficient of determination** for the Pearson's correlation. Computing the coefficient of determination simply involves squaring the *r* value. The r^2 (multiplied by 100%) represents the percentage of variance shared between the two variables (Cohen & Cohen, 1983). In our example, *r* was 0.56, and therefore r^2 was 0.31; this indicates that pain levels and behavioral disturbance shared 31% of the

same variance. More specifically, 31% of the variance in pain levels can be explained by knowing the resident's level of behavioral disturbances, and, vice versa, 31% of the variance in behavioral disturbances can be explained by knowing the resident's pain level (Cipher et al., 2006).

Nonparametric Alternatives

If one or both of your variables do not meet the assumptions for a Pearson's correlation, or if your variables are scaled on an ordinal scale of measurement (rather than interval or ratio), both Spearman's rank-order correlation coefficient and Kendall's tau are more appropriate statistics. The Spearman's rank-order correlation coefficient and Kendall's tau calculations involve converting the data to ranks, discarding any variance or normality issues associated with the original values.

If your data meet the assumptions for the Pearson's correlation coefficient, it is the preferred analysis procedure. You would calculate a nonparametric alternative only if your data violate those assumptions. Because Spearman's correlation and Kendall's tau are based on ranks of the data, the properties of the original data are lost when they are converted to ranks. Because of this fact, most nonparametric statistics of association yield lower statistical power (Daniel, 2000). Grove's (2007) statistical workbook provides examples of Spearman's rank-order correlation coefficient from published studies and provides guidance in the interpretation of these results.

If both of your variables are dichotomous, the phi coefficient is the appropriate statistic to determine an association. If both of your variables are nominal and one or both has more than two categories, Cramer's *V* statistic is the appropriate statistic. Spearman's rank-order correlation coefficient, Kendall's tau, phi, and

Cramer's *V* are addressed in detail by Daniel (2000) and Munro (2005).

Role of Correlation in Understanding Causality

In any situation involving causality, a relationship exists between the factors involved in the causal process. Therefore, the first clue to the possibility of a causal link is the existence of a relationship. However, *a relationship does not mean causality*. For example, blood glucose level may be related to or correlated with body temperature; however, this does not mean that one *causes* the other. Two variables can be highly correlated but have no causal relationship. However, as the strength of a relationship increases, the possibility of a causal link increases. The absence of a relationship precludes the possibility of a causal connection between the two variables being examined, given adequate measurement of the variables and absence of other variables that might mask the relationship (Cohen & Cohen, 1983). A correlational study can be the first step in determining the dynamics important to nursing practice within a particular population. Determining these dynamics can allow us to increase our ability to predict and control the situation studied. However, correlation cannot be used to show causality.

Spurious Correlations

Spurious correlations are relationships between variables that are not logical. In some cases, these significant relationships are a consequence of chance and have no meaning. When you choose a level of significance of $\alpha = 0.05$, 1 in 20 correlations that you compute will be statistically significant by chance alone. There is really no true relationship between the two variables under study in the population; you just happened to draw a sample that showed a relationship where there typically is not one. Other pairs of variables may be correlated because of the influence of other unrelated or confounding variables. For example, you might find a positive correlation between the number of deaths on a nursing unit and the number of nurses working on the unit. The number of deaths cannot be explained as occurring because of increases in the number of nurses. It is more likely that a third variable (units having patients with more critical conditions) explains both the increased number of nurses and the increased number of deaths. In many cases, the "other" variable remains unknown, although the researcher can use reasoning to identify and exclude most of these spurious correlations.

Bland and Altman Plots

Bland and Altman plots are used to examine the extent of agreement between two measurement techniques. In nursing research, Bland and Altman plots are used to display visually the extent of interrater agreement and test-retest agreement (see Chapter 16 for discussion of reliability). For both instances, pairs of data are collected from each subject (from rater 1 and rater 2, or administration 1 and administration 2), and each subject's two values are subtracted from one another. The differences are plotted on a graph, displaying a scatter diagram of the differences plotted against the averages. Limits of agreement are defined as twice the standard deviation above and below the mean. Bland and Altman plots are primarily used to see how many of the values are outside these limits. Acceptable interrater or test-retest agreement is considered to be reflected when at least 95% of the values are within the limits of agreement on the plot (Altman, 1991).

Example

Table 23-3 displays test-retest data obtained from the Clifford and Cipher (2005) study introduced earlier. The GMPI was administered to 22 long-term care residents twice within 48 hours. The score from the GMPI subscale Activity Interference was analyzed for test-retest agreement. This subscale is indicative of the level of functional impairment secondary to pain, rated on a scale of 1 to 10, with 1 representing no impairment and 10 representing extreme impairment (Clifford & Cipher, 2005). Each subject's subscale score at Assessment 1 and Assessment 2 is displayed in Table 23-3, along with the difference between each pair of scores.

A Bland and Altman plot of these data is illustrated in Figure 23-7. The line of perfect agreement is drawn as a dotted line in the exact horizontal middle of the graph, and the limits of agreement are the two outside dotted lines. Only one value is outside of the limits of agreement. Therefore, 21 of the 22 pairs (95.5%) were within the limits of agreement. Incidentally, the *r* between the first and second administrations of the subscale was 0.96. However, the Bland and Altman plot does not always corroborate a Pearson's correlation coefficient, and vice versa, because they are distinctly different methods (Bland & Altman, 1986).

The coefficient of repeatability was created by Bland and Altman (1986) as an indication of the repeatability of a single method of measurement. Because the same method is being measured repeatedly, the mean difference should be zero. Use the following formula to calculate a coefficient of repeatability (*CR*), where $s_{x_1-x_2}$ is the standard deviation of the difference scores.

$$CR = 1.96 \, (s_{x_1-x_2})$$

TABLE 23-3	Test-Retest Data from the Geriatric Multidimensional Pain and Illness Inventory Activity Interference Subscale	
Activity Interference, Time 1	Activity Interference, Time 2	Difference Score
2.0	2.8	0.8
3.0	3.6	0.6
3.8	4.0	0.2
3.6	3.8	0.2
3.2	3.2	0.0
4.4	4.6	0.2
3.6	3.0	−0.6
2.8	2.6	−0.2
3.4	3.4	0.0
5.8	5.6	−0.2
6.8	7.2	0.4
3.0	3.6	0.6
5.0	5.6	0.6
4.8	4.0	−0.8
3.4	3.2	−0.2
6.6	6.0	−0.6
3.0	3.0	0.0
5.8	6.2	0.4
4.8	5.2	0.4
7.0	7.2	0.2
5.8	6.0	0.2
6.0	6.0	0.0

Data from Clifford, P. A., & Cipher, D. J. (2005). The Geriatric Multidimensional Pain and Illness Inventory: A new instrument measuring pain and illness in long-term care. *Clinical Gerontologist, 28*(3), 49.

Table 23-3 displays each difference score, of which $s_{x_1-x_2} = 0.42$. Therefore, the *CR* is calculated as:

$$CR = 1.96 \, (0.42)$$
$$CR = 0.82$$

Interpretation of Results

In their study, Clifford and Cipher (2005) found the *CR* value was 0.82. This value is used to compute lower and upper limits of agreement (Bland & Altman, 1986). The mean difference between the two assessments of Activity Interference was 0.10. In other words, the average difference between the first and second administrations of this subscale was 0.10. A perfect average agreement would be 0, meaning that on average the two sets of scores were exactly the same. The *CR* value, 0.82, is added to and subtracted from the mean difference to create lower and upper limits of acceptable agreement: 0.10 ± 0.82. Differences within 0.10 ± 0.82 would not be deemed clinically important, according to Bland and Altman (2010). Differences between the two administrations that are less than −0.72 and greater than 0.92 are "unacceptable for clinical purposes" (Bland & Altman, 2010). The *CR* is not an inferential statistic, and values of lower and upper limits of agreement are not interpreted the way one would interpret a confidence interval. Rather, they are formulas invented by Bland and Altman for heuristic purposes to make decisions on the extent of agreement between two measurements.

Factor Analysis and Principal Components Analysis

Factor analysis and principal components analysis (PCA) are statistical techniques designed to examine interrelationships among large numbers of variables to

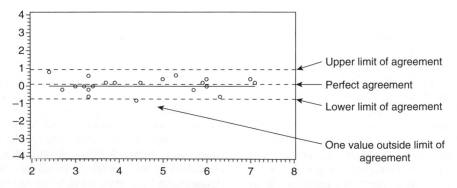

Figure 23-7 Bland and Altman plot of test-retest data.

reduce them to a smaller set of variables and to identify clusters of variables that are most closely linked together (**factors**). Factors are hypothetical constructs created from the original variables. The difference between factor analysis and PCA lies in the method in which the variance of the data is extracted and analyzed (Tabachnick & Fidell, 2006). PCA is the procedure of choice for a researcher who is primarily interested in reducing a large number of variables down to a smaller number of components.

A common reason for performing PCA is to assist with validity investigations of a new measurement method or scale, particularly subjective assessments or instruments that pertain to attitudes, beliefs, values, or opinions. When researchers develop a new instrument, PCA can serve to assist the researcher in investigating its content and construct validity, as described in Chapter 16. The results of PCA assist researchers in understanding which questions are redundant (or assess the same concept), which questions represent subsets of variables, and which items stand alone and reflect unique concepts.

Mathematically, PCA extracts maximum variance (explanatory "power" to predict one variable's value from another's value) from the data set with each "component" (often used interchangeably with "factor"). The first principal component is the linear combination of the variables (or instrument items) that maximizes the variance of their component scores. The second component is formed from residual correlations. Subsequent components are formed from the residual correlations that have not yet been created.

Once the factors have been identified mathematically, the researcher attempts to explain why the variables are grouped as they are. Factor analysis aids in the identification of theoretical constructs. Factor analysis is also used to confirm the accuracy of a theoretically developed construct. For example, a theorist might state that the concept "hope" consists of the elements (1) anticipation of the future, (2) belief that things will work out for the best, and (3) optimism. Instruments could be developed to measure these three elements, and factor analysis could be conducted to determine whether subject responses clustered into these three groupings.

Example

The following example describes how PCA was used to investigate content and construct validity for the GMPI (Clifford & Cipher, 2005). There were 14 items from the GMPI administered to 401 long-term care residents. GMPI, a scale introduced earlier in this chapter, was developed to assess pain experienced

TABLE 23-4 Item Factor Loadings on Three GMPI Subscales

Factor Loading	GMPI Item
Scale 1: Pain and Suffering	
.88	Current level of pain
.86	Level of pain in the last week
.67	Level of suffering in the past week
Scale 2: Activity Interference	
.67	Pain's interference with walking
.60	Pain's interference with sitting up
.84	Pain's interference with leaving room
.91	Pain's interference with social activities
.75	Pain's interference with satisfaction/enjoyment
Scale 3: Emotional Distress	
.85	Lonely because of pain
.63	Irritable due to pain
.69	Anxious due to pain
.73	Coping with problems

Clifford, P. A., & Cipher, D. J. (2005). The Geriatric Multidimensional Pain and Illness Inventory: A new instrument measuring pain and illness in long-term care. *Clinical Gerontologist, 28*(3), 51.

by individuals in long-term care facilities. Of the 14 items, 12 items were retained to be included in the final version of the GMPI scale. Using factor analysis, three factors were identified and are listed in Table 23-4.

The first factor accounted for 40% of the variance extracted from the PCA solution, followed by 16% and 9% from the second and third factors. Table 23-4 lists the factor loadings of each item. **Factor loadings** are the correlations between the item and the new factor. The first factor, named Pain and Suffering by the researchers, was correlated with three of the GMPI items—current level of pain, level of pain in the last week, and level of suffering. All other GMPI items were not highly correlated with factor 1 (the factor loadings were < 0.30) and are not listed in Table 23-4. The second factor, named Activity Interference, was correlated with five of the GMPI items, all of which pertained to life interference secondary to the pain. The factor loadings ranged from 0.60 to 0.91. The third factor, named Emotional Distress, was correlated with four of the GMPI items, all of which pertained to emotional distress secondary to the pain. The factor loadings ranged from 0.63 to 0.85.

In this analysis, the items loaded highly on only one factor, which is not always the case in PCA. For example, the first GMPI item was "How bad is your pain right now?" This item loaded highly on factor 1 (Pain and Suffering) but had low loadings of less than 0.30 on the other two factors. The fourth GMPI item was "How much has your pain interfered with you being able to walk around?" This item loaded highly on factor 2 (Activity Interference) but had low loadings of less than 0.30 on the other two factors. This was the case for all GMPI items, with the exception of two items that did not load highly on any of the factors. Those two items were permanently dropped from the instrument.

"Naming" the Factor

The three factors generated from the PCA were named according to the nature of the items that loaded on those factors. When naming the factor, the researcher must examine the items that cluster together in a factor and seem to explain that clustering. Variables with high loadings on the factor must be included, even if they do not fit the researcher's preconceived theoretical notions of which items "fit" together because they reflect a similar concept. The purpose is to identify the broad construct of meaning that has caused these particular variables to be so strongly intercorrelated. Naming this construct is an important part of the procedure because naming of the factor provides theoretical meaning.

Factor Scores

After the initial factor analysis, additional studies are conducted to examine changes in the phenomenon in various situations and to determine the relationships of the factors with other concepts. **Factor scores** are used during data analysis in these additional studies. To obtain factor scores, the variables included in the factor are identified, and the scores on these variables are summed for each study participant. Thus, each participant has a score for each factor in the instrument. There are several methods of computing factor scores. One of the most common methods involves simply adding the participant's scores on the items that load on a factor. Using the GMPI data as an example, to obtain a factor score for Pain and Suffering, a study participant's scores on current level of pain, pain in the past week, and level of suffering would be summed. For example, if a participant scored an 8 on current pain, 7 on pain the past week, and 9 on level of suffering, the participant's factor score for Pain and Suffering would equal 24.

Individual's factor score for pain
and suffering $= 8 + 7 + 9 = 24$

Another common method of computing a factor score is using the factor loadings to weight each study participant's score. Applying the same hypothetical scores as before, the factor loadings are multiplied by the item scores to create the factor score:

$$(0.88) 8 + (0.86) 7 + (0.67) 9 = 19.09$$

In the first method, each item is weighted equally in the equation because the weight is essentially "1." In the second method, each item is adjusted for the extent to which that item loads on that factor. The advantages and disadvantages of these factor score methods, in addition to descriptions of other methods for obtaining factor scores, are reviewed by DiStefano, Zhu, & and Mîndrilă (2009).

KEY POINTS

- Correlational analyses identify relationships or associations between or among variables.
- The purpose of the analysis is also to clarify relationships among theoretical concepts or help to identify potentially causal relationships, which can be tested by inferential analysis.
- All data for the analysis should have been obtained from a single population from which values are available on all variables to be examined.
- Correlational analysis provides two pieces of information about the data: the nature of a linear relationship (positive or negative) between the two variables and the magnitude (or strength) of the linear relationship.
- Pearson's product-moment correlation coefficient is the preferred computation when investigating the association among two variables measured at the interval or ratio level and when the variables meet the other required statistical assumptions.
- Spearman's rank-order correlation coefficient and Kendall's tau are both nonparametric statistics that are calculated when the assumptions of Pearson's correlation cannot be met, such as variables measured at the ordinal level or non-normal distribution of values for a variable.
- The first clue to the possibility of a causal link is the existence of a relationship, but a relationship does not mean causality.
- Bland and Altman plots are a graphical display of agreement between two administrations of an

instrument or two raters of a clinician-rated instrument.

• The coefficient of repeatability is a value that is used to determine acceptable lower and upper limits of interrater agreement and test-retest agreement.

• Principal components analysis is a procedure that reduces a large number of variables down to a smaller number of components and is most often used during the construction of a new measurement method or scale.

• The results of principal components analysis assist the researcher in understanding which questions assess the same concept and are redundant, which questions represent subsets of variables, and which items stand alone.

REFERENCES

Aberson, C. L. (2010). *Applied power analysis for the behavioral sciences*. New York, NY: Routledge Taylor & Francis Group.

Altman, D. G. (1991). *Practical statistics for medical research* (1st ed.). London, UK: Chapman & Hall.

Bland, J. M., & Altman, D. M. (1986). Statistical methods for assessing agreement between two methods of clinical measurement. *Lancet*, *1*(8476), 307–310.

Bland, J. M., & Altman, D. M. (2010). Statistical methods for assessing agreement between two methods of clinical measurement. *International Journal of Nursing Studies*, *47*(8), 931–936.

Cipher, D. J., Clifford, P. A., & Roper, K. D. (2006). Behavioral manifestations of pain in the demented elderly. *Journal of the American Medical Director's Association*, *7*(6), 355–365.

Cipher, D. J., & Hooker, R. S. (2006). Are patients satisfied with PAs and NPs? *Journal of the American Association of Physician Assistants*, *19*(1), 36–44.

Clifford, P. A., & Cipher, D. J. (2005). The Geriatric Multidimensional Pain and Illness Inventory: A new instrument measuring pain and illness in long-term care. *Clinical Gerontologist*, *28*(3), 45–61.

Clifford, P. A., Cipher, D. J., & Roper, K. D. (2005). Assessing dysfunctional behaviors in long-term care. *Journal of the American Medical Director's Association*, *6*(5), 300–309.

Cohen, J. (1988). *Statistical power analysis for the behavioral sciences* (2nd ed.). Hillsdale, NJ: Lawrence Erlbaum Associates.

Cohen, J., & Cohen, P. (1983). *Applied multiple regression/correlation analysis for the behavioral sciences* (2nd ed.). Hillsdale, NJ: Erlbaum.

Corty, E. W. (2007). *Using and interpreting statistics: A practical text for the health, behavioral, and social sciences*. St. Louis, MO: Mosby.

Daniel, W. W. (2000). *Applied nonparametric statistics* (2nd ed.). Pacific Grove, CA: Duxbury Press.

DiStefano, C., Zhu, M., & Mîndrilă, D. (2009). Understanding and using factor scores: Considerations for the applied researcher. *Practical Assessment, Research & Evaluation*, *14*(20), 1–9.

Grove, S. K. (2007). *Statistics for health care research: A practical workbook*. St. Louis, MO: Saunders.

Lupien, S. J., Maheu, F., Tu, M., Fiocco, A., & Schramek, T. E. (2007). The effects of stress and stress hormones on human cognition: Implications for the field of brain and cognition. *Brain & Cognition*, *65*(3), 209–237.

Munro, B. H. (2005). *Statistical methods for health care research* (5th ed.). Philadelphia, PA: Lippincott Williams, & Wilkins.

Tabachnick, B. G., & Fidell, L. S. (2006). *Using multivariate statistics* (5th ed.). Needham Heights, MA: Allyn & Bacon.

Yerkes, R. M., & Dodson, J. D. (1908). The relation of strength of stimulus to rapidity of habit-formation. *Journal of Comparative Neurology & Psychology*, *18*(5), 459–482.

Zar, J. H. (1999). *Biostatistical analysis* (4th ed.). Upper Saddle River, NJ: Prentice-Hall.

24
CHAPTER

Using Statistics to Predict

In nursing practice, the ability to predict future events is crucial. Clinical researchers might investigate if length of hospital stay of patients can be predicted by severity of illness. Health outcome researchers want to know what factors play an important role in responses of patients to health promotion, illness prevention, and rehabilitation interventions. Educators are interested in knowing what variables are most effective in predicting scores of undergraduate nurses on the registered nurse (RN) licensure examination. Advanced practice nurses are interested in what variables predict their success in passing their national certification examinations.

The statistical procedure most commonly used for prediction is regression analysis. The purpose of a regression analysis is to identify which factor or factors predict or explain the value of a dependent (outcome) variable. In some cases, the analysis is exploratory, and the focus is prediction. In others, selection of variables is based on a theoretical proposition, and the purpose is to develop an explanation that confirms the theoretical proposition.

In **regression analysis**, the independent (predictor) variable or variables influence variation or change in the value of the dependent variable. The goal is to determine how accurately one can predict the value of an outcome (or dependent) variable based on the value or values of one or more predictor (or independent) variables. This chapter describes some common statistical procedures used for prediction. These procedures include simple linear regression, multiple regression, logistic regression, and Cox proportional hazards regression.

Simple Linear Regression

Simple linear regression provides a means to estimate the value of a dependent variable based on the value of an independent variable. Simple linear regression is an effort to explain the dynamics within the scatter plot by drawing a straight line (the **line of best fit**) through the plotted scores. This line is drawn to explain best the **linear relationship** or association between two variables. Knowing that linear relationship, we can, with some degree of accuracy, use regression analysis to predict the value of one variable if we know the value of the other variable (Cohen & Cohen, 1983). Figure 24-1 illustrates the linear relationship between treatment compliance (independent variable) and posttreatment functional impairment (dependent variable) among patients with chronic pain. As shown in the scatter plot, there is a strong inverse relationship between the two variables. Higher levels of treatment compliance are associated with lower levels of functional impairment.

In simple linear regression, the dependent variable is continuous, and the predictor can be any scale of measurement. However, if the predictor is nominal, it must be correctly coded. When the data are ready, the parameters a and b are computed to obtain a regression equation. To understand the mathematical process, recall the algebraic equation for a straight line:

$$y = bx + a$$

where

y = dependent variable (outcome)
x = independent variable (predictor)
b = **slope of the line** (beta, or what the increase in value is along the x-axis for every unit of increase in the y value)
a = **y-intercept** (the point where the regression line intersects the y-axis)

A regression equation can be generated with a data set containing participants' x and y values. When this equation is generated, it can be used to predict y values of future participants, given only their *x* values. In simple or bivariate regression, predictions are made in cases with two variables. The score on variable *y* (dependent variable) is predicted from the same individual's known score on variable *x* (independent variable).

No single regression line can be used to predict with complete accuracy every *y* value from every *x* value. You could draw an infinite number of lines through the scattered paired values. However, the purpose of the regression equation is to develop the line that allows the highest degree of prediction possible—the **line of best fit**. The procedure for developing the line of best fit is the **method of least squares**. The formulas for the beta (*b*) and *y*-intercept (*a*) of the regression equation are computed as follows. Note that when the *b* is calculated, that value is inserted into the formula for *a*.

$$b = \frac{n\Sigma XY - \Sigma X \Sigma Y}{n\Sigma X^2 - (\Sigma X)^2} \qquad a = \frac{\Sigma Y - b\Sigma X}{n}$$

Calculation of Simple Linear Regression

Table 24-1 displays how one would arrange data to perform linear regression by hand. Regression analysis is conducted by a computer for most studies, but this calculation is provided to increase your understanding of the aspects of regression analysis and how to interpret the results. This example uses actual clinical data obtained from adults with a painful injury who received multidisciplinary pain management. The calculation in this chapter includes a subset of the study data belonging to those patients (*n* = 12) with the highest levels of coping skills (Cipher, Fernandez, & Clifford, 2002). A subset was selected for this illustration so that the computation example would be small and manageable. In actuality, studies involving linear regression need to be adequately powered, so they employ a larger sample (Aberson, 2010; Cohen & Cohen, 1983). The strength of this example is that the data are actual, unmodified clinical data from a study.

The first variable in Table 24-1 is the patient's level of treatment compliance—the predictor or independent variable (*x*) in this analysis. The second variable is the patient's posttreatment level of functional impairment—the dependent variable (*y*). Treatment compliance was assessed by patients' scores on the Cognitive Psychophysiological Treatment Clinical Rating Scales (Clifford, Cipher, & Schumacker, 2003), which yields an overall compliance score with higher numbers

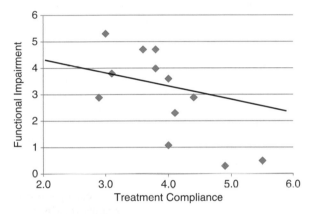

Figure 24-1 Linear relationship between treatment compliance and posttreatment functional impairment.

TABLE 24-1	Computation of Linear Regression Equation			
Patient	X (Compliance)	Y (Functional Impairment)	X²	XY
1	4.9	0.3	24.01	1.47
2	5.5	0.5	30.25	2.75
3	4.0	1.1	16.00	4.40
4	4.1	2.3	16.81	9.43
5	4.4	2.9	19.36	12.76
6	2.9	2.9	8.41	8.41
7	4.0	3.6	16.00	14.40
8	3.1	3.8	9.61	11.78
9	3.8	4.0	14.44	15.20
10	3.6	4.7	12.96	16.92
11	3.8	4.7	14.44	17.86
12	3.0	5.3	9.00	15.90
Σ	47.10	36.10	191.29	131.28

representing better levels of compliance with the pain management treatment regimen. Functional impairment was represented by patients' scores on the Interference subscale of the Multidimensional Pain Inventory (Kerns, Turk, & Rudy, 1985), with higher scores representing more functional impairment. The null hypothesis being tested is: *Treatment compliance is not a significant predictor of posttreatment functional impairment among patients undergoing pain management.* The data in Table 24-1 are arranged in columns, which correspond to the elements of the formula. The summed values in the last row of Table 24-1 are inserted into the appropriate places in the formula.

Calculation Steps

Step 1: Calculate *b*.
From the values in Table 24-1, we know that $n = 12$, $\Sigma X = 47.10$, $\Sigma Y = 36.10$, $\Sigma X^2 = 191.29$, and $\Sigma XY = 131.28$. These values are inserted into the formula for *b*, as follows:

$$b = \frac{12\ (131.28) - (47.10)\ (36.10)}{12\ (191.29) - 47.10^2}$$

$$b = -1.62$$

Step 2: Calculate *a*.
From Step 1, we know that $b = -1.62$, and we plug this value into the formula for *a:*

$$a = \frac{36.10 - (-1.62)\ (47.10)}{12}$$

$$a = 9.37$$

Step 3: Write the new regression equation:

$$y = -1.62X + 9.37$$

Step 4: Calculate *R*
The **multiple *R*** is defined as the correlation between the actual *y* values and the predicted *y* values using the new regression equation. The predicted *y* value using the new equation is represented by the symbol *ŷ* to differentiate it from *y*, which represents the actual *y* values in the data set. We can use our new regression equation from Step 3 to compute predicted functional impairment levels for each participant, the outcome of interest, using his or her compliance rating. For example, the compliance rating of patient no. 1 is 4.9, and the predicted functional impairment for patient no. 1 is calculated as:

$$\hat{y} = -1.62\ (4.9) + 9.37$$

$$\hat{y} = 1.43$$

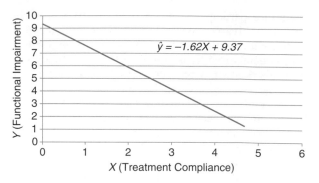

Figure 24-2 Regression line represented by regression equation.

The predicted *ŷ* is 1.43. This procedure would be continued for the rest of the subjects, and the Pearson correlation between the actual functional impairment levels (*y*) and the predicted functional impairment levels (*ŷ*) would yield the multiple *R* value. In this example, $R = 0.75$. The higher *R*, the more likely that the new regression equation accurately predicts *y* because the higher the correlation, the closer the actual *y* values are to the predicted *ŷ* values. Figure 24-2 displays the regression line where the *x*-axis represents possible treatment compliance values, and the *y*-axis represents the predicted functional impairment levels (*ŷ* values).

Step 5: Determine whether the predictor variable significantly predicts *y*.
To know whether the predictor significantly predicts *y*, the value of beta must be tested against zero because zero reflects the presence of no significant association between the variables, or null hypothesis. In simple regression, this is most easily accomplished by using the *R* value from Step 4:

$$t = R\sqrt{\frac{n-2}{1-R^2}}$$

$$t = 0.75\sqrt{\frac{12-2}{1-0.56}}$$

$$t = 3.58$$

The *t* value is compared with the *t* probability distribution table (see Appendix B). The *df* for this *t* statistic is $n - 2$. The critical *t* value at alpha (α) = 0.05, $df = 10$ is 2.23. Our obtained *t* was 3.58, which exceeds the critical value in the table, indicating a significant association between the predictor (*x*) and outcome (*y*).

Step 6: Calculate R^2.

After establishing the statistical significance of the R value, it must be examined for clinical importance. This examination is accomplished by obtaining the **coefficient of determination** for regression—which simply involves squaring the R value. R^2 represents the percentage of variance in y explained by the predictor. In our example, R was 0.75, and R^2 was 0.56. Multiplying $0.56 \times 100\%$ indicates that 56% of the variance in posttreatment functional impairment can be explained by knowing the patients' level of treatment compliance (Cohen & Cohen, 1983).

R^2 is most helpful in testing the contribution of the predictors in explaining an outcome when more than one predictor is included in the regression model. In contrast to R, R^2 for one regression model can be compared with another regression model that contains additional predictors (Cohen & Cohen, 1983). For example, Cipher et al. (2002) added another predictor, the patients' coping style, to the regression model of functional impairment. The R^2 values of both models were compared, the first with treatment compliance as the sole predictor and the second with treatment compliance and copying style as predictors. The R^2 values of the two models were statistically compared to indicate whether the proportion of variance in $\hat{y}$ was significantly increased by including the second predictor of coping style in the model.

Interpretation of Results

The b (beta or slope of the line) was 1.62, indicating an inverse relationship between treatment compliance and posttreatment functional impairment. The t statistic was significant, indicating that we can reject our null hypothesis and conclude that: *Treatment compliance significantly predicted posttreatment functional impairment levels among adults with chronic pain. Higher levels of treatment compliance significantly predicted lower levels of functional impairment.*

Multiple Regression

Multiple regression analysis is an extension of simple linear regression in which more than one independent variable is entered into the analysis (Munro, 2005). Because the relationships between multiple predictors and y are tested simultaneously, the calculations involved in multiple regression analysis are very complex. Multiple regression is best conducted using a statistical software package such as those presented in Table 21-2. However, full explanations and examples of the matrix algebraic computations of multiple regression are presented by Stevens (2009) and Tabachnick and Fidell (2006).

Interpretations of multiple regression findings are the same as with simple regression. The beta (b) values of each predictor are tested for significance, and a multiple R and R^2 are computed. The only difference is that in multiple regression, when all predictors are tested simultaneously, each b has been adjusted for every other predictor in the regression model. The b represents the independent relationship between that predictor and y, even after controlling for (or accounting for) the presence of every other predictor in the model.

Mancuso (2010) conducted a study of 102 subjects with diabetes to develop a predictive model of glycemic control, as measured by glycosylated hemoglobin (HbA_{1c}). The five predictors for HbA_{1c} were health literacy, patient trust, knowledge of diabetes, performance of self-care activities, and depression. The five predictors of glycemic control were tested with multiple regression analysis. The analysis yielded five b values, each with a corresponding p value. As shown in Table 24-2, patient trust and depression were significant predictors of glycemic control (HbA_{1c}), even after adjusting for the presence or contribution of every other predictor in the model. Health literacy, diabetes knowledge, and performance of self-care activities did not significantly predict HbA_{1c} levels. R^2 was 0.285, indicating that patient trust and depression accounted for 28.5% of the variance in HbA_{1c} (the measure of glycemic control).

The findings from this study have potential implications for the management of patients with diabetes. Because lower levels of patient trust were associated with higher HbA_{1c} values, fostering communication and trusting collaboration between the patient and the healthcare provider could directly or indirectly improve glycemic control. Higher levels of depression were also associated with higher HbA_{1c} values, and early interventions or referrals aimed at addressing depressive symptoms could be important in improving glycemic control. Regression analysis is not an indication of cause and effect. However, these results can serve as a benchmark for further research aimed at investigating the influence of patient factors such as trust and depression on glycemic control.

Multicollinearity

Multicollinearity occurs when the independent variables in a multiple regression equation are strongly correlated with one another. The presence of multicollinearity does not affect predictive power (the

TABLE 24-2 Predictors of Hemoglobin A_{1c} in Patients with Diabetes

Independent Variable	Unstandardized Coefficients		Standarized Coefficient		Significance (*p*)
	B	SE	β	t	
Health literacy	−0.063	0.080	−0.070	−0.0782	0.436
Patient trust	−0.873	0.165	−0.459	−5.288	0.000*
Diabetes knowledge	0.012	0.011	0.100	1.116	0.267
Performance of self-care activities	0.005	0.135	0.003	0.040	0.968
Depression	0.036	0.014	0.226	2.589	0.011*

From Mancuso, J. M. (2010). Impact of health literacy and patient trust on glycemic control in an urban USA populations. *Nursing & Health Sciences, 12*(1), 94–104.
*$p < 0.05$, significant.

capacity of the independent variables to predict values of the dependent variable in that specific sample); rather, it causes problems related to generalizability and the stability of the findings. If multicollinearity is present, the equation lacks predictive validity, and the amount of variance explained by each variable in the equation is inflated. Additionally, when cross-validation is performed, the *b* values do not remain consistent across samples (Cohen & Cohen, 1983). Multicollinearity is minimized by carefully selecting the independent variables and thoroughly determining their presence before the regression analysis. If highly correlated independent variables are found, the correlated predictors might be combined into one score or value yielding one predictor, or only one of the measures (scores) might be included in the regression equation.

The first step in identifying multicollinearity is to examine the bivariate correlations among the independent variables. You would perform multiple correlation analyses before conducting the regression analyses. The correlation matrix is carefully examined for evidence of multicollinearity. Most researchers consider multicollinearity to exist if a bivariate correlation is greater than 0.65. However, some researchers use a stronger correlation of 0.80 or greater as an indication of multicollinearity (Schroeder, 1990).

Types of Independent Variables Used in Regression Analyses

Variables in a regression equation can take many forms. Traditionally, as with most multivariate analyses, variables are measured at the interval or ratio level. However, researchers also use categorical or dichotomous variables (referred to as dummy variables), multiplicative terms, and transformed terms. A mixture of types of variables may be used in a single regression equation. The following discussion describes the various terms used as variables in regression equations.

Dummy Variables

To use categorical variables in regression analysis, a coding system is developed to represent group membership. Categorical variables of interest in nursing that might be used in regression analysis include gender, income, ethnicity, social status, level of education, and diagnosis. If the variable is dichotomous, such as gender, members of one category are assigned the number 1, and all others are assigned the number 0. In this case, for gender the coding could be:

1 = female
0 = male

If the categorical variable has three values, two dummy variables are used; for example, social class could be classified as lower class, middle class, or upper class. The first dummy variable (X_1) would be classified as:

1 = lower class
0 = not lower class

The second dummy variable (X_2) would be classified as:

1 = middle class
0 = not middle class

The three social classes would be represented in the data set in the following manner:

Lower class $X_1 = 1$, $X_2 = 0$
Middle class $X_1 = 0$, $X_2 = 1$
Upper class $X_1 = 0$, $X_2 = 0$

The variables lower class and middle class would be entered as predictors in the regression equation, in which both are tested against the reference category, upper class. Specifically, the *b* values for these two variables would represent whether *y* differs by lower class versus upper class and middle class versus upper class. When more than three categories define the values of the variable, increased numbers of dummy

TABLE 24-3	Association between Angiotensin-Converting Enzyme (ACE) Inhibitor Use and Colon Polyps	
	Polyps	No polyps
ACE inhibitor use	251	1508
No ACE inhibitor	603	2284

ACE, Angiotensin-converting enzyme.

TABLE 24-4	Notation in Cells of the Odds Ratio Table	
	Polyps	No polyps
ACE inhibitor use	*a*	*b*
No ACE inhibitor	*c*	*d*

ACE, Angiotensin-converting enzyme.

variables are used. The number of dummy variables is always one less than the number of categories (Aiken & West, 1991). An example of how one might analyze dichotomous dummy variables is presented in the next section.

Odds Ratio

When both the predictor and the dependent variable are dichotomous, the odds ratio (OR) is a commonly used statistic to obtain an indication of association. The odds ratio is defined as the ratio of the odds of an event occurring in one group to the odds of it occurring in another group (Gordis, 2008). Put simply, the OR is a way of comparing whether the odds of a certain event is the same for two groups. For example, the odds of a myocardial infarction occurring in men versus women could be compared. This research evidence would be valuable in predicting myocardial infarctions in men and women in clinical practice (Melnyk & Fineout-Overholt, 2011; Sackett, Straus, Richardson, Rosenberg, & Haynes, 2000).

Calculation

The formula for the OR is:

$$OR = \frac{ad}{bc}$$

A study examining the use of angiotensin-converting enzyme (ACE) inhibitors in 4646 veterans is presented as an example. The use of ACE inhibitors was examined in relation to having advanced adenomatous colon polyps in this population (Kedika et al., 2011). These data are presented in Table 24-3.

The formula for the OR designates the predictor's ratios of 1's to 0's within the positive outcome in the numerator and the predictor's ratios of 1's to 0's within the negative outcome in the denominator. The values must be coded accordingly. Table 24-4 displays the following notation to assist you in calculating the OR:

$$OR = \frac{ad}{bc} = \frac{(251)\,(2284)}{(1508)\,(603)} = \frac{573,284}{909,324} = 0.63$$

$$OR = 0.63$$

Interpretation

An OR of $\cong -1$ indicates that the probability of the event (polyps) is the same for both groups.

An OR of >1 indicates that the probability of the event (polyps) is higher among subjects exposed (to ACE inhibitors).

An OR of <1 indicates that the probability of the event (polyps) is lower among subjects exposed (to ACE inhibitors).

The OR for the study was 0.63, indicating the odds of polyps among veterans using ACE inhibitors is lower than among veterans who did not use ACE inhibitors. We can further note that veterans who used ACE inhibitors were *37% less likely to have polyps* (Kedika et al., 2011). This value was computed by subtracting the OR from 1.00 (1.00 − 0.63 = 0.37 × 100% = 37%). The difference between the obtained OR and 1.00 represents the extent of the lesser or greater likelihood of the event occurring.

Confidence Intervals

OR values are often accompanied by a confidence interval, which consists of a lower and upper limit value. The 95% confidence interval is interpreted as there is a 95% probability that the population value lies between [lower limit] and [upper limit]. If the confidence interval does not include the number 1.00, this would indicate a significant association between the medication use and the polyps. The 95% confidence interval for the OR for ACE inhibitor use and polyps was 0.54 to 0.74; this means that there is a 95% probability that the population value lies between the values of 0.54 and 0.74. Because this interval excludes the value of 1.00, it indicates that there is a statistically significant association between ACE inhibitor use and polyps.

Logistic Regression

Logistic regression replaces linear regression when the researcher wants to test a predictor or predictors of a dichotomous dependent variable. Some common examples of dependent variables that are analyzed with logistic regression are: patient lived or died, responded or did not respond to treatment, and employed or unemployed. The logistic regression model can be considered more flexible than linear regression in the following ways:

1. Logistic regression can have continuous predictors, nominal predictors, or a combination of the two, with no assumptions regarding normality of the distribution.
2. Logistic regression can test predictors with a non-linear relationship between the predictor and the dependent variable.
3. With a logistic regression model, you can compute the odds of a person's outcome. Each predictor is associated with an OR that represents the independent association between that predictor and the outcome y (Tabachnick & Fidell, 2006).

Because the dependent variable is either 1 or 0, logistic regression analysis produces a regression equation that yields probabilities of the outcome occurring for each person. If the predictor is continuous, we can determine the probability of the outcome occurring with a predictor score of some value X. If the predictor is dichotomous, we can determine the probability of the outcome occurring with a predictor value of "1" and a predictor value of "0."

Calculation

Logistic regression is best conducted using a statistical software package such as those presented in Table 21-2. Full explanations and examples of the computations of logistic regression are presented by Tabachnick and Fidell (2006). A brief overview is provided in this chapter, with an example of simple logistic regression using actual clinical data.

Because the dependent variable in logistic regression is dichotomous, the predicted $\hat{y}$ is always in the range of 0 to 1, which is interpreted as a probability. Similar to linear regression, the predicted $\hat{y}$ values are calculated from a b (or more than one b in the case of multiple predictors) and a y-intercept. In contrast to linear regression, the b and y-intercept are the exponents of the number e (2.718). An exponent of e is commonly referred to as the natural logarithm. In other words, the natural logarithm of a given number is the power to which e would have to be raised to equal that number. When the b and y-intercept serve

as natural logarithms, it allows the result to yield a probability (a value between 0 and 1).

Recall the example from the ACE inhibitor and polyps data (Kedika et al., 2011). If a person used ACE inhibitors, the probability of that patient having colon polyps is calculated:

Given: For these data, $b = -0.46$, and the y-intercept (a) is -1.33.

$$\hat{Y} = \frac{e^{-0.46(1)+-1.33}}{1 + e^{-0.46(1)+-1.33}}$$

$$\hat{Y} = \frac{e^{-1.79}}{1 + e^{-1.79}} \qquad \text{so} \qquad \hat{Y} = \frac{0.167}{1.167} = 0.14$$

The probability of having colon polyps if the patient used ACE inhibitors is only 0.14, or 14%. The probability of having colon polyps if the patient did *not* use ACE inhibitors is 21%, as shown next. The risk of having polyps is greater if the patient did not use ACE inhibitors.

$$\hat{Y} = \frac{e^{-0.46(0)+-1.33}}{1 + e^{-0.46(0)+-1.33}}$$

$$\hat{Y} = \frac{e^{-1.33}}{1 + e^{-1.33}} \qquad \text{so} \qquad \hat{Y} = \frac{0.26}{1.26} = 0.21$$

Odds Ratio (OR) in Logistic Regression

Each predictor is associated with an OR in a logistic regression model. If the predictor is dichotomous, the OR is interpreted as: with an X value of "yes," the odds of the outcome occurring is [OR value] times as likely. The ACE inhibitor and polyps example yielded an OR of 0.63. As was stated previously, this OR indicates that veterans using ACE inhibitors were 0.63 times as likely to have polyps. Another way of stating this is that veterans who used ACE inhibitors were *37% less likely to have polyps*. Thus, patients treated with ACE inhibitors to lower their blood pressure have a decreased likelihood of developing colon polyps.

If the predictor is continuous, the OR is interpreted as: for every 1-unit increase in X, the odds of the outcome occurring are [OR value] times as likely. For example, the association between years of education and obtaining employment among persons with a spinal cord injury was investigated (Ottomanelli, Sippel, Cipher, & Goetz, 2011). The predictor was age, and the dependent variable was employment (yes/ no). The OR was 1.10, indicating that for every year older in age, the patient was 1.10 times as likely (or 10% more likely) to have obtained employment.

In the same study, the association between being male and obtaining employment among persons with spinal cord injury was investigated (Ottomanelli et al., 2011). The predictor was being male (yes/no), and the dependent variable was employment (yes/no). The OR was 1.00, indicating that patients who were male were 1.00 times as likely (or just as likely) as females to have obtained employment. In other words, the likelihood of employment was equal among males and females.

Cox Proportional Hazards Regression

When testing predictors of a dependent variable that is time-related, the appropriate statistical procedure is Cox proportional hazards regression (or Cox regression) (Hosmer, Lemeshow, & May, 2008). The dependent variable in Cox regression is called the hazard, a neutral word intended to describe the risk of event occurrence (e.g., risk of obtaining an illness, risk of complications from medications, or risk of relapse). The primary output in a Cox regression analysis represents the relationship between each predictor variable and the *hazard,* or rate of event occurrence.

Cox regression is a type of survival analysis that can answer questions pertaining to the amount of time that elapses until an event occurs. Examples of the types of questions that can be answered using Cox regression follow. A group of nurse practitioners begins a doctoral program. What variables predict how long it will take the students to graduate? A group

of depressed adults completes a cognitive therapy program. What variables predict the time elapsed from the end of treatment until a patient's first relapse?

The major difference between using Cox regression as opposed to linear regression is the ability of survival analysis to handle cases where survival time is unknown. For example, in the study of treatment for streptococcal pharyngitis (strep throat), perhaps only 20% of cases relapse. The other 80% do not relapse by the end of the researcher's study. Thus, it is unknown how long it will be until the patients relapse. Survival times that are known only to exceed a certain value are called censored data. Censored data can also occur when a participant drops out of the study. Cox regression calculations take into account censored data when estimating the relationships between predictors and *y*—in contrast to linear regression analyses, which would delete or exclude those cases from analysis (Hosmer et al., 2008).

Logistic regression yields odds ratios for each predictor to represent the relationship between that predictor and *y,* whereas Cox regression yields hazard ratios. A hazard ratio (*HR*) is interpreted almost identically to an OR with the exception that the *HR* represents the risk of the event occurring *sooner.*

An example of Cox regression used in clinical research is presented in Table 24-5. Predictors of major adverse cardiovascular events (MACE) in a sample of 312 veterans with rheumatoid arthritis were tested with Cox regression (Banerjee et al., 2008). There were 10 predictors of cardiovascular events tested, and the analysis yielded 10 hazard ratios, each

TABLE 24-5   Cox Proportional Hazards Regression Results of Major Adverse Cardiovascular Events in Veterans with Rheumatoid Arthritis

Predictor	Hazard Ratio (Unadjusted)*	p Value	Hazard Ratio (Adjusted)†	p Value
DAS score	1.29	0.02	1.31	0.01
Age	1.01	0.62	0.99	0.83
Hypertension	2.55	0.03	2.43	0.08
Tobacco use	1.37	0.33	1.12	0.78
Diabetes	1.3	0.33	0.99	0.99
Hyperlipidemia	2.63	< 0.01	2.45	0.01
History of vascular disease	2.36	< 0.01	2.54	<0.01
DMARD use	0.63	0.06	0.52	<0.01
aTNF-α use	0.65	0.23	0.81	0.02
DMARD + aTNF-α use	0.68	0.34	0.82	0.83

Note: Full explanations and examples of the computations of Cox regression are presented in Hosmer, Lemeshow, & May (2008).
aTNF-α, Anti–tumor necrosis factor-α medication; *DAS,* disease activity score; *DMARD,* disease-modifying antirheumatic drug.
*Adjusted for all other model predictors.
From Banerjee, S. D., et al. (2008). Cardiovascular outcomes in male veterans with rheumatoid arthritis. *American Journal of Cardiology, 101*(8), 1204.
Hosmer, D. W., Lemeshow, S., & May, S. (2008). *Applied survival analysis: Regression modeling of time to event data* (2nd ed.). Hoboken, NJ: John Wiley & Sons.

with a corresponding *p* value. As shown in Table 24-5, the disease activity score (DAS) for extent of rheumatoid arthritis, hypertension, hyperlipidemia, and history of vascular disease all were significant predictors of a cardiovascular event when each predictor was tested separately. However, when all 10 predictors were tested simultaneously, the hazard ratios were called **adjusted hazard ratios**, which means that each *HR* has been adjusted for every other predictor in the regression model. The results of the adjusted *HR* values indicated that DAS, hyperlipidemia, history of vascular disease, disease-modifying antirheumatic drug (DMARD) use, and anti–tumor necrosis factor (anti-TNF) medication use all were significant predictors of a MACE, even after controlling for the presence of every other predictor in the model. Full explanations and examples of the computations of Cox regression are presented by Hosmer et al. (2008).

The findings from this study could have indications for the treatment of rheumatoid arthritis in clinical practice. Because higher levels of rheumatoid arthritis disease activity were associated with a greater likelihood of MACE, it could be that the successful control of rheumatoid arthritis symptoms could directly or indirectly reduce the risk of MACE. DMARD and anti-TNF use were associated with a lower risk of MACE, and so proper medication management of these patients might be an important factor in reducing the risk of MACE. Traditional cardiovascular risk factors studied in other populations (e.g., age, diabetes, smoking history) did not predict MACE in this sample (D'Agostino et al., 2000; Kannel, McGee, & Gordon, 1976). Therefore, male veterans with rheumatoid arthritis seem to be unique with regard to the experience of MACE and may require tailored treatment specific to their demographics to minimize cardiovascular events.

KEY POINTS

- The purpose of a regression analysis is to predict or explain as much of the variance in the value of the dependent variable as possible.
- The independent (predictor) variable or variables cause variation in the value of the dependent (outcome) variable.
- Simple linear regression provides a means to estimate the value of a dependent variable based on the value of an independent variable.
- Multiple regression analysis is an extension of simple linear regression in which more than one independent variable is entered into the analysis to predict a dependent variable.

- Multicollinearity occurs when the independent variables in a multiple regression equation are strongly correlated and results in unstable findings.
- The odds ratio is a way of comparing whether the odds of a certain event is the same for two groups.
- Logistic regression replaces linear regression when you want to test a predictor or predictors of a dichotomous dependent variable.
- When testing predictors of a dependent variable that is time-related, the appropriate statistical procedure is Cox proportional hazards regression (or Cox regression).
- The hazard ratio represents the risk of the event occurring sooner.

REFERENCES

Aberson, C. L. (2010). *Applied power analysis for the behavioral sciences*. New York, NY: Routledge Taylor & Francis Group.

Aiken, L. S., & West, S. G. (1991). *Multiple regression: Testing and interpreting interactions*. Newbury Park, UK: Sage.

Banerjee, S. B., Compton, A. P., Hooker, R. S., Cipher, D. J., Reimold, A., Brilakis, E. S., et al. (2008). Cardiovascular outcomes in male veterans with rheumatoid arthritis. *American Journal of Cardiology*, *101*(8), 1201–1205.

Cipher, D. J., Fernandez, E., & Clifford, P. A. (2002). Coping style influences compliance with multidisciplinary pain management. *Journal of Health Psychology*, *7*(5), 665–673.

Clifford, P. A., Cipher, D. J., & Schumacker, R. E. (2003). Compliance and stages of change in multidisciplinary pain centers. *The Pain Clinic*, *15*(4), 355–368.

Cohen, J., & Cohen, P. (1983). *Applied multiple regression/correlation analysis for the behavioral sciences* (2nd ed.). Hillsdale, NJ: Erlbaum.

D'Agostino, R. B., Russell, M. W., Huse, D. M., Ellison, R. C., Silbershatz, H., Wilson, P. W., et al. (2000). Primary and subsequent coronary risk appraisal: New results from the Framingham Study. *American Heart Journal*, *139*(2 Pt 1), 272–281.

Gordis, L. (2008). *Epidemiololgy* (4th ed.). Philadelphia, PA: Saunders.

Hosmer, D. W., Lemeshow, S., & May, S. (2008). *Applied survival analysis: Regression modeling of time to event data* (2nd ed.). Hoboken, NJ: John Wiley & Sons.

Kannel, W. B., McGee, D., & Gordon, T. (1976). A general cardiovascular risk profile: The Framingham Study. *American Journal of Cardiology*, *38*(1), 46–51.

Kedika, R., Patel, M., Pena Sahdala, H. N., Mahgoub, A., Cipher, D. J., & Siddiqui, A. A. (2011). Long-term use of angiotensin converting enzyme inhibitors is associated with decreased incidence of advanced adenomatous colon polyps. *Journal of Clinical Gastroenterology*, *45*(2), e12–e16.

Kerns, R. D., Turk, D. C., & Rudy, T. E. (1985). The West-Haven Yale Multidimensional Pain Inventory (WHYMPI). *Pain*, *23*(4), 345–356.

Mancuso, J. M. (2010). Impact of health literacy and patient trust on glycemic control in an urban USA populations. *Nursing & Health Sciences*, *12*(1), 94–104.

Melnyk, B. M., & Fineout-Overholt, E. (2011). *Evidence-based practice in nursing & healthcare: A guide to best practice* (2nd ed.). Philadelphia, PA: Lippincott Williams & Wilkins.

Munro, B. H. (2005). *Statistical methods for health care research* (5th ed.). Philadelphia, PA: Lippincott Williams & Wilkins.

Ottomanelli, L., Sippel, J., Cipher, D. J., & Goetz, L. (2011). Factors associated with employment among veterans with spinal cord injury. *Journal of Vocational Rehabilitation*, *34*(1), 141–150.

Sackett, D. L., Straus, S. E., Richardson, W. S., Rosenberg, W., & Haynes, R. B. (2000). *Evidence-based medicine: How to practice and teach EBM*. London, UK: Churchill Livingstone.

Schroeder, M. A. (1990). Diagnosing and dealing with multicollinearity. *Western Journal of Nursing Research*, *12*(2), 175–187.

Stevens, J. P. (2009). *Applied Multivariate Statistics for the Social Sciences* (5th ed.). London, UK: Psychology Press.

Tabachnick, B. G., & Fidell, L. S. (2006). *Using Multivariate Statistics* (5th ed.). Needham Heights, MA: Allyn & Bacon.

25

CHAPTER

Using Statistics to Determine Differences

The statistical procedures in this chapter examine differences between or among groups. Statistical procedures are available for nominal, ordinal, and interval/ratio level data. The procedures vary considerably in their power to detect differences and in their complexity. How one interprets the results of these statistics depends on the design of the study. If the design is quasi-experimental or experimental and the study is well designed and has no major issues in regard to threats to internal and external validity, causality can be considered, and the results can be inferred to the associated population. If the design is comparative descriptive, differences identified are associated only with the sample under study. The parametric statistics used to determine differences that are discussed in this chapter are the independent samples *t*-test, paired or dependent samples *t*-test, and analysis of variance (ANOVA). If the assumptions for parametric analyses are not achieved or if study data are at the ordinal level, the nonparametric analyses of Mann-Whitney *U*, Wilcoxon signed-rank test, and Kruskal-Wallis *H* are appropriate techniques to use to test the researcher's hypotheses. The chapter concludes with a discussion of the chi-square test of independence, which is a nonparametric analysis technique for analyzing nominal level data.

Choosing Parametric versus Nonparametric Statistics to Determine Differences

Parametric statistics are always associated with a certain set of assumptions that the data must meet; this is because the formulas of parametric statistics yield valid results only when the properties of the data are within the confines of these assumptions (Munro, 2005). If the data do not meet the parametric

assumptions, there are nonparametric alternatives that do not require those assumptions to be met, usually because nonparametric statistical procedures convert the original data to rank-ordered or ordinal level data.

Many statistical tests can assist the researcher in determining whether his or her data meet the assumptions for a given parametric test. The most common assumption (that accompanies all parametric tests) is the assumption that the data are normally distributed. The K^2 test and the Shapiro-Wilk test are formal tests of normality that assess whether distribution of a variable is non-normal—that is, skewed or kurtotic (see Chapter 21) (D'Agostino, Belanger, & D'Agostino, 1990). The Shapiro-Wilk test is used with samples with less than 1000 subjects. When the sample is larger, the Kolmogorov-Smirnov D test is more appropriate. All of these statistics are found in mainstream statistical software packages and are accompanied by a p value. Significant normality tests with $p \leq 0.05$ indicate that the distribution being tested is significantly different from the normal curve, violating the normality assumption. The nonparametric statistical alternative is listed in each section in the event that the data do not meet the assumptions of each parametric test illustrated in this chapter.

t-tests

One of the most common parametric analyses used to test for significant differences between group means of two samples is the *t*-test. The **independent *t*-test analysis technique** was developed to examine differences between two independent groups; the **paired or dependent *t*-test analysis technique** was developed to examine differences between two matched or paired groups, or a comparison of pretest and posttest measurements. The details of the independent and paired *t*-tests are described in this section.

t-test for Independent Samples

The most common parametric analysis technique used in nursing studies to test for significant differences between two independent samples is the **independent samples** *t*-test. The samples are independent if the study participants in one group are unrelated to or different from the participants in the second group. Use of the *t*-test for independent samples involves the following assumptions:

1. Sample means from the population are normally distributed.
2. The dependent or outcome variable is measured at the interval/ratio level.
3. The two samples have equal variance.
4. All observations within each sample are independent.

The *t*-test is robust to moderate violation of its assumptions. **Robustness** means that the results of analysis can still be relied on to be accurate when an assumption has been violated. The *t*-test is not robust with respect to the between-samples or within-samples independence assumptions, and it is not robust with respect to an extreme violation of the normality assumption unless the sample sizes are extremely large. Sample groups do not have to be equal for this analysis—instead, the concern is for equal variance. A variety of *t*-tests have been developed for various types of samples. The formula and calculation of the independent samples *t*-test is presented next.

Calculation

The formula for the *t*-test is:

$$t = \frac{\bar{X}_1 - \bar{X}_2}{s_{\bar{X}_1 - \bar{X}_2}}$$

where
$\bar{X}_1$ = mean of group 1
$\bar{X}_2$ = mean of group 2
$s_{\bar{X}_1 - \bar{X}_2}$ = to the standard error of the difference between the two groups.

To compute the *t*-test, one must compute the denominator in the formula, which is the standard error of the difference between the means. If the two groups have different sample sizes, one must use this formula:

$$s_{\bar{X}_1 - \bar{X}_2} \sqrt{\frac{(n_1 - 1)s_1^2 + (n_2 - 1)s_2^2}{n_1 + n_2 - 2} \left(\frac{1}{n_1} + \frac{1}{n_2}\right)}$$

where
n_1 = group 1 sample size
n_2 = group 2 sample size

s_1 = group 1 variance
s_2 = group 2 variance

If the two groups have the same number of subjects in each group, one can use this simplified formula:

$$s_{\bar{X}_1 - \bar{X}_1} = \sqrt{\frac{s_1^2 + s_2^2}{n}}$$

where
n = sample size in each group and not the total sample of both groups

Using an example from a study examining the levels of depression among 16 elderly long-term care residents, differences between residents with and without dementia were investigated (Cipher & Clifford, 2004). A subset of data for these patients was selected for this example so that the computation would be small and manageable (Table 25-1). In actuality, studies involving *t*-tests need to be adequately powered to identify significant differences between groups accurately (Aberson 2010; Cohen & Cohen, 1983). All data presented in this chapter are actual, unmodified clinical data for a small number of study participants.

The independent variable in this example was level of dementia and included two levels—a "no dementia" group and a "severe dementia" group. The level of dementia was based on clinical ratings of neuropsychologists using the Functional Assessment Staging Tool (Reisberg, Ferris, Deleon, & Crook, 1982). The dependent variable was the score of the long-term care resident on the Geriatric Depression Scale (GDS) (Yesavage, Brink, & Rose, 1983). The GDS assesses

TABLE 25-1 Depression Scores by Dementia Level among Elderly Long-Term Care Residents

Patient No.	No Dementia Group GDS Score	Patient No.	Severe Dementia Group GDS Score
1	5	9	3
2	5	10	6
3	10	11	5
4	11	12	4
5	8	13	9
6	8	14	7
7	10	15	4
8	10	16	7

GDS, Geriatric depression scale.

the level of depression in elderly adults, with higher numbers indicative of more depressive symptoms. The null hypothesis is: *There are no significant differences between elderly adults with dementia and elderly adults without dementia on depression scores.*

The computations for the *t*-test are as follows:

Step 1: Compute means for both groups, which involves the sum of scores for each group divided by the number in the group.
The mean for Group 1, No Dementia: $\bar{X}_1 = 8.38$
The mean for Group 2, Severe Dementia: $\bar{X}_2 = 5.63$

Step 2: Compute the numerator of the *t*-test:

$$\bar{X}_1 - \bar{X}_2 = 2.75$$

Step 3: Compute the standard error of the difference.
a. Compute the variances for each group:
s^2 for Group 1 = 5.41
s^2 for Group 2 = 3.98
b. Plug into the standard error of the difference formula:

$$s_{\bar{X}_1 - \bar{X}_2} = \sqrt{\frac{s_1^2 + s_2^2}{n}}$$

$$s_{\bar{X}_1 - \bar{X}_2} = \sqrt{\frac{5.41 + 3.98}{8}}$$

$$s_{\bar{X}_1 - \bar{X}_2} = 1.08$$

Step 4: Compute *t* value:

$$t = \frac{\bar{X}_1 - \bar{X}_2}{s_{\bar{X}_1 - \bar{X}_2}}$$

$$t = \frac{2.75}{1.08}$$

$$t = 2.55$$

Step 5: Compute degrees of freedom (*df*):

$$df = n_1 + n_2 - 2$$

$$df = 8 + 8 - 2$$

$$df = 14$$

Step 6: Locate the critical *t* value in the *t* distribution table in Appendix B at the back of your textbook and compare the critical *t* value with the obtained *t* value.

The critical *t* value for 14 degrees of freedom at alpha (α) = 0.05 is 2.15. This means that if we viewed the *t* distribution for *df* = 14, the middle 95% of the distribution would be marked by −2.15 and 2.15, as shown in Figure 25-1.

Interpretation of Results

Our obtained *t* is 2.55, exceeding the critical value, which means that our *t*-test is *significant* and represents a real difference between the two groups. We can reject the null hypothesis and state: *An independent samples t-test computed on GDS scores revealed long-term residents with no dementia had significantly higher depression scores than long-term residents who had severe dementia, t (14) = 2.55, p < 0.05; $\bar{X}$ = 8.4 versus 5.6.* Prior research suggests that elderly residents with dementia do not experience less depression, but rather they have difficulty communicating their distress (Ott & Fogel, 2004; Scherder et al., 2005). With additional research in this area, this knowledge might be used to facilitate improvements in methods used by healthcare professionals to assess emotional distress accurately among elderly adults with dementia (Cipher, Clifford, & Roper, 2006; Thakur & Blazer, 2008).

Nonparametric Alternative

If the data do not meet the assumptions involving normality or equal variances for an independent

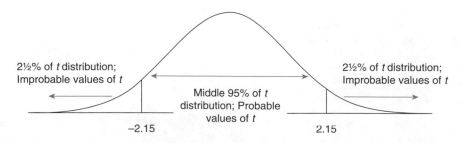

Figure 25-1 **Probability distribution of *t* at *df* = 14.**

samples *t*-test, the nonparametric alternative is the **Mann-Whitney** *U* **test**. Mann-Whitney *U* calculations involve converting the data to ranks, discarding any variance or normality issues associated with the original values. In some studies, the data collected are ordinal level, and the Mann-Whitney *U* test is appropriate for analysis of the data. The Mann-Whitney *U* test is 95% as powerful as the *t*-test in determining differences between two groups. For a more detailed description of the Mann-Whitney *U* test, see the statistical textbooks by Daniel (2000) and Munro (2005). The statistical workbook for healthcare research by Grove (2007) has exercises for expanding your understanding of *t*-tests and Mann-Whitney *U* results from published studies.

t-tests for Paired Samples

When samples are related, the formula used to calculate the *t* statistic is different from the formula previously described for independent groups. One type of **paired samples** refers to a research design that repeatedly assesses the same group of people, a design commonly referred to as a **repeated measures design**. Another research design for which a paired samples *t*-test is appropriate is the case-control research design. **Case-control designs** involve a matching procedure whereby a control subject is matched to each case, in which the cases and controls are different people but matched demographically (Gordis, 2008). Paired or dependent samples *t*-tests can also be applied to a crossover study design, in which subjects receive one kind of treatment and subsequently receive a comparison treatment (Gordis, 2008). However, similar to the independent samples *t*-test, this *t*-test requires that differences between the paired scores be independent and normally or approximately normally distributed.

Calculation

The formula for the paired samples *t*-test is:

$$t = \frac{\bar{D}}{S_{\bar{D}}}$$

where

$\bar{D}$ = mean difference of the paired data
$S_{\bar{D}}$ = standard error of the difference
To compute the *t*-test, one must compute the denominator in the formula, the standard error of the difference:

$$s_{\bar{D}} = \frac{s_{\bar{D}}}{\sqrt{N}}$$

where

$s_{\bar{D}}$ = standard deviation of the differences between the paired data
N = number of subjects in the sample

Using an example from a study examining the level of functional impairment among 10 adults receiving rehabilitation for a painful injury, changes over time were investigated (Cipher, Kurian, Fulda, Snider, & Van Beest, 2007). These data are presented in Table 25-2. A subset was selected for this example so that the computations would be small and manageable. In actuality, studies involving both independent and dependent samples *t*-tests need to be adequately powered (Aberson 2010; Cohen & Cohen, 1983).

The independent variable in this example was treatment over time, meaning that the whole sample received rehabilitation for their injury for 3 weeks. The dependent variable was functional impairment, which was represented by patients' scores on the Interference subscale of the Multidimensional Pain

---

TABLE 25-2   Functional Impairment Levels at Baseline and after Treatment

Subject No.	Baseline Functional Impairment Scores	Post-Treatment Functional Impairment Scores	Difference
1	2.9	1.7	1.2
2	5.7	2.9	2.8
3	2.3	2.9	−0.6
4	3.9	3	0.9
5	3.8	3.1	0.7
6	3.3	3.2	0.1
7	2.9	3.2	−0.3
8	4.7	3.2	1.5
9	3.2	2.1	1.1
10	4.9	3.4	1.5

Inventory (MPI) (Kerns, Turk, & Rudy, 1985), with higher scores representing more functional impairment. The null hypothesis is: *There is no significant reduction in functional impairment from baseline to posttreatment for patients in a rehabilitation program.*

The computations for the *t*-test are as follows:

Step 1: Compute the difference between each subject's pair of data (see last column of Table 25-2).

Step 2: Compute the mean of the difference scores, which becomes the numerator of the *t*-test:

$$\bar{D} = 0.89$$

Step 3: Compute the standard error of the difference.
  a. Compute the standard deviation of the difference scores:

$$s = 0.99$$

  b. Plug into the standard error of the difference formula:

$$s_{\bar{D}} = \frac{s_{\bar{D}}}{\sqrt{N}}$$

$$s_{\bar{D}} = \frac{0.99}{\sqrt{10}}$$

$$s_{\bar{D}} = 0.313$$

Step 4: Compute *t* value:

$$t = \frac{\bar{D}}{s_{\bar{D}}}$$

$$t = \frac{0.89}{0.313}$$

$$t = 2.84$$

Step 5: Compute degrees of freedom:

$$df = n - 1$$

$$df = 10 - 1$$

$$df = 9$$

Step 6: Locate the critical *t* value on the *t* distribution table and compare with our obtained *t* value.

The critical *t* value for 9 degrees of freedom at alpha (α) = 0.05 is 2.26. Our obtained *t* is 2.84, exceeding the critical value (see *t*—Table in Appendix B). This means that if we viewed the *t* distribution for *df* = 9, the middle 95% of the distribution would be marked by −2.26 and 2.26.

Interpretation of Results

Our obtained *t* = 2.84 exceeds the critical *t* value in the table, which means that our *t*-test is statistically significant and represents a real difference between participant's preintervention and postintervention functional impairment scores. We can reject our null hypothesis and state: *A paired samples* t-*test computed on MPI functional impairment scores revealed that the patients undergoing rehabilitation had significantly lower functional impairment levels from baseline to posttreatment,* t (9) = 2.84, p < 0.05; $\bar{X}$ = 3.8 versus 2.9. During the 3-week rehabilitation program, patients successfully reduced their functional impairment levels. With additional research in this area, this knowledge might be used to facilitate evidence-based practice interventions in rehabilitation facilities to improve patients' functional status (Melnyk & Fineout-Overholt, 2011).

Nonparametric Alternative

If the interval/ratio level data do not meet the normality assumptions for a paired samples *t*-test, the nonparametric alternative is the **Wilcoxon signed-rank test**. The Wilcoxon signed-rank test calculations involve converting the data to ranks, discarding any variance or normality issues associated with the original values. This analysis technique is also appropriate when the study data are ordinal level, such as self-care abilities identified as low, moderate, and high based on the Orem Self-Care Model (Orem, 2001). This test is thoroughly addressed by Daniel (2000) and Munro (2005) in their statistical textbooks. Grove (2007) has an exercise for expanding your understanding of the Wilcoxon signed-rank results from published studies.

One-Way Analysis of Variance

Analysis of variance (ANOVA) is a statistical procedure that compares data between two or more groups or conditions to investigate the presence of differences between those groups on some continuous dependent or outcome variable. The formulas for ANOVA compute two estimates of variance: (1) differences among (within) the data and (2) differences between the groups or conditions.

Why perform ANOVA and not a *t*-test? A *t*-test is formulated to compare two sets of data or two groups at one time. Data generated from a clinical trial that has four experimental groups, treatment 1, treatment 2, treatments 1 and 2 combined, and a control, would require six *t*-tests. As a result, the chance of making a Type I error (alpha error) increases substantially (or is inflated) because so many computations are being performed. Specifically, the chance of making a Type I

TABLE 25-3 Monthly Medical Costs of Three Treatment Groups*		
Multidisciplinary Group Costs	**Standard Care Group Costs**	**Pharmacotherapy Group Costs**
74	168	603
748	328	707
433	186	868
422	199	286
297	154	919
Σ = Sum = **1974**	**1035**	**3382**
Grand total = 6392		

*Costs were U.S. dollars averaged monthly.

error is the number of comparisons multiplied by the alpha level. ANOVA is the better statistical technique for examining differences among more than two groups.

ANOVA is a procedure that culminates in a statistic called the **F statistic**. This value is compared against an F distribution (see Appendix D) to determine whether the groups significantly differ from one another on the dependent variable studied. The basic formula for the F is:

$$F = \frac{\text{Mean square between groups}}{\text{Mean square within groups}}$$

The term *mean square* (MS) is used interchangeably with the word "variance." The formulas for ANOVA compute two estimates of variance: the between-groups variance and the within-groups variance. The between-groups variance represents differences between the groups or conditions being compared, and the within-groups variance represents differences among (within) each group's data. The formula is:

$$F = \frac{\text{MS between}}{\text{MS within}}$$

Calculation

Using an example from a study examining medical costs among 15 women receiving treatment for a chronic pain condition, monthly medical costs for 1 year incurred after treatment ended were examined (Cipher, Fernandez, & Clifford, 2001). The data from this study are presented in Table 25-3. A subset of data was selected from the unmodified clinical data of this study for this example so that the computation would be manageable. In actuality, studies involving ANOVA need to be adequately powered to detect differences

accurately among study groups (Aberson 2010; Cohen & Cohen, 1983).

The independent variable in this example was the type of study treatment or intervention. Patients received multidisciplinary treatment, standard care (primary care physician only), or pharmacotherapy by an anesthesiologist. The dependent variable was the medical costs incurred per month during the year after treatment. The null hypothesis was: *There is no significant difference between the treatment groups in posttreatment monthly medical costs.*

The steps to perform an ANOVA are as follows:
Step 1: Compute correction term, C.
Square the grand sum (G), and divide by total N:

$$C = \frac{6392^2}{15} - 2,723,844.3$$

Step 2: Compute total sum of squares.
Square every value in data set, sum, and subtract C:

$$(74^2 + 748^2 + 433^2 + 422^2 + 297^2 + 168^2 + 328^2 \dots$$
$$+ 919^2) - 2,723,844.3 = 3,795,722$$
$$- 2,723,844.3 = 1,071,877.7$$

Step 3: Compute between groups sum of squares.
Square the sum of each column and divide by N. Add each, and then subtract C.

$$\frac{1974^2}{5} + \frac{1035^2}{5} + \frac{3382^2}{5} - 2723,844.3$$
$$(779,335.2 + 214,245 + 2,288,937.8)$$
$$- 2,723,844.3 = 558,673.7$$

Step 4: Compute within groups sum of squares.
Subtract the between groups sum of squares (Step 3) from total sum of squares (Step 2).

TABLE 25-4	Analysis of Variance Summary Table			
Source of Variation	SS	df	MS	F
Between groups	558,673.73	2	279,336.9	6.53
Within groups	513,204	12	42,767	
Total	1,071,877.7	14		

$$1,071,877.7 - 558,673.7 = 513,204$$

Step 5: Create an ANOVA summary table (Table 25-4).

   a. Insert the sum of squares values in the first column.

   b. The degrees of freedom are in the second column. Because the F is a ratio of two separate statistics (mean square between groups and mean square within groups) both have different df formulas—one for the "numerator" and one for the denominator:

> Mean square between groups df
> = number of groups − 1
>
> Mean square within groups df
> = (number of groups − 1) $(n − 1)$

   For this example, the df for the numerator is 3 − 1 = 2. The df for the denominator is (3 − 1) (5 − 1) = 12.

   c. The mean square between groups and mean square within groups are in the third column. These values are computed by dividing the SS by the df. Therefore, the MS between = 558,673.73 ÷ 2 = 279,336.9. The MS within = 513,204 ÷ 12 = 42,767.

   d. The F is the final column and is computed by dividing the MS between by the MS within. Therefore, $F = 279,336.9 ÷ 42,767 = 6.53$.

Step 6: Locate the critical F value on the F distribution table (see Appendix D) and compare our obtained F value with it. The critical F value for 2 and 12 df at alpha $(\alpha) = 0.05$ is 3.88. Our obtained F is 6.53, which exceeds the critical value.

Interpretation of Results

Our obtained $F = 6.53$ exceeds the critical value in the table, which means that our F is statistically significant and that the population means are not equal. We can reject our null hypothesis that the three groups have the same monthly posttreatment medical costs.

However, the F does not tell us which treatment groups differ from one another. Further testing, termed *multiple comparison tests* or *post hoc tests,* are required to complete the ANOVA process and determine all the significant differences among the study groups.

Post hoc tests have been developed specifically to determine the location of group differences after ANOVA is performed on data from more than two groups. These tests were developed to reduce the incidence of a Type I error. Frequently used post hoc tests are the Newman-Keuls test, the Tukey Honestly Significant Difference (HSD) test, the Scheffe test, and the Dunnett test (Munro, 2005). When these tests are calculated, the alpha level is reduced in proportion to the number of additional tests required to locate statistically significant differences. For example, for several of the aforementioned post hoc tests, if many groups' mean values are being compared, the magnitude of the difference is set higher than if only two groups are being compared. Post hoc tests are tedious to perform by hand and are best handled with statistical computer software programs.

After computing post hoc tests for our example, the final interpretation is: *Analysis of variance performed on monthly medical costs revealed significant differences between the three treatment groups, F (2, 12) = 6.53, p < 0.05. Post hoc comparisons using the Tukey HSD comparison test indicated that the patients in the pharmacotherapy group incurred significantly higher medical costs after treatment than the patients in the standard care group ($676.60 versus $207.00). However, there were no significant differences between the monthly medical costs of the multidisciplinary group and the standard care group or between the multidisciplinary group and the pharmacotherapy group.* Grove's (2007) statistical workbook for healthcare research has exercises for expanding your interpretation and understanding of ANOVA and post hoc procedure results from published studies.

Nonparametric Alternative

If the data do not meet the normality assumptions for an ANOVA, the nonparametric alternative is the Kruskal-Wallis test. Calculations for the Kruskal-Wallis test involve converting the data to ranks, discarding any variance or normality issues associated with the original values. Similar to the ANOVA, the **Kruskal-Wallis test** is a nonparametric analysis technique that can accommodate the comparisons of more than two groups. The Kruskal-Wallis test is also the appropriate analysis technique to use if the study data being analyzed are ordinal level. This test is thoroughly addressed in textbooks by Daniel (2000) and Munro (2005).

Other ANOVA Procedures

The ANOVA example presented earlier used equal sample sizes in each group. The calculations for an ANOVA with unequal sample sizes are slightly different. Moreover, there are other kinds of ANOVA that accommodate other research designs involving various numbers of independent and dependent variables, such as factorial ANOVA, repeated measures ANOVA, and mixed factorial ANOVA. These ANOVA procedures are presented and explained in comprehensive statistics textbooks such as Zar's text (2007).

Chi-Square Test of Independence

The chi-square (χ^2) test compares differences in proportions of nominal level variables. When a study requires that researchers compare proportions (percentages) in one category versus another category, the χ^2 is a statistic that reveals if the difference in proportion is statistically improbable. The χ^2 has its own theoretical distribution and associated χ^2 table (see Appendix E).

A one-way chi-square is a statistic that compares different levels of one variable only. For example, a researcher may collect information on gender and compare the proportions of males to females. If the one-way chi-square is statistically significant, it would indicate that proportions of one gender are significantly higher than proportions of the other gender than what would be expected by chance (Daniel, 2000). A two-way chi-square is a statistic that tests whether proportions in levels of one variable are significantly different from proportions of the second variable. For example, the presence of advanced colon polyps was studied in three groups of patients: patients having a normal body mass index (BMI), patients who were overweight, and patients who were obese (Siddiqui et al., 2009). The research question tested was: *Is there a significant difference between the three groups (normal, overweight, and obese) in the presence of advanced colon polyps?* The results of the chi-square analysis indicated that a larger proportion of obese patients fell into the category of having advanced colon polyps compared with normal-weight and overweight patients, suggesting that obesity may be a risk factor for developing advanced colon polyps.

Assumptions

One assumption of the chi-square test is that only one datum entry is made for each subject in the sample. If repeated measures from the same subject are being used for analysis, such as pretests and posttests, chi-square is not an appropriate test (the McNemar test is the appropriate test) (Munro, 2005). Another assumption is that for each variable, the categories are mutually exclusive and exhaustive. No cells may have an expected frequency of zero. However, in the actual data, the observed cell frequency may be zero. Until more recently, each cell was expected to have a frequency of at least five, but this requirement has been mathematically shown to be unnecessary. However, no more than 20% of the cells should have fewer than five (Conover, 1971). The test is distribution-free, or nonparametric, which means that no assumption has been made for a normal distribution of values in the population from which the sample was taken.

Calculation

The computations for a two-way chi-square test are presented in this section. A study examining the presence of candiduria (presence of *Candida* species in the urine) among 97 adults with a spinal cord injury is presented as an example. The differences in the use of antibiotics were investigated using chi-square analysis (Goetz, Howard, Cipher & Revankar, 2010). The data for this study are presented in Table 25-5, as a contingency table. A contingency table is a table that displays the relationship between two or more categorical variables (Daniel, 2000).

The formula for a two-way chi-square is:

$$\chi^2 = \frac{n[(A)(D) - (B)(C)]^2}{(A + B)(C + D)(A + C)(B + D)}$$

where the contingency table is labeled as such:

A	B
C	D

Fitting the cells into the formula would appear as:

TABLE 25-5   Candiduria and Antibiotic Use in Adults with Spinal Cord Injuries

	Candiduria	No candiduria
Antibiotic use	15	43
No antibiotic use	0	39

$$\chi^2 = \frac{97\,[(15)(39) - (43)(0)]^2}{(15 + 43)(0 + 39)(15 + 0)(43 + 39)}$$

$$\chi^2 = \frac{33,195,825}{2,782,260}$$

$$\chi^2 = 11.93$$

With any chi-square analysis, the degrees of freedom (*df*) must be calculated to determine the significance of the value of the statistic. The following formula is used for this calculation:

$$df = (R - 1)(C - 1)$$

where
R = number of rows
C = number of columns

In the example, the chi-square value was 11.93, and *df* was 1, which was calculated as follows:

$$df = (2 - 1)(2 - 1) = 1$$

Interpretation of Results

The chi-square statistic is compared with the chi-square values in the table in Appendix E. The table includes the critical values of chi-square for specific degrees of freedom at selected levels of significance. If the value of the statistic is equal to or greater than the value identified in the chi-square table, the difference between the two variables is statistically significant. The critical χ^2 for *df* = 1 is 3.84, and our obtained χ^2 is 11.93, exceeding the critical value and indicating a significant difference between antibiotic users and nonusers in the presence of candiduria. Subjects who used antibiotics had significantly higher rates of candiduria than subjects who did not use antibiotics (26% versus 0%). This finding suggests that antibiotic use may be a risk factor for developing candiduria, and further research is needed to investigate candiduria as a direct effect of antibiotics.

KEY POINTS

- Parametric statistics used to determine differences are accompanied by certain assumptions, and the data must be tested for whether they meet those assumptions before computing the statistic.
- Many tests of normality can assist the researcher in determining the suitability of the data for the use of parametric statistics.
- In the event that the data do not meet the assumptions of the parametric statistic, there are nonparametric alternatives that do not adhere to the assumptions of the parametric test.
- The *t*-test is one of the most commonly used parametric analyses to test for significant differences between statistical measures of two samples or groups.
- The independent samples *t*-test indicates a difference between two groups of subjects, whereas the paired samples *t*-test indicates a difference in two assessments of the same subjects or two groups matched on selected variables.
- The Mann-Whitney *U* test is the nonparametric alternative to the independent samples *t*-test when the study data violate one or more of the independent samples *t*-test assumptions.
- The Wilcoxon signed-rank test is the nonparametric alternative to the paired or dependent samples *t*-test when the study data violate one or more of the paired samples *t*-test assumptions.
- ANOVA can be used to examine data from two or more groups and compares the variance within each group with the variance between groups.
- ANOVA conducted on three or more groups that is significant requires the use of post hoc analysis procedures to determine the location of group differences.
- The Kruskal-Wallis test is the nonparametric alternative to the ANOVA when the study data violate one or more of the ANOVA assumptions.
- The chi-square test compares proportions (percentages) in one category of a variable of interest with proportions in another category.
- McNemar test is the appropriate statistical test to use when analyzing nominal level data obtained from repeated measures from the same subject, such as pretests and posttests.

REFERENCES

Aberson, C. L. (2010). *Applied power analysis for the behavioral sciences*. New York, NY: Routledge Taylor & Francis Group.

Cipher, D. J., & Clifford, P. A. (2004). Dementia, pain, behavioral disturbances and ADLs: Toward a comprehensive conceptualization of quality of life in long-term care. *International Journal of Geriatric Psychiatry, 19*(8), 741–748.

Cipher, D. J., Clifford, P. A., & Roper, K. D. (2006). Behavioral manifestations of pain in the demented elderly. *Journal of the American Medical Director's Association, 7*(6), 355–365.

Cipher, D. J., Fernandez, E., & Clifford, P. A. (2001). Cost effectiveness of multidisciplinary pain management: Comparison of three treatment groups. *Journal of Clinical Psychology in Medical Settings, 8*(4), 237–244.

Cipher, D. J., Kurian, A. K., Fulda, K. G., Snider, R., & Van Beest, J. (2007). Using the MBMD to delineate treatment outcomes in rehabilitation. *Journal of Clinical Psychology in Medical Settings*, *14*(2), 102–112.

Cohen, J., & Cohen, P. (1983). *Applied multiple regression/correlation analysis for the behavioral sciences.* Hillsdale, NJ: Lawrence Erlbaum.

Conover, W. J. (1971). *Practical nonparametric statistics.* New York, NY: Wiley.

D'Agostino, R. B., Belanger, A., & D'Agostino, R. B., Jr. (1990). A suggestion for using powerful and informative tests of normality. *American Statistician*, *44*(4), 316–321.

Daniel, W. W. (2000). *Applied nonparametric statistics* (2nd ed.). Pacific Grove, CA: Duxbury Press.

Goetz, L., Howard, M., Cipher, D., & Revankar, S. G. (2010). Occurrence of candiduria in a population of chronically catheterized patients with spinal-cord injury. *Spinal Cord*, *48*(1), 51–54.

Gordis, L. (2008). *Epidemiolology* (4th ed.). Philadelphia, PA: Saunders.

Grove, S. K. (2007). *Statistics for health care research: A practical workbook.* St. Louis, MO: Saunders.

Kerns, R. D., Turk, D. C., & Rudy, T. E. (1985). The West-Haven Yale Multidimensional Pain Inventory (WHYMPI). *Pain*, *23*(4), 345–356.

Melnyk, B. M., & Fineout-Overholt, E. (2011). *Evidence-based practice in nursing & healthcare: A guide to best practice* (2nd ed.). Philadelphia, PA: Lippincott Williams & Wilkins.

Munro, B. H. (2005). *Statistical methods for health care research.* Philadelphia: PA: Lippincott Williams & Wilkins.

Orem, D. E. (2001). *Nursing concepts of practice* (6th ed.). St. Louis, MO: Mosby.

Ott, B. R. & Fogel, B. S. (2004). Measurement of depression in dementia: Self vs clinician rating. *International Journal of Geriatric Psychiatry*, *7*(12), 899–904.

Reisberg, B., Ferris, B., Deleon, M. J., & Crook, T. (1982). The global deterioration scale for assessment of primary degenerative dementia. *American Journal of Psychiatry*, *139*(9), 1136–1139.

Scherder, E., Oosterman, J., Swaab, D., Herr, K., Ooms, M., Ribbe, M., et al (2005). Recent developments in pain in dementia. *British Medical Journal*, *330*(7489), 461–464.

Siddiqui, A. A., Nazario, H., Mahgoub, A., Pandove, S., Cipher, D. J., & Spechler, S. J. (2009). Obesity is associated with an increased prevalence of advanced adenomatous colon polyps in a male veteran population. *Digestive Disease & Sciences*, *54*(7), 1560–1564.

Thakur, M., & Blazer, D. G. (2008). Depression in long-term care. *Journal of the American Medical Directors Association*, *9*(2), 82–87.

Yesavage, J., Brink, T., & Rose, T. (1983). Development and validation of a geriatric depression scale: A preliminary report. *Journal of Psychiatry Reserves*, *17*(1), 37–49.

Zar, J. H. (2007). *Biostatistical Analysis* (5th ed.). Upper Saddle River, NJ: Prentice-Hall.

26
CHAPTER

Interpreting Research Outcomes

When data analysis is complete, there is a feeling that the answers are known and the study is finished. However, the results of statistical analysis alone are inadequate to complete a study. The researcher may know the results, but without careful intellectual examination, these results are of little use to others or to the body of nursing knowledge. To be useful, the evidence from data analysis needs to be carefully examined, organized, and given meaning, and the statistical significance and clinical importance need to be assessed with implications for practice and directions for further research. This process is referred to as the interpretation of research outcomes.

Interpretation is one of the most important parts of a study because some of the most profound insights of the entire research process occur during this step of the study. There is a tendency to rush this important step to finish the study, but it is not a step to be minimized or hurried. The process takes time for reflection. Often, a researcher becomes too close to the details to be able to see the big picture. At this point, dialogue with colleagues or mentors can add clarity and expand meaning to the interpretation of study findings and formation of conclusions.

Data collection and analysis are action-oriented activities that require concrete thinking. However, when interpreting the results of the study, one tends to implement abstract thinking, including the creative use of introspection, reasoning, and intuition. In some ways, these last steps in the research process are the most difficult. They require you to synthesize the logic used to develop the research plan, implement the strategies used in the data collection phase, and examine the mathematical logic or insight and pattern formation obtained in data analysis. Evaluating the research process used in the study, producing meaning from the results, and forecasting the usefulness of the findings are all part of interpretation and require high-level intellectual processes.

The interpretation of research outcomes is usually the final chapter of theses or dissertations and the final section of research articles, which is often entitled "Discussion." Presentations of studies often conclude with an interpretation of the research outcomes. This chapter focuses on the interpretation of research outcomes from quantitative, outcomes, and intervention research. The interpretations of research outcomes for qualitative research are presented in Chapter 12. The process of interpreting research outcomes for quantitative, outcomes, and intervention studies includes the following: (1) examining study evidence, (2) determining findings, (3) forming conclusions, (4) identifying limitations, (5) generalizing the findings, (6) considering implications for practice, and (7) suggesting further studies. Each of these activities is discussed in this chapter with examples from a quantitative descriptive, predictive correlational study by Rutkowski and Connelly (2011).

Examining Evidence

The first step in interpretation involves considering the evidence available that supports or contradicts the validity of study results related to the research purpose and objectives, questions, or hypotheses. The process is similar to conducting a critical appraisal of your own study. Your temptation is to ignore flaws—certainly not to point them out. However, an honest completion of this process is essential to build a body of knowledge. It is not a time for confession, remorse, and apology but rather for thoughtful reflection. You need to identify the limitations of your study and consider how these might affect the study findings and conclusions (Fawcett & Garity, 2009).

Evidence from the Research Plan
The initial evidence regarding the validity of the study results is derived from reexamining the research plan.

Reexamination requires that you reexplore the logic of the methodology. Analyze the logical links among the problem statement, purpose, research questions, variables, framework, design, sample, measurement methods, and types of analyses. These elements of the study should logically link together and be consistent with the research problem. Remember the old adage: a chain is only as strong as its weakest link. This saying is also true of research because all studies have limitations. This examination of the study needs to identify its weakest links or limitations as well as its strengths.

You need to examine these limitations in terms of their impact on the results. Could the results, or some of the results, be a consequence of a weakness in the methodology rather than a true test of the hypotheses? Can the research objectives, questions, or hypotheses be answered from the methodology used in the study? Could the results be a consequence of an inappropriate conceptual or operational definition of a variable? Do the research questions clearly emerge from the framework? Can the results be related back to the framework? Are the analyses logically planned to address the research objectives, questions, or hypotheses?

If the types of analyses are inappropriate for examining the research questions, what do the results of analyses mean? For example, if the design failed to control extraneous variables, could some of these variables explain the results, rather than the results being explained by the variables measured and examined through statistical analysis? Was the sample studied a logical group on which to test the hypotheses? The researcher must carefully evaluate each link in the design to determine potential weaknesses. Every link is clearly related to the meaning given to the study results. If the researcher is reviewing a newly completed study and determines that some of the analyses were inappropriate, then these analyses need to be redone. If the study has several weaknesses or breaks in logical links, the findings may need to be seriously questioned.

Evidence from Measurement

One assumption often made in interpreting study results is that the study variables were adequately measured. This adequacy is determined by examining the fit of operational definitions with the framework and through validity and reliability information. Although you should determine the reliability and validity of measurement strategies before using them in your study, you need to reexamine the measures at this point to determine the strength of evidence available from the results (Fawcett & Garity, 2009; Waltz, Strickland, & Lenz, 2010). For example, did the scale

used to measure anxiety truly reflect the anxiety experienced in the study population? What was the effect size? Were the validity and reliability of instruments examined in the present study? Can this information be used to interpret the results? The validity and reliability of measurement methods are critical to the validity of results

A descriptive, predictive correlational study by Rutkowski and Connelly (2011) is presented as an example throughout this chapter. The purpose of this study was "to examine the relationships between parent physical activity, parent-adolescent obesity risk knowledge, and adolescent physical activity" (Rutkowski & Connelly, 2011, p. 52). These researchers based their study on the significant problem of childhood obesity in the United States and the need to determine knowledge of adolescents and their parents of obesity risk and their physical activity. The study included three measurement methods, Obesity Risk Knowledge Scale (ORK-10) (Swift, Glazebrook, & Mcdonald, 2006), International Physical Activity Questionnaire (IPAQ, 2001), and Patient Centered Assessments and Counseling for Exercise Plus Nutrition + Moderate Vigorous Physical Activity (PACE+ MVPA) (Prochaska, Sallis, & Long, 2001). The researchers clearly linked the study variables (obesity risk knowledge, physical activity of adults, and physical activity of adolescents) to the three measurement methods in Table 26-1. The measurement methods, validity, and reliability were addressed in the following study excerpt.

"The ORK-10 (Swift et al., 2006) is a 10-item self-report instrument that measures knowledge regarding the health risks associated with obesity.... Internal consistency reliability estimates have been reported with Cronbach's alpha coefficient [r] of .83 (Swift et al., 2006). The measure has not been tested with children, but Swift encourages its use with children 12 years and older (J. Swift, personal communication, July 10, 2007). In this study, the coefficient alphas for the adolescent scale scores are .53 and .59 for parents....

The PACE+ Adolescent Physical Activity Measure (MVPA; Prochaska et al., 2001) was originally developed as a screening tool for use by clinical staff to measure physical activity levels in adolescents seeking treatment in primary care.... Although brief, this instrument is practical and assesses targeted behavior that offers clinical information to practitioners....

The IPAQ has been developed to provide a set of well-developed instruments that are used

TABLE 26-1	Summary of Study Measures and Scoring
Variable	Measure
Obesity Risk Knowledge	
Adults and adolescents	ORK-10 (data from Swift et al., 2006): includes 10 items that yield responses of either 1 or 0 points. Scores range from 0-10 with higher scores indicating higher levels of knowledge.
Physical Activity	
Adults	IPAQ (http://www.ipaq.ki.se/IPAQ.asp?mnu_sel=EEF&pg_sel=DDE): Data analyzed in minutes/day and sorted into the following three categories: (1) low—no activity is reported *or* some activity is reported but not enough to meet categories 2 or 3; (2) moderate—≥3 days of vigorous activity of at least 20 minutes *or* ≥5 days of moderate-intensity activity or walking of at least 30 minutes per day *or* ≥5 days of any combination of walking, moderate-intensity, or vigorous-intensity activities achieving a minimum of at least 600 MET-minutes/week; (3) high—either vigorous-intensity activity on at least 3 days and accumulating at least 1500 MET-minutes/week *or* ≥7 days of any combination of walking, moderate-intensity, or vigorous-intensity activities accumulating at least 3000 MET-minutes/week.
Adolescents	PACE+ Adolescent Physical Activity Measure (data from Prochaska et al., 2001): each response has a scale of 0-7 days. The scores for each question are added together, and the total is divided by 2. A score of <5 indicates that the Healthy People 2010 guideline for adolescent physical activity is not being met.

MET, Metabolic equivalent of the task.
Rutkowski, E. M., & Connelly, C. D. (2011). Obesity risk knowledge and physical activity in families of adolescents. *Journal of Pediatric Nursing, 26*(1), 53.

internationally to obtain comparable estimates of [adult] physical activity (IPAQ, 2001). This instrument is designed in both a short version including four generic items and a long version that reflects five activity domains (IPAQ). The study presented here incorporates the short version because it is able to capture the general conditions of parental activity without being burdensome to complete.... Validity and reliability evaluation in 14 countries and across six continents has been reported (IPAQ). In this study, coefficient alpha [r] is .80." (Rutkowski & Connelly, 2011, pp. 53-54)

Rutkowski and Connelly (2011) provided a detailed description of their measurement methods and how they were scored (see Table 26-1). The validity and reliability of the IPAQ are very strong because the scale has been used internationally in several countries and had strong reliability in this study ($r = 0.80$). The PACE+ MVPA is recognized to have test-retest reliability and concurrent validity, but no specific information was provided. The ORK-10 has evidence of strong internal consistency reliability with adults in previous studies but has not been used with adolescents and had low internal reliability alpha coefficients in this study ($r = 0.053$ for adolescents and $r = 0.59$ for parents). The discussion of the measurement methods would have been strengthened by an expanded description of the ORK-10 scale validity and the reliability and validity for the PACE+ MVPA. The

reliability of the ORK-10 is a study limitation that might have influenced the study findings. The researchers recognized the limitation of the ORK-10 scale reliability for both adolescents and adults, which is discussed later in this chapter.

Evidence from the Data Collection Process

Many activities that occur during data collection affect the meaning of study results. Did the study have a high refusal rate for subject participation, or was the attrition high? Was the sample size sufficient (Aberson, 2010; Fawcett & Garity, 2009; Thompson, 2002)? Did strategies for acquiring a sample eliminate important groups whose data would have influenced the results? Did the research team achieve intervention fidelity when the treatment was implemented (Stein, Sargent, & Rafaels, 2007)? Did unforeseen events occur during the study that might have changed or had an impact on the data? Were measurement techniques consistent? What impact do inconsistencies have on interpreting results? Sometimes data collection does not proceed as planned. Unforeseen situations alter the collection of data. What were these variations in the study? What impact do they have on interpreting the results? Sometimes someone other than the subject completes data collection forms. Also, variations may occur when scales are administered. For example, an anxiety scale may be given to one subject immediately before a painful procedure and to another subject on awakening in the morning. Values on these measures cannot be considered comparable. Data integrity also depends on the responses of the research participants, which could be compromised by anxiety, time constraints, denial, or other factors not in the direct control of the researcher. The researcher must be on the alert for these subject factors that could compromise the integrity of the data. Values on these measures cannot be considered comparable. These types of differences are seldom reported and sometimes not even recorded. To some extent, only the researcher knows how consistently the measurements were taken. Reporting of this information depends on the integrity of the researcher (Fawcett & Garity, 2009; Kerlinger & Lee, 2000; Pyrczak & Bruce, 2005; Stein et al., 2007).

Rutkowski and Connelly (2011) clearly identified their sampling method as purposive, convenience and noted appropriate inclusion sampling criteria. A power analysis was conducted to determine that the sample size of 94 adolescent/parent dyads was adequate for this study. There was no sample attrition noted in the study, but it would have been helpful if the researchers had discussed the refusal rate of potential participants. The procedures for collecting data in this study were clearly described as indicated in the following excerpt. However, the researchers might have provided a little more detail about the self-administration of the scales by the adults and adolescents.

"All study procedures including protocols for recruiting participants and obtaining informed consent had been reviewed and approved by the appropriate administrative and university institutional review boards for the protection of human subjects prior to study initiation.... The study protocol was presented, questions addressed, and informed consent was obtained from the parent as well as parents' permission to approach their child regarding participation. Next, parents self-administered a survey containing demographic questions and several standardized instruments including the Obesity Risk Knowledge Scale (ORK-10; Swift et al, 2006) and the IPAQ. Surveys were collected by the PI [principal investigator] immediately.

Following the collection of parent surveys, a follow-up meeting was held with those adolescents who met the criteria and whose parents signed consents for their participation. Adolescents who signed assent forms were then asked to self-administer both the demographic survey and several standardized measures including the ORK-10 and PACE+ MVPA (Prochaska et al., 2001)." (Rutkowski & Connelly, 2011, pp. 52-53)

Evidence from the Data Analysis Process

The process of data analysis is an important factor in evaluating the meaning of results. One important part of this examination is to summarize the study weaknesses related to the data analysis process. Ask yourself these questions concerning the meaning of your results: Were the data checked to ensure that limited or no errors occurred during data entry into the computer? How many subjects have missing data, and how was missing data managed to decrease the effects on the study results? Were the analyses accurately implemented and calculated? Were statistical assumptions violated? Were the statistics used appropriate for the data? It is best to address these issues initially before analyses are performed and again when completing the analyses and preparing the final report. Researchers should consult with a biostatistician during the planning of a study and during data analysis to ensure the appropriateness of the statistical tests selected. The biostatistician could also be helpful in interpreting the results. Before submitting a study for publication, we recommend rechecking each analysis reported in the paper. We also encourage reexamining the analysis statements in the article for accuracy and clarity. Are you correctly interpreting the results of the analysis? Documentation on each statistical value or analysis statement reported in the paper is filed with a copy of the article. The documentation includes the date of the analysis, the page number of the computer printout showing the results (the printout is stored in a file by date of analysis), the sample size for the analysis, and the number of missing values (Corty, 2007; Grove, 2007; Fawcett & Garity, 2009). Rutkowski and Connelly (2011) identified their data analysis with a separate heading that is presented in the following excerpt.

"Data Analysis

The sample size for the analysis is 94 dyads, which is sufficient to detect a moderate standardized effect size (*ES*) ($d = 0.32$) using a two-tailed significance test with a power of 0.80 and a significance level of 0.05. Data have been analyzed using the software package *Statistical Package for Social Sciences, Version 15* (SPSS, Inc, 2008). Descriptive and multivariate statistics have been used in this study." (Rutkowski & Connelly, 2011, p. 54)

The data analysis section clearly addressed the sample size of the study, analysis software package used, and the types of analyses conducted. This section would have been strengthened by including a power analysis that discussed the effect size for relationships because the study examined both differences between the adolescents and their parents and relationships of obesity risk knowledge with physical activities for adolescents and adults (Aberson, 2010). This section mentioned the inferential statistic conducted for group differences, the two-tailed *t*-test, but did not mention that relationships were examined with the Pearson product-moment correlation and regression analysis techniques.

Evidence from Data Analysis Results

The outcomes of data analysis are the most direct evidence of the results. The researcher has intimate knowledge of the research and needs to evaluate its strengths and limitations carefully when judging the validity of the results. In descriptive and correlational studies, the validity of the results depends on how accurately the variables were measured in selected samples and settings. Interpretation of results from quasi-experimental and experimental studies is often based on decision theory, with five possible results: (1) significant results that are in keeping with the results predicted by the researcher, (2) nonsignificant results, (3) significant results that oppose the results predicted by the researcher, (4) mixed results, and (5) unexpected results (Shadish, Cook, & Campbell, 2002).

Significant and Predicted Results

Significant results that coincide with the researcher's predictions are the easiest to explain and, unless weaknesses are present, validate the proposed logical links among the elements of the study. These results support the logical links developed by the researcher among the purpose, framework, questions, variables, and measurement methods (Shadish et al., 2002). This outcome is very satisfying to the researcher. However, the researcher needs to consider alternative explanations for the positive findings. What other elements could possibly have led to the significant results?

Nonsignificant Results

Unpredicted nonsignificant or inconclusive results are the most difficult to explain. These results are often referred to as negative results. The negative results could be a true reflection of reality. In this case, the reasoning of the researcher or the theory used by the researcher to develop the hypothesis is in error. If so, the negative findings are an important addition to the body of knowledge. With nonsignificant results, it is important to determine if adequate power of 0.8 or higher was achieved for the data analysis. The researcher needs to conduct a power analysis to determine if the sample size was adequate to prevent the risk of a Type II error (Aberson, 2010; Shadish et al., 2002). A Type II error means that in reality the findings are significant, but because of weaknesses in the methodology, the significance was not detected.

Negative results could also be due to inappropriate methodology, a deviant sample, problems with internal validity, inadequate measurement, use of weak statistical techniques, or faulty analysis. Unless these weak links are detected, the reported results could lead to faulty information in the body of knowledge (Angell, 1989). It is easier for the researcher to blame faulty methodology for nonsignificant findings than to find failures in theoretical or logical reasoning. If faulty methodology is blamed, the researcher needs to explain exactly how the breakdown in methodology led to the negative results. Negative results, in any case, do not mean that there are no relationships among the variables or differences between groups; they indicate that the study failed to find any relationships or differences.

Significant and Not Predicted Results

Significant results that are the opposite of those predicted, if the results are valid, are an important addition to the body of knowledge. An example would be a study in which the researchers proposed that social support and ego strength were positively related. If the study showed that high social support was related to low ego strength, the result would be the opposite of that predicted. Such results, when verified by other studies, indicate that the theory being tested needs modification and refinement. Because these types of studies can affect nursing practice, this information is important.

Mixed Results

Mixed results are probably the most common outcome of studies. In this case, one variable may uphold the characteristics predicted, whereas another does not, or two dependent measures of the same variable may show opposite results. These results might be an accurate reflection of reality but also might be due to study limitations (Shadish et al., 2002). The study limitations might include differing reliability or validity of two methods of measuring variables, varying data collection processes, small sample size, or missing subject data. Additional research is indicated to examine mixed study results.

Mixed results may also indicate a need to modify existing theory.

Unexpected Results

Unexpected results are relationships found between variables that were not hypothesized and not predicted from the framework guiding the study. These unexpected results are also called serendipitous results. Most researchers examine as many elements of data as possible in addition to the elements directed by the research objectives, questions, or hypotheses. The researchers can use these findings to develop or refine theories and to formulate later studies. In addition, serendipitous results are as important as evidence in developing the implications of the study. However, researchers must deal carefully with serendipitous results when considering their meaning because the study was not designed to examine these results.

Evidence from Previous Studies

The results of the present study should always be examined in light of previous findings. It is important for the researcher to know whether the results are consistent with past research. Consistency in findings across studies is important for developing theories and refining scientific knowledge for the nursing profession. Therefore, any inconsistencies need to be explored to determine reasons for the differences. Replication of studies and synthesis of findings from existing studies using meta-analyses and systematic reviews are critical for the development of empirical knowledge for an evidence-based practice (Brown, 2009; Craig & Smyth, 2012; Melnyk & Fineout-Overholt, 2011).

Determining Findings

Findings are developed by evaluating evidence (discussed previously in this chapter) and translating and interpreting study results. Although much of the process of developing findings from results occurs in the mind of the researcher, evidence of such thinking can be found in published research reports (Pyrczak & Bruce, 2005). It is important during this process to talk with colleagues or mentors to clarify meanings or expand implications of the research findings. The study results and findings are presented for Rutkowski and Connelly's (2011) research examining the relationships among the variables parent and adolescent physical activities and parent and adolescent obesity risk knowledge. As part of the study results, the researchers described the participants of the study

TABLE 26-2 Characteristics of the Adolescent-Parent Dyads

	Adolescent	Parent
Age, M (SD), range	12.8 (1.0), 11.8-13.8	44.1 (5.2), 31-60
Ethnicity, n (%)		
Caucasian	70 (74.5)	69 (74.2)
Hispanic	14 (14.9)	16 (17.2)
Asian	5 (5.3)	6 (6.5)
Other	5 (5.3)	2 (2.2)
Gender, n (%)		
Male	56 (59.6)	19 (20.2)
Female	38 (40.4)	75 (79.8)
BMI, M (SD), range	19.4 (2.7), 13.6-32.9	24.1 (4.9), 24.1-43.2
Household size, M (SD), range	4.41 (0.9), 2-6	4.41 (0.9), 2-6
Grade in school, n (%)		
6th	17 (18.3)	
7th	28 (30.1)	
8th	35 (37.6)	
9th	8 (8.6)	
10th	5 (5.4)	
Grade point average, n (%)		
2.0-2.9	10 (11.6)	
3.0-3.9	53 (61.6)	
4.0 or higher	23 (24.5)	
Marital status, n (%)		
Married		85 (91.4)
Single		2 (2.2)
Divorced		5 (5.4)
Widowed		1 (1.1)
Number of years with partner, M (SD), range		17.5 (4.9), 2-31
Education, n (%)		
Less than high school		2 (2.3)
High school diploma		14 (16.1)
College		46 (51.7)
Graduate school		26 (29.9)
Work outside the home, yes, n (%)		31 (33.3)

BMI, Body mass index; *M (SD)*, mean (standard deviation).
From Rutkowski, E. M., & Connelly, C. D. (2011). Obesity risk knowledge and physical activity in families of adolescents. *Journal of Pediatric Nursing, 26*(1), 54.

and presented the sample characteristics of the adolescents and their parents in Table 26-2. Rutkowski and Connelly (2011, p. 55) noted that "This sample is not representative of families living in southern California; however, it is representative of families living in the community sampled." The study objectives (aims), results, and findings are presented in the following excerpt.

Objective 1 was to describe and compare the obesity risk knowledge and physical activity level of the parents and adolescents.

"*Results.* In this sample of adolescent/parent dyads, the mean score for adolescents' obesity risk knowledge (ORK-10) is 4.69 (*SD* = 1.63), and the mean score for the parents is 5.54 (*SD* = 1.84 [Table 26-3]). These scores are based upon 10 being the score that reflects the most knowledge and 0 reflecting the least knowledge. *t*-tests have been conducted to determine whether youth differ significantly from parents on the ORK-10. The results indicated that adolescent obesity risk knowledge is statistically significantly lower than their parents $t_{(1,92)} = 3.45$, $p < .001$.

Both the parents and adolescents are active at levels measured to meet standardized guidelines (U.S. Department of Health and Human Services [USDHHS], 2000). The level of physical activity as measured by the PACE+ indicates that most adolescent participants are meeting the recommended level of daily activity (*M* = 5.33, *SD* = 1.23 [see Table 26-3]). Among the parent participants, IPAQ scores range from 0 to 12,558 (*M* = 3741.07, *SD* = 3135.4); categories of activity levels indicate 61.7% report physical activity at a vigorous level (*M* = 1960, *SD* = 2,164), 18.1% report a moderate level (*M* = 872,

SD = 1,285), and 14.9% report physical activity at a low level [see Table 26-3]." (Rutkowski & Connelly, 2011, p. 55)

"*Findings.* The ORK-10 scores of both the adolescents and parents are low, with adolescent scores statistically lower than parental scores. This is not unexpected because parents have acquired more experiences that would provide insight into some of the questions included in this measure. When selecting the ORK-10 for use in this study, most of the scale items seemed to be relevant.... Despite this perceived relevance, several of the participating youth questioned the measure's content and stated unfamiliarity with some of the questions, particularly those items posed in the negative, for example, 'Obesity does not increase the risk of developing high blood pressure.' These same youth identified words that, if substituted, would increase the level of comprehension of the scale items, which may consequently impact overall scores. An additional finding of interest indicates that in this group of experts, both adolescent and parent mean scores are higher than for the nonexpert group in the Swift et al. (2006) original research." (Rutkowski & Connelly, 2011, pp. 55-56)

TABLE 26-3	Obesity Risk Knowledge and Physical Activity of Family Dyads (*N* = 94)	
Obesity Risk Knowledge,	**Adolescent**	**Parent**
	4.69 (1.63)	5.54 (1.84)
M (*SD*), range	0-10	0-10
Physical Activity		
PACE+, *M* (*SD*)	5.33(1.23)	
IPAQ, *M* (*SD*)		3741.07
		(3135.4)
Vigorous level, *n* (%)		58 (61)
Moderate level, *n* (%)		17 (18.1)
Low walking, *n* (%)		14 (14.9)

From Rutkowski, E. M., & Connelly, C. D. (2011). Obesity risk knowledge and physical activity in families of adolescents. *Journal of Pediatric Nursing, 26*(1), 55.

Objective 2 was to examine the relationships of obesity risk knowledge and physical activities for the parents and adolescents.

"*Results.* A statistically significant inverse relationship has been found between parental 'sitting' activities (including commute time) and the adult ORK scores ($r = -.23$, $p < .05$) as well as parent activity levels and the PACE+ score for activity levels of adolescents ($r = -.23$, $p < .05$). There is no significant relationship between adolescent obesity risk knowledge and adolescent physical activity ($r = .15$, $p > .05$)." (Rutkowski & Connelly, 2011, p. 55)

"*Findings.* Among our sample of adolescent/parent dyads, our findings indicate obesity risk knowledge is not associated with adolescent physical activity. This study does however provide important information on the association between parent physical activity and adolescent physical activity. Especially notable is the inverse relationship between parent activity level and the PACE+ scores of adolescents. This is noteworthy because it is consistent with findings reported a decade earlier by researchers from the School of Public Health at the University of Minnesota (Luepker, 1999). They noted that seriously committed parents who follow exercise routines that are vigorous in nature are frequently engaged in fitness activities that involve only themselves.... Typically these parents do not share their physical activity time with family members, especially younger age children (Luepker, 1999). Many parents participate in their routines outside of 'family time' and in essence exclude children purposefully because they may impede the intensity and duration goals of the parental activity. Luepker concluded that parents who are moderate and less 'serious' are better role models because their children actually see them being physical.... These parents are more apt to include their children in their physical activities. Seriously active parents often work out early in the morning before work, on lunch breaks, after work before returning home, or at night after the children go to bed. Their children never benefit from a role modeling relationship in the area of physical activity (Bandura, 1997). As explained by Luepker, the paradoxical situation of having a very fit, athletic parent and a less than adequately active child is often the result of this absent role model." (Rutkowski & Connelly, 2011, p. 55)

Objective 3 includes the variables of "adolescent and parental obesity risk knowledge, parent physical activity, and selected adolescent characteristics examined to determine their prediction of the adolescent's physical activity" (Rutkowski & Connelly, 2001, p. 52).

"**Results**. Simultaneous multiple regression was conducted to determine the accuracy of the independent variables of parent physical activity, parent ORK-10 score, and adolescent ORK-10 score in predicting adolescent physical activity [dependent variable] while controlling for adolescent gender, ethnicity, and age. Regression results indicate the overall model does not significantly predict adolescent physical activity, $R^2 = 0.116$, $R^2_{adj} = 0.048$, $F_{(6,78)} = 1.70$, $p = 0.13$." (Rutkowski & Connelly, 2011, p. 55)

"**Findings**. The researchers did not discuss the nonsignificant regression analysis results but did address the low Cronbach alpha reliability coefficients for the ORK-10 scale for the adolescents and their parents. The low reliability of this scale for both groups might have had an impact on the study results.

"It should be noted that the data from our sample of family dyads have produced lower internal reliabilities than the Swift et al. (2006) original study. This is not unexpected because inconsistent internal reliabilities are often found for instruments in 'early development' (Frank-Stromborg & Olsen, 2004). In our study, the measure has been used with participants from a different culture and age groups than those of the original research. Based upon our findings, further refinement of the measure is needed to avoid contextual confusion and to increase cultural and international application. Use of the ORK-10 is an initial step in assessing obesity risk knowledge. Further research into the scale refinement, reliability, and validity is warranted." (Rutkowski & Connelly, 2011, p. 56)

Forming Conclusions

Conclusions are derived from the study findings and are a synthesis of findings. Forming **conclusions** for a study requires a combination of logical reasoning, creative formation of a meaningful whole from pieces of information obtained through data analysis and findings from previous studies, receptivity to subtle clues in the data, and use of an open context in considering alternative explanations of the data.

When forming conclusions, it is important to remember that research never proves anything; rather, research offers support for a position. Proof is a logical part of deductive reasoning, but not of the research process. Therefore, formulation of causal statements is risky. For example, the causal statement that *A causes B* (absolutely, in all situations) cannot be scientifically proved. It is more credible to state conclusions in the form of conditional probabilities that are qualified. It would be more appropriate to state in the study that if *A* occurred, then *B* occurred under conditions *x*, *y*, and *z* (Kerlinger & Lee, 2000; Shadish et al., 2002), or that if *A* occurred, then *B* had an 80% probability of occurring. Because this was a descriptive, predictive correlational study and some of the results were nonsignificant, Rutkowski and Connelly (2011) presented only tentative conclusions that are included in the statement of findings. One conclusion is the adults' obesity risk knowledge is related to their physical activity but the adolescents' obesity risk knowledge is not related to their physical activity. The main study conclusion was that parents' activity levels (vigorous, moderate, or low) are inversely related to the adolescents' activity levels. Thus, children's activity levels are most positively impacted when parents role model physical activity and exercise with their children.

One of the risks in developing conclusions in research is going beyond the data—specifically, forming conclusions that the data do not warrant. The most common example is a study that examines relationships between *A* and *B* by correlational analysis and then concludes that *A* causes *B*. Going beyond the data is due to faulty logic and occurs more frequently in published studies than one would like to believe. Be sure to check the validity of arguments related to conclusions before revealing findings.

Identifying Limitations

Limitations are restrictions or problems in a study that may decrease the generalizability of the findings. All studies have limitations, and these might be theoretical or methodological in nature. Theoretical limitations are weaknesses in a study framework and conceptual and operational definitions of variables that restrict the abstract generalization of the findings. At this stage of the research process, theoretical and methodological limitations often overlap. Concerns are raised about the theoretical basis of the study because of unexpected findings. Some of the following theoretical limitations might be identified by researchers:

1. A concept might not be as clearly defined as needed within the theory used as the study framework.
2. The relationships among some concepts from the theory are not presented as clearly as needed in the study framework.
3. A study variable might not be as clearly linked to a concept in the framework as needed.
4. An objective, question, or hypothesis might not be clearly linked to a relationship or proposition in the study framework.

Theoretical limitations are one explanation for study results that are nonsignificant or unexpected. For example, the study framework included a relationship between self-efficacy and health decisions. However, the data analysis did not reveal a statistically significant relationship between these two concepts. The underlying reasons may be that the theory was unclear related to the definitions of concepts or identification of relationships or that the measurements of the concepts were not valid or reliable.

Methodological limitations are weaknesses in the study design that can limit the credibility of the findings and restrict the population to which the findings can be generalized. Methodological limitations result from factors such as nonrepresentative samples, weak designs, single setting, limited control over treatment (intervention) implementation, instruments with limited reliability and validity, limited control over data collection, and improper use of statistical analyses (Fawcett & Garity, 2009; Kerlinger & Lee, 2000; Shadish et al., 2002).

Ideally, the theoretical and methodological limitations are identified before the conduct of the study, and the researchers minimize these limitations as much as possible. However, some limitations are not identified until the study is conducted and are usually identified in the discussion section of the study report with implications of how they might have influenced the study findings. Despite a researcher's higher motives to be objective, subjective judgments and biases sometimes creep into the study conclusions. Researchers need to control subjectivity and biases and recognize any theoretical or methodological limitations of their study before forming conclusions. Limitations and their impact on the study findings must be included in the research report. Rutkowski and Connelly (2011) clearly identified their study limitations, which did limit the conclusions drawn in this study. The reliability limitation of the ORK-10 scale was previously discussed in the findings for Objective 3. In addition, the study would have been strengthened by the conduct of a power analysis for each of the nonsignificant results to determine the power for detecting relationships and the potential for a type II error. The other study limitations are described in the following study excerpt.

> **"Limitations**
> The findings of this study must be considered in relation to the study's limitations. First, the sample is a purposive convenience sample that is relatively homogenous with respect to ethnicity, geographic location, and social economic status (SES), not randomly selected or matched. This nonrandom procedure may influence the findings through self-selection bias. Second, the cross-sectional design disallows for changes over time and may not capture the complex phenomena under study." (Rutkowski & Connelly, 2011, p. 56)

Generalizing the Findings

Generalization extends the implications of the findings from the sample studied to a larger population or from the situation studied to a larger situation. For example, if the study were conducted on diabetic patients, it may be possible to generalize the findings to persons with other chronic illnesses or to well individuals. Studies such as randomized clinical trials usually have large heterogeneous samples, which increase the ability to generalize the findings (Shadish et al., 2002).

How far can generalizations be made? The answer to this question is debatable. From a narrow perspective, one cannot really generalize from the sample on which the study was conducted. Any other sample is likely to be different in some way. The conservative position, represented by Kerlinger and Lee (2000), recommends caution in considering the extent of generalization. Conservatives consider generalization particularly risky if the sample was small, homogeneous, and not randomly selected. However, as discussed in Chapter 15, generalizations are often made to abstract or theoretical populations. Thus, conclusions need to address applications to theory. Judgments about the reasonableness of generalizing need to address issues related to external validity, as discussed in Chapter 10.

Generalizations based on accumulated evidence from many studies are called empirical generalizations. These generalizations are important for verifying theoretical statements or developing new theories. Empirical generalizations are the base of a science and contribute to scientific conceptualization, which provide a basis for generating evidence-based guidelines to manage specific practice problems (Brown, 2009; Craig & Smyth, 2012; Melnyk & Fineout-Overholt, 2011). Chapter 19 provides a detailed discussion of research synthesis processes and strategies for promoting evidence-based nursing practice.

Rutkowski and Connelly (2011) made no generalizations in their study, and their findings were reflective only of the sample studied. Because this is a relatively new area of research that was examined with a descriptive, predictive correlational design, the lack of generalization of findings seems appropriate. In addition, the limitations of the ORK-10 scale reliability, the nonrandom homogeneous sample, and the cross-sectional design would not support generalization of the findings from the study sample to the target population (see Chapter 15 for more details on generalization).

Considering Implications

Implications of research findings for nursing are the meanings of the conclusions for the body of nursing knowledge, theory, and practice. Implications for practices are often based, in part, on whether treatment decisions or outcomes would be different in view of the study findings. A clinically important study should result in altered decisions or actions by nurses that improve patient and family outcomes (Gatchel & Mayer, 2010). The study implications provide specific suggestions for implementing the findings in practice. You need to consider the areas of nursing for which your study findings would be useful. In presenting their implications for practice, Rutkowski and Connelly (2011) discussed the role of nurses in educating parents to be role models to their children regarding physical activity.

> **"Clinical Implications**
>
> "Pediatric nurses, community health nurses, pediatric nurse practitioners, school nurses, and clinical nurse specialists all have opportunities to interface with families of adolescents. Nurses practicing in primary care settings are the first-line defenders against the pandemic of childhood obesity....
>
> "Because prevention is the focus of primary care settings, nurses have opportunities to implement promising strategies with families of adolescents (Larson & Story, 2007). Such encounters are ideal for dissemination of the findings of this study in the area of role modeling by parents for adolescents as a means of impacting behavior change. Discussions regarding the need for parental role modeling should be encouraged.
>
> "It is imperative for parents to acknowledge that taking the time to be physically active with their children may have a positive outcome in increasing the activity levels of their children, which will reduce future chronic health problems.... Children need exemplars to establish lifestyle routines that include physical activity. Parents are in an ideal position to be such role models. The patterns of physical activity developed in adolescents will inoculate them against becoming sedentary adults (Luepker, 1999)." (Rutkowski & Connelly, 2011, p. 56)

Recommending Further Research

Completing a study and examining its implications should culminate in recommendations for further research that emerge from the present study and from previous studies in the same area of interest.

Suggested studies or recommendations for further study may include replications or repeating the design with a different or larger sample or different population. In every study, the researcher gains knowledge and experience that can be used to design "a better study next time." Formulating recommendations for future studies will stimulate you to define more clearly how to improve your study. From a logical or theoretical point of view, the findings should lead you directly to more hypotheses to further test the framework you are using. Improvements could involve an alternative methodology, a refined measurement tool, changes in sampling criteria, or a different setting.

Rutkowski and Connelly (2011) provided the following suggestions for future research:

"Directions for Future Studies

Future research examining obesity risk knowledge in relationship to physical activity is needed to stem the tide of the epidemic of childhood obesity. There is a critical need for a reliable and valid measure to assess the level of knowledge that both children and adults have regarding the consequences of being overweight (Swift et al., 2006). Behavior changes are the remedy for this catastrophic health issue and will not be possible without the development of interventions that are effective in reducing the weight-gaining lifestyles of many Americans, especially children. In addition, research is needed to learn what the public does not know about obesity's risks and its long-term effects. To this end, research is currently being conducted in the refinement of the ORK-10 to enhance its application with multicultural and international populations. A reliable and valid measure could become the impetus in guiding discussion in primary care settings regarding the choices in lifestyle to avoid obesity and the concomitant illnesses that are undermining the healthy futures of adolescents and their families." (Rutkowski & Connelly, 2011, p. 56)

KEY POINTS

- To be useful, evidence from data analysis needs to be carefully examined, organized, and given meaning; and this process is referred to as interpretation.
- Interpretation includes several intellectual activities, such as examining evidence, forming conclusions, identifying study limitations, generalizing the findings, considering implications, and suggesting further research.
- The first step in interpretation is considering all of the evidence available that supports or contradicts the validity of the results. Evidence is obtained from various sources, including the research plan, measurement reliability and validity (or precision and accuracy), data collection process, data analysis process, data analysis results, and previous studies.
- The outcomes of data analysis are the most direct evidence available of the results related to the research purpose and the objectives, questions, or hypotheses.
- Five possible results are (1) significant results that are in keeping with those predicted by the researcher, (2) nonsignificant results, (3) significant results that are opposite those predicted by the researcher, (4) mixed results, and (5) unexpected results.
- Findings are a consequence of evaluating evidence, which includes the findings from previous studies.
- Conclusions are derived from the findings and are a synthesis of the findings.
- The limitations of a study might be theoretical or methodological and need to be clearly identified and discussed in relation to the study conclusions.
- Generalization extends the implications of the findings from the sample studied to a larger target population.
- Implications of the study for nursing are the meanings of study conclusions for the body of nursing knowledge, theory, and practice.
- Completion of a study and examination of implications should culminate in recommending future studies that emerge from the present study and previous studies.

REFERENCES

Aberson, C. L. (2010). *Applied power analysis for the behavioral sciences*. New York, NY: Routledge Taylor & Francis Group.

Angell, M. (1989). Negative studies. *New England Journal of Medicine, 321*(7), 464–466.

Bandura, A. (1997). *Self-efficacy: The exercise of control*. New York, NY: W.H. Freeman & Company.

Brown, S. J. (2009). *Evidence-based nursing: The research-practice connection*. Sudbury, MA: Jones & Bartlett Publishers.

Corty, E. W. (2007). *Using and interpreting statistics: A practical text for the health, behavioral, and social sciences*. St. Louis, MO: Mosby.

Craig, J. V., & Smyth, R. L. (2012). *The evidence-based practice manual for nurses* (3rd ed.). Edinburgh, UK: Churchill Livingstone.

Fawcett, J., & Garity, J. (2009). *Evaluating research for evidence-based nursing practice*. Philadelphia, PA: F. A. Davis.

Frank-Stromborg, M., & Olsen, S. (2004). *Instruments for clinical healthcare research* (3rd ed.). Sudbury, MA: Jones & Bartlett.

Gatchel, R. J., & Mayer, T. G. (2010). Testing minimal clinically important difference: Consensus or conundrum? *The Spine Journal*, *35*(19), 1739–1743.

Grove, S. K. (2007). *Statistics for health care research: A practical workbook*. St. Louis, MO: Saunders.

International Physical Activity Questionnaires (IPAQ). (2001). International Physical Activity Questionnaire. Retrieved from http://www.ipaq.ki.se/ipaq.htm.

Kerlinger, F. N., & Lee, H. P. (2000). *Foundations of behavioral research* (4th ed.). Fort Worth, TX: Harcourt College.

Larson, N., & Story, M. (2007). The pandemic of obesity among children and adolescents: What actions are needed to reverse current trends? [Editorial]. *Journal of Adolescent Health*, *41*, 521–522.

Luepker, R. (1999). How physically active are American children and what can we do about it? *International Journal of Obesity*, *23*(Suppl. 2), S12–S17.

Melnyk, B. M., & Fineout-Overholt, E. (2011). *Evidence-based practice in nursing & healthcare: A guide to best practice* (2nd ed.). Philadelphia, PA: Lippincott Williams & Wilkins.

Prochaska, J., Sallis, J., & Long, D. (2001). A physical activity screening measure for use with adolescents in primary care. *Archives of Pediatric & Adolescent Medicine*, *155*(5), 554–559.

Pyrczak, F., & Bruce, R. R. (2005). *Writing empirical research reports* (5th ed.). Glendale, CA: Pyrczak.

Rutkowski, E. M., & Connelly, C. D. (2011). Obesity risk knowledge and physical activity in families of adolescents. *Journal of Pediatric Nursing*, *26*(1), 51–57.

Shadish, W. R., Cook, T. D., & Campbell, D. T. (2002). *Experimental and quasi-experimental designs for generalization causal inference*. Chicago, IL: Rand McNally.

Statistical Package for the Social Sciences (SPSS), Inc. (2008). *SPSS for windows*. Chicago, IL: SPSS.

Stein, K. F., Sargent, J. T., & Rafaels, N. (2007). Intervention research: Establishing fidelity of the independent variable in nursing clinical trials. *Nursing Research*, *56*(1), 54–62.

Swift, J., Glazebrook, C., & Mcdonald, I. (2006). Validation of a brief, reliable scale to measure knowledge about the health risks associated with obesity. *International Journal of Obesity*, *30*(4), 661–668.

Thompson, S. K. (2002). *Sampling* (2nd ed.). New York, NY: John Wiley & Sons.

U.S. Department of Health and Human Services (USDHHS). (2000). *Health people 2010*. Washington, D.C.: U.S. Government Printing Office.

Waltz, C. F., Strickland, O. L., & Lenz, E. R. (2010). *Measurement in nursing and health research* (4th ed.). New York, NY: Springer Publishing Company.

27

CHAPTER

Disseminating Research Findings

Imagine that as a nurse researcher you are conducting a study in which you describe a unique phenomenon, detect a previously unrecognized relationship, or determine the effectiveness of an intervention. This information might make a difference in nursing practice; however, you feel unskilled in presenting the information and overwhelmed by the idea of publishing. You place the study documents in a drawer with the intent to communicate the findings *someday*. Because many nurses have these types of feelings, many valuable nursing studies are not communicated, and the information is lost. Failure to communicate research findings is considered a violation of ethics and a form of scientific misconduct. After involving members of an institutional review board committee to approve your study, and after subjects consented and participated in your study, you have an ethical obligation to complete your end of the process. Without disseminating the findings, funding is wasted, subject time and data are wasted, and knowledge for nursing practice is not advanced.

Communicating research findings, the final step in the research process, involves developing a research report and disseminating it through presentations and publications to audiences of nurses, healthcare professionals, policy makers, and healthcare consumers. Disseminating study findings provides many advantages for the researcher, the nursing profession, and the consumer of nursing services. By presenting and publishing findings, researchers advance the knowledge of a discipline, which is essential for providing evidence-based practice. For individual researchers, communicating study findings often leads to professional advancement, personal recognition, and other psychological and financial compensations. These rewards are extremely important for the continuation of research in a discipline. By communicating research findings, the researcher also promotes the critical analysis of previous studies, encourages the

replication of studies, and identifies additional research problems. Over time, the findings from many studies are synthesized with the ultimate goal of providing evidence-based health care to patients, families, and communities (Craig & Smyth, 2012; Melnyk & Fineout-Overholt, 2010).

To facilitate the communication of research findings for nurse clinicians and researchers, regardless of whether the research is a primary study, a secondary analysis, or a meta-analysis, this chapter describes the basic content of a research report, the audiences for communicating study findings, and the processes for presenting and publishing research reports.

Content of a Research Report

Both quantitative and qualitative research reports include four major sections or content areas: (1) introduction, (2) methods, (3) results, and (4) discussion of the findings (Pyrczak & Bruce, 2007). The type and depth of information included in these sections depend on the study, the intended audiences, and the mechanisms for disseminating the report. For example, theses and dissertations are research reports, written to demonstrate the student's depth in understanding of the research problem and process to faculty members. Research reports developed for publication in journals are written to communicate study findings efficiently and effectively to nurses and other healthcare professionals. Some journals limit the introduction to two or three brief paragraphs that include a statement about the theoretical framework for the study, a sufficient review of the literature to state what the gap in knowledge is, and the clear purpose of the study. The methods, results, and discussion sections of qualitative studies are usually more detailed than those sections of quantitative studies because of the complex data collection and analysis procedures. Finally, the discussion section briefly acknowledges the limitations of the study, presents the findings in relation to other literature, and discusses the implications of the findings for the intended journal audience.

Quantitative Research Report

This section provides direction to novice researchers writing their first quantitative research report. To begin, the title of your research report needs to indicate what you have studied and attract the attention of interested readers. The title should be concise and consistent with the study purpose and the research objectives, questions, or hypotheses. Often a title includes the major study variables and population and indicates the type of study conducted, but it should not include the results or conclusions of a study (Pyrczak & Bruce, 2007). Heo, Moser, Lennie, Zambroski, and Chung (2007, p. 16) provided the following title for their study: "A Comparison of Health-Related Quality of Life between Older Adults with Heart Failure and Healthy Older Adults." This title is concise, states the focus of the study (comparative descriptive), identifies a key study variable (health-related quality of life [HRQOL]), and includes the populations studied (older adults with heart failure and healthy older adults). However, this study is also predictive, and this is not indicated in the study title. The researchers studied additional independent variables (health perception, functional status, physical symptom status, emotional symptom status, and social support) to predict the dependent variable HRQOL in older adults with and without heart failure. An alternative title would be "Predictors of Health-Related Quality of Life in Older Adults with and without Heart Failure." Some journals limit the length for titles of manuscripts, whereas other journals discourage use of colons.

Most research reports also include an abstract that summarizes the key aspects of the study. An abstract is usually about 200 to 300 words and describes the problem, purpose, framework, methods, sample size, key results, and conclusions (Pyrczak & Bruce, 2007). We provide details for developing an abstract of a study later in this chapter. Heo et al. (2007) included the following abstract for their study.

"*Background:* Health-related quality of life (HRQOL) in older adults with heart failure may be affected by a variety of variables, including aging. It is important to determine the unique impact of heart failure to more effectively improve HRQOL in this population [problem].

Objective: The purpose of this study was to compare HRQOL and physical, psychologic, clinical, and sociodemographic status in older adults with and without heart failure.

Methods: The HRQOL of 90 older adults with heart failure and 116 healthy older adults was compared. The factors best associated with HRQOL in each group were determined using multiple regression model.

Results: HRQOL was substantially worse among older adults with heart failure than among healthy older adults. Older adults with heart failure had more severe physical and emotional symptoms, poorer functional status, and worse health perceptions. Physical symptom status was the strongest predictor of HRQOL in both groups. In addition, in older adults with heart failure, physical symptom status, age, and anxiety were related to HRQOL.

Conclusions: The poor HRQOL seen in patients with heart failure is not just a reflection of aging. Comprehensive interventions targeted toward the factors that specifically negatively impact HRQOL are essential in older adults with heart failure." (Heo et al., 2007, p. 16)

Heo et al. (2007) concisely organized their abstract with headings and clearly indicated the problem (background), sample size (90 older adults with heart failure and 116 healthy older adults), results, and conclusions. The purpose of the study was clearly stated under the heading "Objective" as required in the journal's instructions. The "Methods" section was less clear on the type of study design, variables studied, measurement methods, and data collection process. This abstract is a strong abstract but could have been improved if the authors had been allowed to expand the "Methods" section.

Following the abstract are the four major sections of a research report: introduction, methods, results, and discussion. Table 27-1 provides an outline of the content covered in each of these sections for a quantitative research report. The research report by Heo et al. (2007) is used as an example when discussing these sections. The complete research article can be accessed through the Cumulative Index to Nursing and Allied Health Literature (CINAHL). Also, because Heo et al. (2007) received funding from the National Institutes of Health to conduct the study,

TABLE 27-1	Outline for a Quantitative Research Report

Introduction

Background and significance of the problem
Purpose of study
Brief review of relevant literature (may include theoretical framework and conceptual definitions)
Gap in knowledge study will address
Research objectives, questions, or hypotheses

Methods

Research design and intervention if applicable
Setting
Sampling method, consent process
Measurement methods (instrument descriptions and scoring)
Data collection process
Data analysis

Results

Description of sample (may use tables or figures)
Results organized by objectives, questions, or hypotheses
Use narrative, tables, and figures to present results

Discussion

Major findings compared with previous research
Limitations of study
Conclusions
Implications
Future studies that are needed

References

Include references cited in paper, using format specified by journal

"Despite advances in treatment and care, approximately five million people have heart failure in the United States. The number is increasing each year despite high mortality [*significance*].... In patients with heart failure, health-related quality of life (HRQOL) is an important outcome that is closely related to clinical outcomes including rehospitalization and even mortality [*background*].... It is essential to compare these variables and their effects on HRQOL between older adults with and without heart failure to determine the unique impact of heart failure and more effectively improve HRQOL in older adults with heart failure [*problem statement*].

The purpose of this study was to compare HRQOL between older adults with and without heart failure. The specific aims [*objectives*] were to (1) compare physical, psychologic, and social variables in older adults with heart failure with those in healthy older adults, and (2) determine the best model predicting HRQOL in each group from among the physical, psychologic, and social variables." (Heo et al., 2007, pp. 16-17)

the publication is also available at no cost from PubMed Central (http://www.ncbi.nlm.nih.gov/pmc/articles/).

Introduction

The introduction of a research report discusses the background and significance of the problem; identifies the problem statement and purpose, reviews the relevant empirical and theoretical literature, describes the study framework, and identifies the research purpose (aims, objectives, questions, or hypotheses if applicable). You will have developed this content for the research proposal; you summarize it in the final report. Depending on the type of research report, the review of literature and framework might be separate sections or separate chapters as in a thesis or dissertation. Key content from the introduction of the study by Heo et al. (2007) is presented as an example.

Review of Literature

The review of literature section of a research report documents the current knowledge of the problem investigated. The sources included in the literature review are the sources that you used to develop your study and interpret the findings. A review of literature can be two or three paragraphs or several pages long. In journal articles, the review of literature is concise and usually includes 15 to 20 sources. Theses and dissertations frequently include an extensive literature review to document the student's knowledge of the research problem. The summary of the literature review clearly identifies what is known, what is not known or the gap in knowledge, and the contribution of this study to the current knowledge base. The objectives, questions, or hypotheses that were used to direct the study often are stated at the end of the literature review. Heo et al. (2007) provided a brief summary of the relevant literature and included what is known and not known about the effects of heart failure on HRQOL. See Chapter 6 for more information on writing a review of the literature.

Framework

A research report needs to include an explicitly identified framework. In this section, you identify and define the major concepts in the framework and describe the relationships among the concepts (see Chapter 7). You

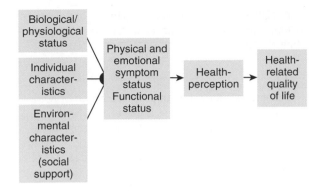

Figure 27-1 Conceptual framework. Factors affecting health-related quality of life. From Heo, S., Moser, D. K., Lennie, T. A., Zambroski, C. H., & Chung, M. L. (2007). A comparison of health-related quality of life between older adults with heart failure and healthy older adults. *Heart & Lung, 36*(1), 107.

can develop a schematic map or model to clarify the logic within the framework. If a particular proposition or relationship is being tested, that proposition should be clearly stated. Developing a framework and identifying the proposition or propositions examined in a study connect the framework and the research purpose to the objectives, questions, or hypotheses. The concepts in the framework need to be linked to the study variables and are used to define the variables conceptually. Heo et al. (2007, p. 17) clearly identified the framework of their study as the Wilson and Cleary (1995) HRQOL model (see Figure 27-1). The variables were conceptually and operationally defined and presented in a table that is included later in this chapter. If the journal allowed more space, the researchers might have expanded the literature review section based on this framework to include effects of age, health perception, functional status, physical symptom status, emotional symptom status, and social support on HRQOL in individuals with and without heart failure.

Methods

The methods section of a research report describes how the study was conducted. This section needs to be concise yet provide sufficient detail for nurses to appraise critically or replicate the study procedures. In this section you will describe the study design, sample, setting, methods of measurement, data collection process, and plan for data analysis. If the research project included a pilot study, the planning, implementation, and results obtained from the pilot study are briefly described. You will also describe any changes made in the research project based on the pilot study (Pyrczak & Bruce, 2007).

Design

The study design should be explicitly stated. Heo et al. (2007) implied a descriptive comparison study by indicating that their purpose was to compare two groups, and this was reinforced with their first aim—to "compare physical, psychologic, and social variables in older adults with heart failure with those in healthy older adults" (Heo et al., 2007, p. 17). The design should match with the stated purpose and link to the planned analysis. For example, it is clear that one group is older adults with heart failure and they will be compared with a group of older adults who are healthy. The two groups will be compared on three types of variables (physical, psychologic, and social). However, the abstract also includes HRQOL as a variable. The second aim—to "determine the best model predicting HRQOL in each group from among the physical, psychologic, and social variables" (Heo et al., 2007, p. 17)—is actually a different study design. It is still a descriptive design rather than an intervention or experiment. However, the word "predictive" assumes a longitudinal design with predictor variables measured at an initial point in time and an outcome variable measured at a later point in time. The type of design is most accurately described as a longitudinal descriptive correlational study. From the way in which the second aim is written, the reader can expect to see two predictive models tested—one for the healthy group and one for the group with heart failure.

A descriptive correlational study design could be longitudinal, as in the case just described, or it could be a cross-sectional descriptive correlational study. A cross-sectional study design includes the same variables and the same type of analysis (correlations and model testing), but data are collected at only one point in time to describe correlates of HRQOL. In both longitudinal and cross-sectional descriptive study designs, the researchers test the correlations or relationships between variables and test models with a particular outcome of interest, but conclusions can be interpreted only as associations or relationships between variables rather than causal.

If your design includes an intervention or treatment, your report needs to describe the treatment, including the protocol for implementing the treatment, training of people (interventionalists) to implement the protocol, and a discussion of the consistency of administration of the treatment (Santacroce, Maccarelli, & Grey, 2004). The reliable and competent implementation of an experimental treatment is referred to as *intervention fidelity*. As discussed in Chapter 14, **intervention fidelity** includes two core components: (1) adherence to the delivery of the prescribed treatment behaviors, session, or course and (2) competence of the researcher or interventionalist in delivering the intervention (Stein, Sargent, & Rafaels, 2007). Santacroce et al. (2004) and Stein et al. (2007) provide detailed directions to promote intervention fidelity in various quasi-experimental studies and clinical trials.

Heo et al. (2007, p. 17) implemented a combined comparative descriptive and predictive design to accomplish the two aims of their study. A more complex study design, such as a randomized clinical trial, might be presented in a table or figure, such as the examples provided in Chapter 11. Most journals require that these more complex studies be depicted in a flow chart using the CONSORT guidelines (Bennett, 2006) as discussed in Chapter 20.

Sample and Setting

This section of the research report should describe the sampling method, criteria for selecting the sample, sample size, and sample characteristics. When a clinical trial or experiment is involved, the report must also address the statistical power analysis used to determine how many subjects per group would be needed to find a statistically significant difference if significance is set at $\alpha \leq 0.05$ or another alpha level. If fewer subjects enroll or complete the study than what was indicated in the original power analysis, the difference may not be statistically significant even if the same group difference is clinically relevant. This is known as a Type 2 statistical error if the researchers conclude that there was no difference between the two groups when the same difference would be statistically significant if the sample had been larger (see Chapter 15).

Details about subject recruitment, including refusal or acceptance rates, should be reported. The number of subjects completing the study should be provided if it differs from the initial sample size, and attrition or retention rate needs to be addressed. If your subjects were divided into groups (experimental and comparison or control groups), identify the method for assigning subjects to groups and the number of subjects in each group. The protection of subjects' rights and the process of informed consent should be explicitly stated. In a published study, the setting is often described in one or two sentences, and agencies are not identified by name unless permission has been obtained. Researchers can present the sample characteristics in narrative format; however, most researchers present the characteristics of their sample in a table (see Chapter 8). Although some researchers report the subject characteristics in this section, these are often presented in the first part of the results section. Heo

et al. (2007) used the heading "Sample and Setting" to introduce the following description of their sampling process.

"Patients hospitalized with an exacerbation of heart failure at one of the three hospitals in a large Midwestern city [*setting*] were screened during admission for inclusion in the study [*convenience sample*]. Patients aged more than 55 years were included. The other inclusion criteria were as follows: (1) a primary diagnosis of heart failure with either preserved or nonpreserved left ventricular systolic function; (2) New York Heart Association (NYHA) functional classification II to IV; (3) discharged home; and (4) living within the greater metropolitan area. Exclusion criteria were as follows: (1) discharged to an extended care facility; (2) referred for hospice or home care; (3) referred to cardiac rehabilitation; or (4) cognitive or psychiatric problems [*inclusion and exclusion criteria*].

"Healthy older adults were recruited from three local senior centers [*setting*] by using flyers and word of mouth [*sample of convenience*]. Individuals aged more than 55 years were included. Those with the following characteristics were excluded from participation: (1) cognitive or psychiatric problems that precluded informed consent; (2) diagnosis of heart disease or heart failure; and (3) other serious chronic illnesses including stroke, chronic lung diseases, and cancer. Older adults with the common comorbidities of hypertension and diabetes were not excluded so individuals with characteristics typical of older adults that are also seen in older adults with heart failure could be included [*inclusion and exclusion criteria*]." (Heo et al., 2007, p. 17)

The researchers identified inclusion and exclusion sample criteria used to determine the target populations for the study (older adults with and without heart failure). They also clearly indicated the sample size of 90 older adults with heart failure and 116 healthy older adults. This sample may be sufficient for a descriptive study, but the adequacy of the sample size would have been better justified for the group comparisons identified in aim 1 if the researchers had conducted a power analysis. By identifying the refusal and attrition rates for the study, the researchers would have increased the readers' understanding about the representativeness of the sample and ability to generalize to the larger population. The more people who refuse or drop out of the study, the less one can generalize to the target population. The sampling method appeared to be a sample of convenience, but it was not clearly stated. A convenience sampling method increases the potential for sampling error and decreases the ability of the researchers to generalize the study findings to the larger population of interest. Recruitment from three local senior centers and three hospital sites increases the likelihood that findings can be generalized to the larger population of older adults, and at least the samples are representative of the local area in the Midwest United States.

Measures

This section of the report describes the measurement methods, which is how variables were operationalized and measured in the study. Details about the measures or instruments used in the data collection process are crucial if nurses are to appraise critically and replicate a study. The details include the measure's scaling and range of scores and the frequency with which the instrument was used; any reliability and validity information previously published on the instrument should also be provided. In addition, the report needs to include the instrument's reliability in the current study and any further support of validity for the current study's sample. If you have used physiological measures, be sure to address their accuracy, precision, selectivity, sensitivity, and sources of error (Pyrczak & Bruce, 2007). In a section titled "Measures," Heo et al. (2007, pp. 17-19) described all of their measures in detail. Each variable was clearly identified, conceptually defined and linked to the framework, and operationally defined to indicate how it was measured. The conceptual and operational definitions (instruments used) were clearly presented in a table (Table 27-2). These researchers provided an excellent link between the framework and the methodology of their study.

Data Collection Process and Procedures

The description of the data collection process in the research report details who collected the data, the procedure for collecting data, and the type and frequency of measurements obtained. In describing who collected the data, your report needs to specify the experience of the data collector and any training provided. If more than one person collected data, describe the precautions taken to ensure consistency and interrater reliability (Pyrczak & Bruce, 2007).

Heo et al. (2007) detailed their data collection process in a section of their report titled "Procedure," which is presented in the following excerpt. The data collection process was clear and concise, institutional review board approval was indicated, subjects' informed consent was described, use of trained data collectors was addressed, and timing and setting were discussed.

TABLE 27-2 Variables and Instruments		
	Instrument	
Variable (Conceptual Definition)	**Older Adults with Heart Failure**	**Healthy Older Adults**
Health-related quality of life (perception of effects of a clinical condition or its treatment on daily life)	Minnesota Living with Heart Failure	
Health perception (perception of overall health)	One item from SF-36	
Functional status (physical functional impairments in daily activities)	Composite measure from New York Heart Association functional class	Composite measure from Duke Activity Status Index
Physical symptom status (dyspnea and fatigue)	Composite measure from Dyspnea and Fatigue Index	Composite measure from two items (dyspnea and fatigue) of Memorial Symptom Assessment Scale
Emotional symptom status (anxiety and depression)	Subscales (depression and anxiety) of Brief Symptom Inventory	
Biological/physiological status (number of comorbidities)	Clinical characteristics questionnaire	
Individual characteristic (age and gender)	Demographic questionnaire	
Environmental characteristics (social support)	Marital status and having a confidant by demographic questionnaire	

SF-36, 36-item short-form health survey.
From Heo, S., Moser, D. K., Lennie, T. A., Zambroski, C. H., & Chung, M. L. (2007). A comparison of health-related quality of life between older adults with heart failure and healthy older adults. *Heart & Lung, 36*(1), 18.

"Procedure

Institutional review board approval was obtained for the conduct of this study. Eligible older adults with heart failure were identified by trained nurse research assistants, and those who gave written, informed consent to participate in the study were included. All data on HRQOL, health perception, functional status, physical symptom status, emotional symptom status, biologic/physiologic status, individual characteristics, and environment characteristics (social support) were collected by nurse research assistants after hospital discharge [see Table 27-2]. Eligible healthy older adults were identified by investigators among older adults who appeared at three senior centers. Investigators explained the research purpose and procedures, obtained informed consent, and answered participants' questions. All gave written, informed consent. Questionnaires were completed at the senior centers [see Table 27-2].

Completion of instruments required 30 to 45 minutes, and trained research nurses were available to assist both older adults with heart failure and healthy older adults. In addition, the instruments were checked to make sure participants did not inadvertently leave any items unanswered. Participants were free to leave items unanswered." (Heo et al., 2007, p. 20)

Analysis Plan

Heo et al. (2007) provided an excellent description of the analysis techniques used to obtain their results.

"Data were analyzed using SPSS (Statistical Packages for the Social Sciences) for Windows (version 12.0, SPSS Inc., Chicago, IL). Descriptive statistics including mean, standard deviation, frequency, and percentage were used to present demographic and clinical characteristics. Mann-Whitney U test, t-test, or chi-square test was used to examine differences in individual characteristics and biologic/physiologic status in older adults with heart failure. To address specific aim 1, the Mann-Whitney U test was used to determine the difference in HRQOL, health perception, functional status, physical and emotional symptom status, and environmental characteristics (social support) because the distribution of each variable in healthy older adults did not show normality. To address specific aim 2, stepwise multiple regression was used to identify variables as a group best associated with HRQOL in each group. A p value of less than 0.05 was considered statistically significant." (Heo et al., 2007, p. 20)

Results

The results section reveals what was learned from the study and includes the results generated from your statistical analyses. The results section is best organized by the research objectives, questions, or hypotheses that are linked to the conceptual framework. Heo et al. (2007) organized their results by characteristics of the sample and the two research aims. Research results can be presented in narrative format and organized into figures and tables. Table 1 is typically the descriptive characteristics of the sample. Because Aim 1 was to compare the healthy group with the heart failure group, the reader would expect to see sample demographic and clinical characteristics described in two columns (healthy group and heart failure group samples). The reader would also expect to see the statistics showing any group differences in these characteristics. The presentation of results depends on the end product of the data analysis and your own preference and any journal instructions. Generally, what is presented in a table is not restated in the text of the narrative. When reporting results in a narrative format, the value of the calculated statistic (t, F, r, or χ^2), the degrees of freedom (df), and probability (p value) should be included. When reporting any nonsignificant results, it is important to include the effect size and power level for that analysis so that readers would be able to evaluate the risk of a Type II error (see Chapter 15).

Students often have difficulty putting all of these Greek-letter statistical findings back into words for the text of the results section. Pallant (2007) provides useful and specific examples of how to translate the Greek symbol results back into English for the text of your report. The *Publication Manual of the American Psychological Association* (American Psychological Association [APA], 2010) provides direction for how to present various statistical results in a research report. The format for reporting chi-square results is a symbol χ^2 with degrees of freedom and sample size in parentheses followed by the χ^2 statistic value and p value. For example, when APA format is required, a chi-square value should be presented in the following format in the text of a research report: χ^2 (4, $N = 90$) = 11.14, $p = 0.025$. Statistical values need to be reported with two decimal digits of accuracy. Although a computer output of data may include results reported to several decimal places, this is unnecessary for the report. For example, reporting the χ^2 value as 11.14 is sufficient even if the computer output says 11.13965 (APA, 2010). The p value should be reported as the exact value, but when the computer output says $p = 0.0000$, it should be reported as $p < 0.001$ because the computer calculates the value only out so far before it rounds off to zero.

Heo et al. (2007) presented their results in narrative and table formats. Some of these results are represented in the next section as example tables. Because journals have space limitations, results are best depicted in tables and should not duplicate what is in the text.

Presentation of Results in Figures and Tables

Figures and tables are used to present a large amount of detailed information concisely and clearly. Researchers use figures and tables to demonstrate relationships, document change over time, and reduce the number of words in the text of the report (APA, 2010; Saver, 2006). However, figures and tables are useful only if they are appropriate for the results you have generated and if they are well constructed (Saver, 2006). Table 27-3 provides guidelines for developing accurate and clear figures and tables for a research report. More extensive guidelines and examples for developing tables and figures for research reports can be found in the *Publication Manual of the American*

TABLE **27-3**	Guidelines for Developing Tables and Figures in Research Reports

Select results to include in report
Identify a few key tables and figures that explain or support major points
Develop simple tables and figures
Ensure tables and figures are complete and clear without referring to the narrative
Give each table or figure a brief title
Tables and figures are numbered separately in the report (e.g., Table 1, 2; Figure 1, 2)
Use descriptive headings, labels, and symbols—may need to provide a key for abbreviations or symbols
Include probability values as actual values or indicate whether less or more stringent by asterisks
Refer to each table and figure in the narrative (e.g., Table 1 presents...)
Use narrative to summarize main ideas, but do not repeat specifics that are in figures and tables

Compiled from APA, 2010; Pallant, 2007; and Pyrczak & Bruce, 2007.

Psychological Association (APA, 2010). For meta-analysis reports that synthesize the results of many studies, particular figures, called forest plots, are very important in the presentation of results (Floyd, Galvin, Roop, Oermann, & Nordstom, 2010).

Figures

Figures are diagrams or pictures that illustrate the results. Researchers often use computer programs to generate sophisticated black-and-white or color figures. Common figures included in nursing research reports are bar graphs and line graphs. Journals often require high-resolution images for reproduction. The APA manual (APA, 2010, p. 167) has a figure checklist for you to review when deciding whether or not to include a figure. Generally, figures require specific formatting and may have less detail than readers want, so potential authors should carefully check with the journal guidelines (Saver, 2006).

Bar graphs typically have horizontal or vertical bars that represent the size or amount of the group or variable studied. The bar graph is also a means of comparing one group with another. Goyal, Gay, and Lee (2010) conducted a study to describe how socioeconomic status influences the risk of postpartum depressive symptoms in first-time mothers. As part of a larger study, the researchers asked women to complete a depression measure, the 20-item Center for Epidemiologic Studies–Depression [CES-D] scale, (see Chapter 17) during their third month of pregnancy and again at 1 month, 2 months, and 3 months postpartum. The researchers compared groups based on prenatal depression risk and presented their results in a vertical bar graph (see Figure 27-2). This figure indicates that the women with high prenatal risk scores (CES-D ≥ 16) were more likely to have high postpartum scores at all three time points. The text indicates that this was significant (χ^2 [1] = 19.9 to 32.5; all $p < 0.001$).

A line graph is developed by joining a series of points with a line and shows how a variable varies over time. In this type of graph, the horizontal scale (x-axis) is used to measure time, and the vertical scale (y-axis) is used to measure number or quantity. A line graph figure needs at least three data points over time on the horizontal axis to show a trend or pattern. However, complexity does not enhance the ability to convey the data in a meaningful way, so it is recommended that no more than 10 time points should be included on a single line graph, and there should be no more than four lines or groups per graph. Figure 27-3 is a line graph developed by Goyal et al. (2010, p. 100) to depict the pattern of depressive symptoms over time by contrasting two groups of childbearing women from their third trimester to their 3-month postpartum assessment. Figure 27-3 is well constructed because it includes four data points per line along the x-axis (mean depressive symptom score at four visits) and two lines representing the study groups (low income and high income) being examined for differences in depressive symptoms after the birth of their first infant. The third dashed line at the value of 16 on the y-axis is helpful for readers to orient the scores for the two groups in context to the score that indicates clinical depression. The discussion of this graph in the text indicated that the pattern of depressive symptoms over the four time points was different for the two groups (F [3192] = 2.76; p = 0.044), with the low-income group improving at 1 month and 2 months postpartum. The figures could be improved by having the sample sizes (n) for each group depicted within the figure or in the legend.

Tables

Tables are used more frequently in research reports than figures and can be developed to present results from numerous statistical analyses without additional software programs. In tables, the results are presented in columns and rows so that the reader can review them easily. The sample tables included in this section present means ($\bar{x}$), standard deviations (SD), t values, chi-square (χ^2) values, Mann-Whitney U values (Z), correlations (r), and regression analysis (R^2) results. Means and standard deviations of the study variables should be included in the published study because of their importance to future research. A variable's mean and standard deviation are essential for (1) providing a basis for comparison across studies, (2) calculating the effect size to determine sample size for future studies, and (3) conducting future meta-analyses (Conn & Rantz, 2003; Sandelowski, 2008). The sample size for each column should be included if the N varies from the total sample.

Heo et al. (2007) presented the results of their study about HRQOL for older adults with and without heart failure in four tables; three are included in this chapter. Table 27-4 compares individual characteristics (demographic variables) and biological and physiological status of the two groups. This table includes means and standard deviations (SDs) for variables measured at the interval or ratio level (age, education in years, and number of comorbidities) and frequencies and percentages (%) for variables measured at the

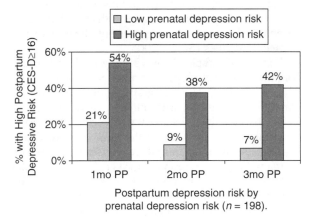

Figure 27-2 Postpartum (PP) depression risk by prenatal depression risk (*n* = 198). *CES-D,* Center for Epidemiologic Studies–Depression. (From Goyal, D., Gay, C., & Lee, K. A. (2010). How much does low socioeconomic status increase the risk of prenatal and postpartum depressive symptoms in first-time mothers? *Women's Health Issues,* 20(2), 101.)

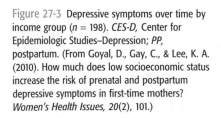

Figure 27-3 Depressive symptoms over time by income group (*n* = 198). *CES-D,* Center for Epidemiologic Studies–Depression; *PP,* postpartum. (From Goyal, D., Gay, C., & Lee, K. A. (2010). How much does low socioeconomic status increase the risk of prenatal and postpartum depressive symptoms in first-time mothers? *Women's Health Issues, 20*(2), 101.)

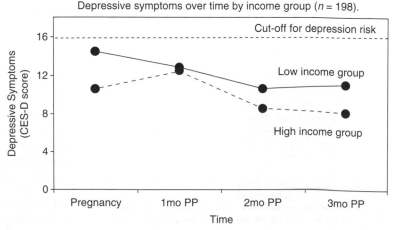

TABLE 27-4 Comparison between Older Adults with Heart Failure and Healthy Older Adults: Individual Characteristics and Biological and Physiological Status

Characteristics	Older Adults with Heart Failure ($N = 90$), no. (%) or M ± SD (Range)	Healthy Older Adults ($N = 116$), no. (%) or M ± SD (Range)	Total ($N = 206$), no. (%) or M ± SD	Statistic	p Value
Age	74.8 ± 8.1 (57-93)	74.2 ± 6.3 (58-92)	74.5 ± 7.1	$t = 0.56$	0.57
Education (yr)	11.7 ± 2.6 (3-20)	13.0 ± 2.7 (4-20)	12.4 ± 2.7	$Z = -3.69$	<0.001
No. comorbidities	2.3 ± 1.2 (0-5)	1.0 ± 0.9 (0-4)	1.6 ± 1.2	$Z = -7.18$	<0.001
Sex (male)	48 (53.3)	27 (23.3)	75 (36.4)	$\chi^2 = 18.26$	<0.001
Marital status					
Married	42 (46.7)	46 (39.7)	88 (42.7)	$\chi^2 = 1.27$	0.74
Divorced/separated	8 (8.9)	13 (11.2)	21 (10.2)		
Widowed	33 (36.6)	45 (38.8)	78 (37.9)		
Other	7 (7.8)	12 (10.3)	19 (9.2)		
Living arrangements (live alone)	48 (53.3)	61 (52.6)	109 (52.9)	$\chi^2 = 0.01$	0.92

M, Mean; *SD,* standard deviation.

From Heo, S., Moser, D. K., Lennie, T. A., Zambroski, C. H., & Chung, M. L. (2007). A comparison of health-related quality of life between older adults with heart failure and healthy older adults. *Heart & Lung, 36*(1), 19.

nominal level (sex, marital status, and living arrangements). The two groups were compared for differences on selected variables using *t*-test (*t*) (variables measured at interval or ratio level), Mann-Whitney *U* (*Z*) (variables measured at ordinal level), and chi-square (χ^2) (variables measured at nominal level). Nonsignificant results ($p > 0.05$) between the two groups in regard to age, marital status, and living arrangements indicate the groups are comparable in these areas. It was expected that the older adults with heart failure would have significantly more comorbidities ($p < 0.001$) than the healthy adults; however, the significant differences for education ($p < 0.001$) and sex ($p < 0.001$) were unexpected. Researchers desire their groups to be comparable on demographic variables, so any differences found between the groups on study outcome variables of interest are less likely to be due to basic demographic differences. Any differences on baseline characteristics need to be controlled in the remaining statistical analyses.

Heo et al. (2007) conducted a Mann-Whitney *U* (*Z*) analysis to address aim 1 to determine differences in two groups for HRQOL, health perception, functional status, physical status, emotional symptoms status (anxiety and depression), and social support (Table 27-5). Older adults with heart failure reported significantly ($p < 0.001$) poorer HRQOL, health perceptions, functional status, physical symptoms status, anxiety, and depression than healthy older adults. Only social support did not significantly differ between the two groups ($p = 0.66$). The results indicate the increased needs of individuals with heart failure and the need to develop evidence based interventions to manage these needs.

Tables are used to identify correlations among variables, and often the table presents a correlation matrix generated from the data analysis. The correlation matrix indicates the correlation values (coefficients) obtained when examining the relationships between variables, two variables at a time (bivariate correlations). The table also includes information about the significance (*p* value) of each correlation coefficient, but the significance will be sample-size dependent. Borge, Wahl, and Moum (2010) conducted a study entitled, "Association of Breathlessness with Multiple Symptoms in Chronic Obstructive Pulmonary Disease." One of the questions in their study was "What are the relationships between … multiple symptoms (breathlessness, depression, anxiety, sleeping difficulties, fatigue and pain)?" (Borge et al., 2010, p. 2690). The researchers presented their results in a correlation matrix, shown in Table 27-6. The six symptom variables are listed horizontally across the top of the table and vertically down the left side of the table. The relationship of Breathlessness with itself (Breathlessness) is always a perfect positive relationship of 1.00. Breathlessness is correlated with Fatigue ($r = 0.51***$). The asterisks (***) indicate that this correlation is significant at $p \leq 0.001$ (some journals would require the exact *p* value). This table identifies the correlation coefficients (Pearson *r* value) between the variables, and the significance of each of these coefficients. Borge et al. (2010) described this table in the text of their article in the following way.

TABLE 27-5	Comparison between Older Adults with Heart Failure and Healthy Older Adults: Health-Related Quality of Life, Health Perception, Functional Status, Physical Symptom Status, Emotional Symptoms Status, and Social Support.			
	Mean ± SD			
Scale	**Older Adults with Heart Failure (N = 90)**	**Healthy Older Adults (N = 116)**	**Statistic**	**p Value**
LHFQ total*	50.8 ± 22.1	14.4 ± 15.9	Z = −9.9	<0.001
LHFQ physical*	23.1 ± 10.4	7.1 ± 8.1	Z = −9.3	<0.001
LHFQ emotional*	11.4 ± 7.2	2.3 ± 3.7	Z = −9.1	<0.001
Health perception*	2.6 ± 0.8	2.1 ± 0.6	Z = −4.9	<0.001
Functional status*	2.6 ± 0.5	1.7 ± 0.6	Z = −8.6	<0.001
Physical symptom status†	4.9 ± 2.2	11.0 ± 1.9	Z = −11.8	<0.001
Emotional symptom status				
Anxiety*	0.9 ± 0.7	0.3 ± 0.5	Z = −6.7	<0.001
Depression*	1.0 ± 0.8	0.4 ± 0.6	Z = −5.7	<0.001
Social support†	2.9 ± 0.8	2.8 ± 1.1	Z = −0.4	0.661

*Higher scores indicate poor status.
†Higher scores mean better status.
LHFQ, Minnesota Living with Heart Failure Questionnaire; *SD,* standard deviation.
From Heo, S., Moser, D. K., Lennie, T. A., Zambroski, C. H., & Chung, M. L. (2007). A comparison of health-related quality of life between older adults with heart failure and healthy older adults. *Heart & Lung, 36*(1), 21.

TABLE 27-6	Correlation Matrix between Symptoms of Patients with Chronic Obstructive Pulmonary Disease (N = 154)					
	Breathlessness	**Fatigue**	**Anxiety**	**Depression**	**Sleeping difficulties**	**Pain intensity**
Breathlessness	1					
Fatigue	0.51***	1				
Anxiety	0.34***	0.45***	1			
Depression	0.38***	0.53***	0.65***	1		
Sleeping difficulties	0.42***	0.58***	0.56***	0.50***	1	
Pain intensity	0.26**	0.48***	0.41***	0.32***	0.51***	1

**Statistically significant at 0.01 level.
***Statistically significant at 0.001 level.
From Borge, C. R., Wahl, A. K., & Moum, T. (2010). Association of breathlessness with multiple symptoms in chronic obstructive pulmonary disease. *Journal of Advanced Nursing, 66*(12), 2695.

"[Table 27-6] shows a significant positive (*p* < 0.001–*p* < 0.01) bivariate relationship between all symptoms... Pearson's *r* ranged from 0.26 (breathlessness-pain intensity) to 0.65 (depression-anxiety)" (Borge et al., 2010, p. 2693).

For many reasons, it would be important to examine this type of correlation matrix before proceeding with other, more complex statistical analyses. Readers should first examine the matrix for the direction of a relationship: is it positive or negative? All of the relationships in this matrix were positive, indicating that the higher a patient's self-reported breathlessness, the higher all other symptom scores will be for that patient. These relationships make sense; a nurse would not see one of these symptoms improve if another symptom worsened (a negative or inverse relationship). Readers should also look for the strength of the relationship (is it > 0.20 or > −0.20 regardless of the direction or the *p* value?). All correlations were greater than 0.20, and all symptoms would likely be considered in the next, more complex analysis using multiple regression models. Readers should also look for multicolinearity between variables (*r* > 0.70), which would indicate that two variables are measuring the same concept. There was no multicolinearity between symptoms, but anxiety and depression were highly correlated (*r* = 0.65) in this sample. If these

TABLE 27-7	Models Best Associated with Health-Related Quality of Life in Older Adults with Heart Failure ($N = 90$)					
Scale	Variables	Beta*	Unique R^2	Accumulated R^2	F	p Value
LHFQ	Physical symptom status	$-0.501^‡$	0.359	0.359	25.050	<0.001
Total	Age	$-0.221^†$	0.071	0.430		
	Anxiety	$0.218^†$	0.037	0.466		

*Standardized slope coefficient.
$^†p < 0.05$.
$^‡p < 0.001$.
LHFQ, Minnesota Living with Heart Failure Questionnaire.
From Heo, S., Moser, D. K., Lennie, T. A., Zambroski, C. H., & Misook, L. C. (2007). A comparison of health-related quality of life between older adults with heart failure and healthy older adults. *Heart & Lung, 36*(1), 21.

two variables were correlated ($r > 0.70$), researchers would need to consider their overlapping variance when testing a multiple regression model. See Chapters 21-25 for additional explanation of specific statistical tests.

Heo et al. (2007, p. 17) conducted a stepwise regression (R^2) to address aim 2 in their study "to determine the best model predicting HRQOL in each group from among the physical, psychologic, and social variables." The researchers reported, "In older adults with heart failure, physical symptom status, age, and one of the emotional symptoms status, anxiety, were associated with HRQOL (F [3, 86] = 25.05, $p < 0.001$)" (Heo et al., 2007, pp. 20-21). The results from the regression analysis are presented in Table 27-7. The table clearly presents the variables included in the regression analysis, the beta result for each variable (physical symptoms status, age, and anxiety), the unique R^2 (percentage of variance in HRQOL explained by each variable), and the accumulated R^2 (0.466 or 46.6% variance in HRQOL explained by the three variables). An analysis of variance (ANOVA) was conducted to determine significance, and the result (F test with df) and significance (p value) are provided (see Table 27-7). To be useful for calculating effect sizes and doing meta-analyses, exact p values are more useful, but some journal formats require this type of asterisk notation. However, when the p value in a computer output is listed as "0.0000," it stops at this point, and the author should report this as $p < 0.001$.

Discussion

The discussion section ties the other sections of your research report together and gives them meaning. It includes your major findings, limitations of the study, conclusions drawn from the findings, implications of the findings for nursing, and recommendations for

further research. Your major findings, which are generated through an interpretation of the results, should be discussed in relation to the overriding conceptual framework as well as the research problem, purpose, and questions or hypotheses. Researchers should compare their findings with the findings from previous research and describe how the new findings extend existing knowledge. Discussion of the findings also includes the limitations that were identified while conducting the study. A study might have limitations related to sample (e.g., size, response rate, attrition), design (e.g., convenience sample, only one clinical site, lack of randomization), or instruments (e.g., measure self-report alcohol intake rather than blood alcohol level). These limitations influence the generalizability of the findings (Pyrczak & Bruce, 2007).

The research report includes the conclusions or the knowledge generated from the findings. Conclusions are frequently stated in tentative or speculative terms because one study by itself does not produce conclusive findings that can be generalized to the larger population. You might provide a brief rationale for accepting certain conclusions and rejecting others. The conclusions need to be discussed in light of their implications for knowledge, theory, and practice. Describe how the findings and conclusions might be implemented in specific practice areas. Conclude your research report with recommendations for further research. Identify specific problems that require investigation, and describe procedures for replicating the study. The discussion section of the report demonstrates the value of conducting the study and stimulates the reader to conduct additional research that is needed to provide evidence-based practice (Craig & Smyth, 2012; Melnyk & Fineout-Overholt, 2010). As is often the case, by the time the study is published, the researchers are conducting the next study to address their own recommendations for future research.

Heo et al. (2007) linked their study findings with findings from previous research, identified the limitations of their study, formed conclusions, indicated areas for future research, and made recommendations for practice. The researchers concluded:

> "Despite marked differences in physical, psychologic, and HRQOL status between the two groups [healthy older adults and older adults with heart failure] physical symptom status was the variable most strongly related to HRQOL in both groups. Both health care providers and patients who often dismiss negative symptomatology as normal signs of aging need to be aware that they are not so appropriate intervention can be undertaken" (Heo et al., 2007, p. 23).

The complete research report for this study can be accessed through CINAHL or PubMed. We recommend you review the study to increase your understanding of the content and organization of a quantitative research report.

Reference Citations

The final section of the research report is the reference list, which includes all sources that were cited in the report. Most of the sources in the reference list are relevant studies that provided a knowledge base for conducting the study. These sources need to have complete citations recorded in a consistent manner. The APA (2010) format is required by the editors of many nursing and psychology journals. Sources need to be cited in the text of the report using a consistent format. It is very important to follow the format guidelines for the journal to which you plan to submit your manuscript for publication. Some journals request that reference citations include only the past 5 years, whereas other journals may limit the number of references to less than 50 (*Nursing Research* limits the number of references to 40 at this time).

Qualitative Research Report

Reports for qualitative research are as diverse as the different types of qualitative studies. The different types of qualitative research are presented in Chapter 4, and methods from specific qualitative studies are presented in Chapter 12. The intent of a qualitative research report is to describe the dynamic implementation of the research project and the unique, creative findings obtained (Marshall & Rossman, 2010). Table 27-8 provides guidelines for developing a qualitative

TABLE 27-8	Outline for a Qualitative Research Report

Introduction
  Background & Significance of the phenomenon to be studied
  Aims or purpose of the study
  Brief review of relevant literature (may include theoretical framework and conceptual definitions)
  Gap in knowledge study will address
  Study questions and qualitative approach to be used
Methods
  Describe qualitative method (phenomenology, historical, grounded theory, ethnographical or exploratory descriptive qualitative)
  Rationale for and basic steps involved in using this method
  Sampling method, consent process
  Setting and researcher access to setting
  Data collection process
  Data analysis plan
Results
  Description of sample (may use table or figure)
  Results organized by question or themes, depending on the method
  Use narrative and quotations to present findings
Discussion
  Major findings compared to previous research
  Limitations of the study
  Conclusions
  Implications
  Future studies that are needed
References
  Include those cited in paper, using format specified by journal

research report. Similar to a quantitative report, a qualitative research report needs a clear, concise title that identifies the focus of the study. A study by Chun, Chesla, and Kwan (2011), titled, "So We Adapt 'Step by Step': Acculturation Experiences Affecting Diabetes Management and Perceived Health for Chinese American Immigrants," is used as an example to present aspects of a qualitative research report.

The abstract for a qualitative research report briefly summarizes the key parts of the study and usually includes the following: (1) aim of the study; (2) qualitative approach (e.g., phenomenology, grounded theory, ethnography, or historical); (3) methods including sample, setting, and methods of data collection; (4) brief synopsis of findings; and (5) implications of the findings (Munhall, 2012). Detailed guidelines for developing an abstract for a qualitative study are presented later in this chapter. The abstract for the study by Chun et al. (2011) follows.

"This study examines how acculturation affects type 2 diabetes management and perceived health for Chinese American immigrants in the U.S. Acculturation experiences or cultural adaptation experiences affecting diabetes management and health were solicited from an informant group of immigrant patients and their spouses ($N = 40$) during group, couple and individual interviews conducted from 2005 to 2008. A separate respondent group of immigrant patients and their spouses ($N = 19$) meeting inclusion criteria reviewed and confirmed themes generated by the informant group. Using interpretive phenomenology, three key themes in patients' and spouses' acculturation experiences were identified: a) utilizing health care, b) maintaining family relations and roles, and c) establishing community ties and groundedness in the U.S. Acculturation experiences reflecting these themes were broad in scope and not fully captured by current self-report and proxy acculturation measures. In the current study, shifting family roles and evaluations of diabetes care and physical environment in the U.S. significantly affected diabetes management and health, yet are overlooked in acculturation and health investigations. Furthermore, the salience and impact of specific acculturation experiences respective to diabetes management and perceived health varied across participants due to individual, family, developmental, and environmental factors. In regards to salience, maintaining filial and interdependent family relations in the U.S. was of particular concern for older participants and coping with inadequate health insurance in the U.S. was especially distressing for self-described lower-middle to middle-class participants. In terms of impact, family separation and relocating to ethnically similar neighborhoods in the U.S. differentially affected diabetes management and health due to participants' varied family relations and pre-migration family support levels and diverse cultural and linguistic backgrounds, respectively. Implications for expanding current conceptualizations and measures of acculturation to better comprehend its dynamic and multidimensional properties and complex effects on health are discussed. Additionally, implications for developing culturally-appropriate diabetes management recommendations for Chinese immigrants and their families are outlined" (Chun et al., 2011, p. 256).

Chun et al.'s (2011) abstract clearly identifies the aim of the study, the type of study conducted (interpretive phenomenology), the population (Chinese immigrants to the United States with type 2 diabetes and their spouses), and sample size (40). The abstract met the word limit for this particular journal but might have been clearer if authors had indicated that their sample was Cantonese-speaking and sample size was 20 couples or dyads. It is not until the methods section that the researchers describe participants as a convenience sample residing in one area of California.

Following the abstract, qualitative research reports usually include four major sections: introduction, methods, results, and discussion. The content included in each of these sections is identified in Table 27-8 and presented next.

Introduction

The introduction section of the report identifies the research topic or life experience under investigation and specifies the type of qualitative study that was conducted. The study aim or purpose and specific research questions flow from the phenomenon, clarify the study focus, and identify expected outcomes of the investigation. The introduction is used to describe the significance of the study topic for nursing knowledge and practice and to provide documentation of the significance by citing current and relevant literature (Sandelowski, 2010). The evolution of the study is described to provide a context for the phenomenon being studied. Provide a rationale for conducting the study, and place the study within both a historical and experiential context. The historical context provides a basis for the study and situates the study in a period of time. The experiential context presents your involvement in the research experience and your understanding of the phenomenon under study.

Some qualitative reports include a brief literature review in the introduction or in a separate section of the report after a brief introduction. Other reports include literature only near the end of the report in the discussion of the findings. The following text was abstracted from the introduction of Chun et al.'s (2011) interpretive phenomenology study of acculturation experiences affecting diabetes management and perceived health for Chinese American immigrants. This study is an example of a multidisciplinary study funded by the National Institute of Nursing Research. The complete article can be accessed through PubMed. Because this research was federally funded by the National Institutes of Health, the article can be accessed at no cost from PubMed Central by searching on the author's name (http://www.ncbi.nlm.nih.gov/pmc/).

Lastly, both proxy and self-report acculturation measures do not directly evaluate the context in which acculturation unfolds, thus important family, cultural and sociopolitical contexts shaping cultural adaptation and health are overlooked. Consequently, fundamental questions concerning the nature of acculturation and its relationship to diabetes management and health—namely, how do Chinese immigrants actually experience acculturation, and how do these experiences complicate or support their diabetes management and health?—largely remain a matter of conjecture.

A primary goal of this study was to articulate the complex ways in which acculturation affects diabetes management and perceived health for first-generation

Chinese immigrants in the U.S. Special attention was given in identifying key acculturation experiences, including instances of stressful or successful cultural adaptation, which respectively complicated or facilitated their diabetes management. Qualitative research methods were utilized to comprehend the multidimensional and dynamic properties of acculturation based on immigrant participants' extended narratives of their cultural adaptation experiences. Qualitative methods also allowed for findings and interpretations that were culturally-anchored in immigrant participants' daily diabetes management and health practices." (Chun et al., 2011, p. 257)

Methods

The methods section includes three parts: general method of inquiry, specific methods of inquiry used in the study, and data analysis plan (Table 27-8). The general methods section includes the specific qualitative approach (e.g., phenomenology, grounded theory, or ethnography) used to conduct the study and provides a brief background or reference to that method. The philosophical basis for and the assumptions of the qualitative method are provided and documented from the current literature. The methodology steps used to conduct a qualitative study vary based on the philosophical basis of the study, the topic studied, and the experiences of the researcher conducting the study. When developing a report of a qualitative study, you need to discuss the steps of the qualitative method, the procedures, and the outcomes and provide a rationale for selecting this qualitative method to guide your investigation (Denzin & Lincoln 2005; Marshall & Rossman, 2010). Chun et al. (2011) described the qualitative method used to conduct their investigation in the following way.

"Method

This interpretive comparative interview study was conducted from 2005 to 2008 with an informant group of 20 foreign-born Chinese American couples in which at least one member was diagnosed with type 2 diabetes....

Narrative and thematic analyses were conducted by a multicultural and multidisciplinary team of Chinese American and European American nurses and psychologists (Benner, 1994; Cohen, Kahn, & Steeves, 2000)." (Chun et al., 2011, pp. 257-258)

In the methods section of a qualitative report, it is helpful to describe your relevant educational and clinical background for conducting the study. This documentation helps evaluate the worth of the study because the researcher serves as a primary data-gathering instrument and analyses occur within the reasoning processes of the researcher (Munhall, 2012). In the report of your qualitative study, you need to describe the site and participants selected for the study. Your unique role as the researcher should also be detailed, including training of project staff, entry into the setting, selection of participants, and ethical considerations extended to the participants during data collection and analysis (see Table 27-8).

The research report includes a description of your data collection tools, such as observation guides, open-ended interviews, direct participation, documents, life histories, audiovisual media (photographs, DVDs, videos, or audiotapes), biographies, and diaries. The flexible, dynamic way in which the researcher collects data is described, including the time spent collecting data, how data were recorded, and amount of data collected. For example, if your data collection involved participant observation, you should describe the number, length, structure, and focus of the observation and participation periods. In addition, you should identify the tools (e.g., audiotapes) for recording the data from these periods of observation and participation. Chun et al. (2011) described the methods applied in their study in the following way.

"A convenience sample was recruited from community clinics, community service organizations and via public notices in the San Francisco Bay Area in

California. Six semi-structured interviews with couples in individual, couple and group contexts focused on illness understandings, perceptions of diabetes care, acculturation histories and concrete positive, negative and memorable narratives of diabetes care. Couples narrated in each other's presence (2 couple interviews) and in group interviews with those who shared their experience as a patient (2 group interviews) or spouse (2 group interviews). A subset of these informants (n = 13) was also interviewed individually if extra time was needed to complete interview questions or if nondisclosure in shared interview settings suggested a private interview would yield more complete data. Interviews were conducted in Cantonese and audiotaped text was simultaneously translated from Cantonese to English and transcribed verbatim by skilled bilingual bicultural staff. Each audiofile was then reviewed and checked for accuracy by a separate bilingual bicultural staff member who had conducted the interview [*procedures and data collection*].

Inclusion criteria included a diabetes diagnosis for at least one year, aged 35 to 75, married for a minimum of 1 year, self-identified as Chinese American or Chinese, immigrated to the U.S. from mainland China or Hong Kong and having a spouse who would agree to participate. Exclusion criteria for patients included major diabetes complications (proliferative retinopathy, cerebrovascular accident or myocardial infarction within the last 12 months, renal insufficiency, or amputations) because our intent was to study patients who were early enough in the disease progression to benefit from behavioral and family interventions [*participant selection*]." (Chun et al., 2011, p. 257)

"… Ethical approval for this study was obtained from the human subjects review boards at University of California, San Francisco and the University of San Francisco [*ethical considerations*]." (Chun et al., 2011, p. 258)

Analysis Plan

The plan for analyzing the data should include who will be coding the data, how they were trained, any issues regarding interrater reliability for coding, and the software product used, if any. Chun et al. (2011) described their analysis plan as follows.

"After all text was coded for thematic codes in Atlas-ti, complete text for two codes—'acculturation positive' and 'acculturation negative'—were reviewed. 'Acculturation positive' included examples of positive cultural adaptation experiences in the U.S. that supported diabetes management, including acculturation buffers or protective factors that mitigated acculturation stress and enhanced positive health perceptions. 'Acculturation negative' included examples of negative cultural adaptation experiences that made diabetes management difficult, including acculturation stressors and challenges that compromised health perceptions. The analyzed text comprised over 465 pages of extracted text, and represented a broad inclusive portion of narratives drawn from interviews conducted in all three contexts (couple, group and individual interviews). Simultaneous to this thematic analysis, summaries for each couple were also constructed. Thus text for this manuscript was analyzed in the context of the holistic analysis of each couple's acculturation experiences.

To address generalizability, findings were presented to a separate respondent group of patients and spouses who met the same inclusion criteria as the informant group, a process known as member checking. Respondents (13 patients and 6 spouses) represented 16 separate families.... Respondents met in separate patient groups and spouse groups for two 2-hour interviews to review themes presented in this manuscript for adequacy, and to add personal variations to the presented themes." (Chun et al., 2011, p. 258)

Results

The results section of the research report includes data analysis procedures and presentation of the findings. The data, in the form of notes, tapes, and other materials from observations and interviews, must be synthesized into meaningful categories or organized into common themes by the researcher. The data analysis procedures are performed during and after the data collection process (Marshall & Rossman, 2010; Munhall, 2012). These analysis procedures and the process for implementing them are described in Chun et al.'s (2011) research report.

"Results

"Acculturation experiences affecting type 2 diabetes management and perceived health were identified from the narratives of Chinese immigrant patients (P) and spouses (S) in the current study. These acculturation experiences centered on three key themes: a) utilizing health care, b) maintaining family relations and roles, and c) establishing community ties and groundedness in the U.S. Participants reported variable acculturative stress levels across these themes that differentially affected their diabetes management practices and perceived health." (Chun et al., 2011, p. 258)

Present your results in a manner that clarifies for the reader the phenomenon under investigation. These results include descriptions, themes, social processes, and theories that emerged from the study of life experiences, cultures, or historical events. Sometimes, these theoretical ideas are organized into conceptual maps, models, or tables. Researchers often gather additional data or reexamine existing data to verify their theoretical conclusions, and this process is described in the report (Denzin & Lincoln, 2005; Marshall & Rossman, 2010). Some qualitative study findings lack clarity and quality, which makes it difficult for practitioners to understand and apply them. Some of the problems with qualitative study findings are misuse of quotes and theory, lack of clarity in identifying patterns and themes in the data, and misrepresentation of data and data analysis procedures in the report (Sandelowski, 2010). Researchers must clearly and accurately develop their findings and present them in a way that a diverse audience of practitioners and researchers can understand.

Chun et al. (2011) presented their results in narrative form. Each of these themes had supporting themes that were extrapolated from the interviews. Each theme was presented with supporting data verbatim to substantiate the researchers' process in identifying themes for the reader to grasp a full understanding of the participant's experience. In the final major theme, "establishing community ties and sense of groundedness," Chun et al. (2011) identified three subthemes substantiated with eight rich quotes from their participant couples. The following excerpt from their report is particularly meaningful, as it served to provide the authors with the title for their manuscript.

"Relocating to ethnically-matched neighborhoods

Participants reported strong community ties and groundedness when relocating to ethnically-matched neighborhoods like San Francisco Chinatown because it diffused language stressors, made them feel at ease and at home, and permitted gradual cultural adjustment to the U.S. It also supported cultural maintenance of valued Chinese dietary practices to manage their diabetes.

Mr. P22 (70-years old): We don't have any big problems ... there are a lot of Chinese here.... People can help and communicate with each other.... So we adapt step by step.... It's as if I'm in my home country and village.... The foods we eat, the living customs are more or less the same...." (Chun et al., 2011, p. 261)

Discussion

The discussion section includes conclusions, study limitations, implications for nursing, and recommendations for further research. The conclusions are a synthesis of the study findings and the relevant theoretical and empirical literature. Limitations are identified and their influence on the formulation of the conclusions is addressed. Conclusions include the study aim and the research questions, which were used to guide the conduct of the study. Implications of the findings for nursing practice and theory development are explored, and suggestions are provided for further research (Denzin & Lincoln, 2005). Chun et al. (2011) formed conclusions with support from the relevant literature, identified study limitations, and provided implications for practice. They also provided direction for further research in the following excerpt.

"The current study's findings reveal a complex and multifaceted relationship between acculturation and diabetes management and perceived health. This was illustrated by the broad scope, varying salience, and differential impact of participants' acculturation experiences. In regard to scope, participants reported a wide range of acculturation experiences covering three key themes.... Such a broad scope of acculturation experiences highlights the need to expand the parameters in which acculturation is conceptualized and measured in health research.

Most studies employ proxy or self-report acculturation measures that do not directly or comprehensively assess such broad acculturation influences on diabetes and health (Chun, 2006; Perez-Escamilla & Putnik, 2007; Salant & Lauderdale, 2003).

Limitations to the current study include the focus on Cantonese-speaking Chinese immigrants. This linguistic dialect is predominant among Chinese immigrants in the San Francisco region where this study was conducted. Future studies should include the growing numbers of Mandarin-speaking Chinese immigrants in the U.S. with distinct sociocultural backgrounds and life experiences. Additionally, future investigations should include the perspectives of other family members such as children, siblings, and extended family in multigenerational immigrant households and the perspectives of widowed or unmarried persons with diabetes. Expanded analyses of different family relationships and structures can deepen our understanding of Chinese immigrant family acculturation processes and their significance to diabetes management and health. Also, potential age-related differences in acculturation experiences were not fully examined in this study and should thus be included in future research. Lastly, future investigations should identify culturally-appropriate diabetes interventions, including bicultural competencies and skills development, that facilitate diabetes management in different cultural settings" (Chun et al., 2011, pp. 262-263).

Theses and Dissertations

Theses and dissertations are research reports that students develop in depth as part of the requirements for a degree. The content included in a thesis or dissertation depends on the university requirements, the research guidelines of the nursing college or school, and the members of the student's research committee. Most theses and dissertations are organized by chapters, with the college or university specifying the content of each chapter. The content included in a thesis follows the general outline of quantitative and qualitative research reports (Tables 27-7 and 27-8). Chapter 28 also provides guidelines for the content of theses and dissertation proposals. Baggs (2011) discussed the option of publishable papers as chapters for a dissertation and issues to consider regarding copyright and intellectual property. The APA (2010) website has a chapter on converting a thesis or dissertation to a journal article (http://supp.apa.org/style/pubman-ch08.pdf).

Audiences for Communication of Research Findings

Before developing a research report, you need to determine who will benefit from knowing the findings. The greatest impact on nursing practice can be achieved by communicating nursing research findings to a variety of audiences, including nurses, other health professionals, healthcare consumers, and policy makers. Nurses, including administrators, educators, practitioners, and researchers, must be aware of research findings for use in practice and as a basis for conducting additional studies. Other health professionals need to be aware of the knowledge generated by nurse researchers and facilitate the use of that knowledge in the healthcare system as part of the delivery of evidence-based practice (Craig & Smyth, 2012). Consumers are interested in research findings about illnesses that they or family members have. Policy makers at the local, state, and federal levels use research findings to generate health policy that has an impact on consumers, individual practitioners, and the healthcare system. Rather than the more common research with individuals as the source of data, Chapman, Wides, and Spetz (2010) provided an excellent example of communicating policy-related research findings using the *Medicare Claims Processing Manual,* reports from the National Council of State Boards of Nursing, and congressional reports as their source of data. They tabulated their data and concluded that more data are needed in these documents about the type of care provided. They also concluded from their analysis that the payment system for advanced practice nurses needs to be remodeled (Chapman et al., 2010).

Strategies for Communicating Research to Different Audiences

Research findings can be communicated or disseminated as oral podium presentations, visual posters, and written reports. Each type of report can reach additional audiences in electronic format. Table 27-9 outlines various strategies for disseminating findings to nurses, healthcare professionals, policy makers, and consumers.

Audience of Nurses

The most common mechanisms nurses use to communicate research findings to their peers are presentations at conferences and meetings. Sigma Theta Tau, the international honor society for nursing, sponsors international, national, regional, and local research conferences. Specialty organizations, such

TABLE 27-9   Audience and Strategies for Communicating Research

| Audience | Strategies for Communicating Research | | |
	Oral and Visual Presentation	Written Report	Electronic Media
Nurses—administrators, educators, clinicians, practitioners, researchers	Nursing research conferences	Nursing-refereed journals	DVD
	Professional nursing meetings and conferences	Nursing books	Podcast
		Monographs	Video and audio recordings
	Collaborative nursing groups	Research newsletters	Websites
	Thesis and dissertation defenses	Theses and dissertations	
		Foundation reports	
		Electronic databases	
Other healthcare professionals	Professional conferences and meetings	Professional journals and books	DVD
		Newsletters	Podcast
	Interdisciplinary collaboration	Foundation reports	Video and audio recordings
		Electronic databases	Websites
Policy makers	Testimony on health problems to state and federal legislators	Written testimony	Video recorded testimony
		Reports to legislators	
		Reports to funding agencies	
		AHRQ and NINR reports and presentations to policy makers	
Healthcare consumers	Television and radio interviews	Newspaper	Websites
	Community meetings	News and popular magazines	Podcast
	Patient and family teaching	Electronic databases	

AHRQ, Agency for Healthcare Research and Quality; *NINR,* National Institute for Nursing Research.

as the American Association of Critical Care Nurses, Oncology Nurses' Society, and Association of Women's Health, Obstetrics, and Neonatal Nursing, sponsor research conferences. Many universities and some healthcare agencies sponsor or cosponsor research conferences. For various reasons, nurses are not always able to attend these research conferences. To increase the communication of research findings and disseminate the new knowledge more diffusely, conference sponsors often provide podcasts or DVDs of the research presentations. Some sponsors publish abstracts of studies with the conference proceedings, publish the abstracts in a research journal supplement, or provide materials electronically on their websites.

The publishing opportunities in nursing continue to increase, with 74 journals currently listed and evaluated by *Journal Citation Reports* (Polit & Northam, 2011). Opportunities to publish research have grown with the expansion of research journals. When deciding on a potential journal for your work, four criteria should be considered: (1) the intended readers you want to reach with your research findings, (2) the fit of your topic to the journal's focus, (3) the journal's

track record for publishing in a timely manner, and (4) the impact factor for the journal. The content for your work may be most applicable to a small specialty group, or perhaps a broader audience would find it interesting and useful to their practice. You should not limit your options to a nursing journal if a wider audience of health professionals needs to know the findings of your research. You can look at your list of reference citations to get an idea of journals that have an interest in publishing on your topic. If it is important for your findings to be reported as soon as possible, consider an online journal or a journal that has monthly issues rather than quarterly issues. Finally, the impact factor for a journal is important to consider (see Publishing Research Findings section of this chapter). The 74 nursing journals listed by Polit and Northam (2011) give you a place to start.

Many researchers disseminate their findings by publishing books or chapters in books. Foundations and federal agencies that sponsor a research project often provide reports of studies that have been conducted or are in progress. The American Nurses' Foundation publishes a newsletter, *Nursing Research*

Report, which identifies studies they funded and includes abstracts of these studies. The National Institute for Nursing Research provides reports on its funded grants, including research project titles, names and addresses of researchers, period of support, a brief description of each project, and any publication citations that result from the research (www.nih.gov/ninr).

Audience of Healthcare Professionals and Policy Makers

Nurse researchers communicate their research to other health professionals at meetings and conferences sponsored by organizations such as the American Heart Association, American Public Health Association, American Cancer Society, American Lung Association, National Hospice Organization, and National Rural Health Association. Nurses must believe in the value of their research and present their findings at conferences that attract a variety of healthcare professionals. Nurse researchers and other health professionals conducting research on the same problem might collaborate to publish an article, a series of articles, a book chapter, or a book. This type of interdisciplinary collaboration increases communication of research findings and facilitates synthesis of research knowledge to promote evidence-based practice.

The Agency for Healthcare Research and Quality (2011) was one of the first national organizations to develop and distribute evidence-based guidelines for practice. The Agency for Healthcare Research and Quality implemented the "Evidence-based Practice Centers (EPC) Program," which includes the awarding of contracts to institutions in the United States and Canada to serve as an EPC. EPCs review all relevant scientific literature on clinical, behavioral, and organization and financing topics to produce evidence reports and technology assessments. These reports are used for informing and developing coverage decisions, quality measures, educational materials and tools, guidelines, and research agendas (Donaldson, Rutledge, & Geiser, 2008). The institutions with EPCs and the activities of these centers can be viewed online at www.ahrq.gov/clinic/epc (see Chapter 19).

Audience of Healthcare Consumers

Healthcare consumers as an audience are frequently neglected by nurse researchers. The findings from nursing studies can be communicated rapidly to the public through news releases. A nursing research article published in a local paper has the potential of being picked up by a national wire service and published in other papers across the United States. Nurse researchers also need to make their findings available through electronic means. An increasing amount of healthcare information is available electronically on various websites, but often this information is not based on research. There is a need to provide consumers with evidence-based guidelines and educational materials to assist them in making quality healthcare decisions.

Nursing research findings should be communicated to consumers by being published in news magazines, such as *Time* and *Newsweek,* or popular health magazines, such as *American Baby* and *Health.* Health articles published for consumer magazines and online distribution reach millions of readers at a time (e.g., webmd.com or *WebMD the Magazine*). Television and radio are other valuable media for communicating research findings to consumers and other healthcare providers. Another important method of communicating research findings to consumers is through patient and family teaching. Nursing interventions and practice protocols based on research are more credible to consumers than unresearched actions, and the ultimate goal is evidence-based practice (Craig & Smyth, 2012). Freelance journalists often contact authors of scientific articles, and these writers have the skills to translate research findings into language for consumers. Lee and Gay (2011) published a study entitled, "Can Modifications to the Bedroom Environment Improve the Sleep of New Parents? Two Randomized Controlled Trials." A skilled journalist writing for *Parenting Magazine* subsequently was able to catch consumers' attention with the title, "Desperately Seeking Sleep," to disseminate the same data contained in the research publication but for a targeted public audience (Bernstein, 2011).

Presenting Research Findings

Research findings are communicated at conferences and meetings through verbal and poster presentations. With **presentations**, researchers have an opportunity to share their preliminary findings, answer questions about their studies, interact with other interested researchers, and receive immediate feedback on their study. Research project findings are frequently presented at conferences as preliminary findings based on the quality of the abstract submitted by the researchers. When research findings are published, the data must not be published elsewhere, and any presentation of these data at a conference should be acknowledged.

Verbal Presentations

Researchers communicate their findings through verbal presentations at local, national, and international conferences. Presenting findings at a conference requires receiving acceptance of your abstract as a presenter, developing a research report, delivering the report, and responding to questions.

Receiving Acceptance as a Presenter

Most research conferences require researchers to submit an abstract, and acceptance as a presenter is based on the quality of the abstract. The abstract should be based on the theme of the conference and the organizers' criteria for reviewing the abstract. As noted earlier, an abstract is a clear, concise summary of a study that is usually limited to 100 to 250 words. The abstract submitted for a verbal presentation is usually based on results from a completed study that is not yet published. Findings from a pilot study or preliminary findings would be acceptable for a poster presentation (Pyrczak & Bruce, 2007). The sponsors of a research conference circulate a call for abstracts 9 months to 1 year before the conference. Many research journals and newsletters publish these requests for abstracts, and they are available electronically. In addition, conference sponsors email requests for abstracts to universities, major healthcare agencies, and known nurse researchers.

The call for abstracts stipulates the format for the abstract. Frequently, abstracts are limited to 1 page, single-spaced, and include the content outlined in Box 27-1 (for an abstract of a quantitative study) and Box 27-2 (for an abstract of a qualitative study). When abstracts are submitted online, you may be limited to a specific number of words or characters. For electronic submissions, write and revise the abstract in a separate document. Depending on the instructions, you may copy and paste the text in a box on the webpage or attach the file.

The title of your abstract must create interest, and the body of your abstract "sells" the study to the reviewers. An example of an abstract is presented in Box 27-3. Names and affiliations would be removed for review. Writing an abstract requires practice; frequently, a researcher rewrites an abstract many times until it meets all the criteria, including the word limit, outlined by the conference sponsors. Careful attention to the criteria of the sponsoring agency should assist you in developing and refining your abstract and increase your chances of having the abstract accepted for either a podium or poster presentation. The Western Institute of Nursing (WIN) has an

---

Box 27-1 **Outline for Quantitative Study Abstract**

I. Title of the Study
II. Introduction
   Statement of the problem and purpose
   Identification of the framework
III. Methodology
   Design
   Sample size
   Identification of data analysis methods
IV. Results
   Major findings
   Conclusions
   Implications for nursing
   Recommendations for further research
   Note: The title and authors with affiliations, a conflict of interest statement, a brief reference list of one or two key citations, and the acknowledgment of funding source are not usually considered in the word limitations for the abstract.

Box 27-2 **Outline for a Qualitative Study Abstract**

I. Title of the Study
II. Introduction
   Identification of phenomenon to be studied
   Statement of the aim of the study
   Identification of the qualitative method used to conduct the study
   Evolution of the study (rationale for conducting the study, historical context, and experiential context)
III. Methodology
   Discussion of the background, philosophy, and assumptions for the method used to conduct the study
   Brief description of the sample, setting, and data collection process
IV. Results
   Brief description of data analysis procedures
   Major findings
   Conclusions
   Implications for nursing
   Recommendations for further research
   Note: The title and authors with affiliations, a conflict of interest statement, a brief reference list of one or two key citations, and the acknowledgment of funding source are not usually considered in the word limitations for the abstract.

| Box 27-3 | **Example of an Abstract: "Sleep Adequacy and Environmental Demands among Racially Diverse Women"** |

Dawn E. Dailey, RN, MSN, APRN, BC
Doctoral Candidate
Department of Family Health Care Nursing
University of California San Francisco
San Francisco, CA

Harvey C. Davis, RN, PhD
Assistant Professor
Department of Health and Human Services
San Francisco State University
San Francisco, CA

Bruce A. Cooper, PhD
Senior Statistician
Office of Research
University of California San Francisco
San Francisco, CA

Kathryn A. Lee, RN, PhD, FAAN
Professor
Department of Family Health Care Nursing
University of California San Francisco
San Francisco, CA

Aim: To describe environmental demands associated with sleep inadequacy among Caucasian and African American women.

Background: Sleep deprivation is purported to affect an individual's health through physiological, cognitive, emotional, and social mechanisms. Regardless of age, women are more likely to suffer from poor sleep. However, little is known about sleep adequacy in subgroups of American women.

Conceptual basis: This study is based on an adaptation of a framework developed by Lee and colleagues (1994) that describes internal and external environmental demands that result in sleep disturbance and daytime fatigue. Internal environmental demands are characterized as physical illness, depression, age, smoking patterns, alcohol use, physical activity, mental health, stress, and energy levels. External environmental demands are characterized as marital status, income, employment status, educational level, number of children, role demands, and life events.

Methods: A secondary analysis was conducted using the Centers for Disease Control and Prevention's (CDC) 2002 Behavioral Risk Factor Surveillance System (BRFSS) database. BRFSS is an ongoing data collection program designed to measure behavioral risk factors in random samples of adults 18 years and older. Of the 32,503 adults surveyed, 29,465 were Caucasian and 3,040 were African American women ranging in age from 18 to 65 years (mean = 42 years). Participants were asked to report the number of days they did not get enough sleep within the last month. Days of inadequate sleep in the past month were re-coded as adequate (0-11 days), moderate (12-23 days), or severe (24-30 days). Comparative analyses (t-test, chi-square) were used to describe differences in health-related characteristics and sleep adequacy between the two groups of women. Multiple regression analysis was used to identify key factors related to insufficient sleep.

Results: While more Caucasian women (32%) reported overall sleep inadequacy (moderate and severe) than African American women (30%), significantly more African American women (22%) compared to Caucasians (16%) reported severe problems with sleep ($X^2 = 61.02$; $p = .0001$). Preliminary findings indicate that sleep inadequacy is associated with specific health behaviors, chronic medical conditions, and psychological symptoms.

Implications: Preliminary results indicate that perception of inadequate sleep permeates the lives of women. Findings suggest that African American women suffer from more severe sleep problems than their Caucasian counterparts. Inadequate sleep has a profound impact on health, functioning, and well-being. These findings build upon existing knowledge of sleep disturbances and can lead to the development of effective interventions to enhance sleep quality in diverse groups of women.

Source: Dailey, D. E., Davis, H. C., Cooper, B.A., & Lee, K. A. (2005). Sleep inadequacy and environmental demands among racially diverse women. Abstract for presentation at Western Institute of Nursing Conference, San Francisco, CA.

excellent tutorial called, "Writing a WINning abstract" by Lentz (2011b) from University of Washington School of Nursing. This tutorial can be accessed at the WIN website (http://www.ohsu.edu/son/win/pcorner.shtml).

Some sponsors ask that you specify whether you want to be considered for an oral podium presentation or a poster presentation, whereas other sponsors decide on a poster versus oral podium presentation based on their own criteria or scoring system. Generally, abstracts that describe smaller sample sizes and read more like a small unfinished pilot work are less likely to be accepted for an oral podium presentation. Some sponsoring agencies require that you submit two versions of your abstract: one with names and affiliations that would be in their program or published abstracts and another that removes all names and affiliations so that the abstract is anonymous and reviewers are blinded. Read the sponsor's instructions carefully because they usually require that content of the abstract has not been published or presented elsewhere. Instructions also indicate whether or not accepted abstracts are published, usually as a supplemental issue of the sponsor's affiliated professional journal.

Developing an Oral Research Presentation

The presentation developed depends on the focus of the conference, the audience, and the time designated for each presentation. Some conferences focus on certain sections of the research report, such as tool development, data collection and analysis, findings, or implications of the findings for nursing practice. It is important to address the major sections of a research report (introduction, methods, results, and discussion) in your presentation. The content of a presentation varies depending on whether the audience consists of mainly researchers or clinical nurses. You would be best prepared for this type of presentation if you attended a previous meeting and if you practice your presentation on a local audience of peers. If you are unsure who your conference audience represents (clinicians or researchers, students or experienced researchers) or how large the audience will be (a concurrent session with an audience that specifically selects your presentation based on the title and their interest or a general session with the entire audience of conference participants), it is important to ask the contact person for the conference. In planning your allotted time for the presentation, it also is helpful to know if questions from the audience will be allowed during your presentation, allowed at the end of your presentation, or held until the end of your entire session when participants direct their questions to any one of the presenters in your session.

Time is probably the most important factor in developing a presentation because many presenters are limited to 10 or 15 minutes, with an additional 5 minutes for questions. As a guideline, you want to aim for one slide per minute. Your title slide, acknowledgment slide, and final slide of references or slide calling for questions from the audience should be included in the formula. These slides are included in the timing because someone will be introducing you after settling the audience, the previous speaker may be running late, and you do not want to be encroaching on the next speaker's time. The WIN website also has a tutorial on how to do a 10-minute oral research presentation developed by Lentz (2011b) (http://www.ohsu.edu/son/win/pcorner.shtml). Your audience is there to hear what is new in your area of research, not to hear all the background review of literature that brought you to this current research. For guidance, you should spend 20% (2 minutes or 2 slides) of your time on the title and introduction, 20% on the methodology, 40% on the results, and 20% on the discussion and implications for practice and research.

Your title slide should provide the audience with the gap in knowledge that you are addressing in your presentation. Your introduction should acknowledge funding sources and collaborators if applicable as well as any conflict of interest. A very brief review of key background literature and a simple diagram of the conceptual framework should lead directly into the research questions or hypotheses that address the gap in knowledge. The methodology content includes a brief identification of the design, sampling method, measurement techniques, and analysis plan. The content covered in the results section should start with a table of your sample characteristics followed by a slide of results for each question or hypothesis. The presentation should conclude with a brief discussion of findings, implications of your findings for clinical practice, and recommendations for future research. Most presenters find that the shorter the presentation time, the greater the preparation time needed. If you are limited to 10 minutes, you must be very selective about which one or two research questions or hypotheses you will focus on. If you have 15 or 20 minutes, you may still limit your presentation to three research questions or hypothesis but allow more time to discuss the details regarding the strengths and limitations of your research.

The longer the presentation, the more important figures and pictures, or some animation, become. The information presented on each slide should be limited to eight lines or fewer, with six or fewer words per line. A single slide should contain information that can be easily read and examined in 30 seconds to 1 minute. Only major points are presented on visuals, so use single words, short phrases, or bulleted points to convey ideas, not complete sentences. Figures such as bar graphs and line graphs usually convey ideas more clearly than tables. Pictures of the research setting, equipment, and photographs of the research team help the audience to visualize the research project better. A laser pointer may be useful to guide the audience to your key point on the slide, but the deliberate and careful use of color is more appealing to the audience, can increase the clarity of the information presented, and can call attention to a particular important statistical test and *p* value without need for a laser pointer. However, avoid using particular shades of red color for bulleted points or highlighted wording, particularly if you have a dark background; red may appear fine on your computer as you develop the slide, but becomes difficult to see when projected to a large audience.

Preparing the script and visuals for a presentation is difficult, so enlist the assistance of an experienced researcher and audiovisual expert. Rehearse your presentation with experienced researchers, and use their comments to refine your script, visuals, and presentation style. If your presentation is too long, synthesize your script and provide handouts for important content. PowerPoint slides provide an excellent format for presenting an oral research report; they include easy-to-read fonts, color, creative backgrounds, visuals or pictures to clarify points, and animation options. However, consulting an audiovisual expert will ensure that your materials are clear and properly constructed, with the print large enough and dark enough for the audience to read. When the PowerPoint slides have been developed, view them from the same vantage point as the audience to ensure that each slide is clear and can be visualized without totally darkening the room.

Delivering a Research Report and Responding to Questions

A novice researcher might attend conferences and examine the presentation style of other researchers before presenting an oral report. Even though each researcher needs to develop his or her own presentation style, observing others can promote an effective style. An effective presentation requires practice. You need to rehearse your presentation several times, with the script, until you are comfortable with the timing, the content, and your presentation style. When practicing, use the visuals so that you are comfortable with the equipment. It is always advantageous to check out the room where you will be presenting to see how chairs are arranged and how the podium and screen are situated.

Most conferences organize their oral presentations by topic into a session moderated by an expert in the field. The session usually includes a presentation by the researcher, a comment by the session's moderator, and a question period before moving to the next speaker. If your presentation is too long for the allotted time, there will be no opportunity for questions from the audience. When preparing for a presentation, try to anticipate the questions that members of the audience might ask and rehearse your answers. Practice your presentation with colleagues and ask them to raise questions. If you practice making clear, concise responses to specific questions, you will be less anxious during your presentation. When giving a presentation, have someone make notes of the audience's questions, suggestions, or comments because they are often useful when preparing a manuscript for publication or developing the next study.

Poster Sessions

Your research abstract may be accepted at a conference as a poster session rather than podium presentation. A poster session is a visual presentation of your study, all on one surface, with either three or four columns. Before developing a poster, follow the conference sponsor's directions for (1) the size limitations or format restrictions for the poster, (2) the size of the poster display area, and (3) the background and potential number of conference participants. Your institution may have a template with the logo that you are required to use for the audience to identify your affiliation more easily. A poster usually includes the following content: the title of the study; investigator and institution names; purpose; research objectives, questions, or hypotheses (if applicable); framework; design; sample; instruments; essential data collection procedures; results; conclusions; implications for nursing; recommendations for further research; a few key references; and acknowledgments.

For clarity and conciseness, a poster often includes pictures, tables, or figures to communicate the study. Figure 27-4 presents the award-winning WIN poster developed by Dr. Dawn Dailey when she was a doctoral student at University of California, San Francisco. This poster was presented at the WIN meeting in 2005, based on acceptance of the abstract presented in Box 27-3. It has a polished, professional look and presents the key aspects of the study using a balance of text, figures, and color in a 3-column format. Conference sponsors often provide boards for displaying posters, so the poster can be rolled to prevent creases and easily transported to the conference in a protective tube. Online services (e.g., Makesigns.com) will ship the poster to your hotel destination for an extra fee; this avoids any problem with airport security or risk of misplacing your poster while traveling.

A quality poster completely presents a study, yet can be comprehended in 5 minutes or less. Bold

UNIVERSITY OF CALIFORNIA SAN FRANCISCO
Sleep Adequacy and Environmental Demands among Racially Diverse Women
DE Dailey, HC Davis, BA Cooper, & KA Lee

University of California San Francisco

UCSF School of Nursing

Introduction

Sleep disturbance is supported to affect an individual's health through physiological, cognitive, emotional, and social mechanisms. Regardless of age, women are more likely to suffer from poor sleep. However, little is known about sleep inadequacy in subgroups of American women.

Purpose
- Describe environmental demands associated with sleep inadequacy among Caucasian and African American women.

This study is based on an adaptation of a framework developed by Lee and colleagues (1994) that describes internal and external environmental demands resulting in sleep disturbances and fatigue (Figure 1 below).

Internal Environmental Demands	External Environmental Demands
Physical illness*	Material status*
Menstrual cycle phase	Income*
Depression*	Occupation
Anxiety*	Employment status*
Self-esteem	Level of education*
Age*	Number of children*
Smoking*	Age of children
Sleeping patterns	Role demands
Diet patterns*	Social support
Weight*	Positive life events
Caffeine/alcohol intake*	Negative life events
Exercise patterns*	

Sleep Adequacy

* Variables in CDC BRFSS 2002 database

Methods

- Secondary analysis using the Center for Disease Control and Prevention's (CDC) 2002 Behavioral Risk Factor Surveillance System (BRFSS) database.
- BRFSS is an ongoing data collection program designed to measure behavioral risk factors in random samples of adults 18 years and older
- Of the 62,341 individuals surveyed, 53% were women with ages ranging from 18 to 65 years.

Sleep Assessment

Sleep adequacy was assessed by asking:
During the past 30 days, for about how many days have your felt you did not get enough rest or sleep?

Recoded categories:
- Adequate= 0-11 days
- Moderately inadequate = 12-23 days
- Severely inadequate = 24-30 days

Results

Table 1: Selected Sample Characteristics

	White n=29465	Black n=3040
Internal		
Age (years)	43	40
Anxiety (days/month)	6.6	6.1
Depression (days/month)	3.8	4.4
Perceived health (days/month)	2.3	2.6
Weight (pounds)	156	172
Smoker	26%	23%
BMI (normal limits)	18%	29%
Physical illness	49%	57%
Alcohol consumption (times/month)	2.6	1.5
External		
<High school	7%	11%
<25,000 per year	24%	45%
Children in home	41%	56%
Married	59%	27%
Employed	68%	67%

Figure 2: Differences in Sleep Severity between Caucasian and African American women

White / Black

Percentage / Sleep Inadequacy (Moderately, Severely)

Table 2: Multiple Regression Procedure, with Sleep Inadequacy Score as the Dependent Variable and 14 Internal and External Demands as Independent Variables

Explanatory Variables	Cummulative R2	R2 Change	beta	p
Race/ethnicity	.147	.146		
Internal Variables	.147			
Physical illness			.080	.0001
Depression			.013	.0001
Anxiety			.019	.0001
Age			-.007	.0001
Smoker			-.063	.0001
Diet patterns			-.001	.840
Weight			.001	.011
Alcohol consumption			-.054	.005
Exercise			-.062	.0001
External Variables	.184	.038		
Marital status			.013	.189
Income			.001	.686
Employment status			.033	.001
Educational level			.008	.118
Children in home			.053	.0001

Summary

1. In this sample of women, African Americans were younger and fewer were married. African American women also had lower incomes, more children in the home, and less education.

2. Whites and Blacks experienced the same percentage of sleep inadequacy. However, a higher percentage of Blacks reported severe sleep inadequacy.

3. Internal variables accounted for 15% of the variance in sleep inadequacy. Very little (<4%) was due to external role demands.

4. In this sample, anxiety, depression, age and perceived health were the strongest predictors of sleep inadequacy. Ethnicity was not a significant predictor of sleep inadequacy. These 3 variable accounted for 15% of the variance in sleep inadequacy.

5. The strongest predictors of sleep inadequacy in the Caucasian sample were anxiety, perceived health, age, depression, and number of children in the home.

6. The strongest predictors of sleep inadequacy in the African American sample were anxiety, depression, age, physical illness and employment.

Conclusions/Further Study

- Sleep inadequacy permeates the lives of women.
- Findings suggest that African American women suffer from more severe sleep inadequacy than Caucasian women.
- Inadequate sleep is associated with health and functioning.
- These finding support existing knowledge of sleep disturbances and its association with anxiety and depression.
- Further research is needed to understand variables that affect sleep in subgroups of women to promote the development of effective interventions to enhance sleep quality.

Reference:
Lee, KA et al (1994). Fatigue as a response to environmental demands in women's lives. Image-Journal of Nursing Scholarship, 26(2),149-154

For additional information contact:
Dawn E. Dailey, RN, MSN, PhD(c)
Department of Family Health Care Nursing
University of California San Francisco

Figure 27-4 Poster of "Sleep Adequacy and Environmental Demands Among Racial Diverse Women." (From University of California San Francisco.)

headings are used for the different parts of the research report, followed by concise narratives or bulleted phrases. Print size on a poster needs to be large enough to be read at 3 feet (approximately 20 font size), but the title or banner should be readable at 20 feet (Shelledy, 2004). There may be an extra cost for glossy finish, but the crisp appearance and readability may be worth the price to you. Poster sessions usually last 1 to 2 hours; you should remain by your poster during this time and offer to answer any questions when a viewer is present. Most researchers provide conference participants with a copy of the 1-page accepted abstract or a 1-page color handout of the poster tacked to the poster board with contact information, particularly if you cannot stand by your poster for the entire allotted time. Websites are available to assist you with research posters. You can also search the Internet for "research poster" to view current websites or a commercially available product (http://www.makesigns.com), or visit the University of Buffalo website at http://ublib.buffalo.edu/libraries/asl/guides/bio/posters.html.

Conferences include both quantitative and qualitative research posters. Narrative content does not lend itself to the crisp presentation required on a poster. The number of words on a poster, even for a qualitative study, should be kept to a minimum, so you must select the most critical information to include. It is recommended that sections of the poster be color-coordinated; research has been conducted on use of color to attract people to a poster (Keegan & Bannister, 2003).

Summary and implications sections are frequently where a viewer looks first, given the limited time for viewing many posters during a session. Because rich narrative text is so meaningful in qualitative studies, authors are advised to bold and enlarge the font for a few particularly meaningful quotes, and use artwork or photos that conceptualize the quote in a visual way. Posters usually take 10 to 20 hours to develop based on the complexity of the study and the experience of the researcher. Novice researchers usually need more than 20 hours to develop a poster. Important points in poster development include planning ahead, seeking the assistance of others, and limiting the information on the poster (Shelledy, 2004). Your school or workplace should have a template and color scheme for you to use with the appropriate logos and colors.

One major advantage of a poster session is the opportunity for one-to-one interaction between the researcher and the viewer. At the end of the poster session, individuals interested in a study frequently stay to speak to the researcher. Have a notepad on hand to record comments and contact information for individuals conducting similar research. Exchanging business cards and writing key information on the back of the card is a useful practice. Poster sessions provide an excellent opportunity to begin networking with other researchers involved in the same area of research. Conference participants occasionally request your study instruments or other items, so it is essential that you keep a record of their contact information and specific requests.

Publishing Research Findings

Oral and poster presentations are a valuable means of rapidly communicating findings, but their impact is limited and the contents should not be previously published. Even if the accepted abstract is published in a supplemental volume of a journal associated with the conference sponsors, you should be planning publication of the full findings for a research journal as you prepare for the oral podium or poster presentation. Published research findings are permanently recorded in a journal or book and usually reach a larger audience than presentations do. There should be an acknowledgment in the published report that the contents of your paper were presented at a particular research conference. The presentation and comments from the audience can provide a basis for finalizing your article for publication. Many journal editors are conference attendees and may request your paper for an article when they hear your oral presentation or see your poster. Many researchers present their findings at a conference and never submit the paper for publication; this could create the impression on a vita that a researcher's efforts are more focused on traveling than on research dissemination. Studies with negative findings (no significant difference or relationship) are frequently not submitted for publication. These negative findings can be as important to the development of knowledge as positive findings because they direct future research, and they should find a venue for publication and broad dissemination. Many authors strategize placing these nonsignificant findings within a publication that does have a key positive finding.

Publishing research findings is a rewarding experience, but the process demands a great deal of time and energy. The manuscript rejections or requests for major revisions that most authors receive can be discouraging. However, you can take certain steps to increase the probability of having a manuscript accepted for publication. While you are developing your study and writing the proposal, outline your plans for publishing the findings. At this time, you and other members of your research team should discuss and determine authorship credit. Authorship can become a complex issue when the research is a collaborative project among individuals from different disciplines. Some researchers develop the entire manuscript and then face the decision of who will be first, second, third, or last author. There are many ways to determine authorship credit, but the decision should be acceptable to all investigators involved. Authorship credit should be given only to the individuals who made substantial contributions to developing and implementing a study and to writing the manuscript (Baggs, 2008). Some journals require that all authors sign a written statement and checklist of their contributions. A novice author may want to consider seeking help from a more experienced author who can either be a coauthor on the manuscript or receive an acknowledgment for their contribution in the acknowledgment section. In many cases, the last author is usually the senior mentor or leader of the team who secured the resources (funding, space, and equipment) for conducting the study.

Publishing a Journal Article

Developing a manuscript for publication includes the following steps: (1) selecting a journal, (2) developing a query letter, (3) preparing a manuscript, (4) submitting the manuscript for review, and (5) revising the manuscript.

Selecting a Journal

Selecting a journal for publication of your study requires knowledge of the basic requirements of the journal, the journal's review process, and recent articles published in the journal. A **refereed journal** is peer-reviewed and uses referees or expert reviewers to determine whether a manuscript is acceptable for publication. In nonrefereed journals, the editor makes the decisions to accept or reject manuscripts, but these decisions are usually made after consultation with a nursing expert. Most refereed journals require manuscripts to be reviewed anonymously, or blinded, by two or three reviewers. In some cases, there are two reviewers for the scientific content and one reviewer for particular attention to the statistical content (Henly, Bennett, & Dougherty, 2010). The reviewers are asked to determine the strengths and weaknesses of a manuscript, and their comments are anonymously sent from the journal editor to the contact author. Most academic institutions support the refereed system and may recognize only publications that appear in peer-reviewed journals for faculty seeking tenure and promotion.

Having a manuscript accepted for publication depends not only on the quality of the manuscript but also on how closely the manuscript matches the goals of the journal and its subscribers or audience (Dougherty, Freda, Kearney, Baggs & Broome, 2011). It is a good idea to review articles recently published in the journal to which you plan to submit a manuscript. This detailed review lets you know whether a research topic has recently been addressed and whether the research findings would be of interest to that journal's readers. This process enables you to identify and prioritize a few journals that would be appropriate for publishing your findings. Checking the references in your own manuscript may reveal certain journals that publish research on your topic. Reviewing the journal's impact factor, the time line for their review process, and the waiting period from acceptance to publication date can also influence your decision on where to submit your manuscript for review and publication.

Journal Impact Factor

Journal Citation Report provides quantitative measures to evaluate scientific journals, including data on journal impact factors. *Journal Citation Report* is produced by Thomson Institute for Scientific Information. The impact factor is a measure of the frequency with which the "average article" in a journal has been cited in a given period of time (Garfield, 2006). A list of selected impact factors can also be found by professional field (e.g., nursing, law, education, economics) at http://www.sciencegateway.org/rank/index.html.

The impact factor for a journal is calculated based on a 3-year period and can be considered to be the average number of times published papers are cited up to 2 years after publication. The impact factor cannot be calculated until all of the year's publications are included; the most current impact factor may be 1 to 2 years old. The impact factor for a journal can usually be found at the journal's website. Here is an example of information found at one journal website in 2011:

2009 IMPACT FACTOR: 4.357
2009 IMPACT FACTOR RANKING: 2nd out of 70 reproductive medicine journals
TIMING: 84% of manuscripts published within 6 months

Generally, specialty journals in nursing have lower impact factors than broad-based journals such as *Journal of the American Medical Association* or *New England Journal of Medicine*. Your work is important to publish, and there is a journal that will match your needs and the needs of its readership, but it would be important to aim for the higher impact nursing journals that command a higher respect for the quality of their reviewers and their review process and hence the quality of their publications.

Developing a Query Letter

A query letter determines an editor's interest in reviewing your manuscript. This letter should be no more than 1 page and usually includes the abstract and the researcher's qualifications for writing the article. The length of the manuscript and the numbers of tables or figures may be useful, and the editor may be interested to know when, if ever, something on this topic was last published in their journal. Some editors appreciate a list of potential reviewers that you might suggest. Address your query letter in an email to the current editor of a journal. Indicate in the letter the title of the manuscript you would like to submit, why publishing the manuscript is important, and why the readers of the journal would be interested in reading the manuscript. Even if a letter is not required by a journal, some researchers send a query letter because the response (positive or negative) enables them to make the final selection of a journal for submitting their manuscript. Often an editor responds that the journal is planning a special issue on a particular topic and provides the due dates so that you can prepare well in advance. Other journals, such as *Advances in Nursing Science,* accept manuscripts submitted only for their special topic issues, and their website will indicate due dates by topic.

Preparing a Manuscript

A manuscript is written according to the format outlined by the journal. Guidelines for developing a manuscript are usually published in the issue of the journal or on the journal's website. Follow these guidelines explicitly to increase the probability of your manuscript being accepted for publication. Information provided for authors includes (1) directions for manuscript preparation, (2) discussion of copyright and conflict of interest, and (3) guidelines for submission of the manuscript.

Writing research reports for publication requires skills in technical writing that are not used in other types of publications. Technical writing condenses information and is stylistic. The *Publication Manual of the American Psychological Association* (APA, 2010); *A Manual for Writers of Research Papers, Theses, Dissertations* (Turabian, Booth, Colomb, & Williams, 2007); and the *Chicago Manual of Style* (University of Chicago Press Staff, 2010) are considered useful sources for quality technical writing. Most journals stipulate the format style required for their

journal. In a review of 65 nursing journals, Northam, Yarbough, Haas, and Duke (2010) noted that 36 (55%) require APA format.

A quality research report has no errors in punctuation, spelling, or sentence structure. It is also important to avoid confusing words, clichés, jargon, and excessive wordiness and abbreviations. Word processing programs have "tools" commands that have the capacity to proofread manuscripts for errors. However, as the author, you still need to respond and correct sentences that the software program has identified as problematic. These program tools also do a word count to ensure that your manuscript adheres to the limitations specified in the journal guidelines.

Knowledge about the author guidelines provided by the journal and a background in technical writing will help you to develop an outline for a proposed manuscript. The brief outlines presented in Tables 27-1 and 27-8 must be expanded in detail to guide your writing of a manuscript. You can use the outline to develop a rough draft of your article, which you will revise numerous times. Present the content of your article logically and concisely under clear headings, and select a title that creates interest and reflects the content. The APA manual (APA, 2010) provides detailed directions regarding appropriate terms to use in describing study results and manuscript preparation. Consider using an article from the journal as a guide or template; this can help you see the general length of an introduction and discussion section, how tables are presented, how references are cited, and how acknowledgments are worded.

Developing a well-written manuscript is difficult. Often, universities and other agencies offer writing seminars to assist students and faculty in preparing a publication. Some faculty members who chair thesis and dissertation committees also assist their students in developing an article for publication. In this situation, the faculty member is almost always the second author for the article. The APA manual (APA, 2010) has a section on how to reduce the content of a thesis or dissertation for publication.

When you are satisfied with your manuscript, ask one or two colleagues to review it for organization, completeness of content, and writing style. Colleagues' comments can guide you in making any final revisions. You may also want to ask a friend or family member to read the paper. Although your friend may not understand the topic or statistical results, he or she should be able to read the paper and understand the message you are trying to communicate. The manuscript should be expertly typed according to the journal's specifications. If the journal has an international focus, it would be important to specify that your sample is from a particular geographic area such as the United States. For example, if the journal is British, appropriate spelling is important (e.g., "labor" would be spelled "labour"); software spell check tools have options for American English, British English, and other languages. The reference list for the manuscript needs to be in a complete and correct format. Computer programs are available with bibliography systems that enable you to compile a consistent reference list formatted in any commonly accepted journal style. With these programs, you can maintain a permanent file of reference citations. When you need a reference list for a manuscript, you can select the appropriate references from the collection and use the program to format for the requirements of a particular journal.

Submitting a Manuscript for Review

Guidelines in each journal indicate the name of the editor and the address for manuscript submission. Submit your manuscript to only one journal at a time; only when you confirm that your manuscript is not accepted should you submit to a different journal. Most journals now accept only manuscripts submitted electronically, and the editor provides a Portable Document Format (PDF) version to reviewers when they accept the offer to review the manuscript. When submitting the manuscript, include your complete mailing address, phone number, fax number, and email address. The corresponding author who submits the manuscript usually receives notification of receipt of the manuscript within 1 to 2 days if sent by email, and in many cases the notification is sent to all authors listed on the title page of the manuscript.

Peer Review

Most journals use some form of peer review process to evaluate the quality of manuscripts submitted for publication. The manuscript is usually sent to two or three reviewers with guidelines from the editor for performing the review. In most cases, the review is "blinded," which means that the reviewers do not know who the author is, and the author does not know who is reviewing the paper. For reviewers to be blinded, journal instructions will indicate that any materials in the manuscript that identify the authors or institutions should be omitted and replaced with brackets to indicate that something was intentionally removed from the text—"[removed for blind review]."

For research papers, reviewers are asked to evaluate the validity of the study. Reviewers consider whether the methodology was adequate to address the research question or hypotheses and whether the findings are trustworthy and correctly interpreted. For example, if results were not statistically significant, was a power analysis performed? Reviewers also evaluate whether the discussion was appropriate given the findings and whether the author adequately discussed the clinical implications of the findings without going beyond the actual data. Reviewers are also asked to comment on the relevancy of the reference citations, the usefulness of any tables or figures, and the consistency between the title, abstract, and text of the manuscript. Reviewers also look for the strengths and limitations of the study, which the authors should convey in their discussion. Every study has its limitations, and a limitation is not a reason for rejecting the manuscript. However, reviewers want to see that the authors have accurately identified and addressed limitations for the readers.

Responding to Requests to Revise a Manuscript

After reviewing your manuscript, the journal editor will reach one of four possible decisions: (1) accept the manuscript as submitted, (2) accept the manuscript pending minor revisions, (3) tentative acceptance of the manuscript pending major revisions, or (4) rejection of the manuscript. Accepting a manuscript as submitted is extremely rare. The editor will send you a letter that indicates acceptance and the likely date of publication.

Most manuscripts are returned to the author for minor or major revisions before they are published. Many of these returned manuscripts are never revised. If a reviewer identifies a major or minor limitation of the study, that limitation should be considered and can be added to your other limitations in the discussion section. An author may also incorrectly interpret the request for revision as a rejection and assume that a revised manuscript would also be rejected. This assumption is not usually true because revising a manuscript based on reviewers' comments improves the quality of the manuscript. When editors return a manuscript for revision, they include the reviewers' actual comments or a summary of the comments to direct the revision. These reviewers and the editor have devoted time to reviewing your manuscript, and you should make the necessary revisions or respond with your rationale for not making a specific change requested by a reviewer and return the revised manuscript to the same journal for reconsideration.

It is important to review each comment from a reviewer carefully and make the revisions that improve the quality of the research report without making inaccurate statements about the study. Often an editor will provide guidance about how to respond to a reviewer if you ask for help. When you have revised your manuscript based on the reviewers' comments, it should be resubmitted with a cover letter explaining exactly how you responded to each review comment or recommendation. It is helpful to number each comment and recommendation, followed by your response and description of your modification as well as page number in your manuscript for that revision. You can also provide a table with a column for the requested changes and a second column with the changes made or the rationale for why a change could not be made. The second column should also include the number of the page where a change was made. Often an editor requests that the changes in the manuscript be identified with "track changes" or highlighting. In some cases, you may disagree with a reviewer's recommendation. If so, provide a rationale for your disagreement, but do not ignore any comment or recommendation. Sometimes the revised manuscript and your cover letter are returned to the reviewers, and still further modification is requested in the paper before it is published. Although these experiences are frustrating, they provide the opportunity to improve your writing skills and logical development of ideas. Frequently, editors request that the final manuscript be submitted electronically as a clean copy with no track changes or highlights.

An author who receives a rejection can feel devastated, but he or she is not alone and should never take it personally. All authors, even experienced ones, have had manuscripts rejected. Manuscripts are rejected for various reasons. When a group of nursing journal editors surveyed manuscript reviewers and asked them to identify the most important indicators for a manuscript's contribution to nursing, there were five key factors (Dougherty et a., 2011). Table 27-10 identifies

TABLE **27-10**	Important Indicators of a Manuscript's Contribution to Nursing	
Factor	Number (%)
Knowledge or research evidence	1404 (83.8%)
Timeliness/topic of current interest	1153 (68.8%)
Newly emerging idea	1141 (68.1%)
Generalizability across population or international boundaries	698 (41.7%)
Contribution to theory	534 (31.9%)

From Dougherty, M. C., Freda, M. C., Kearney, M. H., Baggs, J. G., & Broome, M. (2011). Online survey of nursing journal peer reviewers: Indicators of quality in manuscripts. *Western Journal of Nursing Research, 33*(4), 506–521.

these issues and their mean frequencies. "Timeliness of the topic" was more important than "contribution to theory" and reflected the predominance of reviewers who review for nursing research journals. When you receive a rejection notice, give yourself a cooling-off period and then ask colleagues to help you determine what the reviewers were saying about why the manuscript was rejected. The editor's introductory comments to the author in a rejection letter can often help to guide you in your responses to reviewers' concerns. Most manuscripts, especially those that are poorly written, can be revised and submitted to a different journal that was your second choice.

Publishing Research Findings in Online Journals

Many print journals are moving to online formats. These journals continue to provide their traditional print version but also have a website with access to some or all of the articles in the printed journal. The number of online nursing journals is also growing. These online-only journals have some distinct advantages for authors. Email links from author to editor and editor to reviewer allow papers to be submitted and sent electronically and allow reviewer comments to be sent back to the editor more quickly. Reviewer comments are compiled by the editor more quickly and sent to the author by email. When the author revises the article and resubmits it by email, the editor can ask the same reviewers to evaluate the article again. Once the article is judged to be satisfactory, it is accepted for publication. This process is particularly important for international scientific communications. Online journals use "continuous publication," which means that there is no wait for approved articles to be published because the editor does not have to wait until the next issue is scheduled for publication. The notion of an "issue" is becoming antiquated as a result of electronic publishing. Approved articles are placed online almost immediately, which is important for research reports because there is more rapid access to recent research findings by other researchers and clinicians interested in facilitating evidence-based practice. There may be added fees for publishing in an online format, but the possibilities of dialogue with readers, including other researchers in the same field of study, are great. However, additional work needs to be done to ensure that online publications are secured and that each publication is permanently available with a permanent identifier for citation and linking. Journal publishers have begun to assign a Digital Object Identifier (DOI) to each article. The DOI system is managed by the International DOI

Foundation, and identifiers are assigned to all types of digital work. The DOI will never change, even if the location for that work does change. The use of DOIs is expected to increase and become accepted as the permanent identifier for scientific and scholarly publications (DOI Handbook, 2006).

Not all online journals are refereed or provide peer review. You may wish to check for information on the peer review process at the online journal website. Peer review is essential to scholars in the university tenure track system. Electronic publishing may result in a more open peer review process. Baggs (2011) discussed some issues to be aware of when considering Internet postings, particularly related to multiple versions and intellectual property issues.

Publishing in an online journal has potential advantages. The constraint on length of the manuscript, imposed because of the cost of print publishing, usually does not exist. Multiple tables, figures, graphics, and even streaming audio and video are possibilities with online journals. Animations can be created to assist the reader in visualizing ideas. Links may be established with full-text versions of citations from other online sources. It is possible to track the number of times the article has been accessed to assess its impact on the scientific community. Electronic listservs and chat rooms may be available to discuss the paper. All of these capabilities are not currently available with every online journal. The technology to provide them exists, but online journals with some of these advanced technologies cover their costs by charging subscription fees or obtaining financing through advertisements. Online journals are rapidly emerging, and websites are available (www.medscape.com/pages/public/publications) that provide a listing and electronic access to the online health journals.

Publishing Research Findings in Books

Some qualitative studies and large, complex quantitative studies are published as chapters within books, monographs, or books. Publishing a book requires extensive commitment on the part of the researcher. In addition, the researcher must select a publisher and convince the publisher to support the book project. A prospectus must be developed that identifies the proposed content of the book, describes the market readership for the book, and includes a rationale for publishing the book. The publisher and researcher must negotiate a contract that is mutually acceptable regarding (1) the content and length of the book, (2) the time required to complete the book, (3) the percentage of royalties that the author will receive, (4) any financial coverage to be offered in advance, and

(5) how it will be marketed. The researcher must fulfill the obligations of the contract by producing the proposed book within the agreed time frame. Publishing a book is a significant accomplishment and an effective, but sometimes slow, means of communicating research findings.

Duplicate Publications and Self-Plagiarism

Duplicate publication is the practice of publishing the same article or major portions of the article in two or more print or electronic media without notifying the editors or referencing the other publication in the reference list (Baggs, 2008). Duplicate publication is a form of plagiarism (self-plagiarism) and is not only unethical but also poor practice because it limits an opportunity for others to publish new knowledge, artificially inflates the importance of a study topic, clutters the literature with redundant information, rewards researchers for publishing the same content twice, and may violate copyright law. Many journal editors screen a manuscript for plagiarism using software programs. If portions of the material have been presented at a scientific meeting in the form of an oral podium or poster presentation, this should be acknowledged along with funding sources and any potential conflict of interest.

Journals require the submission of an original manuscript, not previously published, so submitting a manuscript that has been previously published without referencing the duplicate work or notifying the editor of the previous publication is unethical and a form of scientific misconduct (see Chapter 9). Previous publications related to the study must be cited in the text of the manuscript and the reference list. Editors have the responsibility of developing a policy on duplicate publications and informing all authors, reviewers, and readers of this policy. In addition, editors must ensure that readers are informed of duplicate materials by adequate citation of the materials in the article's text and reference list. A duplicate publication can result in retractions and refusal to accept other manuscripts for review from the author (Baggs, 2008; International Committee of Medical Journal Editors, 2011).

KEY POINTS

- Communicating research findings, the final step in the research process, involves developing a research report and disseminating it through presentations and publications to audiences of nurses, healthcare professionals, policy makers, and healthcare consumers.

- Both quantitative and qualitative research reports include four basic sections: (1) introduction, (2) methods, (3) results, and (4) discussion.
- In a quantitative research report, the introduction briefly identifies the problem that was studied and presents an empirical and theoretical basis for the study. The methods section of the report describes how the study was conducted; the results section reveals what was found; and the discussion section includes the limitations, conclusions that support or refute other published work, implications for nursing practice, and recommendations for further research.
- In qualitative research, the introduction section identifies the phenomenon under investigation and describes the type of qualitative study that was conducted. The methods section includes both the general and the applied methods for the study conducted. The results section of the research report includes the data analysis procedures and presentation of the findings, and the discussion section includes conclusions, limitations, implications for nursing, and recommendations for further research.
- The greatest impact on nursing practice can be achieved by communicating nursing research findings to nurses, other health professionals, policy makers, and healthcare consumers.
- Research findings are presented at conferences and meetings through oral podium and poster presentations of selected portions of your research study; the report developed depends on the focus of the conference, the audience, and the time designated for each presentation.
- A poster session is a visual presentation of a study. Conference sponsors provide information concerning (1) size limitations or format restrictions for the poster and (2) the size of the poster display area. The home institution should provide (1) the institution's logo to place with your title and affiliations and (2) any requirements for the color scheme.
- Developing a manuscript for publication includes the following steps: (1) selecting a journal, (2) writing a query letter, (3) preparing an original manuscript, (4) submitting the manuscript for review, and (5) responding to requests for revision of the manuscript.
- Selecting a journal for publication of a study requires knowledge of the basic requirements of the journal, the journal's refereed status, its impact factor, and recent articles published in the journal.
- An increasing area of concern in publishing is the practice of duplicate publications where the same article or major portions of the article are published in two or more print or electronic media without notifying the editors or referencing the other publication in the reference list.

REFERENCES

Agency for Healthcare Research and Quality (AHRQ). (2011). *Evidence-based practice centers: Synthesizing scientific evidence to improve quality and effectiveness in health care.* Retrieved from http://www.ahrq.gov/clinic/epc/.

American Psychological Association (APA). (2010). *Publication manual of the American Psychological Association* (6th ed.). Washington, DC: Author.

Baggs, J. G. (2008). Issues and rules for authors concerning authorship versus acknowledgements, dual publication, self plagiarism, and salami publishing [Editorial]. *Research in Nursing & Health, 31*(4): 295–297.

Baggs, J. G. (2011). The dissertation manuscript option, internet posting, and publication [Editorial]. *Research in Nursing & Health, 34*(2), 89–90.

Benner, P. E. (1994). *Interpretative phenomenology: Embodiment, caring, and ethics in health and illness.* Thousand Oaks, CA: Sage Publications.

Bennett, J. A. (2006). The consolidated standards of reporting trials (CONSORT): Guidelines for reporting randomized trials. *Nursing Research, 54*(2), 128–132.

Bernstein, N. (2011). Desperately seeking sleep. *Parenting Magazine.* Retrieved from http://www.parenting.com/article/desperately-seeking-sleep-21354392?page=0,2.

Borge, C. R., Wahl, A. K., & Moum, T. (2010). Association of breathlessness with multiple symptoms in chronic obstructive pulmonary disease. *Journal of Advanced Nursing, 66*(12), 2688–2700.

Chapman, S. A., Wides, C. D., & Spetz, J. (2010). Payment regulations for advanced practice nurses: implications for primary care. *Policy, Politics, & Nursing Practice, 11*(2), 89–98.

Chun, K. M. (2006). Conceptual and measurement issues in family acculturation research. In M. H. Bornstein & L. R. Cote (Eds.), *Acculturation and parent-child relationships: Measurement and development* (pp. 63e78). Mahwah, N.J: Lawrence Erlbaum Associates.

Chun, K. M., Chesla, C. A., & Kwan, C. M. L. (2011). "So we adapt step by step": Acculturation experiences affecting diabetes management and perceived health for Chinese American immigrants. *Social Science & Medicine, 72*(2), 256–264.

Cohen, M. Z., Kahn, D. L., & Steeves, R. H. (2000). *Hermeneutic phenomenological research: A practical guide for nurse practitioners.* Thousand Oaks, CA: Sage Publications.

Conn, V. S., & Rantz, M. J. (2003). Research methods: Managing primary study quality in meta-analyses. *Research in Nursing & Health, 26*(4), 322–333.

Craig, J. V., & Smyth, R. L. (2012). *The evidence-base practice manual for nurses* (3rd ed.). Edinburgh, UK: Churchill Livingstone.

Dailey, D. E., Davis, H. C., Cooper, B. A., & Lee, K. A. (2005). Sleep inadequacy and environmental demands among racially diverse women. Abstract for presentation at the Western Institute of Nursing Conference, San Francisco, CA. Available from http://hdl.handle.net/10755/158158.

Denzin, N. K., & Lincoln, Y. S. (2005). Introduction: The discipline and practice of qualitative research. In N. K. Denzin & Y. S. Lincoln (Eds.) *The Sage handbook of qualitative research* (3rd ed.) (pp. 1–32). Thousand Oaks, CA: Sage.

Digital Object Identifier (DOI) Handbook. (2006). Retrieved from doi:10.1000/186.

Donaldson, N., Rutledge, D., & Geiser, K. (2008). Role of the external coach in advancing research translation in hospital-based performance improvement. In K. Henriksen, J. B. Battles, M. A. Keyes, & M. L. Grady (Eds.), *Advances in patient safety: New directions and alternative approaches (Vol. 2: Culture and redesign).* Rockville, MD: Agency for Healthcare Research & Quality.

Dougherty, M. C., Freda, M. C., Kearney, M. H., Baggs, J. G., & Broome, M. (2011). Online survey of nursing journal peer reviewers: Indicators of quality in manuscripts. *Western Journal of Nursing Research, 33*(4), 506–521.

Floyd, J. A., Galvin, E. A., Roop, J. C., Oermann, M. H., & Nordstrom, C. K. (2010). Graphics for dissemination of meta-analyses to staff nurses. *Nursing Research, 18*(1), 72–86.

Garfield, E. (2006). The history and meaning of the journal impact factor. *Journal of the American Medical Association, 295*(1), 90–93.

Goyal, D., Gay, C., & Lee, K. A. (2010). How much does low socioeconomic status increase the risk of prenatal and postpartum depressive symptoms in first-time mothers? *Women's Health Issues, 20*(2), 96–104.

Henly, S. J., Bennett, J. A., & Dougherty, M. C. (2010). Scientific and statistical reviews of manuscripts submitted to *Nursing Research*: Comparison of completeness, quality, and usefulness. *Nursing Outlook, 58*(4), 188–199.

Heo, S., Moser, D. K., Lennie, T. A., Zambroski, C. H., & Chung, M. L. (2007). A comparison of health-related quality of life between older adults with heart failure and healthy older adults. *Heart & Lung, 36*(1), 16–24.

International Committee of Medical Journal Editors [ICMJE]. (2011). *Uniform requirements for manuscripts submitted to biomedical journals: Writing and editing for biomedical publication.* Retrieved from http://www.icmje.org/index.html.

Keegan, D. A., & Bannister, S. L. (2003). Effect of colour coordination of attire with poster presentation on poster popularity. *Canadian Medical Association Journal, 169*(12), 1291–1292.

Lee, K. A., Lentz, M. J., Taylor, D. L., Mitchell, E. S., & Woods, N. F. (1994). Fatigue as a response to environmental demands in women's lives. *Image: Journal of Nursing Scholarship, 26*(2), 149-154.

Lee, K. A., & Gay, C. L. (2011). Can modifications to the bedroom environment improve the sleep of new parents? Two randomized controlled trials. *Research in Nursing & Health, 34*(1), 7–19.

Lentz, M. (2011a). *Writing a WINning abstract.* Retrieved from http://www.ohsu.edu/son/win/pcorner.shtml.

Lentz, M. (2011b). *Yes it is possible: A research report in 10 minutes.* Retrieved from http://www.ohsu.edu/son/win/pcorner.shtml .

Marshall, C., & Rossman, G. B. (2010). *Designing qualitative research* (5th ed.). Thousand Oaks, CA: Sage.

Melnyk, B. M., & Fineout-Overholt, E. (2010). *Evidence-based practice in nursing & healthcare: A guide to best practice* (2nd ed.). Philadelphia: Lippincott Williams & Wilkins.

Munhall, P. (2012). *Nursing research: A qualitative perspective* (5th ed.). Sudbury, MA: Jones & Bartlett Learning.

Northam, S., Yarbough, S., Haas, B., & Duke, G. (2010). Journal editor survey: Information to help authors publish. *Nurse Educator, 35*(1), 29–36.

Pallant, J. (2007). *SPSS survival manual.* New York, NY: Open University Press, McGraw-Hill.

Perez-Escamilla, R., & Putnik, P. (2007). The role of acculturation in nutrition, lifestyle, and incidence of type 2 diabetes among Latinos. *The Journal of Nutrition, 137*, 860-870.

Polit, D. F., & Northam, S. (2011). Impact factors in nursing journals. *Nursing Outlook, 59*(1), 18–28.

Pyrczak, F., & Bruce, R. R. (2007). *Writing empirical research reports: A basic guide for students of the social and behavioral sciences* (6th ed.). Los Angeles, CA: Pyrczak.

Salant, T., & Lauderdale, D. S. (2003). Measuring culture: a critical review of acculturation and health in Asian immigrant populations. *Social Science & Medicine, 57*, 71-90.

Sandelowski, M. (2008). Reading, writing and systematic review. *Journal of Advanced Nursing, 64*(1), 104–110.

Sandelowski, M. J. (2010). Getting it right [Editorial]. *Research in Nursing & Health, 33*(1), 1–3.

Santacroce, S. J., Maccarelli, L. M., & Grey, M. (2004). Methods: Intervention fidelity. *Nursing Research, 53*(1), 63–66.

Saver, C. (2006). Tables and figures: Adding vitality to your article. *AORN Journal, 84*(6), 945–950.

Shelledy, D. C. (2004). How to make an effective poster. *Respiratory Care, 49*(10), 1213–1216.

Stein, K. F., Sargent, J. T., & Rafaels, N. (2007). Intervention research: Establishing fidelity of the independent variable in nursing clinical trials. *Nursing Research, 56*(1), 54–62.

Turabian, K. L., Booth, W. C., Colomb, G. G., & Williams, J. M. (2007). *A manual for writers of research papers, theses, dissertations, seventh edition: Chicago style for students and researchers.* Chicago, IL: University of Chicago Press.

University of Chicago Press Staff. (2010). *The Chicago manual of style* (16th ed.). Chicago, IL: University of Chicago Press.

Wilson, I. B., & Cleary, P. D. (1995). Linking clinical variables with health-related quality of life: A conceptual model of patient outcomes. *Journal of the American Medical Association, 273*(1), 59–65.

28

Writing Research Proposals

evolve http://evolve.elsevier.com/Grove/practice/

With a background in the quantitative, qualitative, outcomes, and intervention research methodologies, you are ready to propose a study. A research proposal is a written plan that identifies the major elements of a study, such as the research problem, purpose, and framework, and outlines the methods and procedures to conduct the proposed study. A proposal is a formal way to communicate ideas about a study to seek approval to conduct the study and obtain funding. Researchers who are seeking approval to conduct a study submit the proposal to a select group for review and, in many situations, verbally defend the proposal. Receiving approval to conduct research has become more complicated because of the increasing complexity of nursing studies, the difficulty involved in recruiting study participants, and increasing concerns over legal and ethical issues. In many large hospitals and healthcare corporations, both the lawyer and the institutional review board (IRB) evaluate the research proposals. The expanded number of healthcare studies being conducted has led to conflict among investigators over who has the right to recruit potential research participants. The increased number of proposed studies has resulted in greater difficulty in obtaining funding. Researchers need to develop a quality study proposal to facilitate university and clinical agency IRB approval, obtain funding, and conduct the study successfully. This chapter focuses on writing a research proposal and seeking approval to conduct a study. Chapter 29 presents the process of seeking funding for research.

Writing a Research Proposal

A well-written proposal communicates a significant, carefully planned research project; shows the qualifications of the researchers; and generates support for the project. Conducting research requires precision and rigorous attention to detail. Reviewers often judge a researcher's ability to conduct a study by the quality of the proposal. A quality study proposal is clear, concise, and complete. Writing a quality proposal involves (1) developing ideas logically, (2) determining the depth or detail of the content of the proposal, (3) identifying critical points in the proposal, and (4) developing an esthetically appealing copy (Martin & Fleming, 2010; Merrill, 2011; Offredy & Vickers, 2010).

Developing Ideas Logically

The ideas in a research proposal must logically build on each other to justify or defend a study, just as a lawyer would logically organize information in the defense of a client. The researcher builds a case to justify why a problem should be studied and proposes the appropriate methodology for conducting the study. Each step in the research proposal builds on the problem statement to give a clear picture of the study and its merit (Merrill, 2011). Universities, medical centers, federal funding agencies, and grant writing consultants have developed websites to help researchers write successful proposals for quantitative, qualitative, outcomes, and intervention research. For example, the University of Michigan provides an online guide for proposal development (http://www.drda.umich.edu/proposals/PWG/pwgcomplete.html). The National Institute of Nursing Research (NINR, 2012) provides online training for developing nurse scientists at http://www.ninr.nih.gov/Training/OnlineDevelopingNurseScientists/. You can use a search engine of your choice, such as Google, and search for research proposal development training; proposal writing tips; courses on proposal development; and proposal guidelines for different universities, medical centers, and government agencies. In addition, various publications have been developed to help individuals improve their scientific writing skills (American Psychological Association [APA], 2010; Offredy & Vickers, 2010; Turabian, Booth, Colomb, & Williams, 2007; University of Chicago Press Staff, 2010).

Determining the Depth of a Proposal

The depth or detail of the content of a proposal is determined by guidelines developed by colleges or schools of nursing, funding agencies, and institutions where research is conducted. Guidelines provide specific directions for the development of a proposal and should be followed explicitly. Omission or misinterpretation of a guideline is frequently the basis for rejection or requiring revision. In addition to following the guidelines, you need to determine the amount of information necessary to describe each step of your study clearly. Often the reviewers of your proposal have varied expertise in the area of your study. The content in a proposal needs to be detailed enough to inform different types of readers yet concise enough to be interesting and easily reviewed (Martin & Fleming, 2010). The guidelines often stipulate a page limit, which determines the depth of the proposal. The relevant content of a research proposal is discussed later in this chapter and varies based on the purpose of the proposal.

Identifying Critical Points

The key or critical points in a proposal must be evident, even to a hasty reader. You might highlight your critical points with bold or italicized type. Sometimes researchers create headings to emphasize critical content, or they may organize the content into tables or graphs. It is critical in a proposal to detail the background and significance of the research problem and purpose, study methodology, and research production plans (data collection and analysis plan, personnel, schedule, and budget) (APA, 2010; Offredy & Vickers, 2010; Turabian et al., 2007).

Developing an Esthetically Appealing Copy

An esthetically appealing copy is typed without spelling, punctuation, or grammatical errors. A proposal with excellent content that is poorly typed or formatted is not likely to receive the full attention or respect of the reviewers. The format used in typing the proposal should follow the guidelines developed by the reviewers or organization. If no particular format is requested, researchers commonly follow APA (2010) format. An appealing copy is legible (the print is dark enough to be read) with appropriate tables and figures to communicate essential information. You need to submit the proposal by the means requested as a mailed hard copy, an email attachment, or uploaded file.

Content of a Research Proposal

The content of a proposal is written with the interest and expertise of the reviewers in mind. Proposals are typically reviewed by faculty, clinical agency IRB members, and representatives of funding institutions. The content of a proposal varies with the reviewers, the guidelines developed for the review, and the type of study (quantitative or qualitative) proposed. This section addresses the content of (1) a student proposal for both quantitative and qualitative studies, (2) condensed research proposals, and (3) preproposals.

Content of a Student Proposal

Student researchers develop proposals to communicate their research projects to the faculty and members of university and agency IRBs (see Chapter 9 for details on IRB membership and the approval process). Student proposals are written to satisfy requirements for a degree and are usually developed according to guidelines outlined by the faculty. The faculty member who will be assisting with the research project (the chair of the student's thesis or dissertation committee) generally reviews these guidelines with the student. Each faculty member has a unique way of interpreting and emphasizing aspects of the guidelines. In addition, a student needs to evaluate the faculty member's background regarding a research topic of interest and determine whether a productive working relationship can be developed. Faculty members who are actively involved in their own research have extensive knowledge and expertise that can be helpful to a novice researcher. Both the student and the faculty member benefit when a student becomes involved in an aspect of the faculty member's research. This collaborative relationship can lead to the development of essential knowledge for providing evidenced-based nursing practice (Brown, 2009; Craig & Smyth, 2012; Melnyk & Fineout-Overholt, 2011).

The content of a student proposal usually requires greater detail than a proposal developed for an agency or funding organization. The proposal is often the first three or four chapters of the student's thesis or dissertation, and the proposed study is discussed in the future tense—that is, what the student *will do* in conducting the research. A student research proposal

TABLE 28-1 Quantitative Research Proposal Guidelines for Students

Chapter I	Introduction
	A. Background and significance of the problem
	B. Statement of the problem
	C. Statement of the purpose
Chapter II	Review of Relevant Literature
	A. Review of theoretical literature
	B. Review of relevant research
	C. Summary
Chapter III	Framework
	A. Development of a framework
	(Develop a map of the study framework, define concepts in the map, describe relationships or propositions in the map, indicate the focus of the study, and link concepts to study variables)
	B. Formulation of objectives, questions, or hypotheses
	C. Definitions (conceptual and operational) of study variables
	D. Definition of relevant terms
Chapter IV	Methods and Procedures
	A. Description of the research design
	(Model of the design, strengths and weaknesses of the design validity)
	B. Identification of the population and sample
	(Sample size, use of power analysis, sample criteria, and sampling method including strengths and weaknesses)
	C. Selection of a setting
	(Strengths and weaknesses of the setting)
	D. Presentation of ethical considerations
	(Protection of subjects' rights and university and healthcare agency review processes)
	E. Description of the intervention if appropriate for the type of study
	(Provide a protocol for implementing the intervention, detail who will implement the intervention, and describe how intervention fidelity is ensured)
	F. Selection of measurement methods
	(Reliability, validity, scoring, and level of measurement of the instruments as well as plans for examining reliability and validity of the instruments in the present study; precision and accuracy of physiological measures)
	G. Plan for data collection
	(Data collection process, training of data collectors if appropriate, schedule, data collection forms, and management of data)
	H. Plan for data analysis
	(Analysis of demographic data; analyses for research objectives, questions, or hypotheses; level of significance if appropriate; and other analysis techniques)
	I. Identification of limitations
	(Methodological and theoretical limitations)
	J. Discussion of communication of findings
References	Include references cited in the proposal and follow APA (2010) format
Appendices	Presentation of a study budget and timetable

usually includes a title page with the title of the proposal, the name and credentials of the investigator, university name, and the date. You need to devote time to developing the title so that it accurately reflects the scope and content of the proposed study (Martin & Fleming, 2010).

Content of a Quantitative Research Proposal

A quantitative research proposal usually includes a table of contents that reflects the following chapters or sections: (1) introduction, (2) review of relevant literature, (3) framework, and (4) methods and procedures. Some graduate schools require in-depth development of these sections, whereas others require a condensed version of the same content. Another approach is that proposals for theses and dissertations be written in a format that can be transformed into a publication. Table 28-1 outlines the content often covered in the chapters of a student quantitative research proposal.

Introduction

The introductory chapter identifies the research topic and problem and discusses their significance and background. The significance of the problem addresses its importance in nursing practice and the expected generalizability of the findings. The magnitude of a problem is partly determined by the interest of nurses; other healthcare professionals; policy makers; and healthcare consumers at the local, state, national, or international level. You can document this interest with sources from the literature. The background describes how the problem was identified and historically links the problem to nursing practice. Your background information might also include one or two major studies conducted to resolve the problem, some key theoretical ideas related to the problem, and possible solutions to the problem. The background and significance form the basis for your problem statement, which identifies what is not known and the need for further research. Follow your problem statement with a succinct statement of the research purpose or the goal of the study (see Chapter 5) (Martin & Fleming, 2010; Merrill, 2011).

Review of Relevant Literature

The review of relevant literature provides an overview of the essential information that will guide you as you develop your study and includes relevant theoretical and empirical literature (see Table 28-1). Theoretical literature provides a background for defining and interrelating relevant study concepts, whereas empirical literature includes a summary and critical appraisal of previous studies. Here you will discuss the recommendations made by other researchers, such as changing or expanding a study, in relation to the proposed study. The depth of the literature review varies; it might include only recent studies and theorists' works, or it might be extensive and include a description and critical appraisal of many past and current studies and an in-depth discussion of theorists' works. The literature review might be presented in a narrative format or in a pinch table that summarizes relevant studies (see Chapter 6) (Pinch, 1995). The literature review shows that you have a command of the current empirical and theoretical knowledge regarding the proposed problem (Merrill, 2011; Offredy & Vickers, 2010).

This chapter concludes with a summary. The summary includes a synthesis of the theoretical literature and findings from previous research that describe the current knowledge of a problem (Merrill, 2011). Gaps in the knowledge base are also identified, with a description of how the proposed study is expected to contribute to the nursing knowledge needed for evidence-based practice.

Framework

A framework provides the basis for generating and refining the research problem and purpose and linking them to the relevant theoretical knowledge in nursing or related fields. The framework includes concepts and relationships among concepts or propositions, which are sometimes represented in a model or a map (see Chapter 7). Middle-range theories from nursing and other disciplines are frequently used as frameworks for quantitative studies, and the proposition or propositions to be tested from the theory need to be identified (Smith & Liehr, 2008). The framework needs to include the concepts to be examined in the study, their definitions, and their link to the study variables (see Table 28-1). If you use another theorist's or researcher's model from a journal article or book, letters documenting permission to use this model from the publisher and the theorist or researcher need to be included in your proposal appendices.

In some studies, research objectives, questions, or hypotheses are developed to direct the study (see Chapter 8). The objectives, questions, or hypotheses evolve from the research purpose and study framework, in particular the proposition to be tested, and identify the study variables. The variables are conceptually defined to show the link to the framework, and they are operationally defined to describe the procedures for manipulating or measuring the study variables. You also will need to define any relevant terms and to identify assumptions that provide a basis for your study.

Methods and Procedures

The researcher describes the design or general strategy for conducting the study, sometimes including a diagram of the design (see Chapter 11). Designs for descriptive and correlational studies are flexible and can be unique to the study being conducted (Kerlinger & Lee, 2000). Because of this uniqueness, the descriptions need to include the design's strengths and weaknesses. Presenting designs for quasi-experimental and experimental studies involves (1) describing how the research situation will be structured; (2) detailing the treatment to be implemented (Chlan, Guttormson, & Savik, 2011); (3) explaining how the effect of the treatment will be measured; (4) specifying the variables to be controlled and the methods for controlling them; (5) identifying uncontrolled extraneous variables and determining their impact on the findings; (6) describing the methods for assigning subjects to the treatment group, comparison or control group, or placebo group; and (7) exploring the strengths and weaknesses of the design (Shadish, Cook, & Campbell, 2002). The design needs to account for all the objectives, questions, or hypotheses identified in the proposal. If a pilot study is planned, the design should include the procedure for conducting the pilot and for incorporating the results into the proposed study (see Table 28-1).

Your proposal should identify the target population to which your study findings will be generalized and the accessible population from which the sample will be selected. You need to outline the inclusion and exclusion criteria you will use to select a study participant or subject and present the rationale for these sample criteria. For example, a participant might be selected according to the following sample criteria: female, age 18 to 60 years, hospitalized, and 1 day status post abdominal surgery. The rationale for these criteria might be that the researcher wants to examine the effects of a selected pain management intervention on women who have recently undergone hospitalization and abdominal surgery. The sampling method and the approximate sample size are discussed in terms of their adequacy and limitations in investigating the research purpose (Thompson, 2002). A power analysis usually is conducted to determine an adequate sample size to identify significant relationships and differences in studies (see Chapter 15) (Aberson, 2010).

A proposal includes a description of the proposed study setting, which frequently includes the name of the agency and the structure of the units or sites where the study is to be conducted. The specific setting is often identified in the proposal but not in the final research report. The agency you select should have the potential to generate the type and size of sample required for the study. Your proposal might include the number of individuals who meet the sample criteria and are cared for by the agency in a given time period. In addition, the structure and activities in the agency need to be able to accommodate the proposed design of the study. If you are not affiliated with this agency, it would be helpful if you had a letter of support for your study from the agency.

Ethical considerations in a proposal include the rights of the subjects and the rights of the agency where the study is to be conducted. Describe how you plan to protect subjects' rights as well as the risks and potential benefits of your study. Also, address the steps you will take to reduce any risks that the study might present. Many agencies require a written consent form, and that form is often included in the appendices

of the proposal. With the implementation of the Health Insurance Portability and Accountability Act (HIPAA), healthcare agencies and providers must have a signed authorization form from patients to release their health information for research. You must also address the risks and potential benefits of the study for the institution (Martin & Fleming, 2010; Offredy & Vickers, 2010). If your study places the agency at risk, outline the steps you will take to reduce or eliminate these risks. It is also necessary for you to state that the proposal will be reviewed by the thesis or dissertation committee, university IRB, and agency IRB.

Some quantitative studies are focused on testing the effectiveness of an intervention, such as quasi-experimental studies or randomized controlled trials. In these types of studies, the elements of the intervention and the process for implementing the intervention must be detailed (Bulecheck, Butcher, & Dochterman, 2008). You need to develop a protocol that details the elements of the intervention and the process for implementing them (see Chapter 14 and the example quasi-experimental study proposal at the end of this chapter). Intervention fidelity needs to be ensured during a study so that the intervention is consistently implemented to designated study participants (Chlan et al., 2011; Santacroce, Maccarelli, & Grey, 2004).

Describe the methods you will use to measure study variables, including each instrument's reliability, validity, methods of scoring, and level of measurement (see Chapter 16). A plan for examining the reliability and validity of the instruments in the present study needs to be addressed. If an instrument has no reported reliability and validity, you may need to conduct a pilot study to examine these qualities. If the intent of the proposed study is to develop an instrument, describe the process of instrument development (Waltz, Strickland, & Lenz, 2010). If physiological measures are used, address the accuracy, precision, sensitivity, selectivity, and error rate of the instrument (Ryan-Wenger, 2010). A copy of the interview questions, questionnaires, scales, physiological measures, or other tools to be used in the study is usually included in the proposal appendices (see Chapter 17). You must obtain permission from the authors to use copyrighted instruments, and letters documenting that permission has been obtained must be included in the proposal appendices.

The data collection plan clarifies what data are to be collected and the process for collecting the data. In this plan you will identify the data collectors, describe the data collection procedures, and present a schedule for data collection activities. If more than one person will be involved in data collection, it is important to describe methods used to train your data collectors to ensure consistency. The method of recording data is often described, and sample data recording sheets are placed in the proposal appendices. Also, discuss any special equipment you will use or develop to collect data for the study, and address data security, including the methods of data storage (see Chapter 20).

The plan for data analysis identifies the analysis techniques that will be used to summarize the demographic data and answer the research objectives, questions, or hypotheses. The analysis section is best organized by the study objectives, questions, or hypotheses. The analysis techniques identified need to be appropriate for the type of data collected (Grove, 2007). For example, if an associative hypothesis is developed, correlational analysis is planned. If a researcher plans to determine differences among groups, the analysis techniques might include a t-test or analysis of variance (ANOVA) (Munro, 2005). A level of significance ($\alpha = 0.05, 0.01$, or 0.001) is also identified (see Chapters 21 through 25). Often, a researcher projects the type of results that will be generated from data analysis. Dummy tables, graphs, and charts can be developed to present these results and are included in the proposal appendices if required by the guidelines. The researcher might project possible findings for a study and indicate what support or nonsupport of a proposed hypothesis would mean in light of the study framework and previous research findings.

The methods and procedures chapter of a proposal usually concludes with a discussion of the study's limitations and a plan for communication of the findings. Both methodological and theoretical limitations are addressed. Methodological limitations might include areas of weakness in the design, sampling method, sample size, measurement tools, data collection procedures, or data analysis techniques; theoretical limitations set boundaries for the generalization of study findings. The accuracy with which the conceptual definitions and relational statements in a theory reflect reality has a direct impact on the generalization of study findings. Theory that has withstood frequent testing through research provides a stronger framework for the interpretation and generalization of findings. A plan is included for communicating the research through presentations to audiences of nurses, other health professionals, policy makers, and healthcare consumers and publication (see Chapter 27).

A budget and timetable are frequently included in the proposal appendices. The budget projects the expenses for the study, which might include the cost for data collection tools and procedures; special equipment; consultants for data analysis; computer time; travel related to data collection and analysis; typing; copying; and developing, presenting, and publishing the final report. Study budgets requesting external funding for researchers' time include investigators' salaries and secretarial costs. You need a timetable to direct the steps of your research project and increase the chance that you will complete the project on schedule. A timetable identifies the tasks to be done, who will accomplish these tasks, and when these tasks will be completed. An example proposal for a quasi-experimental study is presented at the end of this chapter to guide you in developing your study proposal.

Content of a Qualitative Research Proposal

Qualitative research proposal guidelines are unique for the development of knowledge and theories using various qualitative research methods. A qualitative proposal usually includes the following content areas: (1) introduction; (2) research philosophy and general method; (3) applied method of inquiry; and (4) current knowledge, limitations, and plans for communication of the study findings (Marshall & Rossman, 2011; Munhall, 2012; Patton, 2002; Sandelowski, Davis, & Harris, 1989). Guidelines are presented in Table 28-2 to assist you in developing a qualitative research proposal.

Introduction

The introduction usually provides a general background for the proposed study by identifying the phenomenon, clinical problem, issue, or situation to be investigated and linking it to nursing knowledge. The general aim or purpose of the study is identified and provides the focus for the qualitative study to be conducted. The study purpose might be followed by research questions that direct the investigation (Munhall, 2012; Offredy & Vickers, 2010). For example, a possible aim or purpose for an ethnographic study might be to "describe the coping processes of Mexican American adults with type 2 diabetes receiving care in a federally funded clinic." The research questions might focus on the influences of real-world problems, cultural elements, and the clinic environment on the coping processes of these adults. Thus, the study questions might include any of the following: How do Mexican American adults respond to a new diagnosis of type 2 diabetes? What is the impact of type 2 diabetes on Mexican American adults and their families over time? What community, clinic, and family types of support exist for Mexican American adults with type 2 diabetes? What does it

TABLE 28-2	**Qualitative Research Proposal Guidelines for Students**
Chapter I	Introduction
	A. Identify the phenomenon to be studied
	B. Identify the study purpose or aim and its significance
	C. State the study questions or objectives
	D. Describe the evolution of the study
	1. Provide a rationale for conducting study
	2. Place the study in context historically
	3. Discuss the researcher's experience with phenomenon
	4. Discuss the relevance of the study to nursing
Chapter II	Philosophical and Conceptual Foundation and General Method for the Proposed Study
	A. Identify the type of qualitative research (phenomenological research, grounded theory research, ethnographic research, exploratory-descriptive qualitative research, and historical research) to be conducted
	B. Describe the philosophical and theoretical basis for the research method
	C. Explain the research assumptions
	D. Discuss the general steps, procedures, and outcomes for this method
	E. Translation of concepts or terms
Chapter III	Method of Inquiry
	A. Demonstrate the researcher's credentials for conducting this qualitative study
	B. Select a site and population
	C. Describe the plan for the researcher's role in the following
	1. Entry into the site and approval to collect data
	2. Selection of study participants
	3. Ethical considerations
	D. Describe the plan for data collection
	1. Data to be collected
	2. Procedures for data collection
	3. Procedures for recording data during data collection
	E. Describe the plan for data analysis conducted with data collection
	1. Steps for coding information
	2. Use of specific data analysis procedures advanced in the specific research method (phenomenology research, grounded theory research, ethnography research, exploratory-descriptive qualitative research, and historical research)
	3. Steps to be taken to verify the information
Chapter IV	Current Knowledge, Limitations, and Plans for Communication of the Study
	A. Summarize and reference relevant literature as appropriate for the type of qualitative study
	B. Disclose anticipated findings, hypotheses, and hunches
	C. Discuss procedures to remain open to unexpected information
	D. Discuss limitations of the study
	E. Identify plans for communication of findings (Marshall & Rossman, 2011; Munhall, 2012)
References	Include references cited in the proposal and follow APA (2010) format
Appendices	Present the study budget and timetable

mean to Mexican American adults to have their diabetes under control?

The introduction also includes the evolution of the study and its significance to nursing practice, patients, the healthcare system, and health policy. The discussion of the evolution of the study often includes how the problem developed (historical context), who or what is affected by the problem, and the researcher's experience with the problem (experiential context). Whenever possible, the significance and evolution of the study purpose needs to be documented from the literature (Munhall, 2012). The significance of a study may include the number of people affected, how this phenomenon affects health and quality of life, and the consequences of not understanding this phenomenon. Marshall and Rossman (2011) identified the following questions to assess the significance of a study: (1) Who has an interest in this domain of inquiry? (2) What do we already know about the topic? (3) What has not been answered adequately in previous research and practice? (4) How will this research add to knowledge, practice, and policy in this area? The introduction section concludes with an overview of the remaining sections that are covered in the proposal.

Philosophical and Conceptual Foundation and General Methods for the Proposed Study

This section introduces the philosophical and conceptual foundation for the qualitative research method (phenomenological research, ethnographic research, grounded theory research, exploratory-descriptive qualitative research, or historical research) selected for the proposed study. The researcher provides a rationale for the qualitative method selected and discusses its ability to generate the knowledge needed in nursing (see Table 28-1). The investigator introduces the philosophy, essential elements of the philosophy, and the assumptions for the specific type of qualitative research to be conducted.

The philosophy varies for the different types of qualitative research and guides the conduct of the study. For example, a proposal for a phenomenological study might indicate the purpose of the study is to understand the experience of young and middle-aged women receiving news about a family *BRCA 1/2* genetic mutation. "The specific study aims are to (a) describe the experiences of women learning about a family *BRCA 1/2* mutation, (b) describe the meaning of genetic risk to female biologic relatives of *BRCA 1/2* mutation carriers, and (3) gain an understanding of practical knowledge used in living with risk" (Crotser & Dickerson, 2010, p. 367). Genetic testing has determined that 5% to 10% of breast cancers are caused by inherited gene mutations such as *BRCA 1* or *BRCA 2*. "Heideggerian hermeneutic phenomenology was selected to guide this study.... By listening to the stories of women who lived the experience, HCPs [healthcare providers] will understand the meaning of living with risk through the language used to express their life view (Heidegger, 1975)" (Crotser & Dickerson, 2010, p. 358). Assumptions about the nature of the knowledge and the reality that underlie the type of qualitative research to be conducted are also identified. The assumptions and philosophy provide a theoretical perspective for the study that influences the focus of the study, data collection and analysis, and articulation of the findings.

Method of Inquiry

Developing and implementing the methodology of qualitative research require an expertise that some believe can be obtained only through a mentorship relationship with an experienced qualitative researcher. The role of the researcher and the intricate techniques of data collection and analysis are thought to be best communicated through a one-to-one relationship. Thus, planning the methods of a qualitative study requires knowledge of relevant sources that describe the different qualitative research techniques and procedures (Marshall & Rossman, 2011; Miles & Huberman, 1994; Munhall, 2012; Patton, 2002), in addition to requiring interaction with a qualitative researcher. The proposal needs to reflect the researcher's credentials for conducting the particular type of qualitative study proposed (see Chapter 12 for details on qualitative research methods).

Identifying the methods for conducting a qualitative study is a difficult task because sometimes the specifics of the study design emerge during the study. In contrast to quantitative research, in which the design is a fixed blueprint for a study, the design in qualitative research emerges or evolves as the study is conducted. You must document the logic and appropriateness of the qualitative method and develop a tentative plan for conducting your study. Because this plan is tentative, researchers reserve the right to modify or change the plan as needed during the conduct of the study (Sandelowski et al., 1989). However, the design or plan must be (1) consistent with the philosophical approach, study purpose, and specific research aims or questions; (2) be well conceived; and (3) address prior criticism, as appropriate (Fawcett & Garity, 2009). The tentative plan describes the process for selecting a site and population and the initial steps taken to gain access to the site. Having access to the site includes establishing relationships that facilitate recruitment of the participants necessary to address the research purpose and answer the research questions. For the research question, "How do Mexican American adults cope with a new diagnosis of type 2 diabetes while receiving care in federally funded clinics?" the participants might be identified in a specific clinic or by contacting particular healthcare providers. Although initial contact might be made through a clinic, the interviews and observations might occur in the community, at family gatherings, or in the participants' homes.

The researcher must gain entry into the setting, develop a rapport with the participants that will facilitate the detailed data collection process, and protect the rights of the participants (Marshall & Rossman, 2011; Sandelowski et al., 1989). You need to address the following questions in describing the researcher's role: (1) What is the best setting for the study? (2) How will I ease my entry into the research site? (3)

How will I gain access to the participants? (4) What actions will I take to encourage the participants to cooperate? (5) What precautions will I take to protect the rights of the participants and to prevent the setting and the participants from being harmed? You need to describe the process you will follow to obtain informed consent and the actions you will take to decrease study risks. The sensitive nature of some qualitative studies increases the risk for participants, which makes ethical concerns and decisions a major focus of the proposal (Munhall, 2012; Patton, 2002).

The primary data collection techniques used in qualitative research are observation and in-depth interviewing. Observations can range from highly detailed, structured notations of behaviors to ambiguous descriptions of behaviors or events. The interview can range from structured, closed-ended questions to unstructured, open-ended questions (Marshall & Rossman, 2011; Munhall, 2012). You need to address the following questions when describing the proposed data collection process: (1) What data will be collected? For example, will the data be field notes from memory, audio recordings of interviews, transcripts of conversations, DVDs of events, or examination of existing documents? (2) What techniques or procedures will the research team use to collect the data? For example, if interviews are to be conducted, will a list of the proposed questions be included in the appendix? (3) Who will collect data and provide any training required for the data collectors? (4) Where will sources of data be located? In historical research, data are collected through an exhaustive review of published and unpublished literature. (5) How will the data be recorded and stored?

The methods section also needs to address how you will document the research process. For example, you might keep a research journal or diary during the course of the study. These notes can document the day-to-day activities, methodological events, decision-making procedures, and personal notes about the informants. This information becomes part of the audit trail that you can provide to ensure the quality of the study (Miles & Huberman, 1994; Munhall, 2012; Patton, 2002).

The methods section of the proposal also includes the analysis techniques and the steps for conducting these techniques. In qualitative research, data collection and analysis often occur simultaneously. The data are usually in the form of notes, digital files, audio recordings, DVDs, and other material obtained from observation, interviews, and completing questionnaires. Through qualitative analysis techniques, these data are organized to promote understanding and determine meaning (see Chapter 12) (Patton, 2002). Researchers also need to identify software programs they plan to use for data analysis.

Current Knowledge Base, Limitations, and Plans for Communication of the Study

This section of the proposal summarizes and documents all relevant literature that was reviewed for the study. Similar to quantitative research, qualitative studies require a literature review to provide a basis for the study purpose and to clarify how this study will expand nursing knowledge (Marshall & Rossman, 2011; Munhall, 2012). This initial literature review is often conducted to establish the significance of the study and to develop research questions to guide the study. In phenomenological and grounded theory research, an additional literature review is usually conducted toward the end of the research project. The findings from a phenomenological study are compared and combined with findings from the literature to contribute to the current knowledge of the phenomenon. In grounded theory research, the literature is used to explain, support, and extend the theory generated in the study (Glaser & Strauss, 1965). In all types of qualitative studies, the findings obtained are examined in light of the existing literature (see Chapter 4).

You need to describe how the literature reviewed has influenced your proposed research methods. Biases and previous experience with the research problem need to be addressed, as does their potential impact on the proposed study. Often, anticipated findings, hypotheses, and hunches are identified before the study is conducted, followed by a discussion of the procedures that might be used to remain open to new information. You will also need to address the limitations of your proposed study in the context of limitations of similar studies.

Conclude your proposal by describing how you plan to communicate your findings to various audiences through presentations and publications. Often, a realistic budget and timetable are provided in the appendix. A qualitative study budget is similar to a quantitative study budget and includes costs for data collection tools, software, and recording devices; consultants for data analysis; travel related to data collection and analysis; transcription of recordings; copying related to data collection and analysis; and developing, presenting, and publishing the final report. However, one of the greatest expenditures in qualitative research is the researcher's time. Develop a timetable to project how long the study will take; often a period of 2 years or more is designated for data collection and analysis (Marshall & Rossman, 2011; Munhall, 2012; Patton,

2002). You can use your budget and timetable to make decisions regarding the need for funding.

Excellent websites have been developed to assist novice researchers in identifying an idea for qualitative study and developing a qualitative research proposal and reports (see www.nova.edu/ssss/QR/qualres.html). The Office of Behavior and Social Sciences Research within the National Institutes of Health has a website to assist researchers in developing qualitative and quantitative research proposals for funding (http://grants.nih.gov/grants/writing_application.htm). You can use these websites and other publications to promote the quality of your qualitative research proposal. The quality of a proposal is based on the potential scientific contribution of the research to nursing knowledge; the research philosophy guiding the study; the research methods; and the knowledge, skills, and resources available to the investigators (Marshall & Rossman, 2011; Munhall, 2012; Patton, 2002).

Content of a Condensed Proposal

The content of proposals developed for review by clinical agencies and funding institutions is usually a condensed version of the student proposal. However, even though these proposals are condensed, the logical links between components of the study need to be clearly shown. A condensed proposal often includes a statement of the problem and purpose; previous research that has been conducted in the area (usually limited to three to five studies); the framework, variables, design, sample, ethical considerations, and plans for data collection and analysis; and plans for dissemination of findings.

A proposal submitted to a clinical agency needs to identify the specific setting clearly, such as the emergency department or intensive care unit, and the projected time span for the study. Members of clinical agencies are particularly interested in the data collection process and involvement of institutional personnel in the study. The researcher needs to identify any expected disruptions in institutional functioning, with plans for preventing these disruptions when possible. The researcher must recognize that anything that slows down or disrupts employee functioning costs the agency money and can interfere with the quality of patient care. By showing that you are aware of these concerns and have proposed ways to minimize their effects, you increase the probability of obtaining approval to conduct your study.

Various companies, corporations, and organizations provide funding for research projects. A proposal developed for these types of funding institutions frequently includes a brief description of the study, the significance of the study to the institution, a timetable, and a budget. Most of these proposals are brief and might contain a 1-page summary sheet or abstract at the beginning of the proposal that summarizes the steps of the study. The salient points of the study are included on this page in easy-to-read, nontechnical terminology. Some proposal reviewers for funding institutions are laypersons with no background in research or nursing. An inability to understand the terminology might put the reviewer on the defensive or create a negative reaction, which could lead to disapproval of the study. When a funding institution is examining multiple studies, the summary sheet is often the basis for final decisions. The summary should be concise, informative, and designed to sell the study.

In proposals for both clinical and funding agencies, the investigator needs to document his or her research background and supply a curriculum vitae if requested. The research review committee for approval of funding will be interested in previous research, research publications, and clinical expertise, especially if a clinical study is proposed. If you are a graduate student, the committee may request the names of the university committee members and verification that your proposal has been approved by the student's thesis or dissertation committee and the university IRB. Chapter 29 provides details on proposals submitted for funding.

Content of a Preproposal

Sometimes a researcher sends a preproposal or query letter rather than a proposal to a funding institution. A preproposal is a short document of 4 to 5 pages plus appendices that explores the funding possibilities for a research project. The parts of the preproposal are logically ordered as follows: "(1) letter of transmittal, (2) proposal for research, (3) personnel, (4) facilities, and (5) budget" (Malasanos, 1976, p. 223). The proposal provides a brief overview of the proposed project, including the research problem, purpose, and methodology (brief description), and, most important, a statement of the significance of the work to knowledge in general and the funding institution in particular. By developing a preproposal, researchers are able to determine the agencies interested in funding their study and limit submission of their proposals to only institutions that indicate an interest.

Seeking Approval for a Study

Seeking approval to conduct a study is an action that should be based on knowledge and guided by purpose.

Obtaining approval for a study from a research review committee or IRB requires understanding the approval process, writing a research proposal for review, and, in many cases, verbally defending the proposal. Little has been written to guide the researcher who is going through the labyrinth of approval mechanisms. This section provides a background for obtaining approval to conduct a study.

Clinical agencies and healthcare corporations review studies for the following reasons: (1) to evaluate the quality of the study, (2) to ensure that adequate measures are being taken to protect human subjects, and (3) to evaluate the impact of the study on the reviewing institution (Merrill, 2011; Offredy & Vickers, 2010). What does the researcher hope to result from this institutional review? Most researchers hope to receive approval to collect data at the reviewing institution and to obtain support for the proposed study. IRB reviews sometime identify potential risks or problems related to studies that can be resolved before the studies are implemented.

Approval Process

An initial step in seeking approval is to determine exactly what committees in which agencies must grant approval before the study can be conducted. You need to take the initiative to determine the formal approval process rather than assume that you will be told if a formal review system exists. Information on the formal research review system might be obtained from administrative personnel, an online website, special projects or grant officers, chairs of IRBs in clinical agencies, clinicians who have previously conducted research, university IRB chairs, and university faculty who are involved in research.

Graduate students usually require approval from their thesis or dissertation committee, the university IRB, and the agency IRB where the data are to be collected. University faculty members conducting research seek approval for the studies from the university IRB and the agency IRB. Nurses conducting research in an agency where they are employed must seek approval only at that agency. If the researcher seeks outside funding, additional review committees are involved. Not all studies require full review by the IRB (see Chapter 9 for the types of studies that qualify for exempt or expedited review). However, the IRB, not the researcher, determines the type of review that the study requires for conduct in that agency.

When multiple committees must review a study, sometimes the respective committees agree that the review for the protection of human subjects will be done by only one of the committees, with the findings of that committee generally being accepted by the other committees. For example, if the university IRB examined and approved a proposal for the protection of human subjects, funding agencies usually recognize that review as sufficient. Reviews in other committees focus on approval to conduct the study within the institution or decisions to provide study funding.

As part of the approval process, the researcher must determine the agency's policy regarding (1) the use of the name of the clinical facility in reporting findings, (2) the presentation and publication of the study, and (3) the authorship of publications. The facility's name is used when presenting or publishing a study only with prior written administrative approval. The researcher may feel freer to report findings that could be interpreted negatively in terms of the institution if the agency is not identified. Some institutions have rules that limit what is presented or published in a study, where it is presented or published, and who is the presenter or author. Before conducting a study, researchers, especially employees of healthcare agencies, must clarify the rules and regulations of the agency regarding authorship, presentations, and publications. In some cases, recognition of these rules must be included in the proposal if it is to be approved.

Preparing Proposals for Review Committees

The initial proposals for theses and dissertations are often developed as part of a formal class. The faculty members teaching the class provide students with specific proposal guidelines approved by the graduate faculty and assist them in developing their initial proposals. If students elect to conduct a thesis, they ask an appropriate faculty member to serve as chair. With the assistance of the chair, the student identifies committee members with expertise in the focus of the proposed study or in conducting research who can work effectively together to refine the final proposal. The number of committee members varies for theses (usually a chair and two members) and dissertations (often a chair and four members) and with the university requirements. This proposal requires approval by the thesis or dissertation committee and the university IRB.

Conducting research in a clinical agency requires approval by the agency IRB. This committee has the responsibility to (1) provide researchers with copies of institutional policies and requirements, (2) screen proposals for conducting research in the agency, and (3) assist the researcher with the IRB process. The approval process policy and proposal guidelines are usually available from the chair of the IRB; and the guidelines should be followed carefully, particularly page limitations. Some committees refuse to review proposals that exceed these limitations. Reviewers on these committees are usually evaluating proposals in addition to other full-time responsibilities, and their time is limited.

Investigators also need to be familiar with the IRB's process for screening proposals. Most agency IRBs screen proposals for (1) scientific merit, (2) protection of human rights, (3) congruence of the study with the agency's research agenda, and (4) impact of the study on patient care (Merrill, 2011). Researchers need to develop their proposal with these ideas in mind. They also need to determine whether the committee requires specific forms to be completed and submitted with the research proposal. Other important information can be gathered by addressing the following questions: (1) How often does the committee meet? (2) How long before the next meeting? (3) What materials should be submitted before the meeting? (4) When should these materials be submitted? (5) How many copies of the proposal are required? (6) What period of time is usually involved in committee review?

Social and Political Factors

Social and political factors play an important role in obtaining approval to conduct a study. You need to treat the review process with as much care as development of the study. The dynamics of the relationships among committee members is important to assess. This detail is especially important in the selection of a thesis or dissertation committee to ensure that the members are willing to work together productively. Thorough assessment of the social and political situation in which the study will be reviewed and implemented may be crucial to success of the study.

Clinical agency IRBs may include nurse clinicians who have never conducted research, nurse researchers, and researchers in other disciplines. The reactions of each of these groups to a study could be very different. Sometimes IRB committees are made up primarily of physicians, which is frequently the case in health science centers. Physicians are often not oriented to nursing research methods and might need additional explanations related to the research methodology. However, most physicians are strong supporters of nursing research, helpful in suggesting changes in design to strengthen the study, and eager to facilitate access to subjects.

The researcher needs to anticipate potential responses of committee members and prepare the proposal to elicit a favorable response. It is wise to meet with the chair of the agency IRB early in the development of a proposal. This meeting could facilitate proposal development, rapport between the researcher and agency personnel, and approval of the research proposal.

In addition to the formal committee approval mechanisms, you will need the tacit approval of the administrative personnel and staff who are affected by the conduct of your study. Obtaining informal approval and support often depends on the way in which a person is approached. Demonstrate interest in the institution and the personnel as well as interest in the research project. The relationships formed with agency personnel should be equal, sharing ones because these people can often provide ideas and strategies for conducting the study that you may not have considered. The support of agency personnel during data collection can also make the difference between a successful and an unsuccessful study (Merrill, 2011).

Conducting nursing research can benefit the institution as well as the researcher. Clinicians have an opportunity to see nursing research in action, which can influence their thinking and clinical practice if the relationship with the researcher is positive. These clinicians may be having their first close contact with a researcher, and interpretation of the researcher's role and the aspects of the study may be necessary. In addition, clinicians tend to be more oriented in the present than researchers are, and they need to see the immediate impact that the study findings can have on nursing practice in their institution. Interactions with researchers might help clinicians see the importance of research in providing evidence-based practice and encourage them to become involved in study activities in the future (Offredy & Vickers, 2010). Conducting research and providing evidence-based practice are essential if a hospital is to achieve and maintain Magnet status. The award of Magnet status from the American Nurses Credentialing Center (ANCC, 2012) is prestigious to an institution and validates the excellence in evidence-based nursing care provided by the facility.

Verbal Presentation of a Proposal

Graduate students writing theses or dissertations are frequently required to present their proposals verbally to university committee members, which are called thesis or dissertation proposal defenses. Most clinical agencies require researchers to meet with the IRB to discuss their proposals. In a verbal presentation of a proposal, reviewers can evaluate the researcher as a person, the researcher's knowledge and understanding of the content of the proposal, and his or her ability to reason and provide logical explanations related to the study. These face-to-face meetings give the researcher the opportunity to encourage committee members to approve his or her study.

Appearance is important in a personal presentation because it can give an impression of competence or incompetence. These presentations are business-like, with logical and rational interactions, so one should dress in a business-like manner. The committee might perceive individuals who are casually dressed as not valuing the review process.

Nonverbal behaviors are important during the meeting as well; appearing calm, in control, and confident projects a positive image. Plan and rehearse your presentation to reduce anxiety. Obtain information on the personalities of committee members, their relationships with each other, the vested interests of each member, and their areas of expertise because this can increase your confidence and provide a sense of control. It is important to arrive at the meeting early to assess the environment for the meeting and select a seat carefully. Because you are the presenter, all members of the committee need to be able to see you. However, selecting a seat on one side of a table with all the committee members on the other side could make you feel uncomfortable and simulate an interrogation rather than a scholarly interaction. Sitting at the side of a table rather than at the head might be a strategic move to elicit support.

The verbal presentation of the proposal usually begins with a brief overview of the study. Your presentation needs to be carefully planned, timed, and rehearsed. Salient points should be highlighted, which you can accomplish with the use of audiovisuals. After the presentation, the reviewers will ask questions, so be prepared to defend or justify the methods and procedures used in your study. Sometimes it is beneficial to practice responding to questions related to the study with a friend; this rehearsal will help you to determine the best way to defend your ideas without appearing defensive. When the meeting ends, you need to thank the members of the committee for their time. If the committee did not make a decision regarding the study during the meeting, ask when the decision will be made.

Revising a Proposal

Reviewers sometimes suggest changes in a proposal that improve the study methodology; however, some of the changes requested may benefit the institution but not the study. Remain receptive to the suggestions, explore with the committee the impact of the changes on the proposed study, and try to resolve any conflicts. Usually reviewers make valuable suggestions that might improve the quality of a study or facilitate the data collection process. Revision of the proposal is often based on these suggestions before the study is implemented.

Sometimes a study requires revision while it is being conducted because of problems with data collection tools or subjects' participation. However, if clinical agency personnel or representatives of funding institutions have approved a proposal, the researcher needs to examine the situation seriously before making major changes in the study. Before revising a proposal, address three questions: (1) What needs to be changed? (2) Why is the change necessary? (3) How will the change affect implementation of the study and the study findings? Students need to seek advice from the faculty before revising their studies. Sometimes it is beneficial for seasoned researchers to discuss their proposed study changes with other researchers or agency personnel for suggestions and additional viewpoints.

If a revision is necessary, revise your proposal and discuss the change with members of the IRB in the agency where the study is being conducted. The IRB members might indicate that the investigators can proceed with the study or that the revised proposal might need additional review. If a study is funded, the study changes must be discussed with the representatives of the funding agency. The funding agency has the power to approve or disapprove the changes. However, realistic changes that are clearly described and backed with a rationale will probably be approved.

Example of a Quantitative Research Proposal

An example proposal of a quasi-experimental study is included to guide you in developing a research proposal for a thesis, dissertation, or research project in your clinical agency. The content of this proposal is brief and does not include the detail normally presented in a thesis or dissertation proposal. However, the example provides you ideas regarding the content areas that would be covered in developing a proposal for a quasi-experimental study. This proposal was developed by Dr. Kathy Daniel (2011), faculty at The University of Texas at Arlington College of Nursing.

"THE EFFECT OF NURSE PRACTITIONER DIRECTED TRANSITIONAL CARE ON MEDICATION ADHERENCE AND READMISSION OUTCOMES OF ELDERLY CONGESTIVE HEART FAILURE PATIENTS"

Kathryn Daniel, PhD, RN, ANP-BC, GNP-BC

Chapter 1

Introduction

Hospitalized patients with chronic health diagnoses such as congestive heart failure (CHF), pneumonia, and stroke are often readmitted to acute care hospitals within a 30 day interval for potentially preventable etiologies. These unnecessary readmissions carry a significant cost to Medicare and have been targeted for non-reimbursement. Hospitals and healthcare systems are eager to implement programs that can safely and effectively reduce unnecessary readmissions. Their interests are also tempered by the realization that either way, whether by administrative non-reimbursement policy or actual prevention of unnecessary readmissions, such admissions will no longer be the source of revenue, but rather a cost to the organization. Even though some readmissions will not be preventable, the burden will likely be on the hospital organization to justify payment (Stauffer et al., 2011).

Estimates of the prevalence of heart failure vary. However, older adults, defined as those 65 years of age and older, have documented higher rates of CHF, 6-10%. The trends over the past decade are an older age at first hospital admission for adults with CHF and an older age at death. This is probably secondary to technological advances and evidence-based guidelines for the care of individuals with heart failure. Despite these trends, the cost for management of CHF in the United States (U.S.) accounts for nearly 2% of the total cost of health care in the country (Mosterd & Hoes, 2007; Solomon et al., 2005).

CHF patients have one of the highest readmission rates to the hospital within 30 days of any diagnosis. Nationally 25% of patients discharged from the hospital after an acute care stay for heart failure, are readmitted to the hospital within 30 days (Jencks, Williams, & Coleman, 2009). Reports are as high as 50% of those readmitted from the community had no follow-up with their primary care provider prior to readmission. When patients are readmitted to the hospital within the 30 day period, hospitals may not be reimbursed for subsequent hospitalizations. In 2004, premature CHF readmissions cost the Medicare system an estimated 17.4 billion dollars (Jencks et al., 2009).

Prognosis remains poor once CHF is diagnosed. From the date of index hospitalization, the 30-day mortality rate is between 10 and 20%. Mortality at one year, and five years is estimated between 30 to 40% and 60 to 70% respectively. Most individuals will die with progressively worsening symptoms while others will succumb to fatal arrhythmias (Mosterd & Hoes, 2007; Solomon et al., 2005). With these high morbidity and mortality rates, individuals with CHF need additional healthcare in the community to manage their disease and decrease their rates of premature hospital readmission.

Chapter 2

Review of Relevant Literature

Care for this population is fragmented and uncoordinated. Systems of care today often are connected to sites of care, so when patients are discharged from acute care settings to home or to other settings and back again, there are many opportunities for gaps in care. Vulnerable complex frail patients with new problems or questions about management of existing problems have few knowledgeable resources to help them navigate the new landscape of their health. More and more hospital care is rendered by hospitalist providers who do not follow patients after discharge from the acute care setting, but refer patients back to their outpatient providers for care after discharge. Communication between inpatient and outpatient silos of care may be absent and is frequently delayed.

Medically complex patients who have multiple chronic diseases and few socioeconomic resources are the most vulnerable within this group and most likely to be readmitted. Silverstein, Qin, Mercer, Fong, and Haydar (2008) found that male African American patients over age 75 with multiple medical comorbidities, admitted for a medicine service admission (not surgical) and who had Medicare only as a payer source have the highest risk of readmission. CHF was the highest single predictor of readmission, but other co-morbidities such as cancer, COPD, or chronic renal failure were also contributing factors. The period of greatest vulnerability for readmission is within the first month after hospitalization and before patients have been seen in the office by their primary care provider (PCP) after hospital discharge.

Adverse drug events are a leading cause of readmission (Morrissey, McElnay, Scott, & McConnell, 2003). Medication reconciliation and adherence are important in the post discharge situation. Patients and families do the best they can to relay their drug information to inpatient providers, but they may forget things or assume the provider knows what they are taking. Because patients have had an acute change in their health, their medication regimens are often modified during their hospital stay. In addition, inpatient medication choices are influenced by hospital formularies. Even when diligent providers discharge patients with prescriptions for their new or modified medications, these choices may not be available on the patients' drug formulary plan. So when they present these prescriptions to their local pharmacy after discharge from the hospital, the new medication may not be available to them or is too costly for them to afford. Inpatient providers may also be unaware of all the medications the patient already has at home and duplicate drugs or drug classes that the patient has on hand (Corbett, Setter, Daratha, Neumiller, & Wood, 2010).

Nurse practitioners (NPs) are educated to manage chronic diseases and understand systems of care. Thus, NPs are in a unique position within the healthcare system to have significant positive effects on patient outcomes, thereby decreasing readmissions, improving patient physical and mental health outcomes, and decreasing the costs of care (Naylor et al., 2004). Trials using the transitional care model have been very favorable, both in controlled research settings and in real world settings. Patients followed by a transitional care NP have had substantial reduction in 30 day readmissions (Naylor et al., 2004; Neff, Madigan, & Narsavage, 2003; Stauffer et al., 2011; Zhao & Wong, 2009). Yet in spite of success in prevention of unnecessary readmissions, balancing the cost of such programs must be weighed against decreasing revenue streams before hospitals will support them (Stauffer et al., 2011).

"Transitional care programs utilizing advanced practice nurses have consistently reduced readmissions of vulnerable patients. Medication management is an important part of the transitional care NP role. What is not known is the effect of a transitional care NP program focused on medication management on readmission rates and medication adherence of elderly individuals with CHF. Thus, the purpose of this study is to examine the effects of an NP directed transitional care program on the hospital readmission rate and medication adherence of elderly CHF patients.

Chapter 3

Framework

The Transitional Care Model provides comprehensive in-hospital planning and home follow-up for chronically ill, high-risk older adults hospitalized for common medical and surgical conditions [see Figure 28-1]. This model was initially developed by Dorothy Brooten in the 1980s with a population of high risk pregnant women and low birth weight infants (Brooten et al., 1987; Brooten et al., 1994). Later Naylor and colleagues (2004) developed it further in high risk elderly populations focusing on patients with CHF (Brooten et al., 2002; Naylor et al., 2004). Multiple randomized controlled trials (RCTs) support its effectiveness in reducing unnecessary readmissions (Naylor et al., 2004; Neff et al., 2003; Ornstein, Smith, Foer, Lopez-Cantor, & Soriano, 2011; Williams, Akroyd, & Burke, 2010; Zhao & Wong, 2009).

The goals of care provided by the transitional care model focus on empowering the patient and family through coordination of care and medical management of disease and co-morbidities as needed with the ability to make changes immediately based on set protocols, health literacy, self-care management, and collaboration with other providers and families to prevent unnecessary hospital readmissions. Figure 28-1 illustrates the inter-relationship of concepts of this model (*Transitional care model—when you or a loved one requires care*). Patients who are more vulnerable, either socially or physically, or complex, would utilize more aspects of the transitional care model, whereas patients with more resources (social and physical) need less support during transitions of care. According to this model's conceptual relationships, when advanced practice nurses educate patients about self-management skills, they are more adherent to the overall plan of care. Thus, these chronically ill individuals have fewer unnecessary readmissions and greater medication adherence (Brooten, Youngblut, Kutcher, & Bobo, 2004).

The purpose of this study is to determine the effect of an NP directed transitional care program on medication adherence and hospital readmission rate of discharged elderly adults with CHF. The independent variable (IV) is the NP directed transitional care program and the dependent variables (DVs) are medication adherence and hospital readmission rates. This study will compare the medication adherence and readmission rate of medically complex elderly CHF patients who receive NP directed transitional care with medication

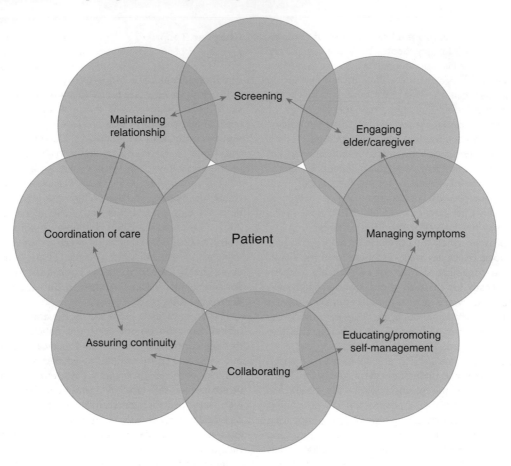

Figure 28-1 Transitional Care Model. (From Transitional Care Model. Retrieved from http://www.transitionalcare.info/)

management, and those who receive standard home health nursing services. The following table summarizes the conceptual and operational definitions for the independent (IV) and dependent variables (DV) in this study.

Variables	Conceptual Definitions	Operational Definitions
IV: nurse practitioner directed transitional care program	Time-limited services delivered by specially trained nurse practitioners to at risk populations designed to ensure continuity and avoid preventable poor outcomes as they move across sites of care and among multiple providers (Brooten et al., 1987; Coleman & Boult, 2003).	Enrollment and participation in a nurse practitioner directed transitional care program including medication management after an acute care hospital stay for CHF (see protocol in Appendix A).
DV: hospital readmission rate	Outcome which reflects inadequate training and preparation of patients/family to manage new/chronic health conditions or breakdown in communication between patient/family and provider (Coleman & Boult, 2003).	Any unplanned readmission to an acute care hospital reported to study investigators within 30 days of hospital discharge. Number of days from hospital discharge to readmission will be measured.

Variables	Conceptual Definitions	Operational Definitions
DV: medication adherence	Adherence to the medical plan of care which reflects shared values, goals, and decision making between patients, families, and providers (Rich, Gray, Beckham, Wittenberg, & Luther, 1996).	Score on the Morisky Medication Adherence Scale measured on intake and at 30 days from index hospitalization discharge (Morisky, Ang, Krousel-Wood, & Ward, 2008).

Hypotheses:

1. CHF patients receiving an NP directed transitional care program with medication management will have greater medication adherence than CHF patients who receive standard home health nursing services after discharge from an acute care hospitalization for CHF.

2. CHF patients receiving an NP directed transitional care program with medication management will have fewer readmissions within 30 days of discharge from index hospitalization and number of days to readmission will be greater than CHF patients who receive standard home health nursing services after discharge from an acute care hospitalization for CHF.

Chapter 4

Methods and Procedures

Design

The design for this study will be a quasi-experimental pretest posttest design comparing readmission outcomes of patients who received NP led transitional care with similar patients who did not receive transitional care at 30 days after index hospitalization discharge (Burns & Grove, 2009). Figure 28-2 provides a model of the study design identifying the implementation of the IV (see Appendix A) and the measurement of the DVs. The study will also compare pretest posttest medication adherence scores between the experimental and standard care groups at 30 days. The protocol for conducting the study is presented in Appendix B. The proposal will be submitted to the Institutional Review Boards (IRBs) of The University of Texas at Arlington (UTA) and a selected healthcare system for approval. After approvals are obtained, patients admitted to one of the participating hospitals in the system who have an admitting diagnosis of CHF will be screened for eligibility. Eligible patients will be approached by study personnel who will

explain the opportunity to participate in the study after discharge from the hospital. Patients who consent to participate will be randomized into either the experimental (intervention) group or the comparison (standard care) group. Demographic information, medical status, and pretest medication adherence will be collected from all patients who consent to be in the study before discharge from the hospital. Outcome measures (hospital readmission rate and posttest medication adherence) will be recorded at 30 days after discharge using the data collection form in Appendix C. The pretest and posttest design with a comparison group has uncontrolled threats to validity due to selection, maturation, instrumentation, and the possible interaction between selection and history (Burns & Grove, 2009; Shadish, Cook, & Campbell, 2002). Randomization of subjects to the treatment, controlled implementation of the study treatment, and quality measurement methods strengthen the study design.

Ethical Considerations

University and Clinical Agency IRB approvals will be obtained. All study personnel who have access to the data or to participants will complete human subject protection training before beginning to participate in study delivery. All participants will have the study explained to them in detail and have all their questions answered before signing consent forms to participate in the study. The consent form for this study is presented in Appendix D. The participants will receive a copy of their signed consent form.

Time frame: This entire study is projected to take one year. Subject recruitment will begin after IRB approval and informational in-services are presented to the nursing and social work staff in the participating hospitals. Data collection and analysis of readmission outcomes and mortality will begin with the recruitment of participants and will end 30 days after the last participant is recruited (see the Study Protocol in Appendix B).

Intervention and Procedures

Patients who consent to participate in the study will be visited by the transitional care NP who will be following them after discharge for an intake visit before they are discharged from the hospital. The same NP will visit the patient in their home within 24 hours of discharge from the hospital to monitor the patient's condition, review the goals of care and plans for care, provide patient education as needed, and manage any new issues as they emerge. The NP will also manage all aspects of the patients' medications. The NP will make at least weekly

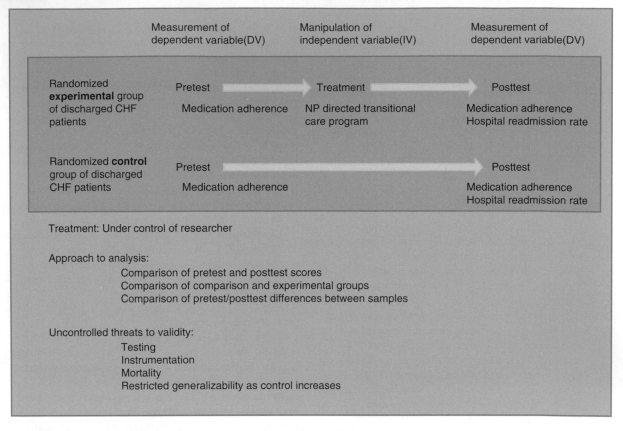

	Measurement of dependent variable(DV)	Manipulation of independent variable(IV)	Measurement of dependent variable(DV)
Randomized **experimental** group of discharged CHF patients	Pretest Medication adherence	Treatment NP directed transitional care program	Posttest Medication adherence Hospital readmission rate
Randomized **control** group of discharged CHF patients	Pretest Medication adherence		Posttest Medication adherence Hospital readmission rate

Treatment: Under control of researcher

Approach to analysis:

        Comparison of pretest and posttest scores
        Comparison of comparison and experimental groups
        Comparison of pretest/posttest differences between samples

Uncontrolled threats to validity:

        Testing
        Instrumentation
        Mortality
        Restricted generalizability as control increases

Figure 28-2 Classic experimental design.

home visits for the entire study period, carefully inquiring about any interval emergency department visits or hospital admissions. Patients who are readmitted to the hospital may be retained in the study for the full study period (30 days) even though they have already reached the end-point of readmission so that medication adherence can be measured. At the end of the 30 days, all patients in the study will be contacted and/or visited at home by study staff to capture outcome measures. The intervention and study protocols were developed to ensure intervention fidelity (see Appendices A and B) (Dumas, Lynch, Laughlin, Smith, & Prinz, 2001; Erlen & Sereika, 2006; Moncher & Prinz, 1991).

NPs who will be delivering transitional care to study patients will receive study related training that explicitly reviews the 2009 Focused Update incorporated into the American College of Cardiology Foundation/American Heart Associated (ACCF/AHA) 2005 Guidelines for the Diagnosis and Management of Heart Failure in Adults (Jessup et al., 2009) as well as training in study protocols

(weekly visits) and study related measures. Since only 40 patients will be in the intervention group, one NP is expected to be able to manage 40 patients over a one year period. To ensure study continuity and coverage for holidays and scheduled absences, a second NP employed in the agency will also be trained. Study recruitment and outcome measures will be accomplished via a study registered nurse who will be trained on study information and procedures (see Appendix B) and the patient consent process.

Subjects and Setting
Sample criteria: An electronic search of the inpatient database each night at midnight will reveal all patients in the participating hospitals with qualifying diagnosis of CHF who are age 75 or older. Other inclusion criteria are the patient must be at least 75 years old, have a minimum of three chronic disease states, male gender, and have Medicare, Medicaid, and or charity status as a payer source. These criteria are selected based on

information from Silverstein and colleagues (2008), which revealed these characteristics specifically increased risk of readmission in a similar population. Study personnel will eliminate any patients who have already been offered participation. Patients who are on ventilator support or vaso-active drips will be deferred until they are stable enough to begin discharge planning. Patients who are being discharged on hospice or who have already participated are not eligible to participate. Patients who are on dialysis will be excluded due to their unique needs and resources.

A power analysis was conducted to determine the desired sample size. Since this intervention is known to be effective in preventing readmission with a moderate effect size, the effect size of 0.45 was chosen with $\alpha = 0.05$ and power of 0.80, indicating a sample size of 70 was required for the study with 35 participants in both the intervention and comparison groups (Aberson, 2010). Ten percent will be added to each group to accommodate for attrition. This leaves a final required sample size of 40 for each group. When the required sample size of 80 has been secured, recruitment will stop. Due to the large population of elderly CHF patients in these hospitals, the sample is hoped to be obtained in 4-6 months.

Demographic variables of interest will be collected to describe the study sample and compare the sample with the population for representativeness. Race, gender, age, chronic illnesses, marital status, educational level, and healthcare insurance will be collected using the data collection form in Appendix C. Socioeconomic status and literacy are known predictors of health status and utilization (Silverstein et al., 2008). Describing relationships between these factors and patient outcomes may be important in explaining study outcomes. The study participants' addresses will be obtained also for contact by NPs following hospital discharge.

Instruments

The Morisky Medication Adherence Scale will be administered to all subjects who agree to participate in the study during intake and at 30 days post initial hospital discharge (Morisky et al., 2008). This tool has established sensitivity of 93% and specificity of 53% when utilized with a similar population of older adults taking anti-hypertensive medications. It consists of eight questions, seven asking for yes/no answers about the patient's self-reported adherence over the preceding two weeks and a final question with a five point Likert style question. High adherence is associated with a score greater than 6 on the scale (see Appendix E). Low/medium adherence was significantly associated with poor blood pressure control, while high adhering patients (80.3%) were more likely to have blood pressure controlled (Morisky et al., 2008). Test-retest procedures were utilized to produce consistency of performance measures from one group of subjects on two separate occasions which were then correlated with the norm reference of actual blood pressure measurements (Waltz, Strickland, & Lenz, 2010). Item-total correlations were >0.30 for each of the eight items in the scale with Cronbach's alpha of 0.83. Confirmatory factor analysis revealed a unidimensional scale with all items loading to a single factor.

The Morisky Medication Adherence Scale is appropriate for the proposed study because it was validated on a similar population of older outpatients who were mostly minority (76.5% black). The questions specifically ask about 'blood pressure medicines' which are the primary medications utilized in CHF management. This eight question instrument is derived from a previously validated four question version (Morisky, Green, & Levine, 1986).

Procedure

Eligible participants will have the study explained to them by the study recruiter who will obtain consent from those who are willing to participate. The recruiter, a registered nurse who is part of the study team, will also capture demographic and medical data, and administer the Morisky Medication Adherence Scale to all participants (see Appendix E). Patients assigned to the transitional care intervention will be visited by a transitional care NP before being discharged home (see Appendix B for Study Protocol).

On the day after discharge, the transitional care NP will visit the patient in their home to evaluate their home situation and resources as well as review the plan of care. For the next 30 days, the transitional care NP will visit the patient on at least a weekly basis. The visit will conform to the transitional care visit guideline in Appendix A so that intervention fidelity will be maintained. At all times a transitional care NP will be available by telephone. Outcome measures (hospital readmissions and medication adherence) will be measured at 30 days after discharge using the data collection form in Appendix C and the Morisky Medication Adherence Scale in Appendix E. The study recruiter will also do these measures to decrease potential for bias.

Plan for Data Management and Analysis

"Demographic data will be analyzed and NP actions and their frequency of use will be examined using descriptive statistics. All encounter content with patients will be recorded in the electronic health record, which all transitional care staff will have access to at all times. The documentation of weekly scheduled visits from the transitional care NP will follow a template so that all areas are consistently addressed with all study participants and intervention fidelity is assured (Erlen & Sereika, 2006). Differences in the interval level data produced by the Morisky Medication Adherence Scale will be examined with t-test at pre-test between the intervention and comparison groups to ensure the groups were similar at the start of the study. Differences will also be examined between pretest and posttest, and at posttest between the intervention and comparison groups. Differences in readmission rates will be examined at 30 days between the intervention and comparison groups. IBM Statistical Package for Social Sciences Statistics 19 will be used to analyze the data. Alpha will be set at 0.05 to conclude statistical difference. The statistical tests will be an independent t-test between two groups and a dependent t-test comparing pre- and posttests. Bonferroni correction for multiple t-tests will be done to reduce the risk of a type I error (Maxwell, & Delaney, 2004).

References

Aberson, C. L. (2010). *Applied power analysis for the behavioral sciences*. New York, NY: Routledge Taylor & Francis Group.

Brooten, D., Kumar, S., Brown, L. P., Butts, P., Finkler, S. A., Bakewell-Sachs, S., et al. (1987). A randomized clinical trial of early hospital discharge and home follow-up of very-low-birth-weight infants. In L. T. Rinke (Ed.), *Outcome measures in home care: Research* (pp. 95–106). New York, NY: National League for Nursing.

Brooten, D., Naylor, M. D., York, R., Brown, L. P., Munro, B. H., Hollingsworth, A. O., et al. (2002). Lessons learned from testing the quality cost model of advanced practice nursing (APN) transitional care. *Journal of Nursing Scholarship, 34*(4), 369–375.

Brooten, D., Roncoli, M., Finkler, S., Arnold, L., Cohen, A., & Mennuti, M. (1994). A randomized trial of early hospital discharge and home follow-up of women having cesarean birth. *Obstetrics and Gynecology, 84*(5), 832–838.

Brooten, D., Youngblut, J. M., Kutcher, J., & Bobo, C. (2004). Quality and the nursing workforce: APNs, patient outcomes and health care costs. *Nursing Outlook, 52*(1), 45–52.

Burns, N., & Grove, S. K. (2009). *The practice of nursing research: Appraisal, synthesis, and generation of evidence* (6th ed.). St. Louis, MO: Saunders.

Coleman, E. A., & Boult, C. (2003). Improving the quality of transitional care for persons with complex care needs. *Journal of the American Geriatrics Society, 51*(4), 556–557.

Corbett, C. F., Setter, S. M., Daratha, K. B., Neumiller, J. J., & Wood, L. D. (2010). Nurse identified hospital to home medication discrepancies: Implications for improving transitional care. *Geriatric Nursing, 31*(3), 188–196.

Dumas, J. E., Lynch, A. M., Laughlin, J. E., Smith, E. P., & Prinz, R. J. (2001). Promoting intervention fidelity. conceptual issues, methods, and preliminary results from the EARLY ALLIANCE prevention trial. *American Journal of Preventive Medicine, 20*(1), 38–47.

Erlen, J. A., & Sereika, S. M. (2006). Fidelity to a 12-week structured medication adherence intervention in patients with HIV. *Nursing Research, 55*(2), S17-S22.

Jencks, S. F., Williams, M. V., & Coleman, E. A. (2009). Rehospitalizations among patients in the Medicare fee-for-service program. *New England Journal of Medicine, 360*(14), 1418–1428. Retrieved from http://dx.doi.org/10.1056/NEJMsa0803563.

Jessup, M., Abraham, W. T., Casey, D. E., Feldman, A. M., Francis, G. S., Ganiats, T. G. et al. (2009). 2009 focused update: ACCF/AHA guidelines for the diagnosis and management of heart failure in adults: A report of the American College of Cardiology Foundation/American Heart Association task force on practice guidelines: Developed in collaboration with the international society for heart and lung transplantation. *Circulation, 119*(14), 1977–2016.

Maxwell, S. E., & Delaney, H. D. (2004). *Designing experiments and analyzing data: A model comparison perspective* (2nd ed.). Mahwah, NJ: Lawrence Erlbaum Associates.

Moncher, F. J., & Prinz, R. J. (1991). Treatment fidelity in outcome studies. *Clinical Psychology Review, 11*(3), 247–266.

Morisky, D. E., Ang, A., Krousel-Wood, M., & Ward, H. J. (2008). Predictive validity of a medication adherence measure in an outpatient setting. *Journal of Clinical Hypertension, 10*(5), 348–354.

Morisky, D. E., Green, L. W., & Levine, D. M. (1986). *Concurrent and predictive validity of a self-reported measure of medication adherence*. Medical Care, 24(1), 67–74.

Morrissey, E. F. R., McElnay, J. C., Scott, M., & McConnell, B. J. (2003). Influence of drugs, demographics and medical history on hospital readmission of elderly patients: A predictive model. *Clinical Drug Investigation, 23*(2), 119–128.

Mosterd, A., & Hoes, A. W. (2007). Clinical epidemiology of heart failure. *Heart, 93*(9), 1137–1146.

Naylor, M. D., Brooten, D. A., Campbell, R. L., Maislin, G., McCauley, K. M., & Schwartz, J. S. (2004). Transitional care of older adults hospitalized with heart failure: A randomized, controlled trial [corrected] [published erratum appears in J Am Geriatr Soc 2004 Jul;52(7):1228]. *Journal of the American Geriatrics Society, 52*(5), 675–684.

Neff, D. F., Madigan, E., & Narsavage, G. (2003). APN-directed transitional home care model: Achieving positive outcomes for patients with COPD. *Home Healthcare Nurse, 21*(8), 543–550.

Ornstein, K., Smith, K. L., Foer, D. H., Lopez-Cantor, M. T., & Soriano, T. (2011). To the hospital and back home again: A nurse practitioner-based transitional care program for hospitalized homebound people. *Journal of the American Geriatrics Society, 59*(3), 544–551.

Rich, M. W., Gray, D. B., Beckham, V., Wittenberg, C., & Luther, P. (1996). Effect of a multidisciplinary intervention on medication compliance in elderly patients with congestive heart failure. *The American Journal of Medicine, 101*(3), 270–276.

Shadish, W. R., Cook, T. D., & Campbell, D. T. (2002). *Experimental and quasi-experimental designs for generalized causal inference.* Boston, MA: Houghton, Mifflin and Company.

Silverstein, M. D., Qin, H., Mercer, S. Q., Fong, J., & Haydar, Z. (2008). Risk factors for 30-day hospital readmission in patients over 65 years of age. *Baylor University Medical Center Proceedings, 21*(4), 363–372.

Solomon, S. D., Zelenkofske, S., McMurray, J. J. V., Finn, P. V., Velazquez, E., Ertl, G., et al. (2005). Sudden death in patients with myocardial infarction and left ventricular dysfunction, heart failure, or both. *New England Journal of Medicine, 352*(25), 2581–2588.

Stauffer, B. D., Fullerton, C., Fleming, N., Ogola, G., Herrin, J., Stafford, P. M., et al. (2011). Effectiveness and cost of a transitional care program for heart failure: A prospective study with concurrent controls. *Archives of Internal Medicine, 14*(14), 1238–1243.

Transitional care model—when you or a loved one requires care. Retrieved 8/8/2011, 2011, from http://www.transitionalcare.info/Abou-1783.html.

Waltz, C. F., Strickland, O. L., & Lenz, E. R. (2010). *Measurement in nursing and health research* (4th ed.). New York, NY: Springer Publishing Company.

Williams, G., Akroyd, K., & Burke, L. (2010). Evaluation of the transitional care model in chronic heart failure. *British Journal of Nursing (BJN), 19*(22), 1402–1407.

Zhao, Y., & Wong, F. K. Y. (2009). Effects of a postdischarge transitional care programme for patients with coronary heart disease in China: A randomised controlled trial. *Journal of Clinical Nursing, 18*(17), 2444–2455.

APPENDIX A: Intervention Protocol for Transitional Care Nurse Practitioner (TCNP) Visit Protocol

1. Patients are visited for their initial visit within 24-48 hours of discharge from the hospital.
2. Only NPs who have been trained on CHF protocols and transitional care protocols and are included on the study IRB protocol may visit/interact with study patients.
3. On the first visit the TCNP will review the hospital discharge plan of care with the patient. A family caregiver is identified on the hospital visit or first home visit. This person should be present and included in all visits and supervise the patient's needs in the home. On every visit the following will be addressed by the TCNP.
   a. Review the plan of care given to the patient on discharge from the hospital.
   b. On all visits after the initial visit, inquire about any unplanned visits to any hospital.
   c. Ask about any new problems, issues, or symptoms that have arisen since hospital discharge.
   d. Conduct a brief review of systems, looking specifically for any changes since discharge from the hospital.
   e. Review log of daily weights/teach if needed to do daily weights before breakfast and after voiding each morning.
   f. Conduct a focused physical exam with careful attention to cardiovascular and respiratory exam on every visit; other systems as indicated by any patient complaints.

g. Review all recommended medications with the patient and caregiver by physically viewing the supply. On the first visit to the home, if the patient does not have a 'medminder,' the TCNP will provide one to the patient/family at no cost and set up the medications for the first week. The available quantities and dosages on hand will be monitored on all medications, not just CHF medications. (Anticipate unexpected problems to arise here with possible duplication of drug classes, unavailable meds, etc.)

h. Review indication, rationale, schedule, and possible side effects of every medication.

i. Provide patient/family education as needed on dietary choices, exercise, as needed medications, etc.

j. When possible and needed the TCNP will adjust medications as required to accommodate individual patient plan formulary.

k. Adjust/titrate meds as indicated to achieve goals of care.

l. Order lab tests necessary to monitor patient response to medication changes.

m. Order any other medications/tests/referrals indicated by patient exam and complaints.

n. Consult immediately with primary care provider (PCP)/cardiologist for any unexpected deterioration in patient condition.

o. Communicate any changes in medication regimen in writing for patient/caregiver.

p. Record visit in electronic health record (EHR); forward copy to patient's PCP for review. Visit template in EHR will include fields to capture the above items 'c-p.'

q. On final home visit at the end of 4th week, collect Morisky Medication Adherence Scale for study.

r. After final visit at the end of the 4th week, compose discharge summary and send to PCP.

Study RN Protocol for Comparison Group

a. The study RN will recruit, consent, and randomize patients. After consent is obtained, she will also obtain demographic information and the pre-test Morisky Medication Adherence Scale on all participants.

b. The study RN will contact all usual care patients by telephone at the end of each week during the study period of four weeks to inquire about any interval hospital admissions.

c. On the final telephone call to the usual care participant at the end of week four, the study RN will also collect the post-test Morisky Medication Adherence Scale.

d. The study RN will also contact all transitional care participants at the end of week four to collect post-test Morisky Medication Adherence Scale.

APPENDIX B: Study Protocol

Recruiting/Intake—Study Registered Nurse (RN)

1. Generate CHF list from hospital IT.
2. Compare list to track daily discharges of patients already recruited.
3. Screening for eligibility: Inclusion sample criteria
   a. Service area is 30 miles from the hospital: Use Internet directions program if you are unsure how far the patient lives from the facility.
   b. Must have heart failure diagnosis
   c. 75 and + in age
   d. African American
   e. Male gender
   f. Medicare, non-funded or Medicaid
   g. Patient resides in a private residence, assisted living facility, or residential care home.

4. Exclusion sample criteria:
   a. Patients discharged home on hospice.
   b. Patients on dialysis.
   c. Patients on ventilators or vaso-active drips should not be approached until they are in the discharge planning stage.
5. If patient meets all above inclusion and exclusion sample criteria: they will be approached for study participation
6. Introduce yourself to the patient and family.
7. Explain the opportunity to participate in the study after discharge from the hospital and what is involved. If patients agree to participate, give them consent to read or read to them if desired.
8. a Ask them to sign consent if they wish to participate.
9. If they decline to participate, thank them for giving you their time. Make a note in the chart that they

were offered study participation and have refused, that they are not in the study.

10. For those patients who consent to participate in the study:
    a. Collect patients' demographic, medical, and educational information.
    b. Administer the Morisky medication adherence scale.
    c. Confirm their address and phone number.
    d. Give them your card and phone number.
    e. Randomize participant to either the intervention or comparison group. Let them know which group they will be in and when to expect contact again.
    f. Intervention group will be visited by NP in hospital and within 24 hours of discharge from hospital in their residence, then weekly throughout study period. Place a transitional care 'sticker' on the chart to alert inpatient staff that we are following the patient who was assigned to the intervention group.
    g. Usual care group will receive weekly phone call from study RN to determine any hospital readmissions, plus one end of study data collection of Morisky medication adherence scale.

Intervention Group:

A transitional care nurse practitioner is preferably certified as an Adult/Gerontology Primary Care Nurse Practitioner, although other nurse practitioners with significant geriatric expertise will be considered. Other types of advanced practice nurses will not be included in this trial although they were included in much of the original studies by Brooten et al. (2004) and Naylor et al. (2004). All transitional care nurse practitioners will complete a standardized orientation and training program focusing on a review of national heart failure guidelines as well as principles of geriatric care, patient and caregiver goal setting, and educational and behavioral strategies focused on patient and caregiver needs.

Scripting for Transitional Care Program Introduction during Inpatient Visit

1. Introduction of yourself to the patient/family
2. You were randomly chosen to be in the Transitional Care group. The goal of the program is to help people (and their families) with heart problems learn how to best manage their illness at home.
   a. Heart failure has more hospital readmissions than any other problem in the United States
   b. 20% of all people discharged with this problem return to the hospital within 30 days
   c. Patients followed in transitional care programs have had lower readmission rates.
3. This is how the program works:
   a. I meet you here in the hospital (probably only one time).
   b. I come to see you very soon after you go home; I will be there within 24-48 hours.
   c. I will see you every week for one month at a minimum; we can add more visits to this if needed for you and your family.
4. I work with your doctors and keep them informed of how things are going at home. I am a nurse practitioner; I am not a home healthcare nurse, although I will work with your home healthcare nurse as needed. Go into more explanation re: differences etc. as needed, give them brochure on 'what is a nurse practitioner.'
   a. Why NPs can do more.
   b. NP can prescribe and make medication changes if necessary and keep your physician informed.
   c. NP can address new problems which might come up.
   d. Your Medicare benefit and supplemental insurance will pay for my visits; you will not be billed for any uncovered co-pays.
5. The goal of the program is not to slow you down, we do not want to interfere with your other activities, and we want you to continue to be able to do as much as you can do.
   a. We will review your medications at every visit.
   b. I will ask you each week about any readmissions to any hospital since the previous visit.
   c. Each week we will review your plan of care, how you are doing, and about any new problems or issues that arise.
   d. The study RN who recruited you to the study will contact you at the end of the study and ask you the same questions that she asked after you initially consented to participate (Morisky Medication Adherence Scale).
6. There will be different levels of coordination involved with each patient.
   a. I may discuss your case with your hospital nurse and hospitalist/cardiologist if needed.

b. I may discuss your case with your primary care
   provider if needed during intervention period;
   he/she will receive a copy of the record for every
   visit.

c. I will provide a comprehensive discharge summary
   to your PCP when discharged from transitional
   care service after one month.

**Study RN—Data Collection on Comparison
Group Patients**

1. Call all usual care patients at 7, 14, 21, and 30 days
   after discharge. On each occasion he/she will

update the database on any hospitalizations that
have occurred since the last interval data collection
(specifically how many days since discharge to
readmission). On the final call, the Morisky
Medication Adherence Scale will also be collected.

APPENDIX C: Data Collection Form

Data Collection Form								Days since Discharge without Readmission				
Study ID	Age	Gender	Race	Years of Education	Pretest Morisky Medication Adherence Score	Heart Failure Diagnosis (ICD-9 Code)	All Other Diagnoses (One Line/ ICD-9 Code)	End of Week 1	End of Week 2	End of Week 3	End of Week 4	Post-test Morisky Medication Adherence Score

APPENDIX D: Informed Consent

Principal Investigator Name:

Kathryn Daniel, PhD, RN, ANP-BC, GNP-BC

Title of Project:

The Effect of Nurse Practitioner Directed Transitional Care on Medication Adherence and Readmission Outcomes of Elderly Congestive Heart Failure Patients

Introduction

You are being asked to participate in a research study. Your participation is voluntary. Please ask questions if there is anything you do not understand.

Purpose

This study is designed to examine the effects of nurse practitioner directed transitional care program on medication adherence and hospital readmission of elderly patients who have congestive heart failure. Nationally, 20% or more of patients who are hospitalized with congestive heart failure are readmitted to the hospital within 30 days, often for reasons that are preventable. Transitional care using nurse practitioners has been shown to have positive benefits for many people like you after they are discharged from the hospital. This study is designed to determine whether medication adherence is also related to decreased hospital readmissions.

Duration

This study will last for 4 weeks after you are discharged from the hospital.

Procedures

After you have read this form and agreed to participate, the intake nurse will gather some basic information from you. Then you will be randomly assigned to receive usual care or transitional care after you are discharged from the hospital.

If you are assigned to the usual care group, you will be given the care your physician orders for you to receive upon discharge from the hospital. In addition, you will be telephoned at your home once per week for 4 weeks by a study nurse who will ask you whether or not you have been back to the hospital. On the 4th and final week's call, she will also ask you some additional questions about how you take your medications.

"If you are assigned to the transitional care nurse practitioner group, your assigned transitional care nurse practitioner will come to your room and introduce herself to you before you are discharged from the hospital. You will also receive the care ordered by your doctor after you are discharged from the hospital including at least weekly visits and telephone support from the transitional care nurse practitioner. The transitional care nurse practitioner will work with you and your doctors to bridge the gap between hospital discharge and your return to your usual primary healthcare provider as you learn to manage the changes in your health.

Possible Benefits

There are no direct benefits to you for participating in this research; however your participation will help us to determine whether or not nurse practitioner led transitional care can decrease unnecessary hospital readmissions and improve medication adherence. It is possible that having direct access to the transitional care nurse practitioner may provide you with more timely evaluation and management of problems that occur during the 4 weeks after discharge from the hospital.

Compensation

You will not receive any compensation for your participation in this study.

Possible Risks/Discomforts

You may return to your usual state of health and activities rapidly and thus not feel the need for a visit from the nurse practitioner or a phone call from the study nurse every week for 4 weeks.

Alternative Procedures/Treatments

There are no alternatives to participation, except not participating. You will always receive the care ordered by your physician.

Withdrawal from the Study

You may discontinue your participation in this study at any time without any penalty or loss of benefits.

Number of Participants

We expect 80 participants to enroll in this study.

Confidentiality

If in the unlikely event it becomes necessary for the Institutional Review Board to review your research records, then The University of Texas at Arlington will protect the confidentiality of those records to the extent permitted by law. Your research records will not be released without your consent unless required by law or a court order. The data resulting from your participation may be made available to other researchers in the future for research purposes not detailed within this consent form. In these cases, the data will contain no identifying information that could associate you with it, or with your participation in any study.

If the results of this research are published or presented at scientific meetings, your identity will not be disclosed.

Contact for Questions

Questions about this research or your rights as a research subject may be directed to Kathryn Daniel at (xxx)xxx-xxxx. You may contact the chairperson of the UT Arlington Institutional Review Board at (xxx)-xxx-xxxx in the event of a research-related injury to the subject.

Consent Signatures

As a representative of this study, I have explained the purpose, the procedures, the benefits, and the risks that are involved in this research study:

_____

_____

Signature and printed name of principal investigator or person obtaining consent/Date

By signing below, you confirm that you have read or had this document read to you.

You have been informed about this study's purpose, procedures, possible benefits and risks, and you have received a copy of this form. You have been given the opportunity to ask questions before you sign, and you have been told that you can ask other questions at any time.

You voluntarily agree to participate in this study. By signing this form, you are not waiving any of your legal rights. Refusal to participate will involve no penalty or loss of benefits to which you are otherwise entitled, and you may discontinue participation at any time without penalty or loss of benefits, to which you are otherwise entitled.

_____

_____
Signature of volunteer/Date

APPENDIX E: Morisky Medication Adherence Scale

Please complete the following scale by circling the best response that fits you.

1. Do you sometimes forget to take your medications? Yes/no
2. Over the past 2 weeks, were there any days when you did not take your medication? Yes/no
3. Have you ever cut back or stopped taking your medication without telling your doctor because you felt worse when you took it? Yes/no
4. When you travel or leave home, do you sometimes forget to bring along your medications? Yes/no
5. Did you take your medicine yesterday? Yes/no
6. When you feel like your blood pressure is under control, do you sometimes stop taking your medication? Yes/no
7. Taking medication everyday is a real inconvenience for some people. Do you ever feel hassled about

sticking to your blood pressure treatment plan? Yes/no
8. How often do you have difficulty remembering to take all your medications? (Select one)
Never
Occasionally, but less than half the time
About half the time
More than half the time
Almost all the time

Morisky, D. E., Ang, A., Krousel-Wood, M., & Ward, H. J. (2008). Predictive validity of a medication adherence measure in an outpatient setting. *Journal of Clinical Hypertension*, *10*(5), 348-354. doi:10.1111/j.1751-7176.2008.07572.x.

KEY POINTS

- This chapter focuses on writing a research proposal and seeking approval to conduct a study.

- A research proposal is a written plan that identifies the major elements of a study, such as the problem, purpose, and framework, and outlines the methods and procedures to conduct a study.

- Writing a quality proposal involves (1) developing the ideas logically, (2) determining the depth or detail of the proposal content, (3) identifying the critical points in the proposal, and (4) developing an esthetically appealing copy.

- A quantitative research proposal usually has four chapters or sections: (1) introduction, (2) review of relevant literature, (3) framework, and (4) methods and procedures.

- A qualitative research proposal generally includes the following chapters or sections: (1) introduction; (2) philosophical and conceptual foundation and general method; (3) method of inquiry; and (4) current knowledge, limitations, and plans to communicate the study.

- Most clinical agencies and funding institutions require a condensed proposal, which usually includes a problem, a purpose, previous research conducted in the area, a framework, variables, design, sample, ethical considerations, plan for data collection and analysis, and plan for dissemination of findings.

- Sometimes a researcher will send a preproposal or query letter to a funding institution rather than a proposal; and the parts of the preproposal are logically ordered as follows: (1) letter of transmittal, (2) proposal for research, (3) personnel, (4) facilities, and (5) budget.

- Seeking approval for the conduct or funding of a study is a process that involves submission of a proposal to a selected group for review and, in many situations, verbally defending that proposal.

- Research proposals are reviewed to (1) evaluate the quality of the study, (2) ensure that adequate measures are being taken to protect human subjects, and (3) evaluate the impact of conducting the study on the reviewing institution.

- Proposals sometimes require revision before or during the implementation of a study; if a change is necessary, the researcher needs to discuss the change with the members of the university and clinical agency IRBs and the funding institution.

- An example of a brief quantitative research proposal of a quasi-experimental study is provided.

REFERENCES

Aberson, C. L. (2010). *Applied power analysis for the behavioral sciences*. New York, NY: Routledge Taylor & Francis Group.

American Nurses Credentialing Center (ANCC). (2012). *Magnet program overview*. Retrieved from http://www.nursecredentialing.org/Magnet/ProgramOverview.aspx.

American Psychological Association (APA). (2010). *Publication manual of the American Psychological Association* (6th ed.). Washington, DC: Author.

Brown, S. J. (2009). *Evidence-based nursing: The research-practice connection*. Sudbury, MA: Jones & Bartlett Publishers.

Bulecheck, G., Butcher, H., & Dochterman, J. (Eds.). (2008). *Nursing interventions classification (NIC)* (5th ed.). St. Louis, MO: Elsevier.

Chlan, L. L., Guttormson, J. L., & Savik, K. (2011). Methods: Tailoring a treatment fidelity framework for an intensive care unit clinical trial. *Nursing Research, 60*(5), 348–353.

Craig, J. V., & Smyth, R. L. (2012). *The evidence-based practice manual for nurses* (3rd ed.). Edinburgh, UK: Churchill Livingstone.

Crotser, C. B., & Dickerson, S. S. (2010). Women receiving news of a family BRCA 1/2 mutation: Messages of fear and empowerment. *Journal of Nursing Scholarship, 42*(4), 367–378.

Daniel, K. (2011). *The effect of nurse practitioner directed transitional care on medication adherence and readmission outcomes of elderly congestive heart failure patients*. Unpublished proposal.

Fawcett, J., & Garity, J. (2009). *Evaluating research for evidence-based nursing practice*. Philadelphia, PA: F. A. Davis Company.

Glaser, B., & Strauss, A. L. (1965). Discovery of substantive theory: A basic strategy underlying qualitative research. *American Behavioral Scientist, 8*(1), 5–12.

Grove, S. K. (2007). *Statistics for health care research: A practical workbook*. St. Louis, MO: Saunders.

Heidegger, M. (1975). *Poetry, language, thought (A. Hofstadter Trans.)*. New York, NY: Harper & Row (original work published 1971).

Kerlinger, F. N., & Lee, H. B. (2000). *Foundations of behavioral research* (4th ed.). Fort Worth, TX: Harcourt College.

Malasanos, L. J. (1976). What is the preproposal? What are its component parts? Is it an effective instrument in assessing funding potential of research ideas? *Nursing Research, 25*(3), 223–224.

Marshall, C., & Rossman, G. B. (2011). *Designing qualitative research* (5th ed.). Los Angeles, CA: Sage.

Martin, C. J. H., & Fleming, V. (2010). A 15-step model for writing a research proposal. *British Journal of Midwifery, 18*(12), 791–798.

Melnyk, B. M., & Fineout-Overholt, E. (2011). *Evidence-based practice in nursing & healthcare: A guide to best practice* (2nd ed.). Philadelphia, PA: Lippincott Williams & Wilkins.

Merrill, K. C. (2011). Developing an effective quantitative research proposal. *The Art & Science of Infusion Nursing, 34*(3), 181–186.

Miles, M. B., & Huberman, A. M. (1994). *Qualitative data analysis: A source book of new methods* (2nd ed.). Beverly Hills, CA: Sage.

Munhall, P. L. (2012). *Nursing research: A qualitative perspective* (5th ed.). Sudbury, MA: Jones & Bartlett.

Munro, B. H. (2005). *Statistical methods for health care research* (5th ed.). Philadelphia, PA: Lippincott.

National Institute of Nursing Research (NINR). (2012). *Online: Developing nurse scientists*. Retrieved from http://www.ninr.nih.gov/Training/OnlineDevelopingNurseScientists/.

Offredy, M., & Vickers, P. (2010). *Developing a healthcare research proposal: An interactive student guide*. Oxford, United Kingdom: Wiley-Blackwell.

Patton, M. Q. (2002). *Qualitative research and evaluation methods* (3rd ed.). Thousand Oaks, CA: Sage.

Pinch, W. J. (1995). Synthesis: Implementing a complex process. *Nurse Educator, 20*(1), 34–40.

Ryan-Wenger, N. A. (2010). Evaluation of measurement precision, accuracy, and error in biophysical data for clinical research and practice. In C. F. Waltz, O. L. Strickland, & E. R. Lenz (Eds.), *Measurement in nursing and health research* (4th ed.) (pp. 371–383). New York, NY: Springer Publishing Company.

Sandelowski, M., Davis, D. H., & Harris, B. G. (1989). Artful design: Writing the proposal for research in the naturalist paradigm. *Research in Nursing & Health, 12*(2), 77–84.

Santacroce, S. J., Maccarelli, L. M., & Grey, M. (2004). Methods: Intervention fidelity. *Nursing Research, 53*(1), 63–66.

Shadish, W. R., Cook, T. D., & Campbell, D. T. (2002). *Experimental and quasi-experimental designs for generalized causal inference*. Chicago, IL: Rand McNally.

Smith, M. J., & Liehr, P. R. (2008). *Middle range theory for nursing* (2nd ed.). New York, NY: Springer Publishing Company.

Thompson, S. K. (2002). *Sampling* (2nd ed.). New York, NY: John Wiley & Sons.

Turabian, K. L., Booth, W. C., Colomb, G. G., & Williams, J. M. (2007). *A manual for writers of research papers, theses, dissertations, seventh edition: Chicago style for students and researchers*. Chicago, IL: University of Chicago Press.

University of Chicago Press Staff. (2010). *The Chicago manual of style* (16th ed.). Chicago, IL: University of Chicago Press.

Waltz, C. F., Strickland, O. L., & Lenz, E. R. (2010). *Measurement in nursing and health research* (4th ed.). New York, NY: Springer Publishing Company.

29
CHAPTER

Seeking Funding for Research

Seeking funding for research is important both for the researcher and for the profession. Well-designed studies can be expensive. As the rigor and complexity of the study design increase, the cost tends to increase. By obtaining funding, the researcher can conduct a complex, well-designed study. Funding indicates that others have reviewed the study and recognize its scientific and social merit. The scientific credibility of the profession is related to the quality of studies conducted by its researchers. Thus, scientific credibility and funding for research are interrelated.

The nursing profession has invested a great deal of energy in increasing the sources of funding and amount of money available for nursing research. Each award of funding enhances the status of the researcher and increases the possibilities of greater funding for later studies. In addition, funding provides practical advantages. For example, funding may reimburse part or all of the researcher's salary and release the researcher from other responsibilities, allowing the researcher to devote time to conducting the study. Funding provides you with the resources to hire research assistants and study coordinators to facilitate data collection and enhance your productivity. Thus, skills in seeking funding for research are as important as skills in the conduct of research.

Building a Program of Research

As a novice researcher, you may have had the dream of writing a grant proposal to the federal government or a national foundation for your first study and receiving a large grant that covers your salary, the salaries of research assistants and secretarial support, equipment, computers, and payments to subjects for their time and effort. In reality, this scenario seldom occurs for an inexperienced researcher. A new researcher is usually caught in the difficult position of needing experience to get funded and needing funding to get the release time to conduct research and gain the needed experience. One way of resolving this dilemma is to design initial studies that can realistically be done without release time and with little or no funding. This approach requires a commitment to put in extra hours of work, which is often unrewarded monetarily or socially. However, when well carried out and published, these types of studies provide the credibility one needs to begin the process toward major grant funding. Guidelines for proposals for federal funding usually include a section of the proposal in which researchers are expected to describe their own research studies that serves as evidence of their ability to conceptualize, implement, and complete a study, including disseminating the findings. Funders want assurance that if they fund a proposal, their money will not be wasted and that the findings of the study will be published.

An aspiring career researcher needs to initiate a program of research in a specific area of study and seek funding in this area. A program of research consists of the studies that a researcher conducts, starting with small, simple studies and moving to larger, complex studies over time. For example, if your research interest is to promote health in rural areas, you need to plan a series of studies that focus on promoting rural health. Early studies may be small with each single successive study building on the findings of the previous study. Finckeissen (2008) described this approach as having a meta-model of research with alternative solutions to a research problem. The findings of each study suggest new solutions or provide evidence that another solution is ineffective. Dr. Jean McSweeney, PhD, RN, FAHA, FAAN, Professor at the College of Nursing, University of Arkansas of Medical Sciences, is an example of a nurse researcher who has built a program of research. Dr. McSweeney's area of clinical practice was critical care, and she became very interested in cardiac patients. To complete her PhD, she

TABLE 29-1 Publications Reflecting a Program of Research: Exemplar of McSweeney's Program of Research in Cardiovascular Health of Women
Citations from Oldest to Most Recent
McSweeney, J. C. (1993). Explanatory models of a myocardial event: Linkages between perceived causes and modifiable health behaviors. *Rehabilitation Nursing Research, 2*(1), 39–49.
McSweeney, J. C. & Crane, P. B. (2001). An act of courage: Women's decision-making processes regarding outpatient cardiac rehabilitation attendance. *Rehabilitation Nursing, 26*(4), 132–140.
Crane, P. B. & McSweeney, J. C. (2003). Exploring older women's lifestyle changes after myocardial infarction. *Medsurg Nursing, 12*(3), 170–076.
McSweeney, J. C., Cody, M., O'Sullivan, P., Elberson, D., Moser, D. K., & Gavin, B. J. (2003). Women's early warning symptoms of acute myocardial infarction. *Circulation, 108*(21), 2619–2623.
McSweeney, J. C., O'Sullivan, P., Cody, M., Crane, P. B. (2004). Development of the McSweeney Acute and Prodromal Myocardial Infarction Symptom Survey. *Journal of Cardiovascular Nursing, 19*(1), 58–67.
McSweeney, J. C. & Coon, S. (2004). Women's inhibitors and facilitators associated with making behavioral changes after myocardial infarction. *Medsurg Nursing, 13*(1), 49–56.
McSweeney, J. C., Lefler, L. L., & Crowder, B. F. (2005). What's wrong with me? Women's coronary heart disease diagnostic experiences. *Progress in Cardiovascular Nursing, 20*(2), 48–57.
McSweeney, J. C., Lefler, L. L., Fischer, E. P., Naylor, A. J., & Evans, L. K. (2007). Women's prehospital delay associated with myocardial infarction: Does race really matter? *The Journal of Cardiovascular Nursing, 22*(4), 279–285.
McSweeney, J. C., Pettey, C. M., Fischer, E. P., & Spellman (2009). Going the distance. *Research in Gerontological Nursing, 2*(4), 256–264.
McSweeney, J. C., Cleves, J. A., Zhao, W., Lefler, L. L., & Yang, S. (2010). Cluster analysis of women's prodromal and acute myocardial infarction by race and other characteristics. *The Journal of Cardiovascular Nursing, 25*(4), 104–110.
McSweeney, J. C., O'Sullivan, P., Cleves, M. A., Lefler, L. L., Cody, M., et al. (2010). Racial differences in women's prodromal and acute symptoms of myocardial infarction. *American Journal of Critical Care, 19*(1), 63–73.
Beck, C., McSweeney, J. C., Richards, K. C., Roberson, P. K., Tsai, P.-F., & Souder, E. (2010). Challenges in tailored intervention research. *Nursing Outlook, 58*(2), 104–110.
McSweeney, J. C., Pettey, C. M., Souder, E., & Rhoads, S. (2011). Disparities in women's cardiovascular health. *Journal of Obstetric, Gynecologic, and Neonatal Nursing, 40*(3), 362–371.

conducted a qualitative study with patients and their significant others to explore behavior changes after a myocardial infarction. Her first post-dissertation study was a qualitative study of women's motivations to change their behavior after a myocardial infarction. She continued by conducting a series of quantitative studies that built on the findings of the previous studies. Table 29-1 lists publications by Dr. McSweeney that indicate the trajectory of her research program. Publication of the studies increased the credibility of the researcher and provided the foundation for future funding.

How do you decide on the focus of your program of research? The ideal focus of a program of research is the intersection of a potential contribution to science, your capacity, and the capital that you can assemble. Figure 29-1 shows the ideal study as overlapping circles of contribution, capacity, and capital.

Contribution

Contribution refers to the gap in knowledge that your research will address. This gap will be identified by

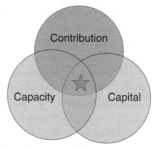

⭐ Indicates the overlap of contribution, capacity, and capital which constitutes an ideal focus for a program of research

Figure 29-1 Ideal focus for a program of research.

reviewing the literature and finding a significant gap in knowledge. Maybe this knowledge is needed to solve a health problem, or it is the evidence needed to advance nursing science. The research focus is broader than a single study. For example, a program of research could be developed related to adherence to antihypertensive medications. The first study might be a qualitative study of the reasons patients give for not taking their antihypertensive medications. Building on that knowledge, the next study might be a descriptive quantitative study of differences in attitudes of men and women toward antihypertensive medications. A later study might measure the outcomes of antihypertensive patients who received an adherence intervention compared with a group of patients who did not receive an intervention. Another consideration related to the research focus is your capacity to study the problem.

Capacity

Capacity consists of the internal resources you possess, such as your intellect, emotional maturity, knowledge, and skills. Because a program of research develops over several years, perseverance and commitment are necessary elements of your capacity. Which areas of nursing and health stimulate your curiosity and sustain your interest? Think about the topics or areas of nursing practice in which you are the most interested. Which patients or clinical areas stimulate your curiosity? Maybe you have a personal connection to a particular area, such as a nurse researcher who is studying autism because she is the mother of a son with autism. Maybe a family member died at a young age from undiagnosed cardiac disease, and now you are passionate to understand the decision-making process related to diagnosis of cardiac disease. Your research focus may evolve over time, but, ideally, your passion for a specific topic or group of patients would provide the basis for a long research career.

Knowledge related to your research area is another element of your capacity related to a specific research topic. This knowledge may come from educational programs, personal study, and clinical experience. If you are interested in genomic research, what is your knowledge of genes and interactions among them and the environment? Have you had a course in genetics or learned the laboratory skills to gather and analyze cellular level data? If you are interested in the effects of positioning on the hemodynamics of unstable, acute patients, have you ever worked in a critical care unit? One aspect of building a research career is to continue to expand your capacity in your focus area, but in the beginning, selecting an area in which you have baseline knowledge is helpful. Your capacity also includes grantsmanship, the knowledge and skill you have related to securing and managing grants.

Capital

People and funding are the capital you need to conduct research over time. The primary purpose of this chapter is to describe how to increase your monetary capital. When a potential contribution to science, your capacity, and available capital overlap, you have found an ideal focus for your research career. This chapter also provides suggestions on how to develop your grantsmanship and increase your capacity in the area in which you believe you can make a meaningful contribution.

Getting Started

Level of Commitment

Developing your capacity as a researcher in a specific area takes a great deal of time and effort. Writing proposals for funding is hard work. Before you begin, reflect on whether your motivation is external or internal. If your motivation is external, you are committed to seeking funding because of the potential to receive rewards from your employer, to earn the high regard of your peers, or to be eligible for a promotion. If your motivation is internal, you are convinced that more knowledge is needed to benefit your patients. Both external and internal motivations are valid reasons to be committed to a program of research; however, an internally motivated researcher will conduct studies with limited funding and continue to seek additional funding even in the absence of external rewards. As an element of capacity, your level of commitment will determine your ability to persevere and develop a program of research.

Support of Other People

Even the most internally motivated person may experience times of discouragement and need the support of peers. Peers who share common values, ways of thinking, and activities can be a reference group for a novice researcher. This occurs when you identify with the group, take on group values and behavior, and evaluate your own values and behavior in relation to those of the group. A new researcher moving into grantsmanship may need to switch from a reference group that views research and grant writing to be either over their heads or not worth their time to a group that values this activity. From this group, you may receive support and feedback necessary to develop grant-writing skills and enact a program of research. In addition, you will have the opportunity to provide similar support and feedback to your peers.

Networking is a process of developing channels of communication among people with common interests who may not work for the same employer or may be geographically scattered. Contacts may be made through social media, computer networks, mail, telephone, or arrangements to meet at a conference (Adegbola, 2011). Strong networks are based on reciprocal relationships. A professional network can provide opportunities for brainstorming, sharing ideas and problems, and discussing grant-writing opportunities. In some cases, networking may lead to the members of a professional network writing a grant that will be a multisite study with data collected in each member's home institution. When a proposal is being developed, the network, which may become a reference group, can provide feedback at various stages of development of the proposal. Adegbola (2011) provides practical tips on how to develop and maintain a professional network.

Through networking, nurses interested in a particular area of study can find peers, content experts, and mentors. A **content expert** may be a clinician or researcher who is known for his or her work in the area in which you are also interested. Through your review of the literature, you identify a researcher who has developed an instrument to measure a variable that you have decided must be included in your proposed study. For example, you want to measure a biological marker of stress and you have read several studies in which an experienced researcher measured the variable using a specific piece of equipment. You can also search the Virginia Henderson International Nursing Library to find funded and unfunded researchers on different topics (http://www.nursinglibrary.org/vhl/pages/aboutus.html). Contact the researcher through email to make a telephone appointment to discuss the strengths and weaknesses of this particular measurement, or you may arrange to meet at an upcoming conference.

A **mentor** is a person who is more experienced professionally and willing to work with a less experienced professional to achieve his or her goals. Because funded nursing researchers are few, the need for mentoring is greater than the number of available mentors (Maas, Conn, Buckwalter, Herr, & Tripp-Reimer, 2009). Finding a mentor may take time and require significant effort. Much of the information needed is transmitted verbally, requires actual participation in grant-writing activities, and is best learned in a mentor relationship. This type of relationship requires a willingness by both professionals to invest time and energy. A mentor relationship has characteristics of both a teacher-learner relationship and a close friendship. Each individual must have an affinity for the other, from which a close working relationship can be developed. The relationship usually continues for a long period.

Grantsmanship

Grantsmanship is not an innate skill; it must be learned. Learning grant-related skills requires a commitment of both time and energy. However, the rewards can be great. Strategies used to learn grantsmanship are described in the following sections and are listed in order of increasing time commitment, involvement, and level of expertise needed. These strategies are attending grantsmanship courses, working with experienced researchers, joining research organizations, and participating on research committees or review panels.

Attending Courses and Workshops

Some universities offer elective courses on grantsmanship. Continuing education programs or professional conferences sometimes offer topics related to grantsmanship. The content of these sessions may include the process of grant writing, techniques for obtaining grant funds, and sources of grant funds. In some cases, representatives of funding agencies are invited to explain funding procedures. This information is useful for developing skill in writing proposals. Not all courses or educational opportunities for learning grantsmanship require attendance at a conference because some seminars are offered as webinars or online courses.

Apprenticeship

Volunteering to assist with the activities of another researcher is an excellent way to learn research and grantsmanship. Graduate students can gain this experience by becoming graduate research assistants. Through an **apprenticeship**, you may gain experience in writing grants and reading proposals that have been funded. Examining proposals that have been rejected can be useful if the comments of the review committee are available. The criticisms of the review committee point out the weaknesses of the study and clarify the reasons why the proposal was rejected. Examining these comments on the proposal can increase your insight as a new grant writer and prepare you for similar experiences. However, some researchers are sensitive about these criticisms and may be reluctant to share them. If an experienced researcher is willing, it is enlightening to hear his or her perceptions and opinions about the criticisms. Ideally, by working closely with an experienced researcher, you have the opportunity to demonstrate your commitment, and the researcher invites you to become a permanent member of a research team.

TABLE 29-2 Regional Nursing Research Organizations		
Region	Website	Email
Eastern Nursing Research Society	http://www.enrs-go.org	info@enrs-go.org
Southern Nursing Research Society	http://www.snrs.org	info@snrs.org
Midwest Nursing Research Society	http://www.mnrs.org	info@mnrs.org
Western Institute of Nursing	http://www.winursing.org/	win@ohsu.edu

Regional Nursing Research Organizations

In the United States, nurse researchers in each region have formed regional research organizations. Table 29-2 lists these organizations and their websites. Each of these regional organizations has an annual conference and provides opportunities for nursing students to display a poster or present a small study of their early research projects. These conferences are an excellent opportunity to network and meet more experienced researchers (Adegbola, 2011).

Serving on Research Committees

Research committees and institutional review boards exist in many healthcare and professional organizations. Through membership on these committees, contacts with researchers can be made. Also, many research committees are involved in reviewing proposals for the funding of small grants or granting approval to collect data in an institution. Often reading proposals for approval for research involving human subjects or for funding can give the novice researcher insight into the importance of clarity and organization in the research proposal. Reviewing proposals and making decisions about funding help researchers become better able to critique and revise their own proposals before submitting them for review.

Identifying Funding Sources

Types of Grants

Two main types of grants are sought in nursing: project grants and research grants. Project grant proposals are written to obtain funding for the development of new educational programs in nursing, such as a program designed to teach nurses to provide a new type of nursing care or as a project to support nursing students seeking advanced degrees. These grants may fund a project manager to achieve the goals of the grant. Although these programs may involve evaluation, they seldom involve research. For example, the effectiveness of a new approach to patient care may be evaluated, but the findings can seldom be generalized beyond the unit or institution in which the patient

care was provided. The emphasis is on implementing the project, not on conducting research. Research grants provide funding to conduct a study. Although the two types of grant proposals have similarities, they have important differences in writing techniques, flow of ideas, and content. This chapter focuses on seeking funding for research. Within research grants, proposals vary depending on the source of funding. Proposals for federal funding are the most complex and include a significant amount of information about your institution's resources and capacity to support the study. The section on Government Funding provides additional information on types of federal proposals.

Nongovernment Funding

Private or Local Funding

The next step is to determine potential sources for small amounts of research money. In some cases, management in the employing institution can supply limited funding for research activities if a good case is presented for the usefulness of the study to the institution. In many universities, funds are available for intramural grants, which you can obtain competitively by submitting a brief proposal to a university committee. Local chapters of nursing organizations have money available for research activities. Sigma Theta Tau International, the honor society for nurses, provides small grants for nursing research that can be obtained through submission to local, regional, national, or international review committees. Another source are organizations, such as the local chapters of the American Cancer Society and the American Heart Association. Although grants from the national offices of these organizations require sophisticated research, local or state levels of the organization may have small amounts of funds available for studies in the organization's area of interest.

Private individuals who are locally active in philanthropy may be willing to provide financial assistance for a small study in an area appealing to them. You need to know who to approach and how and when to make the approach to increase the probability of successful funding. Sometimes this approach requires knowing someone who knows someone who might be willing to provide financial support. Acquiring funds from private individuals requires more assertiveness than other approaches to funding.

Requests for funding need not be limited to a single source. If you need a larger amount of money than one source can supply, seek funds from one source for a specific research need and from another source for another research need. Also, one source may be able to provide funds for a small segment of time; you can then approach another source to seek funding for another phase of the study. You can also combine these two strategies.

Seeking funding from local sources is less demanding in terms of formality and length of the proposal than is the case with other types of grants. Often, the process is informal and may require only a 2- or 3-page description of the study. Provide a clear, straightforward description of the study and how the findings will contribute to practice or future studies. The important thing is to know what funds are available and how to apply for them. Some of these funds go unused each year because nurses are unaware of the existence of the funds or think that they are unlikely to be successful in obtaining the money. This unused money leads granting agencies or potential donors to conclude that nurses do not need more money for research.

Small grants do more than just provide the funds necessary to conduct the research. They are the first step in your being recognized as a credible researcher and in being considered for more substantial grants for later studies. When you receive a grant, no matter how small, include this information on your curriculum vitae. Also, list your participation in funded studies, even if you were not the principal investigator (PI). These entries are evidence of first-level recognition as a researcher.

National Nursing Organizations

Many specialty nursing organizations provide support for studies relevant to their specialty, including nurse practitioner groups. These organizations often provide guidance to budding new researchers who need assistance in beginning the process of planning and seeking funding for research. To determine the resources provided by a particular nursing organization, search the organization's website or contact the organization by email, letter, or phone. Table 29-3 provides information on 10 large specialty nursing organizations that provide grant funding.

Two national nursing organizations that provide small grants not linked to a specialty are the American Nurses Foundation and Sigma Theta Tau International.

TABLE 29-3   National Specialty Nursing Organizations That Fund Research

Organization or Association	Website
Academy of Medical Surgical Nurses	http://www.amsn.org/
American Association of Critical Care Nurses	http://www.aacn.org/
Association of Women's Health, Obstetric, and Neonatal Nurses	http://www.awhonn.org./awhonn/
Emergency Nurses Association	http://www.ena.org/Pages/default.aspx
Hospice and Palliative Care Nurses	http://www.hpna.org/
National Association of Orthopaedic Nurses	http://www.orthonurse.org/
National Gerontological Nursing Association	http://www.ngna.org/
Oncology Nursing Society	http://www.ons.org/
Society of Pediatric Nurses	http://www.pedsnurses.org/index.html
Wound Ostomy and Continence Nurses Society	http://www.wocn.org/

These grants are usually for less than $7500 each year, are very competitive, and are awarded to new investigators with promising ideas. Receiving funding from these organizations is held in high regard. Information regarding these grants is available from the American Nurses Foundation (http://www.anfonline.org/) and Sigma Theta Tau International (http://www.nursingsociety.org/default.aspx).

Industry

Industry may be a good source of funding for nursing studies, particularly if one of their company's products is involved in the study. For example, if a particular type of equipment is being used during an experimental treatment, the company that developed the equipment may be willing to provide equipment for the study or may be willing to fund the study. If a comparison study examining outcomes of one type of dressing versus another is to be conducted, the company that produces one of the products might provide the product or fund the study. Industry-supported research is being scrutinized because of publicized incidents in which possible conflicts of interest resulted in harm to a subject or may have prevented the publication of unfavorable findings (Fry-Revere & Malmstrom, 2009). The ethics of seeking such funding should be carefully considered because there is sometimes a risk that the researcher might not be unbiased in interpreting study results.

Foundations

Many foundations in the United States provide funding for research, but the problem is to determine which foundations have interests in a particular field of study. The board of a foundation may evaluate the foundation's priorities each year, resulting in different priorities each year. You must learn the characteristics of the foundation, such as what it will fund. A foundation may fund only studies by female researchers, or it may be interested only in studies of low-income groups. A foundation may fund only studies being conducted in a specific geographical region. The average amount of money awarded for a single grant and the ranges of awards need to be determined for each foundation. If the average award of a particular foundation is $2500 and if $30,000 is needed, that foundation is not the most desirable source of funds. Identify foundations that match your research topic, geographical location, and funding needs. Review carefully the foundation's guidelines for submitting funding requests. Making a personal visit to the foundation or contacting the staff person responsible for funding is desirable in some cases. You can increase your likelihood of funding by revising your proposal to align with the foundation's priorities.

Several publications list foundations and their interests. If you are affiliated with a university that is a subscriber, a computerized information system, the Sponsored Programs Information Network, can assist you in locating the most appropriate funding sources to support your research interests. The database contains approximately 2000 programs that provide information on federal agencies, private foundations, and corporate foundations. Another useful resource is the *Foundation Directory*, which is available online to subscribers at http://fconline.fdncenter.org. Check with your hospital or university administrators to find out if you have access to this resource.

Government Funding

The largest source of grant monies is the federal government—so much so that the federal government influences what is studied and what is not. Information on funding agencies can be obtained from a document compiled by the federal government, *The Catalog of Federal Domestic Assistance,* which is available online at www.cfda.gov. The National Institutes of Health (NIH), particularly the National Institute for Nursing Research, and Agency for Healthcare Research and Quality are interested in receiving nursing proposals. Each agency has areas of focus and priorities for funding that change over time. It is important to know this information and prepare proposals within these areas to obtain funding. This information is available online at www.grants.gov, a searchable listing of all federal research funding opportunities.

Two approaches can be used to seek federal funding for research. As the researcher, you can identify a significant problem, develop a study to examine it, and submit a proposal for the study to the appropriate federal funding agency. This type of proposal is called an **investigator-initiated research proposal**. Alternatively, an agency within the federal government can identify a significant problem, develop a plan by which the problem can be studied, and publish a **request for proposals (RFP)** or a **request for applications (RFA)** from researchers (Figure 29-2).

Investigator-Initiated Proposals

If the study is initiated by the investigator, it is useful for the researcher to contact an official within the government agency early in the planning process to

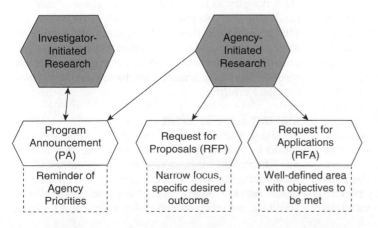

Figure 29-2 Types of federal research proposals.

inform the agency of the intent to submit a proposal. Each agency has established dates, usually three times a year, when proposals are reviewed. You will need to start preparing your proposal months ahead of this deadline, and some agencies are willing to provide assistance and feedback to the researcher during development of the proposal. This assistance may occur through email, telephone conversations, or feedback on a draft of the proposal. Proposals submitted in response to a **program announcement** (PA) are considered investigator-initiated proposals. An agency or group of agencies may release a PA to remind researchers of priority areas and generate interest in a priority area.

Requests for Proposals and Applications

The NIH issues an RFP when scientists advising the institutes have identified a specific need to move an area of knowledge forward. An RFA may be broader than an RFP but will still have a focus and a list of objectives that an institute or center within the NIH has identified. An RFA will have a single application deadline. The amount that has been budgeted for the successful applications is indicated, and the RFA is usually open for several funding cycles.

Submitting a Proposal for a Federal Grant

Ensuring a Unique Proposal

During your review of the literature, you may have read the findings of funded studies, but the literature does not include recently completed or ongoing funded studies. Early in the process of planning a study for which you intend to seek federal funding, it is wise to determine what studies on your topic of interest have been funded previously and what funded studies are currently in process. This information is available on the NIH Research Portfolio Online Reporting Tools—Expenditures and Results (RePORTER), which is maintained by the Office of Extramural Research at the NIH (http://projectreporter.nih.gov/reporter.cfm). The institutes and agencies that fund studies and projects and are included in the RePORTER are listed in Table 29-4. You can search the database by state, subject, type of grant, funding agency, or investigator.

Reviewing proposals that are funded by a particular agency can be helpful. Although the agency cannot provide these proposals, researchers can sometimes obtain them by contacting the PI of the study personally. In some cases, the researcher may travel to

TABLE 29-4 Funding Agencies Included in the National Institutes of Health Research Portfolio Online Reporting Tools—Expenditures and Results (RePORTER)

Agency for Health Care Research and Quality (AHRQ)
Centers for Disease Control and Prevention (CDC)
Food and Drug Administration (FDA)
Health Resources and Services Administration (HRSA)
National Institutes of Health (NIH)
Substance Abuse and Mental Health Services (SAMHSA)
Veterans Affairs

Washington to meet with an agency representative. This type of contact allows the researcher to modify the proposal to fit more closely within agency guidelines, increasing the probability of funding. In many cases, proposals will fit within the interests of more than one government agency at the time of submission. It is permissible and perhaps desirable to request that the proposal be assigned to two agencies for review and potential funding.

Verifying Institutional Support

Grant awards are most commonly made to institutions rather than to individuals. It is important to determine the willingness of the institution to receive the grant and support the study. This willingness needs to be documented in the proposal. Supporting the study involves appropriateness of the study topic; adequacy of facilities and services; availability of space needed for the study; contributions that the institution is willing to make to the study, such as staff time, equipment, or data processing; and provision for overseeing the rights of human subjects. The study's budget will include a category called **indirect costs** to pay the institution's expenses. For federal grants, indirect costs may by as high as 50% of the **direct costs,** the funds necessary to conduct the study. Direct costs are used to pay a portion of the researcher's salary, the salaries of data collectors or other research assistants, obtain equipment for the study, and provide a small payment to study participants to acknowledge their time and effort.

Making Time to Write

Set aside sufficient time to develop your proposal carefully, beginning with a thorough literature review. See Chapter 28 for how to write a proposal. Read the funding agency's guidelines carefully and completely before starting to write. Keep the guidelines nearby as you write so that you can easily refer back to them.

Strictly adhere to the page limitations and required font sizes. The sections of the proposal may be uploaded separately. Be sure that all the sections agree with each other on details such as names of instruments and inclusion criteria for subjects.

Writing your first proposal on a tight deadline is unwise. Proposals require refining the idea and method and rewriting the text several times. Plan on 6 to 12 months for proposal development from the point of early development of your research ideas. As soon as you have a complete draft, ask a peer or mentor to read the proposal to check for errors in logic. As people review your proposal informally, recognize their questions as indications that an idea was not clearly presented and may need to be rewritten. Before submission, it is highly recommended that you have a content expert or other researcher who is not at your institution critique the proposal (Office of Management and Budget, 2011).

Understanding the Review Process

The Center for Scientific Review has the administrative responsibility for ensuring a fair, equitable review of all proposals submitted to NIH or other Public Health Services agencies. After submission, the staff person assigned to your grant will determine which integrated review group will review your proposal for its technical and scientific merit. Within the integrated review group, each grant is assigned to a study section for scientific evaluation. The study section comprises active funded researchers. The study sections have no alignment with the funding agency. Thus, staff persons in the agencies have no influence on the committee's work of judging the scientific merit of the proposal. The proposal is given to two or more reviewers who are considered qualified to evaluate the proposal and have no conflicts of interest. The reviewers rate the proposal on the core criteria and overall impact and submit a written critique of the study. Each member may have 50 to 100 proposals to read in a 1- to 2-month period. A meeting of the full study section is then held. The persons who critiqued the proposal discuss each application, and other members comment or ask questions before recording their scores.

Proposals are assigned a numerical score used to develop a priority rating for funding. A study that is scored is not necessarily funded. The PI may review the progress of the proposal through the stages of review by accessing an online system, called the Electronic Research Administration (eRA) Commons. Funding begins with the proposal that has the highest rank order and continues until available funds are depleted. This process can take 6 months or longer.

Because of this process, researchers may not receive grant money for up to 1 year after submitting the proposal.

Often, researcher-initiated proposals are rejected (or scored but not funded) after the first submission. The critique of the scientific committee, called a summary statement, is available to the researcher via his or her eRA Commons account. Frequently, the agency staff encourages the researcher to rewrite the proposal with guidance from the comments and resubmit it to the same agency. The probability of funding is often greater the second time if the researcher has followed the suggestions.

Responding to Rejected Grant Proposals

The researcher's reaction to a rejected proposal is usually anger and then depression. The frustrated researcher may abandon the proposal, stuff it in a bottom drawer somewhere, and forget it. There seems to be no way to avoid the anger and depression after a rejection because of the significant emotion and time invested in writing it. However, after a few weeks it is advisable to examine the rejection letter again. The comments can be useful in rewriting the proposal for resubmission. The learning experience of rewriting the proposal and evaluating the comments will provide a background for seeking funding for another study.

A skilled grant writer will have approximately one proposal funded for every five submitted. The average is far less than this. Thus, the researcher needs to be committed to submitting proposals repeatedly to achieve grant funding.

Grant Management

Receiving notice that a grant proposal is funded is one of the highlights in a researcher's career and warrants a celebration. However, begin work on the study as soon as possible. You included a detailed plan of activities in the proposal that is ready to be implemented. To avoid problems, you need to consider managing the budget, hiring and training research personnel, maintaining the promised timetable, and coordinating activities of the study.

Managing the Budget

Although the supporting institution is ultimately responsible for dispensing and controlling grant monies, the PI is responsible for monitoring budget expenditures and making decisions about how the money is to be spent (Devine, 2009). If this grant is the first one received, a PI who has no previous administrative experience may need guidance in how to keep records and make reasonable budget decisions. If funding is through a federal agency, the PI will be required to provide interim reports as well as updates on the progress of the study.

Training Research Personnel

When a new grant is initiated, set aside time to interview, hire, and train grant personnel (Martin & Fleming, 2010). The personnel who will be involved in data collection need to learn the process, and then data collection needs to be refined to ensure that each data collector is consistent with the other data collectors. This process helps evaluate interrater reliability. The PI needs to set aside time to oversee the work of personnel hired for the grant.

Maintaining the Study Schedule

The timetable submitted with the proposal needs to be adhered to whenever possible, which requires careful planning. Otherwise, other work activities are likely to take precedence and delay the grant work. Unexpected events do happen. However, careful planning can minimize their impact. The PI needs to refer back to the timetable constantly to evaluate progress. If the project falls behind schedule, action needs to be taken to return to the original schedule or to readjust the timetable.

Coordinating Activities

During a large study with several investigators and other grant personnel, coordinating activities can be a problem. Arrange meetings of all grant workers at intervals to share ideas and solve problems. Keep records of the discussions at these meetings. These actions can lead to a more smoothly functioning team.

Submitting Reports

Federal grants require the submission of interim reports according to preset deadlines. The notice of a grant award sent as a PDF (Portable Document Format) document via email will include guidelines for the content of the reports, which will consist of a description of grant activities. Set aside time to prepare the report, which usually requires compiling figures and tables. In addition to the written reports, it is often useful to maintain contact with the appropriate staff at the federal agency.

Planning Your Next Grant

The researcher should not wait until funding from the first grant has ended to begin seeking funds for a second study because of the length of time required to

obtain funding. It may be wise to have several ongoing studies in various stages of implementation. For example, you could be planning a study, collecting data on a second study, analyzing data on a third study, and writing papers for publication on a fourth study. A full-time researcher could have completed one funded study, be in the last year of funding for a second study, be in the first year of funding for a third study, and be seeking funding for a fourth study. This scenario may sound unrealistic, but with planning, it is not. This strategy not only provides continuous funding for research activities but also facilitates a rhythm of research that prevents time pressures and makes use of lulls in activity in a particular study. To increase the ease of obtaining funding, the studies need to be within the same area of research, each building on previous studies.

KEY POINTS

- Building a program of research requires conducting a series of studies on a topic, with each study building on the findings of the previous one.
- The ideal topic around which to build a research program can be identified by considering topics for which the researcher has or can gain the expertise to conduct studies (capacity), funding is available (capital), and the potential exists for the researcher to make a difference (contribution).
- Writing a grant proposal for funding requires a commitment to working extra hours.
- To receive funding, researchers need to learn grantsmanship skills.
- The first studies are usually conducted with personal funding or small grants.
- Nongovernmental sources of funding include private donors, local organizations, nursing organizations, and foundations.
- Before submitting a proposal to seek federal funding, the researcher should successfully complete two or more small studies and disseminate the findings.
- The researcher identifies a significant problem, develops a study to examine it, and submits a proposal for the study to an appropriate federal funding agency.
- The PI is responsible for keeping within the budget, training research personnel, maintaining the schedule, and coordinating activities.
- Grants require the submission of interim and final reports of expenditures, activities, and achievements.

- A researcher should not wait until funding from one grant ends before seeking funds for the next grant.

REFERENCES

Adegbola, M. (2011). Soar like geese: Building developmental network relationships for scholarship. *Nursing Education Perspectives*, *32*(1), 51–53.

Devine, E. B. (2009). The art of obtaining grants. *American Journal of Health-System Pharmacy*, *66*(6), 580–587.

Finkeissen, E. (2008). Steps from erratic projects toward structured programs of research. *Foundations of Science*, *13*(2), 143–148.

Fry-Revere, S. & Malmstrom, D. B. (2009). More regulation of industry-supported biomedical research: Are we asking the right questions? *Journal of Law, Medicine, and Ethics*, *29*(3), 420–430.

Martin, C. J. H. & Fleming, V. (2010). A 15-step model for writing a research proposal. *British Journal of Midwifery*, *18*(12), 791–798.

Maas, M. L., Conn, V., Buckwalter, K. C., Herr, K., & Tripp-Reimer, T. (2009). Increasing nurse faculty research: The Iowa Gerontological Nurse Research and Regional Research Consortium Strategies. *Journal of Nursing Scholarship*, *41*(4), 411–419.

Office of Management and Budget (2011). Appendix VI: Developing and writing grant proposals (pp. 2700–2702). In: *Catalog of Federal Domestic Assistance*. Retrieved from https://www.cfda.gov/downloads/CFDA_2011.pdf.

Appendix A
Z Values Table

z Score	From Mean to z (%)	z Score	From Mean to z (%)
.00	.00	.46	17.72
.01	.40	.47	18.08
.02	.80	.48	18.44
.03	1.20	.49	18.79
.04	1.60	.50	19.15
.05	1.99	.51	19.50
.06	2.39	.52	19.85
.07	2.79	.53	20.19
.08	3.19	.54	20.54
.09	3.59	.55	20.88
.10	3.98	.56	21.23
.11	4.38	.57	21.57
.12	4.78	.58	21.90
.13	5.17	.59	22.24
.14	5.57	.60	22.57
.15	5.96	.61	22.91
.16	6.36	.62	23.24
.17	6.75	.63	23.57
.18	7.14	.64	23.89
.19	7.53	.65	24.22
.20	7.93	.66	24.54
.21	8.32	.67	24.86
.22	8.71	.68	25.17
.23	9.10	.69	25.49
.24	9.48	.70	25.80
.25	9.87	.71	26.11
.26	10.26	.72	26.42
.27	10.64	.73	26.73
.28	11.03	.74	27.04
.29	11.41	.75	27.34
.30	11.79	.76	27.64
.31	12.17	.77	27.94
.32	12.55	.78	28.23
.33	12.93	.79	28.52
.34	13.31	.80	28.81
.35	13.68	.81	29.10
.36	14.06	.82	29.39
.37	14.43	.83	29.67
.38	14.80	.84	29.95
.39	15.17	.85	30.23
.40	15.54	.86	30.51
.41	15.91	.87	30.78
.42	16.28	.88	31.06
.43	16.64	.89	31.33
.44	17.00	.90	31.59
.45	17.36	.91	31.86

z Score	From Mean to z (%)	z Score	From Mean to z (%)
.92	32.12	1.48	43.06
.93	32.38	1.49	43.19
.94	32.64	1.50	43.32
.95	32.89	1.51	43.45
.96	33.15	1.52	43.57
.97	33.40	1.53	43.70
.98	33.65	1.54	43.82
.99	33.89	1.55	43.94
1.00	34.13	1.56	44.06
1.01	34.38	1.57	44.18
1.02	34.61	1.58	44.29
1.03	34.85	1.59	44.41
1.04	35.08	1.60	44.52
1.05	35.31	1.61	44.63
1.06	35.54	1.62	44.74
1.07	35.77	1.63	44.84
1.08	35.99	1.64	44.95
1.09	36.21	1.65	45.05
1.10	36.43	1.66	45.15
1.11	36.65	1.67	45.25
1.12	36.86	1.68	45.35
1.13	37.08	1.69	45.45
1.14	37.29	1.70	45.54
1.15	37.49	1.71	45.64
1.16	37.70	1.72	45.73
1.17	37.90	1.73	45.82
1.18	38.10	1.74	45.91
1.19	38.30	1.75	45.99
1.20	38.49	1.76	46.08
1.21	38.69	1.77	46.16
1.22	38.88	1.78	46.25
1.23	39.07	1.79	46.33
1.24	39.25	1.80	46.41
1.25	39.44	1.81	46.49
1.26	39.62	1.82	46.56
1.27	39.80	1.83	46.64
1.28	39.97	1.84	46.71
1.29	40.15	1.85	46.78
1.30	40.32	1.86	46.86
1.31	40.49	1.87	46.93
1.32	40.66	1.88	46.99
1.33	40.82	1.89	47.06
1.34	40.99	1.90	47.13
1.35	41.15	1.91	47.19
1.36	41.31	1.92	47.26
1.37	41.47	1.93	47.32
1.38	41.62	1.94	47.38
1.39	41.77	1.95	47.44
1.40	41.92	1.96	47.50
1.41	42.07	1.97	47.56
1.42	42.22	1.98	47.61
1.43	42.36	1.99	47.67
1.44	42.51	2.00	47.72
1.45	42.65	2.01	47.78
1.46	42.79	2.02	47.83
1.47	42.92	2.03	47.88

Continued

z Score	From Mean to z (%)	z Score	From Mean to z (%)
2.04	47.93	2.53	49.43
2.05	47.98	2.54	49.45
2.06	48.03	2.55	49.46
2.07	48.08	2.56	49.48
2.08	48.12	2.57	49.49
2.09	48.17	2.58	49.51
2.10	48.21	2.59	49.52
2.11	48.26	2.60	49.53
2.12	48.30	2.61	49.55
2.13	48.34	2.62	49.56
2.14	48.38	2.63	49.57
2.15	48.42	2.64	49.59
2.16	48.46	2.65	49.60
2.17	48.50	2.66	49.61
2.18	48.54	2.67	49.62
2.19	48.57	2.68	49.63
2.20	48.61	2.69	49.64
2.21	48.64	2.70	49.65
2.22	48.68	2.71	49.66
2.23	48.71	2.72	49.67
2.24	48.75	2.73	49.68
2.25	48.78	2.74	49.69
2.26	48.81	2.75	49.702
2.27	48.84	2.76	49.711
2.28	48.87	2.77	49.720
2.29	48.90	2.78	49.728
2.30	48.93	2.79	49.736
2.31	48.96	2.80	49.744
2.32	48.98	2.81	49.752
2.33	49.01	2.82	49.760
2.34	49.04	2.83	49.767
2.35	49.06	2.84	49.774
2.36	49.09	2.85	49.781
2.37	49.11	2.86	49.788
2.38	49.13	2.87	49.795
2.39	49.16	2.88	49.801
2.40	49.18	2.89	49.807
2.41	49.20	2.90	49.813
2.42	49.22	2.91	49.819
2.43	49.25	2.92	49.825
2.44	49.27	2.93	49.831
2.45	49.29	2.94	49.836
2.46	49.31	2.95	49.841
2.47	49.32	2.96	49.846
2.48	49.34	2.97	49.851
2.49	49.36	2.98	49.856
2.50	49.38	2.99	49.861
2.51	49.40	3.00	49.865
2.52	49.41		

Appendix B
Critical Values for Student's *t* Distribution

Level of Significance (α), One-Tailed Test						
	.001	.005	.01	.025	.05	.10

Level of Significance (α), Two-Tailed Test						
df	.002	.01	.02	.05	.10	.20
2	22.327	9.925	6.965	4.303	2.920	1.886
3	10.215	5.841	4.541	3.182	2.353	1.638
4	7.173	4.604	3.747	2.776	2.132	1.533
5	5.893	4.032	3.365	2.571	2.015	1.476
6	5.208	3.707	3.143	2.447	1.943	1.440
7	4.785	3.499	2.998	2.365	1.895	1.415
8	4.501	3.355	2.896	2.306	1.860	1.397
9	4.297	3.250	2.821	2.262	1.833	1.383
10	4.144	3.169	2.764	2.228	1.812	1.372
11	4.025	3.106	2.718	2.201	1.796	1.363
12	3.930	3.055	2.681	2.179	1.782	1.356
13	3.852	3.012	2.650	2.160	1.771	1.350
14	3.787	2.977	2.624	2.145	1.761	1.345
15	3.733	2.947	2.602	2.131	1.753	1.341
16	3.686	2.921	2.583	2.120	1.746	1.337
17	3.646	2.898	2.567	2.110	1.740	1.333
18	3.610	2.878	2.552	2.101	1.734	1.330
19	3.579	2.861	2.539	2.093	1.729	1.328
20	3.552	2.845	2.528	2.086	1.725	1.325
21	3.527	2.831	2.518	2.080	1.721	1.323
22	3.505	2.819	2.508	2.074	1.717	1.321
23	3.485	2.807	2.500	2.069	1.714	1.319
24	3.467	2.797	2.492	2.064	1.711	1.318
25	3.450	2.787	2.485	2.060	1.708	1.316
26	3.435	2.779	2.479	2.056	1.706	1.315
27	3.421	2.771	2.473	2.052	1.703	1.314
28	3.408	2.763	2.467	2.048	1.701	1.313
29	3.396	2.756	2.462	2.045	1.699	1.311
30	3.385	2.750	2.457	2.042	1.697	1.310
31	3.375	2.744	2.453	2.040	1.696	1.309
32	3.365	2.738	2.449	2.037	1.694	1.309
33	3.356	2.733	2.445	2.035	1.692	1.308
34	3.348	2.728	2.441	2.032	1.691	1.307
35	3.340	2.724	2.438	2.030	1.690	1.306
36	3.333	2.719	2.434	2.028	1.688	1.306
37	3.326	2.715	2.431	2.026	1.687	1.305
38	3.319	2.712	2.429	2.024	1.686	1.304
39	3.313	2.708	2.426	2.023	1.685	1.304
40	3.307	2.704	2.423	2.021	1.684	1.303
45	3.281	2.690	2.412	2.014	1.679	1.301

Continued

Level of Significance (α), Two-Tailed Test—cont'd

df	.002	.01	.02	.05	.10	.20
50	3.261	2.678	2.403	2.009	1.676	1.299
55	3.245	2.668	2.396	2.004	1.673	1.297
60	3.232	2.660	2.390	2.000	1.671	1.296
65	3.220	2.654	2.385	1.997	1.669	1.295
70	3.211	2.648	2.381	1.994	1.667	1.294
75	3.202	2.643	2.377	1.992	1.665	1.293
80	3.195	2.639	2.374	1.990	1.664	1.292
85	3.189	2.635	2.371	1.988	1.663	1.292
90	3.183	2.632	2.368	1.987	1.662	1.291
95	3.178	2.629	2.366	1.985	1.661	1.291
100	3.174	2.626	2.364	1.984	1.660	1.290
200	3.131	2.601	2.345	1.972	1.653	1.286
300	3.118	2.592	2.339	1.968	1.650	1.284
∞	3.1	2.58	2.33	1.96	1.65	1.28

Appendix C

Critical Values of *r* for Pearson Product Moment Correlation Coefficient

Level of Significance (α), One-Tailed Test								
.05	.025	.01	.005		.05	.025	.01	.005

Level of Significance (α), Two-Tailed Test								
df = N − 2	.10	.05	.02	.01	*df = N − 2*	.10	.05	.02	.01
1	.9877	.9969	.9995	.9999	39	.2605	.3081	.3621	.3978
2	.9000	.9500	.9800	.9900	40	.2573	.3044	.3578	.3932
3	.8054	.8783	.9343	.9587	41	.2542	.3008	.3536	.3887
4	.7293	.8114	.8822	.9172	42	.2512	.2973	.3496	.3843
5	.6694	.7545	.8329	.8745	43	.2483	.2940	.3458	.3801
6	.6215	.7067	.7887	.8343	44	.2455	.2907	.3420	.3761
7	.5822	.6664	.7498	.7977	45	.2429	.2876	.3384	.3721
8	.5493	.6319	.7155	.7646	46	.2403	.2845	.3348	.3683
9	.5214	.6021	.6851	.7348	47	.2377	.2816	.3314	.3646
10	.4973	.5760	.6581	.7079	48	.2353	.2787	.3281	.3610
11	.4762	.5529	.6339	.6835	49	.2329	.2759	.3249	.3575
12	.4575	.5324	.6120	.6614	50	.2306	.2732	.3218	.3542
13	.4409	.5140	.5923	.6411	55	.2201	.2609	.3074	.3385
14	.4259	.4973	.5742	.6226	60	.2108	.2500	.2948	.3248
15	.4124	.4821	.5577	.6055	65	.2027	.2404	.2837	.3126
16	.4000	.4683	.5426	.5897	70	.1954	.2319	.2737	.3017
17	.3887	.4555	.5285	.5751	75	.1888	.2242	.2647	.2919
18	.3783	.4438	.5155	.5614	80	.1829	.2172	.2565	.2830
19	.3687	.4329	.5034	.5487	85	.1775	.2108	.2491	.2748
20	.3598	.4227	.4921	.5368	90	.1726	.2050	.2422	.2673
21	.3515	.4132	.4815	.5256	95	.1680	.1996	.2359	.2604
22	.3438	.4044	.4716	.5151	100	.1638	.1946	.2301	.2540
23	.3365	.3961	.4622	.5052	120	.1496	.1779	.2104	.2324
24	.3297	.3882	.4534	.4958	140	.1386	.1648	.1951	.2155
25	.3233	.3809	.4451	.4869	160	.1297	.1543	.1827	.2019
26	.3172	.3739	.4372	.4785	180	.1223	.1455	.1723	.1905
27	.3115	.3673	.4297	.4705	200	.1161	.1381	.1636	.1809
28	.3061	.3610	.4226	.4629	250	.1039	.1236	.1465	.1620
29	.3009	.3550	.4158	.4556	300	.0948	.1129	.1338	.1480
30	.2960	.3494	.4093	.4487	350	.0878	.1046	.1240	.1371
31	.2913	.3440	.4031	.4421	400	.0822	.0978	.1160	.1283
32	.2869	.3388	.3973	.4357	450	.0775	.0922	.1094	.1210
33	.2826	.3338	.3916	.4297	500	.0735	.0875	.1038	.1149
34	.2785	.3291	.3862	.4238	600	.0671	.0799	.0948	.1049
35	.2746	.3246	.3810	.4182	700	.0621	.0740	.0878	.0972
36	.2709	.3202	.3760	.4128	800	.0581	.0692	.0821	.0909
37	.2673	.3160	.3712	.4076	900	.0548	.0653	.0774	.0857
38	.2638	.3120	.3665	.4026	1000	.0520	.0619	.0735	.0813

Appendix D
Critical Values of F for $\alpha = 0.05$ and $\alpha = 0.01$

Please see page 681

Critical Values of F for α = 0.05

df Denominator	\multicolumn{19}{c}{Degrees of Freedom (df) Numerator}																		
	1	2	3	4	5	6	7	8	9	10	12	15	20	24	30	40	60	120	∞
1	161.4	199.5	215.7	224.6	230.2	234.0	236.8	238.9	240.5	241.9	243.9	245.9	248.0	249.1	250.1	251.1	252.2	253.3	254.3
2	18.51	19.00	19.16	19.25	19.30	19.33	19.35	19.37	19.38	19.40	19.41	19.43	19.45	19.45	19.46	19.47	19.48	19.49	19.50
3	10.13	9.55	9.28	9.12	9.01	8.94	8.89	8.85	8.81	8.79	8.74	8.70	8.66	8.64	8.62	8.59	8.57	8.55	8.53
4	7.71	6.94	6.59	6.39	6.26	6.16	6.09	6.04	6.00	5.96	5.91	5.86	5.80	5.77	5.75	5.72	5.69	5.66	5.63
5	6.61	5.79	5.41	5.19	5.05	4.95	4.88	4.82	4.77	4.74	4.68	4.62	4.56	4.53	4.50	4.46	4.43	4.40	4.36
6	5.99	5.14	4.76	4.53	4.39	4.28	4.21	4.15	4.10	4.06	4.00	3.94	3.87	3.84	3.81	3.77	3.74	3.70	3.67
7	5.59	4.74	4.35	4.12	3.97	3.87	3.79	3.73	3.68	3.64	3.57	3.51	3.44	3.41	3.38	3.34	3.30	3.27	3.23
8	5.32	4.46	4.07	3.84	3.69	3.58	3.50	3.44	3.39	3.35	3.28	3.22	3.15	3.12	3.08	3.04	3.01	2.97	2.93
9	5.12	4.26	3.86	3.63	3.48	3.37	3.29	3.23	3.18	3.14	3.07	3.01	2.94	2.90	2.86	2.83	2.79	2.75	2.71
10	4.96	4.10	3.71	3.48	3.33	3.22	3.14	3.07	3.02	2.98	2.91	2.85	2.77	2.74	2.70	2.66	2.62	2.58	2.54
11	4.84	3.98	3.59	3.36	3.20	3.09	3.01	2.95	2.90	2.85	2.79	2.72	2.65	2.61	2.57	2.53	2.49	2.45	2.40
12	4.75	3.89	3.49	3.26	3.11	3.00	2.91	2.85	2.80	2.75	2.69	2.62	2.54	2.51	2.47	2.43	2.38	2.34	2.30
13	4.67	3.81	3.41	3.18	3.03	2.92	2.83	2.77	2.71	2.67	2.60	2.53	2.46	2.42	2.38	2.34	2.30	2.25	2.21
14	4.60	3.74	3.34	3.11	2.96	2.85	2.76	2.70	2.65	2.60	2.53	2.46	2.39	2.35	2.31	2.27	2.22	2.18	2.13
15	4.54	3.68	3.29	3.06	2.90	2.79	2.71	2.64	2.59	2.54	2.48	2.40	2.33	2.29	2.25	2.20	2.16	2.11	2.07
16	4.49	3.63	3.24	3.01	2.85	2.74	2.66	2.59	2.54	2.49	2.42	2.35	2.28	2.24	2.19	2.15	2.11	2.06	2.01
17	4.45	3.59	3.20	2.96	2.81	2.70	2.61	2.55	2.49	2.45	2.38	2.31	2.23	2.19	2.15	2.10	2.06	2.01	1.96
18	4.41	3.55	3.16	2.93	2.77	2.66	2.58	2.51	2.46	2.41	2.34	2.27	2.19	2.15	2.11	2.06	2.02	1.97	1.92
19	4.38	3.52	3.13	2.90	2.74	2.63	2.54	2.48	2.42	2.38	2.31	2.23	2.16	2.11	2.07	2.03	1.98	1.93	1.88
20	4.35	3.49	3.10	2.87	2.71	2.60	2.51	2.45	2.39	2.35	2.28	2.20	2.12	2.08	2.04	1.99	1.95	1.90	1.84
21	4.32	3.47	3.07	2.84	2.68	2.57	2.49	2.42	2.37	2.32	2.25	2.18	2.10	2.05	2.01	1.96	1.92	1.87	1.81
22	4.30	3.44	3.05	2.82	2.66	2.55	2.46	2.40	2.34	2.30	2.23	2.15	2.07	2.03	1.98	1.94	1.89	1.84	1.78
23	4.28	3.42	3.03	2.80	2.64	2.53	2.44	2.37	2.32	2.27	2.20	2.13	2.05	2.01	1.96	1.91	1.86	1.81	1.76
24	4.26	3.40	3.01	2.78	2.62	2.51	2.42	2.36	2.30	2.25	2.18	2.11	2.03	1.98	1.94	1.89	1.84	1.79	1.73
25	4.24	3.39	2.99	2.76	2.60	2.49	2.40	2.34	2.28	2.24	2.16	2.09	2.01	1.96	1.92	1.87	1.82	1.77	1.71
26	4.23	3.37	2.98	2.74	2.59	2.47	2.39	2.32	2.27	2.22	2.15	2.07	1.99	1.95	1.90	1.85	1.80	1.75	1.69
27	4.21	3.35	2.96	2.73	2.57	2.46	2.37	2.31	2.25	2.20	2.13	2.06	1.97	1.93	1.88	1.84	1.79	1.73	1.67
28	4.20	3.34	2.95	2.71	2.56	2.45	2.36	2.29	2.24	2.19	2.12	2.04	1.96	1.91	1.87	1.82	1.77	1.71	1.65
29	4.18	3.33	2.93	2.70	2.55	2.43	2.35	2.28	2.22	2.18	2.10	2.03	1.94	1.90	1.85	1.81	1.75	1.70	1.64
30	4.17	3.32	2.92	2.69	2.53	2.42	2.33	2.27	2.21	2.16	2.09	2.01	1.93	1.89	1.84	1.79	1.74	1.68	1.62
40	4.08	3.23	2.84	2.61	2.45	2.34	2.25	2.18	2.12	2.08	2.00	1.92	1.84	1.79	1.74	1.69	1.64	1.58	1.51
60	4.00	3.15	2.76	2.53	2.37	2.25	2.17	2.10	2.04	1.99	1.92	1.84	1.75	1.70	1.65	1.59	1.53	1.47	1.39
120	3.92	3.07	2.68	2.45	2.29	2.17	2.09	2.02	1.96	1.91	1.83	1.75	1.66	1.61	1.55	1.50	1.43	1.35	1.25
∞	3.84	3.00	2.60	2.37	2.21	2.10	2.01	1.94	1.88	1.83	1.75	1.67	1.57	1.52	1.46	1.39	1.32	1.22	1.00

From Merrington, M., and Thompson, C.M. (1943). Tables of percentage points of the inverted beta (F) distribution. *Biometrika, 33*(1), 73–78.

Critical Values of F for α = 0.01

df Denominator	df Numerator																		
	1	2	3	4	5	6	7	8	9	10	12	15	20	24	30	40	60	120	∞
1	4052	4999.5	5403	5625	5764	5859	5928	5982	6022	6056	6106	6157	6209	6235	6261	6287	6313	6339	6366
2	98.50	99.00	99.17	99.25	99.30	99.33	99.36	99.37	99.39	99.40	99.42	99.43	99.45	99.46	99.47	99.47	99.48	99.49	99.50
3	34.12	30.82	29.46	28.71	28.24	27.91	27.67	27.49	27.35	27.23	27.05	26.87	26.69	26.60	26.50	26.41	26.32	26.22	26.13
4	21.20	18.00	16.69	15.98	15.52	15.21	14.98	14.80	14.66	14.55	14.37	14.20	14.02	13.93	13.84	13.75	13.65	13.56	13.46
5	16.26	13.27	12.06	11.39	10.97	10.67	10.46	10.29	10.16	10.05	9.89	9.72	9.55	9.47	9.38	9.29	9.20	9.11	9.02
6	13.75	10.92	9.78	9.15	8.75	8.47	8.26	8.10	7.98	7.87	7.72	7.56	7.40	7.31	7.23	7.14	7.06	6.97	6.88
7	12.25	9.55	8.45	7.85	7.46	7.19	6.99	6.84	6.72	6.62	6.47	6.31	6.16	6.07	5.99	5.91	5.82	5.74	5.65
8	11.26	8.65	7.59	7.01	6.63	6.37	6.18	6.03	5.91	5.81	5.67	5.52	5.36	5.28	5.20	5.12	5.03	4.95	4.86
9	10.56	8.02	6.99	6.42	6.06	5.80	5.61	5.47	5.35	5.26	5.11	4.96	4.81	4.73	4.65	4.57	4.48	4.40	4.31
10	10.04	7.56	6.55	5.99	5.64	5.39	5.20	5.06	4.94	4.85	4.71	4.56	4.41	4.33	4.25	4.17	4.08	4.00	3.91
11	9.65	7.21	6.22	5.67	5.32	5.07	4.89	4.74	4.63	4.54	4.40	4.25	4.10	4.02	3.94	3.86	3.78	3.69	3.60
12	9.33	6.93	5.95	5.41	5.06	4.82	4.64	4.50	4.39	4.30	4.16	4.01	3.86	3.78	3.70	3.62	3.54	3.45	3.36
13	9.07	6.70	5.74	5.21	4.86	4.62	4.44	4.30	4.19	4.10	3.96	3.82	3.66	3.59	3.51	3.43	3.34	3.25	3.17
14	8.86	6.51	5.56	5.04	4.69	4.46	4.28	4.14	4.03	3.94	3.80	3.66	3.51	3.43	3.35	3.27	3.18	3.09	3.00
15	8.68	6.36	5.42	4.89	4.56	4.32	4.14	4.00	3.89	3.80	3.67	3.52	3.37	3.29	3.21	3.13	3.05	2.96	2.87
16	8.53	6.23	5.29	4.77	4.44	4.20	4.03	3.89	3.78	3.69	3.55	3.41	3.26	3.18	3.10	3.02	2.93	2.84	2.75
17	8.40	6.11	5.18	4.67	4.34	4.10	3.93	3.79	3.68	3.59	3.46	3.31	3.16	3.08	3.00	2.92	2.83	2.75	2.65
18	8.29	6.01	5.09	4.58	4.25	4.01	3.84	3.71	3.60	3.51	3.37	3.23	3.08	3.00	2.92	2.84	2.75	2.66	2.57
19	8.18	5.93	5.01	4.50	4.17	3.94	3.77	3.63	3.52	3.43	3.30	3.15	3.00	2.92	2.84	2.76	2.67	2.58	2.49
20	8.10	5.85	4.94	4.43	4.10	3.87	3.70	3.56	3.46	3.37	3.23	3.09	2.94	2.86	2.78	2.69	2.61	2.52	2.42
21	8.02	5.78	4.87	4.37	4.04	3.81	3.64	3.51	3.40	3.31	3.17	3.03	2.88	2.80	2.72	2.64	2.55	2.46	2.36
22	7.95	5.72	4.82	4.31	3.99	3.76	3.59	3.45	3.35	3.26	3.12	2.98	2.83	2.75	2.67	2.58	2.50	2.40	2.31
23	7.88	5.66	4.76	4.26	3.94	3.71	3.54	3.41	3.30	3.21	3.07	2.93	2.78	2.70	2.62	2.54	2.45	2.35	2.26
24	7.82	5.61	4.72	4.22	3.90	3.67	3.50	3.36	3.26	3.17	3.03	2.89	2.74	2.66	2.58	2.49	2.40	2.31	2.21
25	7.77	5.57	4.68	4.18	3.85	3.63	3.46	3.32	3.22	3.13	2.99	2.85	2.70	2.62	2.54	2.45	2.36	2.27	2.17
26	7.72	5.53	4.64	4.14	3.82	3.59	3.42	3.29	3.18	3.09	2.96	2.81	2.66	2.58	2.50	2.42	2.33	2.23	2.13
27	7.68	5.49	4.60	4.11	3.78	3.56	3.39	3.26	3.15	3.06	2.93	2.78	2.63	2.55	2.47	2.38	2.29	2.20	2.10
28	7.64	5.45	4.57	4.07	3.75	3.53	3.36	3.23	3.12	3.03	2.90	2.75	2.60	2.52	2.44	2.35	2.26	2.17	2.06
29	7.60	5.42	4.54	4.04	3.73	3.50	3.33	3.20	3.09	3.00	2.87	2.73	2.57	2.49	2.41	2.33	2.23	2.14	2.03
30	7.56	5.39	4.51	4.02	3.70	3.47	3.30	3.17	3.07	2.98	2.84	2.70	2.55	2.47	2.39	2.30	2.21	2.11	2.01
40	7.31	5.18	4.31	3.83	3.51	3.29	3.12	2.99	2.89	2.80	2.66	2.52	2.37	2.29	2.20	2.11	2.02	1.92	1.80
60	7.08	4.98	4.13	3.65	3.34	3.12	2.95	2.82	2.72	2.63	2.50	2.35	2.20	2.12	2.03	1.94	1.84	1.73	1.60
120	6.85	4.79	3.95	3.48	3.17	2.96	2.79	2.66	2.56	2.47	2.34	2.19	2.03	1.95	1.86	1.76	1.66	1.53	1.38
∞	6.63	4.61	3.78	3.32	3.02	2.80	2.64	2.51	2.41	2.32	2.18	2.04	1.88	1.79	1.70	1.59	1.47	1.32	1.00

From Merrington, M., and Thompson, C.M. (1943). Tables of percentage points of the inverted beta (F) distribution. *Biometrika*, 33(1), 73–78.

Appendix E
Critical Values of the χ^2 Distribution

df	Alpha (α) Level				
	.10	.05	.025	.01	.001
1	2.7055	3.8415	5.0239	6.6349	10.8276
2	4.6052	5.9915	7.3778	9.2103	13.8155
3	6.2514	7.8147	9.3484	11.3449	16.2662
4	7.7794	9.4877	11.1433	13.2767	18.4668
5	9.2364	11.0705	12.8325	15.0863	20.5150
6	10.6446	12.5916	14.4494	16.8119	22.4577
7	12.0170	14.0671	16.0128	18.4753	24.3219
8	13.3616	15.5073	17.5345	20.0902	26.1245
9	14.6837	16.9190	19.0228	21.6660	27.8772
10	15.9872	18.3070	20.4832	23.2093	29.5883
11	17.2750	19.6751	21.9200	24.7250	31.2641
12	18.5493	21.0261	23.3367	26.2170	32.9095
13	19.8119	22.3620	24.7356	27.6882	34.5282
14	21.0641	23.6848	26.1189	29.1412	36.1233
15	22.3071	24.9958	27.4884	30.5779	37.6973
16	23.5418	26.2962	28.8454	31.9999	39.2524
17	24.7690	27.5871	30.1910	33.4087	40.7902
18	25.9894	28.8693	31.5264	34.8053	42.3124
19	27.2036	30.1435	32.8523	36.1909	43.8202
20	28.4120	31.4104	34.1696	37.5662	45.3147
21	29.6151	32.6706	35.4789	38.9322	46.7970
22	30.8133	33.9244	36.7807	40.2894	48.2679
23	32.0069	35.1725	38.0756	41.6384	49.7282
24	33.1962	36.4150	39.3641	42.9798	51.1786
25	34.3816	37.6525	40.6465	44.3141	52.6197
26	35.5632	38.8851	41.9232	45.6417	54.0520
27	36.7412	40.1133	43.1945	46.9629	55.4760
28	37.9159	41.3371	44.4608	48.2782	56.8923
29	39.0875	42.5570	45.7223	49.5879	58.3012
30	40.2560	43.7730	46.9792	50.8922	59.7031
31	41.4217	44.9853	48.2319	52.1914	61.0983
32	42.5847	46.1943	49.4804	53.4858	62.4872
33	43.7452	47.3999	50.7251	54.7755	63.8701
34	44.9032	48.6024	51.9660	56.0609	65.2472
35	46.0588	49.8018	53.2033	57.3421	66.6188
36	47.2122	50.9985	54.4373	58.6192	67.9852
37	48.3634	52.1923	55.6680	59.8925	69.3465
38	49.5126	53.3835	56.8955	61.1621	70.7029
39	50.6598	54.5722	58.1201	62.4281	72.0547
40	51.8051	55.7585	59.3417	63.6907	73.4020
41	52.9485	56.9424	60.5606	64.9501	74.7449
42	54.0902	58.1240	61.7768	66.2062	76.0838
43	55.2302	59.3035	62.9904	67.4593	77.4186
44	56.3685	60.4809	64.2015	68.7095	78.7495
45	57.5053	61.6562	65.4102	69.9568	80.0767

From Corty, E. (2007). *A Practical Text for the Health, Behavioral and Social Sciences.* St. Louis, MO: Mosby.

Appendix F
Statistical Power Tables (Δ = Effect Size)

5% Level, One-Tailed Test

Δ	Power 99	95	90	80	70	60	50	40	30	20	10
0.01	157695	108215	85634	61823	47055	36031	27055	19363	12555	6453	1321
0.02	39417	27050	21405	15454	11763	9007	6764	4841	3139	1614	331
0.03	17514	12019	9511	6867	5227	4003	3006	2152	1396	718	148
0.04	9848	6578	5348	3861	2939	2251	1691	1210	785	404	84
0.05	6299	4323	3421	2470	1881	1440	1082	775	503	259	54
0.06	4372	3000	2375	1715	1305	1000	751	538	349	180	38
0.07	3209	2203	1744	1259	959	734	552	395	257	133	29
0.08	2455	1685	1334	963	734	562	422	303	197	102	23
0.09	1938	1330	1053	761	579	444	334	239	156	81	18
0.10	1568	1076	852	616	469	359	270	194	126	66	15
0.11	1294	889	704	508	387	297	223	160	104	54	13
0.12	1086	746	590	427	325	249	188	135	88	46	11
0.13	924	635	503	363	277	212	160	115	75	39	10
0.14	796	546	433	313	238	183	138	99	65	34	*
0.15	692	475	376	272	207	159	120	86	56	30	*
0.16	607	417	330	239	182	140	105	76	50	27	*
0.17	537	369	292	211	161	124	93	67	44	24	*
0.18	478	328	260	188	144	110	83	60	39	21	*
0.19	428	294	233	169	129	99	75	54	35	19	*
0.20	385	265	210	152	116	89	67	49	32	17	*
0.22	317	218	173	125	96	74	56	40	27	15	*
0.24	265	182	144	105	80	62	47	34	23	12	*
0.26	224	154	122	89	68	52	40	29	19	11	*
0.28	192	132	105	76	58	45	34	25	17	10	*
0.30	166	114	91	66	51	39	30	22	15	*	*
0.32	145	100	79	58	44	34	26	19	13	*	*
0.34	127	88	70	51	39	30	23	17	12	*	*
0.36	113	78	62	45	35	27	20	15	10	*	*
0.38	100	69	55	40	31	24	18	14	*	*	*
0.40	89	62	49	36	28	21	16	12	*	*	*
0.45	69	48	38	28	21	17	13	10	*	*	*
0.50	54	37	30	22	17	13	10	*	*	*	*
0.55	43	30	24	17	14	11	*	*	*	*	*
0.60	34	24	19	14	11	*	*	*	*	*	*
0.65	28	19	16	12	*	*	*	*	*	*	*
0.70	23	16	13	10	*	*	*	*	*	*	*
0.75	18	13	10	*	*	*	*	*	*	*	*
0.80	15	10	*	*	*	*	*	*	*	*	*
0.85	12	*	*	*	*	*	*	*	*	*	*
0.90	*	*	*	*	*	*	*	*	*	*	*

From Kraemer, H.C., and Thiemann, S. (1987). *How Many Subjects: Statistical Power Analysis in Research*. Newbury Park, CA: Sage.

1% Level, One-Tailed Test

					Power						
Δ	99	95	90	80	70	60	50	40	30	20	10
0.01	216463	157695	130162	100355	81264	66545	54117	42972	32469	22044	10917
0.02	54106	39417	32535	25085	2031	16634	13528	10742	8117	5511	2730
0.03	24040	17514	14456	11146	9026	7391	6011	4773	3607	2449	1214
0.04	13517	9848	8128	6267	5075	4156	3380	2684	2029	1378	683
0.05	8646	6299	5200	4009	3247	2659	2163	1718	1298	882	437
0.06	6000	4372	3609	2783	2254	1846	1501	1192	901	612	304
0.07	4405	3209	2649	2043	1655	1355	1102	876	662	450	224
0.08	3369	2455	2027	1563	1266	1037	843	670	507	344	171
0.09	2660	1938	1600	1234	999	819	666	529	400	272	136
0.10	2152	1568	1295	998	809	663	539	428	324	220	110
0.11	1776	1294	1069	824	668	547	445	354	268	182	91
0.12	1490	1086	897	692	560	459	374	297	225	153	77
0.13	1268	924	763	589	477	391	318	253	191	130	65
0.14	1092	796	657	507	411	337	274	218	165	112	56
0.15	949	692	571	441	357	293	238	190	144	98	49
0.16	833	607	501	387	314	257	209	166	126	86	43
0.17	736	537	443	342	277	277	185	147	112	76	39
0.18	655	478	395	305	247	202	165	131	100	68	34
0.19	587	428	353	273	221	181	148	118	89	61	31
0.20	528	385	318	246	199	163	133	106	81	55	29
0.22	434	317	262	202	164	135	110	87	66	46	24
0.24	363	265	219	169	137	113	92	73	56	38	21
0.26	307	224	185	143	116	95	78	62	47	33	18
0.28	263	192	159	123	100	82	67	53	41	29	16
0.30	227	166	137	106	86	71	58	46	35	25	14
0.32	198	145	120	93	75	62	51	41	31	22	12
0.34	174	127	105	82	66	55	45	36	28	20	11
0.36	154	113	93	72	59	48	40	32	25	18	10
0.38	137	100	83	64	52	43	35	29	22	16	*
0.40	122	89	74	57	47	39	32	26	20	15	*
0.45	94	69	57	44	36	30	25	20	16	12	*
0.50	73	54	45	35	29	24	20	16	13	*	*
0.55	58	43	36	28	23	19	16	13	11	*	*
0.60	47	34	29	23	19	16	13	11	*	*	*
0.65	38	28	23	18	15	13	11	*	*	*	*
0.70	30	23	19	15	12	11	*	*	*	*	*
0.75	25	18	15	12	10	*	*	*	*	*	*
0.80	20	15	12	10	*	*	*	*	*	*	*
0.85	16	12	10	*	*	*	*	*	*	*	*
0.90	12	*	*	*	*	*	*	*	*	*	*

From Kraemer, H.C., and Thiemann, S. (1987). *How Many Subjects: Statistical Power Analysis in Research*. Newbury Park, CA: Sage.

Glossary

A

absolute zero point   Point at which a value of zero indicates the absence of the property being measured. Ratio-level measurements, such as weight scales, vital signs, and laboratory values, have an absolute zero point.

abstract   Clear, concise summary of a study, usually limited to 100 to 250 words.

abstract thinking   Oriented toward the development of an idea without application to or association with a particular instance, and independent of time and space. Abstract thinkers tend to look for meaning, patterns, relationships, and philosophical implications.

abstract thought processes   Enable both science and theories to be blended into a cohesive body of knowledge, guided by a philosophical framework and applied to clinical practice.

acceptance rate   Number or percentage of the subjects who agree to participate in a study. The percentage is calculated by dividing the number of subjects agreeing to participate by the number of subjects approached. For example, if 100 subjects are approached and 90 agree to participate, the acceptance rate is 90% (90 ÷ 100 × 100% = 90%).

accessible population   Portion of a target population to which the researcher has reasonable access.

accidental or convenience sampling   Nonprobability sampling technique in which subjects are included in the study because they happened to be in the right place at the right time. Available subjects are simply entered into the study until the desired sample size is reached.

accuracy   The closeness of the agreement between the measured value and the true value of the quantity being measured.

accuracy in physiological measures   Comparable to validity in that it addresses the extent to which the instrument measured the domain that is defined in the study.

accuracy of a screening test   Test used to confirm a diagnosis, evaluating it in terms of its ability to correctly assess the presence or absence of a disease or condition in comparison with a gold standard.

adjusted   Term used when each hazard ratio (*HR*) has been adjusted for every other predictor in the regression model.

administrative databases   Databases with standardized sets of data for enormous numbers of patients and providers that are created by insurance companies, government agencies, and others not directly involved in providing patient care.

Agency for Healthcare Research and Quality (AHRQ)   Federal government agency created in 1989 to carry out research, demonstration projects, evidence-based guideline development, training, and research dissemination activities with respect to healthcare services and systems. Focus of this agency is to promote evidence-based health care; see the website for details at www.ahrq.gov. AHRQ was previously named Agency for Health Care Policy and Research, with a name change in 1999.

alpha (α)   Level of significance or cutoff point used to determine whether the samples being tested are members of the same population (nonsignificant) or different populations (significant); alpha is commonly set at 0.05, 0.01, or 0.001. Alpha is also the probability of making a type I error.

alternate-forms reliability   Also referred to as *parallel forms reliability*, which involves comparing the equivalence of two versions of the same paper-and-pencil instruments.

analysis of covariance (ANCOVA)   Statistical procedure designed to reduce the error term (or variance within groups) by partialing out the variance resulting from a confounding variable by performing regression analysis before performing analysis of variance (ANOVA).

analysis of sources   Process of determining the value of a reference for a particular study. The source is critically appraised and then compared with that of other studies to determine the existing body of knowledge in relation to the research problem.

analysis of variance (ANOVA)   Statistical technique used to examine differences among two or more groups by comparing the variability between the groups with the variability within the groups.

ancestry searches   Use of citations in relevant studies to identify additional studies. Especially important in conducting a systematic review of research.

anonymity   In research, the condition in which a subject's identity cannot be linked, even by the researcher, with his or her individual responses.

applied or practical research   Scientific investigations conducted to generate knowledge that will directly influence or improve practice.

apprenticeship A volunteer position in which one works closely with an experienced researcher in order to develop one's research skills.

assent A child's affirmative agreement to participate in research.

associative hypothesis Identifies or predicts the relationship between or among variables that occur or exist together in the real world. It is usually developed to guide a correlational study.

associative relationship Identifies concepts that occur or exist together in the real world; thus, when one concept changes, the other concept changes. These relationships are part of theory and can be tested through research.

assumptions Statements taken for granted or considered true, even though they have not been scientifically tested.

asymmetrical relationship If A occurs (or changes), then B will occur (or change), but there may be no indication that if B occurs (or changes), A will occur (or change). delete A_B; A—B.

attrition rate The number and percentage of subjects or study participants who drop out of a study before completion, which creates a threat to the study's internal validity.

authority Person with expertise and power who is able to influence opinion and behavior.

autoethnography The formal study of one's own culture or social context.

B

background for a research problem Part of the research problem that indicates what is known or the key research that has been done in the problem area to be studied.

bar graphs Figures or illustrations that provide a picture of the results from a study. These graphs can be horizontal or vertical bars that represent the size or amount of the group or variable studied.

basic or pure research Scientific investigations for the pursuit of knowledge for knowledge's sake or for the pleasure of learning and finding truth.

being A term in phenomenological research whereby a person's experiences of the world are unique to that person.

being-in-time Term from phenomenological research that indicates that a person experiences life situations within the framework of time and that the past and the future influence the now and thus are part of being-in-time.

beneficence, principle of Encourages the researcher to do good and, above all, to do no harm.

benefit-risk ratio Means by which researchers and reviewers of research judge the potential benefits and risks in a study to promote the conduct of ethical research.

best interest standard In determining whether an individual should participate in a study, the researcher needs to do what is best for the individual on the basis of balancing risks and benefits in a study.

best research evidence The strongest empirical knowledge available that is generated from the synthesis of quality study findings to address a practice problem.

between-group variance Variance of the group means around the grand mean (the mean of the total sample) that is examined in analysis of variance (ANOVA).

bias Any influence or action in a study that distorts the findings or slants them away from the true or expected.

biased coin design Technique used to randomly assign subjects to groups in which selection of the group to which a particular subject will be assigned is biased in favor of groups that have smaller sample sizes at the point of the assignment of that subject.

bibliographical database Database that either consists of citations relevant to a specific discipline or is a broad collection of citations from a variety of disciplines.

bimodal Distribution of scores from a study has two modes (or most frequently occurring scores), which usually means that the researcher has not adequately defined the study population.

bivariate analysis Statistical procedures that involve comparison of summary values from two groups of the same variable or from two variables within a single group.

bivariate correlation analysis Analysis techniques that measure the extent of the linear relationship between two variables.

Bland and Altman plot Analysis technique for examining the extent of agreement between two physiological measurement techniques. Generally used to compare a new technique with an established one.

blinding Structure of a design whereby either the patient or those providing care to the patient are unaware whether the patient is in the experimental group or the control group.

blocking Part of the randomized block design, in which the subjects are rank ordered in relation to the blocking variable to control the effects of this variable, thus improving the validity of study findings.

body of knowledge Information, principles, theories, and empirical evidence that are organized by the beliefs accepted in a discipline at a given time.

Bonferroni procedure Parametric analysis technique that controls for escalation of significance and that can be used if various t-tests must be performed on different aspects of the same data.

borrowing Appropriation and use of knowledge from other disciplines to guide nursing practice.

bracketing Qualitative research technique of suspending or laying aside what is known about an experience being studied.

breach of confidentiality Accidental or direct action that allows an unauthorized person to have access to raw study data or subject identity information.

C

calculated variable A variable used in the analysis is not collected but calculated from other variables.

canonical correlation Extension of multiple regression with more than one dependent variable.

care bundles Combinations of interrelated nursing actions.

care maps Type of map developed in intervention research of the intervention theory that illustrates the elements of the intervention and the causal links among them, and that should show all the causal pathways described in the intervention theory.

carryover effect Application of one treatment can influence the response to following treatments.

case-control design Involves a matching procedure whereby a control subject is matched to each case, so that the cases and controls are different people matched demographically.

case study design A design that guides the intensive exploration of a single unit of study, such as a person, family, group, community, or institution.

causal connection The link between the independent variable (cause) and the dependent variable (outcome or effect) that is examined in quasi-experimental, experimental, and intervention research.

causal explanation The description or explanation of the effect(s) of the independent variable (cause or intervention) on the dependent variable (outcome).

causal hypothesis or relationship Relationship between two variables in which one variable (independent variable) is thought to cause or determine the presence of the other variable (dependent variable). Some causal hypotheses include more than one independent or dependent variable.

causality Has three conditions: (1) there must be a strong relationship between the proposed cause and effect, (2) the proposed cause must precede the effect in time, and (3) the cause has to be present whenever the effect occurs.

cell Intersection between the row and column in a table where a specific numerical value is inserted.

censored data Survival times that are known only to exceed a certain value.

central limit theorem States that even when statistics, such as means, come from a population with a skewed (asymmetrical) distribution, the sampling distribution developed from multiple means obtained from that skewed population will tend to fit the pattern of the normal curve.

chi-square test of independence (χ^2) Used to analyze nominal data to determine significant differences between observed frequencies within the data and frequencies that were expected.

citation Act of quoting a source, using it as an example, or presenting it as support for a position taken.

citation bias Occurs when certain studies are cited more often than others and are more likely to be identified in database searches.

classical hypothesis testing Refers to the process of testing a hypothesis to infer the reality of an effect.

cleaning data Checking raw data to determine errors in data recording, coding, or entry.

client treatment matching Also called *treatment matching*; is used in intervention research to compare the relative effectiveness of various treatments when the following conditions are met: (1) there is no clearly superior treatment for individuals with a problem, (2) a number of treatments have some proven efficacy for undifferentiated subjects, and (3) there is evidence of differential outcomes with and among treatments for defined subtypes of patients.

clinical databases Databases of patient, provider, and healthcare agency information that are developed by healthcare agencies and sometimes providers to document care delivery and outcomes.

clinical expertise Consists of a practitioner's knowledge, skills, and past experience in accurately assessing, diagnosing, and managing an individual's health needs.

clinical guidelines Standardized, current national and international guidelines for the assessment, diagnosis, and management of patient conditions that are developed by clinical guideline panels or professional groups to improve the outcomes of care and promote evidence-based health care (see www.guideline.gov).

clinical judgment The use of clinical expertise to make sound decisions in the provision of evidence-based health care.

clinical pathways Critical pathways or guidelines developed by healthcare agencies to define the expected care activities and outcomes of care in specific patient care situations. These pathways are developed on the basis of previous research, agency data, and clinical experience to provide evidence-based practice.

clinical trial A study conducted to determine the effect of a selected intervention (such as a drug or nursing or medical procedure) on identified patient outcomes using a structured experimental design. Produces a strong type of research evidence that can be synthesized with other study findings to determine the current best research evidence in a practice area.

cluster sampling A sampling frame is developed that includes a list of all the states, cities, institutions, or organizations (clusters) that could be used in a study, and a randomized sample is drawn from this list. Cluster sampling is used when it is not possible to use simple random sampling or the individual elements of the population are unknown, preventing development of the sampling frame.

code A symbol or abbreviation used to label words or phrases in the data.

codebook Identifies and defines each variable in a study and includes an abbreviated variable name, a descriptive variable label, and the range of possible numerical values of every variable entered into a computer file.

coding In quantitative studies, the process of transforming qualitative data into numerical symbols that can be computerized. In qualitative studies, the process of labeling phrases and quotations to identify themes and patterns.

coefficient of determination (R^2) Computed from a matrix of correlation coefficients; provides important information on multicollinearity. This value indicates the degree of linear dependencies among the variables.

coefficient of stability Result of a correlational analysis of the scores of two educational tests or scales given two to four weeks apart.

coercion Overt threat of harm or excessive reward intentionally presented by one person to another to obtain compliance, such as offering subjects a large sum of money to participate in a dangerous research project.

cognitive application of research Use of research-based knowledge to affect a person's way of thinking about, approaching, and observing situations.

cohorts Samples in time-dimensional studies within the field of epidemiology.

communicating research findings Developing a research report and disseminating it through presentations and publications to a variety of audiences.

comparative analysis Involves examining methodology and findings across studies for similarities and differences. The frequency of similar findings might be recorded.

comparative descriptive design Used to describe differences in variables in two or more groups in a natural setting.

comparative evaluation Has four parts: (1) substantiation of the evidence, (2) fit of the evidence with the healthcare setting, (3) feasibility of using research findings, and (4) concerns with current practice.

comparative experimental design Less rigorous experimental design in which random sampling is difficult if not impossible. The studies include convenience samples with random assignment to groups.

comparison group A group of subjects that is not selected through random sampling and usually does not receive a treatment. There are four types of comparison groups: (1) groups that receive no treatment, (2) groups that receive a placebo treatment, (3) groups that receive standard or usual healthcare, and (4) groups that receive a second experimental treatment or a different treatment dose for comparison with the first experimental treatment.

complete IRB review Extensive review by an institutional review board (IRB) for studies with greater than minimal risk.

complete observation The researcher is passive and has no direct social interaction in the setting.

complete participation The researcher becomes a member of the group and conceals the researcher role.

complex hypothesis Predicts the relationship (associative or causal) among three or more variables; thus, the hypothesis could include two (or more) independent and two (or more) dependent variables.

comprehending a source Involves reading the entire source carefully and focusing on understanding the major concepts and the logical flow of ideas within the source.

computer searches Conducted to scan the citations in different databases and identify sources relevant to a research problem.

computerized database Structured compilation of information that can be scanned, retrieved, and analyzed by computer and can be used for decisions, reports, and research.

concept Term that abstractly describes and names an object or phenomenon, thus providing it with a separate identity or meaning.

concept analysis Strategy through which a set of attributes or characteristics essential to the connotative meaning or conceptual definition of a concept are identified.

concept derivation Process of extracting and defining concepts from theories in other disciplines. May require a concept analysis that examines the use of the concept in the nursing literature, compares the results with the existing conceptual definition, and, if the two are different, modifies the definition to be consistent with nursing usage.

concept synthesis Process of describing and naming a previously unrecognized concept.

conceptual definition Provides a variable or concept with connotative (abstract, comprehensive, theoretical) meaning and is established through concept analysis, concept derivation, or concept synthesis. The conceptual definition of a variable in a study is often developed from the study framework and is the link between the study framework and the operational definition of the variable.

conceptual map Strategy for expressing a framework of a study that diagrammatically shows the interrelationships of the concepts and statements.

conceptual model Set of highly abstract, related constructs that broadly explains phenomena of interest, expresses assumptions, and reflects a philosophical stance.

conclusions   Synthesis and clarification of the meaning of study findings.

concrete thinking   Thinking that is oriented toward and limited by tangible things or events observed and experienced in reality.

concurrent relationship   Relationship in which both variables and concepts occur simultaneously.

concurrent triangulation strategy   This design model is selected when a researcher wishes to use quantitative and qualitative methods in an attempt to confirm, cross-validate, or corroborate findings within a single study.

condensed proposal   A brief or shortened proposal developed for review by clinical agencies and funding institutions.

confidence interval   Range in which the value of the population parameter is estimated to be.

confidentiality   Management of private data in research so that subjects' identities are not linked with their responses.

confirmatory data analysis   Use of inferential statistics to confirm expectations regarding the data that are expressed as hypotheses.

confirmatory studies   Conducted only after a large body of knowledge has been generated with exploratory studies; are expected to have large samples and to use random sampling techniques.

confounding variables   Variables that have the potential to affect the outcome of a study, which are recognized before the study is initiated but that cannot be controlled, or variables not recognized until the study is in process.

consensus knowledge building   Outcomes design that requires critical appraisal and synthesis of an extensive international search of the literature on the topic of concern, including unpublished studies, studies in progress, dissertations, and theses.

consent form   Written form, audio recording, or video recording used to document a subject's agreement to participate in a study.

concurrent validity   Ability to predict the current value of one measure on the basis of the value obtained on the measure of another concept.

construct validity   Examines the fit between conceptual and operational definitions of variables and determines whether the instrument actually measures the theoretical construct that it purports to measure.

constructs   Concepts at very high levels of abstraction that have general meanings.

content analysis   Qualitative analysis technique used to classify words in a text into a few categories chosen because of their theoretical importance.

content expert   A clinician or researcher who is known for his or her work in a specific area.

content validity   Examines the extent to which the measurement method includes all the major elements relevant to the construct being measured. Evidence for content-related validity is obtained from the literature, representatives of the relevant populations, and content experts.

content validity ratio   Calculated by researchers for each item on a scale by rating it a 0 (not necessary), 1 (useful), or 3 (essential).

content validity index   Developed to obtain a numerical value that reflects the level of content-related validity evidence for a measurement method.

contingent relationship   Occurs only if a third variable or concept is present.

continuous variable   Variable in which higher numbers represent more of that variable and the lower numbers represent less of that variable.

control   Imposing of rules by the researcher to decrease the possibility of error and increase the probability that the study's findings are an accurate reflection of reality.

control group   Group of elements or subjects not exposed to the experimental treatment. The term *control group* is used in studies with random sampling methods.

convenience sampling   See *accidental sampling*.

convergent validity   Type of measurement validity obtained by using two instruments to measure the same variable, such as depression, and correlating the results from these instruments. Evidence of validity from examining convergence is achieved if the data from the two instruments have a moderate to strong positive correlation.

correlational analysis   Statistical procedure conducted to determine the direction (positive or negative) and magnitude (or strength) of the relationship between two variables.

correlational coefficient   Indicates the degree of relationship between two variables; coefficients range in value from +1.00 (perfect positive relationship) to 0.00 (no relationship) to −1.00 (perfect negative or inverse relationship).

correlational matrix   A table of the bivariate correlations of every pair of variables in a data set. Along the diagonal through the matrix the variables are correlated with themselves, with the left and right sides of the table being mirror images of each other.

correlational research   Systematic investigation of relationships between two or more variables to explain the type (positive or negative) and strength of relationships in the world and not to examine cause and effect.

correlational study designs   Variety of study designs developed to examine relationships among variables.

counterbalancing   Administration of various treatments in random order rather than consistently in the same sequence.

covert data collection   Occurs when subjects are unaware that research data are being collected.

criterion-referenced testing Comparison of a subject's score with a criterion of achievement that includes the definition of target behaviors. When the subject has mastered the behaviors, he or she is considered proficient in these behaviors, such as being proficient in the behaviors of a nurse practitioner.

critical appraisal of research Systematic, unbiased, careful examination of all aspects of a study to judge the merits, limitations, meaning, and significance based on previous research experience and knowledge of the topic.

critical appraisal process for qualitative research Evaluating the quality of a qualitative study by examining its philosophical congruence, methodological coherence, intuitive comprehension, and intellectual contribution.

critical appraisal process for quantitative research Examination of the quality of a quantitative study using the following three steps: (1) identifying the steps of the research process, (2) determining the study's strengths and weaknesses, and (3) evaluating the credibility and meaning of a study to nursing knowledge and practice.

critical cases Cases that make a point clearly or are extremely important in understanding the purpose of the study and are identified through purposive sampling.

critical pathways See *clinical pathways*.

critical value In quantitative data analysis, the value at which statistical significance is achieved in a study.

crossover or counterbalanced design Includes the administration of more than one treatment to each subject, and the treatments are provided sequentially rather than concurrently; comparisons are then made of the effects of the different treatments on the same subject.

cross-sectional designs Used to examine groups of subjects in various stages of development simultaneously with the intent of inferring trends over time.

cultural immersion The spending of extended periods in the culture one is studying using ethnographic methods to gain increased familiarity with such things as language, sociocultural norms, and traditions in a culture.

curvilinear relationship A relationship between two variables that varies depending on the relative values of the variables. The graph of the relationship is a curved line rather than a straight one.

cutoff point In factor analysis, variables' factor loading must be at least 0.30 to explain a meaningful portion of the variance within a factor, and these variables are included as elements of the factor.

D

data (plural) Pieces of information that are collected during a study (singular: datum).

data analysis Conducted to reduce, organize, and give meaning to data.

data coding sheet A sheet for organizing and recording data for rapid entry into a computer.

data collection Precise, systematic gathering of information relevant to the research purpose or the specific objectives, questions, or hypotheses of a study.

data collection forms Forms developed or modified for a study to use for recording demographic data, information from patient records, observations, or values from physiological measures.

data collection plan Details on how a study will be implemented.

data saturation In qualitative research, occurs when additional sampling provides no new information, only redundancy of previous collected data.

data use agreement Limits how the data set for a study may be used and how it will be protected to meet Health Insurance Portability and Accountability Act (HIPAA) requirements.

datum Single piece of information collected for research.

debriefing Complete disclosure of the study purpose and results at the end of a study.

deception Misinforming subjects for research purposes.

decision making Cognitive process of assessing a situation and deciding on a course of action, which is important for conducting research and providing health care.

Declaration of Helsinki Ethical code based on the Nuremberg Code that differentiated therapeutic from non-therapeutic research.

deductive reasoning Reasoning from the general to the specific, or from a general premise to a particular situation.

deductive thinking Thinking that begins with a theory or abstract principle that guides the selection of methods to gather data to support or refute the theory or principle.

degrees of freedom (*df*) Freedom of a score's value to vary given the other existing scores' values and the established sum of these scores ($df = N - 1$).

de-identifying health data Involves removing the 18 elements that could be used to identify an individual or his or her relatives, employer, or household members; this term is part of the Health Insurance Portability and Accountability Act (HIPAA).

Delphi technique Method of measuring the judgments of a group of experts for assessing priorities or making forecasts.

demographic or attribute variables Specific variables such as age, gender, and ethnicity that are collected in a study to describe the sample.

denominator The number on the bottom part of a fraction

denotative definition Dictionary definition of a word.

dependent groups Groups in which the subjects or observations selected for data collection are in some way related to the selection of other subjects or observations. For example, if subjects serve as their own control by using the pretest as a control, the observations (and therefore the groups) are dependent. Use of twins in a study or matching subjects on a selected variable, such as medical diagnosis or age, results in dependent groups.

dependent variable Response, behavior, or outcome that is predicted and measured in research; changes in the dependent variable are presumed to be caused by the independent variable.

description Involves identifying and understanding the nature and attributes of nursing phenomena and sometimes the relationships among these phenomena. This is an outcome of research.

descriptive correlational design Used to describe variables and examine relationships that exist in a study situation.

descriptive design Used to identify a phenomenon of interest, identify variables within the phenomenon, develop conceptual and operational definitions of variables, and describe variables in a study situation.

descriptive research Provides an accurate portrayal or account of the characteristics of a particular individual, event, or group in real-life situations for the purpose of discovering new meaning, describing what exists, determining the frequency with which something occurs, and categorizing information.

descriptive statistics Summary statistics that allow the researcher to organize the data in ways that give meaning and facilitate insight, such as frequency distributions and measures of central tendency and dispersion.

descriptive study designs Variety of designs developed to gain more information about characteristics within a particular field of study and to provide a picture of situations as they naturally happen.

descriptive theory Describes the causal process occurring in intervention research.

design Blueprint for conducting a study that maximizes control over factors that could interfere with the validity of the findings.

design validity Strength of a design to produce accurate results, which is determined by examining statistical conclusion validity, internal validity, construct validity, and external validity.

deterministic relationship Causal statement of what always occurs in a particular situation, such as a scientific law.

deviation score Difference score, which is obtained by subtracting the mean from each score; indicates the extent to which a score deviates from the mean.

dialectic reasoning Involves the holistic perspective, in which the whole is greater than the sum of the parts, and examining factors that are opposites and making sense of

them by merging them into a single unit or idea that is greater than either alone.

diary Record of events kept by a subject over time that is collected and analyzed by a researcher.

difference scores See *deviation score*.

diminished autonomy Describes subjects with decreased ability to voluntarily give informed consent because of legal or mental incompetence, terminal illness, or confinement to an institution.

direct costs Specific costs for materials and equipment to conduct a study that are identified in a grant proposal.

direct measurement Measurement object and measurement strategies are specific and straightforward, such as those for measuring the concrete variables of height, weight, or temperature.

direction of a relationship The direction of a relationship can be positive or negative. With a positive relationship, the two variables change in the same direction (increase or decrease together). With a negative relationship, the variables change in opposite directions; thus, as one variable increases, the other decreases.

directional hypothesis Predicts the specific nature of the interaction or relationship between two or more variables.

disproportionate sampling In stratification, when each stratum has an equivalent number of subjects in the sample, versus each stratum having a number of subjects in proportion to its occurrence in the population, which is proportionate sampling.

dissemination of research findings Diffusion or communication of research findings by presentations and publications to a variety of audiences, such as nurses, other health professionals, policy developers, and consumers.

dissertation Extensive, usually original, research project that is completed as the final requirement for a doctoral degree.

distribution-free No assumption has been made for a normal distribution of values in the population from which the sample was taken.

distribution Spread of scores in a study or database.

divergent validity Type of measurement validity obtained by finding an instrument that measures the opposite of the concept or variable being studied and correlating the data collected with an instrument that measures the concept or variable studied. For example, if the focus of a study is to measure hope, one instrument would measure hope and another would measure despair.

dose-intensity The amount of the intervention delivered in terms of the (1) components of the intervention, (2) duration of a single session for the intervention, (3) frequency with which the intervention is delivered (e.g., daily, times per week, times per month), and (4) cumulative intervention intensity (number of treatments received and duration).

double-blinding in a study design Structure of a design in which neither the patient nor the caregivers are aware of the group (experimental or control) to which the patient is assigned during a study.

dummy variables Categorical or dichotomous variables used in regression analysis.

duplicate publication bias Practice of publishing the same article or major portions of the article in two or more print or electronic media without notifying the editors or referencing the other publication in the reference list.

duration of an intervention The time required to deliver a treatment in a study, which includes examining the time for each individual treatment and the total time the treatment is delivered during the study.

dwelling with the data Immersion in the data as part of the process of data management and reduction in phenomenology.

E

ebooks Books available in a digital or electronic format.

effect size Degree to which the phenomenon is present in the population or to which the null hypothesis is false.

effectiveness A treatment or intervention indicates that it is capable of producing positive results in a usual or routine care condition.

element Person (subject or participant), event, behavior, or any other single unit of a study.

eligibility criteria See *sampling criteria*.

eliminative induction Qualitative data analysis technique that is part of a process referred to as *analytic induction* and requires that the hypothesis generated from the analysis be tested against alternatives.

embodied Heideggerian phenomenologist's belief that the person is a self within a body; thus the person is referred to as embodied.

embodiment The unity of body and mind that eliminates the idea of a subjective and objective world.

emic view Anthropological research approach of studying behavior from within the culture.

empirical generalizations Statements that have been repeatedly tested through research and have not been disproved. Scientific theories have empirical generalizations.

empirical literature Includes relevant studies published in journals, in books, and online, as well as unpublished studies, such as master's theses and doctoral dissertations.

empirical world Experienced through our senses; the concrete portion of our existence.

endogenous variables Variables whose variations are explained within the theoretical model as part of a study with a model-testing design.

environmental variable Type of extraneous variable related to the setting in which a study is conducted.

epistemology A view of knowing and knowledge.

equivalence reliability Compares two versions of the same paper-and-pencil instrument or two observers measuring the same event.

error score Amount of random error in the measurement process.

errors in physiological measures Sources of erroneous measurement with physiological instruments; include environment, user, subject, machine, and interpretation errors.

escalates significance During analysis of study data, there is an increased identification of significant findings that might not be an accurate reflection of reality and might be a type I error (saying something is significant when it is not). For example, performing multiple *t*-tests to analyze study data can cause an increase or escalation of significant findings and an increased incidence of type I error.

estimator Statistic that produces a value as a function of the scores in a sample. Much of inferential statistical analysis involves the use of point estimation to evaluate the fit between the estimator (a statistic) and the population parameter.

ethical principles Principles of respect for persons, beneficence, and justice relevant to the conduct of research.

ethnographic research Qualitative research methodology developed within the discipline of anthropology for investigating cultures that involves collection, description, and analysis of data to develop a theory of cultural behavior.

ethnographies The written reports of a culture from the perspective of insiders. These reports were initially the products of anthropologists who studied primitive, foreign, or remote cultures.

ethnography A word derived by combining the Greek roots of *ethno* (folk or people) and *graphos* (picture or portrait).

ethnonursing research Emerged from Leininger's theory of transcultural nursing and focuses mainly on observing and documenting interactions with people to determine how daily life conditions and patterns are influencing human care, health, and nursing care practices.

etic approach Anthropological research approach of studying behavior from outside the culture and examining similarities and differences across cultures.

evaluation step of critical appraisal Determining the validity, credibility, significance, and meaning of the study by examining the links among the study process, study findings, and previous studies.

evaluation apprehension Shown when subject's responses in the experiment are due to apprehension rather than the effects of the independent variable.

event-partitioning designs Merger of the longitudinal and trend designs to increase sample size and avoid the effects of history on the validity of findings.

evidence-based practice (EBP) Conscientious integration of best research evidence with clinical expertise and patient values and needs in the delivery of quality, cost-effective health care.

evidence-based practice centers Universities and healthcare agencies identified by the Agency for Healthcare Research and Quality (AHRQ) as centers for the conduct, communication, and synthesis of research knowledge in selected areas to promote evidence-based health care.

evidence-based practice guidelines Rigorous, explicit clinical guidelines developed on the basis of the best research evidence available (such as findings from systematic reviews, metaanalyses, mixed-methods systematic reviews, meta-syntheses, and extensive clinical trials); supported by consensus from recognized national experts and affirmed by outcomes obtained by clinicians.

exclusion sampling criteria Sampling requirements identified by the researcher that prevent an element or subject from being in a sample.

execution errors Errors that occur because of a defect in the data collection procedure.

exempt from review Studies that have no apparent risks for the research subjects might be designated as exempt from review by the chair of the institutional review board (IRB).

existence statement Declares that a given concept exists or that a given relationship occurs.

exogenous variables Variables within the theoretical model that are caused by factors from outside the model; these variables are examined in a study with a model-testing design.

expedited IRB review Review process for studies that have some risks, which are minimal or no greater than those ordinarily encountered in daily life or during the performance of routine physical or psychological examinations.

experimental group Subjects who are exposed to the experimental treatment or intervention.

experimental research Objective, systematic, controlled investigation to examine probability and causality among selected independent and dependent variables for the purpose of predicting and controlling phenomena.

experimental study designs Designs that provide the greatest amount of control possible to examine causality more closely.

experimenter expectancy Researcher's belief or projection of the outcome of a study.

explanation Achieved when research clarifies the relationships among phenomena and identifies why certain events occur.

exploratory data analysis Examining the data descriptively to become as familiar as possible with the nature of the data and to search for hidden structures and models.

exploratory-descriptive qualitative research Research conducted to address an issue or problem in need of a solution and/or understanding using qualitative methodology.

exploratory factor analysis Similar to stepwise regression, in which the variance of the first factor is partialed out before analysis is begun on the second factor. It is performed when the researcher has few prior expectations about the factor structure.

exploratory regression analysis Used when the researcher may not have sufficient information to determine which independent variables are effective predictors of the dependent variable; thus, many variables may be entered into the analysis simultaneously. This type is the most commonly used regression analysis strategy in nursing studies.

exploratory studies Designed to increase the knowledge of a field of study and not intended for generalization to large populations. Exploratory studies provide the basis for confirmatory studies.

external criticism Method of determining the validity of source materials in historical research that involves knowing where, when, why, and by whom a document was written.

external validity Extent to which study findings can be generalized beyond the sample used in the study.

extraneous variables Exist in all studies and can affect the measurement of study variables and the relationships among these variables.

F

***F* statistic** Value or result obtained from conducting a type of analysis of variance.

fabrication in research Type of misconduct in research that involves making up study results and recording or reporting them.

face validity Verifies that the instrument looked like or gave the appearance of measuring the content desired for a study.

factor Hypothetical construct created by factor analysis and includes the clustering of like variables that are named based on the focus of the clustered variables.

factor analysis Analysis that examines interrelationships among large numbers of variables and disentangles those relationships to identify clusters of variables that are most closely linked together. Two types of factor analysis are exploratory and confirmatory.

factor loading The regression coefficient for the variable on the factor determined by factor analysis.

factor scores Variables included in a factor are identified, and the scores on these variables are summed for each subject; thus, each subject will have a score for each factor in the instrument.

factorial analysis of variance Mathematically, the analysis technique is simply a specialized version of multiple regression; a number of types of factorial ANOVA have been developed to analyze data from specific experimental designs.

factorial design Study design that includes two or more different characteristics, treatments, or events that are independently varied within a study.

fair treatment Ethical principle that promotes fair selection and treatment of subjects during the course of a study.

false negative Result of a diagnostic or screening test that indicates a disease is not present when it is.

false positive Result of a diagnostic or screening test that indicates a disease is present when it is not.

falsification of research Type of research misconduct that involves either manipulating research materials, equipment, or processes or changing or omitting data or results such that the research is not accurately represented in the research record.

fatigue effect When a subject becomes tired or bored with a study; can affect the findings from the study.

feasibility of a study Determined by examining the time and money commitment; the researcher's expertise; availability of subjects, facility, and equipment; cooperation of others; and the study's ethical considerations.

field notes Notes made during and immediately following the observations.

field work Data collection process for a qualitative study.

findings Translated and interpreted results from a study.

fishing Conducting multiple statistical analyses of relationships or differences searching for significant study findings; can increase the risk for type I error.

fixed-effect model Model used when each study is estimating the exact same quality

focus groups Groups that are designed to obtain participants' perceptions in a specific (or focused) area in a setting that is permissive and nonthreatening.

forced choice Response set for items in a scale that have an even number of choices, such as four or six, in which the respondents cannot choose an uncertain or neutral response and must indicate support for or against the topic measured.

forest plots Particular figures that are very important in the presentation of results in meta-analysis reports that synthesize the results of many studies.

framework The abstract, logical structure of meaning that guides development of the study and enables the researcher to link the findings to the body of knowledge for nursing.

frequency distribution Statistical procedure that involves listing all possible measures of a variable and tallying each datum on the listing. The two types of frequency distributions are ungrouped and grouped.

frequency table A way of organizing the data by listing every possible value in the first column of numbers and the frequency (tally) of each value in the second column of numbers.

funnel plot Provides graphic representations of possible effect sizes (ESs) or odds ratios (ORs) for interventions in selected studies

G

general proposition Highly abstract statement of the relationship between two or more concepts that is found in a conceptual model.

generalization Extends the implications of the findings from the sample that was studied to the larger population or from the situation studied to a larger situation.

geographical analyses Used to examine variations in health status, health services, patterns of care, or patterns of use by geographical area.

going native In ethnographic research, when the researcher becomes part of the culture and loses all objectivity and, with it, the ability to observe clearly.

gold standard Most accurate means of currently diagnosing a particular disease; serves as a basis for comparison with newly developed diagnostic or screening tests.

government report Document with facts that can be used to develop the significance and background section of a research proposal or report.

grant Research funding from private or public institutions to support the conduct of a study.

grantsmanship Expertise and skill in successfully developing proposals to obtain funding for selected studies.

grey literature Studies that have limited distributions, such as theses and dissertations, unpublished research reports, articles in obscure journals, some online journals, conference papers and abstracts, conference proceedings, research reports to funding agencies, and technical reports.

grounded theory research Qualitative, inductive research technique based on symbolic interaction theory that is conducted to discover what problems exist in a social scene and the processes people use to handle them. The research process involves formulation, testing, and redevelopment of propositions until a theory is developed.

grouped frequency distribution Presents a count of patient characteristics that are divided by subsets. For example, instead of providing number of subjects for all ages, provides number of subjects from ages 20 to 29 and 30 to 39.

Grove Model for Implementing Evidence-Based Guidelines in Practice Model developed by one of the textbook authors (Grove) to promote the use of national, standardized evidence-based guidelines in clinical practice.

H

Hawthorne effect Psychological response in which subjects change their behavior simply because they are subjects in a study, not because of the research treatment.

hazard A neutral word intended to describe the risk of event occurrence.

hazard ratio (HR) Interpreted almost identically to an odds ratio (*OR*), with the exception that the *HR* represents the risk of the event's occurring *sooner.*

heterogeneity Researcher's attempt to obtain subjects with a wide variety of characteristics to reduce the risk of bias in studies not using random sampling.

hierarchical statement sets Composed of a general proposition, specific proposition, and hypothesis or research question, moving from abstract statements to more concrete statements proposition and a hypothesis or research question.

highly controlled settings Artificially constructed environments that are developed for the sole purpose of conducting research, such as laboratories, experimental centers, and research medical units.

HIPAA Privacy Rule Federal regulations implemented in 2003 to protect an individual's health information. The HIPAA Privacy Rule affects not only the healthcare environment but also the research conducted in this environment.

historical research Qualitative research method that includes a narrative description or analysis of events that occurred in the remote or recent past.

history An event that is not related to the planned study but that occurs during the time of the study.

history effect Event that is not related to the planned study but occurs during the time of the study and could influence the responses of subjects to the treatment.

homogeneity Degree to which objects are similar or a form of equivalence, such as limiting subjects to only one level of an extraneous variable to reduce its impact on the study findings.

homogeneity reliability Type of reliability testing used with paper-and-pencil tests that addresses the correlation of various items within the instrument. Also referred to as internal consistency reliability.

homoscedastic Data are evenly dispersed both above and below the regression line, which indicates a linear relationship on a scatter diagram (plot).

horizontal axis The *x* axis in a scatterplot or graph of a regression line.

human rights Claims and demands that have been justified in the eyes of an individual or by the consensus of a group of individuals and are protected in research.

hypothesis Formal statement of the expected relationship(s) between two or more variables in a specified population.

hypothesis guessing Occurs when subjects within a study guess the hypothesis of the researcher.

hypothetical population A population that cannot be defined according to sampling theory rules, which require a list of all members of the population.

I

immersed Being fully invested in the data and spending extensive amounts of time reading and thinking about the data.

immersion in the data Initial phase of qualitative data analysis when researchers become very familiar with the data by reading and rereading notes and transcripts, recalling observations and experiences, listening to audio tapes, and viewing videos.

implications of research findings for nursing Meaning of research conclusions for the body of knowledge, theory, and practice in nursing.

inclusion sampling criteria Sampling requirements identified by the researcher that must be present for the element or subject to be included in the sample.

incomplete disclosure Subjects are not completely informed about the purpose of a study because that knowledge might alter the subjects' actions. After the study, the subjects must be debriefed about the complete purpose of the study and the findings.

independent groups Groups in which the selection of one subject is totally unrelated to the selection of other subjects. An example is when subjects are randomly selected and assigned to the treatment and control groups.

independent samples *t*-test The most common parametric analysis technique used in nursing studies to test for significant differences between two independent samples.

independent variable Treatment, intervention, or experimental activity that is manipulated or varied by the researcher to create an effect on the dependent variable.

indirect costs Expenses related to a research project but not specifically part of the implementation of the steps of the study, such as administrative costs. Grants that fund indirect costs provide researchers greater freedom to conduct studies.

indirect measurement Used with abstract concepts; the concepts are not measured directly, but instead, indicators or attributes of the concepts are used to represent the abstraction, such as a perception of pain scale to measure chronic pain.

individually identifiable health information (IIHI) Any information collected from an individual, including demographic information, that is created or received by healthcare providers, a health plan, or a healthcare clearinghouse, that is related to the past, present, or future physical or mental health or condition of an individual, and that identifies the individual.

inductive reasoning Reasoning from the specific to the general in which particular instances are observed and then combined into a larger whole or general statement.

inference Use of inductive reasoning to move from a specific case to a general truth. Thus, statistics are used to infer from the specific study results to a general statement about the larger population.

inferential statistics   Statistics designed to allow inference from a sample statistic to a population parameter; commonly used to test hypotheses of similarities and differences in subsets of the sample under study.

inferred causality   Cause-and-effect relationship is identified from numerous studies conducted over time to determine risk factors or causal factors in selected situations.

informants   People interviewed to learn more about the meaning of observations.

information-rich cases   Cases selected during the purposive sampling process from which qualitative researchers can learn a great deal about the central focus of their study.

informed consent   Prospective subject's agreement to voluntarily participate in a study, which is reached after the subject assimilates essential information about the study.

inherent variability   Data can be naturally expected to have a few random observations included in the extreme ends of the tails.

institutional review   Process of examining studies for ethical concerns by a committee of peers to determine if the study can be conducted in a selected agency.

institutional review board (IRB)   Committee that reviews research to ensure that the investigator is conducting the research ethically. Universities, hospital corporations, and many managed care centers have IRBs to promote the conduct of ethical research and to protect the rights of prospective subjects at their institutions.

instrumentation   A component of measurement that involves the application of specific rules to develop a measurement device or instrument.

integration   Making connections between ideas, theories, and experience.

intention to treat   An analysis based on the principle that participant data are analyzed according to the groups into which they were randomly assigned regardless of what happens to them in the study.

interaction effects   Influence on the design validity by the interaction of different facets of the study, such as selection of subjects and treatment, setting and treatment, or history and treatment.

interaction of different treatments   A threat to construct validity; occurs when subjects receive more than one treatment in a study.

intercept   The point where the regression line crosses (or intercepts) the y axis; is represented by the letter a.

intermediate end points   Events or markers that act as precursors to the final outcome.

intermediate outcome   Mediating variables in theory-guided intervention research.

intermediate mediation   Level of casual assertion that considers causal factors operating between molar and micro levels.

internal consistency   Maintaining the integrity of the different steps of the research process, such as sample selection, measurement of study variables, implementation of study treatment, and data collection.

internal consistency reliability   See homogeneity reliability.

internal criticism   Involves examination of the reliability of historical documents.

internal validity   Extent to which the effects detected in the study are a true reflection of reality rather than being the result of the effects of extraneous variables.

interpretation   Process of information that occurs in the mind of the reader.

interpretation of research outcomes   Involves examining the results of data analysis, forming conclusions, considering the implications for nursing, exploring the significance of the findings, generalizing the findings, and suggesting further studies.

interrater reliability   Degree of consistency between two raters who are independently assigning ratings to a variable or attribute being investigated.

interrupted time-series designs   Designs similar to descriptive time designs except that a treatment is applied at some point in the observations.

interval data   Numerical information collected during a study that has equal distances between a continuum of values and the data also follows the rules of mutually exclusive categories, exhaustive categories, and rank ordering, which influences the type of statistical analyses that can be conducted.

interval estimate   Researcher identifies a range of values on a number line where the population parameter is thought to be.

interval level of measurement   Interval scales have equal numerical distances between intervals or values of the scale in addition to following rules of mutually exclusive categories, exhaustive categories, and rank ordering, such as temperature.

intervening variable   Mediating variable that can affect the occurrence, strength, or direction of a relationship.

intervention fidelity   Reliable and competent implementation of an experimental treatment that includes two core components: (1) adherence to the delivery of the prescribed treatment behaviors, session, or course, and (2) competence in the researcher or interventionalist's skillfulness in delivery of the intervention.

intervention research   Methodology for investigating the effectiveness of a nursing intervention in achieving the desired outcome or outcomes in a natural setting.

intervention taxonomy An organized categorization of interventions performed by nurses.

intervention theory This theory includes a careful description of the problem that the intervention will address, intervening actions that must be implemented to address the problem, moderating variables that might change the impact of the intervention, mediating variables that might alter the effect of the intervention, and expected outcomes of the intervention.

interventionist In intervention research, a person who has been formally prepared to provide a particular intervention and is accountable for the fidelity of the intervention.

interventions Treatments, therapies, procedures, or actions that are implemented by researchers to determine their outcomes in a study, and if effective, are implemented by healthcare professionals to and with patients, in a particular situation, to move the patients' conditions toward desired health outcomes that are beneficial to them.

intervention reliability Ensures that the research treatment is standardized and applied consistently each time it is administered in a study.

interview Structured or unstructured verbal communication between the researcher and subject during which information is obtained for a study.

introspection Process of turning your attention inward toward your own thoughts to provide increased awareness and understanding of the flow and interplay of feelings and ideas.

intuition Insight or understanding of a situation or event as a whole that usually cannot be logically explained.

intuitive comprehension Reader recognizes the findings of a qualitative study as being a credible representation of reality.

invasion of privacy When private information is shared without an individual's knowledge or against his or her will.

investigator-initiated research proposal Researcher identifies a significant problem, develops a study to examine it, and submits a proposal for the study to the appropriate federal funding agency.

inverse linear relationship Indicates that as one variable or concept changes, the other variable or concept changes in the opposite direction; also referred to as a *negative linear relationship*.

Iowa Model of Evidence-Based Practice Model developed in 1994 and revised in 2001 by Titler and colleagues to promote evidence-based practice in clinical agencies.

J

justice, principle of States that human subjects should be treated fairly.

K

key informants Participants in qualitative studies who provide quality information during the conduct of the study.

keywords Major concepts or variables that must be included in your literature search. Keywords or terms can be identified by determining the concepts relevant to your study, the populations of particular interest in your study, interventions to be implemented, and measurement methods to be used in the study, or possible outcomes for the study.

knowledge Essential content or body of information for a discipline that is acquired through traditions, authority, borrowing, trial and error, personal experience, role-modeling and mentorship, intuition, reasoning, and research.

Kolmogorov-Smirnov two-sample test Nonparametric test used to determine whether two independent samples have been drawn from the same population.

kurtosis Degree of peakedness (platykurtic, mesokurtic, or leptokurtic) of the curve shape that is related to the spread or variance of scores.

L

landmark studies Major projects that generate knowledge that influences a discipline and sometimes society in general and marks an important stage of development or a turning point in a field of research.

language bias Can occur if searches focus just on studies in English and important studies exist in other languages.

latent transition analysis (LTA) Outcomes research strategy used in situations in which stages or categories of recovery have been defined and transitions across stages can be identified. To use this analysis method, each member of the population is placed in a single category or stage for a given point of time.

least-squares The fact that when deviations from the mean are squared, the sum is smaller than the sum of squared deviations from any other value in a sampling distribution.

least-squares regression line A line drawn through a scatterplot that represents the smallest deviation of each value from the line.

legally authorized representative Individual or other body authorized under applicable law to consent on behalf of a prospective subject to the subject's participation in the procedures involved in the research.

leptokurtic Term used to describe an extremely peaked-shape distribution of a curve, which means that the scores in the distribution are similar and have limited variance.

level of significance See *alpha (α)*.

levels of measurement The rules for assigning numbers to objects so that a hierarchy in measurement was established, and the levels of measurement from lower to higher are nominal, ordinal, interval, and ratio.

Likert scale   Instrument designed to determine the opinion or attitude of a subject; it contains a number of declarative statements with a scale after each statement.

limitations   Theoretical and methodological restrictions or weaknesses in a study that may decrease the generalizability of the findings.

line graphs   Figures or illustrations that are used to represent the results from studies. Often line graphs are used to show changes in different groups over time.

line of best fit   The use of a regression equation to develop the line that allows the highest degree of prediction possible in a predictive correlational study, in which independent variables are used to predict the dependent variable.

linear relationship   Relationship between two variables or concepts will remain consistent regardless of the values of each of the variables or concepts.

literature review   See *review of relevant literature*.

location bias   Can occur if studies are published in lower-impact journals and indexed in less searched databases.

logic   Science that involves valid ways of relating ideas to promote human understanding; includes abstract and concrete thinking and logistic, inductive, and deductive reasoning.

logical positivism   Branch of philosophy that operates on strict rules of logic, truth, laws, axioms, and predictions. Quantitative research emerged from logical positivism.

logistic reasoning   Used to break the whole into parts that can be carefully examined, as can the relationships among the parts; one can understand the whole by examining the parts.

longitudinal designs   Panel designs used to examine changes in the same subjects over an extended period.

low statistical power   When the strength or power of a study to detect relationships between variables of differences between groups is below the acceptable standard power (0.8) needed to conduct a study. Low statistical power increases the likelihood of a type II error.

M

manipulation   Implementation or controlled movement of a treatment or an independent variable in a study to determine its effect on the study dependent variable.

Mann-Whitney *U* test   Used to analyze ordinal data with 95% of the power of the *t*-test to detect differences between groups of normally distributed populations.

matching   Technique used when an experimental subject is randomly selected and a subject similar in relation to important extraneous variables is randomly selected for inclusion in the control or comparison group. This process results in dependent or related groups.

maturation   Unplanned and unrecognized changes experienced during a study, such as subjects growing older, wiser, stronger, hungrier, or more tired, that can influence the findings of a study.

mean   Value obtained by summing all the scores and dividing that total by the number of scores being summed.

mean deviation   The average difference score, using the absolute values.

mean difference   A standard statistic that is calculated to determine the absolute difference between two groups.

measurement   Process of assigning numbers to objects, events, or situations in accord with some rule.

measurement error   Difference between what exists in reality and what is measured by a research instrument.

measures of central tendency   Statistical procedures (mode, median, and mean) for determining the center of a distribution of scores.

measures of dispersion   Statistical procedures (range, difference scores, sum of squares, variance, and standard deviation) for examining how scores vary or are dispersed around the mean.

median   Score at the exact center of the ungrouped frequency distribution.

mediator variables   Variables that bring about the effects of the intervention after it has occurred and thus influence the outcomes of an intervention study.

memo   Developed by the researcher to record insights or ideas related to notes, transcripts, or codes during qualitative data analysis.

mentee   The protégé who is guided by a mentor in the mentorship process.

mentor   Someone who serves as a teacher, sponsor, guide, exemplar, or counselor for a novice or protégé. For example, an expert nurse serves as a guide or role model for a novice nurse or mentee.

mentorship   Intense form of role-modeling in which an expert nurse serves as a teacher, sponsor, guide, exemplar, or counselor for a novice nurse.

mesokurtic   Term that describes a normal curve with an intermediate degree of kurtosis and intermediate variance of scores.

meta-analysis   Involves the statistical pooling of the results from several previous studies into a single quantitative analysis that provides one of the highest levels of evidence for an intervention's efficacy.

metasummary, qualitative   Synthesis or summing of findings across qualitative reports to determine the current knowledge in an area.

meta-synthesis, qualitative   Synthesis of qualitative studies that provides a fully integrated, novel description or explanation of a target event or experience versus a summary view of that event or experience. Meta-synthesis requires more complex, integrative thought in developing a new perspective or theory based on the findings of previous qualitative studies.

method of least squares   Procedure in regression analysis for developing the line of best fit.

methodological designs   Used to develop the validity and reliability of instruments to measure research concepts and variables.

methodological limitations   Restrictions or weaknesses in the study design that limit the credibility of the findings and the population to which the findings can be generalized.

metric ordinal scale   Scale that has unequal intervals; its use to collect data during a study results in ordinal data.

micromediation   Examines causal connections at the level of small particles such as atoms; is part of multicausality theory.

middle-range theories   Theories that are less abstract and address more specific phenomena than grand theories, that are directly applicable to practice, and that focus on explanation and implementation.

minimal risk   Risk of harm anticipated in the proposed research is not greater, with regard to probability and magnitude, than that ordinarily encountered in daily life or during the performance of routine physical or psychological examinations.

mixed-method approach   Offers investigators the opportunity to utilize the strengths of both qualitative and quantitative research designs in the conduct of a study.

mixed-method systematic review   Synthesis of any of a variety of study designs, such as qualitative research and quasi-experimental, correlational, and/or descriptive study, to determine the current knowledge in an area.

mixed results   Study results including a combination of significant and nonsignificant outcomes, which are probably the most common results of studies.

modal percentage   Appropriate for nominal data; indicates the relationship of the number of data scores represented by the mode with the total number of data scores.

mode   Numerical value or score that occurs with the greatest frequency in a distribution; however, it does not necessarily indicate the center of the data set.

model-testing designs   Used to test the accuracy of a hypothesized causal model or map.

moderator variable   Variable that occurs with the intervention (independent variable) and alters the causal relationship between the intervention and outcomes. It includes characteristics of the subjects and the person implementing the intervention.

molar   Causal laws related to large and complex objects that are part of the theory of multicausality.

monographs   Books, booklets of conference proceedings, or pamphlets, which are usually written once and may be updated with a new edition.

monomethod bias   More than one measure of a variable is used in a study, but all measures use the same method of recording, such as using two paper-and-pencil scales to measure depression in a study.

mono-operation bias   Occurs when only one method of measurement is used to measure a variable or concept in a study, such as the use of one paper-and-pencil scale to measure chronic pain.

multicausality   Recognition that a number of interrelating variables can be involved in having a particular effect.

multicollinearity   Occurs when the independent variables in a regression equation are strongly correlated.

multidimensional scaling   A measurement method that was developed to examine many aspects or elements of a concept or variable.

multilevel analysis   Used in epidemiology to study how environmental factors and individual attributes and behavior interact to influence individual-level health behavior and disease risk.

multilevel synthesis   Involves synthesizing the findings from quantitative studies separate from qualitative studies and then integrating the findings from these two syntheses in the final report.

multimethod-multitrait technique   When a variety of data collection methods, such as interview and observation, are used and different measurement methods are used for each concept in a study.

multitrait-multimethod   The approach of combining convergent and divergent validity testing of instruments.

multimodal   A distribution of scores that has more than two modes or most frequently occurring scores.

multiple regression analysis   Extension of simple linear regression with more than one independent variable entered into the analysis.

multistage cluster sampling   Type of cluster sampling when the random selection of the sample continues through several stages.

N

narrative analysis   Qualitative means of formally analyzing text including stories.

natural settings   Field settings or uncontrolled, real-life settings where research is conducted, such as subjects' homes, worksites, or schools.

necessary relationship   One variable or concept must occur for the second variable or concept to occur.

negative likelihood ratio   Ratio of true-negative results to false-negative results; is calculated as follows: Negative likelihood ratio = 100% − Sensitivity ÷ Specificity.

negative linear relationship   See *inverse linear relationship*.

negative results Unpredicted nonsignificant or inclusive results from a study that are often the most difficult to explain.

negatively skewed Data are not normally distributed in a study; characterized by a curve in which the largest portion of data is above the mean.

nested design Design that allows the researcher to consider the effect of variables that are found only at some levels of the independent variables being studied.

nested variables Variables found only at certain levels of the independent variable, such as gender, race, socioeconomic status, and education.

naturalistic inquiry encompasses studies designed to study people and situations in their natural states.

network sampling Nonprobability sampling method that includes a snowballing technique that takes advantage of social networks and the fact that friends tend to hold characteristics in common. Subjects meeting the sample criteria are asked to assist in locating others with similar characteristics.

networking Process of developing channels of communication between people with common research interests throughout the country.

nominal data Lowest level of data that can only be organized into categories that are exclusive and exhaustive, but the categories cannot be compared or rank ordered and can only be analyzed by the lowest level of statistical analyses.

nominal level of measurement Lowest level of measurement that is used when data can be organized into categories that are exclusive and exhaustive, but the categories cannot be compared or rank ordered, such as gender, race, marital status, and diagnoses.

noncoercive disclaimer A statement that participation is voluntary and refusal to participate will involve no penalty or loss of benefits to which the subject is entitled.

nondirectional hypothesis States that a relationship exists but does not predict the exact nature of the relationship.

nonequivalent control group designs Designs in which the control group is not selected by random means, such as the one-group posttest-only design, posttest-only design with nonequivalent groups, and one-group pretest-posttest design.

nonparametric statistical analysis Statistical techniques used when the assumptions of parametric statistics are not met, and most commonly used to analyze nominal- and ordinal-level data.

nonprobability sampling Nonrandom sampling in which not every element of the population has an opportunity for selection in the sample, such as convenience (accidental) sampling, quota sampling, purposive sampling, and network sampling.

nonsignificant results Negative results or results contrary to the researcher's hypotheses that can be an accurate reflection of reality or can be caused by study weaknesses. Also see *negative results*.

nontherapeutic research Research conducted to generate knowledge for a discipline and in which the results from the study might benefit future patients but will probably not benefit those acting as research subjects.

normal curve A symmetrical, unimodal bell-shaped curve that is a theoretical distribution of all possible scores, but no real distribution exactly fits the normal curve.

normally distributed Data points that follow the spread or distribution of a normal curve.

norm-referenced testing Test performance standards that have been carefully developed over years with large, representative samples through the use of standardized tests with extensive reliability and validity.

null hypothesis States that there is no relationship between the variables being studied; a statistical hypothesis used for statistical testing and interpreting statistical outcomes.

number needed to treat A metric that is defined as the number of patients who would have to be treated with the new intervention to avoid one event that might have occurred with standard treatment.

Nuremberg Code Ethical code of conduct to guide investigators when conducting research.

numerator The number on the top part of a fraction.

Nursing Care Report Card Evaluation of hospital nursing care using 10 indicators (2 structure indicators, 2 process indicators, and 6 outcome indicators). This report card could facilitate benchmarking or setting a desired standard that would allow comparisons of hospitals in terms of their nursing care quality.

nursing interventions Deliberative cognitive, physical, or verbal activities performed with or on behalf of individuals and their families that are directed toward accomplishing particular therapeutic objectives relative to individuals' health and well-being.

nursing research Scientific process that validates and refines existing knowledge and generates new knowledge that directly and indirectly influences the delivery of evidence-based nursing practice.

nursing-sensitive patient outcomes Patient outcomes that are influenced by or associated with nursing.

O

oblique rotation Type of rotation in factor analysis used to accomplish the best fit (best-factor solution) and in which the factors are allowed to be correlated.

observation Collection of data through listening, smelling, touching, and seeing, with an emphasis on what is seen.

observational checklist Form used to record whether a behavior occurred.

observational measurement Use of structured and unstructured observation to measure study variables.

observed level of significance The actual level of significance that is achieved or observed in a study.

observed score Actual score or value obtained for a subject on a measurement tool.

observer as participant Researcher's time is spent mainly observing and interviewing subjects and less in the participation role.

odds ratio (OR) The ratio of the odds of an event occurring in one group, such as the treatment group, with the odds of it occurring in another group, such as the standard care group.

one-group posttest-only design Preexperimental design with numerous threats to validity that is inadequate for making causal references.

one-group pretest-posttest design Quasi-experimental design in which the pretest scores serve as the comparison group and the posttest scores after the treatment serve as the experimental group.

one-tailed test of significance Analysis used with directional hypotheses in which extreme statistical values of interest are thought to occur in a single tail of the curve.

one-way chi-square A statistic that compares different levels of one variable only measured at the nominal level.

open-label extension A term that usually applies to randomized controlled trials or other clinical trials whereby participants in the active treatment group are offered an opportunity to continue treatment and those in the placebo or control group are given the option to transition to the active treatment at the conclusion of the intervention period.

operational definition Description of how variables or concepts will be measured or manipulated in a study.

operational reasoning Involves identification and discrimination among many alternatives or viewpoints and focuses on the process of debating alternatives.

operationalizing a variable or concept Development of the conceptual definition of a concept or variable to link it to the study framework and the operational definition of a concept or variable so it can be measured or manipulated in a study.

operator Permits grouping of ideas, selection of places to search in a database record, and ways to show relationships within a database record, sentence, or paragraph. The most common operators are Boolean, locational, and positional.

operator, Boolean The three words AND, OR, and NOT are used with the researcher's identified concepts in conducting searches of databases.

operator, locational Search operator that identifies terms in specific areas or fields of a record, such as article title, author, and journal name.

operator, positional Search operator used to look for requested terms within certain distance of one another. Common positional operators are NEAR, WITH, and ADJ.

ordinal data Data that can be ranked, but the intervals between the ranked data are not necessarily equal, such as military ranks. This level of data is analyzed by nonparametric statistical techniques.

ordinal level measurement Measurement that yields data that can be ranked, but the intervals between the ranked data are not necessarily equal, such as levels of coping.

outcomes of care The dependent variables or clinical results of health care that are measured to determine the impact of the process of care management techniques. The outcomes from the Medical Outcomes Study Framework include clinical end points, functional status, general well-being, and satisfaction with care.

outcome reporting bias Occurs when study results are not reported clearly and with complete accuracy.

outcomes research Important scientific methodology that was developed to examine the end results of patient care. The strategies used in outcomes research are a departure from traditional scientific endeavors and incorporate evaluation research, epidemiology, and economic theory perspectives.

outliers Extreme scores or values in a set of data that are exceptions to the overall findings.

out-of-pocket costs Those expenses incurred by the patient, family, or both that are not reimbursable by the insurance company; they might include costs of buying supplies, dressings, selected medications, or special foods.

P

paired or dependent samples Samples that are related or matched in some way. See dependent groups.

paradigm Particular way of viewing a phenomenon in the world.

parallel-forms reliability See *alternate-forms reliability*.

parallel synthesis Involves the separate synthesis of quantitative and qualitative studies, but the findings from the qualitative synthesis are used in interpreting the synthesized quantitative studies.

parameter Measure or numerical value of a population.

parametric statistical analyses Statistical techniques used when three assumptions are met: (1) the sample was drawn from a population for which the variance can be calculated, and the distribution is expected to be normal or approximately normal, (2) the level of measurement should be interval or ratio with an approximately normal distribution, and (3) the data can be treated as though they were obtained from random samples.

paraphrasing Involves expressing clearly and concisely the ideas of an author in your own words.

partially controlled setting Environment that the researcher manipulates or modifies in some way when it is used as a setting for a study.

participant observervation Special form of observation in which researchers immerse themselves in the setting so they can hear, see, and experience the reality as the participants do. However, the participants are aware of the dual roles of the researcher (participant and observer).

participants Individuals who participate in qualitative and quantitative research; also referred to as *subjects* in quantitative research.

path coefficient Effect of the independent variable on the dependent variable that is determined through path analysis.

patient Someone who has already gained access to care.

pattern Analysis of qualitative data to determine the trends and links among the facets of the data that can become the meaningful findings from the study.

Pearson's product-moment correlation coefficient (r) Parametric test used to determine the relationship between two variables.

percentage distribution Indicates the percentage of the sample with scores falling within a specific group or range.

percentage of variance Amount of variability explained by a linear relationship; the value is obtained by squaring Pearson's correlation coefficient (r). For example, if an r = 0.5 in a study, the percentage of variance explained is r^2 = 0.25, or 25%.

periodicals Subset of serials with predictable publication dates, such as journals that are published over time and are numbered sequentially for the years published.

permission to participate in a study Agreement of parents or guardians to the participation of their child or ward in research.

person Someone who may or may not have gained access to care.

personal experience Gaining of knowledge by being personally involved in an event, situation, or circumstance.

phenomena experiences that cannot be explained by examining causal relations but need to be studied as the very things they are.

phenomenological research Inductive, descriptive qualitative methodology developed from phenomenological philosophy for the purpose of describing experiences as they are lived by the study participants.

phenomenological researcher Researcher who focuses on describing experiences as they are lived by the study participants rather than large samples with generalizable findings.

philosophy Broad, global explanation of the world that gives meaning to the world of nursing and provides a framework within which thinking, knowing, with doing occur.

physiological measures Techniques used to measure physiological variables either directly or indirectly, such as techniques to measure heart rate or mean arterial pressure.

philosophical perspective The worldview of the researcher that guides the questions asked and the methods selected for conducting a specific study.

PICOS Format An abbreviation that stands for Population or participants of interest; Intervention needed for practice; Comparisons of the intervention with control, placebo, standard care, variations of the same intervention, or different therapies; Outcomes needed for practice; and Study design. PICOS is one of the most common formats used to develop a relevant clinical question to guide a systematic review of research.

pilot study Smaller version of a proposed study conducted to develop or refine the methodology, such as the treatment, instrument, or data collection process.

placebo An intervention intended to have no effect; however, it is like the test intervention or is experienced like the real study intervention to account for how study participants would respond without actually receiving the real intervention.

plagiarism Type of research misconduct that involves the appropriation of another person's ideas, processes, results, or words without giving appropriate credit, including those obtained through confidential review of others' research proposals and manuscripts.

platykurtic Term that indicates a relatively flat curve with the scores having large variance among them.

population All elements (individuals, objects, events, or substances) that meet the sample criteria for inclusion in a study; sometimes referred to as a *target population*.

population-based studies Important type of outcomes research that involves studying health conditions in the context of the community rather than the context of the medical system.

population parameter A true but unknown numerical characteristic of a population. Parameters of the population are estimated with statistics.

population studies Studies that target the entire population.

position papers Papers disseminated by professional organizations and government agencies to promote a particular viewpoint on a debatable issue.

positive likelihood ratio Likelihood ratio calculated to determine the likelihood that a positive test result is a true positive and a negative test result is a true negative. Positive Likelihood Ratio = Sensitivity ÷ (100% − Specificity).

positive linear relationship Indicates that as one variable changes (value of the variable increases or decreases), the second variable will also change in the same direction.

positively skewed Data from a study having a non-normal distribution that is characterized by a curve that has the largest portion of data below the mean.

post hoc tests Statistical tests developed specifically to determine the location of differences in studies with more than two groups, such as when ANOVA results are significant in a study that has three or more groups. Frequently used post hoc tests are Bonferroni's procedure, the Newman-Keuls test, the Tukey HSD test, the Scheffé test, and Dunnett's test.

poster session Visual presentation of a study by using pictures, tables, and illustrations on a display board.

posttest-only design with comparison group Preexperimental design conducted to examine the difference between the experimental group that receives a treatment and the comparison group that does not.

power Probability that a statistical test will detect a significant difference or relationship that exists, which is the capacity to correctly reject a null hypothesis. Standard power of 0.8 is used to conduct power analysis to determine the sample size for a study.

power analysis Used to determine the risk of a type II error so that the study can be modified to decrease the risk, if necessary. Conducting a power analysis involves alpha, effect size, and standard power of 0.8 to determine the sample size for a study. Power analysis is also conducted when nonsignficant results are obtained to determine the power of the analysis conducted.

practical or clinical significance Associated with its importance to the body of knowledge that applies to nursing; sometimes referred to as clinical significance.

practice effect Occurs when subjects improve as they become more familiar with the experimental protocol.

practice pattern Usual care that is provided on a unit or in a setting.

practice pattern profiling Epidemiological technique used in outcomes research that focuses on patterns of care rather than individual occurrences of care.

practice styles Particular ways to implement health care that affect health outcomes and are examined in outcomes research. Practice styles are part of the construct process of care from Donabedian's theory of health care.

practice theories Another name for middle-range theories that are usefulness in practice.

precision Accuracy with which the population parameters have been estimated within a study. Also used to describe the degree of consistency or reproducibility of measurements with physiological instruments.

prediction Ability to estimate the probability of a specific outcome in a given situation that can be achieved through research.

prediction equation Outcome of regression analysis whereby a formula or equation is developed to predict a dependent variable.

predictive design Developed to predict the value of the dependent variable on the basis of values obtained from the independent variables; one approach to examining causal relationships between variables.

predictive validity Type of construct instrument validity in which future performance or attitudes are proposed or predicted on the basis of an instrument's scores—for example, measuring health-related behaviors with an instrument to predict future health status of individuals.

premise Statement that identifies the proposed relationship between two or more variables or concepts.

preproposal Short document (four to five pages plus appendices) written to explore the funding possibilities for a research project.

prescriptive theory Specifies what must be done to achieve the desired effects, including (1) the components, intensity, and duration required, (2) the human and material resources needed, and (3) the procedures to be followed to produce the desired outcomes.

presentation The sharing of research findings verbally by delivering a research report and responding to questions, or by displaying a poster of a study at a conference or meeting.

pretest and posttest design with a comparison group Type of quasi-experimental design frequently implemented to determine the effect of a treatment by comparing the experimental group (treatment group) with the comparison group.

pretest-posttest control group design Classic experimental design in which two randomized groups—one receiving the experimental treatment and one receiving no treatment, a placebo treatment, or usual or standard care—are examined for differences to determine the impact of a treatment.

primary prevention studies Specially designed studies that attempt to measure things that do not happen. Changes in a community are examined and inferred to be a consequence of the effectiveness of the prevention program (treatment).

primary source Source that is written by the person who originated or is responsible for generating the ideas published.

primary theoretical source Source that is written by the theorist who developed the theory or conceptual content.

primordial cell Concept from Donabedian's framework that is the physical-physiological function of the individual patient being cared for by the individual practitioner.

principal component analysis Second step in exploratory factor analysis that provides preliminary information that the researcher needs so that decisions can be made before the final factoring.

principal investigator (PI) In a research grant, the individual who will have primary responsibility for administering the grant and interacting with the funding agency.

privacy The freedom an individual has to determine the time, extent, and general circumstances under which private information will be shared with or withheld from others.

probability Addresses relative, rather than absolute, causality. Probability of a relationship and significance of interventions are examined in research.

probability distributions Distributions of values for different statistical analysis techniques, such as tables of *r* values for Pearson Product Moment Correlation, *t* values for *t* test, or *F* values for analysis of variance. Some common probability distribution tables are found in the appendices of this text.

probability sampling method Random sampling techniques in which each member (element) in the population should have a greater than zero opportunity to be selected for the sample; examples are simple random sampling, stratified random sampling, cluster sampling, and systematic sampling.

probability statement Expresses the likelihood that something will happen in a given situation and addresses relative rather than absolute causality.

probability theory Theory that addresses relative rather than absolute causality. Thus, from a probability perspective, a cause will not produce a specific effect each time that particular cause occurs, but the probability value indicates how frequently the effect might occur with the cause.

probing Technique interviewers use to obtain more information in a specific area of the interview.

problem statement Single statement that follows the significance and background of a problem and identifies the gap in the knowledge base needed for practice.

problematic reasoning Involves identifying a problem, selecting solutions to the problem, and resolving the problem.

procedural rigor In critical appraisal of qualitative studies, the standard of methodological congruence includes procedural rigor, which involves examining a study for the researcher's detail in applying selected procedures or steps of a qualitative study.

process of care Construct that includes mechanisms for delivering health care; is one of three constructs (structure, process, and outcomes of care) in Donabedian's theory of health care.

project grant proposal Paper written to obtain funding for the development of new educational programs in nursing, such as a program designed to teach nurses to provide a new type of nursing care or as a project to support nursing students seeking advanced degrees.

proportionate sampling In stratification, each stratum should have numbers of subjects selected in proportion to their occurrence in the population.

proposal, research Written plan identifying the major elements of a study, such as the problem, purpose, and framework, and outlining the methods to conduct the study; a formal way to communicate ideas about a proposed study to receive approval to conduct the study and to seek funding.

proposition Abstract, formal statement of the relationship between two concepts.

prospective cohort study Epidemiological study in which a group of people are identified who are at risk for experiencing a particular event.

protection from discomfort and harm A right of research subjects based on the ethical principle of beneficence, which holds that one should do good and, above all, do no harm. The levels of discomfort and harm are (1) no anticipated effects, (2) temporary discomfort, (3) unusual levels of temporary discomfort, (4) risk of permanent damage, and (5) certainty of permanent damage.

providers of care Individuals responsible for delivering care, such as nurse practitioners and physicians, who are part of the structure of care of Donabedian's theory of health care.

publication bias Bias that occurs when studies with positive results are more likely to be published than studies with negative or inconclusive results.

published research Studies that are permanently recorded in hard copies of journals or books or are posted online for readers to access.

purposive sampling Judgmental or selective sampling method that involves conscious selection by the researcher of certain subjects or elements to include in a study. Purposive sampling is a type of nonprobability sampling.

Q

Q-sort methodology Technique of comparative rating in which a subject sorts cards with statements on them into designated piles (usually 7-10 piles in the distribution of a normal curve) that might range from best to worst.

qualitative research Systematic, interactive, subjective approach used to describe life experiences and give them meaning.

qualitative research proposal A document developed by a researcher of a proposed qualitative study that often includes an introduction, philosophical base, and methodology for conducting the study.

qualitative research synthesis Process and product of systematically reviewing and formally integrating the findings from qualitative studies. Qualitative research synthesis consists of two categories, metasummary and meta-synthesis.

qualitative research reports The intent of a qualitative research report is to describe the dynamic implementation of the research project and the unique, creative findings obtained. The report usually includes introduction, methods, results, and discussion sections.

quantitative research Formal, objective, systematic study process to describe and test relationships and to examine cause-and-effect interactions among variables.

quantitative research proposal A document developed by a researcher of a proposed quantitative study that often includes the introduction, review of the literature, framework, and methodology proposed for the study.

quantitative research report Report that includes an introduction, methods, results, and a discussion of findings for a quantitative study.

quasi-experimental research Type of quantitative research conducted to explain relationships, clarify why certain events happen, and examine causality between selected independent and dependent variables.

quasi-experimental study designs Designs with limited control that were developed to provide alternative means of examining causality in situations not conducive to experimental controls.

query letter Letter sent to an editor of a journal to determine interest in publishing an article, or a letter sent to a funding agency to determine interest in funding a study.

questionnaire Printed self-report form designed to elicit information that can be obtained through written responses of the subject.

quota sampling Nonprobability convenience sampling technique with an added strategy to ensure the inclusion of subject types likely to be underrepresented in the convenience sample, such as women, minority groups, and the undereducated.

R

random assignment to groups Procedure used to assign subjects to treatment or comparison groups in which the subjects have an equal opportunity to be assigned to either group.

random-effect model A method of analyzing studies that are not all estimating the same intervention effect but related effect over studies that follows a distribution across studies.

random error Error that causes individuals' observed scores to vary haphazardly around their true score without a pattern.

random heterogeneity Subjects in a treatment or intervention group differing in ways that correlate with the dependent variable.

random sampling methods See *probability sampling method*.

random variation Expected difference in values that occurs when one examines different subjects from the same sample.

randomization From a sampling theory point of view, each individual in the population should have a greater than zero opportunity to be selected for a sample, which is achieved by random sampling. The methods of assigning subjects to groups can also be random and promote randomization in the final study groups.

randomized blocking design Experimental design in which the researcher includes subjects with various levels of an extraneous variable in the sample but controls the numbers of subjects at each level of the variable and their random assignment to groups within the study.

randomized controlled trials (RCTs) Classic means of examining the effects of various treatments in which the effects of a treatment are examined by comparing the treatment group with the no-treatment group.

range Simplest measure of dispersion, obtained by subtracting the lowest score from the highest score or just identifying the lowest and highest scores in a distribution of scores.

rating scales Crudest form of measure using scaling techniques; ratings are chosen from an ordered series of categories of a variable assumed to be based on an underlying continuum—for example, rating acute pain on a scale from 1 to 10, with 1 being minimal pain and 10 being extreme pain.

ratio level of measurement Highest measurement form that meets all the rules of other forms of measure: mutually exclusive categories, exhaustive categories, rank ordering, equal spacing between intervals, and a continuum of values; also has an absolute zero, such as weight.

readability The degree of difficulty of a text to be read and comprehended; can be determined by a readability formula such as the Fog Index. The readability of a scale can influence the reliability and validity of a scale used in a study.

repeated measures design A research design that repeatedly assesses or measures study variables for the same group of people.

reasoning Processing and organizing ideas to reach conclusions; examples are problematic, operational, dialectic, and logistic types of reasoning.

recommendations for further research Ideas that emerged from the present study and previous studies in the same area that provide directions for future studies.

recruiting research participants The process of obtaining subjects or participants for a study that includes identifying potential subjects, approaching them to participate in the study, and gaining their acceptance to participate.

refereed journal Publication that uses expert reviewers (referees) to determine whether a manuscript will be accepted for publication.

reference group Group of individuals who constitute the standard against which individual subjects' scores are compared.

referencing Comparing a subject's score against a standard; used in norm-referenced and criterion-referenced testing.

reflexivity Self-awareness and critical examination of the interaction between self and the data during collection and analysis of qualitative data. May lead the researcher to explore personal feelings and experiences that influence the study.

refusal rate Percentage of potential subjects who decide not to participate in a study. The refusal rate is calculated by dividing the number refusing to participate by the number of potential subjects approached. For example, if 100 subjects are approached and 15 refuse to participate, the refusal rate is $15 \div 100 = 0.15$, or 15%.

regression analysis Analysis wherein the independent (predictor) variable or variables influence variation or change in the value of the dependent variable.

regression coefficient R Statistic for regression analysis.

regression line Line that best represents the values of the raw scores plotted on a scatter diagram. The procedure for developing the line of best fit is the method of least squares.

relational statement Declares that a relationship or link of some kind (positive or negative) exists between two or more concepts. Relational statements are also called propositions in theory and become the focus of testing in quantitative research.

relative risk Type of risk associated with conducting any diagnostic and screening test for determining the health problems of patients.

relevant literature Sources that are pertinent or highly important in providing the in-depth knowledge needed to make changes in practice or to study a selected problem.

reliability Represents the consistency of the measure obtained. Also see *reliability testing*.

reliability testing Measure of the amount of random error in the measurement technique. Reliability testing of measurement methods focuses on the following three aspects of reliability: stability, equivalence, and internal consistency or homogeneity.

reliable measure A measurement method used in research that provides consistent data from subjects.

replication Reproducing or repeating a study to determine whether similar findings will be obtained.

replication, approximate Operational replication that involves repeating the original study under similar conditions and following the methods as closely as possible.

replication, concurrent Involves collection of data for the original study and simultaneous replication of the data to provide a check of the reliability of the original study. Confirmation of the original study findings through replication is part of the original study's design.

replication, exact Involves precise or exact duplication of the initial researcher's study to confirm the original findings.

replication, systematic Constructive replication that is done under distinctly new conditions in which the researchers conducting the replication do not follow the design or methods of the original researchers; instead, the second investigative team begins with a similar problem statement but formulates new means to verify the first investigator's findings.

representativeness of the sample Sample must be like the population in as many ways as possible.

request for applications (RFA) Similar to an RFP except that the government agency not only identifies the problem of concern but also describes the design of the study. Researchers bid for this contract.

request for proposals (RFP) An opportunity for funding where an agency within the federal government seeks proposals from researchers dealing with a specific problem. *Federal Register* publishes opportunities for funding that usually have deadlines that are only a few weeks after the publication, and researchers need to have a strong background in the area of concern to submit a proposal.

research Diligent, systematic inquiry or investigation to validate and refine existing knowledge and generate new knowledge.

research benefit Something of health-related, psychosocial, or other value to an individual research subject, or something that will contribute to the acquisition of generalizable knowledge. Assessing research benefits is part of the ethical process of balancing benefits and risks for a study.

research design See *design*.

research grant Funding awarded specifically for conducting a study.

research hypothesis Alternative hypothesis to the null hypothesis, stating that there is a relationship or a difference between two or more variables.

research methodology The process or plan for conducting the specific steps of the study.

research misconduct   Fabrication, falsification, or plagiarism in processing, performing, or reviewing research, or in reporting research results; it does not include honest error or differences in opinion.

research objectives (or aims)   Clear, concise, declarative statements that are expressed to direct a study and are focused on identification and description of variables or determination of the relationships among variables, or both.

research problem   Area of concern where there is a gap in the knowledge base needed for nursing practice. Research is conducted to generate essential knowledge to address the practice concern, with the ultimate goal of providing evidence-based nursing care.

research proposal   See *proposal, research.*

research purpose   Concise, clear statement of the specific goal or aim of the study that is generated from the problem.

research questions   Concise, interrogative statements developed to direct studies that are focused on description of variables, examination of relationships among variables, determination of differences between two or more groups, and prediction of dependent variable using independent variables.

research topics   Concepts or broad problem areas that indicate the foci of essential research knowledge needed to provide evidence-based nursing practice. Research topics include numerous potential research problems.

research utilization   Process of synthesizing, disseminating, and using research-generated knowledge to make an impact on or a change in the existing practices in society.

research variables or concepts   Qualities, properties, or characteristics identified in the research purpose and objectives or questions that are observed or measured in a study. Research variables or concepts are often used in qualitative studies or descriptive and correlational quantitative studies, in which the intent is to observe or measure variables as they exist in a natural setting without the implementation of a treatment.

research participants or informants   See *subjects.*

researcher-participant relationships   In qualitative research, the specific interactions between the researcher and the study participants to accomplish the purpose of the study.

residual variables   Type of variable in a model testing design that indicates the effect of unmeasured variables not included in the model. These variables explain some of the variance found in the data but not the variance within the model.

respect for persons, principle of   Indicates that persons have the right to self-determination and the freedom to participate or not participate in research.

responder analysis   An additional technique to identify variables associated with a beneficial response to an intervention or to determine outcomes of potential importance to the treatment.

response set   Parameters within which the question or item is to be answered in a questionnaire.

results   Outcomes from data analysis that are generated for each research objective, question, or hypothesis.

retention rate   The number and percentage of subjects completing the study.

retaining research participants   Specific actions taken by the researcher to keep subjects participating in a study and to prevent their attrition; provides a more representative sample for the study and decreases the threats to design validity.

retrospective study   Epidemiological study in which a group of people are identified who have experienced a particular event—for example, studying occupational exposure to chemicals to determine cause-and-effect relationships.

review of relevant literature   Analysis and synthesis of research sources to generate a picture of what is known and not known about a particular situation or research problem.

right to self-determination   See *self-determination, right to.*

rigor   Striving for excellence in research through the use of discipline, scrupulous adherence to detail, and strict accuracy.

risk ratio   The ratio of the risk of those subjects in the intervention group to the risk of those in the control group for having a particular health outcome.

rival hypothesis   Alternate explanation of cause in a study.

robustness   Analysis procedure that will yield accurate results even if some of the assumptions are violated by the data being analyzed.

role-modeling   Learning by imitating the behavior of an exemplar or role model.

S

sample   Subset of the population that is selected for a study.

sample attrition   See *attrition rate.*

sample characteristics   Description of the research subjects obtained by analyzing data acquired from the measurement of the demographic variables (e.g., age, gender, ethnicity, medical diagnoses).

sample size   Number of subjects or participants recruited and consenting to take part in a study.

sampling   Selecting groups of people, events, behaviors, or other elements with which to conduct a study.

sampling criteria   List of the characteristics essential for membership in the target population. Sampling criteria consist of both inclusion and exclusion criteria.

sampling error   Difference between a sample statistic used to estimate a population parameter and the actual but unknown value of the parameter.

sampling frame   Listing of every member of the population with membership defined by the sampling criteria.

sampling method   Process of selecting a group of people, events, behaviors, or other elements that are representative of the population being studied; includes probability or random and nonprobability or nonrandom sampling methods.

sampling plan   Describes the strategies that will be used to obtain a sample for a study and may include either probability or nonprobability sampling methods.

scale   Self-report form of measurement composed of several items that are thought to measure the construct being studied, in which the subject responds to each item on the continuum or scale provided, such as a pain perception scale or state anxiety scale.

scatter diagrams or scatterplots   Figures that provide useful preliminary information about the nature of the relationship between variables that should be developed and examined before correlational analysis is performed.

science   Coherent body of knowledge composed of research findings, tested theories, scientific principles, and laws for a discipline.

scientific method   All procedures that scientists have used, currently use, or may use in the future to pursue knowledge, such as quantitative, qualitative, outcomes, and intervention research.

scientific theory   Theory with valid and reliable methods of measuring each concept and relational statements that have been repeatedly tested through research and demonstrated to be valid.

secondary analysis design   Involves studying data previously collected in another study, but using different methods of organization of the data and different statistical analyses to reexamine the data.

secondary source   Source that summarizes or quotes content from primary sources.

seeking approval to conduct a study   Process that involves submission of a research proposal to a selected group for review and often verbally defending that proposal.

selection   The process by which subjects are chosen to take part in a study and how subjects are grouped within a study.

selectivity in physiological measures   Element of accuracy that involves the ability to identify the signal under study correctly to distinguish it from other signals.

self-determination, right to   Based on the ethical principle of respect for persons, which states that humans are capable of controlling their own destiny. The right to self-determination is violated through the use of coercion, covert data collection, and deception in the research process.

semantic differential scale   Instrument that consists of two opposite adjectives with a seven-point scale between them. The subject selects one point on the scale that best describes his or her view of the concept being examined on the opposite adjectives.

seminal study   Study that prompted the initiation of a field of research.

sensitivity of physiological measures   Related to the amount of change of a parameter that can be measured precisely.

sensitivity of screening or diagnostic test   The accuracy of a screening or diagnostic test; the proportion of patients with the disease who have a positive test result or true positive.

sequential explanatory strategy   Method whereby the researcher collects and analyzes quantitative data followed by the collection and analysis of qualitative data.

sequential exploratory strategy   Method in which the collection and analysis of qualitative data precedes the collection of quantitative data.

sequential transformative strategy   Strategy in which either qualitative or quantitative data collection and analysis can come first. The results are integrated during the interpretation phase.

sequential relationship   Relationship in which one concept occurs later than the other.

serendipitous results   Unexpected results from a study that were not the original focus of the study.

serendipity   Accidental discovery of something valuable or useful during the conduct of a study.

serials   Literature published over time or in multiple volumes; serials do not necessarily have a predictable publication date.

setting   Location for conducting research; may be natural, partially controlled, or highly controlled.

sham   Interventions are often used with procedures, and are a variation of a "fake" intervention that omits the essential therapeutic element of the intervention.

Shapiro-Wilk's *W* test   A formal test of normality that assesses whether a variable's distribution is skewed and/or kurtotic.

significance of a problem   Part of the research problem that indicates the importance of the problem to nursing and to the health of individuals, families, and communities.

significant results   Results that are in keeping with those identified by the researcher.

simple hypothesis Predicts the relationship (associative or causal) between two variables.

simple interrupted time-series design Similar to the descriptive time-series design, with the addition of a treatment that occurs or is applied (interrupts the time series) at a given point in time.

simple linear regression Parametric analysis technique that provides a means to estimate the value of a dependent variable based on the value of an independent variable.

simple random sampling Selection of elements at random from the sampling frame for inclusion in a study. Each study element has a probability greater than zero of being selected for inclusion in the study.

situated The way a person is in a specific context and time that shapes his or her experiences, paradoxically freeing and constraining the person's ability to establish meanings through language, culture, history, purposes, and values.

situated freedom The amount of freedom a patient has in healthcare options as a result of his or her specific circumstance.

skewed A curve that is asymmetrical (positively or negatively skewed) because of an asymmetrical distribution of scores from a study.

skimming a source Quickly reviewing a source to gain a broad overview of the content.

slope Determines the direction and angle of the regression line within the graph. The value is represented by the letter *b*.

small area analyses Geographical analyses used to examine variations in health status, health services, patterns of care, or patterns of use by geographical areas.

Spearman rank-order correlation coefficient Nonparametric analysis technique for ordinal data that is an adaptation of the Pearson's product-moment correlation used to examine relationships among variables in a study.

specific propositions Statements found in theories that are at a moderate level of abstraction and provide the basis for the generation of hypotheses to guide a study.

specificity of a screening or diagnostic test Proportion of patients without disease who have a negative test result or true negative. Specificity indicates the accuracy of a screening or diagnostic test.

split-half reliability Process used to determine the homogeneity of an instrument's items; the items are split in half, and a correlational procedure is performed between the two halves.

spurious correlations Relationships between variables that are not logical. In some cases, these significant relationships are a consequence of chance and have no meaning.

stability reliability Concerned with the consistency of repeated measures of the same attribute with the use of the same scale or instrument over time.

stage-based interventions Interventions tailored to a specific phase of recovery, response to treatment, or change in behavior.

standard deviation (*SD*) Measure of dispersion that is calculated by taking the square root of the variance.

standard of care The national designation of the type of care that patients should receive from healthcare agencies and providers.

standard scores Used to express deviations from the mean (difference scores) in terms of standard deviation units, such as *Z* scores, in which the mean is 0 and the standard deviation is 1.

standardized mean difference Calculated in a meta-analysis when the same outcome, such as depression, is measured by different scales or methods.

standardized mortality ratio Observed number of deaths divided by the expected number of deaths and multiplied by 100.

statement synthesis Development of statements proposing specific relationships among the concepts being studied. This step is a part of developing a framework for a study.

statistic Numerical value obtained from a sample that is used to estimate the parameters of a population.

statistical conclusion validity Concerned with whether the conclusions about relationships and differences drawn from statistical analyses are an accurate reflection of reality.

statistical hypothesis See *null hypothesis*.

statistical regression Movement or regression of extreme scores toward the mean in studies using a pretest-posttest design.

statistical significance Results are unlikely to be due to chance; thus, there is a difference between groups, or there is a significant relationship between variables.

Stetler model Model developed by Stetler that provides a comprehensive framework to enhance the use of research findings by nurses to facilitate evidence-based practice.

stratification Used in a design so that subjects are distributed throughout the sample by using sampling techniques similar to those used in blocking, but the purpose of the procedure is even distribution throughout the sample.

stratified random sampling Used when the researcher knows some of the variables in the population, which are critical to achieving representativeness. These identified variables are used to divide the sample into strata or groups.

strength of a relationship Amount of variation explained by the relationship.

structured interviews Use of strategies that give the researcher an increasing amount of control over the content of the interview.

structured observation   Clearly identifying what is to be observed and precisely defining how the observations are to be made, recorded, and coded.

structures of care   The elements of organization and administration, as well as provider and patient characteristics, that guide the processes of care.

study validity   Measure of the truth or accuracy of a claim that is an important concern throughout the research process.

study variables   Concepts at various levels of abstraction that are measured, manipulated, or controlled in a study.

subject attrition   See *attrition rate.*

subjects   Individuals participating in a study.

subject term   Term included in a database thesaurus that one needs identified.

substantive theory   Theory of social process developed by the discovery mode to explain a particular social world.

substitutable relationship   Relationship in which a similar concept can be substituted for the first concept and the second concept will occur.

substituted judgment standard   In the ethical conduct of research, it is a standard concerned with determining the course of action that incompetent individuals would take if they were capable of making a choice.

sufficient relationship   States that when the first variable or concept occurs, the second will occur regardless of the presence or absence of other factors.

sum of squares   Mathematical manipulation involving summing the squares of the difference scores that is used as part of the analysis process for calculating the standard deviation.

summary statistics   See *descriptive statistics.*

summated scales   Scales in which various items are summed to obtain a single score.

survey   Data collection technique in which questionnaires or personal interviews are used to gather data about an identified population.

symbolic meanings   In qualitative data analysis, the meaning attached to particular ideas or clusters of data.

symmetrical curve   A curve in which the left side is a mirror image of the right side.

symmetrical relationship   Complex relationship that consists of two statements: If A occurs (or changes), B will occur (or change); if B occurs (or changes), A will occur (or change); A $\leftrightarrow$ B.

synthesis of sources   Clustering and interrelating ideas from several sources to form a gestalt or new, complete picture of what is known and not known in an area.

systematic bias or variation   Consequence of selecting subjects whose measurement values are different or vary in some way from the population.

systematic error   Measurement error that is not random but occurs consistently, such as a scale that inaccurately weighs subjects 3 pounds heavier than they are.

systematic review   Structured, comprehensive synthesis of quantitative studies in a particular healthcare area to determine the best research evidence available for expert clinicians to use to promote an evidence-based practice.

systematic sampling   Conducted when an ordered list of all members of the population is available and involves selecting every *k*th individual on the list, starting from a point that is selected randomly.

T

table   Presentation of the results of a study in columns and rows for easy review by the reader.

tails   Extremes of the normal curve where significant statistical values can be found.

target population   Group of individuals who meet the sampling criteria and to which the study findings will be generalized.

tentative theory   Theory that is newly proposed, has had minimal exposure to critical appraisal by the discipline, and has had little testing.

testable hypothesis   Contains variables that are measurable or can be manipulated in the real world.

test-retest reliability   Determination of the stability or consistency of a measurement technique by correlating the scores obtained from repeated measures.

textbooks   Monographs written to be used in formal educational programs

themes   In qualitative data analysis, the concepts or patterns that emerge after researchers have spent extensive time examining the data.

theoretical limitations   Weaknesses in the study framework and conceptual and operational definitions that restrict abstract generalization of the findings.

theoretical literature   Concept analyses, maps, theories, and conceptual frameworks that support a selected research problem and purpose.

theoretical sampling   Often used in grounded theory research to advance the development of a theory throughout the research process. The researcher gathers data from any individual or group that can provide relevant data for theory generation.

theory   An integrated set of defined concepts, existence statements, and relational statements that present a view of a phenomenon and can be used to describe, explain, predict, or control that phenomenon.

therapeutic research   Research that provides the patient an opportunity to receive an experimental treatment that might have beneficial results.

thesis   Research project completed by a master's student as part of the requirements for a master's degree.

threats to statistical conclusion validity   The reasons for the false conclusions that might be obtained from the results of data analyses.

time-lag bias   A type of publication bias. Occurs because studies with negative results are usually published later, sometimes 2 or 3 years later, than studies with positive results.

time-dimensional designs   Designs used to examine the sequence and patterns of change, growth, or trends over time.

total variance   The sum of the within-group variance and the between-group variance; determined by conducting analysis of variance (ANOVA).

traditions   Truths or beliefs that are based on customs and past trends and provide a way of acquiring knowledge.

translation/application   Transforming from one language to another to facilitate understanding; part of the process of interpreting research outcomes in which results are translated and interpreted into findings.

translational research   An evolving concept that is defined by the National Institutes of Health as the translation of basic scientific discoveries into practical applications.

treatment   Independent variable or intervention that is manipulated in a study to produce an effect on the dependent variable. The treatment or independent variable is usually detailed in a protocol to ensure consistent implementation in the study.

treatment diffusion   Occurs when the control group subjects communicate with the experimental subjects and are exposed to aspects of the study treatment.

treatment fidelity   The accuracy, consistency, and thoroughness in how an intervention is delivered according to the specified protocol, treatment program, or intervention model.

treatment standardization   A process of ensuring that the research treatment is applied consistently each time the treatment is administered; part of intervention fidelity.

trend designs   Designs used to examine changes in the general population in relation to a particular phenomenon.

trial and error   An approach with unknown outcomes that is used in a situation of uncertainty when other sources of knowledge are unavailable.

triple-blinded   Type of study in which participants, researchers, and those involved in data management are unaware of group assignment.

truncated   In correlational designs, if the range of scores is truncated, the obtained correlational value will be artificially depressed. The lowest values and the highest values for a variable either are not measured or are condensed and merged with less extreme values.

true negative   Result of a diagnostic or screening test that indicates accurately when a disease is not present.

true positive   Result of a diagnostic or screening test that indicates accurate identification of the presence of a disease.

true score   Score that would be obtained if there were no error in measurement; some measurement error always occurs.

t-test   A parametric analysis technique used to determine significant differences between measures of two samples; t-test analysis techniques exist for dependent and independent groups.

two-tailed test of significance   Type of analysis used for a nondirectional hypothesis in which the researcher assumes that an extreme score can occur in either tail.

two-way chi-square   A statistic that tests whether proportions in levels of one variable are significantly different from proportions of the second variable.

type I error   Error that occurs when the researcher concludes that the samples tested are from different populations (the difference between groups is significant) when, in fact, the samples are from the same population (the difference between groups is not significant). The null hypothesis is rejected when it is true.

type II error   Error that occurs when the researcher concludes that there is no significant difference between the samples examined when, in fact, a difference exists. The null hypothesis is regarded as true when it is false.

U

unexpected results   Relationships found between variables or differences between groups that were not hypothesized or predicted from the framework guiding the study.

ungrouped frequency distribution   Process whereby researchers list all categories of the variable on which they have data and tally each datum on the listing.

unimodal   Distribution of scores in a sample has one mode or most frequently occurring score.

unstructured interview   Interview initiated with a broad question, after which subjects are usually encouraged to elaborate on particular dimensions of a topic.

unstructured observations   Spontaneously observing and recording what is seen with a minimum of planning.

V

validation   Phase in which the research reports are critically appraised to determine their scientific soundness.

validity of instrument   The extent to which an instrument actually reflects or is able to measure the construct being examined.

variables   Qualities, properties, or characteristics of persons, things, or situations that change or (vary) and are manipulated, measured, or controlled in research.

variance Measure of dispersion that is the mean or average of the sum of squares.

variance analysis Outcomes research strategy to track individual and group variance from a specific critical pathway. The goal is to decrease preventable variance in the process, thus helping patients and their families achieve optimal outcomes.

vary To be different; numerical values associated with variables will change from one instance to another.

verbal presentation The communication of a research report at a professional conference or meeting.

vertical axis The *y* axis in a graph of a regression line or scatterplot.

visual analog scale A line 100 mm in length with right-angle stops at each end on which subjects are asked to record their response to a study variable. Also referred to as *magnitude scale*.

volunteer sample Those willing to participate in the study. All samples with human subjects must be volunteer samples.

voluntary consent Indication that prospective subject has decided to take part in a study of his or her own volition without coercion or any undue influence.

W

Wilcoxon matched-pairs signed-ranks test Nonparametric analysis technique used to examine changes that occur in pretest-posttest measures or matched-pairs measures.

within-group variance Variance that results when individual scores in a group vary from the group mean.

Y

y intercept Point where the regression line crosses (or intercepts) the *y* axis. At this point on the regression line, $x = 0$.

Z

Z scores Standardized scores developed from the normal curve.

Index

Page numbers followed by "f" indicate figures, "t" indicate tables, and "b" indicate boxes.